Clinical Hematology and Hemato-Oncology

Hara Prasad Pati • Renu Saxena
Maitreyee Bhattacharyya • Tuphan Kanti Dolai
Editors

Clinical Hematology and Hemato-Oncology

Diagnosis, Management, and Advances

Springer

Editors
Hara Prasad Pati
Former Professor, Department of Haematology
All India Institute of Medical Sciences (AIIMS)
New Delhi, India

Maitreyee Bhattacharyya
Institute of Haematology & Transfusion Medicine (IHTM)
Medical College
Kolkata, West Bengal, India

Renu Saxena
Department of Hematopathology
Medanta, The Medicity
Gurugram, Haryana, India

Tuphan Kanti Dolai
Department of Hematology
Nil Ratan Sircar Medical College and Hospital (NRSMCH)
Kolkata, West Bengal, India

ISBN 978-981-92-1166-1 ISBN 978-981-92-1167-8 (eBook)
https://doi.org/10.1007/978-981-92-1167-8

This Springer imprint is published by the registered company Springer Nature Singapore Pte Ltd.
The registered company address is: 152 Beach Road, #21-01/04 Gateway East, Singapore 189721, Singapore

Contents

About the Editors

Dr. Hara Prasad Pati completed his MD in pathology from the All India Institute of Medical Sciences (AIIMS), New Delhi, and was a former professor of hematology, Department of Haematology, at AIIMS, New Delhi, India. With 33 years of experience in the field, his areas of research interest include acute leukemia, chronic leukemia (CML), MDS, drug trials (deferiprone), hemostasis, functional platelet disorders, venous thrombosis, particularly splanchnic venous thrombosis, red cell enzymology, hematopoietic cell colony culture, electron microscopy, angiogenesis, immunohistochemistry, and flow cytometry. He has been honored with several orations, fellowships, vising professorship, and life time achievements. He has published over 220 papers in peer-reviewed national and international journals and co-edited 9 hematology books.

Dr. Renu Saxena is Senior Director of Path and Lab medicine and Head of Hematopathology at Medanta, The Medicity, Gurgaon, India. She is a former professor and head of the department of hematology at All India Institute of Medical Sciences, New Delhi, India. Her areas of research interest include diagnosis and molecular genetics of hemostasis, thrombosis, thalassemia, hemoglobinopathies, hemolytic disorders, and acute and chronic leukemias, DNA analysis for hemophilia A linkage studies, intron 22 and 1 inversion, von Willebrand disease characterization, F V Leiden, prothrombin 20210, and MTHFR gene mutations. She is recipient of several national and international awards, including the prestigious B C Roy Award. She has published over 600 papers in peer-reviewed national and international journals, edited 9 books, and is a fellow of the National Academy of Medical Sciences (FNAMS) and the International Medical Sciences Academy.

Dr. Maitreyee Bhattacharyya completed her DM in clinical hematology from the All India Institute of Medical Sciences. Currently, she is director at the Institute of Hematology and Transfusion Medicine, Medical College, Kolkata, India. Her areas of interest include hematological malignancies and bone marrow transplants. She is the nodal officer for the West Bengal state thalassemia control program and the state technical expert for comprehensive hemophilia care. She is also an advisory board member of the Bengal Medical Genomic Center. She has published over 112 papers in peer-reviewed national and international journals.

Dr. Tuphan Kanti Dolai (DM, MD, DNB, MBBS, FICP, FICH) completed his DM in clinical hematology from the All India Institute of Medical Sciences, New Delhi, India. Currently, he is working as a professor and head of the hematology department at NRS Medical College and Hospital, Kolkata, West Bengal, India. He has published over 135 papers in peer-reviewed national and international journals. He is also the honorary secretary of the Indian Society of Hematology and Blood Transfusion.

Part I
Hereditary & Acquired Anemias Including of Nutritional Causes

Chapter 1
Vitamin B12 and Folic Acid: Biochemistry, and Burden of Disease in India

Somanath Padhi, RajLaxmi Sarangi, and Hara Prasad Pati

Abstract Vitamin B12 (B12) and folic acid (FA) are two key, interdependent, B-group vitamins that are essential for carrying out several cellular reactions essential for vital systemic functions in humans. While it is important to understand the available natural sources of both B12 and FA, their modes of absorption, the factors that influence these, and subsequent biochemical reactions to diagnose clinically *overt* deficiency syndromes, the subclinical deficiency states can easily be missed in routine practice, with potential clinical ramifications. While FA deficiency states are relatively uncommon, thanks to the already existing food fortification policies in India, the B12 deficiency syndrome continues to remain as just a "tip of the iceberg" phenomenon, both at the community and hospital setting at large. This chapter aims to present a comprehensive overview of these two micronutrients, from their biochemistry to the burden of clinical/subclinical disease out of their deficiency in the Indian scenario.

Keywords Micronutrients · B12 · Folate · Bioavailability · Disease burden · Fortification

S. Padhi
Department of Pathology and Laboratory Medicine, All India Institute of Medical Sciences, Bhubaneswar, Odisha, India

R. Sarangi
Department of Biochemistry, Kalinga Institute of Medical Sciences, Bhubaneswar, Odisha, India

H. P. Pati (✉)
Former Professor, Department of Haematology, All India Institute of Medical Sciences (AIIMS), New Delhi, India

H. P. Pati et al. (eds.), *Clinical Hematology and Hemato-Oncology*,
https://doi.org/10.1007/978-981-92-1167-8_1

Learning Objectives

- To have a sound idea of sources and daily requirements of vitamin B12 (B12) and folic acid (FA).
- To have a thorough understanding of the important biochemical reactions involving B12 and FA.
- To have an update on the epidemiology of B12 and FA deficiency in the Indian subcontinent, underlying contributing factors, and the way forward in food fortification policies.

1.1 Introduction

Vitamin B12 [also called cobalamin, Castle's "extrinsic factor"] (B12), and folic acid (FA) (also known as folate, pteroylglutamic acid, vitamin B9) are two essential interdependent micronutrients that belong to the B-group of vitamins. These two are the key players in "one carbon moity transfer" biochemical functions that are implicated in DNA synthesis, normal hematopoietic and non-hematopoietic cellular function, myelination of the nervous system, and many more [1]. The clinical syndrome of B12 and/or FA deficiency states may vary from vague, non-specific, clinically innocuous signs to more clinically significant multisystemic syndrome of megaloblastic anemia (MA), and potentially irreversible neuropsychiatric and cardiovascular syndromes [2]. There is a paucity of knowledge among all strata of health care providers regarding the ever-increasing prevalence of "B12 deficiency states" and its potential multisystemic impact, which continues to affect all ages of life; starting from pre-conception, conception, intrauterine, to post-partum, all decades of life. Although existing food fortification policies have somewhat ameliorated the burden of Iron-FA deficiency states in India, the B12 deficiency remains a "tip of the iceberg" state, and continues to emerge as a potential National Health Issue requiring urgent attention at all levels in the days to come [3]. This chapter is an overview of creating awareness regarding the bioavailability and biochemistry of the above two essential micronutrients; creating awareness among readers regarding the growing menace of health care issues out of deficiency states; and the way forward in the existing health care policy.

1.2 Biochemistry

1.2.1 Folic Acid

1.2.1.1 Source and Daily Requirements

The main dietary source of FA includes green leafy vegetables such as spinach, lettuce, broccoli, as well as fruits like lemons, bananas, oranges, etc. It is also found in cereals, grains, nuts, beans, beef, fish, liver, and kidneys. The recommended dietary allowances (RDA) for children-adolescents, lactating mothers, pregnant women, and adults (including those of childbearing age) are 50 to 200, 500, 600, and 400 micrograms (mcg), respectively. The RDA for an average adult is *higher* than the usual minimal requirement of 50–100 mcg, as the bioavailability is solely dependent upon the hydroxylation-dependent conversion of *poly* to *mono* glutamate forms of FA that facilitate intestinal absorption (*see below*). Liver is the primary site of storage of FA, and the body can store up to 5 mg of FA for a period ranging from 3 to 5 months. Prolonged storage or overwashing in abundant water can significantly reduce the folate content of the food [1, 4, 5].

1.2.1.2 Absorption, Transport, Bioavailability (Fig. 1.1)

Folic acid or folate, the *inactive* form of the coenzyme, is rarely found in nature; and hence needs to be supplemented in the form of fortified food products because of its higher bioavailability, chemical stability, and ready conversion to its active coenzyme form while passing through the brush border enterocytes (BBE). FA is mainly absorbed from the "jejunum and upper ileum" through a passive transport mechanism following the concentration gradient in a neutral (pH = 7.4) gut luminal environment. Prior to its absorption across the BBE, one of the two enzymes, *glutamate carboxypeptidase* or *polyglutamate hydrolase (*also called *intestinal folate conjugase),* present in the luminal surface of jejunum-ileum, hydrolyses the reduced/*polyglutamate* form (commonly present in the food or supplements) to its more readily absorbable *monoglutamate* (FA-MG) form. The FA-MG forms

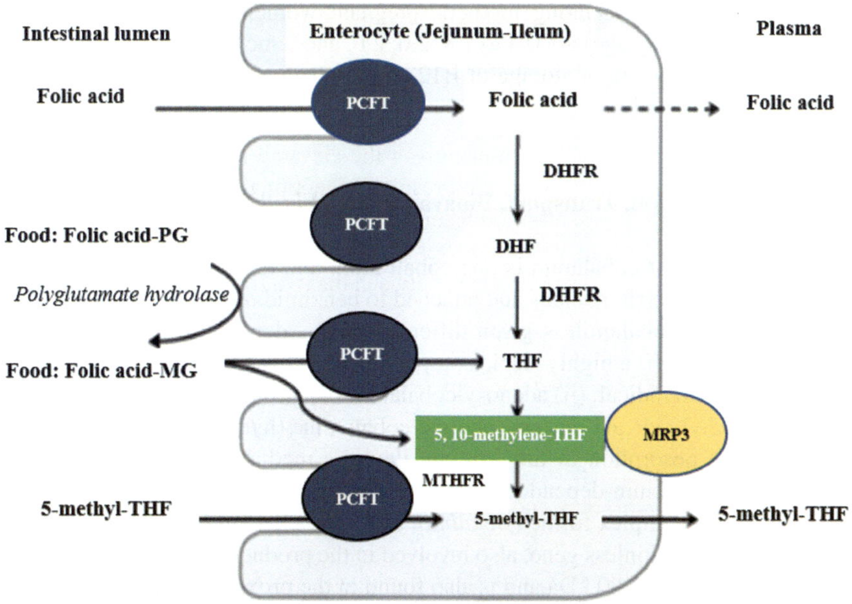

Fig. 1.1 Intestinal absorption of folic acid. (Modified and adopted from Torrez [2] and Shane [5])

are then absorbed across the BBE through pH-sensitive proton-coupled folate transporter (PCFT).

Once taken up by the enterocyte, the enzyme *dihydrofolate reductase* (DHFR) converts the FA-MG through a two-step reaction to 5-methyl tetrahydrofolate (5-MTHF), which then exits the enterocyte through the multidrug resistant protein 3 (MRP3) located on the basolateral membrane of the enterocyte to enter either the systemic or enterohepatic circulation (liver, bile acid, intestine). In the systemic circulation, 66% bind to albumin, 33% remains free, and roughly 1% bind to folate binding protein (FBP). It enters the cells (where it is to be used) either by binding to reduced-folate transporter 1 and 2 (RTF-1 or RTF-2). Intracellular folate transport is mediated by clathrin-mediated endocytosis. Once inside the cell (methyl tetrahydrofolate), it must be demethylated to become tetrahydrofolate (functional folate that can accept glutamic acid chains; these in turn prevent it from exiting the cell, in other words, they "anchor" it inside the cell). Excess intracellular FA can pass into the bloodstream and then be filtered through the glomerulus, secreted into the proximal tubule, and eliminated in the urine at a rate of 2–5 mcg/day [4, 5].

1.2.2 Vitamin B12

1.2.2.1 Source and Daily Requirements

The main dietary source of B12 includes animal food such as meat, fish, and dairy products, and plant-derived food products literally do not contain this micronutrient. The RDA recommended in the literature ranges from 2 to 5 mcg per day: for children-adolescents, lactating mothers, pregnant women, and adults (including those of childbearing age) are 0.4 to 1.8, 2.6, 2.6, and 2 mcg, respectively. Like FA, liver is the primary site of storage of B12 and the body can store up to 2–5 mg of B12 for 3–4 months [1, 4, 5].

1.2.2.2 Absorption, Transport, Bioavailability (Fig. 1.2) [2, 6, 7]

Chemically, B12 or cobalamin is one cobalt atom and tetrapyrole rings located at the center of the corrin nucleus and attached to benzimidazole ribonucleosides 5, 6 through cobalt. Cobalamin is given different names, depending on the radical to which it is bound: (i) a highly stable compound called cyanocobalamin (B12) when bound to a cyano radical, (ii) adenosylcobalamin (adenosyl radical), (iii) methylcobalamin (methyl radical), and (iv) hydroxycobalamine (hydroxyl radical).

Cobalamin absorption in the terminal ileum is mediated by a receptor called *cubilin* using a calcium-dependent *passive* transport mechanism. The cubilin receptor is actually a complex formed of *cubilin* and 2 proteins—*megalin* and AMN (the product of the amnionless gene, also involved in the production of amnion). It has a molecular weight of 460 kDa and is also found in the proximal renal tubule, where it mediates the absorption of B12 itself.

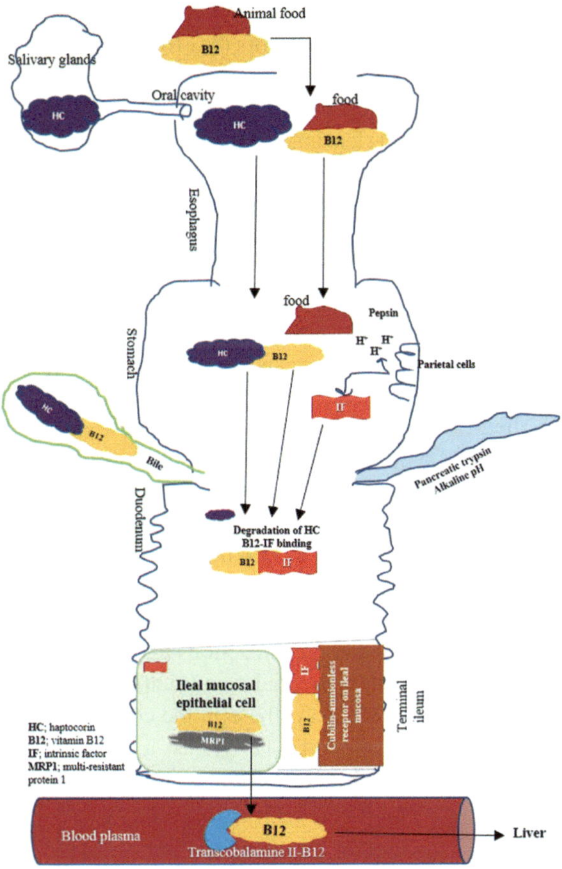

Fig. 1.2 Absorption of vitamin B12 in the gastrointestinal tract. (Modified and adopted from Torez [2], Green [6], and Kumar [7])

In the gastric acidic environment, B12 in food gets dissociated from the food-associated proteins by the action of pepsin and then binds to the B12-binding protein called transcobalamine 1, haptocorin (HC), or R binder, secreted into saliva (also bile, breast milk). This binding protects B12 from the acidic environment of the stomach. The HC-B12 complex reaches the *upper part* of the small intestine, where B12 gets dissociated from HC in an alkaline pH (contributed by pancreatic juice and bile), and then taken up by the Castle intrinsic factor (IF) secreted by the gastric parietal epithelial cells. The B12-IF complex is then transported to the terminal ileal mucosa, where it binds to *cubilin* and is taken up into the BBE by means of a calcium-dependent passive transport mechanism [6, 7].

Once inside the enterocyte, the B12-IF complex is engulfed by lysosomes, where enzymes degrade the IF and release the B12. The B12 then exits to the cytoplasm, where it is taken up by transcobalamine II (TC II, the main B12 binding carrier protein). In this way, the TC II-B12 complex exits the enterocyte through MRP3 located at its basolateral membrane and is released into the systemic circulation or the enterohepatic cycle (liver, bile acids, intestine). In the systemic circulation,

TC II transports it to the cells, where it will be used. It is taken up into the cells by binding to either TC II receptors (TC IIR) or megalin (at the renal proximal tubules). Cobalamin is taken up by cells by means of clathrin-mediated endocytosis, the same intracellular transport mechanisms used in FA uptake. Once inside the cells, TC II is degraded, thus releasing the B12 [6, 7].

1.3 Biochemical Functions of FA and B12 (Fig. 1.3) [2, 7, 8]

Folate coenzymes participate in three major interrelated metabolic cycles in the cell cytosols: purine biosynthesis (purine cycle), and more importantly, thymidylate (thymidylate cycle) and methionine synthesis (methionine cycle). 5,10-methylene-tetrahydrofolate plays a central role in these cycles, as it can be used directly for thymidylate synthesis, or it can be reduced to 5-methyltetrahydrofolate in the methionine synthesis cycle, or can be oxidized to 10-formyl-tetrahydrofolate to be used in purine synthesis. Although these synthetic cycles are located in the cytosol, mammalian cells also contain a large mitochondrial folate pool, which is also involved in the provision of one-carbon precursors for cytosolic one-carbon metabolism (Fig. 1.3a) [2, 5, 7, 8].

Three major biochemical reactions in humans are known to involve B12 (cobalamin) [5]. In *one*, methyl-cobalamin (methyl-B12) serves as an essential cofactor for the enzyme methionine synthase in the conversion of homocysteine to methionine. In this process, methyl-B12 yields a methyl group that is recovered from 5-methylTHF, the principal form of FA in plasma. THF is crucial because this,

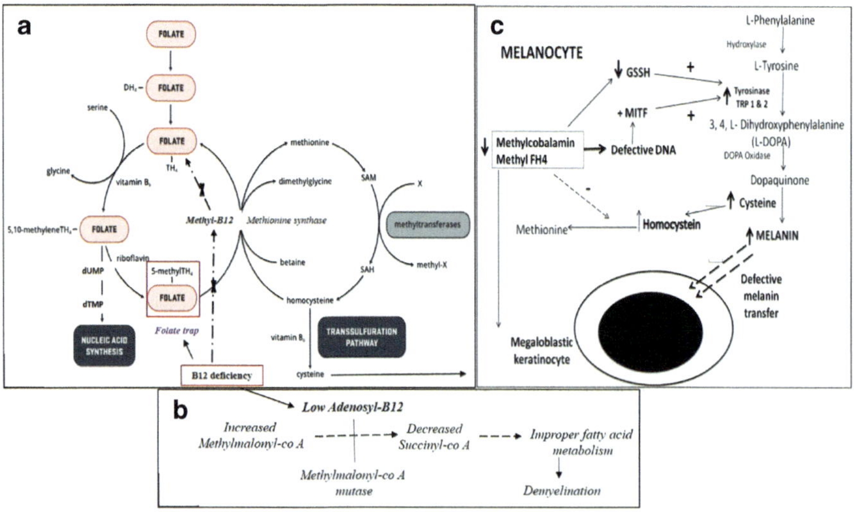

Fig. 1.3 Biochemical functions of B12 and folate. (Modified and adopted from Torez [2], Kumar [7], and Padhi [8])

through its derivative 5, 10, methyleneTHF, is essential for the conversion of deoxyuridine monophosphate (dUMP) to deoxythymidine monophosphate (dTMP), a vital step in DNA synthesis. It is postulated that the fundamental cause of the defective DNA synthesis in B12 deficiency is secondary to the reduced availability of THF, most of which is "trapped" as 5-methylTHF (Fig. 1.3a). The already existing negative FA balance can only exacerbate the situation. Therefore, supplementation with combined FA and B12 can only improve the above scenario. The *second* important biochemical pathway involves adenosyl-B12 in the conversion of methylmalonyl-CoA to succinyl-CoA in the presence of the cofactor methylmalonyl co A mutase [2, 7]. This step is important for fatty acid metabolism and the subsequent incorporation of the correct fatty acid into the myelin lipid coat of the nervous system (Fig. 1.3b). Therefore, B12 deficiency may lead to peripheral neuropathy and, when remain undiagnosed and untreated for a prolonged period, to its more severe form, sub-acute combined degeneration (SACD) of the spinal cord; a condition which do not require FA supplementation; rather can even be aggravated by FA therapy [7]. The *third* important biochemical function involves the role played by methyl-B12 in the conversion of reduced glutathione to melanin through DOPA-tyrosinase-DOPA oxidase-cysteine pathway; an important pathway implicated in the pathogenesis of mucocutaneous (Addisonian type) hyperpigmentation in patients with B12 deficiency (Fig. 1.3c) [8].

1.4 Vitamin B12 and FA Deficiency in India: An Overview

Vitamin B12 and folic acid (FA) deficiency is common in the Indian subcontinent, with millions at risk for both [9]. This trend is postulated to be multifactorial in origin; the *lack* of intake of a balanced diet, blended with socioeconomic-cultural practices and unhealthy lifestyle, are primary reasons. Additionally, malabsorption secondary to gastrointestinal factors, as well as intake of drugs/toxins, may also play a substantial role. A balanced diet should ideally contain one source of calories (cereal), one source of protein, high intake of fresh green leafy vegetables as well as fresh fruits (rich source of B12), and adequate water (2–2.5 L/day to produce at least 1.5 L of urine output). India has the maximum number of vegetarians in the world; however, they hardly take any vegetables, including green leafy vegetables, and fresh fruits. Even if they consume green leafy vegetables, it is often thoroughly washed for fear of pesticide residues or to remove the dirt, which in fact removes the harmless bacteria as the only source of B12, and it is always cooked before consumption, resulting in loss of FA too. The lack of *regular* consumption of fish, meat, and eggs by non-vegetarian people, combined with faulty cooking practices (deep-frying), contributes to these micronutrient deficiencies [10]. Ileocecal tuberculosis (with a prevalence of up to 20% in some parts) is a major cause of impaired B12 absorption among Indians, whereas atrophic gastritis of pernicious anemia, and intake of drugs such as metformin in diabetics and proton pump inhibitors, etc., are also frequently implicated (Fig. 1.4) [10]. The myriad of clinical manifestations is diverse, and can be multisystemic, and it may involve wide age groups like pregnant mothers, newborn babies, children, adolescents/adults, and the elderly [11].

1.4.1 Prevalence of Anemia and Micronutrient Deficiency (B12 and FA) (CNNS 2016–18 India): The Summary of Findings from CNNS 2016–18 Is Presented in Fig. 1.5 [12]

The Key Findings from the Above Survey Were as Follows

The prevalence of anemia among 1–4 years, 5–9 years, and 10–19 years' age groups was 40.5%, 95% CI: 38.6–42.6, 23.4%, 21.8–25.2, and 28.4%, 26.8–30.0, respectively. The prevalence of *severe* anemia [Hb < 7.0 g/dl (1–4 years), <8.0 g/dl (5–19 years)] in all three groups was 1%. The prevalence of B12 deficiency among three age groups was 17.6%, 13.2–23.2, 17.5%, 12.6–23.7, and 27.6%, 17.6–25.0, respectively. The prevalence of folate deficiency among the same age groups was 17.9%, 14.7–21.7, 21.1%, 23.6–31.9, and 25.9%, 22.5–29.6, respectively (Fig. 1.5a). The prevalence of folate or B12 deficiency anemia was also *lower* among female

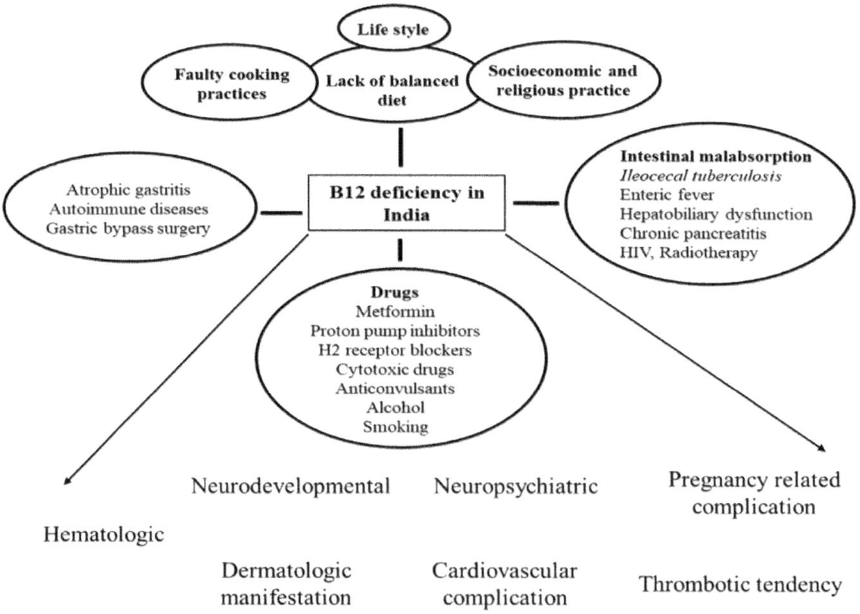

Fig. 1.4 A flow chart depicting the common underlying causes leading to vitamin B12 deficiency with its antecedent complications in India [9–11]

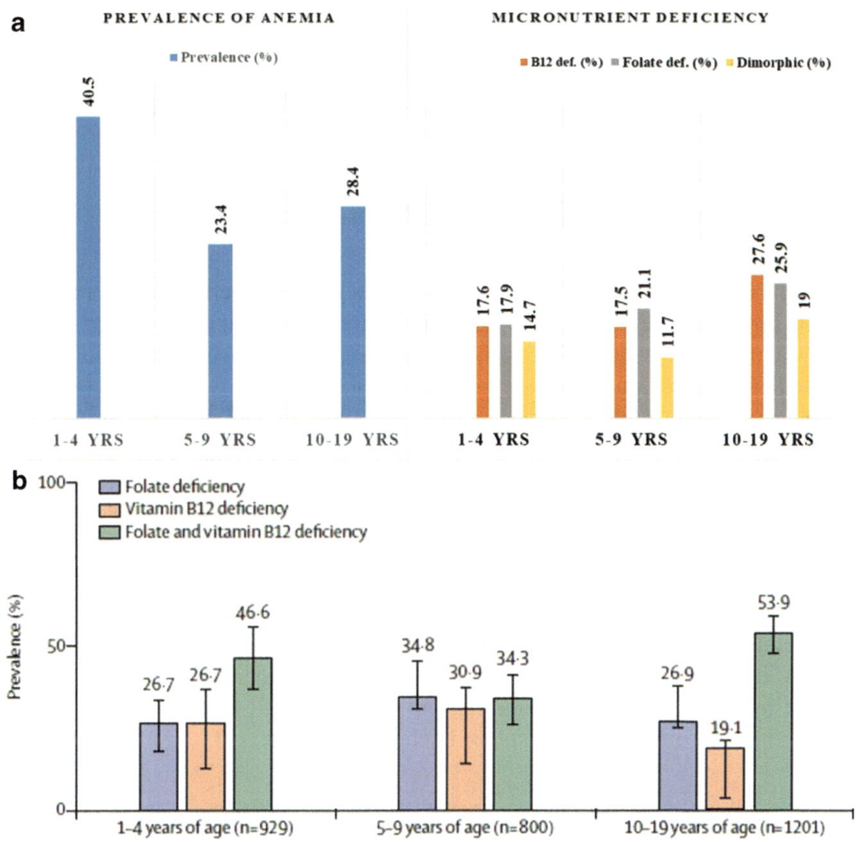

Fig. 1.5 Prevalence of anemia and micronutrient deficiency among children 1–19 years of age in India. (Data extracted from CNNS 2016–18 India [12])

adolescents compared to their male counterparts (22.2% vs. 33.5%, respectively; $p < 0.0001$). Among participants with folate or B12 deficiency anemia (folate or B12 deficiency anemia alone and dimorphic anemia), *combined folate and B12 deficiency was most common in all three age groups* (46.6%, 34.3%, 53.9%, respectively, Fig. 1.5b) [12].

The majority (54–56%) of participants in the three age groups were vegetarian, more than one-third (36–39%) were non-vegetarian, and a small proportion (6–9%) consumed eggs along with a vegetarian diet. More than 85% consumed dark green leafy vegetables and pulses or beans at least once per week; one-third consumed eggs, fish, or chicken or meat at least once per week; and 60% consumed milk or curd at least once per week [12].

A recent systematic review and meta-analysis [13] [data extrapolated from 270 studies, 2015 to 2020] has reported that the prevalence of B12 deficiency of 53% (95% CI: 41–64%) [57% (<18 years) (25–89%), 48% (>18 years) (35–62%), 68% (nonspecific age groups) (38–98%)]. Similarly, the prevalence of FA deficiency was reported to be 37% (27–46%) [39% (<18 years) (22–57%), 41% (>18 years) (24–58%), 25% (nonspecific age group) (12–38%)]. The overall prevalence data matches that from both southern and northern Indian studies. This high prevalence data suggests amendment of already existing food fortification policies [13].

1.4.2 B12 and FA Deficiency in Pregnancy

The summary of a systematic review of 46 studies on B12 deficiency in pregnancy and its impact on the health status of the offspring is summarized in Table 1.1 [14, 15]. The majority of the Indian women of the reproductive age group were already B12 deficient at the time of conception. Overall prevalence of B12 deficiency among pregnant women (both rural and urban, community and hospital-based) was 40–70%; a higher prevalence of 50–70% reported from Western, Southern, and Northern parts of India (70–74%). Prevalence from eastern and north-eastern India was not reported. B12 deficiency was higher during the *third* trimester of pregnancy (29%) as compared to early pregnancy (21%). FA deficiency was lower (20%, cut off <3 ng/ml) compared to that of B12, and this has been reported to be constant as per world standards due to already existing food fortification policies [14, 15].

Overall, maternal B12 deficiency was linked to low birth weight, neural tube defects, intrauterine growth retardation, small for gestational age among new born babies; maternal gestational diabetes; low levels of B12, neurocognitive impairment, adiposity, and insulin resistance in childhood period [13].

Table 1.1 Vitamin B12 deficiency in pregnancy and associated health-related risks [13]

	Level of evidence
Intrauterine	
Preeclampsia Macrocytic anemia Recurrent pregnancy loss Preterm delivery	Low
Gestational diabetes	Moderate
New-born	
Low birthweight Neural tube defects	High
Higher intrauterine growth retardation/small for gestational age	Moderate
Small neonatal size Neonatal morbidity	Low
Childhood	
Low offspring B12 Neurocognitive impairment Adiposity Insulin resistance	Moderate
Cardiovascular stress response	Low

1.4.3 B12 Deficiency: The Burden of Disease in Hospital Setting

A PubMed and Google Scholar database search on B12 deficiency in India yielded nearly 600 articles, which were further refined to include original studies. A comprehensive summary of various Indian hospital-based studies on B12 and folate deficiencies is presented in Table 1.2 and the same pertaining to the aging/elderly population is summarized in Table 1.3 [8, 14, 16–34].

The middle-aged to elderly/aging Indian population is vulnerable to B12 and/or FA deficiency. Chronic hyperhomocysteinaemia secondary to B12 and/or FA insufficiency is a major risk factor in occlusive vascular diseases—particularly increased small-vessel cerebrovascular disease–related strokes, and subsequent neurodegenerative diseases. There are reports among elderly patients to suggest that homocysteine-lowering therapy can significantly slow down the accelerated rate of brain atrophy and improve cognition [35].

1.4.4 Food Fortification: A Potential Way Forward in Combating Deficiency

Both CNNS 2016–18 India, as well as several systematic review and meta-analyses-based studies, have suggested amending the already existing fortification policies of the National Programs to combat the increasing prevalence of micronutrient deficiencies; specifically, B12 and FA deficiency. Food Safety and Standards Authority of India (FSSAI) has initiated several measures to improve/eliminate micronutrient deficiencies in the vulnerable Indian population through food supplementation and dietary diversification [36]. India, being the second top tea producer in the world (next to China), widespread usage of B12-folate fortified *tea* could be an acceptable, practically feasible, and efficacious means to improve the essential micronutrient deficiency among the vulnerable Indian population [35–37].

1.4.5 Summary and Conclusion

Vitamin B12 and folic acid are two essential micronutrients that are central to many important cellular biochemical functions in humans. It is essential to understand their natural sources, their modes of absorption, transport, and the factors influencing their bioavailability. The major factors contributing to B12-folate deficiency in India have been attributed mainly to lack of a "balanced diet," inadequate nutrition, socio-cultural practices, malabsorption, alcoholism, drugs, cancer, etc. B12 deficiency in India continues to show a higher trend, even surpassing iron deficiency in highly prevalent regions with an overall national prevalence of 53%. The majority

Table 1.2 Vitamin B12, folate deficiency in hospital setting: summary of hospital-based data from India [8, 14, 16–28]

Author, year [ref.]	Place	Age, yrs.	Number	Prevalence	Cutoff	Presentation	Remark
Bansal, 2024 [16]	PGIMER, Chandigarh	Pregnant women (24–29 years) 89%; 3rd trimester	500	B12; 65% (325/500) Isolated; 32% B12 + iron: 28% FA; 1.9%	< 150 pg/ml <2 mcg/l	Anemia	Low socioeconomic status Nutritional
Aher, 2023 [17]	GMC, Nagpur, Maharashtra	13–67	100	–	<250 pg/ml	Symptomatic anemia Neuropsychiatric Skin pigmentation	Vegetarian diet Alcoholic Male gender
Singh, 2022 [18]	Multicentre, Uttar Pradesh	All age groups, male and female	220	Low B12; 209/220 (95%) 51% (35–65 years) 40/52 (77%); MA (on BM)	<145 pg/ml	Mucocutaneous Neurological Psychiatric Hematologic	Urban males, Vegans, T2DM on therapy, PPIs, malabsorption
Aggarwal, 2022 [19]	RML, Delhi	57	688 CHF	B12; 15% Folate; 7.5%			
Mishra, 2022 [20]	KIMS, Odisha	6–14	150	B12 + FA; 74% B12; 16.7% FA; 9.3%	200 pg/ml	Symptomatic anemia Skin pigmentation	Nutritional
Behere, 2021 [14]	KEM, Pune	Pregnant mothers	46 studies	B12; 40–70% 1st, 2nd, 3rd trimester: 21%,19%, 29%	200 pg/ml	–	Maternal B12 is linked to neural tube defects, pregnancy complications, LBW, and long-term complications in offspring

Bandopadhyay, 2021 [21]	West Bengal	20–80	478	B12: Females: 27% Males: 28%	200 pg/ml	Neurological Hematological Gastrointestinal Dermatological	–
Umashankar, 2020 [22]	AIIMS, Rishikesh	1–18	111	B12; 65%		Lethargy, weight loss, pigmentation, hypotonia	Neurological manifestation is common in <6 years; hematological manifestation is common in >6 years of age.
Pattnaik, 2020 [23]	JIPMER, Pondicherry	–	105 (ALL on maintenance)	B12; 8% FA; 45%			The prevalence of anemia is linked to relapse
Azad, 2020 [24]	PGI, Chandigarh, AIIMS, New Delhi	<1 year	200	B12; 22%	211 pg/ml		>50% of developmental delay in infants is attributed to B12 deficiency
Singla, 2019 [25]	New Delhi	50	11,913	B12; 47% Pre diabetes: 37.8% Diabetes: 18%	200 pg/ml		B12 in females > males
Sharma,2019 [26] (review of studies on geriatric anemia between 2004–2015)	PGI, Chandigarh	≥60 (Geriatric)	105 Review of other studies	B12, folate; 1.9% (3–38%)		Fatigue, weakness, shortness of breath. Vertigo common in ≥80 years	>50% were vegetarians Upper GI malignancy, nutritional deficiency-common etiologies.

(continued)

Table 1.2 (continued)

Author, year [ref.]	Place	Age, yrs.	Number	Prevalence	Cutoff	Presentation	Remark
Sowndarya, 2019 [27]	KMC, Mangalore	18–70	2661	B12; 28% FA; 18.8%	<200 pg/ml		More prevalent in 18–30 years Poor nutrition Pregnancy Thyroid disorders, cancer
Deepankar, 2018 [28]	RML, PGIMER, New Delhi	15–95 years	97	B12; 54% FA; 26% B12 + FA; 21% MA; 78% (BM examination)		Symptomatic anemia Skin hyperpigmentation (48%)	63% non- vegans Alcohol Drugs Malabsorption
Padhi, 2016 [8]	PIMS, Pondicherry	Adults	198	B12; 13%	190 pg/ml	Symptomatic anemia Skin hyperpigmentation	Pigmentation linked to pancytopenia, macrocytosis, severe B12 deficiency

Table 1.3 B12 and/or FA deficiency in elderly/aging Indian population [29–34]

Author, year [ref.]	Setting	Place	Number	Age group	Prevalence	Remarks
Sundarakumar, 2021 [29]	Rural community	Bengaluru	776; males 872; females	58 ± 10.2 years	B12; 42.3% FA; 11.1%	Low socioeconomic status, dietary practice, vegan, lack of fortification programs
Sucharita, 2016 [30]		Bengaluru	47	>60 years	B12; 61.7%	Parasitic infestation, *H pylori* infection, tropical sprue were common among elderly. Low B12 is linked to poorer cognitive performance.
Gupta, 2020 [31]	Rural community	Uttarakhand	958	60–70 years	FA; high B12; not reported	Lack of recommended daily intake of FA secondary to poor socioeconomic status and faulty dietary practices
Gonmei, 2018 [32]	Slum community	New Delhi	77	≥60 years	B12; 36.4% FA; 12%	Poor socioeconomic status, malnourishment
Shobha, 2011 [33]	Urban	Bengaluru	175	>60 years	B12 (<150 pg/ml); 16%	Adequate nutritional intake
Sharma, 2024 [34]		St. John's, Bengaluru	28	≥60 years	B12 (<148 pg/ml); 20/28	Low B12 level was linked to poor skeletal mass (sarcopenia) ($R = 0.510$, $P = 0.007$)

of the Indian women of reproductive age group are already B12 deficient at the time of conception, and the prevalence of B12 deficiency is higher during the third trimester. The aging/elderly population is highly vulnerable to B12 deficiency-related cardiovascular and neurodegenerative diseases, which warrants urgent attention.

References

1. Roberts AB, Taylor A, Sodi R. Vitamins and trace elements. In: Rifai N, Horvath AR, Wittwer CT, editors. Tietz textbook of clinical chemistry and molecular diagnostics. 6th ed. New Delhi: Elsevier; 2018. p. 669–79. isbn:978-0-323-35921-4.
2. Torrez M, Chabot-Richards D, Babu D, Lockhart E, Foucar K. How I investigate acquired megaloblastic anemia. Int J Lab Hematol. 2022;44:236–47.
3. Kar R, Padhi S, Jayalakshmy R. Prevalence of anemia and burden of disease in India. In: Sasidharan PK, editor. ICH Nutritional anemias in India. Guidelines for diagnosis and management. 1st ed. New Delhi: Jaypee Brothers Medical Publishers Pvt. Ltd; 2024. p. 1–15. isbn:978-9-356-96934-6.
4. Castellanos-Sinco HB, Ramos-Peñafiel CO, Santoyo-Sánchezc A, Collazo-Jalomaa J, Martínez-Murilloa C, Montaño-Figueroaa E, Sinco-Ángeles A. Megaloblastic anaemia: folic acid and vitamin B12 metabolism. Rev Med Hosp Gen Méx. 2015;78:135–43.
5. Shane B. Folate and vitamin B12 metabolism: overview and interaction with riboflavin, vitamin B6, and polymorphisms. Food Nutr Bull. 2008;29(2 (supplement)):S5–S16.
6. Green R. Vitamin B12 deficiency from the perspective of a practicing haematologist. Blood. 2017;129:2603–11.
7. Kumar V, Abbas AK, Aster JC. Red blood cell and bleeding disorders. In: Robbins and Cotran pathologic basis of disease. 10th ed. New Delhi: Elsevier; 2020. isbn:978-0-323-53113-9.
8. Padhi S, Sarangi R, Ramdas A, Ravichandran K, Varghese RG, Alexander T, et al. Cutaneous hyperpigmentation in megaloblastic anemia: a five-year retrospective review. Mediterr J Hematol Infect Dis. 2016;8:e2016021.
9. Thomas L, Sasidharan PK. Clinical profile of vitamin B12 deficiency and response to treatment. Ann Clin Med Res. 2021;2:1052.
10. Sasidharan PK. B12 deficiency in India. Arch Med Health Sci. 2017;5:261–8.
11. Yajnik C, Deshmukh U, Katre P, Limaye T. Vitamin B12 deficiency in developing and newly industrialising countries. In: Vitamin B12, Advances and insights. 1st ed. Taylor & Francis Group; 2017. https://doi.org/10.1201/9781315119540-7.
12. Shalini T, Pullakhandam R, Ghosh S, Kulkarni B, Rajkumar H, Sachdev HS, et al. Prevalence of vitamin B12 and folate deficiencies in Indian children and adolescents. Nutrients. 2023;15:3026.
13. Venkatesh U, Sharma A, Ananthan VA, Subbiah P, Durga R, CSIR Summer Research training team. Micronutrient's deficiency in India: a systematic review and meta-analysis. J Nutr Sci. 2021;10:e110.
14. Behere RV, Deshmukh AS, Otiv S, Gupte MD, Yajnik CS. Maternal vitamin B12 status during pregnancy and its association with outcomes of pregnancy and health of the offspring: a systematic review and implications for policy in India. Front Endocrinol (Lausanne). 2021;12:619176.
15. Finkelstein JL, Fothergill A, Krisher JT, Thomas T, Kurpad AV, Dwarkanath P. Maternal vitamin B12 deficiency and perinatal outcomes in southern India. PLoS One. 2021;16:e0248145.
16. Bansal A, Suri V, Sikka P, Attri SV, Varma N, Saini SS, et al. B12 deficiency is the commonest cause of anaemia during pregnancy in northern India: study from a tertiary care institute. Indian J Hematol Blood Transfus. 2024;40:78–82.
17. Aher A, Navghare P, Zawar S. Study of clinical and haematological profile of vitamin B12 deficiency and to check response to vitamin B12 therapy. Vidarbha J Intern Med. 2023;33:73–6.

18. Singh J, Dinkar A, Gupta P, Atam V. Vitamin B12 deficiency in northern India tertiary care: prevalence, risk factors and clinical characteristics. J Family Med Prim Care. 2022;11:2381–8.
19. Aggarwal P, Sinha SK, Khanra D, Razi M, Nath RK, Shrivastava A. Hematinic deficiency in patients with heart failure with reduced ejection fraction (HFrEF). Ann Cardiol Angeiol (Paris). 2022;71:153–9.
20. Mishra R, Madduri MV, Pradhan S. Megaloblastic anemia in children from Eastern Odisha, India: a clinical and hematological profile analysis. Natl J Physiol Pharm Pharmacol. 2022;12:1493–6.
21. Bandopadhyay D, Choudhury JR, Mukherjee K. Vitamin B12 deficiency in Eastern India: a hospital based cross-sectional study. J Clin Diagn Res. 2021;15:BC01–4.
22. Umasanker S, Bhakat R, Mehta S, Rathaur VK, Verma PK, Bhat NK, et al. Vitamin B12 deficiency in children from Northern India: time to reconsider nutritional handicaps. J Family Med Prim Care. 2020;9:4985–91.
23. Pattnaik J, Kayal S, Dubashi B, Basu D, Vinod KV, Nandeesha H, et al. Profile of anemia in acute lymphoblastic leukemia patients on maintenance therapy and the effect of micronutrient supplementation. Support Care Cancer. 2020;28:731–8.
24. Azad C, Jat KR, Kaur J, Guglani V, Palta A, Tiwari A, et al. Vitamin B12 status and neurodevelopmental delay in Indian infants: a hospital-based cross-sectional study. Paediatr Int Child Health. 2020;40:78–84.
25. Singla R, Garg A, Surana V, Aggarwal S, Gupta G, Singla S. Vitamin B12 deficiency is endemic in Indian population: a perspective from North India. Indian J Endocrinol Metab. 2019;23:211–4.
26. Sharma D, Suri V, Pannu AK, Attri SV, Varma N, Kochhar R, et al. Patterns of geriatric anemia: a hospital-based observational study in North India. J Family Med Prim Care. 2019;8:976–80.
27. Sowndarya K, Basavaiah SH, Shenoy R, Hegde A. Proportion and associated factors of vitamin B12 deficiency - a retrospective laboratory-based study. Curr Res Nutr Food Sci. 2019;7(3).
28. Deepankar P, Roshan R, Gupta HK, Buxi G. Relative prevalence of vitamin B12 and folic acid in megaloblastic anemia and its clinical – etiological profile in a tertiary care center. Int J Sci Stud. 2018;6:23–30.
29. Sundarakumar JS, Shahul Hameed SK, SANSCOG Study Team, Ravindranath V. Burden of vitamin D, vitamin B12 and folic acid deficiencies in an aging, rural Indian community. Front Public Health. 2021;9:707036.
30. Sucharita S, Thomas T, Sowmya S, Krishnamachari S, Kurpad VA, Vaz M. Subclinical vitamin B12 deficiency and heart rate variability across life cycle. Curr Aging Sci. 2016;9:217–23.
31. Gupta A, Ramakrishnan L, Pandey R, Sati H, Khandelwal R, Khenduja P, et al. Risk factors of anemia amongst elderly population living at high-altitude region of India. J Family Med Prim Care. 2020;9:673.
32. Gonmei Z, Dwivedi S, Toteja GS, Singh K, Vikram NK, Bansal PG. Anaemia and vitamin B12 deficiency in elderly. Asian J Pharm Clin Res. 2018;11:402–4.
33. Shobha V, Tarey SD, Singh RG, Shetty P, Unni US, Srinivasan K, et al. Vitamin B12 deficiency and levels of metabolites in an apparently normal urban South Indian elderly population. Indian J Med Res. 2011;134:432–9.
34. Sharma S, Bhadra R, Selvam S, Sambashivaiah S. Vitamin B12 status and skeletal muscle function among elderly: a literature review and pilot study on the effect of oral vitamin B12 supplementation in improving muscle function. Aging Med (Milton). 2024;7:480–9.
35. Vora RM, Alappattu MJ, Zarkar AD, Soni MS, Karmarkar SJ, Antony AC. Potential for elimination of folate and vitamin B12 deficiency in India using vitamin-fortified tea: a preliminary study. BMJ Nutr Prev Health. 2021;4:293–306.
36. Food Safety and Standards Authority of India (FSSAI). Food safety and standards authority of India: joint Declaration on food fortification. Available: http://www.old.fssai.gov.in/Portals/0/Pdf/Joint_Declaration_Food_Fortification_21_10_2016.pdf. Accessed 9 Sept 2019.
37. Goh YE, Manger MS, Duggal M, Das R, Saklani S, Agarwal S, et al. Women in selected communities of Punjab, India have a high prevalence of iron, zinc, vitamin B12, and folate deficiencies: implications for a multiply-fortified salt intervention. Nutrients. 2023;15:3024.

Chapter 2
Iron Metabolism and Inherited Causes of Iron Deficiency Anemia

Vinu Balraam KV and Jasmita

Abstract Iron metabolism is crucial for oxygen transport and enzymatic functions, with disruptions leading to iron deficiency anemia (IDA). While acquired IDA is common, inherited forms arise from genetic mutations affecting iron absorption, transport, and utilization. These include iron-refractory iron deficiency anemia (IRIDA), hypotransferrinemia, DMT1 deficiency, ferroportin disease, and congenital sideroblastic anemias, which often mimic acquired IDA.

This chapter highlights the molecular mechanisms regulating iron homeostasis, emphasizing transferrin, DMT1, ferroportin, and hepcidin. Genetic mutations in *TMPRSS6*, *TF*, *SLC11A2*, *ALAS2*, and *SLC25A38* disrupt iron balance, leading to anemia. A structured diagnostic approach incorporating iron markers (serum iron, ferritin, transferrin saturation [TSAT], soluble transferrin receptor [sTFR]), hepcidin levels, and genetic testing is essential for distinguishing between inherited iron deficiency anemia (IDA) and acquired cases.

Management requires individualized treatment. IRIDA is refractory to oral iron and necessitates intravenous (IV) iron therapy, while hypotransferrinemia may need plasma or apotransferrin (apoTf) therapy. Vitamin B6 benefits some cases of sideroblastic anemia, and hematopoietic stem cell transplantation (HSCT) is curative for severe cases. Emerging therapies, such as hepcidin modulators, CRISPR-based gene therapy, and AI-driven precision medicine, may become promising alternatives.

Future research focuses on genomic sequencing, non-invasive iron monitoring, and personalized iron chelation. Advances in gene-editing technologies and stem cell therapies may revolutionize treatment, improving patient outcomes. A deeper understanding of iron regulatory pathways and genetic determinants is key to early diagnosis and targeted therapy.

Vinu Balraam KV (✉)
Command Hospital Chandimandir, Panchkula, India

Jasmita
All India Institute of Medical Sciences, New Delhi, India
e-mail: jasmita@aiims.edu

H. P. Pati et al. (eds.), *Clinical Hematology and Hemato-Oncology*,
https://doi.org/10.1007/978-981-92-1167-8_2

Keywords Genetic mutations · Hepcidin regulation · Iron deficiency · Iron metabolism · Microcytic anemia

Learning Objectives

- *Understand Iron Metabolism:* Appreciate the key pathways involved in iron absorption, transport, storage, and utilization, highlighting regulatory mechanisms such as hepcidin, transferrin, and ferroportin.
- *Differentiate Between Inherited and Acquired IDA:* Identify the genetic mutations affecting iron homeostasis and differentiate them from acquired causes of microcytic anemia.
- *Diagnose Genetic Iron Deficiency Disorders:* Implement a structured diagnostic approach using biochemical markers (serum iron, ferritin, transferrin saturation, soluble transferrin receptor), hepcidin levels, and genetic testing.
- *Classify Different Types of Inherited IDA:* Recognize the clinical and laboratory features of IRIDA (*TMPRSS6* mutations), hypotransferrinemia (*TF* mutations), sideroblastic anemias (*SLC25A38*, *ALAS2* mutations), and *DMT1* deficiency (*SLC11A2* mutations).
- *Optimize Treatment Strategies:* Learn about tailored treatment plans using IV iron therapy, plasma transfusions, pyridoxine, iron chelation, erythropoietin (EPO) therapy, and HSCT.

2.1 Introduction

From the dawn of human civilization during the Iron Age, when iron was prized for its utility in tools, weapons, and even early medicinal applications, to its modern characterization as a vital element in cellular processes, our understanding of iron has undergone a dramatic evolution. Early observations of iron's role in human blood laid the groundwork for later discoveries that defined its essential function in hemoglobin (Hb). At the same time, advances in biochemistry revealed the sophisticated mechanisms governing its absorption, transport, and storage—most notably through proteins like transferrin (Tf) and ferritin and regulatory systems such as the iron regulatory proteins/elements (IRP/IRE) network. Today, research into iron metabolism sheds light on fundamental aspects of human physiology and informs strategies for managing disorders ranging from anemia to iron overload.

It was as early eighteenth century that the presence of iron was established in the red blood cells (RBCs) by an Italian Physician and Scientist, Dr. Vincenzo Menghini, which even preceded the discovery of Hb [1]. In the clinical context, iron deficiency has been widely recognized since the medieval ages. Claimed to be hysterical and known by various names, *Chlorosis*, or green sickness, or De morbo virgineo, was a disease thought to affect mainly adolescent/teenage girls as early as 1554 [2]. This was followed by a gradual decline in the prevalence of this disease, coinciding with a trend of general improvement in hygiene and nutrition, increasing acceptance of meat consumption, and various other unknown factors [3]. Today, menstruating women and pregnant ladies, closely followed by children of growing age, are the ones who are most likely to develop iron deficiency owing to a mismatch between demand and supply. Understanding this requires exploring iron metabolism, one of the most tightly regulated processes in the human body.

2.2 Clinical Case

In this section, we will discuss a clinical case scenario wherein a 5-year-old boy is brought to the clinic by his parents due to persistent fatigue, pale skin, and slow growth. He was previously diagnosed with IDA and was on oral iron supplements for the past 6 months with minimal improvement in Hb levels.

On initial evaluation, there was a history of chronic blood loss, gastrointestinal issues, or dietary iron deficiency. Family history reveals a sibling with similar anemia but without any clear diagnosis. On physical examination, he had pallor with mild tachycardia. No jaundice or organomegaly was appreciated. Lab workup revealed microcytic hypochromic anemia (MHA) with Hb 8.5 g/dL, mean corpuscular volume (MCV) of 55 fL, serum iron 15 μg/dL, 10% TSAT, serum ferritin of 80 ng/mL, normal soluble transferrin receptor (sTfR) levels, and high hepcidin levels. There was no history of any chronic disease, and the autoimmune workup was negative. Hb electrophoresis did not reveal any abnormality, and the workup for common alpha and beta thalassemia mutations returned negative. Next-generation sequencing (NGS) revealed a homozygous variant in the *TMPRSS6* gene c.939del (p.Phe314fs). The sibling was also tested subsequently and found to be positive for the same mutation. A final diagnosis was IRIDA, which highlights the importance of a careful algorithmic approach to identify unexplained microcytic anemia.

2.3 Iron Metabolism: The Essential Blueprint

Iron is an indispensable micronutrient that supports numerous critical physiological processes, including oxygen transport, cellular respiration, DNA synthesis, and various enzymatic reactions. As a transition metal, iron alternates between ferrous (Fe^{2+}) and ferric (Fe^{3+}) states, a property that underlies its utility in redox reactions but also its potential for toxicity through the generation of reactive oxygen species (ROS) [4, 5]. The human body carefully regulates iron levels to ensure sufficient availability for vital functions while preventing excess accumulation that can lead to cellular damage. Unlike other nutrients, iron cannot be actively excreted from the body; instead, it is recycled and stored efficiently. This regulation depends on the intestinal absorption of iron from the duodenum, transport via transferrin (Tf), storage in ferritin, recycling from senescent red blood cells (RBCs), and systemic regulation by hepcidin [6]. This chapter provides a comprehensive overview of the

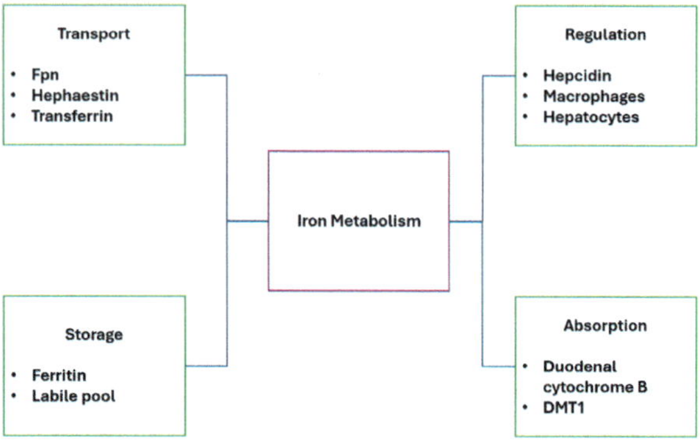

Fig. 2.1 Iron metabolism is tightly regulated by factors governing iron absorption, transport, storage, and recycling via various regulatory pathways. (Image generated from Napkin AI—Available from: https://www.napkin.ai). DMT1 divalent metal transporter 1; Fpn ferroportin

mechanisms governing iron absorption, transport, storage, and recycling, as well as the regulatory pathways that maintain systemic iron balance (Fig. 2.1).

2.3.1 *Iron Absorption and Distribution*

The total body iron content in an average adult ranges between 3 and 4 g. This iron is distributed among several compartments:

(a) Hemoglobin: Approximately 65–70% of body iron is found in Hb within RBCs. This form of iron is critical for the reversible binding of oxygen and its delivery to tissues.
(b) Myoglobin and Enzymes: Around 5–10% of iron is present in myoglobin (which stores oxygen in muscle) and various enzymes involved in mitochondrial respiration, catalysis, and DNA synthesis.
(c) Storage Forms: About 20–30% of iron is stored in the liver, spleen, and bone marrow (BM) as ferritin or hemosiderin. Ferritin is a protein complex that can store up to 4500 iron atoms per molecule in a redox-inactive state.
(d) Plasma Transport Pool: A small fraction (<0.1%) circulates in plasma, bound to Tf, which safeguards against iron-induced oxidative damage and facilitates cell delivery.

This compartmentalization ensures that iron is readily available for critical cellular functions while limiting the concentration of free iron that could catalyze harmful oxidative reactions. This distribution varies with age, sex, and physiological conditions. Newborns and menstruating women have higher iron demands [4].

Dietary sources of iron include both heme and non-heme iron [5]. Heme iron is predominantly found in animal-based foods (e.g., red meat, poultry, and fish) and is highly bioavailable due to its intact porphyrin ring structure. Despite constituting only about 10–15% of the total dietary iron, heme iron accounts for nearly two-thirds of the absorbed iron in omnivorous diets. On the contrary, non-heme iron, present in plant-based foods and iron-fortified products, is less readily absorbed. Its absorption is highly variable, ranging from approximately 5–12% in vegetarian diets to 14–18% in mixed diets, and is influenced by several factors [6].

2.3.2 Molecular Mechanisms of Iron Absorption [5]

Iron absorption occurs primarily in the duodenum and proximal jejunum, where enterocytes serve as the gatekeepers of systemic iron intake. The process involves several key steps:

1. Reduction of Non-heme Iron: Most non-heme iron is ingested in the Fe^{3+} state, which is insoluble and poorly absorbed. To facilitate absorption, Fe^{3+} must be reduced to Fe^{2+}. This reduction is mediated by duodenal cytochrome b (Dcytb), an enzyme localized to the brush border of enterocytes. Dcytb utilizes electrons from dietary ascorbic acid and other reducing agents to convert Fe^{3+} into the more soluble Fe^{2+}.
2. Transport Across the Apical Membrane: Once reduced, enterocytes take up Fe^{2+} via divalent metal transporter 1 (DMT1). DMT1 is a proton-coupled symporter that relies on an acidic microenvironment for optimal function. The Na^+/H^+ exchanger-3 (NHE3) in the duodenum helps maintain this acidic pH, thereby indirectly supporting iron uptake.
3. Heme Iron Absorption: Uptake of heme iron by duodenal enterocytes is still unknown, but a mechanism that involves the heme carrier protein 1 (HCP1) protein, encoded by the *SLC46A1* gene, has been proposed [7]. Once inside the cell, heme oxygenase-1 (HO-1) degrades the heme molecule, releasing Fe^{2+}, which follows the same intracellular pathways as non-heme iron.
4. Intracellular Fate of Absorbed Iron: Within enterocytes, absorbed iron has two possible fates:
   (a) Storage: Iron may be stored bound to ferritin. This is a protective mechanism that temporarily sequesters iron and prevents the formation of free radicals.
   (b) Export: Iron destined for systemic circulation is exported from the basolateral side of the enterocyte by ferroportin (FPN1), the only known iron exporter. Before export, Fe^{2+} must be oxidized to Fe^{3+} to facilitate its binding to Tf in the plasma. This oxidation is carried out by hephaestin or ceruloplasmin

2.3.3 Regulation of Absorption

The efficiency of dietary iron absorption is finely tuned based on the body's iron status:

(a) Enhancers: Vitamin C (ascorbate) significantly increases non-heme iron absorption by acting as a reducing agent.
(b) Inhibitors: Dietary components like phytates, polyphenols, and calcium can impede absorption.
(c) Adaptive Mechanisms: In states of iron deficiency, the expression of DMT1 is upregulated, and absorptive efficiency can increase several-fold (up to 3–5 times), ensuring that even low dietary iron can meet physiological needs [6].

2.3.4 *Iron Transport and Cellular Uptake*

1. Role of Transferrin in Iron Transport: Once iron is exported from enterocytes, it is oxidized to Fe^{3+} and binds to Tf, a plasma glycoprotein [5]. Tf transports iron in the blood in a non-reactive state, protecting tissues from potential oxidative damage. Under normal conditions, Tf is about 30% saturated with iron, which allows a buffer capacity to accommodate fluctuations in iron levels.
2. Transferrin Receptors and Endocytosis: Cells that require iron express transferrin receptors (TfR1 and TfR2) on their surfaces. Erythroid precursors are particularly rich in TfR1 [5]. Diferric transferrin (Fe^{3+}-Tf) binding to TfR1 triggers receptor-mediated endocytosis, forming an endocytic vesicle. Within the acidic environment of the endosome, Fe^{3+} is reduced to Fe^{2+} by the enzyme STEAP3 Ferrireductase, and DMT1 then transports Fe^{2+} into the cytosol, where it becomes available for metabolic processes such as heme synthesis and the production of iron-sulfur (Fe/S) clusters essential for mitochondrial function. The apoTf-TfR complex is recycled back to the plasma membrane, where apoTf is released at neutral pH to bind more iron. The excess iron is stored as ferritin and hemosiderin.
3. Non-Transferrin Bound Iron (NTBI): In cases of iron overload, when Tf is nearly saturated, excess iron exists as NTBI, which is taken up by tissues through alternate pathways (e.g., ZIP14 transporter in hepatocytes) and is associated with cellular toxicity due to its propensity to generate ROS [8].

2.3.5 *Iron Storage and Recycling*

1. Intracellular Iron Storage in Ferritin: Ferritin is the primary intracellular iron storage protein and comprises 24 subunits forming a hollow sphere capable of storing up to 4500 iron atoms in a soluble, non-toxic form. Ferritin has two distinct forms, and its composition can vary:

   (a) *H-ferritin* contains ferroxidase activity and facilitates the rapid oxidation of Fe^{2+} to Fe^{3+}.
   (b) *L-ferritin* promotes efficient nucleation and storage of iron.

When iron is in excess, it is sequestered within ferritin to protect cells from iron-induced oxidative damage. Additionally, hemosiderin serves as a long-term storage form in cases of iron overload.

2. Recycling Iron Through Macrophages: The majority of iron used daily is not derived from dietary absorption but from the recycling of senescent RBCs. Macrophages of the reticuloendothelial system (RES), primarily in the spleen, liver, and BM, are responsible for this recycling process. Macrophages engulf old or damaged RBCs, following which the enzyme heme oxygenase-1 (HO-1) breaks down heme into biliverdin, carbon monoxide, and free iron. Iron is then either stored in ferritin or exported from macrophages by ferroportin. The exported Fe^{2+} is oxidized by hephaestin or ceruloplasmin, allowing binding to transferrin and re-entry into the plasma iron pool [5].

This recycling process is highly efficient, with approximately 20–25 mg of iron recycled daily, far exceeding the 1–2 mg absorbed from the diet [4]. This makes recycling the predominant source of iron for ongoing physiological functions, especially for erythropoiesis.

2.3.6 Regulation of Iron Homeostasis: The Hepcidin-Ferroportin Axis

1. Hepcidin: The Central Regulator [6]: Hepcidin is a small peptide hormone produced mainly in the liver and is considered the master regulator of systemic iron homeostasis. It controls iron levels by binding to ferroportin on the surface of enterocytes, macrophages, and hepatocytes, inducing its internalization and subsequent degradation. This action limits iron release into the bloodstream and reduces intestinal iron absorption.
2. Factors Influencing Hepcidin Expression [6]: Several physiological signals finely tune hepcidin synthesis:

   (a) Iron Status: Elevated body iron levels stimulate hepcidin production via the bone morphogenic protein (BMP)-SMAD signaling pathway. Key molecules in this pathway include BMP6, hemojuvelin (HJV), and the HFE protein. Mutations in these components can lead to abnormal hepcidin expression and iron overload.

   (b) Erythropoietic Activity: Increased erythropoietic demand, such as during hemorrhage or growth spurts, suppresses hepcidin production. Erythroblasts secrete erythroferrone (ERFE), which inhibits hepcidin synthesis, thereby promoting iron release for hemoglobin synthesis.

   (c) Inflammation: Pro-inflammatory cytokines, notably interleukin-6 (IL-6), induce hepcidin transcription through the JAK-STAT3 pathway. This response helps limit iron availability to pathogens during infections but may contribute to anemia of chronic disease.

(d) Hypoxia: Hypoxia-inducible factors (HIFs) modulate iron absorption under low oxygen conditions. HIF2α enhances iron uptake by increasing the expression of DMT1 and ferroportin in enterocytes.

3. Molecular Signaling in Hepcidin Regulation: At the molecular level, the regulation of hepcidin transcription involves several interconnected pathways:

   (a) BMP-SMAD Pathway: BMP6 binds to its receptors (BMPR) on hepatocytes in conjunction with the co-receptor HJV. This binding triggers the phosphorylation of SMAD1/5/8 proteins, which form complexes with SMAD4 and translocate to the nucleus. The SMAD complex binds to the promoter region of the *HAMP* gene (encoding hepcidin), increasing its transcription.
   (b) HFE-TfR2 Axis: The interaction between HFE and transferrin receptor 2 (TfR2), modulated by the levels of diferric transferrin, also influences hepcidin synthesis. This complex is enhanced when plasma iron is high, leading to increased hepcidin production.
   (c) Erythropoietic Suppression via ERFE: ERFE is secreted by erythroid precursors in response to EPO stimulation. It acts as a decoy, binding BMP6 and dampening BMP-SMAD signaling, resulting in reduced hepcidin transcription [5].

These pathways underscore the dynamic and responsive nature of hepcidin regulation, ensuring that iron absorption and recycling are closely matched to the body's needs.

2.3.7 *Intracellular Iron Regulation: The IRP/IRE System*

Beyond systemic regulation, iron metabolism is also controlled at the cellular level by the IRP/IRE system. This post-transcriptional mechanism adjusts the expression of key iron metabolism proteins in response to intracellular iron levels [9].

1. Mechanism of the IRP/IRE System

IRPs (IRP1 and IRP2) are RNA-binding proteins that interact with IREs, specific stem-loop structures located in mRNA's untranslated regions (UTRs). Under low iron conditions, IRPs bind to IREs. Bindings to the 3′ UTRs (e.g., TfR1 mRNA) stabilize the mRNA, thus increasing the synthesis of iron uptake proteins. On the contrary, binding to the 5′ UTRs (e.g., ferritin, ferroportin mRNAs) inhibits translation, reducing iron storage and export [3].

When intracellular iron is sufficient, IRP binding diminishes, leading to degradation of TfR1 mRNA, thereby reducing iron uptake. Simultaneously, ferritin and ferroportin translation increases, promoting iron storage and export [3].

2. Regulation of IRP Activity

IRP1 exists in two forms—an active RNA-binding form when iron is scarce and an inactive aconitase form when it binds a [4Fe-4S] cluster under iron-replete conditions [9]. IRP2 is regulated by iron-dependent degradation via the ubiquitin-proteasome pathway. In iron-replete cells, IRP2 is ubiquitinated and degraded, leading to decreased IRE binding [10]. This fine-tuning ensures that cellular iron uptake, storage, and export are adjusted dynamically according to intracellular iron concentrations.

2.3.8 Integration of Iron Metabolism: A Dynamic Network

The coordination of iron absorption, transport, storage, and recycling involves an intricate network of molecular signals. Enterocytes, hepatocytes, and macrophages communicate through hormonal signals such as hepcidin and regulatory proteins like IRPs to maintain iron balance. For instance, when iron stores are low, enterocytes upregulate DMT1 expression, and ferroportin remains active, while low hepcidin levels permit maximum iron export from both enterocytes and macrophages. In states of iron overload, increased hepcidin levels lead to ferroportin degradation, limiting both dietary absorption and iron release from storage sites. Erythropoietic signals, primarily mediated by ERFE, further fine-tune this balance by suppressing hepcidin in response to increased red blood cell production demands.

The dynamic interplay between these systems ensures that iron supply is continuously matched to the metabolic and developmental needs of the organism.

2.3.9 Iron in Heme Synthesis: The Final Integration

Heme synthesis, primarily occurring in erythroid precursor cells, is a tightly regulated process requiring iron as a crucial cofactor (Fig. 2.2). It begins in the mitochondria with succinyl-CoA and glycine, catalyzed by aminolevulinate synthase (ALAS2), whose translation is controlled by the IRE/IRP system to synchronize heme production with iron availability [11]. Aminolevulinic acid (ALA) undergoes cytosolic enzymatic reactions, forming protoporphyrin IX, which is converted to heme by ferrochelatase (FECH) via Fe^{2+} insertion [11]. Iron also regulates gene expression and enzyme activity in heme synthesis. Transferrin receptor 1 (TfR1) facilitates iron uptake into mitochondria via mitoferrin-1 (MFRN1) and ABCB10 transporters. An impaired iron supply disrupts heme production, leading to anemia [12]. Heme-regulated inhibitor (HRI) kinase balances heme and globin synthesis, preventing excess globin production [11]. This intricate regulation ensures efficient erythropoiesis and hemoglobin function, emphasizing the necessity of iron homeostasis.

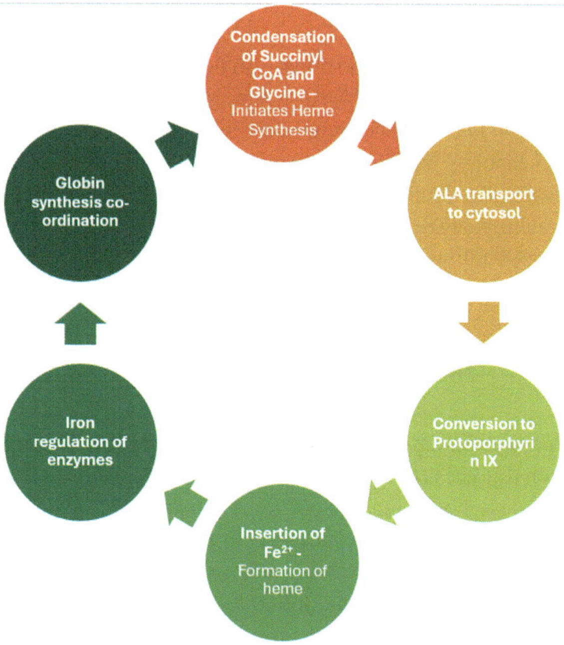

Fig. 2.2 Heme synthesis and iron regulation cycle. (Image generated from Napkin AI—Available from: https://www.napkin.ai)

2.4 Overview of Iron Deficiency Anemia

Iron deficiency (ID) and iron deficiency anemia (IDA) impose a substantial disease burden worldwide. Globally, there were over 1.2 billion cases of IDA in 2016 [13]. According to WHO estimates, 42% of anemia cases in children and 50% in women can be effectively managed with iron supplementation, though the impact varies across different regions [14].

Reduced iron availability for RBC production leads to iron-deficient erythropoiesis, characterized by hypochromia, microcytosis, and anemia. IDA impacts erythropoiesis by altering renal EPO production and modulating erythroblast sensitivity to EPO through TfR2. In cases of absolute ID, erythroblasts and RBCs contribute to maintaining plasma iron levels by donating iron through ferroportin, which helps counteract serum iron depletion and shields red blood cells from oxidative stress. These findings challenge the conventional view that microcytic anemia is the primary consequence of absolute iron deficiency. Instead, erythroid cells actively release iron to ensure an adequate supply for other physiological functions [15].

The primary causes of absolute ID include excessive blood loss and insufficient dietary iron intake or absorption, which fail to meet the body's physiological demands (Fig. 2.3). Few important causes of IDA are listed in Table 2.1.

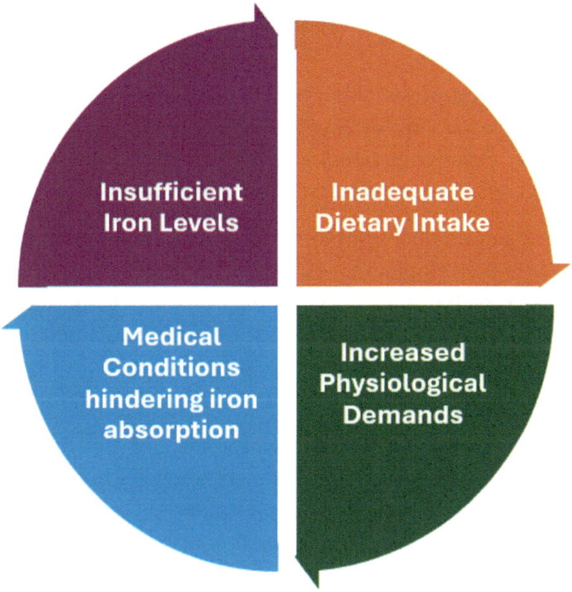

Fig. 2.3 Most important causes of iron deficiency include inadequate dietary intake and excessive blood loss, failing to meet the increased physiological demands. (Image generated from Napkin AI—Available from: https://www.napkin.ai)

Table 2.1 Causes of absolute iron deficiency **(list includes but is not limited to)**

Category	Subcategory	Causes
Inadequate iron uptake	Inadequate nutritional iron intake	Low heme iron diet, food insecurity, poor diet diversity, and prolonged breastfeeding
	Inadequate nutritional iron absorption	Use of antacids, gastric bypass surgery, atrophic gastritis, *H. pylori* infection, and inflammatory bowel disease
	Obesity and genetic factors	Increased hepcidin in chronic inflammation, and iron-refractory anemia (*TMPRSS6* mutations)
Increased iron requirements	Growth, pregnancy, blood loss	Early childhood growth, pregnancy, heavy menstruation, and erythropoiesis-stimulating therapy
Blood loss	Gastrointestinal blood loss	Varices, ulcers, carcinoma, reflux esophagitis, NSAID use, and inflammatory bowel disease
	Gynecological bleeding	Heavy menstruation, bleeding disorders (von Willebrand, hemophilia), fibroids, and intrauterine devices
	Urinary tract bleeding	Renal or bladder cancer, schistosomiasis, and intravascular hemolysis
	Respiratory and other blood loss	Severe hemoptysis (lung cancer, infections), blood donation, and hemodialysis-related iron losses
Exercise	Physical activity and hemolysis	Iron loss in sweat, reduced dietary iron intake, gastrointestinal bleeding, and hemolysis

H. pylori Helicobacter pylori, *NSAID* non-steroidal anti-inflammatory drug

2.4.1 *Clinical Manifestations and Diagnosis*

The clinical presentation of IDA varies depending on the severity of iron depletion. Early stages may be asymptomatic, but as the condition progresses, patients commonly experience fatigue, pallor, weakness, and reduced exercise tolerance due to impaired oxygen delivery. Other manifestations include:

(a) Neurological symptoms: Cognitive impairment, poor concentration, irritability, and developmental delays in children.
(b) Epithelial changes: Dry skin, brittle nails, and koilonychia (spoon-shaped nails).
(c) Gastrointestinal symptoms: Glossitis (inflamed tongue), angular stomatitis, and dysphagia.
(d) Pica: A craving for non-nutritive substances like ice, dirt, or starch.

Apart from these classic symptoms, many of the inherited causes of IDA present with features of iron overload and target organ damage. In the subsequent sections, we will be discussing the various inherited causes of IDA, its pathophysiology, clinical manifestations, treatment options, and implications as far as future research trends are concerned.

2.5 Inherited Causes of Iron Deficiency Anemia, Pathophysiology, and Clinical Features

Unlike acquired iron deficiency anemia (IDA), which is commonly caused by nutritional deficiencies, chronic blood loss, or malabsorption, inherited forms of IDA result from genetic mutations that impair iron absorption, transport, storage, or utilization. These conditions are rare and often present as MHAs that do not respond to conventional oral iron therapy. Inherited IDA disorders can be classified based on the affected genes and biological pathways involved in iron metabolism:

1. *Defects in Iron Transport and Uptake*

   (a) Hypotransferrinemia (*TF* gene mutations): Causes a deficiency of transferrin, the protein responsible for iron transport.
   (b) DMT1 mutations (*SLC11A2* gene): Impair the iron transporter involved in intestinal iron absorption and erythroid iron uptake.
   (c) *STEAP3* mutations: Affect ferrireductase activity, impairing iron reduction and uptake.

2. *Defects in Iron Absorption*
   Iron-Refractory Iron Deficiency Anemia (IRIDA, *TMPRSS6* mutations): Leads to inappropriately high hepcidin levels, blocking dietary iron absorption.
3. *Defects in Iron Recycling*
   Aceruloplasminemia (*CP* gene mutations): Affects iron mobilization from stores, leading to systemic iron dysregulation.

4. *Defects in Mitochondrial Iron Utilization*

   X-linked and autosomal recessive sideroblastic anemias (*ALAS2*, *ABCB7*, *SLC25A38*, *GLRX5* mutations): Impair iron incorporation into heme, leading to ring sideroblasts (RS).

These rare genetic conditions require specialized genetic testing and targeted management strategies to distinguish them from acquired iron deficiency anemia (IDA). Table 2.2 provides a comprehensive list of inherited causes of IDA.

Table 2.2 Inherited causes of iron deficiency anemia [18–21]

Category of defect and *disease*	Gene	Pathophysiology and genetic basis	Clinical features
Iron absorption-*IRIDA*	*TMPRSS6*	Mutations in *TMPRSS6* lead to defective Matriptase-2 protein, which fails to suppress hepcidin, reducing iron absorption and resulting in iron deficiency despite adequate intake Autosomal recessive (Chromosome 22q12-q13) 20 missense mutations 5 nonsense mutations 10 frameshift mutations 1 large in-frame deletion 9 intronic mutations (milder phenotype) High frequency of *TMPRSS6* variations in Indian ethnicity	Symptoms in early childhood (may ameliorate into adulthood due to reduced iron requirement) MHA with low TSAT and normal/high levels of hepcidin No improvement with oral iron supplements (slow response to IV iron) Misdiagnosis is common in India due to limited genetic testing and low awareness
Iron transport *Congenital hypotransferrinemia/ hereditary atransferrinemia*	*TF*	Lack of transferrin, defective iron transport Extremely rare disorder, reported in only around 16 cases from 14 families worldwide Genetic basis is not fully understood, with a handful of case reports describing polymorphisms at various nucleotide positions	Pallor, fatigue, and increased sensitivity to infections Severe hepatic, pancreatic, and cardiac iron overload due to the presence of NTBI, compounded by enhanced intestinal iron absorption due to decreased hepatic hepcidin production
Iron uptake *DMT1-related anemia*	*SLC11A2* (DMT1)	Defective iron uptake from intestine and endosomes Very rare disorder (only a few cases)	Birth-young adulthood age of presentation Microcytic anemia, milder increase in ferritin and visceral iron overload

(continued)

Table 2.2 (continued)

Category of defect and *disease*	Gene	Pathophysiology and genetic basis	Clinical features
Iron export *Ferroportin-related anemia/type 4A hemochromatosis*	*SLC40A1*	Failure of iron export, iron trapping in enterocytes and macrophages Autosomal dominant Iron retention mainly within the macrophages	Iron-restricted erythropoiesis affects adults mainly No anemia in the basal state (although plasma iron and TSAT may be decreased) Anemia can occur during venesection therapy due to a defective iron recycling process
Iron export- *Aceruloplasminemia*	CP gene	Autosomal recessive Iron overload in CP mutations is primarily due to the absence of CP-related ferroxidase activity, which disrupts ferroportin-mediated iron export, causing iron accumulation in cells.	Adulthood Low plasma iron and TSAT Visceral iron overload in liver and basal ganglia (extra-pyramidal symptoms) Absence of spleen iron overload
Iron export-*STEAP3/ TSAP6-related anemia*	*STEAP3/TSAP6*	Defect in iron egress from the endosome Loss of ferrireductase activity leads to trapping of Fe^{3+} in the endocytic vesicles	Mild MHA RS in BM
Iron utilization *CSA*	*SLC25A38*	Autosomal recessive (one of the most frequent causes of CSA) *SLC25A38* gene encodes the erythroid-specific mitochondrial carrier protein Defective mitochondrial iron incorporation leading to impaired heme synthesis	Young age Severe transfusion dependent microcytic anemia, increased serum iron, visceral iron overload and presence of RS in BM
Iron utilization-*X-linked sideroblastic anemia*	*ALAS2*	80 different mutations reported till date Enzyme exclusively expressed in erythroid cells Mutations lead to defective heme synthesis	Varying age of presentation Moderate MHA (non-transfusion dependent) Visceral iron overload RS in BM

(continued)

Table 2.2 (continued)

Category of defect and *disease*	Gene	Pathophysiology and genetic basis	Clinical features
Iron utilization *-Erythropoietic protoporphyria*	*FECH*	Ferrochelatase catalyzes final step of heme synthesis. Mutations in *FECH* gene leads to excess of protoporphyrin IX and impaired iron incorporation leading to blighted heme assembly	Childhood MHA along with photosensitivity Hepatic failure and RS in BM
Iron-Sulphur cluster *GLRX 5-related CSA*	GLRX5	*GLRX5* is a mitochondrial protein highly expressed in erythroid cells. It is part of the assembly machinery of Fe/S clusters and ensures the maintenance of normal mitochondrial and cytosolic homeostasis Mutation leads to iron accumulation in mitochondria	Only 2 cases reported so far Severe microcytic anemia, RS and mitochondrial iron overload Marked iron overload

ALAS2 5′-aminolevulinate synthase, *BM* bone marrow, *CP* ceruloplasmin, *CSA* congenital sideroblastic anemia, *DMT1* divalent metal transporter 1, *FECH* ferrochelatase, *GLRX5* glutaredoxin5, *IRIDA* iron-refractory iron deficiency anemia, *NTBI* non-transferrin bound iron, *RS* ring sideroblasts, *TSAT* transferrin saturation, *TF* transferrin

A study by Bhatia et al. systematically screened 550 pediatric cases of anemia and found that 11% (60 cases) were refractory to oral iron therapy. Among these, 23 cases exhibited the IRIDA phenotype, characterized by low plasma iron, normal ferritin, and elevated hepcidin levels. Genetic sequencing of 20 cases identified TMPRSS6 mutations in 60% (12/20), reinforcing the autosomal recessive nature of IRIDA [16].

Another study by Athiyarath et al. (2015) investigated pregnant women with anemia unresponsive to oral iron supplements, using NGS. The study identified rare and novel variations in iron metabolism-related genes (*TMPRSS6*, *TF*, *TRF2*, *SLC11A2*, and *HAMP*), suggesting that intronic variations may contribute to anemia severity. A comprehensive genomic study (2019–2021) further analyzed 290 anemia cases, detecting pathogenic genetic variants in 56% (23/41) of tested cases, with 41% (17/41) showing inherited iron defects. These findings emphasize the need for genetic screening, targeted therapies, and public health initiatives to manage inherited iron disorders in India's iron-deficient endemic population [17].

2.6 Diagnostic and Therapeutic Approaches

Iron metabolism plays a pivotal role in diagnosing microcytic anemia, necessitating iron status assessment in all cases. Advancements in iron metabolism research have refined our understanding, highlighting not only acquired IDA but also hereditary iron disorders as critical considerations in unexplained microcytic anemias, hence necessitating a high index of suspicion in all unexplained cases of microcytic anemias. A stepwise approach is recommended for approaching a case of IDA. Most importantly, the common cause of ID needs to be excluded before exploring for the rarer inherited causes (Fig. 2.4).

The diagnostic approach to hereditary microcytic anemia follows a stepwise protocol. The initial step begins with a careful history and physical examination, including assessment of familial history to look for a pattern of inheritance. The main cornerstone of evaluation begins with excluding the common causes of IDA

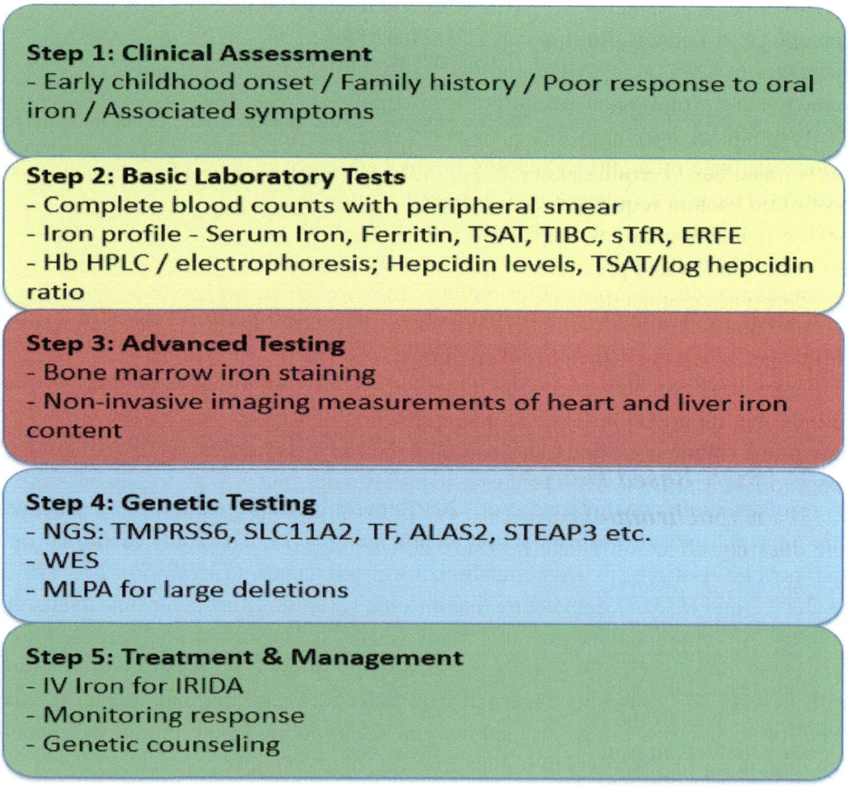

Fig. 2.4 Stepwise systematic approach to diagnosing a case of iron deficiency anemia. ERFE erythroferrone; IRIDA iron-refractory iron deficiency anemia MPLA Multiplex ligation-dependent probe amplification; NGS next-generation sequencing; sTfR soluble Transferrin Receptor; TIBC total iron binding capacity; TSAT transferrin saturation; WES whole exome sequencing

and its mimickers in all cases, i.e., acquired IDA and beta/alpha thalassemia trait (BTT/ATT). Next step: additional biochemical markers such as zinc protoporphyrin (ZPP), plasma hepcidin, and sTfR levels, along with BM examination, are reserved for suspected sideroblastic anemia. Imaging is recommended for patients with suspected iron overload disorders to quantify the iron content in organs like the heart and liver. In many cases, a combination of iron-related biochemical markers with a careful history and response to iron therapy can guide us to a probable cause of inherited IDA (Table 2.3). Next step consists of confirmatory tests as guided by the preceding steps viz., genetic testing, which is even more important for cases with unexplained anemia after biochemical evaluation. NGS offers a powerful approach to diagnosing overlapping or atypical phenotypes, providing crucial insights for prognosis and treatment decisions. Depending on disease heterogeneity and clinical presentation, either targeted single-gene testing or broad-spectrum multigene panels may be used.

Not so long back, the Structured Approach to Diagnosing IRIDA (SAID) model was developed to streamline early suspicion, targeted biochemical testing, and genetic confirmation to improve IRIDA diagnosis [16]. It elaborately explains to consider IRIDA in the differential when anemia presents in infancy or early childhood; family history suggests persistent, unexplained anemia; severe microcytosis and hypochromia are present out of proportion to the severity of anemia; no classical ID symptoms are noted, and there is no organomegaly or systemic signs of another disorder. Overall, distinguishing between acquired and hereditary causes of microcytic anemia requires an integrated diagnostic approach, combining clinical history, hematological parameters, iron status markers, and genetic evaluation. Early recognition and precise molecular diagnosis are critical for optimizing treatment, preventing unnecessary iron supplementation, and guiding personalized management strategies. Herein, we present a concise algorithmic approach to diagnose a case of unexplained inherited cause of microcytic anemia (Fig. 2.5).

2.6.1 NGS-Based Detection of Inherited Microcytic Hypochromic Anemias

With the advent of NGS, the diagnostic approach to inherited microcytic anemias has significantly improved. NGS allows for a simultaneous and comprehensive analysis of multiple genes, making it an invaluable tool in diagnosing these complex disorders, especially when clinical features overlap between different subtypes. We restrict ourselves to the NGS-based detection of inherited microcytic anemias due to genetic defects in iron metabolism in this chapter, viz. IRIDA, CSAs, and disorders of iron transport and storage.

Given the genetic heterogeneity of these inherited anemias, traditional diagnostic methods such as hemoglobin electrophoresis, iron studies, and biochemical assays often fail to provide a conclusive diagnosis. NGS panels overcome this challenge by enabling:

Table 2.3 Differentiating features of various microcytic anemias [20–23]

Condition/parameters	RBC	Hb	MCV	RDW	Reticulocyte response to anemia	Serum iron	Ferritin	TSAT	FEP	Hepcidin	RS on BM
IDA	Low	Low	Low	High	Low	Low	Low	Very low	High	Low	Absent
BTT	High	Low	Low	Normal	Low	Normal	Normal	Normal	Normal		Absent
AI	Low	Low	Low	Normal	Low	Low	Normal/ high	Normal	Normal	High	Absent
IRIDA	Very low	Low/ very low	Very low	Normal	Low	Low	Normal/ low	Very low	Very high	High[a]	Absent
DMT1-related anemia	Low	Very low	Very low	Normal	Low	High	High	Very high	High	Normal/ low	Absent
Erythropoietic porphyria	Low	Low	Very low	Normal	Low	Normal	Normal	High	Very high	Low	Present
STEAP3/TSAP6 related anemia	Low	Very low	Low	High	Low	Normal/ high	Normal/ high	Very high	Normal	Normal/ high	Present
SLC25A38 CSA	Low	Very low	Low	Normal/ high	Low	Normal/ high	High	High	Normal	No data	Prominent
ALAS2 XLR CSA	Low	Low	Low	Normal/ high	Low	Normal/ high	High	High	Normal/ low	No data	Prominent
GLRX5-related CSA	Low	Very low	Very low	Normal	Low	Normal	High	High	Normal	No data	Present
Congenital hypotransferrinemia	Low	Low	Very low	Normal	Low	Low[b]	Normal	Fully saturated	Normal	Low	Absent

AI anemia of inflammation, *ALAS* 5′-aminolevulinate synthase, *BM* bone marrow, *BTT* beta thalassemia trait, *CSA* congenital sideroblastic anemia, *FEP* free erythrocyte porphyrin, *Hb* hemoglobin, *IDA* iron deficiency anemia, *MCV* mean corpuscular volume, *RBC* red blood cells, *RDW* red cell distribution width, *RS* ring sideroblasts, *TSAT* transferrin saturation

[a]In the absence of inflammation, an elevated hepcidin-to-TSAT ratio serves as a highly specific marker for IRIDA

[b]Low concentrations of transferrin-bound iron with iron-deficient erythropoiesis and high concentrations of NTBI with subsequent iron overload in visceral organs

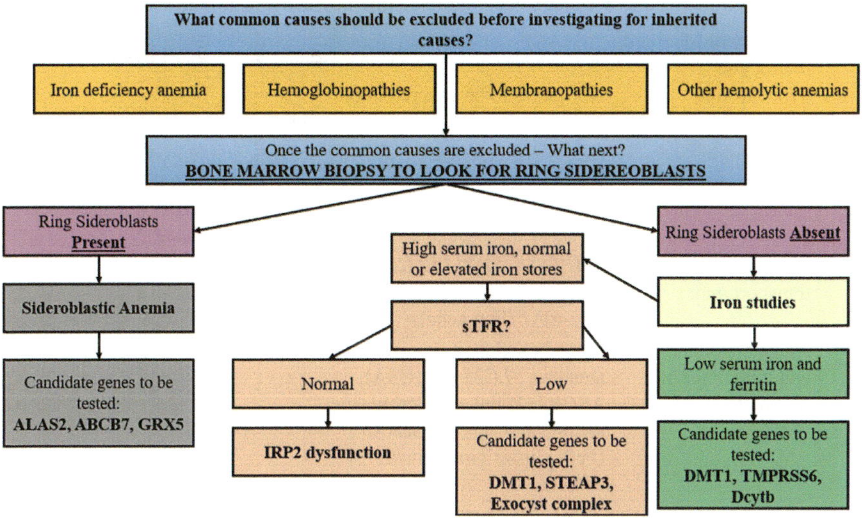

Fig. 2.5 Decoding microcytic hypochromic anemia: a stepwise genetic approach [20]. Before diving into genetic investigations, common causes like iron deficiency, hemoglobinopathies, membrane disorders, and hemolytic anemias must be ruled out. Once excluded, a bone marrow biopsy helps distinguish sideroblastic vs. non-sideroblastic anemia. Further assessment of iron levels and utilization reveals underlying defects in iron absorption or erythroid iron metabolism, pointing toward specific candidate genes responsible for the condition. ALAS2 5′-aminolevulinate synthase, ABCB7 ATP binding cassette subfamily B member 7, DMT1 divalent metal transporter 1, Dcytb duodenal cytochrome b, sTfR soluble transferrin receptor

Comprehensive Detection of Mutations: Simultaneous analysis of multiple genes associated with MHAs.

(a) Differentiation of Overlapping Disorders: Many inherited anemias have similar clinical presentations. NGS helps in accurately distinguishing conditions like IRIDA, sideroblastic anemias, and thalassemia's.
(b) Identification of Rare and Novel Variants: NGS facilitates the discovery of previously unrecognized mutations, broadening the spectrum of known genetic causes.
(c) Cost-Effective and Time-Saving Approach: Traditional sequential testing of individual genes is time-consuming and expensive, whereas NGS can analyze multiple genes in a single test.

2.6.2 Minimum NGS Panel for Diagnosing Inherited Microcytic Hypochromic Anemias (Table 2.4)

To effectively diagnose inherited MHAs, a targeted NGS panel needs to be employed, which includes the following key genes as enumerated in Table 2.4.

Table 2.4 Minimum panel for diagnosing inherited microcytic hypochromic anemias

S no	Category of inherited microcytic hypochromic anemias gene panel	Key genes to be covered in the NGS panel	Remarks
1	Hemoglobin synthesis genes	*HBA1*, *HBA2*, *HBB*	Hemoglobinopathies are much more common than inherited causes of MHAs due to defects in iron metabolism
2	Iron metabolism and transport genes	*TMPRSS6*, *SLC11A2* (DMT1 gene), *TF* (Transferrin gene), *SLC40A1* (Fpn gene)	
3	Heme biosynthesis and mitochondrial iron metabolism genes	*ALAS2* (X-linked sideroblastic anemia), *SLC25A38* (CSA), *ABCB7* (X-linked sideroblastic anemia and ataxia), *GLRX5* (Fe/S cluster biosynthesis defect)	
4	Ferritin and iron storage genes	*FTH1*, *FL* (Ferritin heavy and light chain mutations affecting iron storage)	
5	Additional regulatory genes	*HAMP* (hepcidin gene), *GATA1*	HAMP regulates iron homeostasis and *GATA1* gene affects erythroid differentiation and heme metabolism

2.6.3 Clinical Application of NGS in Diagnosis: Step-by-Step Approach to NGS-Based Diagnosis

1. Clinical Evaluation and 1st Line Laboratory Investigations: Identify patients with persistent MHA that do not improve with iron therapy. Perform baseline CBC, ferritin, serum iron, transferrin saturation, and Hb electrophoresis.
2. NGS Panel Testing: Use an NGS-based iron metabolism and hemoglobinopathy gene panel to detect mutations. Analyze deletions, point mutations, copy number variations (CNVs), and splice-site mutations.
3. Interpretation of Results: If known pathogenic mutations are detected, confirm the diagnosis and guide treatment. If variants of uncertain significance (VUS) are found, perform family segregation studies or functional validation.
4. Post-Test Clinical Decision Making: If a diagnosis is confirmed, implement targeted management strategies (e.g., transfusions, chelation, iron supplementation, or bone marrow transplantation). If no mutations are detected, consider alternative non-genetic causes or novel genetic variants requiring further study.

2.6.4 Therapeutic Approach

The treatment of microcytic anemias caused by genetic disorders requires a targeted and individualized approach based on the specific underlying mutation, aiming to correct the anemia, prevent complications, and effectively manage iron homeostasis. In IRIDA, the primary treatment objective is to bypass hepcidin-mediated iron restriction. Oral iron supplementation is largely ineffective, and IV iron therapy is preferred, although it rarely normalizes Hb levels. Some cases may show partial responsiveness to high-dose oral iron with vitamin C, but regular IV iron infusions are often necessary. The goal is to maintain functional iron availability while avoiding iron overload, which requires closely monitoring serum ferritin levels [23].

Hypotransferrinemia, which results in defective iron transport, is treated with plasma transfusions or apoTf therapy to restore iron transport capacity. In severe cases, blood transfusions may be required to maintain Hb levels. The primary goal in these disorders is to ensure adequate iron delivery to erythropoiesis while preventing iron toxicity [23].

For sideroblastic anemias, treatment strategies vary based on the specific genetic defect. X-linked sideroblastic anemia (*ALAS2* mutations) often responds to pyridoxine (Vitamin B6) therapy, improving Hb production. However, other sideroblastic anemias, such as those caused by *SLC25A38* or *GLRX5* mutations, require lifelong transfusions combined with iron chelation therapy to prevent iron overload. In severe cases, hematopoietic stem cell transplantation (HSCT) may be considered as a curative option. The main treatment objective is to enhance erythropoiesis, minimize ineffective red cell production, and prevent systemic iron accumulation.

In erythropoietic protoporphyrias, which impair heme synthesis and cause photosensitivity, treatment involves avoiding sun exposure and managing anemia. In severe cases, HSCT remains the only curative therapy. Anemias associated with *SLC11A2 (DMT1)* and *STEAP3* mutations, which disrupt iron transport into erythroid precursors, are managed with EPO therapy combined with iron chelation therapy to stimulate red blood cell production and prevent systemic iron overload, respectively. Blood transfusions may be required in severe cases [23].

Ultimately, early recognition and a structured diagnostic approach are crucial in determining the most effective treatment strategy for genetic microcytic anemias. The overarching treatment objectives are optimizing erythropoiesis, correcting iron imbalances, preventing iron toxicity, and improving overall patient outcomes. Genetic testing plays a key role in guiding therapy, ensuring that treatment is precisely tailored to the underlying pathophysiology of each disorder. Emerging therapies, such as hepcidin modulators, enzyme inhibitors, and gene therapy, hold promise for more effective long-term management and potential cures in the future [22].

2.7 Summary

Iron metabolism is a tightly regulated process critical for oxygen transport and cellular functions. While acquired IDA is widespread, inherited forms result from genetic mutations affecting iron absorption, transport, and utilization. This chapter outlines the molecular mechanisms regulating iron homeostasis, with a focus on transferrin, DMT1, ferroportin, and hepcidin. Disorders such as IRIDA, congenital hypotransferrinemia, sideroblastic anemia, and DMT1-related anemia often mimic acquired IDA, making accurate diagnosis essential.

A structured diagnostic approach is emphasized, integrating serum iron studies, hepcidin levels, genetic testing, and functional biomarkers to differentiate inherited anemias from acquired conditions. Treatment strategies vary based on the underlying defect: IV iron therapy is essential for IRIDA, plasma transfusions are used in hypotransferrinemia, and pyridoxine supplementation benefits certain sideroblastic anemias. For severe cases, HSCT remains the only curative option. Emerging therapies, including hepcidin modulators, CRISPR gene therapy, and AI-driven personalized medicine, hold promise for more effective and targeted treatments.

Future research is focused on refining genomic screening, non-invasive iron monitoring, and targeted therapies. The integration of precision medicine and AI-based diagnostics is expected to revolutionize the management of inherited microcytic anemias, ensuring earlier detection, individualized treatment, and improved patient outcomes.

References

1. Busacchi V. [Vincenzo Menghini and the discovery of iron in the blood]. Bull Sci Med (Bologna). 1958;130(2):202–5.
2. Brumberg JJ. Chlorotic girls, 1870-1920: a historical perspective on female adolescence. Child Dev. 1982;53(6):1468–77.
3. Sheftel AD, Mason AB, Ponka P. The long history of iron in the universe and in health and disease. Biochim Biophys Acta. 2012;1820(3):161–87.
4. Utkurovich NA. An overview of iron metabolism in health and disease. J Adv Med Res. 2021;33(8):70-78. https://doi.org/10.9734/jammr/2021/v33i830888.
5. Roemhild K, Von Maltzahn F, Weiskirchen R, Knüchel R, Von Stillfried S, Lammers T. Iron metabolism: pathophysiology and pharmacology. Trends Pharmacol Sci. 2021;42(8):640–56.
6. Yiannikourides A, Latunde-Dada G. A short review of iron metabolism and pathophysiology of iron disorders. Medicine. 2019;6(3):85.
7. Shayeghi M, Latunde-Dada GO, Oakhill JS, Laftah AH, Takeuchi K, Halliday N, et al. Identification of an intestinal heme transporter. Cell. 2005;122(5):789–801.
8. Liuzzi JP, Aydemir F, Nam H, Knutson MD, Cousins RJ. Zip14 (Slc39a14) mediates non-transferrin bound iron uptake into cells. Proc Natl Acad Sci USA. 2006;103(37):13612–7.
9. Aisen P, Wessling-Resnick M, Leibold EA. Iron metabolism. Curr Opin Chem Biol. 1999;3(2):200–6.
10. Camaschella C, Nai A, Silvestri L. Iron metabolism and iron disorders revisited in the hepcidin era. Haematologica. 2020;105(2):260–72.

11. Chiabrando D, Mercurio S, Tolosano E. Heme and erythropoieis: more than a structural role. Haematologica. 2014;99(6):973–83.
12. Silvestri L, Nai A. Iron and erythropoiesis: a mutual alliance. Semin Hematol. 2021;58(3):145–52.
13. GBD 2016 Disease and Injury Incidence and Prevalence Collaborators. Global, regional, and national incidence, prevalence, and years lived with disability for 328 diseases and injuries for 195 countries, 1990-2016: a systematic analysis for the Global Burden of Disease Study 2016. Lancet Lond Engl. 2017;390(10100):1211–59.
14. WHO [Internet]. World Health Organization; [cited 2025 Mar 3]. GHO | By category | Anaemia in children < 5 years - Estimates by WHO region. Available from: https://apps.who.int/gho/data/view.main.ANEMIACHILDRENREGv.
15. Pasricha SR, Tye-Din J, Muckenthaler MU, Swinkels DW. Iron deficiency. Lancet. 2021;397(10270):233–48.
16. Bhatia P, Jain R, Singh A. A structured approach to iron refractory iron deficiency anemia (IRIDA) diagnosis (SAID): the more is "SAID" about iron, the less it is. Pediatr Hematol Oncol J. 2017;2(2):48–53.
17. Athiyarath R, Shaktivel K, Abraham V, Singh D, Bondu JD, Chapla A, et al. Association of genetic variants with response to iron supplements in pregnancy. Genes Nutr. 2015;10(4):25.
18. Tripathi P, Hariharan R, Kapoor U. IRIDA- an Indian perspective. Indian J Pathol Oncol. 2024;11(2):108–18.
19. Nazir H, Al-Khabori MK, Kohistani N, Puchalka J, Klein C. A rare case of congenital atransferrinemia: international collaboration for genetic diagnosis. Blood. 2014;124(21):4883.
20. Iolascon A, De Falco L, Beaumont C. Molecular basis of inherited microcytic anemia due to defects in iron acquisition or heme synthesis. Haematologica. 2009;94(3):395–408.
21. Brissot P, Bernard DG, Brissot E, Loréal O, Troadec MB. Rare anemias due to genetic iron metabolism defects. Mutat Res Rev Mutat Res. 2018;777:52–63.
22. Cappellini MD, Russo R, Andolfo I, Iolascon A. Inherited microcytic anemias. Hematology. 2020;2020(1):465–70.
23. Donker AE, Raymakers Reinier AP, Vlasveld LT, van Barneveld T, Terink R, Dors N, et al. Practice guidelines for the diagnosis and management of microcytic anemias due to genetic disorders of iron metabolism or heme synthesis. Blood. 2014;123(25):3873–86.

Chapter 3
Iron Deficiency Anemia: Newer Iron Formulations and Their Advantages

Kartikey Saini, Saurabh Rasal, and Mukul Aggarwal

Abstract Iron deficiency anemia (IDA) remains a significant global health concern, necessitating the development of effective management strategies to replenish iron stores and enhance clinical outcomes. This chapter reviews the evolution of iron therapy, from traditional oral iron formulations (ferrous and ferric salts) to modern intravenous (IV) iron preparations, such as ferric carboxymaltose and ferric derisomaltose. Key considerations include bioavailability, dosing strategies, and adverse effects such as gastrointestinal intolerance (oral iron) and hypersensitivity reactions (IV iron). Emerging oral formulations (sucrosomial iron, ferric maltol) and IV options with enhanced safety profiles are discussed. Optimal management involves individualized therapy based on etiology, severity, and patient tolerance, with monitoring of hemoglobin, ferritin, and transferrin saturation to assess treatment response.

Keywords Iron deficiency anemia (IDA) · Intravenous iron supplementation · Oral iron therapy · Hypophosphatemia · Alternate-day iron dosing · Complement activation-related pseudo-allergy · CARPA

K. Saini · S. Rasal · M. Aggarwal (✉)
Department of Haematology, AIIMS, New Delhi, India

H. P. Pati et al. (eds.), *Clinical Hematology and Hemato-Oncology*,
https://doi.org/10.1007/978-981-92-1167-8_3

Learning Objectives

At the end of the chapter, the reader must be able to understand:

- *Historical development* of oral and IV iron therapies, including key advancements in formulation safety and efficacy.
- *Comparison of oral iron preparations*, including ferrous salts, ferric complexes, and newer agents (e.g., sucrosomial iron), in terms of bioavailability, dosing, and tolerability.
- *Indications for IV iron therapy*, such as malabsorption, CKD, and refractory IDA, and differentiate between available IV formulations (FCM, FDI, ferumoxytol).
- *Ideal dosing strategies* for oral iron (e.g., alternate-day dosing) and IV iron (e.g., single high-dose infusions) to optimize absorption and minimize side effects.
- *Identify and management of adverse effects*, including GI intolerance (oral iron), hypophosphatemia (FCM), and hypersensitivity reactions (CARPA).
- *Assessment of treatment response* using hemoglobin trends, ferritin levels, and transferrin saturation, and define criteria for oral iron refractoriness.

3.1 Introduction

Iron deficiency (ID) anemia continues to contribute to significant comorbidity and public health issues. The management of iron deficiency anemia includes oral and intravenous (IV) supplementation, apart from management of the underlying etiology. Iron salts have been utilized for over 300 years, following the discovery of iron as a key component of blood in the seventeenth century. Initially, their use was rooted in the belief that iron consumption enhanced strength. The field of iron therapy was revolutionized in the early nineteenth century by Pierre Blaud, who introduced iron pills—combinations of ferrous sulphate and potassium carbonate—for oral ingestion. Over time, numerous oral iron formulations were developed, though many faced limitations such as reduced efficacy in malabsorptive disorders and reliance on patient compliance.

Ferric oxyhydroxide was the first parenteral iron; it had high toxicity and was withdrawn soon after launch in 1932. The introduction of high molecular weight (HMW) iron dextran in the 1950s allowed for higher-dose delivery but may cause hypersensitivity reactions. Later advancements in biotechnology led to safer formulations like low molecular weight (LMW) iron dextran, iron sucrose, and ferric gluconate, which required multiple infusions for adequate dosing. The introduction of ferric carboxymaltose (FCM), ferric derisomaltose (FDI), and ferumoxytol in the twenty-first century revolutionized IV iron therapy by offering high-dose capacity with better safety and tolerability [1].

Iron replacement therapy aims to correct anemia, improve red cell indices, and replete iron stores. Oral iron is commonly used initially due to the convenience of administration, easy availability, and low costs. Elemental iron @ 50–200 mg daily for at least 3 months, of which around 10% is absorbed by the gut [2, 3]. Excess iron can cause alterations in the gut microbiota with a shift to pathogenic bacteria, leading to susceptibility to infections and local inflammation. IV iron increases Hb levels and iron stores quickly, though some side effects are unique.

3.2 Oral Iron Supplements

Oral iron supplements mostly include ferrous (Fe^{2+}) or ferric (Fe^{3+}) complexes and carbonyl iron and heme iron polypeptide. (Table 3.1).

3.2.1 *Ferrous Salts*

These include ferrous salts with sulphate, fumarate, or gluconate as well as citrate, glycine sulphate, iodine, bisglycinate, carbonate, chloride, aspartate, ascorbate, succinate, or tartrate in tablet or syrup forms. Dissolved Fe^{2+} is oxidized readily to insoluble Fe^{3+}, Sodium bisulfite may be added to keep ferrous in the reduced form.

Table 3.1 Comparison of oral iron formulations

Formulation	Type	Key features	Advantages	Disadvantages
Ferrous salts	Ferrous sulphate	Most common, low-cost, gold standard	High bioavailability; widely available	GI side effects: poor absorption in malabsorption
	Ferrous fumarate	High elemental iron content	Effective for iron repletion	Similar GI side effects to ferrous sulfate
	Ferrous gluconate	Lower elemental iron content	Better tolerated than ferrous sulfate	Less effective for severe anemia
Ferric complexes	Ferric maltol	Lipophilic Fe^{3+} complex with maltol	Can be taken with food; fewer GI side effects	Higher cost, lower bioavailability than ferrous salts
	Sucrosomial iron	Ferric pyrophosphate encapsulated in phospholipid-sucrose matrix	Efficient absorption via paracellular/transcellular routes; reduced GI effects	May not fully replenish iron stores; higher cost
Other formulations	Carbonyl iron	Elemental iron in microscopic spheres	Less GI irritation	Slower absorption; limited clinical superiority
	Heme iron polypeptide	Derived from bovine hemoglobin	Better absorption than non-heme iron	Limited evidence of clinical superiority; potential cancer risk

Enteric-coated slow-release formulations can potentially have reduced gastrointestinal side effects. However, iron absorption past the duodenum and upper jejunum is minimal.

Ferrous sulfate is the most economical, frequently prescribed, and is considered the gold standard oral supplement.

3.2.2 *Ferric Complexes*

Ferric polysaccharide complexes release iron and saccharides in gastric fluid, enhancing iron bioavailability by converting Fe^{3+} to Fe^{2+}. Newer ferric supplements are citrate, maltol, and sucrosomial compounds. Their bioavailability is lower than ferrous salts but improves iron stores as well as Hb. The BESTIRON study found that ferrous sulfate was more effective than ferric polysaccharide. A systematic review of over 8400 patients indicated that iron protein succinylate matched or exceeded the efficacy of other iron treatments [4].

Iron absorption is better on an empty stomach. Sucrosomial iron and ferric polysaccharide may also be taken with meals.

3.2.3 *Efficacy of Oral Iron Supplements*

Serum iron is considered a poor marker of IDA as well as an efficacy measure of iron supplementation.

An Hb rise of 1–2 g/dL within a month of initiation of therapy can be considered a reasonable response. Repletion of body iron stores, reflected by serum ferritin >50 μg/L, usually takes longer and sometimes is not achieved if the underlying cause for IDA is not addressed or patient compliance with therapy is poor. Oral iron refractoriness is defined as failure to increase in Hb >1 gm/dl at a dose of at least 100 mg per day for 4–6 weeks [5].

3.3 Newer Preparations

3.3.1 *Ferric Citrate*

Ferric citrate therapy for a year increases iron stores, improves red cell parameters, and reduces the requirements for IV iron and erythropoietin for dialysis-dependent CKD patients. It is also used to reduce hyperphosphatemia in these patients, as well as to correct IDA non-dialysis CKD patients. It forms oligomeric complexes that neutralize phosphate anions and form insoluble precipitates at acidic gastric pH. It predominates in monomeric complexes at a more basic duodenal pH, where iron is bioavailable [6].

3.3.2 *Ferric Maltol*

Maltol forms a lipophilic complex with Fe^{3+} in a 3:1 ratio, creating a redox-inert form of iron that remains unabsorbed. Before absorption, iron dissociates from the maltol complex through the DMT1 transporter in enterocytes. Meanwhile, free maltol is absorbed and excreted by the kidneys. It achieves a significant increase in Hb, non-inferior to IV iron by week 12 in IDA due to IBD, CKD, and was approved by the FDA in 2019 [7].

3.3.3 *Sucrosomial Iron*

This consists of a matrix of sucrose esters of fatty acids (called sucresters) and phospholipids that encapsulate ferric pyrophosphate. Sucrosome is formed when tricalcium phosphate coats and stabilizes the phospholipid bilayer of this matrix and protects the iron. Sucresters enhance absorption by reducing the resistance of the intestinal barrier. Sucrosomial iron is absorbed as intact nanoparticles via transcellular (Peyer's patches microfold cells) and paracellular routes, independent of DMT1. It improves Hb but does not always replenish iron stores fully [8].

3.4 Carbonyl Iron and Heme Iron

"Carbonyl" refers to controlled heating of vaporized iron pentacarbonyl that leads to the deposition of uncharged, elemental iron as sub-microscopic crystals forming microscopic spheres (<5 µm diameter). The conversion of particulate carbonyl iron into soluble and absorbable ionized iron relies on the stomach's acidic environment. It does not offer an added advantage over iron salts.

Heme iron is absorbed directly into enterocytes in a non-competitive manner with non-heme iron, and hence without the influence of hepcidin. It is produced by the enzymatic hydrolysis of bovine hemoglobin. Peptides and amino acids produced during the hydrolysis of hemoglobin maintain the solubility of heme even in the acidic pH of the stomach. There are potential but unproven risks of colon cancer with heme-iron [9]. It does not offer superiority over iron salts in the trials.

3.4.1 *Newer Experimental Formulations (Table 3.2)*

A new iron formulation, Fe-ASP, has been developed from an N-acetyl-aspartylated derivative of casein. The casein coating helps prevent iron from converting into insoluble salts in the stomach, allowing more iron to be absorbed in the duodenum and reducing gastrointestinal side effects.

Table 3.2 Newer iron preparations and their applications

Formulation	Mechanism	Indications	Key Benefits	Limitations
Ferric citrate	Binds phosphate in the stomach; releases iron in the duodenum	Non-dialysis CKD, hyperphosphatemia in dialysis-dependent CKD	Reduces phosphate levels; improves iron stores	Limited to specific patient populations
Ferric maltol	Fe^{3+}-maltol complex dissociates at enterocytes	IDA due to IBD, CKD	Can be taken with food; non-inferior to IV iron	Higher cost; not superior to ferrous salts
Sucrosomial iron	Ferric pyrophosphate encapsulated in phospholipid-sucrose matrix	IDA in diverse etiologies (e.g., pregnancy, IBD, CKD)	Efficient absorption; reduced GI side effects	May not fully replenish iron stores; higher cost
Iron hydroxide adipate tartrate (IHAT)	Absorbed as nanoparticles via endocytosis	Experimental; potential alternative to ferrous sulphate	Reduced GI toxicity; improved efficacy	Still in clinical trials
Iron amino acid chelates	Chelated iron (e.g., ferrous bisglycinate) resists dietary inhibitors	General IDA	Less affected by dietary inhibitors, reduced GI side effects	Limited evidence of superiority over ferrous salts

The ACCESS trial compared Fe-ASP to ferrous sulfate for treating IDA and found that Fe-ASP was non-inferior in increasing baseline Hb. Additionally, key measures of erythropoiesis, such as changes in Hb, red blood cells, and reticulocyte counts, showed greater improvement with Fe-ASP than with $FeSO_4$ [10].

Microencapsulated iron pyrophosphate-fortified fruit juice has been studied in iron-deficient females at 500 ml/day for 16 weeks. It provides 18 mg Fe/day.

Iron hydroxide adipate tartrate (IHAT) is a nano-dispersed Fe^{3+} (III) oxo-hydroxide, which is tartrate-modified and does not need to be solubilized in the stomach for absorption. It is absorbed as nanoparticles via endocytosis by duodenal enterocytes. Tentatively less GI toxic, it is currently under trial.

Iron amino acid chelates (ferrous bisglycinate, ferric Tris glycinate) appear to be absorbed like non-heme iron preparations. It is less susceptible to interactions with phosphates, phytates, and fibers in the meals. There is little data to support its superiority to iron salts.

Polysaccharide iron complex (PIC) is a synthetic complex of carbohydrate with ferric iron. It is spherical, 3–10 nm in diameter, and contains a ferrihydrite core like ferritin. PIC may taste better, with lower GI toxicity; however, a randomized trial in children found that it is less efficacious with similar GI toxicity compared to ferrous sulfate [1].

3.5 How to Dose Iron Therapy?

Higher doses of oral iron exhibit suboptimal absorption due to the induction of hepcidin expression and increased gastrointestinal side effects. Consequently, it is advisable to limit oral iron administration to a single dose daily or alternate days. Every other day (QOD) dosing minimizes the expression of hepcidin and enhances the percentage absorption of iron. It has been shown to have an equivalent effect on a rise in Hb and ferritin [11, 12]. Although the total quantity of iron absorbed with QOD dosing is marginally lower than that with daily dosing, daily supplementation may be appropriate for individuals who tolerate the side effects well.

Plasma hepcidin concentrations adhere to a circadian rhythm, typically increasing throughout the day; therefore, it is optimal to administer oral iron during the morning. Doses exceeding 60–120 mg of elemental iron per day or every other day do not confer considerable advantages with respect to repletion of iron stores and may lead to unintended adverse effects. In contrast, lower dosages of iron should be considered for patients experiencing negative side effects.

3.5.1 Oral Iron Refractoriness

Iron repletion is defined as a ferritin level ≥50 ng/mL, at which there is complete resolution of ID symptoms. Ferritin responses should be assessed at 12 weeks after initiating oral iron therapy. Patients who do not replete iron by 3 months are candidates for parenteral iron administration. In patients with significant anemia, a Hb rise of less than 1.0 g/dl at day 14 can potentially identify refractoriness, earlier during treatment. (Table 3.3).

Table 3.3 Efficacy monitoring of oral iron therapy

Parameter	Optimal response	Suboptimal response	Refractoriness
Hemoglobin (Hb)	Increase of ≥2 g/dL within 3–4 weeks	Increase of 1–2 g/dL within 4 weeks	Increase of <1 g/dL after 4–6 weeks of treatment (at ≥100 mg/day elemental iron)
Ferritin	>100 μg/L indicates repletion of iron stores	20–50 μg/L indicates partial repletion	<20 μg/mL indicates persistent iron deficiency
Transferrin saturation	>20% indicates adequate iron availability	10–20% indicates partial improvement	<10% indicates ongoing iron deficiency

3.6 Intravenous Iron

IV iron has modified the treatment landscape of IDA. The major complication of the previous generation IV formulations was the high rates of severe anaphylactic reactions linked with the presence of labile iron in the preparation [1].

3.6.1 Indications for IV Iron

1. Iron deficiency: Patients with confirmed iron deficiency (low ferritin and transferrin saturation) who do not tolerate oral iron or are refractory to oral iron.
2. Patients requiring quick iron repletion, i.e., Preoperative patients.
3. Chronic kidney disease (CKD): Patients with IDA and to improve response to erythropoietin.
4. Chronic inflammation (e.g., inflammatory bowel disease, heart failure, or malignancy) where oral iron absorption is impaired due to high hepcidin levels.
5. In non-anemic heart failure patients with biochemical iron deficiency, to improve quality of life and enhance physical performance.
6. Pregnant or postpartum women with iron deficiency anemia when oral iron is ineffective or poorly tolerated, especially when a quicker response is warranted, as in the late second and third trimesters.
7. Patients with GI malabsorption syndromes, celiac disease, gastric or duodenal surgeries.
8. Cancer patients with iron deficiency anemia due to limited oral iron absorption, due to inflammation, chemotherapy, or ongoing losses [13].

3.7 IV Preparations and Their Clinical Implications (Table 3.4)

3.7.1 Ferric Carboxymaltose (FCM)

FCM consists of a ferric hydroxide core that is stabilized by a carboxymaltose shell. This unique structure facilitates controlled and gradual iron release, reducing the risk of free iron toxicity. FCM facilitates single doses of up to 1000 mg, to be repeated after at least a week. It corrects anemia and replenishes Fe stores quickly; thus it is beneficial in conditions such as postpartum anemia or chronic diseases like CKD, heavy uterine bleeding, IBD, and congestive heart failure (CHF). It was associated with a smaller number of cardiac events or hospitalizations in patients with CHF and ID.

FCM can cause hypophosphatemia in up to 50% of patients (10% severe cases), due to elevated levels of fibroblast growth factor 23 (FGF 23). FCM promotes the

Table 3.4 Comparison of IV iron preparations

Iron formulation	Core size	Labile-free iron content	CARPA risk	Dosing frequency and administration
Iron sucrose (IS)	Small	High	Higher	100–200 mg per dose, requiring 5–10 doses. Given 1–3 times per week
Ferric carboxymaltose (FCM)	Medium	Moderate	Lower	750–1000 mg per dose, allowing for 1–2 doses for full repletion. Given every 1–2 weeks
Iron derisomaltoside (IDM)	Large	Very low	Lowest	500–2000 mg single infusion
Iron isomaltoside (IIM)	Large	Very low	Lowest	Up to 1500 mg per infusion, allowing for single or fewer doses. Given every few weeks as needed
Ferumoxytol (FMX)	Large	Low	Lower	510 mg per dose, given as two infusions 3–8 days apart. Can be infused rapidly (over ~15 minutes)

cleavage of biologically inactive fragments of FGF23. However, formulations with certain properties (e.g., high iron release rates) transiently elevate iFGF23, which drives phosphate loss.

Hypophosphatemia stimulates the secretion of parathyroid hormone (PTH). PTH exacerbates phosphate loss by increasing urinary excretion and may lead to a calcium-phosphate imbalance. Hypophosphatemia is often asymptomatic or can be associated with vague symptoms like fatigue, weakness, and muscle cramps. Severe hypophosphatemia (<1 mg/dL) can be associated with neurological symptoms, including paraesthesia, confusion, or irritability, musculoskeletal symptoms, bone pain, fractures, or osteomalacia (softening of bones), as well as arrhythmias or reduced myocardial contractility in extreme cases [14].

3.7.2 *Ferric Derisomaltose (FDI)*

FDI has a highly stable carbohydrate matrix composed of a linear glucose polymer that tightly binds elemental iron, ensuring controlled release while minimizing labile iron levels (<1%). It has a significantly lower incidence of hypophosphatemia (<8%). FDI showed a statistically significant decrease in cardiac event mortality in patients with CHF. It can be administered up to 1000 mg infused over 20 minutes, enhancing patient convenience and adherence.

Evidence from large-scale trials confirms its robust safety profile with reduced hypersensitivity reactions. FDI has been extensively studied in populations with CKD, IBD, and PPA, demonstrating superior safety and comparable efficacy to FCM and iron sucrose [15].

3.7.3 Ferumoxytol

Ferumoxytol is a super-paramagnetic iron oxide linked to poly-glucose sorbitol carboxymethyl ether. It is a semi-synthetic iron oxide nanoparticle coated with carbohydrates, which enables rapid infusion without test dosing. Its unique structure reduces labile iron levels, minimizing oxidative stress and toxicity. It was introduced with the advantage of rapid infusion of up to a 510 mg dose in under a minute, but had high rates of infusion reactions. Subsequently, dosing duration was changed to at least 15 min in two divided doses, at a gap of a week, reducing the severe events to rarity and minor infusion reactions in 1–3% of patients. Ferumoxytol may interfere with MRI imaging and has been associated with cardiovascular risks in susceptible populations [16].

3.7.4 Iron Isomaltoside

Iron Isomaltoside has a linear carbohydrate chain that provides a stable iron complex, allowing controlled release and low immunogenicity, and can be delivered up to 2000 mg in a single session, making it ideal for patients with significant iron deficits, reducing the frequency of hospital visits, and enhancing treatment adherence [17]. It can cause a fishbane-like reaction in up to 5% of patients, early during infusion, that warrants holding the infusion for a few minutes, after which it can be safely administered.

3.7.5 CARPA

Complement activation-related pseudo-allergy (CARPA) is characterized by complement-mediated activation by nanoparticles of labile/free iron that do not bind transferrin quickly. It can trigger mast cells and basophils, resembling IgE-mediated allergy. CARPAs are infusion rate-dependent events that can occur at any time and do not require prior sensitization. They are not life-threatening and resolve quickly, and are characterized by back pain, myalgias, flushing, arthralgias, and chest heaviness. These reactions are self-limited, and diphenhydramine should be avoided as it can worsen symptoms. After the subsidence of symptoms, rechallenge at a slower rate is usually considered [18] (Table 3.5).

3.7.6 Management of Acute Allergic Reactions

For minor infusion reactions, immediately stop the infusion, switch to hydration fluid (e.g., normal saline), and closely monitor the patient. Most of them are self-limiting and resolve spontaneously without further intervention. If symptoms persist or worsen after 15 minutes, IV corticosteroid (e.g., hydrocortisone 200 mg/equivalent)

Table 3.5 Differences between CARPA and IgE hypersensitivity reactions

	Complement activation-related pseudo-allergy	IgE-mediated allergy
Mediated by	Complement proteins	IgE
Need for prior exposure	+/−	Almost always
Duration	Self-limiting	Persistent
Symptoms	Pruritic, urticaria, flushing, chest tightness, arthralgia	Hypotension, angioedema, generalized urticaria, stridor and bronchospasm, vomiting
Treatment	Hold infusion, hydrocortisone	Hold infusion, hydrocortisone, antihistamine, epinephrine
Prognosis	Generally good	Life threatening
Rechallenge with the drug	Can be done easily	Best avoided

can be administered. Symptomatic therapy is also added, i.e., for nausea, ondansetron 4–8 mg IV, for urticaria, a second-generation antihistaminic such as cetirizine 10 mg oral. First-generation antihistamines (e.g., diphenhydramine) and vasopressors should be avoided, as they may exacerbate hypotension, tachycardia, sedation, or even lead to shock. Mild hypotension can often be managed with IV hydration.

For patients whose symptoms resolve completely, rechallenge may be considered, with reinitiation at 50% of the initial rate and monitoring for 15 minutes. If well tolerated, increase the infusion rate to the desired level. Recurrence of symptoms should be managed as previously described. Although package inserts recommend monitoring for 30 minutes post-infusion, this is seldom required, as delayed reactions are exceedingly rare.

Common symptoms include flu-like symptoms, myalgias, arthralgias, and fever, which typically resolve within 24 hours and can be managed with NSAIDs. Symptoms persisting beyond a few days should be evaluated for other causes, such as hypophosphatemia.

Severe or life-threatening reactions, though extremely rare, require immediate management as anaphylaxis with epinephrine, an antihistaminic agent, and hydrocortisone. For patients requiring subsequent IV iron therapy, consider premedication or alternative formulations to minimize the risk of recurrence. Proper documentation of symptoms and management is essential for future reference (Table 3.5).

3.7.7 Response Assessment After IV Iron

Following IV iron treatment, CBC, ferritin, and percent transferrin saturation (TSAT) should be conducted after 4–8 weeks. Circulating iron can interfere with the assay if conducted earlier, leading to inaccurate results. Hemoglobin levels are expected to begin increasing within a period of 1–2 weeks following the initiation of treatment. Ideally, these levels should rise by approximately 1–2 g/dL within 4–8 weeks, indicating a positive response to the intervention [18]. In the absence of inflammation, the target ferritin level is 50 ng/mL, irrespective of sex.

3.7.8 Oral Iron Plus IV Iron

Several large meta-analyses have suggested that long-term oral iron therapy potentially leads to improvement in the quality of life of IDA patients, especially young women. If the patient intends to avoid more doses of IV iron and is tolerating oral iron well without major side effects, oral iron can be continued indefinitely, or until menopause in females. Obviously, for malabsorption and post-gastro-duodenal surgery patients, oral iron therapy is of no use.

3.7.9 Management of Iron Deficiency in Pregnancy

Iron deficiency during pregnancy, with or without anemia, is a significant challenge and impacts both maternal and fetal outcomes. Current ACOG guidelines define iron deficiency without anemia as ferritin <30 ng/mL with hemoglobin ≥11 g/dL, but routine treatment is not recommended due to insufficient evidence linking it to adverse neonatal outcomes.

For iron deficiency anemia (hemoglobin <11 g/dL), oral iron (typically ferrous sulfate) is the first-line therapy, although it is associated with high rates of gastrointestinal intolerance (up to 70%). Alternate-day dosing improves absorption and reduces side effects by avoiding hepcidin suppression. Intravenous (IV) iron (e.g., ferric derisomaltose, ferric carboxymaltose) offers an alternative, particularly for severe or refractory cases, with faster hemoglobin correction and improved neonatal ferritin levels. Routine iron supplementation with 30 mg of ferrous iron per day, in conjunction with a balanced diet, is recommended starting at around week 12 of gestation. In females with anemia, treatment with higher doses of iron (60–120 mg daily) is recommended.

In severe cases of anemia (Hb < 70 g/l) or advanced gestation (>34 weeks), intravenous iron is recommended.

Trials continue to evaluate the role of IV iron in reducing perinatal complications, including postpartum hemorrhage and neurodevelopmental delays in offspring. Treatment in pregnancy should be individualized, balancing efficacy, tolerability, and gestational timing, with close monitoring of maternal and fetal iron status [19].

3.7.10 Case Study

A 28-year-old woman presents with generalized weakness, shortness of breath, and easy fatigability. She is seeking a second opinion for her symptoms. Previously, she was diagnosed with iron deficiency anemia (IDA), showing a hemoglobin (Hb) level of 6.9 g/dL, red blood cells were microcytic and hypochromic, and serum ferritin was 1 ng/mL.

After experiencing gastric intolerance with oral iron (ferrous sulfate), she received intravenous ferric carboxymaltose (FCM), which had to be stopped due to severe anaphylaxis. She now seeks further management options.

3.7.11 Case Continued

Our patient intolerant to oral iron supplementation and anaphylactic to ferric carboxymaltose can be prescribed newer oral supplementation, including sucrosomial iron with better GI tolerability, and even newer IV iron supplementation, including Iron Derisomaltoside and Isomaltoside.

3.8 Conclusion

Efficacy and tolerability of the preparation, when selecting an iron dosing regimen, are the most important considerations. A comprehensive approach involving dynamics of hepcidin metabolism, the severity of anemia, the type of formulation, and patient preference, is the need of the hour [20].

References

1. Pantopoulos K. Oral iron supplementation: new formulations, old questions. Haematologica. 2024;109(9):2790–801. Published 2024 Sep 1. https://doi.org/10.3324/haematol.2024.284967.
2. Stoffel NU, et al. Oral iron supplementation in iron-deficient women: how much and how often? Mol Asp Med. 2020;75:100865. https://doi.org/10.1016/j.mam.2020.100865.
3. Stoffel NU, von Siebenthal HK, Moretti D, Zimmermann MB. Oral iron supplementation in iron-deficient women: how much and how often? Mol Asp Med. 2020;75:100865. https://doi.org/10.1016/j.mam.2020.100865.
4. Cancelo-Hidalgo MJ, Castelo-Branco C, Palacios S, et al. Tolerability of different oral iron supplements: a systematic review. Curr Med Res Opin. 2013;29(4):291–303. https://doi.org/10.1185/03007995.2012.761599.
5. Lo JO, Benson AE, Martens KL, et al. The role of oral iron in the treatment of adults with iron deficiency. Eur J Haematol. 2023;110(2):123–30. https://doi.org/10.1111/ejh.13892.

6. Bazeley JW, Wish JB. Recent and emerging therapies for iron deficiency in anemia of CKD: a review. Am J Kidney Dis. 2022;79(6):868–76. https://doi.org/10.1053/j.ajkd.2021.09.017.
7. Pergola PE, Fishbane S, Tom Pergola PE, Fishbane S, Ganz T. Novel oral iron therapies for iron deficiency anemia in chronic kidney disease. Adv Chronic Kidney Dis. 2019;26(4):272–91. https://doi.org/10.1053/j.ackd.2019.05.002.
8. Gómez-Ramírez S, Brilli E, Tarantino G, Girelli D, Muñoz M. Sucrosomial® iron: an updated review of its clinical efficacy for the treatment of iron deficiency. Pharmaceuticals (Basel). 2023;16(6):847. Published 2023 Jun 6. https://doi.org/10.3390/ph16060847.
9. Lo JO, et al. Oral iron treatment in adult iron deficiency. Eur J Haematol. 2023;110(2):123–30. https://doi.org/10.1111/ejh.13892.
10. Tsilika M, Mitrou J, Antonakos N, et al. An active new formulation of iron carried by aspartyl casein for iron-deficiency anemia: results of the ACCESS trial. Ann Hematol. 2023;102(6):1341–9. https://doi.org/10.1007/s00277-023-05197-3.
11. Dhanush M, Vinod KV, Manivannan P, et al. Daily versus alternate day oral iron replacement for women with iron deficiency anaemia: a randomized controlled trial. Indian J Hematol Blood Transfus. 2024. https://doi.org/10.1007/s12288-024-01816-9.
12. Beyler O, Demir C, Demircan V, et al. Effects of different doses of oral iron on hepcidin and treatment response in iron deficiency anemia. Indian J Hematol Blood Transfus. 2024. https://doi.org/10.1007/s12288-024-01844-5.
13. Intravenous (IV) iron for severe iron deficiency. In: Perry T, ed. Therapeutics letter. Vancouver: Therapeutics Initiative; 2015.
14. Ponikowski P, Kirwan BA, Anker SD, et al. Ferric carboxymaltose for iron deficiency at discharge after acute heart failure: a multicentre, double-blind, randomised, controlled trial [published correction appears in Lancet. 2021 Nov 27;398(10315):1964. doi:10.1016/S0140-6736(21)02492-2.]. Lancet. 2020;396(10266):1895–904. https://doi.org/10.1016/S0140-6736(20)32339-4.
15. Auerbach M, Achebe MM, Thomsen LL, Derman RJ. Efficacy and safety of ferric derisomaltose (FDI) compared with iron sucrose (IS) in patients with iron deficiency anemia after bariatric surgery. Obes Surg. 2022;32(3):810–8. https://doi.org/10.1007/s11695-021-05858-0.
16. Spinowitz BS, Kausz AT, Baptista J, et al. Ferumoxytol for treating iron deficiency anemia in CKD. J Am Soc Nephrol. 2008;19(8):1599–605. https://doi.org/10.1681/ASN.2007101156.
17. Spinowitz BS, et al. Ferumoxytol for treating iron deficiency anemia in CKD. J Am Soc Nephrol. 2008;19(8):1599–605. https://doi.org/10.1681/ASN.2007101156.
18. Van Doren L, Steinheiser M, Boykin K, Taylor KJ, Menendez M, Auerbach M. Expert consensus guidelines: intravenous iron uses, formulations, administration, and management of reactions. Am J Hematol. 2024;99(7):1338–48. https://doi.org/10.1002/ajh.27220.
19. Lewkowitz AK, Tuuli MG. Identifying and treating iron deficiency anemia in pregnancy. Hematology Am Soc Hematol Educ Program. 2023;2023(1):223–8. https://doi.org/10.1182/hematology.2023000474.
20. Aggarwal M, Kar R. Iron deficiency anemia therapy: hepcidin, dosing, formulations and adjuvants. Indian J Hematol Blood Transfus. 2025;41:225–7. https://doi.org/10.1007/s12288-025-02018-7.

Chapter 4
Diagnostic Approach to Non-spherocytic Haemolytic Anaemia (NSHA)

Poonam Rani and Mrinalini Kotru

Abstract Non-spherocytic haemolytic anaemias (NSHA) are constellations of inherited and acquired haemolytic anaemias with *haemolysis as the primary presentation*. The diagnosis is based on the *absence of spherocytes on the PS examination (PS)*. The hereditary group is mainly constituted by enzymopathies and some surface membrane disorders with subtle RBC changes; while the acquired group comprises mainly of fragmentation syndromes, Paroxysmal nocturnal haemoglobinuria (PNH), and heavy metal toxicity due to Lead or Arsenic.

The hereditary NSHA often presents either as chronic or acute haemolytic anaemias of unknown aetiology. The biochemical and haematological investigations favour haemolytic anaemia; however, the underlying aetiology is not clearly obvious and requires an exhaustive workup to reach the final diagnosis. Similarly, disorders like PNH, drugs, and toxins may have an obscure clinical presentation and may require an extensive workup for arriving at a diagnosis. Most of the other causes, like non-immune haemolytic anaemias, secondary to infections, burns, or thrombotic microangiopathies, do not have haemolysis as the primary clinical presentation. Only a very few of them will present as haemolysis primarily, the rest present with very characteristic clinical features, making diagnosis straightforward.

The diagnostic algorithm for NSHA begins with a *careful examination of PS* to rule out the presence of spherocytes *and demonstrate a negative Coombs test.* Identifying any other specific red cell morphology like elliptocytes, stomatocytes, acanthocytes, echinocytes, sickle cells, fragmented cells, bite cells or basophilic stippling, enable a specific diagnosis on PS itself. The presence of a microcytic hypochromic blood picture and typical clinical presentation enables further workup of Thalassemia and other haemoglobinopathies. Similarly, the presence of bite or blister cells in G6PD deficiency, basophilic stippling in pyrimidine deficiency aids

P. Rani · M. Kotru (✉)
Department of Pathology, UCMS & GTBH, Delhi, India

H. P. Pati et al. (eds.), *Clinical Hematology and Hemato-Oncology*,
https://doi.org/10.1007/978-981-92-1167-8_4

in giving direction to further workup. On the contrary, in the absence of a specific morphology, a careful review of all the clinical and laboratory findings and following a diagnostic algorithm helps in arriving at a diagnosis.

Keywords Non-spherocytic haemolytic anaemia · Enzymopathies · Membranopathies

Learning Objectives
- The causes of non-spherocytic haemolytic anaemia (NSHA)
- To follow the diagnostic algorithm for arriving at a diagnosis

4.1 Introduction

Haemolytic anaemia (HA) means anaemia due to the lysis of red blood cells. There are various aetiologies for haemolysis which can be due to intracorpuscular or extracorpuscular defect resulting from hereditary or acquired causes, resulting in haemolysis at intravascular or extravascular sites. In spite of this gamut of causes, there are classical hallmarks common to all HA. These include anaemia, jaundice, splenomegaly (variable), reticulocytosis, and raised lactate dehydrogenase (LDH). Despite these commonalities, there is a huge clinical heterogeneity, making the diagnosis challenging. *The presence of spherocytes in the smear, along with a decisive Coombs test*, helps in narrowing the diagnosis to a few conditions resulting in spherocytic HA. However, a large number of HbS do not show the presence of spherocytes and are grouped into Non-Spherocytic Haemolytic anaemia (NSHA). Although the absence of spherocytes seems a good starting point for extensive workup, the diagnosis of this extremely heterogeneous group of disorders is complex and requires a careful, systematic approach.

Like all haemolytic anaemias, NSHA is also caused by intracorpuscular and extracorpuscular defects. Amongst the intracorpuscular defects, surface membrane disorders (SMDs) like hereditary elliptocytosis (HE) have a typical morphology, making diagnosis easy. On the other hand, hemoglobinopathies and thalassemia have a very characteristic presentation and laboratory workup. Only some of the above cases, and mainly the enzymopathies actually result in a diagnostic dilemma and require extensive work-up. Amongst the acquired causes, PNH is another entity that may have an obscure presentation, making diagnosis difficult. Amongst the extracorpuscular defects, non-immune haemolytic anemias comprise a significant proportion of acquired NSHA. The presence of schistocytes clinches the diagnosis of this group of disorders. The Haemolysis secondary to heavy metal toxicity and drugs have a subtle presentation and needs an extensive workup to arrive at a diagnosis. Table 4.1 enlists the causes of hereditary as well as acquired NSHA.

Table 4.1 Causes of non-spherocytic haemolytic anaemia

Hereditary NSHA	Thalassemia and haemoglobinopathies
	Enzymopathies Glycolytic pathway enzymopathies: PKD, HKD, GPID, PFKD, aldolase deficiency, TPI deficiency, PGKD Hexose monophosphate shunt pathway enzymopathies: G6PD deficiency; few cases, GSD, GPxD Purine and pyrimidine metabolism defect: Pyrimidine 5′nucleotidase deficiency, adenosine deaminase excess, adenylate kinase deficiency
	Surface membrane disorders (SMDs): Hereditary eliptocytosis (HE), hereditary stomatocytosis. McLeod phenomenon, neuroacanthocytosis syndrome, abetalipoproteinemia
Acquired NSHA	Paroxysmal nocturnal haemoglobinuria
	Fragmentation syndromes: TTP, D+ HUS, aHUS, DIC, HELLP
	Associated with systemic disorders Spur cell anaemia Zieve syndrome Infections: Malaria, babesiosis
	Heavy metal toxicity, such as lead, arsenic

Abbreviations: *PKD* pyruvate kinase deficiency, *HKD* hexokinase deficiency, *GPID* glucose phosphate isomerase deficiency, *PFKD* phosphofructokinase deficiency, *TPI* triose phosphate isomerase deficiency, *PGKD* phosphoglycerate kinase deficiency, *GSD* glutathione synthetase deficiency, *GPxD* glutathione peroxidase deficiency

The diagnosis of haemolytic anaemia requires a step-by-step approach to arrive at a definitive cause. The following discussion involves the step-by-step approach to the diagnosis of NSHA.

4.1.1 Clinical Clues for the Presence of HA

HA has a varied clinical presentation. Whenever a patient presents with features of *anaemia, jaundice with or without splenomegaly*, haematological and biochemical workup for haemolytic anaemia should be done. Apart from this classic presentation, many times HA may present as an *acute, rapidly worsening anaemia* along with a systemic disease, like infection or high fever. On the other hand, it may be very *insidious*, compensated, and accidentally detected during the work-up of a systemic illness or a syndrome. Careful evaluation of the history, including past, travel, family, and drug intake, along with the changes in the haematological and biochemical parameters, will help identify haemolysis. History should specifically be directed to establishing the hereditary vs acquired nature of the haemolysis. A negative family history may not always rule out a hereditary cause. Additionally, the need for repeated blood transfusion, the presence of neonatal hyperbilirubinemia or neuromuscular disorders, and gallbladder disease should also be looked for as these are helpful clues to the underlying aetiology.

Hence, patients with jaundice along with anaemia and/or rapidly worsening anaemia in the absence of haemorrhage are strong indicators of underlying haemolysis and require further workup for establishing haemolysis.

4.1.2 Laboratory Work Up for Evidence of Haemolysis

Laboratory evidence of haemolysis is paramount in confirming the clinical suspicion. The workup is aimed at proving the *presence of increased red cell breakdown and corresponding increased marrow turnover of red cells*. Isolated indirect hyperbilirubinemia, along with increased urine urobilinogen and serum LDH levels, confirms increased RBC breakdown. Reticulocytosis indicates hyperproliferation, a response of normal bone marrow to increased RBC breakdown. Hence, *worsening anaemia on CBC, reticulocytosis, indirect hyperbilirubinemia, and raised LDH* suggest a possibility of HA.

4.1.3 Baseline Screening for Understanding the Nature of Haemolysis

The presence of raised plasma haemoglobin with reduced or absent Serum Haptoglobin and/or haemoglobinuria /haemosiderinuria is definitive evidence for intravascular haemolysis. In addition, the haemosiderinuria also indicates the chronicity of haemolysis. On the other hand, *extravascular haemolysis* mainly has mildly reduced Serum Haptoglobin and normal Plasma Haemoglobin. Splenomegaly is more characteristic of extravascular haemolysis.

The next step in the diagnostic workup includes a careful review of the peripheral smear (PS). *The absence of spherocytes on PS* is extremely vital in considering the possibility of NSHA.

- Specific morphologic abnormality, like the presence of *stomatocytes, acanthocytes, or elliptocytes*, suggests a SMD other than HS. The presence of *acanthocytes and echinocytes* directs the workup towards liver and kidney disorders, respectively. Acanthocytes are also seen in neuroacanthocytosis and abetalipoproteinemia (ABL).
- *Marked anisopoikilocytosis* may suggest an underlying haemoglobinopathy or enzymopathy. In such cases, a commonly available Haemoglobin HPLC is done to detect underlying haemoglobinopathy. Normal HPLC directs the further work-up to other causes, especially enzymopathies.
- *Schistocytes or fragmented cells* are characteristically seen in fragmentation syndromes, mainly DIC, HUS, TTP, HELLP syndrome, etc. Clinical presentation, along with the presence of schistocytes, gives vital clues facilitating a definitive diagnosis.

- There are, however, so many cases where PS may not be helpful and warrants an extensive workup. Patients with the presence of neutropenia and thrombocytopenia along with haemolytic anaemia may require workup of autoimmune disease, including Coombs' Test. Coombs negative anaemia may then require a workup for PNH.

4.1.4 Arriving at a Specific Diagnosis

On the basis of the clinical and laboratory clues, further workup of NSHA is suggested (Fig. 4.1). Although spherocyte is integral to the diagnosis of Autoimmune haemolytic anaemia, many cases may show absence of the same and still be Autoimmune HA. Hence, before proceeding to labour-intensive and less available

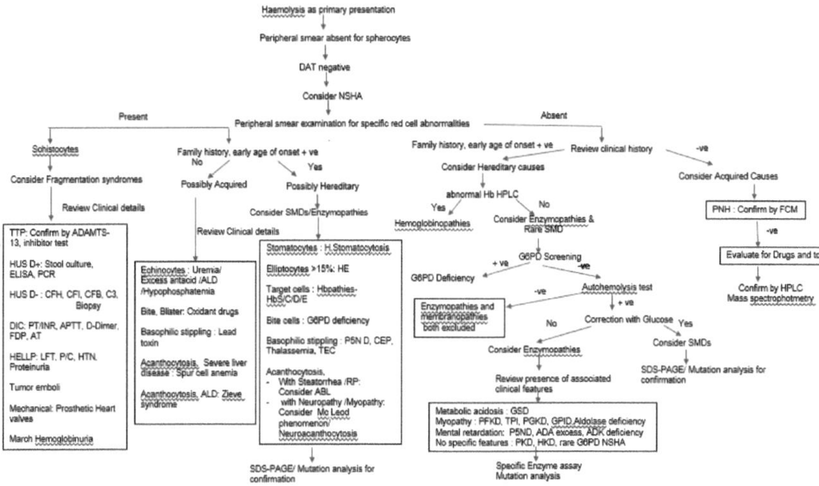

Fig. 4.1 Diagnostic algorithm for NSHA. DAT direct antiglobulin test, NSHA non spherocytic hemolytic anemia, TTP thrombotic thrombocytopenic purpura, ADAMTS A disintegrin and metalloproteinase with thrombospondin motifs, HUS D+ hemolytic uremic syndrome with diarrhea, HUS D- hemolytic uremic syndrome without diarrhea, ELISA enzyme linked immunosorbent assay, PCR polymerase chain reaction, CFH complement factor H, CFI complement factor I, CFB complement factor B, DIC disseminated intravascular coagulation, PT prothrombin time, APTT activated partial thromboplastin time, FDP fibrin degradation product, AT anti thrombin, HELLP hemolysis, elevated liver enzyme, low platelet count, P/C platelet count, HTN hypertension, ALD alcoholic liver disease, SMDs surface membrane disorders, HE hereditary elliptocytosis, P5ND pyrimidine 5′ nucleotidase deficiency, CEP congenital erythropoietic porphyria, TEC transient erythroblastopenia of childhood, RP retinitis pigmentosa, ABL abetalipoproteinemia, GSD glutathione synthetase deficiency, PFKD phosphofructokinase deficiency, PGKD phosphoglycerate kinase deficiency, GPID glucose phosphate isomerase deficiency, ADA excess adenosine deaminase excess, ADK adenylate kinase, PKD pyruvate kinase deficiency, HKD hexokinase deficiency, PNH paroxysmal nocturnal hemoglobinuria, FCM flowcytometry, HPLC high performance liquid chromatography

tests, it's important to *confirm the absence of an immune origin of haemolysis by performing a Direct and indirect Coomb's test.* This is also necessary as identifying the immune origin of haemolysis opens the gates to entirely different and potentially curable causes of haemolysis.

Further course of action is decided by various clues identified on clinical presentation, examination, and initial laboratory workup, which is discussed as follows-

4.1.4.1 Hereditary NSHA

Work Up for Suspected NSHA Caused by Haemoglobinopathies

Thalassaemia and haemoglobinopathies causing haemolysis usually present early in life and are associated with splenomegaly. On PS examination, they are characterized by anisopoikilocyosis and the presence of a variable number of nucleated erythroid precursors in PS (Fig. 4.2). Sickle cells can be observed in variable numbers in sickle cell syndromes. Microcytes, when presence support a diagnosis of thalassaemia. However, many haemoglobinopathies may not have a characteristic feature. Hence, for all cases of NSHA, the next investigation to be done to diagnose or rule out Haemoglobinopathies is Hb HPLC. Tests for workup are briefly discussed.

- Hb HPLC: It is a very quick and efficient way of screening and confirming haemoglobinopathies. However, many a time, diagnosis is elusive and needs molecular testing for confirmation.
- Capillary electrophoresis: It separates various types of haemoglobin and is particularly useful in distinguishing Hb A2 and Hb E. However, molecular testing is required to resolve uncommon haemoglobinopathies.

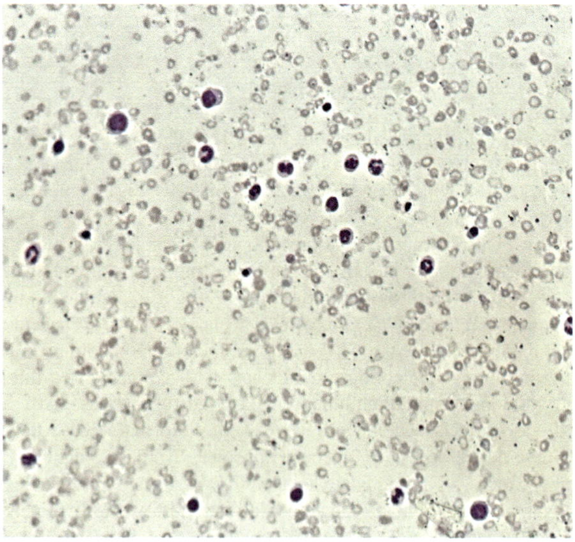

Fig. 4.2 PS of β-Thalassemia major. PS of β-Thalassemia major showing marked anisopoikilocytosis, microcytic hypochromic red cells, many nucleated red cells and some polychromatophils

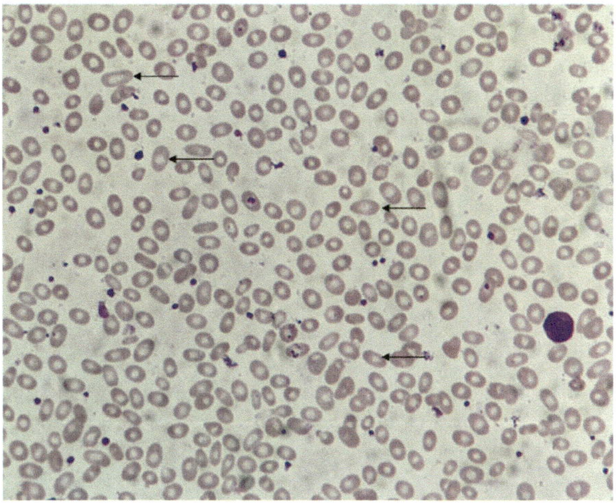

Fig. 4.3 PS of hereditary elliptocytosis. PS of HE showing moderate to marked anisopoikilocytosis with presence of many oval shape (elliptical) red cells called elliptocytes (black arrows)

- Molecular testing: PCR, e.g., ARMS—PCR, GAP PCR, is helpful in detecting the presence of known suspected mutations. They are particularly useful in prenatal testing as the parents' mutational profile is also known. Sanger's sequencing and NGS, however, are used when cases are not resolved by any of the above.

Work Up for Suspected NSHA Caused by Red Cell SMDs

Non-spherocytic SMDs are very rare and hence, the specific tests for diagnosis are not easily available. HE, hereditary stomatocytosis (HSt), and ABL are few of the relatively commoner forms of SMDs after Hereditary Spherocytosis (HS). Family history gives an important clue. While HE and HSt are mainly autosomal dominant, ABL is Autosomal recessive. In addition, ABL is also associated with malabsorption of fat and fat-soluble vitamins, absence of plasma apoB-lipoprotein, hypotriglyceridemia, and hypocholesterolemia [1]. However, empirical diagnosis can be made on examining the specific morphology of red cells on PS (Figs. 4.3 and 4.4). However, the following tests can be done for confirmation.

- Incubated OFT: The results of OFT are variable; however, when abnormal in the patient and family, it provides conclusive evidence of SMDs. In HE, the abnormal OFT correlates with the severity of haemolysis. In non-haemolytic HE, OFT may be completely normal.
- SDS–PAGE: It can quantify various band proteins and highlight their deficiency, like Spectrin, protein 4.1R, and band 3 abnormalities in HE [2]. Similarly, it can quantify Band 7.2b and human Stomatin-like protein 2 (SLP2) in HSt [3].
- Next-generation sequencing (NGS): Exact genotypic diagnosis can be done [4].

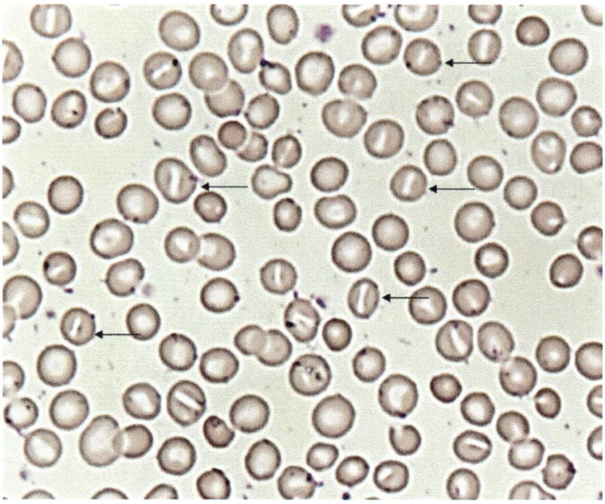

Fig. 4.4 PS of hereditary stomatocytosis. PS of HSt showing moderate to marked anisopoikilocytosis with presence of many red cells with slit like opening called stomatocytes (black arrows)

Work Up for Suspected Enzymopathies

The enzymopathies generally present early in age with a variable clinical presentation which may vary from frank haemolysis to well-compensated chronic haemolytic anaemia. These patients have clinical and biochemical features of haemolysis with normal haemoglobin electrophoresis, direct and indirect coombs test, osmotic fragility, normal lipid profile, and kidney and liver function tests (except indirect hyperbilirubinemia). Enzymopathies can be due to a deficiency of enzymes involved in the pentose phosphate pathway (e.g., G6PD) or glycolytic pathway (e.g., PKD) or enzymes for nucleotide metabolism (e.g., P5ND). PS usually does not show any specific red cell morphology except the presence of bite cells in G6PD deficiency (Fig. 4.5), echinocytes in PKD, and Basophilic stippling in P5ND. The following screening tests are done with the aim of first excluding G6PD deficiency, followed by PKD and P5ND in order of their frequency [5, 6].

Screening Tests

- OFT: It is normal in enzymopathies, except sometimes a tail of fragile cells is seen.
- Autohaemolysis test: The SMDs and metabolic defects can be differentiated by autohaemolysis test. It is a very informative test but because it is labour intensive, hence not widely available. It is increased in both SMDs as well as enzymopathies however addition of Glucose reduces the rate of Haemolysis in SMDs (Type I Haemolysis) as opposed to disorders of glycolytic pathway like Pyruvate kinase deficiency (PKD) where there is failure to correct haemolysis (Type II haemolysis). *The normal autohaemolysis test virtually rules out membrane and enzyme abnormalities* [7].

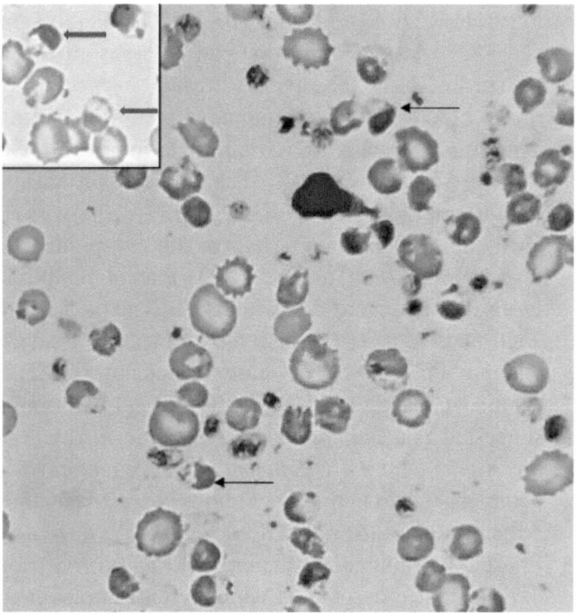

Fig. 4.5 PS of G6PD deficiency. PS of G6PD deficiency showing marked anisopoikilocytosis with presence of blister cells with haemoglobin at one end of red cell (arrow) and polychromatophils. Inset shows Blister cells (blue arrow)

- Methaemoglobin reduction test (MRT)/fluorescent spot test/cytochemical formazan granule test: These tests are used for screening of glucose 6 phosphate dehydrogenase (G6PD). If this is negative, then further tests are done to find out the cause. Point of care testing (POCT) is available, which measures G6PD enzyme activity by electrochemical quantification of NADPH [8–10].
- Red cell 2, 3 DPG levels: Its levels are increased in PKD; however, decreased in HKD. The rest of the enzymopathies yield normal results [11].

Specific Diagnostic Work-Up

This is done mostly in cases where a clear diagnosis is not available from the above methods. Specific diagnostic workup for various enzymopathies is discussed in brief

- G6PD deficiency: It is the commonest enzymopathy. It has three main presentation—chronic NSHA, neonatal jaundice, and acute HA exaggerated by fava beans, infections, or drugs. Most of the cases of G6PD have spherocytes, but *some cases do not show very obvious spherocytes* and hence are categorized as NSHA. As per the current WHO classification, the class A G6PD variant with enzyme activity <20%, chronic HA, and absence of favism, infections, or oxidative drugs fall into the G6PD, CNSHA group [8, 9]. The quantitative estimation of G6PD enzyme activity is done by spectrophotometric analysis. It is important to remember that the enzyme activity should not be measured during an acute haemolytic episode due to enough G6PD enzyme in reticulocytes than older RBCs. The specific diagnosis is established by molecular techniques [12].

- Pyruvate Kinase Deficiency (PKD): The final diagnosis of PKD is based on red cell PK enzyme activity that can be assessed by spectrophotometry. However, similar to G6PD, false positive results may be generated due to reticulocytosis, recent blood transfusion, or incomplete removal of WBC's and platelets from hemolysate. The PK to hexokinase ratio or PK to G6PD ratio may be performed to improve sensitivity [13]. The molecular confirmation is attained by genotyping for mutations in the PKLR gene [14].
- Hexokinase Deficiency (HKD): The end-point enzyme assay is performed to reveal reduced enzymatic activity. Exceptionally, some cases show normal HK levels despite severe HA, which brings up the need for kinetic assays and genetic confirmation of HKI mutation by molecular assays [15].
- Glucose Phosphate Isomerase Deficiency (GPID): These patients may show echinocytes and acanthocytes on PS and neuromuscular impairment [16]. It is suggested that *patients with NSHA and neuromuscular impairment should be investigated for GPI deficiency*. The quantitative enzyme assays on red cell hemolysate help in diagnosis; however, confirmatory diagnosis is made by DNA sequence analysis of the GPI gene [16, 17].
- Phosphofructokinase Deficiency (PFKD) or Glycogen Storage Disease (GSD) Type VII: It is associated with exercise intolerance and myopathy. Family history, classical muscular symptoms, exercise intolerance, rhabdomyolysis panel (comprising of Creatinine kinase, myoglobinuria, and hyperuricemia), PFK enzyme deficiency in muscle biopsy, followed by genetic testing for PFKM deficiency, complete the diagnostic algorithm [18].
- Aldolase A Deficiency: It is a childhood Glycogen Storage Disease, type XII, characterized by NSHA, myopathy, rhabdomyolysis, and developmental delay. Investigations supporting HA, Rhabdomyolysis, Red cell Aldolase enzyme activity, muscle biopsy, and exome sequencing of ALDOA gene confirm the diagnosis [19, 20].
- Triose Phosphate Isomerase (TPI) Deficiency: This childhood NSHA is accompanied by myopathy, recurrent infections, developmental delay, or neurodegenerative disorders. The acylcarnitine analysis reveals raised C3 carnitine levels. The enzyme assays and molecular testing for mutation in the TPI gene are confirmatory diagnostic modalities [21].
- Phosphoglycerate Kinase (PGK) Deficiency: The patients present with Chronic NSHA, myopathy, and neurological manifestations. Workup for HA, tests for rhabdomyolysis (Creatinine kinase, myoglobinuria, and hyperuricemia) are done. It is confirmed by PGK enzyme assays for activity and molecular analysis for mutations in the PGK gene [22, 23].
- Glutathione synthetase deficiency (GSD): The mild variants present with NSHA and splenomegaly; however, moderate and severe cases are complicated by metabolic acidosis due to 5-oxoprolinuria. Investigate for metabolic acidosis, 5-oxoprolinuria, and glutathione levels in urine and blood, and confirm the diagnosis. False positive 5-Oxoprolinuria is also due to severe burns, cystinosis, Stevens—Johnson syndrome, 5-Oxoprolinase deficiency, Tyrosinemia,

Homocystinuria, and drugs like paracetamol, Vigabatrin, or some antibiotics, and should be excluded before final interpretation [24, 25].

- Glutathione Peroxidase Deficiency (GPxD): These patients might remain asymptomatic throughout life or may experience severe chronic NSHA. This enzyme is a selenoprotein; hence, reduced selenium levels affect the antioxidative property of GPX as well as the metabolic function of the thyroid [26]. Demonstrating a selenium deficiency supports the diagnosis. Molecular studies provide a confirmatory diagnosis [27].
- P5N deficiency: This is the third most common enzymopathy, characterized by severe HA to fully compensated chronic NSHA and basophilic stippling on PS. Other causes of basophilic stippling, such as lead poisoning, megaloblastic anaemia, sideroblastic anaemia, some haemoglobin variants, and beta thalassemia trait should be excluded. The false positive results can be seen in transient erythroblastopenia of childhood in which the P5N enzyme is reduced due the presence of many old red blood cells.
  Normal RBCs contain a large number of purines while pyrimidines are found in very small amounts. There is increased concentration of pyrimidine nucleotides and glutathione (GSH) in red blood cells in P5N Deficiency with reduced activity of P5'N1 enzyme in RBC's. Hence, this issue serves as a screening test for P5ND in NSHA cases, especially when basophilic stippling is seen on PS. The purine to pyrimidine ratio (OD 260: OD 280) is markedly reduced. This test is specific for P5'N deficiency and can be used as a screening test as per ICSH 1989. Gene expression analysis of the NT5C3A gene by quantitative PCR for confirmed diagnosis [28].
- Adenine Deaminase (ADA) Excess: These patients have mild to moderate chronic NSHA. Reduced red cell ATP levels and increased red cell ADA activity confirm the diagnosis [29].
- Adenylate Kinase Deficiency (AKD): The clinical presentation varies from Neonatal jaundice, hepatosplenomegaly, unexplained moderate to severe NSHA, developmental delay, and mental retardation in some cases. Enzyme activity of AK1 and molecular analysis for mutations are confirmatory [30].

4.1.4.2 Acquired NSHA

Work Up for Suspected PNH

It is an acquired stem cell disorder with characteristic features of chronic intravascular haemolytic anaemia, thrombotic manifestations, and bone marrow failure; however, all the features might not be present at the same time. It occurs due to acquired mutations in the PIGA gene required for the synthesis of glycosylphosphatidylinositol (GPI) anchor molecules such as CD55, CD59, etc. The deficiency of these regulatory proteins in PNH cells leads to uncontrolled complement activation and membrane attack complex formation, responsible for intravascular haemolysis.

PNH is suspected when a patient presents with macroscopic haemoglobinuria or low-grade chronic intravascular HA precipitated by underlying infections, surgery, or trauma, or history of thromboembolism or pancytopenia, primarily due to bone marrow failure without any obvious evidence of haemolysis. Diagnostic workup of PNH is done when the patient presents with either of the above features or *DCT-negative HA* (especially intravascular haemolysis), not being classified by other tests. Radiological investigations may reveal venous thromboembolism at unusual sites. CBC may show pancytopenia with mild reticulocytosis, and bone marrow done for the workup of pancytopenia may reveal pockets of erythroid precursors, suggesting the presence of PNH. A patient with unexplained iron deficiency anaemia should also be worked up for PNH. The following diagnostic tests are done for confirmation.

- Hams test and sucrose lysis test: It is a method of detecting increased fragility of PNH red cells in acidified serum. However, it is obsolete as it is less sensitive and specific. Also, it can detect PNH in red cells only. If PNH type III cells are <5% or PNH type II cells are <20%, the Hams test gives false-negative results. The test may also be negative when the patient has received a recent transfusion [31].
- Neutrophil alkaline phosphatase: It is low or absent in PNH.
- Gel card test: It is an easy, quick, and cost-effective screening test. However, it is a qualitative test, unable to detect small clones of PNH cells. It is also affected by recent blood transfusion and haemolytic crisis.
- Immunophenotyping by flowcytometry: It is a gold standard test for confirming diagnosis. Moreover, it is a quantitative method. *PNH clone >1% is considered positive, seen in at least two different lineages and on at least 2 different GPI-linked proteins* [32, 33]. The red cells, granulocytes, and monocytes are analysed for expression of GPI-associated proteins CD 55, CD59, FLAER, CD24, CD14, and/or CD157.
- The RBC's are gated with glycophorin or CD235a, then analysed for CD55, CD59 and FLAER expression. Based on the percentage of PNH clones, the disease is classified into Type 1 (normal expression), Type II (partial expression), and Type III (absent expression). The major limitation of analysing red cells is the complement-mediated destruction of PNH-sensitive red cells. A recent blood transfusion and haemolytic crisis may result in a false negative test.
- *FLAER assay:* FLAER directly binds to GPI anchor ankyrin proteins. The absence of fluorescence depicts a deficiency of these GPI proteins on the cell surface. FLAER binds with all the GPI-anchor proteins; hence, it is not affected by the PNH type and variable expression of these proteins on RBCs and WBCs. It is very sensitive at detecting small PNH clones on granulocytes and monocytes, and also, there is no effect of transfusion or haemolysis on FLAER expression [34]. The FLAER expression on neutrophils and monocytes is a highly sensitive flowcytometric method for the diagnosis of PNH [35].
- The granulocytes are considered best for analysis of GPI anchor proteins as they don't undergo complement-mediated lysis. The granulocytes can be gated with

CD15 or CD24. A combination of FLAER and CD24/CD157 is recommended for granulocyte analysis [36].

- The monocytes are mainly gated with CD14 or CD64 and clone identified on combination of FLAER and CD14/CD157 combination [37].

Workup of Fragmentation Syndromes

There is haemolysis of red blood cells, high shear stress in fragmentation syndromes, also called Microangiopathic HA (MAHA). This syndrome is associated with disorders based on five different pathologies: *vWF–rich thrombi, Thrombotic microangiopathy (endothelial injury), fibrin-rich platelet thrombi, vasculitis/vasculopathy, and tumour emboli* [38]. It is suspected in patients of NSHA with the presence of *schistocytes* and thrombocytopenia (TCP) in PS (Fig. 4.6).

- vWF-rich thrombi: Thrombotic thrombocytopenic purpura (TTP) is characterised by widespread hyaline vWF-platelet thrombi in multiple organs, MAHA, TCP, and <10% ADAMTS13 levels. It can be hereditary or acquired (inhibitory antibodies). Full-blown TTP is a pentad of MAHA, TCP, fever, neurologic deficit, and renal abnormalities. However, it may begin as a diad of MAHA with TCP and then progress to a pentad. A confirmatory diagnosis can be made by ascertaining plasma ADAMTS-13 activity. Values <10% is diagnostic of TTP. Acquired TTP shows a positive inhibitor test for Anti-ADAMTS13 IgG (75% of TTP during an acute phase) or IgM and IgA (rarely). Hereditary TTP is suspected when the ADAMTS-13 inhibitor test is negative, and family members show severe or partial deficiency of ADAMTS-13 [38].

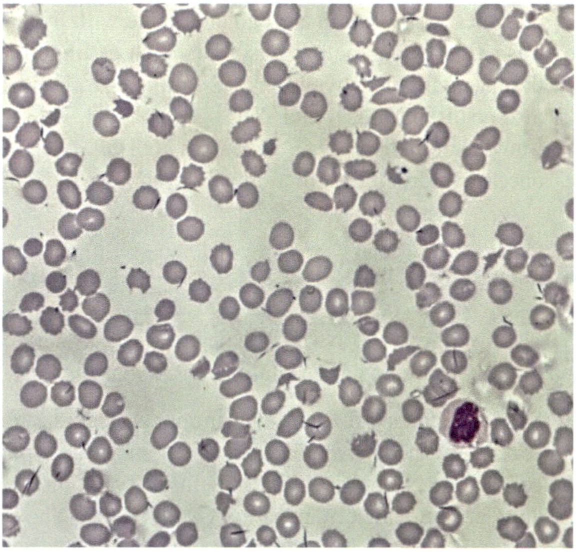

Fig. 4.6 PS of fragmentation syndrome. PS of fragmentation syndrome showing marked anisopoikilocytosis with presence of many red cells which are helmet shaped or have sharp projections called schistocytes (black arrows)

- Thrombotic microangiopathy (TMA-endothelial injury): TMA starts with endothelial injury, progressing to widespread microthrombi formation in many organs, leading to MAHA and TCP. The disorders that fall in the TMA category are Shiga toxin haemolytic uremic syndrome (STx HUS), atypical HUS (aHUS), pneumococcal HUS, anti-VEGF drugs, Antiphospholipid antibody syndrome, diacylglycerol kinase Epsilon (DGKE) nephropathy, and cobalamine C disease. Diagnosis of this heterogenous group is based on a variety of tests guided by clinical presentation.
- Diagnosis of diarrhoea +(D+) STx HUS is done by demonstration of positive stool culture for *Escherichia coli* and Shiga toxin by enzyme immunoassay. Molecular tests like PCR for *E. coli*, confirm the diagnosis [39].
- Diagnosis of aHUS is primarily done in patients who don't have diarrhoea as the primary complaint and STx HUS and TTP are excluded. TMA in renal biopsy provides the supportive evidence. Mutation analysis of complement factor H, I, B, C3, membrane cofactor protein, thrombomodulin, and complement factor H-related protein (Musalem P) confirm the diagnosis [40].
- Fibrin-rich platelet thrombi: Exaggerated uncontrolled activation of the coagulation cascade results in fibrin-rich platelet thrombi in disorders such as disseminated intravascular coagulation, catastrophic antiphospholipid antibody (CAPS) syndrome, Heparin-induced thrombocytopenia, paroxysmal nocturnal haemoglobinuria, and HELLP syndrome of pregnancy. CAPS results in spherocytic/DCT positive HA and hence not discussed in this chapter. Like other NSHA, the confirmatory diagnosis is guided by the clinical features supported by laboratory investigations.
- DIC: Laboratory diagnosis is made by the presence of TCP, raised prothrombin time and activated partial thromboplastin time, hypofibrinogenemia, raised D-Dimer, and fibrin degradation products (FDP) [41, 42]
- HELLP is mainly a clinical diagnosis supported by the presence of altered liver enzymes, HA, TCP in a pregnant female with hypertension and proteinuria.
- Vasculitis/vasculopathy: Disorders such as immune complex vasculitis, scleroderma, malignant hypertension, various viral and fungal infections result can also result in MAHA and TCP.
- Tumour emboli result in MAHA with TCP. Association with tumour and presence of a normal coagulation profile support the diagnosis.

Workup of Miscellaneous NSHA Associated with Acquired Systemic Diseases

These are a group of NSHA associated with systemic disorders; heterogenous in pathogenesis, clinical presentation, and diagnosis.

- Spur cell anaemia: It is a non-immune moderate to severe HA in patients with severe advanced liver disease, splenomegaly, hyperlipidaemia, and $\geq 5\%$ Spur cells in the peripheral blood. The most common aetiology is alcoholic liver disease, accompanied by hepatitis viruses rarely. The excess cholesterol deposits in the red cell membrane are responsible for the spur cell morphology. Spur cells have variable-sized spicules (5–10) with irregular spacing on the red cell surface, and their percentage >5% is an independent adverse prognostic marker [43].

- Zieve syndrome: The episodic HA with transient hyperlipidaemia in alcoholic liver disease patients is known as Zieve syndrome. It has overlapping features with Spur cell anaemia; however, splenomegaly and spur cells >5% are not seen in this condition [44].
- Heavy metal toxicity: The metals such as lead and arsenic lead to NSHA. The diagnosis is difficult and requires a very strong clinical suspicion. The confirmed diagnosis is made by chromatography or mass spectrophotometry.
- Arsenic toxicity leads to acute intravascular haemolytic anaemia as it forms haemoglobin adducts that get attached to the red cell surface, thereby leading to HA. The diagnosis is made by mass spectrophotometry [45].
- Lead poisoning: It results in NSHA, hypertension, and abdominal colic after prolonged exposure to Lead. It is an acquired cause of P5N enzyme deficiency. The PS shows characteristic basophilic stippling. To differentiate from hereditary causes, enzyme assays and mutation analysis are useful. The diagnosis is confirmed by a history of prolonged exposure to Lead, increased Lead levels in blood and urine, along with radiological examination of bones [46].
- Infections: Infections like malaria and babesiosis may lead to NSHA, and the diagnosis of the underlying condition helps in the diagnosis and cure of HA.

4.2 Learning Through a Case

A 12-year-old male presented with a history of severe pallor and jaundice requiring transfusion in the past 7 months. The requirement of transfusion increased in the last 2.5 months. He had a history of recurrent fever requiring multiple hospital admissions. His parents and four siblings revealed no similar complaints. There was no cyanosis, lymphadenopathy, organomegaly, or thrombotic evidence. Investigations show Hb 7.9 g/dl, TLC 3.5×10^9/l & Platelet count 80×10^9/L. The corrected reticulocyte count was 1.5%. Serum bilirubin, total bilirubin 2.4 mg/dl, direct bilirubin 0.4 mg/dl, serum lactate dehydrogenase (LDH) 460 U/L. PS showed pancytopenia, predominantly normocytic normochromic red cells, with occasional poikilocyte, and thrombocytopenia (TCP). The differential leucocyte count was 25% polymorphs, 69% lymphocytes, 5% monocytes, and 1% eosinophils. He was also investigated for HIV, HBV, and typhoid fever, which yielded negative results. Workup for indirect hyperbilirubinemia was advised. Liver function tests showed SGOT-35 U/l, SGPT-40 U/l, & alkaline phosphatase- 120 U/L. Urine examination revealed the presence of Urobilinogen and Hemosiderin. The presence of Hemosiderin in urine indicated the presence of chronic intravascular haemolysis. This finding was supported by raised plasma haemoglobin (11.4 mg/dl). The direct antiglobulin test was negative. Hb HPLC was within normal limits; however, HbF was mildly increased (1.4%).

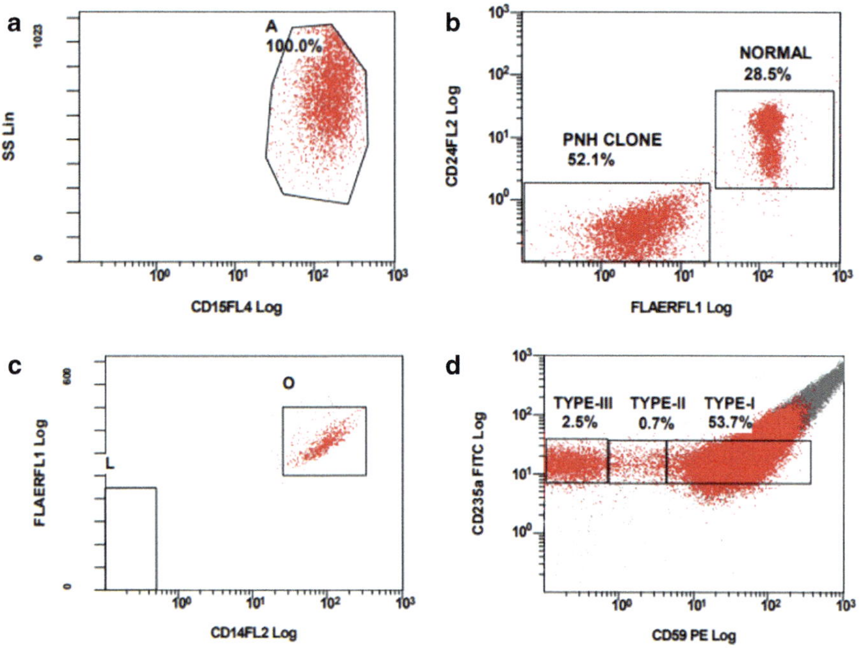

Fig. 4.7 Immunophenotypic diagnosis of PNH. Immunophenotypic diagnosis of PNH: Neutrophils gated with CD15 show PNH clone; 52.1% PNH clone which is negative for CD24 & FLAER (**a** & **b**), Monocytes gated with CD45 and stained with CD14 and FLAER show no PNH clone (**c**), Red cells gated with CD235a and stained with CD59 show mosaic of PNH Type III and Type II cells along with normal Type I red cells (**d**)

The clues to the further workup were the presence of pancytopenia without splenomegaly and a Coombs-negative chronic haemolytic anaemia. The Bone marrow examination was done to explore the cause of pancytopenia. The bone marrow biopsy showed less than 20% cellularity. There were few pockets of erythroid colonies. Given the presence of few erythroid colonies in a hypocellular marrow and chronic intravascular haemolysis, the patient was investigated for paroxysmal nocturnal haemoglobinuria (PNH). The radiological investigations did not reveal any evidence of thrombosis.

Flow cytometric analysis was used to evaluate red blood cells and white blood cells for the GPI-linked proteins. The red blood cells tagged with CD235a, CD55, and CD59 demonstrated 1.5% PNH II clone and an 11% PNH III clone. The CD15-gated granulocytes evaluated in various combinations with CD24 and fluorescently labelled aerolysin (FLAER) antibodies demonstrated a 24.8% PNH clone. The monocytes did not reveal any PNH clone. (Fig. 4.7). The presence of a PNH clone >1% in two lineages confirmed the diagnosis. The patient was given component replacement therapy and immunosuppressants. The family was counselled for haematopoietic stem cell transplantation and referred to a higher centre.

Summary/Learning Objectives
To summarise, NSHA is a *DCT negative HA with the absence of spherocytes* on PS. It encompasses a heterogenous group of both hereditary and acquired causes. Careful history is essential to ascertain the hereditary aetiology or any association with syndromes. Establishing haemolysis, identifying the intravascular or extravascular cause of haemolysis and picking up relevant clues on the peripheral smear are the cornerstones for accurate diagnosis. If a hereditary cause is suspected then Hb HPLC, incubated osmotic fragility test/auto haemolysis test, and methaemoglobin reduction test for G6PD screening form the battery of tests which help identify most of the haemoglobinopathies, SMDs, and G6PD deficiency (the most common enzymopathy). A very few causes, which are not picked up by the above, especially the enzymopathies, need more cumbersome assays and molecular tests for diagnosis. Similarly, in suspected acquired HA, PNH, and fragmentation syndromes should be considered. Characteristic clinical presentation along with the presence of schistocytes, confirms the latter. In absence of any clue on history or peripheral smear with /without the presence of other cytopenia or history of thrombosis, all patients should always be worked up for PNH by flow cytometry.

To conclude, the diagnostic approach requires careful step-by-step exclusion of common conditions and selection of tests guided by the clinical presentation of the patient, until the final diagnosis is reached.

References

1. Sasaki K, Tada H, Komatsu T, Terada H, Endo Y, Ikewaki K, et al. A new case of abetalipoproteinemia caused by novel compound heterozygote mutations in the MTTP gene without fat or vitamin malabsorption. J Atheroscler Thromb. 2024;31(11):1634–40.
2. Dosunmu A, Uche E, Osikomaiya B, Ismail A, Akinbami A, Akanmu A. Red cell membrane protein abnormalities as defined by sds-page among patients with anemia in a West African region hospital practice. Caspian J Intern Med. 2020;11(3):283–9.
3. Wang Y, Morrow JS. Identification and characterization of human SLP-2, a novel homologue of stomatin (band 7.2b) present in erythrocytes and other tissues. J Biol Chem. 2000;275(11):8062–71.
4. Ma S, Qin J, Wei A, Li X, Qin Y, Liao L, et al. Novel compound heterozygous SPTA1 mutations in a patient with hereditary elliptocytosis. Mol Med Rep. 2018;17(4):5903–11.
5. Nkhoma ET, Poole C, Vannappagari V, Hall SA, Beutler E. The global prevalence of glucose-6-phosphate dehydrogenase deficiency: a systematic review and meta-analysis. Blood Cell Mol Dis. 2009;42(3):267–78.
6. Secrest MH, Storm M, Carrington C, Casso D, Gilroy K, Pladson L, et al. Prevalence of pyruvate kinase deficiency: a systematic literature review. Eur J Haematol. 2020;105(2):173–84.
7. Young LE, Izzo MJ, Altman KI, Swisher SN. Studies on spontaneous in vitro autohemolysis in hemolytic disorders. Blood. 1956;11(11):977–97.
8. Luzzatto L, Bancone G, Dugué PA, Jiang W, Minucci A, Nannelli C, et al. New WHO classification of genetic variants causing G6PD deficiency. Bull World Health Organ. 2024;102(8):615–7.
9. Nannelli C, Bosman A, Cunningham J, Dugué PA, Luzzatto L. Genetic variants causing G6PD deficiency: clinical and biochemical data support new WHO classification. Br J Haematol. 2023;202(5):1024–32.

10. Bancone G, Gornsawun G, Chu CS, Porn P, Pal S, Bansil P, et al. Validation of the quantitative point-of-care CareStart biosensor for assessment of G6PD activity in venous blood. PLoS One. 2018;13(5):e0196716.
11. Delivoria-Papadopoulos M, Oski FA, Gottlieb AJ. Oxygen-hemoglobulin dissociation curves: effect of inherited enzyme defects of the red cell. Science. 1969;165(3893):601–2.
12. Geck RC, Powell NR, Dunham MJ. Functional interpretation, cataloging, and analysis of 1,341 glucose-6-phosphate dehydrogenase variants. Am J Hum Genet. 2023;110(2):228–39.
13. Al-Samkari H, Van Beers EJ, Kuo KHM, Barcellini W, Bianchi P, Glenthøj A, et al. The variable manifestations of disease in pyruvate kinase deficiency and their management. Haematologica. 2020;105(9):2229–39.
14. Bianchi P, Fermo E, Glader B, Kanno H, Agarwal A, Barcellini W, et al. Addressing the diagnostic gaps in pyruvate kinase deficiency: consensus recommendations on the diagnosis of pyruvate kinase deficiency. Am J Hematol. 2019;94(1):149–61.
15. Ukonmaanaho EM, Dell'Anna S, Hakonen A, Wartiovaara-Kautto U, Kakko S, Rab MAE, et al. Biallelic hexokinase 1 (HK1) variants causative of non-spherocytic haemolytic anaemia: a case series with emphasis on the HK1 promoter variant and literature review. Br J Haematol. 2024;204(5):2040–8.
16. Dhankar M, Mandal P, Singh R. Unusual cause of haemolytic anaemia: glucose phosphate isomerase deficiency. Pediatr Hematol Oncol. 2024;9(4):283–6.
17. Fermo E, Vercellati C, Marcello AP, Zaninoni A, Aytac S, Cetin M, et al. Clinical and molecular spectrum of glucose-6-phosphate isomerase deficiency. Report of 12 new cases. Front Physiol. 2019;10:467.
18. Lucia A, Martinuzzi A, Nogales-Gadea G, Quinlivan R, Reason S, International Association for Muscle Glycogen Storage Disease study group. Clinical practice guidelines for glycogen storage disease V & VII (McArdle disease and Tarui disease) from an international study group. Neuromuscul Disord. 2021;31(12):1296–310.
19. Sun YB, Li CY, Chen M. [Onset of glycogen storage disease type XII in two brothers in the neonatal period]. Zhongguo Yi Xue Ke Xue Yuan Xue Bao. 2024;46(4):636–40.
20. Santoro L, Pjetraj D, Velmishi V, Campana C, Catassi C, Dionisi-Vici C, et al. A new phenotype of aldolase a deficiency in a 14 year-old boy with epilepsy and rhabdomyolysis - case report. Ital J Pediatr. 2022;48(1):39.
21. Selamioğlu A, Karaca M, Balcı MC, Körbeyli HK, Durmuş A, Yıldız EP, et al. Triosephosphate isomerase deficiency: E105D mutation in unrelated patients and review of the literature. Mol Syndromol. 2023;14(3):231–8.
22. Hierholzer A, Mador J, Guntu R, Schafernak K, Grebe TA. First report of phosphoglycerate kinase deficiency in a Dinè child with review of current literature. Am J Med Genet A. 2025;197(7):e64034.
23. Zhou X, Liu Q, Huang M. An atypical case of phosphoglycerate kinase deficiency with a novel PGK1 variant. Seizure. 2024;117:161–3.
24. Wu X, Jiao J, Xia Y, Yan X, Liu Z, Cao Y, et al. Case report: a Chinese patient with glutathione synthetase deficiency and a novel glutathione synthase mutation. Front Pediatr. 2023;11:1212405.
25. Signolet I, Chenouard R, Oca F, Barth M, Reynier P, Denis MC, et al. Recurrent isolated neonatal hemolytic anemia: think about glutathione synthetase deficiency. Pediatrics. 2016;138(3):e20154324.
26. Souza LSL, Campos RO, Braga JSF, Jesus JDS, Ramos HE, Anunciação SM, et al. Selenium nutritional status and thyroid dysfunction. Arch Endocrinol Metab. 2025;69(1):e230348.
27. Perona G, Guidi GC, Piga A, Cellerino R, Milani G, Colautti P, et al. Neonatal erythrocyte glutathione peroxidase deficiency as a consequence of selenium imbalance during pregnancy. Br J Haematol. 1979;42(4):567–74.
28. Patir DC, Gunes A, Durmaz B, Karaca E, Soyer N. Pyrimidine-5′-nucleotidase deficiency: a new homozygous NT5C3A mutation (c.693+1G>A variant). Clin Lab. 2025;71(2).

29. Chottiner EG, Cloft HJ, Tartaglia AP, Mitchell BS. Elevated adenosine deaminase activity and hereditary hemolytic anemia. Evidence for abnormal translational control of protein synthesis. J Clin Invest. 1987;79(3):1001–5.
30. Dongerdiye R, Sampagar A, Devendra R, Warang P, Kedar P. Rare hereditary nonspherocytic hemolytic anemia caused by a novel homozygous mutation, c.301C>A, (Q101K), in the AK1 gene in an Indian family. BMC Med Genet. 2021;14(1):191.
31. Bain B, Bates I, Laffan M, Lewis S. Dacie and Lewis practical haematology. 10th ed. Churchill Livingstone: London: Elsevier; 2017. p. 239–66.
32. Sutherland DR, Illingworth A, Marinov I, Ortiz F, Andreasen J, Payne D, et al. ICCS/ESCCA consensus guidelines to detect GPI-deficient cells in paroxysmal nocturnal hemoglobinuria (PNH) and related disorders part 2 - reagent selection and assay optimization for high-sensitivity testing. Cytometry B Clin Cytom. 2018;94(1):23–48.
33. Group CF, Group RB, Cell Analysis Committee, Blood Immune Committee, Chinese Medical Association. Chinese expert consensus on paroxysmal nocturnal hemoglobinuria detection via flow cytometry (2021). Zhonghua Xue Ye Xue Za Zhi. 2021;42(4):281–7.
34. Lima M. Laboratory studies for paroxysmal nocturnal hemoglobinuria, with emphasis on flow cytometry. Pract Lab Med. 2020;20:e00158.
35. Red Blood Cell Disease (Anemia) Group, Chinese Society of Hematology, Chinese Medical Association. [Guidelines for the diagnosis and management of paroxysmal nocturnal hemoglobinuria (2024)]. Zhonghua Xue Ye Xue Za Zhi. 2024;45(8):727–37.
36. Athota S, Gopalan S, Arthur P, Jayaram A, Satish A. Deciphering paroxysmal nocturnal hemoglobinuria: an unusual paradigm of hemolytic anemia. Cureus. 2024;16(8):e67194.
37. Bahroun S, Lakhal FB, ElBorgi W, Salem SF, Achour M, Gouider E. [Contribution and limits of CD157 in the detection of the paroxysmal nocturnal hemoglobinuria clone: a case report]. Ann Biol Clin (Paris). 2021;79(4):356–60.
38. Means RT Jr, Rodgers GM, Glader B, Arber DA, Appelbaum FR, Dispenzieri A, et al. Wintrobe's clinical hematology. 15th ed. Lippincott Williams & Wilkins: Wolters Kluwer; 2024. p. 4027–99.
39. Zengin O, Göre B, Öztürk O, Göv M, Şahiner ES, İnan O, et al. Shiga toxin-producing E. coli and hemolytic uremic syndrome: a study of the 2022 outbreak in Turkey. Med Sci Monit. 2024;30:e946033.
40. Musalem P. Ten tips for managing complement-mediated thrombotic microangiopathies (formerly atypical hemolytic uremic syndrome): narrative review. BMC Nephrol. 2025;26(1):158.
41. Botero JP, McIntosh JJ. Labor and delivery: DIC, HELLP, preeclampsia. Hematology Am Soc Hematol Educ Program. 2023;2023(1):737–44.
42. Nimura T, Aomura D, Harada M, Yamaguchi A, Yamaka K, Nakajima T, et al. Investigation of clinical features and association between vascular endothelial injury markers and cytomegalovirus infection associated with thrombotic microangiopathy in patients with anti-neutrophil cytoplasmic antibody (ANCA)-associated vasculitis: case-based research. Int J Mol Sci. 2024;25(2):812.
43. Alexopoulou A, Vasilieva L, Kanellopoulou T, Pouriki S, Soultati A, Dourakis SP. Presence of spur cells as a highly predictive factor of mortality in patients with cirrhosis. J Gastroenterol Hepatol. 2014;29:830–4.
44. Gremida A, Paleti S, Perez ET, McCarthy D. Hemolysis in alcoholic liver disease: Zieve's syndrome. Dig Dis Sci. 2018;63:601–4.
45. Balali-Mood M, Eizadi-Mood N, Hassanian-Moghaddam H, Etemad L, Moshiri M, Vahabzadeh M, et al. Recent advances in the clinical management of intoxication by five heavy metals: mercury, lead, chromium, cadmium and arsenic. Heliyon. 2025;11(4):e42696.
46. Valentine WN, Paglia DE, Fink K, Madokoro G. Lead poisoning: association with hemolytic anemia, basophilic stippling, erythrocyte pyrimidine 5′-nucleotidase deficiency, and intraerythrocytic accumulation of pyrimidines. J Clin Invest. 1976;58(4):926–32.

Chapter 5
Management of Anemia of Renal Failure

Rachit Agrawal, Mehak Trehan, and Rishi Dhawan

Abstract With the rising burden of non-communicable diseases and increased longevity, the prevalence of chronic kidney disease (CKD) has surged globally. Anemia, a common and debilitating complication of CKD, significantly contributes to morbidity and mortality. The pathogenesis is multifactorial, primarily involving inadequate erythropoietin production and iron dysregulation. This chapter delineates the epidemiology, diagnostic framework, and current management strategies of anemia in CKD. Special emphasis is placed on distinguishing between absolute and functional iron deficiency, in alignment with the latest KDIGO guidelines. The utility of various iron formulations, indications for erythropoiesis-stimulating agents (ESAs), and emerging therapies like HIF prolyl hydroxylase inhibitors (HIF-PHI) are reviewed in depth. Blood transfusion—while limited in scope—retains a role in specific clinical contexts. Through a case-based approach and evidence-backed recommendations, this chapter aims to guide hematologists in optimizing anemia care in CKD.

R. Agrawal
Fortis Memorial Research Institute, Gurugram, India

M. Trehan (✉) · R. Dhawan
AIIMS, New Delhi, India

H. P. Pati et al. (eds.), *Clinical Hematology and Hemato-Oncology*,
https://doi.org/10.1007/978-981-92-1167-8_5

Learning Objectives
By the end of this chapter, you will be able to:

- Describe the epidemiology and multifactorial pathogenesis of anemia in chronic kidney disease (CKD), including erythropoietin deficiency, iron dysregulation, and inflammation.
- Outline a systematic diagnostic approach to anemia in CKD, including initial laboratory evaluation, interpretation of iron indices, and identification of contributing comorbidities.
- Evaluate the indications, efficacy, and safety of various therapeutic modalities—including oral and intravenous iron, erythropoiesis-stimulating agents (ESAs), and HIF-prolyl hydroxylase inhibitors (HIF-PHIs).
- Recognize the role and limitations of red blood cell transfusions, including appropriate clinical indications and strategies to minimize transfusions in transplant-eligible patients.

5.1 Introduction

Anemia is a pervasive and clinically significant consequence of CKD, often becoming evident as renal function deteriorates—typically below an estimated glomerular filtration rate (eGFR) of 60 mL/min/1.73 m^2 (stage 3 CKD and beyond), though hematological abnormalities may occur earlier [1].

Globally, 10–15% of adults are estimated to have CKD, with anemia affecting nearly 50% of patients with stage 3 disease and up to 90% in stage 4–5 CKD [2]. In dialysis-dependent individuals, anemia is nearly universal. The KDIGO guidelines define anemia in CKD as hemoglobin <13 g/dL in men or <12 g/dL in women [3].

The NHANES (1999–2016) data corroborate this gradient, reporting anemia in 15% of stage 3, 52% of stage 4, and 89% of stage 5 CKD patients [4]. Elderly individuals face heightened anemia risk due to declining renal function, inflammation, and bone marrow suppression [5].

Diabetes, the leading global cause of CKD, exacerbates this risk. The CRIC study showed diabetic patients with CKD were nearly twice as likely to be anemic compared to their non-diabetic counterparts, driven by chronic inflammation, tubular injury, and impaired erythropoietin signaling [6].

Ethnic disparities are evident. African American and Hispanic populations often exhibit more severe anemia compared to Caucasians at similar CKD stages—attributable to genetic factors (e.g., APOL1 variants), healthcare access, and socioeconomic determinants [7].

Gender also plays a role—women tend to develop anemia earlier, influenced by lower baseline hemoglobin and menstrual losses. Postmenopausal convergence of anemia rates suggests hormonal influence [8].

Despite its prevalence, anemia in CKD is often underdiagnosed and undertreated—particularly in early stages or resource-limited settings. The CKD Outcomes and Practice Patterns Study (CKDopps) revealed that fewer than 40% of non-dialysis CKD patients with anemia received any form of treatment [9]. This under-treatment contributes to fatigue, reduced quality of life, faster CKD progression, and increased cardiovascular risk [10].

In low- and middle-income countries, the burden is magnified by nutritional deficiencies, infections, poor laboratory access, and delayed nephrology referrals. Studies from South Asia and sub-Saharan Africa report anemia rates exceeding 80% in advanced CKD—with most patients untreated [11].

Typically, renal anemia is normocytic and normochromic. Inadequate red cell production, rather than reduced survival, is the principal driver. Serum erythropoietin (EPO) levels remain inappropriately low for the degree of anemia. EPO, produced by interstitial fibroblasts in the renal cortex near peritubular capillaries, is reduced in CKD due to cortical injury.

EPO synthesis is governed by oxygen-sensing pathways involving hypoxia-inducible factors (HIF-1α and HIF-2α). These heterodimeric transcription factors are regulated by oxygen-dependent hydroxylation, targeting HIF-α for proteasomal degradation. HIF-2α predominantly regulates EPO and iron metabolism genes like transferrin and DMT1.

Although EPO-producing capacity is retained in ESRD, the blunted response to hypoxia and uremic inhibition of erythroid progenitors (BFU-e, CFU-e) limits compensatory erythropoiesis. Initiation of dialysis may improve anemia in some patients.

CKD also promotes a pro-inflammatory milieu, with hepcidin—a hepatic peptide—inhibiting gastrointestinal iron absorption and promoting iron sequestration in macrophages, leading to functional iron deficiency. Recurrent blood draws, uremic bleeding, and dialyzer-related losses contribute to absolute iron deficiency [12, 13].

5.2 Diagnosis and Evaluation: [14–20]

Systematic evaluation of anemia in CKD hinges on timely screening and careful distinction between absolute and functional iron deficiency, as well as exclusion of non-renal causes. The patient of CKD, depending on the stage, should be periodically screened for anemia as mentioned in Table 5.1.

Table 5.1 Recommended screening frequency by CKD stage [18]

CKD stage	Frequency
G3	Annually
G4	6 monthly
G5	3 monthly

Initial laboratory evaluation should include:

- Complete blood count (CBC)
- Reticulocyte count
- Serum ferritin
- Transferrin saturation (TSAT)

Table 5.2 shows the ferritin and TSAT thresholds for distinguishing between absolute and functional iron deficiency.

When diagnosis remains elusive, or anemia is disproportionate to CKD stage, extend the workup:

1. Peripheral blood smear (Fig. 5.1 shows the classical findings of renal anemia)
2. Reticulocyte count and absolute reticulocyte number
3. Haptoglobin, LDH, bilirubin (for hemolysis)
4. CRP (inflammatory milieu)
5. Vitamin B12, folate
6. Liver function tests
7. TSH
8. Serum protein electrophoresis with immunofixation + free light chains (rule out plasma cell dyscrasias)
9. Stool occult blood/gastrointestinal evaluation where relevant

Table 5.2 Iron deficiency classification in CKD (18)

Type	Ferritin threshold	TSAT threshold
Absolute iron deficiency	<100 μg/L (non-HD); <200 μg/L (HD)	<20%
Functional iron deficiency (iron-restricted erythropoiesis)	>100 μg/L	<20%

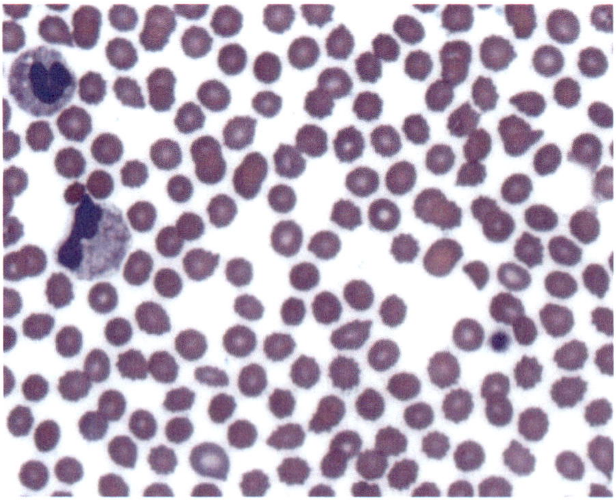

Fig. 5.1 Classical normocytic normochromic anemia of CKD with many burr cells

In patients with severe microcytic anemia and ferritin <45 μg/L, evaluation for chronic blood loss (especially GI and gynecologic) is warranted—even if CKD is present.

Newer parameters as per NICE guidelines

- Hypochromic red cells (%HRC) >6%: Associated with iron deficiency and ESA response
- Reticulocyte hemoglobin content (CHr) <29 pg: Reliable indicator of functional iron deficiency
- HRC and CHr together provide a dynamic overview of iron availability, erythropoiesis, and inflammation.

Limitations

- CHr and HRC require timely analysis (within 6 hours) to avoid artifacts.
- Not reliable in hemoglobinopathies or advanced hematologic malignancies.
- They do not reliably differentiate between functional and absolute iron deficiency.

5.2.1 Not Recommended for Routine Evaluation

1. Serum Epo levels: The deficiency in renal anemia is relative, not absolute, and levels vary widely across individuals with similar hemoglobin concentrations.
2. Hepcidin: Although pathophysiologically important, it is not routinely measured as it does not guide management directly
3. Bone Marrow Examination
   Reserved for selected scenarios
   - ESA hyporesponsiveness
   - Suspected pure red cell aplasia (PRCA)
   - Suspicion of underlying hematologic malignancy

Findings may include erythroid hypoplasia, absent stainable iron, or atypical clonal cells.

5.3 Treatment

5.3.1 Iron Therapy [21–24]

Iron replacement remains the cornerstone of anemia management in CKD—both for restoring hematologic parameters and optimizing erythropoiesis-stimulating agent (ESA) responsiveness. Iron deficiency is extremely prevalent in CKD and may be absolute or functional, both of which require correction prior to or concurrently with ESA initiation.

Table 5.3 Comparison of routes of iron administration in CKD [18]

Feature	Oral iron	Intravenous iron
Hemoglobin response	Slower	Rapid, sustained
Tolerability	GI upset is common (nausea, constipation)	Hypersensitivity reactions possible (rare)
Cost and convenience	Less expensive, self-administered	Costlier, requires a clinical setup
Absorption	Impaired in CKD (↑ hepcidin)	Not affected by GI factors
Use in malabsorption	Limited	Preferred

5.3.1.1 When to Start Iron Therapy

- *Hemodialysis (HD) patients*: Initiate IV iron if ferritin <500 ng/mL or TSAT <30%
- *Non-dialysis (ND) CKD patients*: Initiate if:
  - Ferritin <100 ng/mL and TSAT <40%
  - Ferritin 100–300 ng/mL and TSAT <25

The preferred route is intravenous, given the elevated hepcidin levels in CKD, which impair oral iron absorption and result in functional iron deficiency. Lately, there has been a paradigm shift in iron supplementation for the management of IDA in general. This can be attributed to better access to relatively safer iv formulations and better compliance. The comparison between the two routes of administration of iron is shown in Table 5.3.

5.4 Evidence-Based Strategy: The PIVOTAL Trial [25]

The landmark *PIVOTAL trial* compared proactive high-dose vs. reactive low-dose IV iron in HD patients:

- *Proactive arm*: 400 mg IV iron sucrose/month, continued until ferritin >700 ng/mL or TSAT >40%
- *Reactive arm*: 0–400 mg/month only if ferritin <200 ng/mL or TSAT <20%

Result The proactive arm showed:

- Lower risk of cardiovascular events
- Fewer ESA requirements
- Reduced transfusion need

Table 5.4 Oral iron formulations [18]

Compound	Elemental iron per tablet	Dose per tablet	Usual dose	Comments
Ferric citrate	210 mg	1 g	1–2 tablets TID	Also acts as phosphate binder
Ferric maltol	30 mg	30 mg	1 tablet BID	Better GI tolerability, studied in AEGIS CKD trial
Ferrous fumarate	106 mg	325 mg	1 tablet BID	Moderate GI side effects
Ferrous sulfate	65 mg	325 mg	1 tablet TID	Common, but often poorly tolerated
Ferrous gluconate	35 mg	300 mg	4–6 tablets/day	Better tolerability
Sucrosomial iron	30 mg	30 mg	1 tablet/day	Absorbed via vesicular transport (DMT-1 independent)
Heme iron polypeptide	12 mg	12 mg	1 tablet 3–4×/day	Good bioavailability

Table 5.5 IV iron preparations [18]

Formulation	Max dose	Infusion time	Considerations
Iron sucrose	200 mg	15 min	Weekly 200 mg over 5 weeks
Ferric carboxymaltose	1000 mg	15 min	2 doses 1 week apart; risk of hypophosphatemia
Ferric derisomaltose	1000 mg	20 min	Full dose in 1 sitting
Ferumoxytol	510 mg	15 min	2 doses; black box warning for hypersensitivity
Low molecular weight dextran	20 mg/kg	15 min	Rarely used due to higher adverse event rate

Maintaining high iron stores helps reduce the total dose of ESA and thereby results in a significant reduction in the cost of management of DD CKD patients.

Tables 5.4 and 5.5 briefly describe the different oral and iv iron formulations available for use in CKD patients.

Hypophosphatemia Risk Ferric carboxymaltose and iron isomaltose may activate FGF23 and may cause treatment-emergent hypophosphatemia in kidney transplant recipients and patients with early-stage CKD. This is attributed to the carbohydrate shell of the iron salt. It should be closely monitored in individuals who are receiving multiple doses and may necessitate either oral phosphate supplementation or delaying the iron administration.

5.5 Mitigation of Hazards of Hypersensitivity Reactions

1. Intravenous iron should only be administered in settings capable of managing anaphylactic reactions.
2. Routine pretreatment with steroids or antihistaminics is not recommended.
3. No reaction to the test dose does not preclude hypersensitivity, hence not recommended.
4. Appropriate dose, route, frequency, and dilution of each formulation should be reviewed and followed.

5.6 Ferric Pyrophosphate Citrate (FPC), i.e., Triferic [26]

A newer formulation, FDA-approved in 2015, FPC:

- Is added to dialysate (delivers ~7 mg iron/session)
- Bypasses the reticuloendothelial system and delivers iron directly to circulating transferrin
- Associated with less tissue iron overload

Efficacy confirmed in CRUISE 1 and 2 trials

5.7 Monitoring Strategy

Iron stores should be periodically assessed and replenished as needed (Table 5.6).

Additional Monitoring:

- After ESA dose changes
- Following hospitalization or major blood loss
- If ferritin >700 ng/mL or TSAT >40%, pause supplementation

IV iron should be withheld during active infections due to the theoretical risk of promoting microbial growth.

Table 5.6 Frequency of iron monitoring in CKD

ND CKD	Every 3 months
DD CKD	Monthly

5.8 Clinical Case

Mr. RK, a 52-year-old gentleman with long-standing diabetes, had been under follow-up for Stage 4 chronic kidney disease at AIIMS Delhi. He came to our OPD complaining of overwhelming fatigue, shortness of breath even on mild exertion, and a general sense of not feeling himself. He had been on oral iron (ferrous ascorbate 100 mg daily), folic acid, and subcutaneous erythropoietin (epoetin beta 4000 IU twice weekly) for over 6 weeks. Despite this, his hemoglobin stayed low, fluctuating between 6.7 and 7.1 g/dL, and he needed two units of blood transfusion in the preceding month.

5.9 Initial Workup

The baseline investigations of the patient are summarized in Table 5.7 and the peripheral blood smear morphology shown in Fig. 5.2.

Table 5.7 Lab workup of the patient

Parameter	Result
Hemoglobin (g/dL)	6.9
MCV (fL)	78
Reticulocyte count (%)	0.9
Ferritin (ng/mL)	35
Transferrin saturation (%)	11
Serum iron (mcg/dL)	21
TIBC (mcg/dL)	460
CRP (mg/L)	8

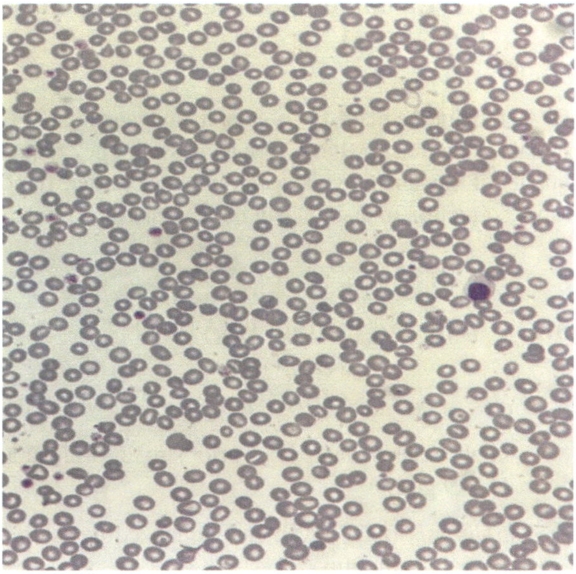

Fig. 5.2 Peripheral smear examination of the patient showing predominantly normocytic normochromic RBC with some hypochromic RBC

5.10 Clinical Interpretation

The persistent anemia despite ESA therapy raised a red flag. A closer look at his labs revealed a low ferritin and transferrin saturation, confirming what we suspected—iron deficiency. In this case, it was absolute iron deficiency, compounded by inflammation (CRP 8 mg/L). Without enough iron on board, even the best EPO can't do its job. This is a classic scenario in CKD patients, where the iron stores are quietly depleted or functionally restricted, and the ESA doses keep climbing.

5.11 Management and Outcome

We promptly switched him to intravenous ferric carboxymaltose (1000 mg), repeated after a week. Oral iron was stopped. Within 4 weeks, his hemoglobin began to rise—touching 9.3 g/dL. We tapered his ESA dose to once weekly. No more transfusions—and Mr. R reported that he finally felt like "his old self again."

Key Learning Points

- Don't chase hemoglobin with EPO alone—**check the iron status first**.
- Ferritin <100 ng/mL and TSAT <20% in CKD almost always signals iron deficiency, and **parenteral iron is the way to go**.
- ESA resistance is often a reflection of what's missing beneath the surface.
- A well-timed IV iron dose can do more than just raise the hemoglobin—it can restore quality of life.

5.12 Erythropoiesis-Stimulating Agent (ESA) Therapy [18, 27–31]

ESAs remain the mainstay of anemia management in CKD once absolute and functional iron deficiency have been addressed. They reduce transfusion needs, improve quality of life, and may modestly improve cardiac remodeling. However, overuse or rapid correction of anemia can increase cardiovascular risk.

5.13 When to Initiate ESA

- *Dialysis-dependent (DD) CKD*: Consider when Hb <9–10 g/dL
  - Higher-risk patients (e.g., prior stroke, vascular access thrombosis): Initiate at Hb <9 g/dL
- *Non-dialysis (ND) CKD*: Individualized decision based on anemia symptoms and risk-benefit ratio

- *Transplant recipients and children*: More nuanced, based on clinical context
- *Target hemoglobin*: ~11.5 g/dL (not to exceed 12 g/dL)

5.14 Major Trials and Cautionary Evidence

- *TREAT Trial*: Darbepoetin to target Hb 13 g/dL did not reduce CV events, but *increased stroke risk* [32].
- *CHOIR Trial*: Epoetin alfa targeting Hb 13.5 vs. 11.3 g/dL led to a higher incidence of MI, stroke, and death [33].
- *CREATE Trial*: Normalization of Hb (13–15 g/dL) did not reduce CV events, compared to a 10.5–11.5 g/dL target [34].

Key Message The severity of anemia is associated with poor outcomes, but full correction does not improve survival and may cause harm.

Dosing strategy for ESA has been summarized in Table 5.8. ESA doses should not be adjusted more frequently than every 4 weeks—unless Hb rises by >1 g/dL within 2 weeks (in which case reduce dose by 25–50%).

Both subcutaneous and intravenous routes of administration have been used (Table 5.9).

Use of ESA may be associated with several adverse effects as well iron depletion and needs to be monitored (Table 5.10).

ESA therapy is often withheld during acute illness, stroke, thromboembolic events, or active cancer—restart requires shared decision-making.

Table 5.8 ESA dosing and adjustments

ESA agent	Initial dose (ND CKD)	Initial dose (DD CKD)	Dose adjustments
Epoetin alfa/beta	4000–10,000 IU weekly or every 2 weeks	50–100 IU/kg thrice weekly	↑ by 25% if Hb rise <1 g/dL in 4 weeks; ↓ by 25% if rise >2 g/dL
Darbepoetin alfa	40–100 μg SC every 2–4 weeks	0.45 μg/kg weekly or 0.75 μg/kg every 2 weeks	↑ or ↓ by 25% based on Hb response
CERA (methoxy PEG-epoetin β)	50–120 μg every 2 weeks or 120–200 μg every 4 wks	0.6 μg/kg every 2 weeks	↑ or ↓ by 30–50 μg based on 4-week response

Table 5.9 Route of administration of ESA

Route	Preferred in	Notes
Subcutaneous	ND CKD	Lower dose needed (~30% less than IV), preferred for long-term maintenance
Intravenous	DD CKD	Convenient in HD units, but requires higher doses

Table 5.10 Monitoring during ESA therapy

Parameter	Frequency
Hemoglobin	Every 2–4 weeks after initiation or dose change; every 3 months during maintenance
Blood pressure	Monitor regularly (ESA can worsen hypertension, often responds to dose reduction)
Iron status (TSAT, ferritin)	Monthly (DD CKD); every 3 months (ND CKD)

5.15 ESA Hyporesponsiveness

5.15.1 Definition

1. *KDIGO 2012*
    - *Initial*: No Hb increase after 1 month of weight-based ESA dosing
    - *Subsequent*: Need to increase ESA dose by ≥50% over baseline to maintain Hb
2. *ESA resistance Index (ERI)*: [35]
    - ESA responsiveness index (Riscavid index): weekly ESA dose/body weight x hemoglobin
    - ESA resistance: ERI >15.4 IU/kg × g/dl (quartile IV)a
    - *Prevalence*: Seen in 12.5–30.3% of HD patients
    - *Risks*: Higher CV events, mortality, and hospitalization

It is often transient and improves after correction of the underlying illness. The causes have been summarized in Table 5.11.

5.15.2 Pure Red Cell Aplasia (PRCA)

A rare but serious complication of ESA therapy—first noted with subcutaneous epoetin-α (non-human albumin formulations) in 2002. It results in the use of albumin-free, polysorbate 80-containing formulations. The development of neutralizing antibodies against both endogenous and recombinant erythropoietin results in loss of response and transfusion dependence.

Clinical Clues

1. Rapid Hb drop (≥1 g/dL/week), transfusion dependence despite high ESA doses
2. Reticulocytopenia (<10,000/μL)
3. Normal leukocyte and platelet counts
4. Bone marrow: <5% erythroid precursors
5. High TSAT/ferritin (EPO not working)
6. *Presence of anti-EPO antibodies* (confirmatory)

Table 5.11 Common causes of ESA resistance

Category	Causes
Iron deficiency	Absolute or functional
Inflammation	Infection, autoimmune disease (↑CRP)
Blood loss	Dialysis tubing, occult GI bleed, menses, hemolysis
Nutrient deficiency	Folate, B12, zinc, copper, vitamin E, carnitine
Inadequate dialysis	Uremic toxins suppress erythropoiesis
Endocrine	Hypothyroidism, secondary hyperparathyroidism
Bone marrow disease	MDS, myeloma, PRCA, hemoglobinopathies
Toxins	Aluminum toxicity (rare today)
Malignancy	Often an underdiagnosed cause of poor ESA response

Management

- Discontinue ESA
- Immunosuppression (e.g., corticosteroids, cyclosporine, cyclophosphamide)
- Consider plasma exchange
- Rechallenge with IV ESA only after antibody clearance

PRCA is exceedingly rare with newer agents like darbepoetin and methoxy-PEG-epoetin beta

5.16 HIF-Prolyl Hydroxylase Inhibitors (HIF-PHI) [36–40]

In response to concerns over high-dose ESA toxicity—especially cardiovascular risks—HIF-PHI have emerged as novel oral agents for anemia in CKD. These drugs stimulate endogenous erythropoietin (EPO) production by stabilizing hypoxia-inducible factors (HIF-1α and HIF-2α) via inhibition of prolyl hydroxylase (PHD), the enzyme responsible for HIF degradation.

They not only enhance erythropoiesis but also improve iron metabolism through hepcidin suppression, facilitating iron absorption and mobilization.

5.17 Mechanism of Action

- *Stabilization of HIF-α* → ↑ EPO gene transcription (primarily renal > hepatic)
- ↑ Expression of iron transporters: *DMT-1, DCYTB, transferrin*
- ↓ Hepcidin synthesis → ↑ duodenal absorption and mobilization of macrophage iron

Currently approved agents have been summarized in Table 5.12.

Table 5.12 Approved agents and key trials

Agent	Dosing frequency	Approved for	Major trials
Daprodustat	Once daily	DD-CKD (FDA approved 2023)	ASCEND-ND, ASCEND-D
Vadadustat	Once daily	DD-CKD (EU/JP only)	PRO2TECT (ND), INNO2VATE (DD)
Roxadustat	Thrice weekly	Approved in China, the EU	ANDES, OLYMPUS, DOLOMITES, SIERRAS
Desidustat	Thrice weekly	India	DREAM-ND, DREAM-D
Enarodustat	Once daily	Japan	SYMPHONY ND, SYMPHONY HD
Molidustat	Once daily	Japan	MIYABI program

Key Insights

- All agents increased hemoglobin in both ESA-naïve and ESA-switched patients
- Efficacy was consistent regardless of baseline CRP, highlighting potential utility in inflammation-driven ESA hyporesponsiveness
- Some trials demonstrated non-inferiority to ESA, particularly in dialysis-dependent settings
- However, HIF-PHI have not demonstrated superiority in cardiovascular safety and have restricted approvals (DD-CKD only in many regions)
- The ability to augment endogenous EPO production is inversely related to the severity of fibrosis and the degree of myofibroblast transdifferentiation of kidney interstitial cells.
- The bioavailability of these oral agents is affected by iron supplements as well as phosphate binders. The agents may have interactions with the multitude of drugs used in CKD patients, which should be checked before prescribing.

5.18 Iron Metabolism Effects

HIF-PHIs improve iron availability via:

- ↓ Hepcidin
- ↑ TIBC
- Variable ↑ or ↓ in TSAT
- ↑ MCV and MCHC

They reduce IV iron requirement and enhance oral iron absorption, which is particularly useful in ND CKD and resource-limited settings.

Iron indices were not primary endpoints in phase 3 trials; more data needed to draw conclusions on long-term effects on iron balance

These newer agents have been linked to a number of side effects as discussed in Table 5.13.

Table 5.13 Safety concerns and black box alerts

Risk	Comments
Thromboembolism	↑ Vascular access thrombosis, DVT, PE—especially with Roxadustat, probably related to an increase in PAI-1 and hemoglobin
MACE	ASCEND-ND: Daprodustat had higher MACE rates than darbepoetin
Cancer progression	HIF may theoretically promote tumor growth; ASCEND-ND showed ↑ risk, needs long term follow-up to draw conclusions
Retinal neovascularization	VEGF upregulation possible at high doses (esp. daprodustat)
Off-target effects	HIF pathway affects genes regulating collagen synthesis, angiogenesis
Thyroid dysfunction	Roxadustat linked to central hypothyroidism; TSH monitoring recommended

Table 5.14 Dosing summary of HIF-PHI

Agent	Starting dose	Maximum dose	Frequency
Daprodustat	2–4 mg QD	24 mg QD	Daily
Vadadustat	300 mg QD	600 mg QD	Daily
Roxadustat	50–100 mg TIW	3 mg/kg	Thrice weekly
Desidustat	100–150 mg TIW	150 mg	Thrice weekly

These concerns have led the *US FDA* to restrict daprodustat and vadadustat to patients on maintenance dialysis for 4 and 3 months, respectively.

Dosing must be titrated every 4 weeks to maintain Hb in the target range.

Table 5.14 describes the dosing strategy for these agents.

5.19 Clinical Recommendations for Use

1. *Correct iron deficiency first*; HIF-PHI will be ineffective in severe IDA
2. *ESA remains first-line*; HIF-PHI for ESA intolerance or resistance
3. *Contraindications (*Table 5.15*)*
4. Do not combine ESA + HIF-PHI
5. TSH monitoring advised 4 weeks after starting roxadustat
6. Discontinue if no Hb response after 3–4 months
7. Immediately discontinue in MACE, thrombosis, or new cancer diagnosis
8. Limited data on hemoglobin targets, reasonable to maintain as recommended for ESA
9. To be used at the lowest effective dose

Sierra's study, including the CKD patients on maintenance dialysis, suggested that weekly doses of Roxadustat were the same for patients irrespective of baseline hsCRP levels. However, higher doses of epoetin were required when hsCRP was elevated, suggesting the potential benefit of HIF-PHI in ESA hyporesponsive patients.

Table 5.15 Contraindications for use of HIF-PHI

Risk based on experiments	Risk based on clinical trials	Insufficient data for risk assessment
Active cancer or with a history of cancer not in complete remission for at least 2–5 years Polycystic kidney disease Proliferative retinal disease Pulmonary arterial hypertension	Prior thromboembolic events Prior cardiovascular events Prior vascular access thrombosis Hepatic impairment Seizures, exfoliative dermatitis, hypothyroidism	Post-kidney transplant anemia Children

Table 5.16 Indications for RBC transfusion in CKD

Clinical scenario	Consider transfusion?
ESA/HIF-PHI ineffective (e.g., PRCA, ESA hyporesponsiveness, marrow failure)	Yes
ESA/HIF-PHI contraindicated (e.g., active cancer, recent stroke, DVT)	Yes
Acute bleeding, hemodynamic instability, or acute CAD	Yes
Preoperative optimization (e.g., urgent cardiac or orthopedic surgery)	Yes
Asymptomatic anemia in a transplant candidate	*Avoid if possible*

5.20 Future Therapies: Ziltevekimab

- Humanized monoclonal antibody targeting IL-6, a key driver of inflammation-induced anemia
- RESCUE trial: Showed Hb improvement in Stage 3–5 CKD and better iron indices at 12 weeks follow-up
- Promising agent, especially in ESA-resistant inflammatory anemia, though still under investigation

5.21 Red Blood Cell (RBC) Transfusions [41–44]

While iron therapy and ESAs (or HIF-PHIs) form the cornerstone of CKD-related anemia management, red cell transfusions remain a valid therapeutic option in select cases. Their primary role is to rapidly restore oxygen delivery in acutely symptomatic patients or when other therapies are contraindicated or ineffective. The indications of blood transfusion have been summarized in Table 5.16.

Hemoglobin alone should not dictate transfusion; symptom burden, rate of Hb decline, and comorbidities must be considered. Transfusion targets depend on the clinical context (Table 5.17).

Table 5.17 Transfusion targets

Patient context	Suggested Hb threshold
Stable patients	<7 g/dL
Cardiac surgery	<7.5 g/dL
Heart disease/CAD	<8 g/dL
Symptomatic anemia (dyspnea, fatigue, angina)	Individualized

5.22 Risks of RBC Transfusion

While transfusion provides immediate symptom relief, it is not disease-modifying and carries important short- and long-term risks:

- *Alloimmunization*: Particularly detrimental in transplant-eligible patients.
  - *Opelz* et al: Allosensitization rate ~28% in CKD patients receiving transfusions
  - Result: Longer transplant wait times, increased graft rejection risk
- *Iron overload*
- *Volume overload* (esp. in ESRD or CHF)
- *Febrile non-hemolytic or hemolytic reactions*
- *Infectious risk* (though rare with current testing protocols)

5.23 Strategies to Minimize Transfusion Need

- Maximize iron, ESA, or HIF-PHI therapy when feasible
- Use minimally invasive procedures in CKD
- Avoid unnecessary frequent blood draws ("phlebotomy anemia")
- Review Hb trends rather than relying on single values
- Prioritize alternatives in transplant-eligible patients

A multidisciplinary approach involving nephrologists, hematologists, and transplant teams is essential to ensure judicious transfusion practices. A comprehensive approach in management of CKD patients is given in Fig. 5.3.

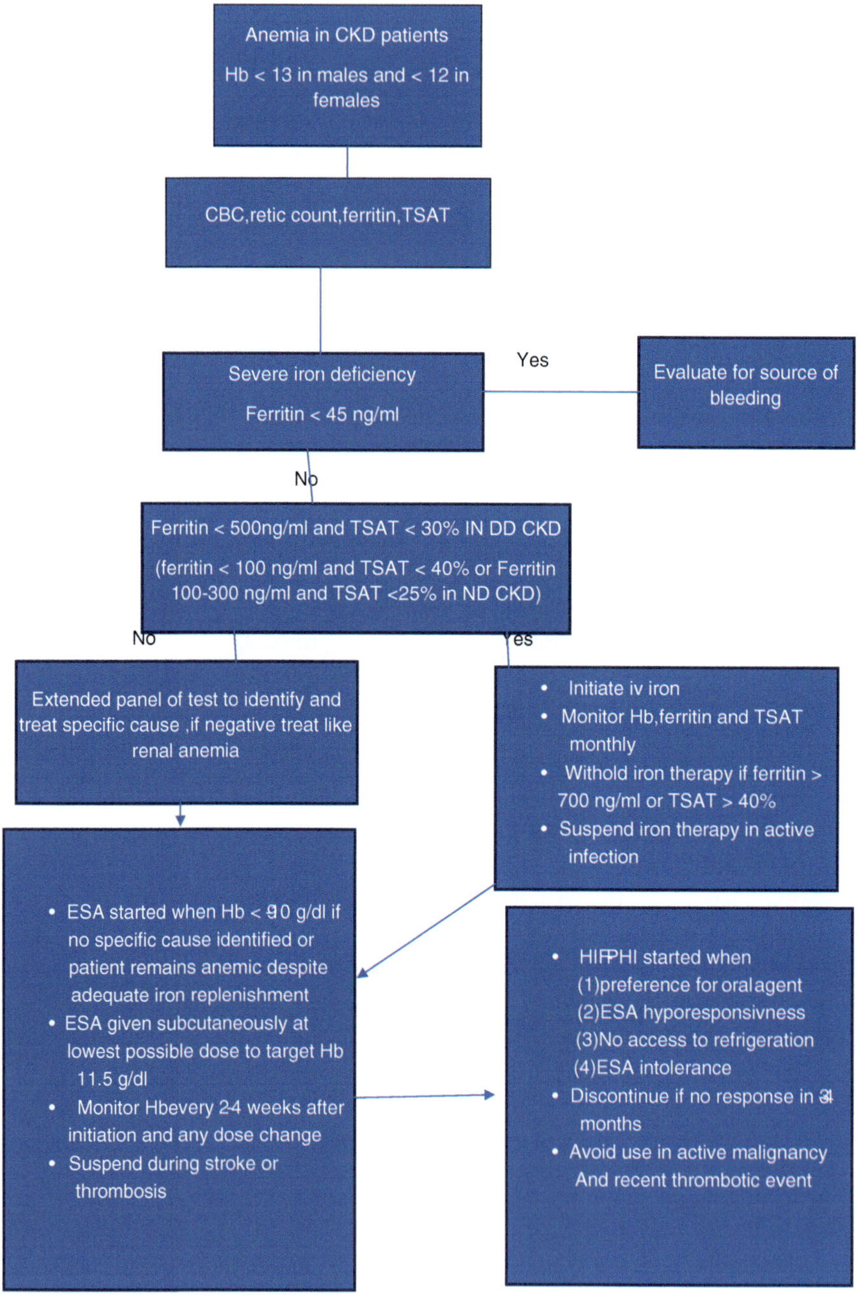

Fig. 5.3 Algorithm for the management of anemia in CKD patient

5.24 Summary

Anemia is a common and progressive complication of CKD, associated with reduced quality of life, increased cardiovascular morbidity, and higher mortality. The pathophysiology is multifactorial—relative erythropoietin deficiency, iron dysregulation, chronic inflammation, and occasionally marrow suppression.

A stepwise and structured diagnostic approach is essential, starting with CBC, iron indices, and ruling out other reversible causes. Functional and absolute iron deficiencies are highly prevalent and must be addressed prior to ESA initiation.

Intravenous iron is preferred over oral formulations in most CKD settings due to elevated hepcidin levels. Proactive iron strategies, as supported by the PIVOTAL trial, reduce ESA needs and cardiovascular events in HD patients. Newer oral iron agents like ferric maltol and sucrosomial iron show promise in ND CKD.

ESAs remain the first-line agents for anemia correction once iron repletion is ensured. Overzealous hemoglobin correction is associated with thrombotic risk and must be avoided. ESA hyporesponsiveness warrants evaluation for inflammation, iron status, nutrient deficiencies, and marrow pathology. Rarely, pure red cell aplasia may complicate ESA use.

HIF-prolyl hydroxylase inhibitors offer an oral alternative, especially in ESA-resistant or inflammatory anemia. Their use, however, is currently limited to dialysis-dependent CKD due to safety concerns—including thromboembolic and cardiovascular risk.

Transfusions are reserved for specific scenarios such as acute bleeding, symptomatic severe anemia, or ESA contraindication. Allosensitization is a major concern in transplant candidates and mandates careful decision-making.

Overall, management of anemia in CKD demands a personalized, multidisciplinary approach—balancing efficacy, safety, transplant eligibility, and cost.

Key Clinical Takeaways

- Anemia in CKD is multifactorial—primarily due to relative erythropoietin deficiency, iron dysregulation (absolute or functional), chronic inflammation, and uremic marrow suppression.
- Regular anemia screening is essential: annually in Stage 3, semiannually in Stage 4, and quarterly in Stage 5 CKD.
- Serum erythropoietin levels are not reliable for diagnosis; focus instead on CBC, reticulocyte count, ferritin, TSAT, and inflammatory markers.
- Parenteral iron is the preferred mode of repletion, especially in dialysis-dependent patients. Proactive iron therapy (e.g., PIVOTAL strategy) improves outcomes.
- ESAs should be used judiciously—initiate when Hb <9–10 g/dL (trigger) and avoid exceeding 11.5 g/dL (target) due to increased thrombotic risk.
- ESA hyporesponsiveness should prompt evaluation for iron deficiency, inflammation, nutrient deficiencies, marrow pathology, and inadequate dialysis.
- HIF-prolyl hydroxylase inhibitors are emerging oral agents approved primarily for dialysis-dependent patients. They are not superior to ESAs in safety and must be used with caution in high-risk patients.

- Red cell transfusions are reserved for acute symptomatic anemia or contraindications to ESA/HIF-PHI. Allosensitization remains a concern in transplant candidates.
- Management must be individualized, guided by symptom burden, comorbidity profile, transplant eligibility, and shared decision-making.
- Optimal anemia management in CKD requires collaboration between hematologists, nephrologists, and internists, and careful balance of efficacy, safety, and patient-centered goals.

References

1. KDIGO clinical practice guideline for anemia in chronic kidney disease. Kidney Int Suppl. 2012;2(4):279–335.
2. Stauffer ME, Fan T. Prevalence of anemia in CKD in the United States. PLoS One. 2014;9(1):e84943.
3. National Institute for Health and Care Excellence (NICE). Chronic kidney disease: managing anemia. NICE guideline NG8.
4. Hsu CY, et al. The NHANES experience: anemia across CKD stages. Am J Kidney Dis. 2002;40(1):20–7.
5. Babitt JL, Lin HY. Mechanisms of anemia in CKD. Nat Rev Nephrol. 2012;8(11):701–14.
6. Astor BC, et al. Association of kidney function with anemia: the CRIC study. Am J Kidney Dis. 2008;51(2):213–23.
7. Parsa A, et al. APOL1 risk variants, race, and anemia in CKD. J Am Soc Nephrol. 2013;24(9):1471–7.
8. Astor BC, et al. Anemia and sex differences in CKD. Kidney Int. 2004;66(6):2329–36.
9. Lopes MB, et al. International variation in anemia management: CKDopps study. Nephrol Dial Transplant. 2019;34(7):1184–96.
10. Singh AK, et al. Emerging therapies and management of anemia in CKD: ASH Educational Book 2022. Hematology Am Soc Hematol Educ Program. 2022;2022(1):102–15.
11. Stanifer JW, et al. The burden of anemia and CKD in Africa and South Asia. Lancet Glob Health. 2014;2(3):e177–84.
12. Feehally J, editor. Comprehensive clinical nephrology. Sixth ed. Edinburgh; New York: Elsevier; 2019. 1333 p.
13. Hoffman R, Benz EJ, Silberstein LE, Heslop HE, Weitz JI, Salama ME, et al., editors. Hematology: basic principles and practice. Eighth ed. Philadelphia: Elsevier; 2023. 2476 p
14. Guedes M, Muenz DG, Zee J, et al. Serum biomarkers of iron stores are associated with increased risk of all-cause mortality and cardiovascular events in nondialysis CKD patients, with or without anemia. J Am Soc Nephrol. 2021;32:2020–30.
15. Coyne D. Iron indices: what do they really mean? Kidney Int Suppl. 2006;(101):S4–8.
16. Eisenga MF, Nolte IM, van der Meer P, et al. Association of different iron deficiency cutoffs with adverse outcomes in chronic kidney disease. BMC Nephrol. 2018;19:225.
17. Iimori S, Naito S, Noda Y, et al. Anaemia management and mortality risk in newly visiting patients with chronic kidney disease in Japan: the CKD-ROUTE study. Nephrology (Carlton). 2015;20:601–8.
18. KDIGO 2025 Clinical practice guideline for anemia in Chronic Kidney Disease (CKD).
19. Ratcliffe LEK, Thomas W, Glen J, Padhi S, Pordes BAJ, Wonderling D, et al. Diagnosis and management of iron deficiency in CKD: a summary of the NICE guideline recommendations and their rationale. Am J Kidney Dis. 2016;67(4):548–58.
20. Girelli D, Nemeth E, Swinkels DW. Hepcidin in the diagnosis of iron disorders. Blood. 2016;127:2809–13.

21. Lee CT, Wu IW, Chiang SS, et al. Effect of oral ferric citrate on serum phosphorus in hemodialysis patients: multicenter, randomized, double-blind, placebo-controlled study. J Nephrol. 2015;28:105–13.
22. Markowitz GS, Kahn GA, Feingold RE, et al. An evaluation of the effectiveness of oral iron therapy in hemodialysis patients receiving recombinant human erythropoietin. Clin Nephrol. 1997;48:34–40.
23. Charytan C, Bernardo MV, Koch TA, et al. Intravenous ferric carboxymaltose versus standard medical care in the treatment of iron deficiency anemia in patients with chronic kidney disease: a randomized, active-controlled, multi-center study. Nephrol Dial Transplant. 2013;28:953–64.
24. Gupta A, Lin V, Guss C, et al. Ferric pyrophosphate citrate administered via dialysate reduces erythropoiesis-stimulating agent use and maintains hemoglobin in hemodialysis patients. Kidney Int. 2015;88:1187–94.
25. Macdougall IC, White C, Anker SD, Bhandari S, Farrington K, Kalra PA, et al. Intravenous iron in patients undergoing maintenance hemodialysis. N Engl J Med. 2019;380(5):447–58.
26. Fishbane SN, Singh AK, Cournoyer SH, Jindal KK, Fanti P, Guss CD, et al. Ferric pyrophosphate citrate (Triferic™) administration via the dialysate maintains hemoglobin and iron balance in chronic hemodialysis patients. Nephrol Dial Transplant. 2015;30(12):2019–26.
27. Aggarwal HK, Nand N, Singh S, et al. Comparison of oral versus intravenous iron therapy in predialysis patients of chronic renal failure receiving recombinant human erythropoietin. J Assoc Physicians India. 2003;51:170–4.
28. Babitt JL, Eisenga MF, Haase VH, et al. Controversies in optimal anemia management: conclusions from a Kidney Disease: Improving Global Outcomes (KDIGO) conference. Kidney Int. 2021;99:1280–95.
29. Cullis JO. Diagnosis and management of anaemia of chronic dis ease: current status. Br J Haematol. 2011;154(3):289–300. An excellent review of the anemia of chronic disease.
30. Association between recombinant human erythropoietin and quality of life and exercise capacity of patients receiving haemodialysis. Canadian Erythropoietin Study Group. BMJ. 1990;300:573–8.
31. Laupacis A. Changes in quality of life and functional capacity in hemodialysis patients treated with recombinant human erythropoietin. The Canadian Erythropoietin Study Group. Semin Nephrol. 1990;10:11–9.
32. Pfeffer MA, Burdmann EA, Chen CY, Cooper ME, De Zeeuw D, Eckardt KU, et al. A trial of darbepoetin alfa in type 2 diabetes and chronic kidney disease. N Engl J Med. 2009;361(21):2019–32.
33. Singh AK, Szczech L, Tang KL, Barnhart H, Sapp S, Wolfson M, et al. Correction of anemia with epoetin alfa in chronic kidney disease. N Engl J Med. 2006;355(20):2085–98.
34. Drüeke TB, Locatelli F, Clyne N, Eckardt KU, Macdougall IC, Tsakiris D, et al. Normalization of hemoglobin level in patients with chronic kidney disease and anemia. N Engl J Med. 2006;355(20):2071–84.
35. Panichi V, Rizza GM, Paoletti S, Bigazzi R, Aloisi M, Barsotti G, et al. Chronic inflammation and mortality in haemodialysis: effect of different renal replacement therapies. Results from the RISCAVID study. Nephrol Dial Transplant. 2008;23(7):2337–43.
36. Haase VH. Hypoxia-inducible factor-prolyl hydroxylase inhibitors in the treatment of anemia of chronic kidney disease. Kidney Int Suppl. 2011;2021(11):8–25.
37. Locatelli F, Del Vecchio L. Hypoxia-inducible fac tor-prolyl hydroxyl domain inhibitors: from theoretical superiority to clinical noninferiority compared with current ESAs? J Am Soc Nephrol. 2022;33(11):1966–79.
38. Maxwell PH, Eckardt KU. HIF prolyl hydroxylase inhibitors for the treatment of renal anaemia and beyond. Nat Rev Nephrol. 2016;12(3):157–68.
39. Raichoudhury R, Spinowitz BS. Treatment of anemia in difficult-to-manage patients with chronic kidney disease. Kidney Int Suppl. 2021;11(1):26–34.

40. Mikhail A, Brown C, Williams JA, et al. Renal association clinical practice guideline on Anaemia of Chronic Kidney Disease. BMC Nephrol. 2017;18:345.
41. Consensus conference. Perioperative red blood cell transfusion. JAMA. 1988;260(2700):2703.
42. Leffell MS, Kim D, Vega RM, et al. Red blood cell transfusions and the risk of allosensitization in patients awaiting primary kidney transplantation. Transplantation. 2014;97:525–33.
43. Brenner N, Kommalapati A, Ahsan M, et al. Red cell transfusion in chronic kidney disease in the United States in the current era of erythropoiesis stimulating agents. J Nephrol. 2020;33:267–75.
44. Chapter 4: Red cell transfusion to treat anemia in CKD. Kidney Int Suppl. 2012;2(4):311–6.

Chapter 6
Management of Aplastic Anemia

Manoranjan Mahapatra and Mehak Trehan

Abstract Acquired aplastic anemia (AA) is a rare but potentially fatal condition characterized by pancytopenia and a hypocellular marrow. Its prevalence is significantly higher in Asia, including India. The major challenge in treating AA in developing countries is the long interval between disease onset and diagnosis and from diagnosis to treatment. So early recognition and referral to a specialist hematology center is critical because timely intervention with stem cell transplant (SCT) or immunosuppressive therapy (IST) significantly improves survival.

In the last few decades, the survival of the AA has been improved substantially due to the availability of better supportive care and definitive management options in both children and adults. The definitive management of AA includes allogenic hematopoietic stem cell transplant (HSCT) and immunosuppressive therapy (IST), including anti-thymocyte globulin with Cyclosporine-A. The integration of Eltrombopag, an oral TPO-RA, into first-line IST is a recent development in the management of AA. Patients who recover from AA require regular follow-up, as around 10–15% of acquired AA patients may develop clonal evolution to develop conditions like myelodysplastic syndrome (MDS), acute leukaemia.

With the addition of eltrombopag to IST, growing experience with haplo-HSCT, and refined diagnostics enabling accurate classification, aplastic anemia has become a largely curable disease, if diagnosed and treated early.

Keywords Aplastic anemia · Bone marrow failure · Immunosupressive therapy · Stem cell transplant

M. Mahapatra (✉) · M. Trehan
Department of Hematology, AIIMS, New Delhi, India

H. P. Pati et al. (eds.), *Clinical Hematology and Hemato-Oncology*,
https://doi.org/10.1007/978-981-92-1167-8_6

Learning Objectives
- To understand the diagnostic workup of aplastic anemia
- To understand the challenges in the management of aplastic anemia in developing countries
- To know the initial treatment algorithm in patients with aplastic anemia
- Recent advances in immunosuppressive therapy (IST) in aplastic anemia

6.1 Introduction

Acquired aplastic anemia (AA) is a rare but potentially fatal condition with bone marrow failure characterized by pancytopenia and a hypocellular marrow without infiltration, dysplasia, or fibrosis. Though uncommon globally, its prevalence is significantly higher in Asia, including India, where it constitutes a major proportion of non-malignant hematological conditions.

Once considered uniformly fatal, its prognosis has dramatically improved over the past two decades owing to refined diagnostic modalities, advances in immunosuppressive therapy (IST), wider applicability of hematopoietic stem cell transplantation (HSCT), and incorporation of thrombopoietin receptor agonists (TPO-RAs)with IST. With survival rates now exceeding 80–90% in optimal settings, the management of AA is undergoing a paradigm shift, moving toward individualized therapy based upon genetics, molecular risk markers, and donor availability [1, 2].

6.2 Challenges in Management of AA in Developing Countries

Although the prevalence of AA is significantly higher in Asian countries, the precise incidence of AA in India is not known due to a lack of epidemiological studies. However, in a hospital-based study, it is known that 20–40% of pancytopenic patients are diagnosed as AA in referral centres [3]. The major challenges in treating AA in developing countries are:

- Long interval between disease onset and diagnosis and from diagnosis to treatment
- Majority of patients have infections, including fungal infections at the time of diagnosis
- Only 20–30 percent of patients receive standard of care (HSCT or ATG)
- Cost of therapy and socioeconomic issues
- Lack of a patient support group

Although the supportive care facilities have significantly improved over the years, the above-mentioned challenges are the major barrier for the successful outcome of aplastic anemic patients in developing countries [4].

6.3 Pathophysiology and Diagnostic Advances

AA results from immune-mediated destruction of hematopoietic stem cells (HSCs), predominantly driven by activated cytotoxic T cells and interferon-gamma. Approximately 70–80% of adult cases are idiopathic, while the rest are secondary to drug exposures, viral infections (notably hepatitis), or inherited bone marrow failure syndromes (IBMFS) such as Fanconi anemia (FA), dyskeratosis congenita (DKC), and GATA2 deficiency [5, 6].

6.4 Diagnostic Workup in Aplastic Anemia

A patient with bicytopenia or pancytopenia is required to undergo various investigations not only to confirm the diagnosis but also to exclude other causes of pancytopenia. Bone marrow biopsy is an essential investigation to look for the cellularity of the bone marrow and to exclude other causes of pancytopenia with hypocellular marrow, like Hypocellular MDS/leukemia. Below are important differentials and key distinguishing features of pancytopenia (Table 6.1).

Once the diagnosis of aplastic anemia is confirmed, it is essential to exclude inherited bone marrow failure syndromes(IBMFSs) like Fanconi anemia and telomeropathies. The initial diagnostic workup is discussed in Table 6.2.

The diagnostic landscape has advanced significantly, allowing better discrimination between AA, hypocellular myelodysplastic syndromes (h-MDS), and IBMFS. Following investigations can be added to the diagnostic workup for a better understanding of disease biology.

- *NGS panels*: It is sometimes essential to exclude inherited bone marrow failure syndromes. It also routinely detects somatic mutations in DNMT3A, ASXL1, PIGA, and BCOR/BCORL1. Mutations at low variant allele frequencies (<10%) are common in idiopathic AA and do not imply MDS transformation [7, 8].
- *Cytogenetic abnormalities*, once thought to define MDS, may occur transiently in AA. Up to 12% of patients with typical AA harbor clones like del(13q), trisomy 8, or monosomy 7 [9].
- *Telomere length testing* is essential in younger patients <40 years or those with suggestive features. Extremely short telomeres point toward telomeropathies such as DKC [10].

Table 6.1 Differential diagnosis of pancytopenia with diagnostic features

Diagnosis	Key diagnostic features	Investigations
Hypocellular bone marrow		
IBMFS (Fanconi anemia, DKC, GATA2 deficiency)	Young age, stigmata (short stature, skin changes, nail dystrophy), family history	Stress cytogenetics, telomere length, NGS panel
Hypoplastic MDS	Bone marrow dysplasia, macrocytosis, abnormal cytogenetics, clonal somatic mutations	Marrow morphology, karyotype, NGS panel
Hypoplastic leukemia	Marrow blasts	Flow cytometry, peripheral smear, immunophenotyping
Drugs/toxins	History of recent drug exposure (chloramphenicol, NSAIDs, anticonvulsants), or toxin (benzene)	Clinical history, drug withdrawal trial
Cellular bone marrow with systemic disorders		
Vitamin B12/folate deficiency	Macrocytosis, hypersegmented neutrophils, neurologic signs (B12)	Serum B12, folate, MMA, homocysteine
Hypersplenism	Pancytopenia with splenomegaly, preserved marrow	Ultrasound abdomen, gastroenterology referral
Viral infections (HIV, EBV, parvovirus B19, Hepatitis)	Acute/subacute pancytopenia, history of viral prodrome	Viral serologies, PCR tests
Cellular bone marrow with primary marrow disease		
Acute leukemia	Marrow blasts	Flow cytometry, peripheral smear, immunophenotyping
Infiltrative disorders (e.g., TB, lymphoma)	Fever, night sweats, weight loss, organomegaly	Bone marrow biopsy, PET-CT, acid-fast staining
Hairy cell leukemia	Middle-aged males, splenomegaly, dry tap marrow	TRAP stain, BRAF V600E mutation, flow cytometry
PNH	Intravascular hemolysis, thrombosis, hemoglobinuria	FLAER-based flow cytometry

Table 6.2 Initial diagnostic tests for aplastic anemia

Test	Purpose
CBC with reticulocyte count	Confirm pancytopenia and marrow failure
Bone marrow aspiration + biopsy	Establish hypocellular marrow without dysplasia
Viral serology	Rule out hepatitis, HIV, EBV
Stress cytogenetics	To exclude Fanconi anemia
HLA typing	Required for all patients <40 years for transplant planning

- *PNH clone detection* via FLAER-based flow cytometry is crucial. A small PNH clone is found in up to 50% of AA cases and confirms immune pathogenesis [11].

The newer guidelines emphasize an integrated approach combining marrow histology, cytogenetics, flow cytometry, and molecular testing to rule out MDS, IBMFS, or leukemia mimics before confirming a diagnosis of AA [12].

6.5 Treatment of Aplastic Anemia

The optimal management of AA includes early diagnosis and timely initiation of definitive treatment as per the age, performance status, and severity of aplastic anemia. The severity of AA is based upon the *Camitta criteria*, first described in 1976 and still globally adopted to stratify aplastic anemia into severe, very severe, and non-severe [1]. The severity of the disease is directly related to the overall survival (OS) and treatment decisions, with VSAA & SAA having a worse prognosis requiring urgent treatment. In the last few decades, the survival of the AA has been improved substantially due to the availability of better supportive care and definitive management options in both children and adults.

6.6 Supportive Care

Supportive care is the cornerstone of management of AA, which is essential to maintain quality of life and to prevent early mortality. It includes a safe and ideal blood product transfusion strategy, prophylaxis, and early management of infections, along with treatment of the iron overload. The important supportive care strategy is discussed in Table 6.3.

Table 6.3 Supportive care in patients with aplastic anemia

Blood product support
RBC transfusion threshold: Hb <70–80 g/L (individualized in outpatient settings)
Platelets: Prophylaxis <10,000/μL; <20,000/μL if febrile/bleeding or on ATG
Use leukodepleted, irradiated, and HLA-matched (if alloimmunized) components
Antimicrobial prophylaxis
Bacterial: Fluoroquinolones may be used in neutropenia
Fungal: Posaconazole (>Fluconazole) preferred for mold coverage
Viral: Acyclovir in transplant settings, monitor CMV with PCR during ATG and post-HSCT
PCP: Not routinely recommended, but can be added if steroids are used >2 weeks or during IST or post-HSCT [13].
Iron chelation therapy
Ferritin >1000 ng/mL or >20 RBC units → start deferasirox (preferred over deferiprone)
Venesection preferred post-HSCT or in responders
Monitor renal function when combined with CSA [14]
G-CSF
Not routinely recommended
May be used temporarily in profound neutropenia with infection

6.7 Definitive Management

The definitive management of AA includes allogenic hematopoietic stem cell transplant (HSCT) and immunosuppressive therapy (IST), including anti-thymocyte globulin with cyclosporine-A. Both IST and HSCT have the potential to restore hematopoiesis but only HSCT has the curative potential. The factors to consider before deciding on the definitive therapy include age, disease severity, comorbidities, HLA-MSD availability, and patient affordability. Figure 6.1 shows the treatment algorithm for SAA/VSAA.

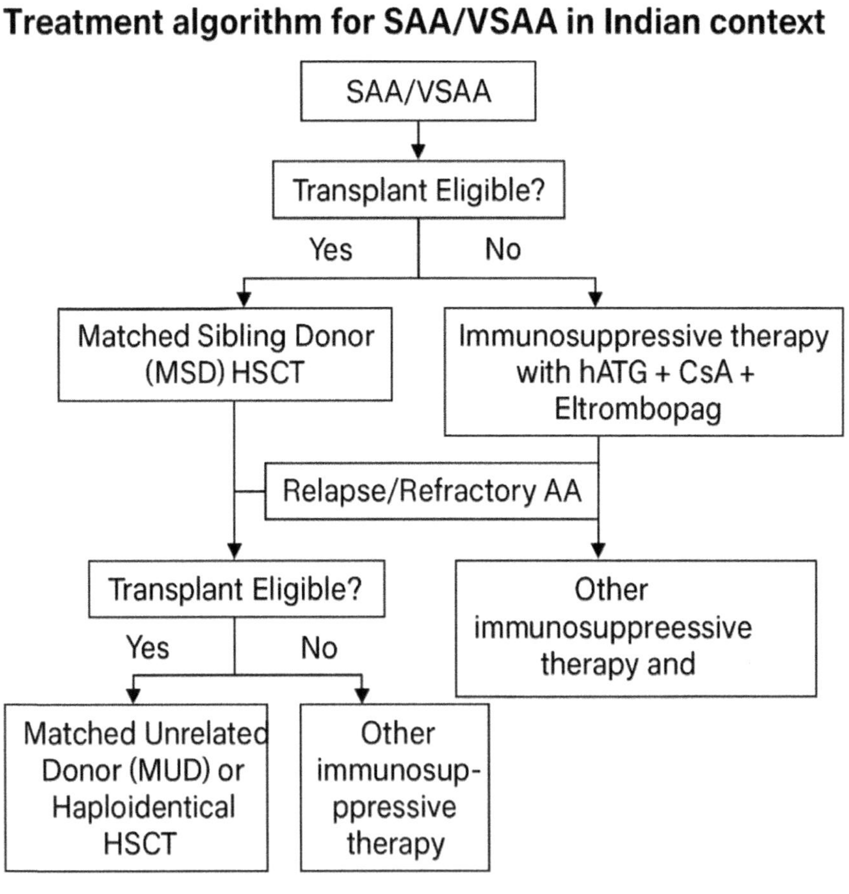

Fig. 6.1 Treatment algorithm for SAA/VSAA in Indian context

6.7.1 *Stem Cell Transplant (SCT)*

Matched sibling HSCT is the only curative treatment of choice for young (≤40 years) fit SAA/VSAA patients. For patients refractory to one course of IST (refractory AA), matched unrelated donor (MUD) HSCT can be considered. Alternative donor-HSCT, including haploidentical or umbilical-cord blood, may be considered in patients with refractory AA who lack MSD or a suitable MUD.

The indications of SCT in Aplastic anemia are as follows:

- SAA/VSAA with MSD and age <40 years: First-line treatment is HSCT
- Failure of IST at 6 months
- Clonal evolution: MDS cytogenetics, TP53 mutation, blasts
- Hypocellular MDS with multilineage dysplasia

For the successful outcome of HSCT in AA patients, the following parameters are of importance [15–17]:

- Patients' age (strongest impact)
- Selection of an appropriate donor by HLA matching at high resolution
- Comorbidities assessment
- Lack of clonal evolution of AA
- Absence of donor-directed antibodies
- Conditioning regimen used
- Source of the stem cells (PBSC or bone marrow)
- Interval between diagnosis and transplant.

6.7.1.1 Source of Stem Cells

It is usually preferred to use bone marrow as a stem cell source over peripheral blood in all age groups because of an overall survival advantage [18]. However, various studies from developing countries have shown that with improved conditioning and immunosuppression, G-CSF mobilized peripheral blood stem cells could be a practical solution, compared to bone marrow [19–21].

6.7.1.2 Conditioning Regimens

For matched sibling transplants, the standard conditioning regimen is cyclophosphamide 200 mg/kg (CY 200) and ATG. It is usual practice to include adding FLU with CY and ATG (FCA) or alemtuzumab (FCC) for multi-transfused SAA patients receiving MSD-HSCT [19, 22]. The conditioning regimen recommended for MUD-HSCT includes FCA and low-dose TBI (2–4 Gy) or FCC for a haploidentical donor [23, 24].

Table 6.4 Summarizes the initial treatment plan for aplastic anemia

Parameters to assess before treatment decision
Age (<40 years or >40 years)
Severity (SAA and VSAA vs non-severe AA)
Donor availability (especially MSD in younger patients)
Transplant eligibility (assess the comorbidities)
Initial treatment strategy
Age <40 years + MSD available: Upfront HSCT is the preferred choice
No MSD available or age >40 years: IST (Horse ATG + CSA ± Eltrombopag) is preferred choice
Relapsed/Refractory AA: 2nd course of IST or MUD/Haplo-HSCT depending on donor availability and patient status
Non-severe AA: Patient can be observed, cyclosporin alone or in combination with androgens/Eltromopag

6.7.1.3 GVHD Prophylaxis

The standard GVHD prophylaxis includes methotrexate with CsA for MSD and high dose post-transplant cyclophosphamide (PTCy) for haplo-matched HSCT [23].

6.7.2 Immunosuppressive Therapy (IST): Evolving Landscape

Immunosuppressive therapy (IST) is the standard of treatment for SAA and VSAA patients who lack a suitably matched sibling donor (MSD), age >40 years, medically unfit, and as bridging therapy while waiting for the HSCT. The standard effective first-line IST regimen includes a combination of anti-thymocyte globulin (ATG) with cyclosporin (CSA) ± Eltromopag (EPAG). The preparation of ATG includes equine-ATG (hATG) and Rabbit-ATG (rATG). Horse ATG is preferred over rabbit ATG due to superior outcomes shown in NIH and EBMT trials. Horse ATG leads to higher ORR (60–75%) and lower relapse compared to rabbit ATG (ORR ~37–50%) [10].

The standard regimen of triple therapy (ATG + CSA + EPAG) is as follows:

- Horse ATG (hATG): 40 mg/kg/day IV for 4 days
- Cyclosporine A (CSA): 5 mg/kg/day PO, adjusted to trough levels 150–250 ng/mL
- Eltrombopag (EPAG): 150 mg/day orally, start Day 1 or Day 14

There are few predictors of the response to IST in AA patients, which include:

- Young age patients (<18 years)
- Less severe disease (SAA vs VSAA)
- Absolute reticulocyte count $\geq 25 \times 10^9$/L
- Absolute lymphocyte count $\geq 1 \times 10^9$/L
- Telomere length (TL)

- Presence of a PNH clone and mutations including PIGA, BCOR, and BCORL1
- Median interval between diagnosis and therapy

6.7.2.1 Addition of Eltrombopag to IST

The integration of Eltrombopag, an oral TPO-RA, into first-line IST is a recent development in the management of AA. A study from *NIH* demonstrated 80% hematologic response, including trilineage recovery [11]. In the *RACE Trial* (2022), addition of Eltrombopag to standard IST (ATG + CSA) showed complete response (CR) at 3 months: 22% vs 10% and Overall response (OR) at 6 months: 68% vs 41% [12]. Eltromopag is now the standard of care in adult IST protocols globally and is increasingly adopted in developing countries like India despite cost constraints [25].

6.7.3 Management of AA in Special Clinical Scenarios

The management of AA in various clinical scenarios, such as in elderly patients and in pregnancy, is really challenging. Table 6.5 summarizes the management of AA in special clinical conditions.

Table 6.5 Management of aplastic anemia with special clinical scenarios

Elderly patient with AA
IST with ATG + CSA ± Eltrombopag can be used safely, but high risk of infections and arrhythmias, should be monitored carefully
Cyclosporin±Eltromopag/danazol: is another good option
Danazol alone may offer hematologic improvement
AA with pregnancy
Avoid ATG, HSCT, and Eltrombopag
CSA is safe and effective
Maintain platelet count >20 × 10^9/L around delivery
PNH clone requires anticoagulation; eculizumab if hemolysis present [26, 27]
Inherited Bone Marrow Failure Syndromes (IBMFS)
Fanconi anemia (FA) and dyskeratosis congenita (DKC): two most common inherited BMFS
Stress cytogenetics, telomere length, preferably NGS panel for IBMFS
Donor screening for IBMFS is necessary if matched sibling donor SCT is planned
Significant modification of containing regimens for SCT: Avoid TBI, use reduced intensity
Presence of PNH clone
Treatment AA as per standard protocol
Consider eculizumab if hemolysis or thrombosis
Hepatitis associated AA
Treatment with IST once viral load resolves;
Good response rates

Table 6.6 Newer updates in management of aplastic anemia

Innovation	Status
Gene therapy	Under trial for telomeropathies (DKC) using lentiviral and CRISPR strategies
Pegcetacoplan (C3 inhibitor)	In PNH-Aplastic syndrome with complement activation (phase II)
Improved Haplo-HSCT	Post-transplant cyclophosphamide with G-CSF priming reducing GVHD
MRD/NGS Monitoring	Helps detect early clonal escape
Novel TPO-R agonists	Romiplostim and avatrombopag under evaluation for refractory AA

6.7.4 Long-Term Follow-Up

Patients who recover from AA (whether via IST or transplant) require regular follow-up. About 10–15% of acquired AA patients may develop clonal evolution to develop conditions like myelodysplastic syndrome (MDS), acute leukaemia, or PNH over a decade. Any new cytopenia or abnormal blood cells should prompt evaluation for MDS/leukaemia. Flow cytometry for PNH clones should be repeated if hemolysis signs appear, since an AA/PNH overlap syndrome can emerge (every 6–12 months).

6.7.5 Future Directions in Management of Aplastic Anemia

There are few newer updates in the management of aplastic anemia, which are summarized in Table 6.6.

6.8 Illustrative Clinical Cases

6.8.1 Case 1

A previously healthy 24-year-old presented with progressive fatigue, gum bleeding, and fever. Clinical examination revealed pallor and mild petechiae but no lymphadenopathy or organomegaly. Hemogram revealed pancytopenia (Hb 5.2 g/dL, ANC 0.3×10^9/L, Platelets 9×10^9/L) with reticulocyte count <0.5%. Bone marrow biopsy showed severe hypocellularity (<10%) with no evidence of dysplasia or infiltration. Flow cytometry using the FLAER assay detected a minor PNH clone (Type III granulocytes 12%). Viral serologies were negative. Stress cytogenetics was normal.

Since there was no HLA match with a sibling, he was managed with immunosuppressive therapy (horse ATG, Cyclosporine A) and Eltrombopag. He demonstrated early signs of hematologic recovery by Day 60, achieved partial response at

3 months, and complete trilineage response by 6 months. He remains in remission on tapering CSA.

He was alright for 6 years without any medication. On routine follow up, he presented with bicytopenia(Hb: 13.4 g/dL; ANC: 0.9×10^9/L; 82×10^9/L). He was started again with cyclosporin and eltromopag, and advised for bone marrow examination. Bone marrow examination revealed the diagnosis of acute myeloid leukemia (AML).

Key Learning Points

- A small PNH clone in AA is a common finding and reinforces immune-mediated pathogenesis. Its presence correlates with a higher likelihood of a favorable response to IST, particularly with the addition of eltrombopag.
- Clonal evolution is a major challenge in patients with aplastic anemia, who respond to IST. A bone marrow examination is necessary whenever there is cytopenia in follow-up.

6.8.2 Case 2

A 14-year-old presented with anemia and recurrent epistaxis. There was a history of frequent infections and mild pancytopenia over the past year. On examination, there was pallor and echymosis. There were no physical abnormalities of inherited bone marrow failures. Hemogram showed Hb 7.1 g/dL, Platelets 22×10^9/L, ANC 0.6×10^9/L. Bone marrow biopsy: hypocellular marrow with no dysplasia or blasts. Stress cytogenetics showed chromosomal breakage with the diepoxybutane (DEB) test, confirming Fanconi anemia. NGS revealed a mutation in the FANCA gene.

Patient was managed with Supportive transfusion support, infection prophylaxis, and androgen therapy. The patient had an HLA-matched sibling. The matched sibling was screened for the Fanconi gene before taking a transplant. The patient was managed with reduced-intensity conditioning (Fludarabine + low-dose Cyclophosphamide + ATG) bone marrow transplant. GVHD prophylaxis with CSA and methotrexate. Engraftment occurred by Day +16. Mild grade I GVHD resolved with steroids.

Key Learning Points

- Inherited bone marrow failure syndromes (IBMFS) should be excluded in young aplastic anemia patients.
- Fanconi anemia (FA) is the most common IBMFS. The phenotypic features of FA are variable and not present in all patients.
- We should do stress cytogenetics and genetic study, even if no phenotypic features in young AA patients.
- Donor screening is an essential component before a matched sibling stem cell transplant. The dose of cytotoxic drugs should be reduced in conditioning regimens.

6.9 Conclusion

Aplastic anemia management is undergoing a transformative evolution. In both adult and pediatric populations, the management of aplastic anemia requires a combination of accurate diagnosis, timely definitive therapy, and meticulous supportive care. With the addition of eltrombopag to IST, growing experience with haplo-HSCT, and refined diagnostics enabling accurate classification, aplastic anemia has become a largely curable disease, if diagnosed and treated early.

References

1. Marsh JC, Ball SE, Cavenagh J, Darbyshire P, Dokal I, Gordon-Smith EC, et al. Guidelines for the diagnosis and management of aplastic anaemia. Br J Haematol. 2009;147(1):43–70. https://doi.org/10.1111/j.1365-2141.2009.07842.x.
2. Kulasekararaj A, Cavenagh J, Dokal I, Foukaneli T, Gandhi S, Garg M, et al. Guidelines for the diagnosis and management of adult aplastic anaemia: a British Society for Haematology guideline. Br J Haematol. 2024;204(3):784–804. https://doi.org/10.1111/bjh.19236.
3. Mahapatra M. Chapter 6: Pancytopenia: aplastic Anemia. In: deGruchy's clinical hematology in medical practice. 6th ed. Wiley India edition; 2013. p. 106–19.
4. Mahapatra M, Singh PK, Agarwal M, et al. Epidemiology, clinicohematological profile and management of aplastic anemia: AIIMS experience. J Assoc Physicians India. 2015;63:30–5.
5. Townsley DM, Dumitriu B, Young NS. Bone marrow failure and the telomeropathies. Blood. 2014;124(18):2775–83. https://doi.org/10.1182/blood-2014-07-526855.
6. Afable MG II, Wlodarski M, Makishima H, Shaik M, Sekeres MA, Tiu RV, et al. SNP array-based karyotyping: differences and similarities between aplastic anemia and hypocellular myelodysplastic syndromes. Blood. 2011;117(25):6876–84. https://doi.org/10.1182/blood-2011-01-330209.
7. Yoshizato T, Dumitriu B, Hosokawa K, Makishima H, Yoshida K, Townsley D, et al. Somatic mutations and clonal hematopoiesis in aplastic anemia. N Engl J Med. 2015;373(1):35–47. https://doi.org/10.1056/NEJMoa1414799.
8. Brodsky RA, Mukhina GL, Li S, Nelson KL, Chiurazzi PL, Buckley JT, et al. Improved detection and characterization of paroxysmal nocturnal hemoglobinuria using fluorescent aerolysin. Am J Clin Pathol. 2000;114(3):459–66. https://doi.org/10.1309/X9T8-WENF-KTUP-1YM1.
9. Bono E, McLornan D, Travaglino E, Gandhi S, Galli A, Khan AA, et al. Clinical, histopathological and molecular characterization of hypoplastic myelodysplastic syndrome. Leukemia. 2019;33(10):2495–505. https://doi.org/10.1038/s41375-019-0479-6.
10. Scheinberg P, Nunez O, Weinstein B, Biancotto A, Wu CO, Young NS. Horse versus rabbit antithymocyte globulin in acquired aplastic anemia. N Engl J Med. 2011;365(5):430–8. https://doi.org/10.1056/NEJMoa1103975.
11. Peffault de Latour R, Kulasekararaj A, Iacobelli S, Terwel SR, Cook R, Griffin M, et al. Eltrombopag added to immunosuppression in severe aplastic anemia. N Engl J Med. 2022;386(1):11–23. https://doi.org/10.1056/NEJMoa2113707.

12. Townsley DM, Scheinberg P, Winkler T, Desmond R, Dumitriu B, Rios O, et al. Eltrombopag added to standard immunosuppression for aplastic anemia. N Engl J Med. 2017;376(16):1540–50. https://doi.org/10.1056/NEJMoa1613878.
13. NICE Clinical Guideline CG151. Neutropenic sepsis: prevention and management in people with cancer. National Institute for Health and Care Excellence (NICE); 2012. Available at: https://www.nice.org.uk/guidance/cg151.
14. Lee JW, Yoon SS, Shen ZX, Ganser A, Hsu HC, Habr D, et al. Iron chelation therapy with deferasirox in patients with aplastic anemia: a subgroup analysis of 116 patients from the EPIC trial. Blood. 2010;116(14):2448–54. https://doi.org/10.1182/blood-2009-12-256040.
15. Dolai T, Jain M, Mahapatra M. Idiopathic aplastic anemia: Indian perspective. Indian J Hematol Blood Transfus. 2023;39(1):1–12. https://doi.org/10.1007/s12288-022-01592-3.
16. Narita A, Kojima S. Biomarkers for predicting clinical response to immunosuppressive therapy in aplastic anemia. Int J Hematol. 2016;104:153–8.
17. Scheinberg P, Young NS. How I treat acquired aplastic anemia. Blood. 2012;120(6):1185–96. https://doi.org/10.1182/blood-2012-03-384453.
18. Bacigalupo A, Socié G, Schrezenmeier H, et al. Bone marrow versus peripheral blood as the stem cell source for sibling transplants in acquired aplastic anemia: survival advantage for bone marrow in all age groups. Haematologica. 2012;97:1142.
19. Kumar R, Prem S, Mahapatra M, Seth T, Chowdhary DR, Mishra P, et al. Fludarabine, cyclophosphamide and horse antithymocyte globulin conditioning regimen for allogeneic peripheral blood stem cell transplantation performed in non-HEPA filter rooms for multiply transfused patients with severe aplastic anemia. Bone Marrow Transplant. 2006;37:745–9.
20. Seth T, Kanga U, Sood P, Sharma V, Mishra P, Mahapatra M. Audit of peripheral stem cell transplantation for aplastic anemia in multitransfused infected patients. Transplant Proc. 2012;44:922–4.
21. Chandy V. Stem cell transplantation in India. Bone Marrow Transplant. 2008;42:S81–4.
22. George B, Mathews V, Viswabandya A, et al. Fludarabine and cyclophosphamide based reduced intensity conditioning (RIC) regimens reduce rejection and improve outcome in Indian patients undergoing allogeneic stem cell transplantation for severe aplastic anemia. Bone Marrow Transplant. 2007;40:13–8.
23. Prata PH, Eikema DJ, Afanasyev B, Bosman P, Smiers F, Diez-Martin JL, et al. Haploidentical transplantation and posttransplant cyclophosphamide for treating aplastic anemia patients: a report from the EBMT Severe Aplastic Anemia Working Party. Bone Marrow Transplant. 2020;55(6):1050–8. https://doi.org/10.1038/s41409-019-0747-9.
24. Sheth VS, Potter V, Gandhi SA, Kulasekararaj AG, de Lavallade H, Muus P, et al. Similar outcomes of alemtuzumab-based hematopoietic cell transplantation for SAA patients older or younger than 50 years. Blood Adv. 2019;3(20):3070–9. https://doi.org/10.1182/bloodadvances.2019000731.
25. Gudala SP, Dhawan R, Aggarwal M, Kumar P, Seth T, Mahapatra M. Additionof eltrombopag to immunosuppressive therapy (ATG, cyclosporine) in acquired aplastic anemia: a tertiary care center experience. Indian J Hematol Blood Transfus. 2020;36(suppl 1):S11.
26. McGowan KE, Malinowski AK, Schuh AC, Whittle W, Shehata N. Aplastic anaemia in pregnancy – a single centre, North American series. Br J Haematol. 2019;184(3):436–9. https://doi.org/10.1111/bjh.15745.
27. Kelly RJ, Hochsmann B, Szer J, Kulasekararaj A, de Guibert S, Roth A, et al. Eculizumab in pregnant patients with paroxysmal nocturnal hemoglobinuria. N Engl J Med. 2015;373(11):1032–9. https://doi.org/10.1056/NEJMoa1502950.

Chapter 7
Comprehensive Management of Thalassemic Patients Including Pregnancy

Tuphan Kanti Dolai, Shipla Roy, and Kaustav Ghosh

Abstract Thalassemia comprises a spectrum of inherited hematologic disorders transmitted in an autosomal recessive pattern, resulting from decreased or absent synthesis of one or more globin chains. Owing to its broad clinical heterogeneity, affected individuals may present with severe anemia necessitating regular blood transfusions, characteristic of transfusion-dependent thalassemia (TDT), or exhibit mild to minimal symptoms, as observed in non-transfusion-dependent thalassemia (NTDT), often permitting normal growth without ongoing transfusion support. These two categories require distinctly different therapeutic approaches. Iron overload represents a key complication in both TDT and NTDT, with the potential to cause significant injury to vital organs such as the heart, liver, and endocrine glands, thereby emphasizing the need for systematic surveillance to avert long-term sequelae. Advances in management strategies, including the availability of oral iron chelation therapy and non-invasive modalities for assessing iron burden, have markedly enhanced survival outcomes and overall quality of life. As a result, many patients now experience improved reproductive prospects and are increasingly able to pursue pregnancy and parenthood. This highlights the necessity for holistic management and ongoing follow-up across the continuum of care.

Keywords Thalassemia · Iron overload · Pregnancy · Management · Regular monitoring

T. K. Dolai (✉) · S. Roy · K. Ghosh
Department of Hematology, Nil Ratan Sircar Medical College and Hospital (NRSMCH), Kolkata, West Bengal, India

H. P. Pati et al. (eds.), *Clinical Hematology and Hemato-Oncology*,
https://doi.org/10.1007/978-981-92-1167-8_7

Learning Objectives

- To ensure that individuals with both transfusion-dependent and non-transfusion-dependent thalassemia have access to suitable and effective therapeutic interventions.
- To establish comprehensive and regular monitoring protocols for all individuals with thalassemia
- To raise awareness among patients and their families about reproductive health and related concerns
- To support a good quality of life that includes a healthy reproductive experience and the potential for delivering healthy children
- To ensure regular monitoring and appropriate management of pregnant women with thalassemia
- To decrease the incidence of thalassemia in future generations through preventive strategies

7.1 Illustrative Clinical Case

A 26-year-old female diagnosed as transfusion-dependent β-thalassemia major since 3 years of age presented with progressively worsening exertional dyspnea over one-year, chronic back pain for 6 months (with a history of NSAID use), and intermittent right upper abdominal pain for 3 months. She had a splenectomy at the age of 7 and has been receiving 2–3 units of packed red blood cells (PRBCs) per month, with a mean pre-transfusion hemoglobin level of approximately 7 g/dL. She was initiated on oral iron chelation therapy at the age of 5; however, adherence and monitoring were inconsistent over the years.

On Physical Examination she had severe pallor, mild icterus, and raised jugular venous pressure (JVP). Her pulse was 110 bpm, blood pressure was 130/70 mmHg, and auscultation revealed bilateral vesicular breath sounds and a prominently loud pulmonary component of the second heart sound, accompanied by a split. Abdominal examination showed hepatomegaly (liver palpable 2 cm below the costal margin) and a splenectomy scar. She was conscious and oriented neurologically.

Laboratory Evaluation Revealed Hemoglobin: 9.2 g/dL, platelets: 850,000/cu mm, total bilirubin: 3.2 mg/dL (direct 1.4 mg/dL), AST: 200 IU/L, ALT: 157 IU/L, corrected calcium: 7.9 mg/dL, Vitamin D3: 10 IU/dL, serum ferritin: 1520 ng/mL, transferrin saturation: 92% with normal renal function and coagulation profile. Abdominal ultrasonography confirmed mild hepatomegaly. Cardiac assessment using Doppler transthoracic echocardiography demonstrated a peak tricuspid regurgitation velocity (TRV) of 3.5 m/s and a left ventricular ejection fraction (LVEF) of 48%, indicative of pulmonary hypertension with evolving left ventricular dysfunction. Cardiac MRI showed a T2* value of 8.3 ms, and liver iron concentration (LIC) was severely elevated at 16.7 mg Fe/g dry weight. Pancreatic MRI T2* was 12.3 ms.

FibroScan elastography indicated liver stiffness of 10.5 kPa, consistent with a METAVIR score of F2 (moderate fibrosis). Viral hepatitis panel (HBV, HCV, CMV, EBV) was negative. A bone density scan revealed a lumbar spine T-score of −4.5, indicative of severe osteoporosis.

Management and Follow-Up The patient was initiated on combined iron chelation therapy with subcutaneous deferoxamine (50 mg/kg) and oral deferasirox (30 mg/kg/day). After 6 months of treatment, deferasirox monotherapy was continued, and the patient was counseled to maintain adequate pre-transfusion hemoglobin levels (≥9 g/dL). To address right-sided heart failure and pulmonary hypertension, she was prescribed oral torsemide (40 mg daily) and tadalafil (40 mg daily), respectively. For hypocalcemia and vitamin D deficiency, she was given calcium + vitamin D3 tablets twice daily and high-dose vitamin D3 (60,000 IU weekly for 8 weeks). Alendronate (70 mg once weekly) was started for osteoporosis. Additionally, levothyroxine was initiated at 1.6 μg/kg for newly diagnosed hypothyroidism.

This case highlights the long-term complications of suboptimally managed thalassemia major, including iron overload, cardiopulmonary issues, liver fibrosis, osteoporosis, and endocrine dysfunction. It emphasizes the importance of regular monitoring, compliance with iron chelation therapy, and a multidisciplinary approach to prevent and manage organ damage in these patients.

7.2 Introduction

Fetal hemoglobin (HbF, α2γ2) is the primary form of hemoglobin responsible for oxygen transport during fetal development. After birth, the adult hemoglobin (HbA, α2β2) gradually replaces it, which makes up about 97% of total hemoglobin in adults, while HbF drops to less than 1%. When the beta-globin chain is defective, it often leads to a noticeable increase in HbF levels. Thalassemia comprises a spectrum of autosomal recessive inherited hematologic disorders characterized by diminished or absent synthesis of one or more globin chains. These disorders are now broadly categorized without separating pure quantitative deficiencies from structural variants that are synthesized at reduced levels, such as hemoglobin E and hemoglobin Lepore. Individuals who are homozygous, compound heterozygous, or carry co-inheritance of thalassemia with other hemoglobinopathies—like Hb E, Hb C, or Hb S—can develop what is known as thalassemia syndromes [1].

Globally, approximately half of all thalassemia cases result from compound heterozygosity for hemoglobin E and β-thalassemia. Hb E/β-thalassemia is particularly common in Southeast Asia and certain regions of the Indian subcontinent [2]. Owing to its marked clinical variability, affected individuals may present with features resembling transfusion-dependent thalassemia major or may exhibit normal growth and development without requiring regular transfusion support. Common symptoms resemble those of severe beta thalassemia and include anemia, jaundice, enlargement of the liver and spleen (hepatosplenomegaly), growth delays, and characteristic facial changes due to bone marrow expansion. In many cases, the clinical picture is indistinguishable from that of thalassemia major, with symptoms beginning in infancy and the need for regular blood transfusions to manage anemia, prevent organ enlargement, suppress abnormal marrow activity, and support normal development. However, some individuals with Hb E/β-thalassemia experience much milder symptoms and may survive well with minimal or infrequent transfusions. Due to this broad clinical heterogeneity and the limited availability of robust long-term data on outcomes and complications, there is still no standardized or universally agreed-upon treatment strategy for Hb E/β-thalassemia [3].

Both transfusion-dependent thalassemia (TDT) and non-transfusion-dependent thalassemia (NTDT) may result in considerable morbidity and mortality if inadequately treated. Optimal therapy combined with vigilant surveillance for complications is essential in both entities. A key complication in TDT and NTDT is iron overload, which can compromise critical organs, including the endocrine glands, heart, and liver—thereby necessitating periodic assessment to avert chronic organ injury. These two phenotypes are clinically distinct and demand tailored management strategies. Recent therapeutic advances, particularly the availability of oral iron chelation agents and non-invasive modalities for early identification and control of iron burden, have substantially improved survival outcomes as well as overall quality of life in individuals with thalassemia [4, 5]. Consequently, many patients now demonstrate enhanced reproductive capacity and a greater inclination toward parenthood. Multiple reports of successful pregnancies indicate that, with appropriate preconception counselling and care, women can achieve favorable pregnancy outcomes through either spontaneous conception or assisted reproductive techniques. Comprehensive management requires a coordinated multidisciplinary approach, generally involving a cardiologist, endocrinologist, and gynecologist under the supervision of a beta-thalassemia specialist. Continuous monitoring of maternal well-being and fetal growth throughout gestation remains critical [6]. Since Walker described the first successful pregnancy in a woman with thalassemia major in 1969, more than 400 successful pregnancies have been documented in the literature [7].

Accordingly, meticulous long-term management and consistent follow-up are fundamental components of care for individuals with thalassemia across the disease trajectory.

7.3 Clinical Manifestations

Thalassemia presents with a broad and varied clinical spectrum, ranging from individuals with no symptoms to those with NTDT or TDT. In infancy, symptoms are usually absent due to the protective effect of high HbF levels. However, in beta thalassemia, where HbF production remains elevated, and in Hb E beta thalassemia, where HbF is replaced by Hb E between 6 and 12 months of age, anemia and enlarged spleen commonly develop. Growth issues typically become noticeable during the first

10 years of life. The frequent initial signs are pallor and an enlarged spleen. In more severe cases, symptoms include anemia, jaundice, characteristic facial changes due to bone marrow expansion, leg ulcers, enlarged liver and spleen, stunted growth, and signs of extramedullary blood formation. Cardiac failure and infections secondary to iron overload represent the predominant causes of mortality. Furthermore, persistent platelet activation may increase susceptibility to vascular complications, including pulmonary hypertension, thromboembolism, cerebrovascular and peripheral thrombotic events. Other complications can include effects of iron overload, prolonged low oxygen levels, and hormonal imbalances due to pituitary dysfunction, leading to conditions like hypothyroidism, delayed puberty or infertility, and osteoporosis. Assessment of a child's health status should incorporate details such as the age at onset of symptoms, family history of hemoglobin disorders, trends in appetite and weight gain, activity and energy levels, overall sense of well-being, irritability, frequency of both minor and major infections, and comparison of daily functioning with that of siblings. During the baseline and all subsequent follow-up evaluations, the physical examination should include identification of features suggestive of bone marrow expansion—particularly changes in facial and cranial morphology documented using a standardized 4-point grading system or serial photographic comparison—along with measurement of spleen and liver dimensions, comprehensive cardiovascular assessment, and tracking of growth parameters through serial height and weight measurements [8]. Pathophysiology of complications in thalassemia is summarized in Fig. 7.1.

Women with TDT have been documented to encounter pregnancy-related complications, including placental insufficiency, placental abruption, gestational hypertension, nephrolithiasis, cholelithiasis, and urinary tract infections [9, 10]. Nevertheless, available evidence does not indicate that women with thalassemia

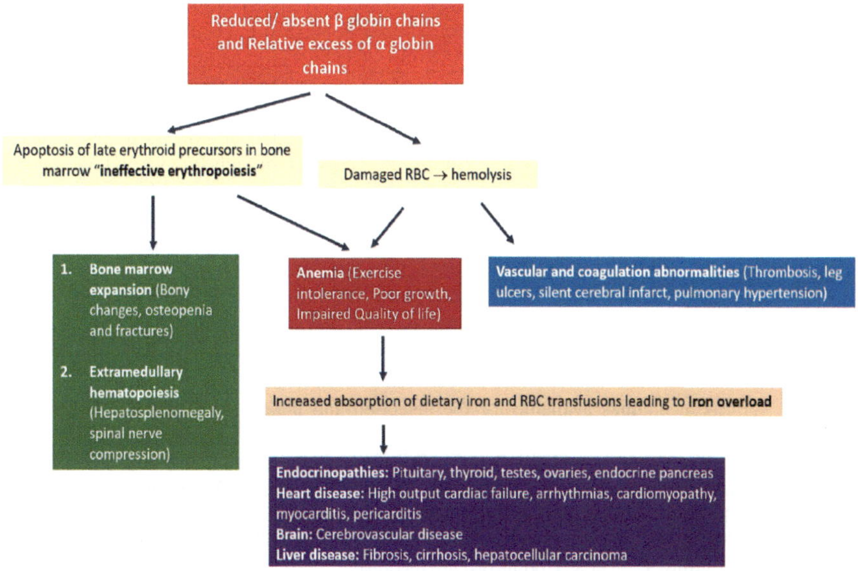

Fig. 7.1 Mechanisms underlying the development of complications in thalassemia

have a greater overall risk of obstetric complications compared with the general population. Pregnancy itself, however, is associated with a three- to fourfold increase in the risk of thrombotic events. Venous thromboembolism represents a significant cause of maternal morbidity, occurring in approximately 0.76 to 1.72 per 1000 pregnancies, while pulmonary embolism continues to be a major contributor to maternal mortality. The heightened prothrombotic state of pregnancy, or hypercoagulability, is thought to serve as a physiological safeguard against excessive bleeding during miscarriage or delivery. Thalassemia further predisposes individuals to a hypercoagulable condition, particularly among individuals who have undergone splenectomy, thereby increasing susceptibility to thromboembolic complications. This risk is partly attributed to the procoagulant properties of negatively charged phospholipids expressed on the membranes of abnormal erythrocytes and immature red cells (erythroblasts), levels of which rise markedly after splenectomy and in patients receiving minimal or no transfusion therapy. Moreover, women with

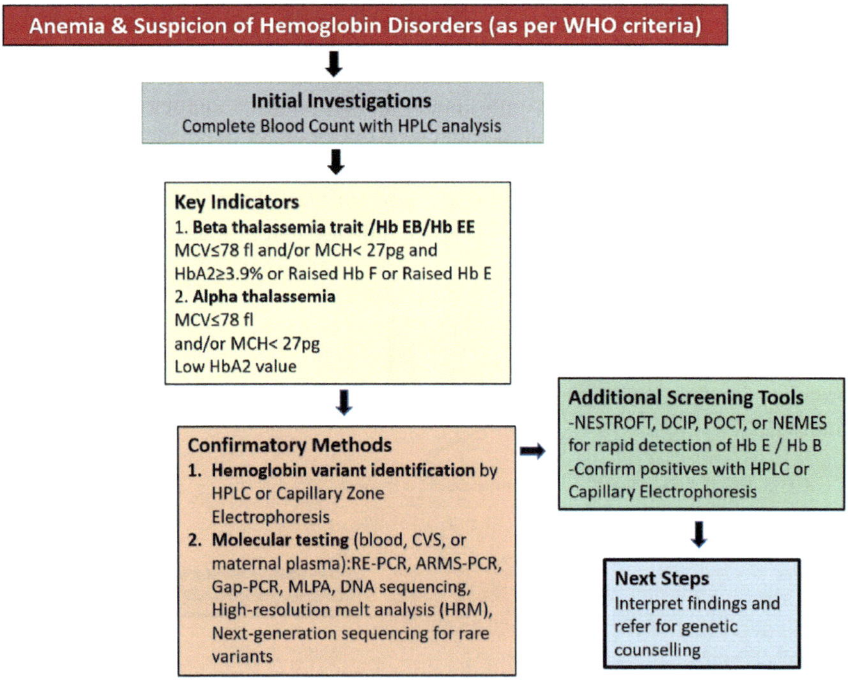

Fig. 7.2 Various techniques available for the detection and diagnosis of hemoglobinopathies. (Abbreviations: ARMS PCR amplification refractory mutation system polymerase chain reaction, CVS chorionic villus sampling, DCIP dichlorophenolindophenol precipitation test, HPLC high-performance liquid chromatography, HRM high-resolution melting, MCH mean corpuscular hemoglobin, MCV mean corpuscular volume, MLPA multiple ligation-dependent probe amplification, NEMES Naked Eye Microcolumn for HbE Screen, NESTROFT Naked Eye Single Tube Red Cell Osmotic Fragility Test, POCT point-of-care testing)

non-transfusion-dependent thalassemia who have seldom or never received transfusions may be at increased risk of developing severe alloimmune anemia if transfusion becomes necessary during pregnancy [11, 12].

7.4 Diagnosis

The approach to diagnosis of thalassemia is summarized in Fig. 7.2.

7.5 Management of Thalassemia

Management of thalassemia is individualized according to disease severity. In patients with E–beta thalassemia, a pre-transfusion hemoglobin level of approximately 7 g/dL is recommended, whereas in beta thalassemia major, a higher target of around 9 g/dL is advised, as these levels aid in suppressing ineffective erythropoiesis [8].

1. *Mild to Moderate Thalassemia*—Cases with hemoglobin levels between 9 and 12 g/dL (mild) and 6–8 g/dL (moderate) are categorized and treated as NTDT [13].

   A. Blood transfusion: The decision to initiate transfusion therapy is guided by clearly defined goals and safety considerations. Key objectives of transfusion therapy include:

      (a) Maintaining the viability and functional integrity of stored red blood cells to support optimal oxygen transport
      (b) Maintaining adequate hemoglobin levels
      (c) Ensuring a normal red cell lifespan in the recipient
      (d) Minimizing the risk of transfusion-transmitted infections

7.5.1 Indication of Blood Transfusion

- Established diagnosis of thalassemia
- Hb value <7 gm/dl on two separate measurements taken at least 2 weeks apart, after excluding other contributing causes such as infection
- Clinical indications regardless of Hb level
  - Marked symptomatic anemia
  - Inadequate growth or failure to thrive
  - Sequelae of intramedullary hematopoiesis, such as pathological fractures and bony changes
  - Clinically relevant extramedullary hematopoiesis

7.5.2 Essential Requirements for Blood Transfusion

- Conduct extended red cell antigen phenotyping prior to the initial transfusion, covering at minimum D, C, c, E, e, and Kell antigens.
- Administer leukocyte-reduced, fresh-packed red blood cells—preferably stored for no longer than 1 week in CPD-A or up to 2 weeks when preserved in an additive solution.
- Keep comprehensive documentation of prior alloimmunization and monitor the patient's yearly transfusion requirements.

  B. Hydroxyurea: It is an S-phase-specific agent that does not cause DNA hypomethylation. It works by blocking the enzyme ribonucleotide reductase, which is responsible for converting ribonucleotide diphosphates into deoxyribonucleotides, thereby inhibiting DNA synthesis. HU promotes the production of HbF, which helps relieve symptoms in patients with beta-thalassemia. The γ-globin chains produced as part of HbF pair with excess α-globin chains, thereby decreasing globin chain imbalance and ameliorating ineffective erythropoiesis. Hydroxyurea (HU) appears to be more beneficial in thalassemia intermedia, where the disparity between α- and β-globin chain synthesis is comparatively milder [14]. In a study by Bohara et al., 61 patients with HbE/β-thalassemia who were either transfusion-dependent or intermittently transfused received varying doses of HU. The results indicated that a higher dose (20 mg/kg/day) was more likely to cause bone marrow suppression than to produce a meaningful rise in HbF levels [15].

  C. Role of iron chelation: Iron chelation therapy is recommended when serum ferritin levels exceed 800 ng/mL or when liver iron concentration is greater than 7 mg/g dry weight. The most frequently prescribed oral chelator is deferasirox, administered at a dose of 20–40 mg/kg/day. Alternative agents include deferiprone at 75–100 mg/kg/day and deferoxamine at 25–60 mg/kg/day [8]. Stepwise approach to iron chelation management in NTDT is shown in Fig. 7.3.

2. *Severe thalassemia:* Individuals with severe forms of thalassemia need ongoing lifelong red blood cell transfusions, iron chelation, and regular surveillance for complications; hence, they should be managed as TDT [16].

   A. *Standard therapy* [8]*:* Red blood cell transfusions and iron chelation. Stepwise approach to iron chelation management in TDT is summarized in Fig. 7.4.

   B. Indications for *splenectomy* [8]:

      - Escalating transfusion needs that make iron chelation insufficient for optimal control (an annual red cell transfusion volume of 200–275 mL/kg/year is considered indicative of increased requirement)
      - Hypersplenism associated with clinically significant cytopenia's

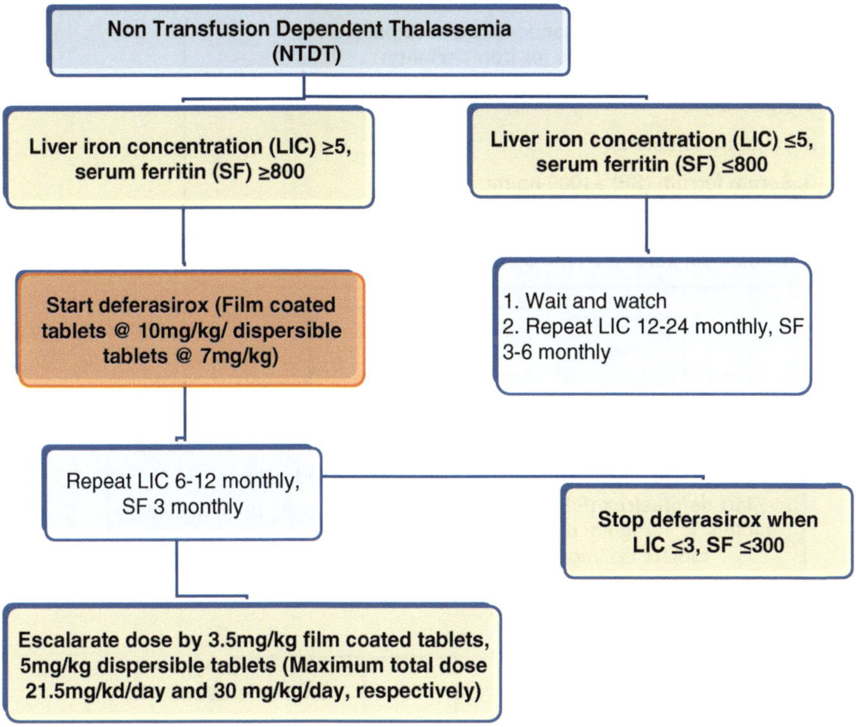

Fig. 7.3 Stepwise approach to iron chelation management in non-transfusion dependent thalassemia

- Symptomatic splenomegaly, presenting with features such as left upper quadrant discomfort, early satiety, or marked splenic enlargement, raising concern for potential rupture

C. *HbF inducer drugs*: The precise mechanism of action of thalidomide is not fully understood. It is thought to exert its effect by inhibiting NF-κB activation stimulated by pro-inflammatory cytokines such as TNF-α, VEGF, and PGE2, along with promoting the generation of reactive oxygen species (ROS). These ROS may activate the p38 MAPK signaling pathway, which has been linked to increased HbF production. Frequently reported adverse effects include somnolence, constipation, gynecomastia, and deep vein thrombosis. Thalidomide is contraindicated during pregnancy because of its teratogenic potential, including defects like phocomelia. The usual initial dose is 1 mg/kg/day, which may be increased up to a maximum of 2 mg/kg/day [17]. In a study conducted by Jain et al., thalidomide was evaluated against hydroxyurea for its safety and efficacy as an HbF inducer in 45 patients with HbE–β thalassemia. Participants were assigned to receive thalidomide with folic acid, hydroxyurea with folic acid, or folic acid alone.

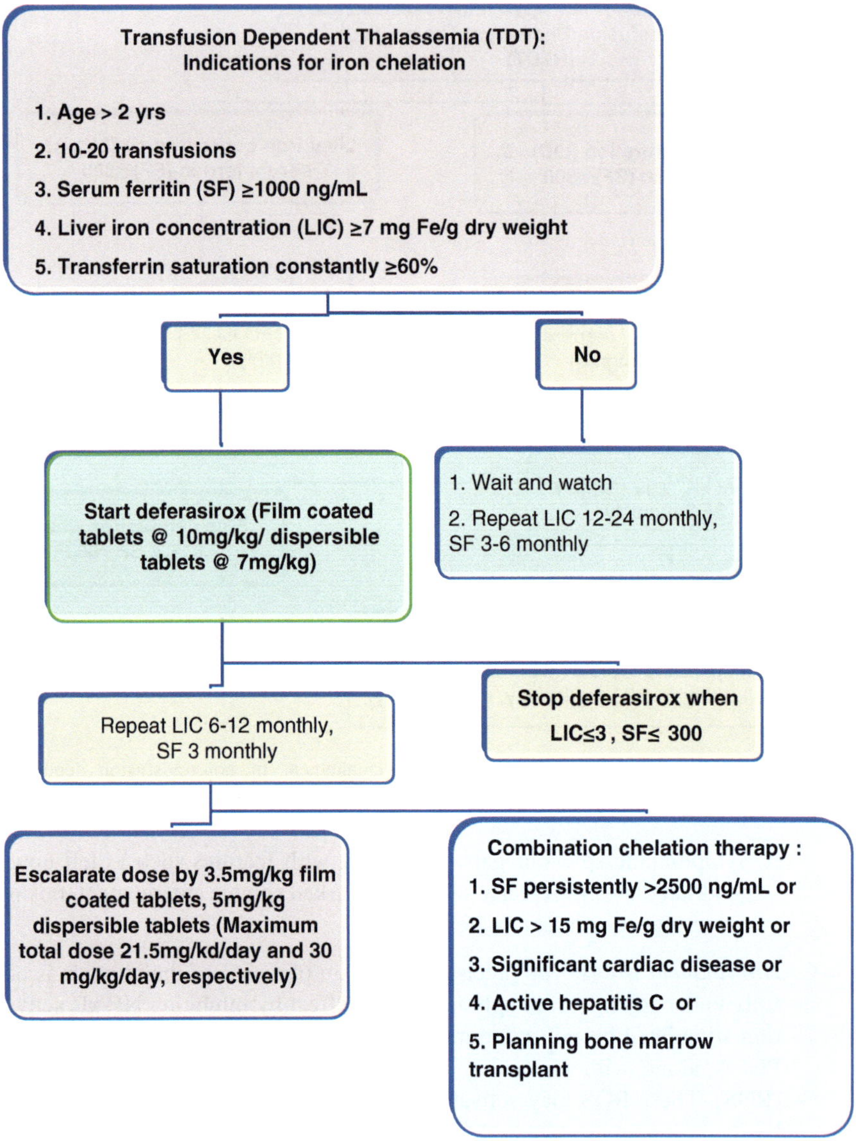

Fig. 7.4 Stepwise approach to iron chelation management in transfusion dependent thalassemia

Follow-up demonstrated that patients treated with thalidomide achieved a significantly greater rise in hemoglobin levels than those receiving hydroxyurea ($p < 0.0001$). This benefit correlated with increased HbF levels and a reduction in ineffective erythropoiesis. Moreover, the thalidomide group experienced a more pronounced decrease in transfusion requirements. No serious adverse events were observed in any treatment arm. The authors concluded that thalidomide resulted in a substantial and sustained hemoglobin improvement and enhanced transfusion independence compared with hydroxyurea in individuals with HbE–β thalassemia [18].

D. *Management of complications* [8]

1. Iron overload: Treatment with iron chelating agents such as deferasirox, deferoxamine, or deferiprone.
2. Pulmonary hypertension: Use of PDE5 inhibitors (e.g., sildenafil) or endothelin receptor antagonists (e.g., bosentan).
3. Thrombosis: Prophylaxis with aspirin and management with low molecular weight heparin.
4. Extramedullary hematopoiesis: Managed with radiotherapy, surgical intervention, or hypertransfusion.
5. Skeletal complications: Calcium and vitamin D3 supplementation, along with bisphosphonates such as alendronate.
6. Endocrine dysfunction: Hormone replacement therapy and optimal iron chelation.
7. Cholelithiasis: Surgical removal of the gallbladder (cholecystectomy).
8. Leg ulcers: Management with topical growth factors, zinc supplementation, and hypertransfusion therapy.

E. *Role of hematopoietic stem cell transplantation (HSCT)* [8]: Matched family donor (MFD) allogeneic HSCT is presently regarded as the only definitive curative treatment for TDT. Transplantation should ideally be performed early in life, prior to the onset of iron overload–related complications, when an HLA-identical sibling donor is available. Stem cells may be sourced from either bone marrow or cord blood of the matched sibling. A matched unrelated donor may also be considered if stringent compatibility for both HLA class I and II loci is ensured. Haploidentical HSCT may be undertaken in specialized, experienced transplant centers within structured clinical protocols. Risk stratification using the Lucarelli classification is recommended, and the standard conditioning regimen typically includes busulfan combined with cyclophosphamide. Overall, HSCT is considered more cost-effective than conventional supportive therapy.

F. *Role of haploidentical HSCT*: Allogeneic HSCT remains the only proven potentially curative option; however, its application is often restricted by donor availability and patient-related factors. To expand the donor pool to include haploidentical related donors, Anurathapan et al. introduced a protocol incorporating pharmacologic pre-transplant immunosuppression (PTIS), along with two cycles of dexamethasone and fludarabine. This was followed by conditioning with intravenous fludarabine and busulfan, and post-transplant graft-versus-host disease (GVHD) prophylaxis using cyclophosphamide, tacrolimus, and mycophenolate mofetil. In their cohort of 83 consecutive TDT patients, the projected 3-year overall survival and event-free survival exceeded 96%, with no cases of secondary graft failure.

Subsequent protocol modifications—including the addition of bortezomib and rituximab for patients with elevated anti-DSA titers and pharmacokinetically guided busulfan dosing—resulted in zero graft failures among the next 52 patients. Severe GVHD occurred in 6 of 83 patients (7%). Overall, this haploidentical HSCT strategy appears to be both safe and efficacious for thalassemia management [19].

G. *Gene therapy* [20, 21]*:* Following Gene therapy works by introducing functional copies of the defective gene into a patient's own hematopoietic stem cells, enabling near-normal hemoglobin production in red blood cells. In contrast, gene editing directly alters the genome—often through homologous recombination—though this approach has comparatively lower efficiency. It employs engineered endonucleases to induce targeted double-stranded DNA breaks, which are subsequently repaired by intrinsic cellular repair mechanisms. The principal endonuclease platforms include zinc finger nucleases (ZFNs), transcription activator-like effector nucleases (TALENs), and CRISPR-Cas9 systems. Recent innovations in CRISPR technology, such as base editors and prime editors, allow for more accurate and efficient genomic modifications.

In TDT, gene therapy primarily aims to enhance fetal hemoglobin (HbF) production. This may be achieved through several gene-editing–based strategies:

- Disrupting the β-globin gene promoter by introducing small deletions within regions where BCL11A binds.
- Inducing point mutations in the promoter region of the γ-globin gene.
- Creating targeted mutations in transcription factors such as KLF1, MYB, SOX6, and GATA-1 to reduce their suppressive effect on γ-globin expression and globin switching.

Compared with conventional therapy, gene therapy has the potential to decrease complications related to chronic transfusions and iron overload. CRISPR/Cas9-mediated gene editing for β-thalassemia has demonstrated promising efficacy.

Recommended eligibility criteria for gene therapy include

- Adolescents (>12 to <17 years) with a β^+ genotype who lack an HLA-matched sibling donor.
- Adults (>17 to ≤55 years) with a β^+ genotype without significant comorbidities who are unsuitable candidates for allogeneic HSCT but are fit for autologous gene therapy with acceptable risk.

Mirza et al. [22] reported the first real-world European experience with betibeglogene autotemcel (beti-cel; Zynteglo) between January 2020 and March 2022 in patients aged ≥12 years without a β^0/β^0 genotype and without an HLA-matched sibling donor. Among 15 screened patients, 4 declined

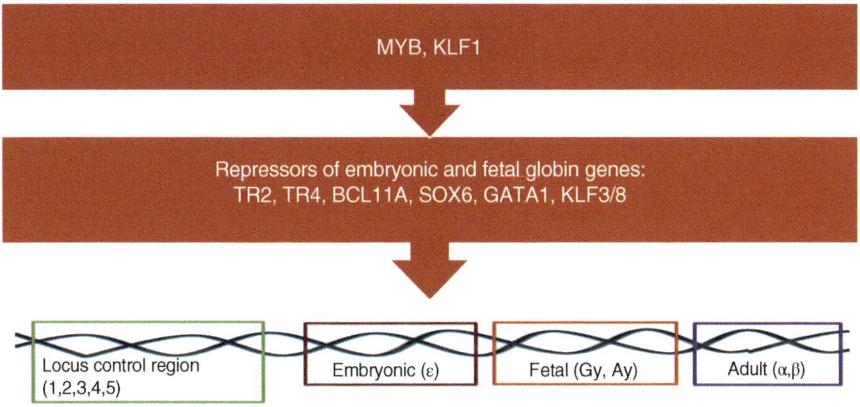

Fig. 7.5 Targets of gene therapy in thalassemia (MYB, KLF1, TR2, TR4, BCL11A, SOX6, GATA1, KLF 3/8)

treatment due to concerns regarding fertility and safety, 2 were excluded owing to severe hepatic iron overload, and 1 was unable to undergo apheresis because of collection failure. The remaining 8 patients received beti-cel after myeloablative busulfan conditioning, and all achieved transfusion independence within 8–59 days. Post-treatment hemoglobin levels ranged from 11.3 to 19.3 g/dL. No deaths occurred, although acute toxicities were consistent with known busulfan-related effects. Platelet support was challenging in 3 patients due to HLA antibodies. During follow-up of up to 24 months, pituitary–gonadal endocrine dysfunction developed in all 3 female patients and in 2 of 5 male patients.

Figure 7.5 shows targets of gene therapy in thalassemia.

H. *Emerging therapies* [23]

- JAK2 inhibitor—Ruxolitinib
- Activin type II inhibitor—Luspatercept, sotatercept
- Rapmycin—motor inhibitor
- Resveratrol, metformin-Fox3 activation, antioxidant
- Minihepcidins
- TMPRSS6 inhibitors
- Exogenous transferrin
- Mitavipat—pyruvate kinase activator

A Phase IV study assessing the safety and efficacy of luspatercept in the management of transfusion-dependent anemia related to myelodysplastic syndromes (MDS) and beta-thalassemia (including β-thalassemia and Eβ-thalassemia) in India is currently underway [24].

Summary of treatment targets in thalassemia is outlined in Fig. 7.6.

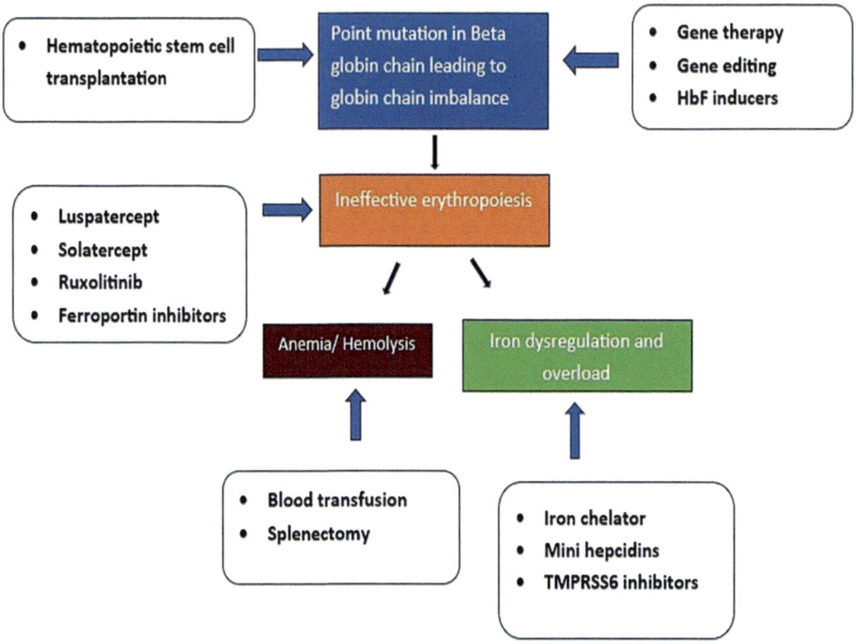

Fig. 7.6 Summary of mechanism of actions of different treatment modalities in thalassemia

7.5.3 Management in Pregnancy

Accordingly, the management of pregnancy in women with thalassemia syndromes necessitates a coordinated multidisciplinary approach to optimize maternal and fetal outcomes.

7.5.4 Preconception Optimization in Patients with Thalassaemia [25–27]

(a) Optimization of patient health
(b) Individuals with TDT and NTDT should be encouraged to seek preconception counseling to discuss their reproductive plans and to recognize the significance of screening their partner for hemoglobinopathy carrier status.

7.5.5 Transfusion-Dependent Patients

Fertility preservation and the importance of effective iron chelation should be addressed, as patients who are well-chelated have pregnancy outcomes similar to those without thalassemia.

- From adolescence onward, routine consultations with patients and their families should emphasize that effective iron chelation may preserve fertility, while restoration of fertility after impairment remains uncertain and inadequately supported by evidence.
- Outside pregnancy, standard iron chelation options include deferoxamine (DFO), deferiprone (DFP), and deferasirox (DFX), used either as monotherapy or in combination.
- Before attempting conception, it is advisable to transition from DFP or DFX to DFO approximately 6–12 weeks in advance.
- Preconception targets should include normalization of cardiac T2* values (>20 ms) and, where feasible, reduction of liver iron concentration to below 7 mg/g dry weight.
- Male patients with infertility requiring hormone replacement therapy (HRT) should focus on maintaining controlled iron levels and can continue their iron chelation therapy during sperm production induction

7.5.6 *Non-transfusion-Dependent Patients*

- The majority of these individuals retain normal fertility and typically do not encounter significant thalassemia-related difficulties with conception
- For women who may become pregnant, the potential need for red blood cell transfusions during pregnancy should be carefully evaluated
- Red cell genotyping and phenotyping, along with a review of any previously formed antibodies, are essential. If alloantibodies are present, more precise blood matching should be considered to minimize the risk of developing additional antibodies during pregnancy

7.5.7 *Pregnancy in Patients Who Have Received Allogeneic Stem Cell Transplant [28, 29]*

- Individuals and families evaluating allogeneic stem cell transplantation (ASCT) should be counseled regarding the possible effects on fertility and referred to reproductive specialists to discuss fertility preservation strategies.
- Female patients may consider oocyte vitrification, embryo freezing, or ovarian tissue preservation before undergoing ASCT.
- Sperm cryopreservation is an option for post-pubertal males prior to initiation of transplant conditioning; preservation of testicular tissue is currently under investigation as a potential future fertility-preserving strategy.
- Patients who have undergone HSCT should be offered genetic counseling, as they remain capable of transmitting the thalassemia gene to their children.
- Because late complications such as diabetes mellitus and thyroid dysfunction may occur following HSCT, ongoing surveillance in dedicated long-term follow-up clinics is recommended.

7.5.8 Evaluation and Management of Patients with Hypogonadism Requiring Induction of Spermatogenesis [30]

- Evaluation of gonadal function should be undertaken in all individuals with thalassemia beginning at puberty, preferably in coordination with pediatric endocrinology specialists.
- To initiate puberty, combined gonadotropin therapy may be used and is often preferred over testosterone replacement, as it better supports testicular growth and improves quality of life. Testosterone can be introduced later if needed.
- For patients undergoing gonadotropin therapy to stimulate sperm production, treatment response should be closely monitored and the dosages may need to be adjusted, or additional therapies added based on progress.
- If spermatogenesis has been achieved but pregnancy does not occur within 12 months—earlier if the female partner is aged 35 years or above—assisted reproductive technologies should be explored.
- In cases where azoospermia persists after 24 months of combined hCG and hMG therapy, and microsurgical testicular sperm extraction (microTESE) is not being considered, gonadotropin therapy may be discontinued and testosterone replacement initiated.

7.5.9 Evaluation and Management of Patients with Hypogonadism Requiring Induction of Ovulation [31]

- A detailed evaluation of fertility in both partners should be performed prior to initiating ovulation induction.
- Patients should receive comprehensive counseling regarding their individualized risk profile, including risks associated with assisted reproduction, the specific thalassemia phenotype, and any coexisting medical conditions.
- If conception does not occur after six treatment cycles, the case should be reviewed by a multidisciplinary team (MDT).
- There is always a risk of multiple pregnancies, so a trigger injection should not be given if more than two follicles larger than 14 mm are seen on the day of the trigger—unless the patient has received detailed and documented counseling.

7.5.10 Management of Pregnant Patients [6, 32, 33]

- Pregnant women with thalassemia should be reviewed monthly up to 28 weeks of gestation, after which follow-up visits should be scheduled every 2 weeks.
- A multidisciplinary team (MDT) should oversee both routine and specialized antenatal care.

- Initiate folic acid supplementation at 5 mg daily prior to conception to reduce the risk of neural tube defects, and maintain it throughout pregnancy.
- Begin low-dose aspirin (75–150 mg daily) starting at 12 weeks of gestation.
- Provide an early viability ultrasound between 7 and 9 weeks.
- Perform fetal growth scans every 4 weeks beginning at 24 weeks of gestation.
- Arrange for an anesthetic evaluation during the third trimester.

7.5.11 Blood Transfusion [6, 8]

- The aim is to keep pre-transfusion hemoglobin levels above 100 g/L to help prevent complications for both mother and baby.
- In some cases, early intervention may help lower the risk of fetal growth restriction (FGR), though this is not guaranteed for all patients.
- For asymptomatic patients with non-transfusion-dependent thalassemia (NTDT), it's important to have a clearly defined transfusion plan included in their obstetric care plan for the later stages of pregnancy.

7.5.12 Thromboprophylaxis [34]

- Patients with thalassemia who have had a splenectomy or present with a platelet count above 600×10^9/L should receive thromboprophylaxis with low-molecular-weight heparin (LMWH) in addition to daily low-dose aspirin (75–150 mg).
- LMWH prophylaxis should be considered from 28 weeks of gestation until 6 weeks after delivery, or throughout pregnancy if there are additional risk factors.
- All pregnant women with thalassemia should receive LMWH during any hospital stays.

7.5.13 Iron Chelation Therapy [35]

- Pregnant patients with known myocardial iron overload should have a cardiology evaluation during the first trimester.
- If no imaging has been done in the year before conception, assessments of iron levels and heart function should be performed.
- Women with myocardial iron accumulation should have ongoing cardiology follow-up throughout pregnancy, with close monitoring of ejection fraction, as any signs of heart failure may require chelation treatment.
- For patients without myocardial iron overload, a cardiology review should take place early in the third trimester to help plan for delivery.

- Any pregnant woman experiencing palpitations should be assessed for possible arrhythmias.
- Pregnant patients at high risk for heart failure (cardiac T2* <10 ms) should begin low-dose subcutaneous desferrioxamine (20 mg/kg/day) 4–5 days per week, starting between 20 and 24 weeks of gestation, under combined supervision of hematology and cardiology teams.

7.5.14 Intrapartum Care [36, 37]

- Inform the multidisciplinary team (MDT)—including senior midwife, obstetrician, anesthetist, and hematology staff—upon admission to the delivery suite.
- If red cell antibodies are present or hemoglobin is below 10 g/dL, perform a blood cross-match on admission; otherwise, a blood group and save sample is sufficient.
- For patients with transfusion-dependent thalassemia (TDT), administer 2 g of IV deferoxamine (DFO) over 24 hours during labor.
- Continuous electronic fetal heart rate monitoring is recommended throughout labor.
- Actively manage the third stage of labor to minimize blood loss.

7.5.15 Postpartum Care [38]

- Breastfeeding should be promoted, since DFO is not absorbed orally, and DFO infusions should be continued postpartum until hospital discharge.
- Administer subcutaneous DFO at 40–60 mg/kg/day, 5 days per week, during the first 6 weeks after delivery.
- If the patient is not breastfeeding, resume the pre-pregnancy chelation regimen as soon as possible.
- Women who have had a splenectomy should receive LMWH for 6 weeks following delivery.
- For hypogonadal patients, consider prescribing low-dose estradiol-only hormone replacement therapy (HRT) to support breastfeeding.

7.5.16 Contraception

All contraceptive methods are generally suitable, and the selection should be personalized to ensure optimal effectiveness and adherence.

7.6 Monitoring [8]

Routine monitoring of thalassemia patients is summarized in Table 7.1.

Table 7.1 Routine monitoring of thalassemia patients

Children and adolescents	
Frequency	*Evaluation/investigation*
Monthly	CBC with PBS
Every 3 months	Height, weight, growth velocity, Tanner staging (after 11 years)
Every 6 months	Serum ferritin, LFT, urea, creatinine, HBsAg, anti-HCV Ab, HIV 1/2 Ab
Annually	FT4, TSH, LH, FSH, GH, serum calcium, vitamin D3, bone age, assessment for skeletal deformities
Every 2 years	Bone mineral density (after 10 years of age)
If clinically indicated	MRI of the hypothalamic–pituitary region
Adults	
Monthly	CBC with PBS, monitoring for transfusion reactions, BP, pulse, SpO_2
Every 3 months	Serum ferritin, LFT, urea, creatinine, HBsAg, anti-HCV Ab, HIV 1/2 Ab
Every 6 months	Vitamin D3, serum calcium, uric acid, FT4, TSH
Annually	Audiometry, ophthalmoscopy, USG whole abdomen, ECG, echocardiography, liver FibroScan, cardiac MRI T2*, estradiol/testosterone, LH, FSH, OGTT
Every 2 years	DXA scan, echocardiographic TRV
If clinically indicated	Lateral spine X-ray (MRI spine if extramedullary hematopoiesis suspected), HAV & HEV Ab, anti-HBs Ab titer (pre-vaccination), PT, APTT, fibrinogen, D-dimer, CRP, blood & urine examination, AFP, MRI hypothalamic–pituitary region, DCT

Abbreviations: *AFP* alpha-fetoprotein, *APTT* activated partial thromboplastin time, *BP* blood pressure, *CBC* complete blood count, *CRP* C-reactive protein, *DCT* direct Coombs test, *D-dimer* fibrin degradation product, *DXA* dual-energy X-ray absorptiometry, *ECG* electrocardiogram, *FSH* follicle-stimulating hormone, *FT4* free thyroxine, *GH* growth hormone, *HAV* hepatitis A virus, *HBsAb* hepatitis B surface antibody, *HBsAg* hepatitis B surface antigen, *HCV* hepatitis C virus, *HEV* hepatitis E virus, *HIV* human immunodeficiency virus, *LH* luteinizing hormone, *LFT* liver function test, *MRI* magnetic resonance imaging, *OGTT* oral glucose tolerance test, *PBS* peripheral blood smear, *PT* prothrombin time, SpO_2 peripheral oxygen saturation, *TRV* tricuspid regurgitant velocity, *TSH* thyroid-stimulating hormone, *USG* ultrasonography

7.6.1 *Monitoring During Pregnancy [39]*

A. *Preconception*

- Cardiac function—Electrocardiogram, echocardiogram
- Liver function—Serum ferritin, alanine/aspartate aminotransferase, bilirubin
- Iron burden—Liver MRI with iron quantification in mg/gram dry weight, Cardiac MRI with T2* in ms
- Gallstones screen—Abdominal ultrasound
- Endocrinopathies—Calcium and vitamin D levels, Bone DXA scan, Glucose tolerance test, fructosamine, thyroid function
- Infections—Screen for hepatitis B, hepatitis C, and HIV infection; assess rubella antibody status; and review immunization records with administration of any indicated vaccines
- Partner screening—test partner and offer genetic counselling where indicated
- Fertility evaluation—referral to fertility expert

B. *Antenatal care:* Summarized in Table 7.2

Table 7.2 Scheme of antenatal care in thalassemia patients

Early pregnancy	Multidisciplinary team (MDT) consultation, including an obstetrician, hematologist, cardiologist, and endocrinologist: Evaluate the patient's endocrine function, liver health, and heart condition Provide education on pregnancy management in thalassemia Review the partner's test results If applicable, discuss prenatal diagnostic options based on partner screening Perform initial blood work and screen for any infections Recommend daily folic acid supplementation (5 mg) and prescribe penicillin prophylaxis for patients without a spleen Assess risk for venous thromboembolism (VTE) and initiate low-dose aspirin therapy Review and update immunization records as needed
7–9 weeks	Viability scan to confirm pregnancy
11–14 weeks	First-trimester ultrasound scan, including nuchal translucency
16 weeks	MDT evaluation Standard antenatal care in accordance with NICE guidelines [36] Perform glucose tolerance test (GTT)
20 weeks	MDT review Second-trimester ultrasound for fetal anatomy
20–24 weeks	Assess cardiac iron overload If cardiac MRI T2* <10 ms, start low-dose deferoxamine If cardiac MRI T2* >20 ms, continue monitoring without deferoxamine Assess thyroid function
24 weeks	MDT evaluation Ultrasound assessment for fetal biometric measurements

(continued)

Table 7.2 (continued)

26–28 weeks	GTT for non-diabetic patients If diabetic Obtain monthly fructosamine level Aim for fructosamine level <300 nmol/L
28 weeks	MDT evaluation Ultrasound assessment for fetal biometric measurements Cardiology evaluation to assist in delivery planning Consideration of venous thromboembolism prophylaxis
30 weeks	Standard antenatal care in accordance with NICE guidelines [36]
32 weeks	Ultrasound assessment to monitor fetal growth and amniotic fluid levels
34 weeks	Routine assessment
36 weeks	MDT evaluation Ultrasound assessment to monitor fetal growth and amniotic fluid levels Determination of the optimal timing and mode of delivery, along with appropriate analgesia planning Obstetric anesthetic review for potential complications during delivery, especially in patients with skeletal deformities that may impact epidural anesthesia Cross-match blood and prepare for delivery Discontinue aspirin
38 weeks	Routine review, consider induction of labor if diabetic
40 weeks	Routine review and discussion on induction if not yet delivered

7.7 Summary

Effective thalassemia care requires a lifelong, multidisciplinary strategy aimed at enhancing quality of life, minimizing complications, and promoting sustained overall health. Key components include

- Accurate diagnosis and classification into TDT or NTDT forms
- Regular blood transfusions for TDT patients to maintain adequate hemoglobin levels
- Iron overload management through iron chelation therapy to protect vital organs (heart, liver, endocrine glands)
- Routine monitoring of cardiac, hepatic, and endocrine functions
- Infection prevention, including vaccinations and prophylactic antibiotics when needed
- Psychosocial support and patient education for self-care and treatment adherence
- Genetic counseling and reproductive health support to prevent transmission and guide family planning
- Multidisciplinary care involving hematologists, cardiologists, endocrinologists, and other specialists

During pregnancy, a multidisciplinary approach aimed at improving patient outcomes and ensuring safe maternal and fetal health is of utmost importance. Care includes tailored treatment for both TDT and NTDT, regular monitoring for complications—especially iron overload—and maintaining organ function (cardiac, hepatic, and endocrine). Pre-pregnancy planning is crucial, with assessments of the patient's health status and partner screening to evaluate genetic risk. Patients are educated on reproductive health, and prenatal diagnostic options are discussed when appropriate. Throughout pregnancy, ongoing monitoring by a team including obstetricians, hematologists, cardiologists, and endocrinologists is essential. Preventive measures such as folic acid supplementation, infection screening, thrombosis risk management, and vaccination updates are also important. Recent therapeutic advances, including the availability of oral iron chelators and non-invasive monitoring modalities, have enhanced survival and overall well-being, allowing an increasing number of women with thalassemia to pursue and achieve successful pregnancies. The overall goal is to support safe pregnancies, deliver healthy babies, and reduce the risk of thalassemia in future generations through education and genetic counseling.

References

1. Weatherall DJ, Clegg JB. Thalassemia: a global public health problem. Nat Med. 1996;2:847–9.
2. Olivieri NF, Pakbaz Z, Vichinsky E. Hb E/beta-thalassaemia: a common & clinically diverse disorder. Indian J Med Res. 2011;134(4):522–31.
3. Rees DC, Styles L, Vichinsky EP, Clegg JB, Weatherall DJ. The hemoglobin E syndromes. Ann N Y Acad Sci. 1998;850:334–43.
4. Cunningham MJ, Macklin EA, Neufeld EJ, Cohen AR, Thalassemia Clinical Research Network. Complications of β-thalassemia major in North America. Blood. 2004;104(1):34–9.
5. Borgna-Pignatti CA, Rugolotto SI, De Stefano P, Zhao HU, Cappellini MD, Del Vecchio GC, et al. Survival and complications in patients with thalassemia major treated with transfusion and deferoxamine. Haematologica. 2004;89(10):1187–93.
6. Shah FT, Nicolle S, Garg M, Pancham S, Lieberman G, Anthony K, et al. Guideline for the management of conception and pregnancy in thalassaemia syndromes: a British society for haematology guideline. Br J Haematol. 2024;204(6):2194–209.
7. Walker EH, Whelton MJ, Beaven GH. Successful pregnancy in a patient with thalassaemia major. BJOG Int J Obstet Gynaecol. 1969;76(6):549–53.
8. Farmakis D, Porter J, Taher A, Cappellini MD, Angastiniotis M, Eleftheriou A. 2021 Thalassaemia International Federation guidelines for the management of transfusion-dependent thalassemia. Hema. 2022;6(8):e732.
9. Origa R, Piga A, Quarta G, Forni GL, Longo F, Melpignano A, et al. Pregnancy and β-thalassemia: an Italian multicenter experience. Haematologica. 2009;95(3):376.
10. Voskaridou E, Balassopoulou A, Boutou E, Komninaka V, Christoulas D, Dimopoulou M, et al. Pregnancy in beta-thalassemia intermedia: 20-year experience of a Greek thalassemia center. Eur J Haematol. 2014;93(6):492–9.
11. Brenner B. Haemostatic changes in pregnancy. Thromb Res. 2004;114(5–6):409–14.
12. James AH. Thrombosis in pregnancy and maternal outcomes. Birth Defects Res C Embryo Today. 2015;105(3):159–66.
13. Cappellini M-D, Cohen A, Eleftheriou A, Piga A, Porter J, Taher A. Guidelines for the clinical management of thalassaemia. Nicosia: Thalassaemia International Federation; 2013.
14. Karimi M. Hydroxyurea in the management of thalassemia intermedia. Hemoglobin. 2009;33(sup1):S177–82.

15. Bohara VV, Ray S, Chakrabarti P, Ray SS, Nath UK, Chaudhuri U. Optimizing the dose of hydroxyurea therapy for patients with β-thalassemia intermedia (Hb E-β-thalassemia): a single center study from eastern India. Hemoglobin. 2014;38(1):44–8.
16. Olivieri NF. Treatment strategies for hemoglobin E beta-thalassemia. Blood Rev. 2012;26:S28–30.
17. Ramanan V, Kelkar K. Role of thalidomide in treatment of beta thalassemia. J Blood Disord Med. 2017;3(1):8–10.
18. Jain M, Chakrabarti P, Dolai TK, Ghosh P, Mandal PK, Baul SN, et al. Comparison of efficacy and safety of thalidomide vs hydroxyurea in patients with Hb E-β thalassemia-a pilot study from a tertiary care Centre of India. Blood Cell Mol Dis. 2021;88:102544.
19. Anurathapan U, Pakakasama S, Songdej D, Pongphitcha P, Chuansumrit A, Andersson BS, et al. Haploidentical hematopoietic stem cell transplantation in thalassemia. Hemoglobin. 2022;46(1):2–6.
20. Breda L, Rivella S, Zuccato C, Gambari R. Combining gene therapy and fetal hemoglobin induction for treatment of β-thalassemia. Expert Rev Hematol. 2013;6(3):255–64.
21. Canver MC, Orkin SH. Customizing the genome as therapy for the β-hemoglobinopathies. Blood. 2016;127(21):2536–45.
22. Mirza A, Ritsert ML, Tao G, Thakar H, Lobitz S, Heine S, et al. Gene therapy in transfusion-dependent non-β0/β0 genotype β-thalassemia: first real-world experience of beti-cel. Blood Adv. 2025;9(1):29–38.
23. El-Beshlawy A, El-Ghamrawy M. Recent trends in treatment of thalassemia. Blood Cell Mol Dis. 2019;76:53–8.
24. https://www.centerwatch.com/clinical-trials/listings/NCT05891249/a-study-to-evaluate-the-safety-and-effectiveness-of-luspatercept-for-the-treatment-of-transfusion-dependent-td-anemia-associated-with-myelodysplastic-syndromes-mds-beta-thalassemia-b-thal-in-india
25. Aessopos A, Karabatsos F, Farmakis D, Katsantoni A, Hatziliami A, Youssef J, et al. Pregnancy in patients with well-treated β-thalassemia: outcome for mothers and newborn infants. Am J Obstet Gynecol. 1999;180(2):360–5.
26. Vlachodimitropoulou E, Thomas A, Shah F, Kyei-Mensah A. Pregnancy and iron status in β-thalassaemia major and intermedia: six years' experience in a North London Hospital. J Obstet Gynaecol. 2018;38(4):567–70.
27. Singer ST, Vichinsky EP. Deferoxamine treatment during pregnancy: is it harmful? Am J Hematol. 1999;60(1):24–6.
28. Picton HM, Wyns C, Anderson RA, Goossens E, Jahnukainen K, Kliesch S, et al. A European perspective on testicular tissue cryopreservation for fertility preservation in prepubertal and adolescent boys. Hum Reprod. 2015;30(11):2463–75.
29. Rahal I, Galambrun C, Bertrand Y, Garnier N, Paillard C, Frange P, et al. Late effects after hematopoietic stem cell transplantation for β-thalassemia major: the French national experience. Haematologica. 2018;103(7):1143.
30. Liu PY, Baker HG, Jayadev V, Zacharin M, Conway AJ, Handelsman DJ. Induction of spermatogenesis and fertility during gonadotropin treatment of gonadotropin-deficient infertile men: predictors of fertility outcome. J Clin Endocrinol Metabol. 2009;94(3):801–8.
31. Yasmin E, Davies M, Conway G, Balen AH. British Fertility Society: 'Ovulation induction in WHO Type 1 anovulation: guidelines for practice' Produced on behalf of the BFS Policy and Practice Committee. Hum Fertil. 2013;16(4):228–34.
32. De-Regil LM, Peña-Rosas JP, Fernández-Gaxiola AC, Rayco-Solon P. Effects and safety of periconceptional oral folate supplementation for preventing birth defects. Cochrane Database Syst Rev. 2015;2015(12):CD007950.
33. Hoffman MK, Goudar SS, Kodkany BS, Metgud M, Somannavar M, Okitawutshu J, et al. Low-dose aspirin for the prevention of preterm delivery in nulliparous women with a singleton pregnancy (ASPIRIN): a randomised, double-blind, placebo-controlled trial. Lancet. 2020;395(10220):285–93.

34. Sultan AA, West J, Tata LJ, Fleming KM, Nelson-Piercy C, Grainge MJ. Risk of first venous thromboembolism in pregnant women in hospital: population based cohort study from England. BMJ. 2013;347:f6099.
35. Davis BA, Porter JB. Long-term outcome of continuous 24-hour deferoxamine infusion via indwelling intravenous catheters in high-risk β-thalassemia. Blood. 2000;95:1229–36.
36. guideline NG201 NI. Antenatal care. Health economics. 2021.
37. Ansari S, Kivan AA, Tabaroki A. Pregnancy in patients treated for beta thalassemia major in two centers (Ali Asghar Children's Hospital and Thalassemia Clinic): outcome for mothers and newborn infants. Pediatr Hematol Oncol. 2006;23(1):33–7.
38. Macdonald C, Sharma S, Kallioinen M, Jewell D. Postnatal care: new NICE guideline for the 'Cinderella service'. Br J Gen Pract. 2021;71(710):394–5.
39. Musallam KM, Cappellini MD, Porter JB, Farmakis D, Eleftheriou A, Angastiniotis M, et al. TIF guidelines for the management of transfusion-dependent β-thalassemia. HemaSphere. 2025;9(3):e70095.

Chapter 8
Comprehensive Management of Sickle Cell Disorders

Amiya Ranjan Nayak and R. K. Jena

Abstract Sickle cell disease is a lifelong, multisystem disorder that affects far more than just the blood. Because of its wide-ranging complications, it requires thoughtful, individualized care delivered by a coordinated multidisciplinary team. Early diagnosis, along with preventive and supportive measures—such as vaccination, infection prophylaxis, hydroxyurea therapy, and appropriate transfusion strategies—can substantially reduce both complications and early mortality. These foundational treatments have transformed outcomes over the past few decades. For some patients, potentially curative options like hematopoietic stem cell transplantation and newer gene-based therapies offer real hope, although issues related to cost, access, and long-term safety remain important considerations. At the same time, prompt and effective management of acute complications—such as vaso-occlusive crises, acute chest syndrome, and transfusion-related problems—is essential to preserving organ function and improving survival. Special situations, including pregnancy and stroke prevention, further highlight the need for structured long-term follow-up and careful planning. Continued research, strong public health initiatives, and equitable access to emerging therapies will be critical to improving the lives of individuals living with sickle cell disease worldwide.

Keywords Sickle cell disease · Vaso-occlusive crisis · Hydroxyurea · Red cell transfusion · Bone marrow transplantation

---

A. R. Nayak · R. K. Jena (✉)
Department of Clinical Hematology, BMT & Cellular Therapy, Utkal Hospital, Bhubaneswar, India

H. P. Pati et al. (eds.), *Clinical Hematology and Hemato-Oncology*,
https://doi.org/10.1007/978-981-92-1167-8_8

Learning Objectives
- Diagnosis and confirmation of sickle cell disease (SCD)
- Clinical presentation and complications
- Management in stable condition
- Disease-modifying agents, including hydroxyurea
- Management for vaso-occlusive crisis and special situations
- Current status of red cell transfusion
- Management during high-risk situations like pregnancy, surgery, etc.
- Curative treatment like bone marrow transplantation

8.1 Introduction

Sickle cell disease (SCD) is a group of inherited blood disorders caused by a mutation in the β-globin gene. In this mutation, the amino acid glutamic acid is replaced by valine in the β-globin chain, producing hemoglobin S (HbS). According to updated HGVS nomenclature, the variant previously described as p.Glu6Val is now referred to as p.Glu7Val, reflecting revised numbering conventions that include the initial methionine residue [1]. The mutation results from a single nucleotide substitution (GAG to GTG) and follows an autosomal recessive pattern of inheritance. Individuals who carry one copy of the mutation (HbAS), commonly referred to as having sickle cell trait, are usually asymptomatic. Interestingly, this carrier state provides partial protection against severe malaria, which explains the high frequency of the mutation in malaria-endemic regions such as sub-Saharan Africa, central India, Saudi Arabia, and some parts of the Mediterranean [2]. The term sickle cell disease is reserved for individuals with genotypes that produce clinical manifestations, including chronic hemolytic anemia and recurrent vaso-occlusive crises. These include homozygous HbSS and compound heterozygous states such as HbSC, HbS/β^0-thalassemia (HbSβ^0), and HbS/β^+-thalassemia (HbSβ^+). The term sickle cell anemia is generally used for the more severe forms, particularly HbSS and HbSβ^0.

8.2 Diagnostic Overview

Chronic hemolytic anemia is the hallmark of SCD, which often manifests as mildly to moderately decreased hemoglobin and hematocrit levels along with a compensatory reticulocytosis that ranges from 3% to 15%. Elevated levels of unconjugated (indirect) bilirubin, lactate dehydrogenase (LDH), and low or nonexistent haptoglobin are laboratory markers of hemolysis. Vaso-occlusive events (VOEs) cause these indicators to deteriorate, indicating increased hemolysis. Because of functional hyposplenia or asplenia, peripheral blood smears usually show sickled red blood cells, target cells, polychromasia, and Howell-Jolly bodies.

Increased white blood cells and platelets are common in HbSS and compound heterozygous HbS β^0-thalassemia, especially in younger patients. In contrast, these counts remain normal in milder forms like HbSC and HbS β^+-thalassemia.

Hemoglobin electrophoresis or high-performance liquid chromatography (HPLC) is necessary for a definitive diagnosis of SCD in order to distinguish between types such HbS, HbC, and others [3]. Solubility tests like Sickledex are positive in both SCD and sickle cell trait but cannot distinguish between them. Electrophoresis patterns help identify specific syndromes—HbSS and HbS β^0-thalassemia show HbS predominantly, while HbSC disease presents with equal parts HbS and HbC. Microcytosis, anemia, and HbA levels aid in differentiating sickle cell trait from HbS β^+-thalassemia. Additionally, co-inheritance of alpha-thalassemia requires genetic testing. Fetal hemoglobin (HbF) levels are variably elevated and influenced by genetic background and therapies like hydroxyurea, with certain βS-haplotypes (e.g., Arab–Indian, Senegal) associated with higher baseline HbF levels [4].

8.3 General Management

8.3.1 Infection Prevention and Vaccination

Functional asplenia puts people with SCD at high risk for serious infections, particularly in those with HbSS and HbS-β^0 thalassemia from birth. Key preventive strategies include complete immunization and penicillin prophylaxis in young children. Immunization should include annual influenza vaccination, PCV-13 (one lifetime dose at age $\geq$ 18), and PPV-23 (at least two doses 5 years apart, with a third dose at age 65). Meningococcal vaccination involves at least two doses of quadrivalent conjugate vaccine with boosters every 5 years, and serogroup B vaccine as per schedule. Hepatitis B vaccine is given in three doses (0, 1, and 4 months), though routine antibody titer monitoring is not well defined. COVID-19 vaccination is also strongly advised due to higher morbidity and mortality, though exact booster intervals are evolving. Hydroxyurea does not impair vaccine response. Prophylactic penicillin is advised from 3 months to 5 years (125–250 mg twice daily), though some continue it into adulthood due to lifelong splenic dysfunction. Patients who are allergic to penicillins are treated with alternatives such as erythromycin. Every family should have a fever response strategy in place because fevers above 38.5 °C are medical emergencies that call for immediate antibiotics and blood cultures [5].

8.3.2 Nutrition

In SCD, chronic hemolysis increases the demand for folic acid, making a 1 mg/day folic acid supplementation routine [6]. Folate deficiency may lead to megaloblastic crises and elevated homocysteine, especially in children. B12 deficiency is detected in about 60% of the Indian population and should be supplemented routinely unless there is any contraindication or the level is high. Deficiencies in nutrients like zinc, vitamin D, and calcium are common, with about half of children showing signs of osteopenia or osteoporosis. Supplementation with vitamin D, calcium, and zinc supports growth and bone health [7]. Multivitamins without iron are generally recommended.

Although iron overload from transfusions is a concern, iron deficiency still affects around 20% of children and must be diagnosed carefully, as chronic hemolysis can falsely elevate serum iron markers.

8.3.3 Blood Transfusion

Blood transfusion is not the primary modality of treatment, especially in stable conditions. The majority of patients (about 90%) can be managed with no or occasional transfusion when treated with hydroxyurea or other supportive therapies. Because of the high incidence of all-antibodies production and other complications peculiar to SCD, it should be administered judiciously in approved indications following extended cross-matching and other standard operating procedures.

In SCD, blood transfusion improves oxygen delivery, dilutes sickled red cells, and suppresses HbS production. It is used in both acute events (like acute chest syndrome, VOCs, splenic sequestration, or perioperative care) and for chronic indications such as stroke prevention. Simple (top-up) or exchange (manual or automated) transfusions can be administered sporadically or often. In order to prevent stroke, HbS levels should be kept below 30%, and for other issues, below 50%. Hb should be kept between 10 and 11 g/dL. A straightforward transfusion to increase hemoglobin to 10 g/dL is typically advised for surgical procedures in patients with HbSS or HbS-β^0 thalassemia [8]. If the baseline Hb is already >10 g/dL, exchange transfusion (often via RBC apheresis) is preferred to avoid hyperviscosity. Chronic transfusions, particularly partial exchanges, help limit iron overload. However, transfusion-related risks include alloimmunization, delayed hemolytic reactions, iron overload, and infections. Alloimmunization affects up to 30% of patients and is reduced by transfusing leukoreduced, extended phenotype-matched blood (matched for antigens such as C, D, E, Kell, Kidd, and Duffy) [9]. RH genotype diversity and ethnic mismatches complicate compatibility, sometimes requiring molecular-level matching. Despite better blood screening, infection risks still exist, and leukoreduction remains essential.

8.3.4 Hydroxyurea (HU) Therapy

Hydroxyurea (also known as hydroxycarbamide) remains the cornerstone of treatment for patients with stable sickle cell disease. It works by increasing fetal hemoglobin levels, which helps reduce red blood cell sickling and decreases inflammation-driven vaso-occlusion. As a result, patients experience fewer painful crises and other complications, leading to better quality of life and improved survival—particularly in those with more severe genotypes such as HbSS and sickle β-thalassemia.

Hydroxyurea is the first medication to get FDA approval for sickle cell disease in 1998, after showing a reduction in pain crises in adults. It inhibits ribonucleotide reductase and lowers HbS% by increasing β-globin production, which raises fetal hemoglobin (HbF) levels. Initial adult trials [10], followed by the Baby HUG trial in children and later in infants, confirmed its efficacy [11].

The Multicenter Study of Hydroxyurea (MSH), which included 299 patients, showed clear long-term survival benefits with hydroxyurea therapy over 17 years of follow-up [12]. Mortality rates steadily declined with longer exposure to the drug. Patients who had never received hydroxyurea had 5 deaths per 100 person-years, while those treated for less than 5 years had 6.8 deaths. With 5–10 years of therapy, the rate dropped to 4.4 deaths, and further declined to 1.8 deaths among those treated for 10–15 years. Notably, no deaths were reported in patients who had received hydroxyurea for 15 years or more, highlighting the substantial long-term survival advantage associated with sustained therapy.

The research confirmed a clear survival benefit with hydroxyurea, later supported by other research. A 17-year prospective study from Greece in SCD patients over 16 showed similar outcomes—fewer pain and ACS episodes, reduced transfusions and hospitalizations, and improved survival compared to standard care. Pediatric data over 15 years also support its safety and effectiveness, showing no major risks to growth, development, fertility, or cancer risk [11].

Evidence from 21 observational studies (3378 adults, 24–96 months follow-up) consistently showed 60–90% fewer pain crises, 90–100% fewer hospitalizations, and a 4–20% rise in HbF. A meta-analysis in children found HbF increased from 5–10% to 15–20%, hemoglobin levels rose, hospitalizations dropped by 56–87%, and pain episodes significantly reduced [13]. By reducing increased cerebral blood flow, hydroxyurea decreased the risk of stroke in children, according to a phase III multinational trial. After 10.1 months, TCD velocities increased by 10.2 cm/sec in the observation group and decreased by 15.5 cm/sec with hydroxyurea ($P = 0.02$) [14].

8.3.4.1 Dose of HU

Hydroxyurea is usually started at a dose calculated according to body weight and then increased gradually, typically every 8 weeks, by about 5 mg/kg/day until either a good clinical response is achieved or the maximum tolerated dose (MTD) is reached. In most patients, the dose can be increased up to around 35 mg/kg/day with careful monitoring. The aim is to identify the lowest dose that provides meaningful benefit, although many clinicians prefer to escalate to the MTD to maximize response. Studies from India have shown that even a starting dose of 10 mg/kg/day can be highly effective, reducing pain episodes in about 92% of patients and lowering transfusion requirements in 87% [15–17]. This dose is commonly recommended as the initial starting point, with a 50% dose reduction advised for patients with chronic kidney disease. In infants and young children who cannot swallow capsules, the capsule can be opened and mixed with a small amount of food to facilitate administration.

8.3.4.2 HU Dose Escalation and Toxicity

When increasing the dose of hydroxyurea, it is important to ensure that blood counts remain within safe limits. Before any dose escalation, the absolute neutrophil count (ANC) should be above 1000/μL, the absolute reticulocyte count (ARC) above 100,000/μL, and the platelet count above 150,000/μL. The maximum tolerated dose (MTD) is generally considered to be reached when mild, stable marrow suppression is achieved—typically reflected by an ANC between 1500 and 3000/μL, an ARC between 80,000 and 100,000/μL, or a platelet count between 80,000 and 100,000/μL.

Hydroxyurea toxicity should be suspected if counts fall below safe thresholds: an ANC below 1500/μL (or below 1000/μL in children under 2 years), an ARC below 80,000/μL, or platelets below 80,000/μL. In such cases, the drug is usually withheld temporarily and resumed once counts recover.

Interestingly, a study from Odisha reported that a fixed low dose of 10 mg/kg/day without dose escalation was both effective and well tolerated. This approach required less frequent laboratory monitoring, was more economical, and showed good patient adherence without significant adverse effects [15], making it a practical option in resource-limited settings.

8.3.4.3 Monitoring of Patient While on HU Therapy

Patients receiving hydroxyurea should undergo regular monitoring to ensure both safety and effectiveness of therapy. A complete blood count (CBC) with differential, platelet count, and reticulocyte count is typically checked every 2–3 months. Kidney function (serum creatinine) and liver function tests are usually monitored every 6–12 months. Serum ferritin and HbF levels are generally assessed once a year to evaluate iron status and treatment response. Pregnancy testing should be performed when clinically appropriate. If signs of hematologic toxicity develop, such as significant cytopenia's, the CBC should be monitored weekly until blood counts recover. Once stable, hydroxyurea can be restarted at a lower dose with continued careful follow-up.

8.3.4.4 Duration of HU Therapy

HU can be continued long term if it is well tolerated and providing benefit. If the response is inadequate, adherence should be carefully reviewed, and the patient should have received the MTD for at least 6 months before considering discontinuation. Before labeling a patient as a non-responder, compliance, dose, and duration must be confirmed, reversible causes such as iron or vitamin B12 deficiency should be excluded, and addition of erythropoiesis-stimulating agents may be considered. If there is still no response, hydroxyurea can then be stopped.

8.3.4.5 Barriers for Use of Hydroxyurea

Despite its well-established benefits in sickle cell disease, hydroxyurea remains underutilized, and addressing barriers to its optimal use is essential. Common challenges include hesitancy among healthcare providers regarding long-term safety, patient fears about potential carcinogenic or teratogenic effects, and difficulties with daily adherence. Regular laboratory monitoring requirements, lack of child-friendly formulations, cost, and limited availability in remote areas also contribute to suboptimal use. Removing these barriers is crucial to ensuring that more patients can benefit from this effective therapy.

8.3.5 Adjuvant Drugs with Benefits

For sickle cell disease patients older than five who still have vaso-occlusive crises (VOCs) after using hydroxyurea, or who are unable to take it, L-glutamine (Endari), an oral medication, was licensed in 2017. It is believed to reduce oxidative stress in red blood cells and is taken twice daily, with dosage adjusted by body weight [18]. Regardless of concurrent hydroxyurea treatment, a large clinical trial showed that it decreased the risk of acute chest syndrome, hospital stays, and pain episodes. With only a few minor gastrointestinal side effects, the medication is usually well taken. However, its long-term benefits remain unclear, and practical challenges such as high cost and the need to mix it with food or drink may limit its use.

If hydroxyurea or L-glutamine are not effective, those with SCD who are 16 years of age or older and have recurrent VOCs may be eligible for Crizanlizumab, a monoclonal antibody that targets P-selectin. In weeks 0 and 2, as well as thereafter every 4 weeks, it is administered intravenously at a dose of 5 mg/kg. The SUSTAIN trial demonstrated a significant reduction in VOC frequency (1.63 episodes/year vs. 2.98 with placebo) [19]. However, the STAND trial questioned its benefit, reporting only a slight difference from placebo [20]. Despite a 2023 recommendation by the European Medicines Agency to withdraw its approval, crizanlizumab may still be used pending final trial outcomes.

Voxelotor, a hemoglobin affinity modifier, is now voluntarily withdrawn from the market by the company.

8.4 Curative Therapies

8.4.1 Allogeneic Hematopoietic Stem Cell Transplantation

Patients with SCD who exhibit severe symptoms, including recurring vaso-occlusive crises, acute chest syndrome, stroke, progressive organ destruction, or transfusion-related problems such as alloimmunization are usually candidates for HSCT, a potentially curative but risky treatment. Decision-making must be personalized and involves careful discussion between patients, families, and specialists. Early referral by primary hematologists to expert transplant centers is vital to optimize timing and outcomes. Matched sibling donor (MSD) transplants remain the gold standard, particularly in children, with overall survival rates exceeding 95% and event-free survival above 85% [21]. For patients lacking MSDs, recent trials have demonstrated encouraging results with haploidentical related donor HCT using non-myeloablative regimens (e.g., fludarabine, thiotepa, ATG, cyclophosphamide, & reduced-dose total body irradiation), achieving 1- and 2-year overall survival rates of 96% & 94%, respectively, in a 2024 study involving 70 patients, with graft failure mostly limited to younger children [22].

Another 2025 study on 42 adolescents and adults showed similar success with 2-year survival of 95% and event-free survival of 88%, and low rates of severe GvHD [23]. Meanwhile, matched unrelated donor (MUD) transplants have traditionally carried high risks of mortality and chronic GvHD, though newer pilot studies incorporating abatacept and reduced intensity conditioning have yielded promising outcomes, with 100% survival and 93% SCD-free survival in a small cohort [24].

8.4.2 Gene Therapy

By altering a patient's own hematopoietic stem cells (HSCs), gene therapy provides a revolutionary way to treat sickle cell disease (SCD) without the need for donor cells and without the dangers of graft-versus-host disease. Two FDA-approved therapies—*lovotibeglogene autotemcel* (Lyfgenia), which introduces an anti-sickling beta globin gene (T87Q variant), and *exagamglogene autotemcel* (Casgevy), which disrupts BCL11A to increase fetal hemoglobin (Hb F)—represent the two major strategies: gene addition and gene editing. Both therapies require myeloablative conditioning (typically busulfan) and autologous transplantation. These interventions aim to increase anti-sickling hemoglobins like Hb F or Hb A2, thereby reducing vaso-occlusive episodes and improving hemoglobin levels [25, 26]. However, potential risks—particularly the unclear risk of myeloid malignancy and transplant-related toxicity—remain concerns. Additionally, cost, access, and equity considerations are crucial in implementing these therapies. The optimal approach must be individualized based on clinical context, genetic background (e.g., alpha thalassemia, baseline Hb F), and shared decision-making with the patient.

8.5 Management of Specific Scenarios

8.5.1 Management of Acute Vaso-occlusive Crisis

A vaso-occlusive crisis (VOC), as defined by the Cooperative Study of Sickle Cell Disease (CSSCD), is a pain episode lasting at least 2 hours that leads to a clinic visit or hospitalization. It is often one of the earliest clinical manifestations of sickle cell disease, occurring in more than 25% of patients and becoming increasingly common after the age of 2 years. VOCs are more frequent in individuals with the HbSS genotype, lower fetal hemoglobin (HbF), and higher baseline hemoglobin. Peak incidence is observed between ages 19 and 39 [27]. The abdomen, arms, chest, and back are common places to experience pain. Dactylitis can manifest in infants and toddlers [28]. As there are no specific lab or clinical signs of VOC, diagnosis relies heavily on patient history and symptom recognition.

Initial evaluation should focus on identifying triggers and excluding complications like infection, dehydration, acute chest syndrome, anemia, stroke, cholecystitis, splenic sequestration, or priapism. Age-appropriate pain assessment instruments should be used, such as a visual analog scale for elderly patients or the Wong-Baker FACES scale for youngsters [29]. The treatment should be adjusted based on severity.

Management of pain during VOC is mainly by non-opioid analgesics. Opioid analgesics are not readily available in most parts of the country due to their regulatory restrictions and thus, should be considered as reserved drugs for resistant cases in tertiary care centers. For mild to moderate pain, NSAIDs and acetaminophen are first-line options. Ketorolac is an effective NSAID but must be used cautiously in patients with renal dysfunction, peptic ulcers, asthma, or bleeding risk. Opioids are essential for moderate to severe pain, with morphine as the preferred agent. A loading dose of 0.1 mg/kg can be given every 20 minutes until pain is controlled, followed by maintenance doses (0.05–0.15 mg/kg) every 2–4 hours, with additional rescue doses if needed. Monitoring for respiratory depression is critical, and naloxone should be available in severe cases. Opioids should be tapered once pain is controlled and transitioned to oral formulations. Pethidine (meperidine) must be avoided due to its neurotoxic metabolite and seizure risk. Hydration is key, as patients with SCD are susceptible to dehydration due to impaired urine concentration. Adults should maintain an oral intake of at least 60 mL/kg/day; IV fluids are indicated when oral intake is insufficient. Urine specific gravity should ideally remain under 1.010. Although hemoglobin may drop during VOC, transfusions are not routinely necessary unless complications arise. Before discharge, patients should be prescribed oral analgesics to prevent recurrence, with tapering by 15–20% daily in those at risk for opioid dependence.

Illustrative Clinical Case 1

A 22-year-old woman with sickle cell disease was admitted for a vaso-occlusive crisis involving severe back and thigh pain. Her baseline hemoglobin was 8.5 g/dL, but on admission had dropped to 6.2 g/dL. She was transfused with two units of crossmatch-compatible, phenotype-matched packed red blood cells. Her pain improved, and she was discharged after 4 days. However, 7 days post-transfusion, she returned with fatigue, dark urine, jaundice, and worsening anemia (Hb 5.1 g/dL), with a drop below her pre-transfusion level. Laboratory evaluation revealed elevated LDH, indirect hyperbilirubinemia, a high reticulocyte count, and a newly positive direct coomb's test (DCT), suggestive of a delayed hemolytic transfusion reaction (DHTR). Extended RBC antibody testing identified a new alloantibody not detected during initial crossmatching. She was managed conservatively with hydration, folic acid, and close monitoring, while avoiding further transfusions due to the risk of hyperhemolysis. However, in critical cases, IVIG can be administered to halt further hemolysis. This case illustrates the importance of vigilance for DHTR in SCD patients, even after apparently uncomplicated transfusions.

8.5.2 Management of Anemia Exacerbation

8.5.2.1 Aplastic Crisis

Aplastic crisis is a transient halt in erythropoiesis, presenting with sudden anemia and marked reticulocytopenia (<1% or <10,000/μL), without a rise in LDH. It results in severe anemia due to ongoing hemolysis without compensatory RBC production and may cause cardiac decompensation if not promptly recognized. Parvovirus B19 is the leading cause, especially in children, accounting for up to 68% of cases. It selectively infects and destroys erythroid precursors. Bone marrow examination typically shows giant pronormoblasts with intranuclear viral inclusions, which are characteristic of parvovirus infection. Diagnosis is confirmed by parvovirus B19 PCR or serology. Other infections (e.g., *Streptococcus pneumoniae*, *Salmonella*, *EBV*) and bone marrow necrosis can also cause transient aplasia. Management involves PRBC transfusion, often a single unit, as marrow recovery usually begins within 7–10 days. In refractory parvovirus B19 cases, IVIG (intravenous immunoglobulin) can be given.

8.5.2.2 Sequestration Crisis

Acute splenic sequestration is a serious and potentially life-threatening complication of sickle cell disease. It presents with a sudden drop in hemoglobin, ongoing reticulocytosis, and a rapidly enlarging, tender spleen, sometimes accompanied by signs of hypovolemia. Platelet counts are often low, and LDH levels may be normal or elevated. It is most commonly seen in young children with HbSS, but can also occur in adults with HbSC or sickle cell–β^+ thalassemia who retain splenic function. Sequestration can occur as early as infancy and may be fatal before SCD is diagnosed, with studies reporting a 30% occurrence rate and 15% fatality among children over 10 years [30]. Management involves prompt restoration of blood volume and RBC mass to prevent hypovolemic shock. Given a 50% recurrence rate, long-term strategies include splenectomy in children over 2–3 years or chronic transfusion in younger children to delay surgery, though recurrence may still occur [31].

8.5.2.3 Delayed Hemolytic Transfusion Reaction (DHTR) and Hyperhemolysis

Delayed hemolytic transfusion reactions (DHTRs) are serious, often overlooked complications in sickle cell disease that resemble vaso-occlusive crises, making diagnosis difficult. They typically occur 4–10 days after transfusion in alloimmunized patients—about 30%—due to RH antigen diversity despite extended matching. Features include sudden hemoglobin drop, high LDH and bilirubin, hemoglobinuria, and sometimes reticulocytopenia. Severe cases may cause hyperhemolysis, worsening anemia, and organ failure. Further transfusions can aggravate hemolysis, so they should be avoided unless essential [32]. High-dose steroids, IVIG, erythropoietin, IV iron, and eculizumab are therapeutic options. Prevention depends on extended antigen matching and detailed transfusion histories.

8.5.2.4 Miscellaneous Causes

Acute infections, especially bacterial sepsis, malaria, and viral illnesses, can suppress erythropoiesis or increase hemolysis. Nutritional deficiencies, particularly of folate, vitamin B12, or iron, may contribute, although iron deficiency is uncommon due to chronic transfusions and hemolysis. Renal dysfunction, commonly seen in older SCD patients, can impair erythropoietin production and worsen anemia. Bone marrow necrosis, a rare but severe complication, presents with bone pain, leukoerythroblastic blood picture, and reticulocytopenia.

Clinical Case 2

An 18-year-old male with known homozygous sickle cell disease, on regular hydroxyurea, presented with a 2-day history of high-grade fever, left-sided pleuritic chest pain, dry cough, and dyspnea. On examination, he was febrile (101.8 °F), tachypneic (RR 28/min), hypoxic (SpO_2 89% on room air), and had reduced breath sounds with crepitations in the left lower lung zone. Investigations revealed anemia (Hb 7.2 g/dL), leukocytosis, elevated LDH and indirect bilirubin, reticulocytosis, and a new infiltrate in the left lower lobe on chest X-ray. He was diagnosed with acute chest syndrome (ACS) and started on oxygen, IV antibiotics (ceftriaxone and azithromycin), IV fluids, and analgesia. However, his clinical condition deteriorated over the next 24 hours, with worsening hypoxia and respiratory distress. In view of progressive symptoms and radiological worsening, he underwent urgent exchange transfusion, following which his oxygenation and overall clinical status significantly improved.

8.5.2.5 Acute Chest Syndrome

About 30% of people with sickle cell disease (SCD) develop acute chest syndrome (ACS), a dangerous and sometimes fatal consequence. When a new infiltrate shows up on chest imaging with symptoms including fever, chest pain, coughing, difficulty breathing, low oxygen levels, or rapid breathing, it is identified. Patients with the HbSS genotype, low fetal hemoglobin levels, elevated baseline hemoglobin, or leukocytosis are more susceptible. In adults, ACS often follows a vaso-occlusive crisis, while in children, it usually occurs after a febrile illness. The condition results from both infection and sickling-related lung injury, with pulmonary fat embolism—present in nearly half of cases—being a key factor in severe presentations. Early indicators of ACS include a drop in hemoglobin, a platelet count below 200,000/μL, and neurological signs. Due to its potential for rapid deterioration, ACS requires prompt hospital-based treatment.

Management focuses on supportive care and early intervention. Oxygen should be given to maintain saturation above 95%, along with adequate pain control and regular incentive spirometry (every 2 hours) to reduce the risk of atelectasis. Broad-spectrum antibiotics covering both typical and atypical organisms should be started promptly. In more severe cases, respiratory support may need to be escalated to noninvasive or mechanical ventilation. Transfusion therapy is crucial—simple transfusion is recommended if oxygenation worsens, hemoglobin falls below 5 g/dL, or the patient deteriorates clinically, with a target hemoglobin of about 10 g/dL (not exceeding 11 g/dL to avoid hyperviscosity).

In order to lower HbS to less than 30%, exchange transfusion is advised for patients with severe or progressive ACS, multilobar involvement, a history of severe episodes, or chronic hypoxia (oxygen saturation ≤85% or PaO_2 ≤55 mmHg).In critical cases, intensive care, repeat imaging, blood gas monitoring, and supportive measures like bronchoscopy or ECMO may be necessary. Careful fluid management is also important to maintain adequate hydration while avoiding overload.

8.5.3 Management of Neurological Complications

Neurologic complications are seen in more than 25% of SCD patients and include ischemic and hemorrhagic strokes, silent cerebral infarcts, seizures, coma, and sensorineural hearing loss. Children with SCD are 200–400 times more likely to experience a stroke than their healthy peers. Around 11% have overt strokes, while silent infarcts—seen on MRI—can be found in over half of adults and are associated with neurocognitive impairment [33]. Infarctive strokes tend to occur in children and older adults, while hemorrhagic strokes are more frequent in those aged 20–30.

Stroke prevention in SCD relies heavily on early identification and timely intervention. Transcranial Doppler (TCD) screening is used to detect elevated cerebral blood flow velocities—indicative of increased stroke risk—in children. The STOP trials demonstrated that chronic transfusion therapy in such high-risk children can reduce stroke incidence by more than 90% [34]. However, long-term transfusions come with challenges like iron overload and alloimmunization. The TWiTCH trial demonstrated that switching to HU was safe for kids who had been receiving regular transfusions for at least a year and whose TCD velocities were stabilized. With no rise in stroke or silent infarct events over a 24-month period, HU was found to be equally effective as transfusion in preserving low TCD velocities [35]. Thus, hydroxyurea is a suitable alternative for selected children with stable disease, good adherence, and access to close monitoring, particularly after initial transfusion-based stroke risk reduction.

Acute strokes in SCD require prompt neuroimaging to differentiate ischemic from hemorrhagic events, followed by partial-exchange transfusion. For secondary prevention, maintaining HbS below 30% through regular transfusion significantly reduces the risk of recurrence from 70% to around 13% [36]. Hydroxyurea may be considered in patients who cannot continue transfusions.

8.5.4 Management in Pregnancy

Preconception counseling and careful medication management are critical for optimizing pregnancy outcomes in individuals with SCD. Comprehensive evaluation should begin before conception, with multidisciplinary involvement including hematology, obstetrics, and genetics teams.

Counseling should include reproductive risk assessment based on partner hemoglobinopathy status, discussion of inheritance patterns, genetic counseling, and reproductive options such as IVF (in vitro fertilization) with preimplantation genetic testing, donor gametes, or adoption. A thorough clinical evaluation should include assessment of kidney and liver function, blood pressure measurement, screening for proteinuria, and echocardiography to look for pulmonary hypertension or elevated tricuspid regurgitation velocity. Pregnancy is generally contraindicated in women with severe pulmonary hypertension because of the high risk of maternal mortality. Immunizations should also be reviewed and updated according to current CDC and WHO recommendations. Live vaccines should be avoided during pregnancy. Hydroxyurea, a key disease-modifying agent in SCD, poses complex decisions—while animal studies suggest teratogenicity, human data are inconclusive. Some studies show increased miscarriage and low birth weight risks if continued during pregnancy, but no consistent rise in congenital anomalies. Decisions regarding continuation should be individualized using shared decision-making; those with severe disease may benefit from continuation, while those with mild SCD may choose to stop hydroxyurea prior to conception or upon pregnancy confirmation. For males, hydroxyurea's impact on fertility is reversible, and fetal risks are negligible [37]. If hydroxyurea is discontinued, regular transfusions may serve as an alternative, provided alloimmunization risks are manageable. All medications should be reviewed: ACE inhibitors, ARBs, and iron chelators should be stopped; folic acid should be supplemented at 4 mg/day throughout pregnancy due to high red cell turnover; iron should only be added if deficiency is evident. Pain must be managed effectively, with NSAIDs avoided in the third trimester. Safe analgesics, prenatal vitamins without iron (unless indicated), and malaria prophylaxis in endemic areas are essential.

Low-dose aspirin from 12 to 36 weeks helps prevent preeclampsia, and thromboprophylaxis is recommended from 28 weeks until 6 weeks postpartum [38]. Regular fetal growth monitoring and consideration for prophylactic transfusion in selected patients help mitigate risks like anemia, fetal hypoxia, and vaso-occlusive crises. During pregnancy, transfusion decisions must balance benefits—like reducing sickling and fetal hypoxia—against risks such as alloimmunization. Blood should be Rh-matched, HbS-negative, and CMV-negative. Prophylactic transfusions are reserved for women with severe symptoms or a prior poor obstetric history. Pain management is critical, and standardized protocols should be followed, avoiding pethidine due to seizure risk. Acute episodes warrant rapid assessment, proper hydration, oxygen support, and multidisciplinary input.

Intrapartum and postpartum care in SCD must be meticulously planned and multidisciplinary. Given the heightened risk of perinatal mortality, labor induction between 38 and 40 weeks is often recommended, with decisions on delivery mode based on obstetric indications and patient preferences. Continuous fetal monitoring, epidural analgesia, and antenatal anesthetic planning are vital to reduce complications. Postpartum, nearly one-fourth of women experience pain episodes; thus, hydration, oxygenation, and thromboprophylaxis with low-molecular-weight heparin are crucial [39]. Breastfeeding is encouraged, and non-estrogen contraceptive options should be discussed.

8.5.5 *Perioperative Management of Sickle Cell Disease Patients*

Patients with sickle cell disease have a higher risk of surgical complications compared with the general population. These include postoperative acute chest syndrome, infections, vaso-occlusive crises, and even increased 30-day mortality. Preoperative planning should involve a multidisciplinary team, including a hematologist familiar with SCD, an anesthesiologist, a transfusion specialist, and the surgical team. With careful optimization before surgery and close monitoring afterward, outcomes can be significantly improved.

1. Preoperative Assessment

   Before surgery, the physician should

- Confirm that all conservative treatments have been exhausted
- Evaluate the necessity of the surgical procedure
- Weigh the risks of surgery against continuing conservative care
- Consider less invasive alternatives
- Assess if surgery will help achieve the patient's personal goals and improve quality of life

Table 8.1 Risk categories of surgical procedures

Low risk	Moderate risk	High risk
Dental surgery Ocular surgery Repair of hernia Dilatation and curettage Debridement of wound Endoscopic procedure Biopsy of superficial tissues	Head and neck surgery Orthopedic procedures Urologic procedures Gall bladder surgery C-section Splenectomy and appendectomy	Thoracic surgery Surgeries with >4 hours' anesthesia requirement Major vascular procedures Spinal surgeries Neurosurgery Heart valve repairs Transplant surgeries

Decisions about surgery in patients with sickle cell disease should be made jointly by the patient and the healthcare team. The key objectives are to optimize the patient medically, assess the risk of perioperative complications, and prepare a clear management plan. Currently, no surgical risk calculators are specifically validated for SCD. Preoperative evaluation should include the patient's genotype, frequency and severity of crises, prior hospitalizations, known triggers, baseline functional status and opioid use, steady-state blood counts, and transfusion history. Surgical procedures are generally categorized as low, moderate, or high risk based on expected blood loss and potential postoperative complications (Table 8.1).

A history of stroke, acute chest syndrome, obstructive sleep apnea (OSA), prior adverse reactions to sedation, or recurrent venous thromboembolism (VTE) should be carefully documented, as these conditions increase the risk of perioperative complications. Functional status should also be assessed, typically using metabolic equivalent tasks (METs); patients unable to perform activities requiring at least 4 METs, such as climbing a flight of stairs, are considered to have higher cardiac risk [40].

2. Preoperative Transfusion

Preoperative transfusion in sickle cell disease (SCD) is intended to lower the risk of postoperative complications by raising hemoglobin levels and reducing the proportion of HbS. Because patients with SCD are at higher risk of acute chest syndrome, vaso-occlusive crises, and even perioperative mortality, transfusion—either as simple transfusion or red cell exchange (RCE)—is often considered before surgery [41]. Evidence, however, has been mixed. The TAPS trial, a multicenter randomized study of 67 patients with HbSS and HbSβ^0 thalassemia, showed significantly fewer complications in transfused patients undergoing moderate-risk surgery (15% vs. 39%, $p = 0.02$) [42]. In contrast, a smaller Saudi trial in patients undergoing cholecystectomy reported more immediate postoperative adverse events in those who received transfusion [43], and a meta-analysis found no clear overall difference in mortality or complications between transfused and non-transfused groups [44]. These findings highlight the need for an individualized approach, taking into account genotype, baseline hemoglobin, cardiopulmonary status, and surgical risk. When transfusion is used, phenotypically matched blood is recommended to reduce alloimmunization, and in patients with baseline hemoglobin above 9 g/dL, exchange

Table 8.2 Summary of pre-operative transfusion recommendations in SCD patients [7]

Genotype	Hb(g/dL)	Surgical risk	Recommendation
HbSS/ HbSβ^0	<9	Low/moderate	Simple transfusion/partial exchange/RCE
HbSS/HbSβ^0	>9	Low/moderate	Partial exchange/RCE
HbSC/HbSβ^{+}/HbSS on hydroxyurea with elevated HbF without severe phenotype	>9	Low	No transfusion
HbSC/HbSβ^{+}	>9	Moderate	Partial exchange/RCE
All genotypes		High	RCE

transfusion may be preferred to avoid exceeding 10 g/dL and increasing blood viscosity [41, 43]. Table 8.2 shows the summary of pre-operative transfusion recommendations in SCD patients.

3. Intraoperative Period

During surgery in patients with sickle cell disease, the main goal is to keep the internal environment as stable as possible. Adequate hydration, normal body temperature, stable blood pressure, proper oxygenation, and balanced acid–base status are all essential, as disturbances in any of these can trigger red cell sickling and lead to complications such as vaso-occlusive crisis, acute chest syndrome, acute kidney injury, or even stroke. To maintain good volume status, prolonged fasting without intravenous fluids should be avoided, fluid intake and output should be carefully monitored, and IV fluids should be tapered once the patient is able to drink adequately. Temperature control is equally important—extreme cold or heat should be avoided before, during, and after surgery, and active warming measures should be used when needed. Respiratory depressants should be minimized, and intubation is usually performed after paralysis with a short-acting agent to reduce stress. Induction of anesthesia should aim to avoid breath-holding, laryngospasm, or agitation. The choice between general and regional anesthesia depends on the patient's age, comorbidities, and type of surgery. While regional anesthesia may reduce oxygen delivery in some settings due to hypoperfusion or venous stasis, it can also improve oxygen tension in the anesthetized area through redistribution of blood flow, making the decision individualized for each case [45].

4. Postoperative Period

Postoperative infections are a common trigger for complications in sickle cell disease and require vigilant monitoring. Any fever of 38 °C or higher should prompt a thorough evaluation, including blood and urine cultures, careful wound examination, and a chest X-ray to identify a possible source. A fall in oxygen saturation by 2% or more from baseline, or a reading of 94% or lower, should raise concern and prompt oxygen supplementation along with evaluation for complications such as acute chest syndrome or pulmonary embolism. This assessment may include clinical examination, arterial blood gas analysis, and appropriate imaging. In addition, all patients with SCD should be encouraged to use an incentive spirometer after surgery to reduce the risk of atelectasis and acute chest syndrome [46].

8.6 Conclusion

SCD is the most common genetic hematologic disease prevalent in most parts of India; 2nd largest reservoir in the world after Africa. It is considered a major public health problem with a significant socioeconomic burden. There are many approved low-cost screening PoCT (Point-of-Care Test) available at present. Hb variant analysis by HPLC, Automated Capillary Zone Electrophoresis, and Microchip Electrophoresis are three confirmatory tests that will detect all common types of Hb Pathies. Molecular investigations may be required in certain controversial/borderline cases. There is a remarkable variability in the clinical presentation, starting from asymptomatic phenotype, vaso-occlusive type, hemolytic type, and mixed phenotype (features of vaso-occlusive and hemolytic). Every organ can be affected by SCD. Thus, regular monitoring at least once a year should be done. HU is the principal disease-modifying agent, should be administered to all the patients regardless of symptoms at low dose of 10 mg/kg/day, which can be gradually increased to the maximum tolerated dose (35 mg/kg/day) if required. Folic acid, Vit B12, calcium, Vit D should be added as supportive therapy. Red cell transfusion with extended antibody cross-matching should be given judiciously in approved indications only. VOC should be managed aggressively with NSAIDs in most of the cases. Preventive measures for VOC should be adopted. High-risk situations like pregnancy and surgery should be managed in tertiary care centers as a team approach following the SOPs. Curative options like Allogenic BMT should benefit high-risk patients only. Gene therapy is in the evolving stage.

References

1. NM_000518.5(HBB):c.20A>T (p.Glu7Val) and Hb SS disease. National Library of Medicine.
2. Piel FB, Patil AP, Howes RE, Nyangiri OA, Gething PW, Williams TN, et al. Global distribution of the sickle cell gene and geographical confirmation of the malaria hypothesis. Nat Commun. 2010;1:104.
3. Lorey F, Cunningham G, Shafer F, et al. Universal screening for hemoglobinopathies using high-performance liquid chromatography: clinical results of 2.2 million screens. Eur J Hum Genet. 1994;2:262.
4. Dover GJ, Boyer SH, Charache S, et al. Individual variation in the production and survival of F cells in sickle-cell disease. N Engl J Med. 1978;299:1428.
5. Yawn BP, Buchanan GR, Afenyi-Annan AN, et al. Management of sickle cell disease: summary of the 2014 evidence-based report by expert panel members. JAMA. 2014;312:1033.
6. Pearson HA, Cobb WT. Folic acid studies in sickle-cell anemia. J Lab Clin Med. 1964;64:913.

7. ICH – ICMR National Guidelines on Management and Control of Sickle Cell Disease, 2022; 1–157.
8. Alexy T, Pais E, Armstrong JK, et al. Rheologic behavior of sickle and normal red blood cell mixtures in sickle plasma: implications for transfusion therapy. Transfusion. 2006;46:912.
9. Chou ST, Jackson T, Vege S, Smith-Whitley K, Friedman DF, Westhoff CM, et al. High prevalence of red blood cell alloimmunization in sickle cell disease despite transfusion from Rh-matched minority donors. Blood. 2013;122:1062–71.
10. Charache S, Terrin ML, Moore RD, et al. Effect of hydroxyurea on the frequency of painful crises in sickle cell anemia. N Engl J Med. 1995;332:1317.
11. Ware RE. How I use hydroxyurea to treat young patients with sickle cell anemia. Blood. 2010;115:5300.
12. Steinberg MH, McCarthy WF, Castro O, Ballas SK, Armstrong FD, Smith W, et al. The risks and benefits of long-term use of hydroxyurea in sickle cell anemia: a 17.5 year follow-up. Am J Hematol. 2010;85(6):403–8.
13. Heeney MM, Ware RE. Hydroxyurea for children with sickle cell disease. Pediatr Clin N Am. 2008;55(2):483–501.
14. Strouse JJ, Lanzkron S, Beach MC, Haywood C, Park H, Witkop C, et al. Hydroxyurea for sickle cell disease: a systematic review for efficacy and toxicity in children. Pediatrics. 2008;122(6):1332–42.
15. Sethy S, Panda T, Jena RK. Beneficial effect of low fixed dose of hydroxyurea in vaso-occlusive crisis and transfusion requirements in adult HbSS patients: a prospective study in a tertiary care center. Indian J Hematol Blood Transfus. 2018;34(2):294–8.
16. Patel DK, Mashon RS, Patel S, Das BS, Purohit P, Bishwal SC. Low dose hydroxyurea is effective in reducing the incidence of painful crisis and frequency of blood transfusion in sickle cell anemia patients from eastern India. Hemoglobin. 2012;36(5):409–20.
17. Jain D, Sarathi V, Desai S, Bhatnagar M, Lodha A. Low fixed-dose hydroxyurea in severely affected Indian children with sickle cell disease. Hemoglobin. 2012;36(4):323–32.
18. Quinn CT. l-Glutamine for sickle cell anemia: more questions than answers. Blood. 2018;132:689.
19. Ataga KI, Kutlar A, Kanter J, et al. Crizanlizumab for the prevention of pain crises in sickle cell disease. N Engl J Med. 2017;376:429.
20. Kutlar A, Kanter J, Liles DK, et al. Effect of crizanlizumab on pain crises in subgroups of patients with sickle cell disease: a SUSTAIN study analysis. Am J Hematol. 2019;94:55.
21. Gluckman E, Cappelli B, Bernaudin F, et al. Sickle cell disease: an international survey of results of HLA-identical sibling hematopoietic stem cell transplantation. Blood. 2017;129:1548.
22. Kassim AA, de la Fuente J, Nur E, et al. An international learning collaborative phase 2 trial for haploidentical bone marrow transplant in sickle cell disease. Blood. 2024;143:2654.
23. Kassim AA, Walters MC, Eapen M, et al. Haploidentical bone marrow transplantation for sickle cell disease. NEJM Evid. 2025;4:EVIDoa2400192.
24. Ngwube A, Shah N, Godder K, et al. Abatacept is effective as GVHD prophylaxis in unrelated donor stem cell transplantation for children with severe sickle cell disease. Blood Adv. 2020;4:3894.
25. Casgevy and Lyfgenia: Two gene therapies for sickle cell disease. Med Lett Drugs Ther. 2024;66:9.
26. Frangoul H, Altshuler D, Cappellini MD, Chen YS, Domm J, Eustace BK, et al. CRISPR-cas9 gene editing for sickle cell disease and beta-thalassemia. N Engl J Med. 2021;384:252–60.
27. Sidman JD, Fry TL. Exacerbation of sickle cell disease by obstructive sleep apnea. Arch Otolaryngol Head Neck Surg. 1988;114:916.
28. Wilkie DJ, Molokie R, Boyd-Seal D, et al. Patient-reported outcomes: descriptors of nociceptive and neuropathic pain and barriers to effective pain management in adult outpatients with sickle cell disease. J Natl Med Assoc. 2010;102:18.
29. Ho K, Spence J, Murphy MF. Review of pain-measurement tools. Ann Emerg Med. 1996;27:427.
30. Emond AM, Collis R, Darvill D, et al. Acute splenic sequestration in homozygous sickle cell disease: natural history and management. J Pediatr. 1985;107:201.

31. Brousse V, Elie C, Benkerrou M, Odievre MH, Lesprit E, Bernaudin F, et al. Acute splenic sequestration crisis in sickle cell disease: cohort study of 190 paediatric patients. Br J Haematol. 2012;156:643–8.
32. Dean CL, Maier CL, Chonat S, et al. Challenges in the treatment and prevention of delayed hemolytic transfusion reactions with hyperhemolysis in sickle cell disease patients. Transfusion. 2019;59(5):1698–705.
33. Kassim AA, Pruthi S, Day M, Rodeghier M, Gindville MC, Brodsky MA, et al. Silent cerebral infarcts and cerebral aneurysms are prevalent in adults with sickle cell anemia. Blood. 2016;127:2038–40.
34. Adams RJ, McKie VC, Hsu L, et al. Prevention of a first stroke by transfusions in children with sickle cell anemia and abnormal results on transcranial Doppler ultrasonography. N Engl J Med. 1998;339:5.
35. Ware RE, Davis BR, Schultz WH, et al. Hydroxycarbamide versus chronic transfusion for maintenance of transcranial doppler flow velocities in children with sickle cell anemia-TCD With Transfusions Changing to Hydroxyurea (TWiTCH): a multicentre, open-label, phase 3, non inferiority trial. Lancet. 2016;387(10019):661.
36. Adams RJ, Brambilla D. Discontinuing prophylactic transfusions used to prevent stroke in sickle cell disease. N Engl J Med. 2005;353:2769.
37. Kroner BL, Hankins JS, Pugh N, et al.; Sickle Cell Disease Implementation Consortium. Pregnancy outcomes with hydroxyurea use in women with sickle cell disease. Am J Hematol. 2022;97(5):603612.
38. Rolnik DL, Wright D, Poon LC, et al. Aspirin versus placebo in pregnancies at high risk for preterm preeclampsia. N Engl J Med. 2017;377(7):613622.
39. Gnanasambanthan S, Datta S. Sickle cell disease in pregnancy. Obstet Gynaecol Reprod Med. 2021;31(12):351354.
40. Weinstein AS, Sigurdsson MI, Bader AM. Comparison of preoperative assessment of patient's metabolic equivalents (METs) estimated from history versus measured by exercise cardiac stress testing. Anesthesiol Res Pract. 2018;2018(September):5912726.
41. Chou ST, Alsawas M, Fasano RM, et al. American Society of Hematology 2020 guidelines for sickle cell disease: transfusion support. Blood Adv. 2020;4(2):327–55.
42. Howard J, Malfroy M, Llewelyn C, et al. The Transfusion Alternatives Preoperatively in Sickle Cell Disease (TAPS) study: a randomised, controlled, multicentre clinical trial. Lancet. 2013;381(9870):930–8.
43. Al-Samak ZM, Al-Falaki MM, Pasha AA. Assessment of perioperative transfusion therapy and complications in sickle cell disease patients undergoing surgery. Middle East J Anesthesiol. 2008;19(5):983–95. PMid:18637600
44. Alotaibi GS, Alsaleh K, Bolster L, Sean McMurtry M, Wu C. Preoperative transfusion in patients with sickle cell disease to prevent perioperative complications: a systematic review and meta-analysis. Hematology. 2014;19(8):463–71.
45. Gross ML, Schwedler M, Bischoff RJ, Kerstein MD. Impact of anesthetic agents on patients with sickle cell disease. Am Surg. 1993;59(4):261–4.
46. Niss O, ColeJenkins C, Davis B, et al. Prevention of acute chest syndrome by implementing a standardized process to improve incentive spirometry use in hospitalized patients with sickle cell disease. Blood. 2017;130(Suppl 1):132.

Part II
Advanced Cutting-Edge Technology in Hematology

Chapter 9
Gene Therapy for Hemoglobinopathy Current Status and Future Direction

Kanjaksha Ghosh and Kinjalka Ghosh

Abstract Management of symptomatic hemoglobinopathies, as exemplified by transfusion-dependent beta thalassemia (TDT), non-transfusion-dependent severe beta thalassemia (NTD), and sickle cell disease (SCD), have been evolving over the last seven decades, but unmet needs to manage this severe disease in the form of gene therapy remain. Success of allogenic stem cell transfusion in symptomatic haemoglobinopathies as a form of allogenic gene replacement therapy started in the 1980s, soon brought to the fore its limitations, e.g., limited applicability, morbidity, and mortality.

Relapse back into the original condition after the procedure. However, the procedure produced long-term amelioration of the disease in a substantial number of patients on whom this therapy was applied.

Gene replacement, gene correction, gene deletion, etc., as a therapeutic modality evolved over the last 35 years through the construction of better transgene, suitable vectors, improved collection techniques for autologous stem cells, and ex vivo gene therapy through successful animal model experimentation and careful clinical trials. These trials, which started from 2010, became successful and have now entered phase 3 of the program. However, a hurdle for gene therapy still remains. Quest for suitable means of providing in vivo gene therapy and non-chemo conditioning protocols is avidly sought after.

Keywords Hemoglobinopathy-transfusion dependent beta thalassemia · Sickle cell disease · Gene therapy · Viral vector · Gene editing · ShRNA-based therapy · Fetal hemoglobin · Ex vivo gene therapy · Stem cell transplantation

---

K. Ghosh (✉)
National Institute of Immunohaematology (ICMR), Mumbai, India

K. Ghosh
Tata Cancer Centre and HomiBhaba National Institute, Mumbai, India

H. P. Pati et al. (eds.), *Clinical Hematology and Hemato-Oncology*,
https://doi.org/10.1007/978-981-92-1167-8_9

Learning Points

- Gene therapy is a burning requirement for the cure of symptomatic haemoglobinopathy.
- Allogenic hemopoietic stem cell transplantation is a form of successful gene therapy with severe limitations.
- Gene therapy trials evolved over the construction of suitable transgenes and viral vectors.
- Self-inactivating lentiviral sequences are an important advance in this area.
- Human trials on gene therapy started with severe diseases like ADA SCID in the 1990s and had to be halted because of post-therapy leukemogenesis.
- Careful investigations and planning paved the way for successful gene therapy in human beings with symptomatic beta hemoglobinopathy.
- The process of ex vivo gene therapy is now well established.
- There is continuing concern for post-treatment leukemogenesis in SCID for which this therapy was halted and, after thorough investigation, restarted.
- Though the therapy is successful, it is still available only in clinical trial mode.
- This trial has not yet started in India but is expected to start soon.
- Final quest is for in vivo gene therapy without integrative leukemogenesis.

9.1 Introduction

Symptomatic hemoglobinopathy, like transfusion-dependent and non-transfusion-dependent beta thalassemia (TDT and NTDT), along with sickle cell disease (SCD), constitutes the commonest monogenic disease across the world and is responsible for substantial morbidity, mortality, lowered quality of life, drain on blood transfusion services, and increased cost of health care across the world [1].

Management of these conditions has evolved overtime and included better pain and crises management in sickle cell disease, judicious leucocyte reduced red cell transfusion (regular transfusion in TDT), proper selection of red cells in terms of antigen selection, prevention of transfusion transmitted vital infection, proper immunization, improved iron chelation (regular in TDT and when required in other conditions), red cell apheresis in certain SCD related condition, replacement therapy folic acid and different hormones as required, etc.

This conservative management is still the bedrock of treating symptomatic haemoglobinopathy across the world [2].

Many chemical entities were evaluated from the later part of the 1980s as fetal hemoglobin inducers (HbF), as it was observed that beta thalassemia syndromes and SCD mostly become symptomatic as the HBF levels steeply fall as the newborn grows in the succeeding few months. From a large number of drugs tested, hydroxyurea is now regularly used in SCD and was found to be moderately effective in raising clinically useful hemoglobin in a small subset of TDT and in a good number of NTDT.

Several new drugs have now been developed and are being used for raising hemoglobin in TDT/NTDT, e.g., Luspatercept and for reducing crises in sickle cell disease, e.g., voxeletor [3–5]. Voxeletor for SCD has now been withdrawn because of increased side effects and mortality.

However, all these developments did not address the basic genetic defect in the symptomatic hemoglobinopathies and there has been a persistent demand for replacement of the defective gene, or addition/deletion of genes that will address the defective function in the hemopoietic stem cells. So gene therapy has been the holy grail in the development of the ultimate management of these conditions. Modern advancements in transplantation technology and molecular biology have made this eminently feasible.

As the management of patients affected by various other genetic conditions evolved through gene therapy and the use of simple measures used extensively in society, i.e., screening for career, marriage counseling, prenatal diagnosis, preconception genetic diagnosis, adoption service, etc., evolved for hemoglobinopathies to cut down newer births of these symptomatic disorders [6].

Present chapter focuses on gene therapy for these two major conditions as it is evolved today and what could be possible direction in future with this kind of therapy.

9.2 Allogenic Stem Cell Transplantation; The First Effective Gene Therapy in Symptomatic Hemoglobinopathy

Allogenic bone marrow/stem cell transplantation allows allogenic hemopoietic stem cells to be engrafted in a properly selected donor to a patient, and after engraftment, the donor hemopoietic stem cells take over red cell production of the donor hemoglobin type. Essentially it is a type of gene therapy and today, the most extensively used treatment to cure TDT or SCD across many centers in the world [7].

Started for transfusion-dependent thalassemia patients in Italy in a big way in the 1980s [7]. A series of studies conducted by the center established the classification of TDT into three risk groups. In group 1, where there is minimum iron overload, a low number of transfused red cells, and minimum hepatosplenomegaly, more than 90% of patients did well and engrafted to become transfusion-free and were cured of thalassemia. These patients were called ex-thalassemic. However, those with a higher number of red cell transfusions, higher iron overload, and significant hepatosplenomegaly, which is the case even to this day in most of our TDT patients, did not do so well with around a 60% success rate and a good amount of mortality and morbidity after transplantation [8]. In these subsets, a large number of transplanted patients relapsed to become thalassemic again.

For sickle cell disease, stem cell transplantation was more difficult due to preexisting morbidity and continued vaso-occlusion during the peri-transplant period. However, with proper selection of patients and using methods to reduce the HbS in the circulation, improved conditioning regimen, and improved post transplantation care and immune-modulations allowed a large number of SCD patients have been able to receive stem cell transplantation and are now ex SCD.

Previously, stem cell donors were restricted to fully HLA-matched sibling donors, which severely restricted the number of patients that could be transplanted. However, with the establishment of many unrelated stem cell registries across the countries and the establishment of registries with collected umbilical cord cells, now this trans plantation can be achieved with a similar risk as completely matched related donor transplantation. Umbilical cord stem cells can also be transplanted with some mismatch in HLA antigen between the donor and the recipient. To improve the outcome, a combination of multiple cord blood stem cells from different donors with similar HLA composition has also been considered.

Haploidentical transplantation outcomes have improved substantially now, but have not been applied to a great extent in the management of hemoglobinopathy. However, as the results are improving, this source of haemopoietic stem cells is also getting attention [9, 10].

When all these permutations and combinations of type of patients, their underlying morbidity, and available donor cells are considered, not more than 50% of all symptomatic hemoglobinopathies are able to receive gene therapy through allogenic stem cell transplantation.

Side effects and mortality of the procedure are also substantial, which has forced a continued search for gene therapy protocols that will use only autologous haemopoietic stem cells.

Table 9.1 Types of gene modification in haemoglobinopathy gene therapy

Lentiviral Vector
Generally used Lentiviral gut less self-inactivating vector:
(a) Gene addition (modified or wild)
(b) ShRNA-mediated BCL11A Knock Down.
(c) Forced Looping of LCR with the y globin promoter area.
(d) Gene Editing:
(i) Gene correction (CRISPR/Cas9 or Zinc finger nuclease)
(ii) BCL11A (Chr 2) disruption with enhancer interaction (+62, +58, +55.nucleotide of enhancer region of betaglobin gene)
(iii) Generation of HPFH mutation.
(e) Base editing technology.

9.3 Types of Gene Therapy Being Considered

Several types of ex vivo gene therapy for symptomatic beta haemoglobinopathy are now considered (Table 9.1)

(i) Lentiviral-based complete wild beta globin gene.
(ii) Lentiviral-based modified beta globin gene for SCD. It is also used to treat TDT as it helps in the easy tracking of the transgene product from the peripheral blood.
(iii) Prevention of fetal hemoglobin switching off using the BCL11A gene-based approach (gene silencing).
(iv) Activation of the fetal hemoglobin gene through improving the beta globin enhancer with the HbF promoter region.
(v) Inducing pancellular HPFH by deletion of the 3.5 KB region near the promoter region of the delta globin gene.
(vi) Editing of the mutation site of the sickling gene using CRISPER/Cas9 or other nucleases.
(vii) Nucleotide editing technologies through homing deaminases converting T to A and C to G (base editing technology).

9.4 Theoretical Development and Application of the Gene Therapy Protocols in Animal Models of Hemoglobinopathy

Broadly, two types of gene therapy are envisaged. (i) Here, the transgene-containing stem cells, as it is developed outside the host by processing and selection, are introduced in the recipient in an adequate number and allow a marrow-conditioned recipient an adequate recovery with transgene containing cell. This is called ex vivo gene therapy and is presently the most commonly used form of gene therapy for haemoglobinopathy [11]. (ii) Other form of gene therapy involves direct injection of the suitably produced trans gene product directly into the host intravenously or into the bone marrow cavity. The transgene is such that it seeks and enters the cells of interest without affecting other cells, specifically cells of the gonads. This form of gene therapy, which is simpler to introduce, is called in vivo gene therapy and has been perfected for severe hemophilia but is still under experimental consideration for hemoglobinopathies [12].

For gene therapy in any form to be successful, a transgene construct incorporating the healthy wild gene or suitably modified gene, which will correct the clinical manifestation of the disease, needs to be converted into a suitable form for transfer into autologous hemopoietic stem cells (HSC). For modified hemopoietic stem cells to have a growth advantage over diseased existing stem cells, the host needs to be conditioned through therapy. After transfusion of an adequate number of modified

Table 9.2 Animal models of hemoglobinopathy

1. Mice:
A. Thalassemia model
$Hbb^{th1/th2./th3}$
Hbb^{th4} (IVS-2 = 654 mutation. Transgenic)
B. Sickle cell disease model
Berkeley mice
SAD mice (Hbs/Hb antillies/Hb D) (transgenic)
C. Transgenic in different animals using CRISPER/Cas9 technology
Rabbit: HBB2 targeting to produce NTDT
Monkey: HBB2 targeting to produce severe NTDT

autologous HSC, there should be some waiting time with possible stimulation of these cells.

Once the patient recovers, the transplanted HSC degree of modified cells in the patient's circulation should be assessed for recovery of the patient/animal [13].

Follow-up of sufficient time is required to establish that the transplantation produces a stable state with the modified gene, and there is no significant post transplantation evolution of MDS/neoplasia, etc., and there is no relapse back into the previous disease condition

9.4.1 Animal Models

Several humanized animal models of beta thalassemia and sickle cell anemia have been used to perfect gene therapy before its use in real-life patients. $Hb^{th3/4}$ mice for beta thalassemia and transgenic SAD (HbS, HbAntilis HbD) and Berkeley mice for sickle cell disease have been extensively used to perfect the process (Table 9.2) [14, 15].

9.4.2 Transgene

Construction of the transgene for gene therapy is done in various ways. The beta globin transgene could be wild type or Recombinant gene containing variant hemoglobin, which can not only be easily detected following gene therapy as a gene product, but also this hemoglobin can directly prevent sickling by disrupting axial and lateral polymerization of HbS in the case of SCD. The beta globin gene has a complex control system with its enhancer, also called LCR, far away from the beta globin gene promoter, and has a complex and long structure and promoter area 5′ to the beta globin gene. It was difficult to package LCR of beta globin in LCR because of its complexity and size, so a portion of alpha globin LCR, i.e., HS 2-3-4, was

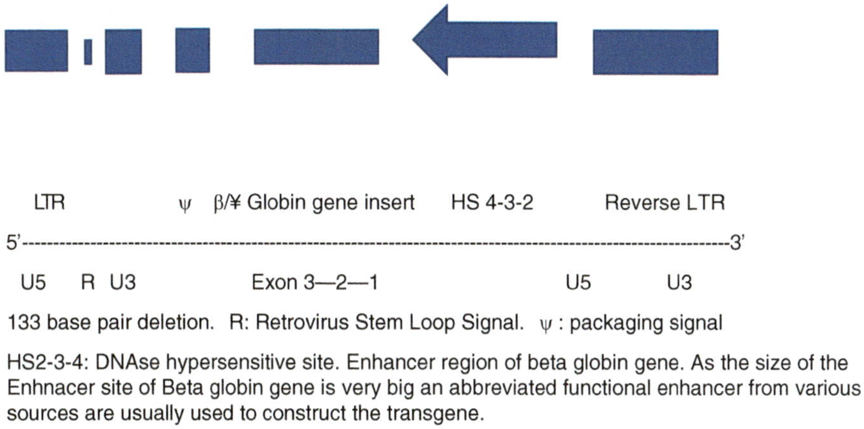

Fig. 9.1 Minimum structure of lentiviral vector for transduction in beta hemoglobinopathy

used to construct the transgene. Theoretically, this transgene can be introduced into the haemopoietic stem cells using Chemical, Physical (electroporation), or viral vectors. Chemical and physical methods are not so effective, and the transgene gets into a small percentage of cells, while transgenes transmitted through viral vectors are very efficient. Two broad types of viral vectors are used using adeno associated viruses or retroviruses. AAV-associated transduced genes are not normally integrated in the host genome but stay there as episomes, which are less prone to cause neoplastic transformation of the cells, but their stability and immune reaction are issues. Retroviral vectors are either human retrovirus sequences or Lentiviral sequences. Generally, for therapeutic purposes involving ex vivo gene therapy for hemoglobinopathy, murine retrovirus is used as a vector. This vector, called gutless and self-inactivating sequence vectors, is produced by removing most of the structural genes of the virus; the space so vacated is now filled by the Hb beta gene and LCR sequences HS 2-3-4. This is flanked by 5′ LTR containing R element and 133 bp deletion to make itself-inactivating (SIN), followed by Ψ gene for packaging the insert. The R element helps the recombinant Hb gene to be packed properly in the cytoplasm in the 3′ end is a reverse LTR (long terminal repeat) to complete the vector material (Fig. 9.1).

The advantage of the lentiviral vector is a high rate of transduction, irrespective of the cell cycle status and integration in the host genome, mainly in the noncoding area of the gene. Though this transduction becomes higher in the proliferating cells. Integration sites are often in the areas of active genes.

The lentiviral vector, though essentially of similar structure, varies in its details for various clinical trials.

For activating the fetal hemoglobin switch as one of the major gene therapy protocols to treat both thalassemia syndrome and SCD, three basic approaches are tested. (i) Here, a zinc finger nuclease is anchored with GATA1-LDB1, a transcription factor, to develop a linkage between the enhancer HS2-3-4 region of the

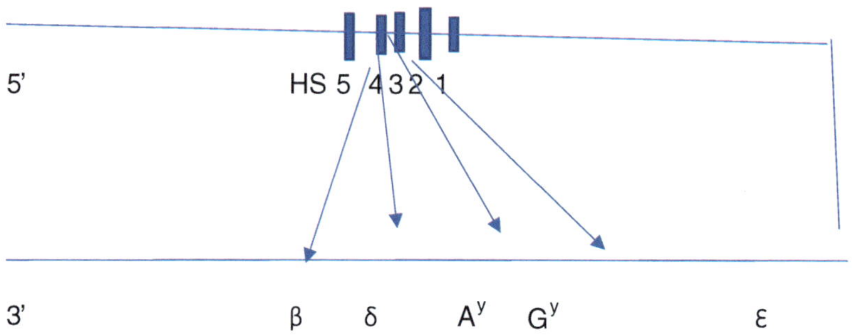

Fig. 9.2 Chromosome 11: Beta globin gene cluster

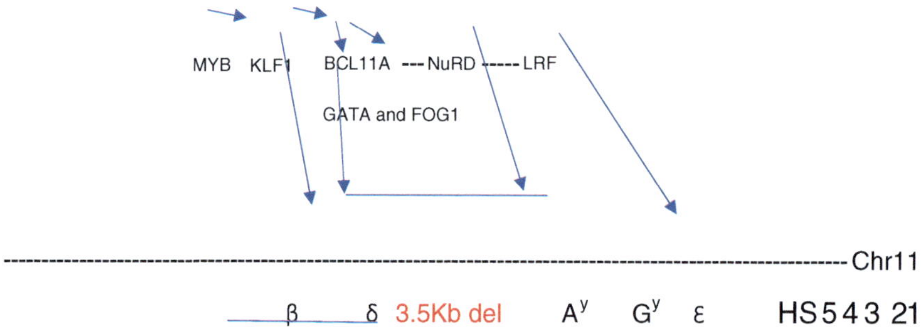

Fig. 9.3 Fetal hemoglobin switching

transgene with G^y promoter region of the globin gene complex (transgene). (ii) A BCL11A inactivating mutation is introduced in the BCL11A gene in chromosome 2. (iii) A 3.5 Kb deletion from the beta hemoglobin gene complex near the promoter of the δ gene for producing PAN cellular HPFH.

Figures 9.1, 9.2, and 9.3 show the structure of the modified beta globin gene complex, how LCR engages with different promoter regions of this gene complex and causes switching off HbF production in early infancy, BCL11A and its inhibition of HBF production, and finally, the minimum structure of a self-inactivating lentiviral vector containing the transgene.

Many other novel ideas have evolved to be tested in the future in the field of Gene editing in different manners and ways [16].

9.4.3 *Types of globin genes incorporated in various trials*

Apart from using the wild beta globin gene in a transgene, a recombinant gene with structural variation has been mostly incorporated for two reasons. (i) The altered hemoglobin molecules could be easily detected in peripheral blood by using the commonly employed HPLC technique, showing the degree of success of engraftment of altered haemopoietic stem cells and thus the success of gene therapy. (ii) For the treatment of sickle cell disease, the recombinant beta globin gene was made to produce a globin chain with the ability to disrupt the sickling process, i.e., $Hb^{T\text{-}87Q}$, a change akin to the amino acid of HBF y chain in a similar position. This change disrupts β^s-β lateral linkages. Similarly, changes in the β chain in position 22 from glutamic acid to alanine additionally disrupt the linkage between β^s-α linkage. In position 16, a change of glycine to aspartic acid increases the affinity of the α chain with adjoining hemoglobin, excluding HbS from the axial polymerization of HbS. In a similar way, AS3, i.e., the beta globin gene with all three amino acid

Table 9.3 Clinical trials for gene therapy of beta haemoglobinopathies (transfusion-dependent thalassemia and sickle cell anemia)

Therapy product	NCT trial no.	Indication	Strategy
1. Lenti/G-beta AS3-FB	02247843	SCD	Lentiviral betagene addition
2. GLOBE	02453477	TDT	As above
3. Zynteglo	032070009 & 02906202	TDT	As above
4. BB305	02140554 & 04293185	SCD	As above
5. ARU1801	02186418	SCD	Lentiviral gamma gene addition
6. CSL 200	04091737	SCD	As above
7. TNS 9.3.55	01639690	TDT	Lentiviral beta gene addition
	04205435	TDT	Gene editing for activating HBF (CRISPER/ Cas9)
8. CTX001	03655679	SCD	HbF activation. Zn finger nuclease
	03745287	TDT	As above
9. ST 400	03432364	TDT	As above
10. BIVV 003	03653247	SCD	As above
11. BIVV	03282656	SCD	Transcriptome Editing with Lentiviral shRNA of BCL11A

TDT transfusion-dependent beta thalassemia, *SCD* sickle cell disease

Exvivo gene transfer (1990- Lymphocyte)	ADA–SCID (1995)	Clonal T cell proliferation. (2003)	SCID & WAS Leukaemia (2008,2014).
Gene Therapyin TDT (2010, Lentivirial)	TDT pt series (2018)	SCD pt (2020)	Many clincal trials. (2025)

Fig. 9.4 Flow diagram: milestones in ex vivo gene therapy

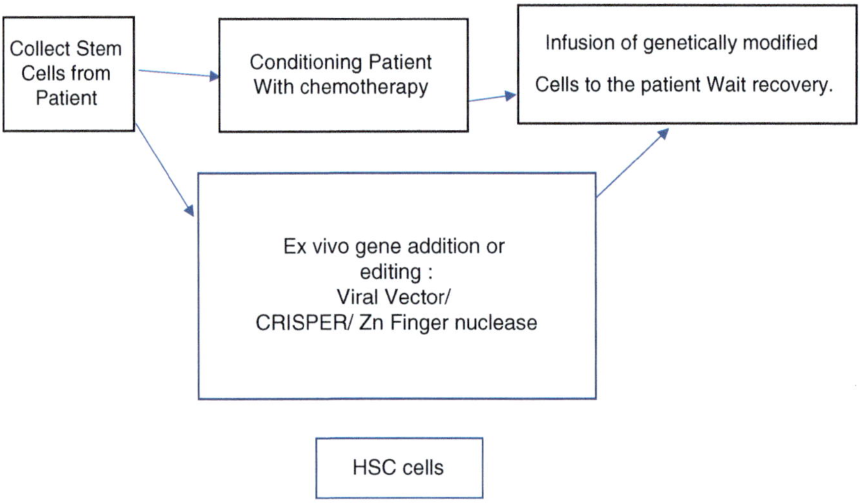

Fig. 9.5 Flow diagram of ex vivo gene therapy procedure for hemoglobinopathy

changes in position 87 (T to Q), 22(D to A), and 16 (G to E), has been created as a major molecule to disrupt the sickling process [13, 16–18].

9.5 Historical Landmarks in Gene Therapy

Serious attempts for gene therapy started in 1989s with ADA deficiency SCID babies. Though successful, it was stopped as some of the patients developed hematological malignancy due to activation of the LMO2 oncogene, due to integration of the transgene. Then, over the years, Vector architecture was improved, as well as screening of the cells to be transplanted after transduction for integration could be developed and regularly undertaken. Meanwhile, in vivo gene therapy for hemophilia B and hemophilia A came of age by using an AAV vector, which normally remains non-integrated in the cell as an episome. For hemoglobinopathy, after proper animal models were developed and tested (Table 9.2) and the lentiviral vector was refined, gene therapy trials for hemoglobinopathy continuously improved since 2010, and from 2018, clinical trials were started. Finally, several clinical trials for TDT and SCD were started, and some of them were successfully concluded in phase 2 and phase 3 trials (Table 9.3). A flow diagram (Fig. 9.4) briefly depicts the historical progress of gene therapy.

9.6 Process of Ex Vivo Gene Therapy in TDT and SCD

The process is similar to autologous stem cell transplantation. Only the transplantable cells are genetically modified autologous haemopoietic stem cells and are presented in Fig. 9.5. Briefly, the procedure starts with the selection of the patients who should be transfusion-dependent, with beta thalassemia or a patient with sickle cell disease who is not a candidate for allogenic bone marrow transplantation because of the lack of a proper stem cell donor, or the organ damage precludes its use.

Transfusion-transmitted viral infection is a contraindication at present, but after the procedure is well established, many of these contraindications will be relative contraindications.

Autologous haemopoietic stem cells are mobilized with G-Csf (Peg filgrastim) and or Plerixafor. For SCD, many prefer using plerixafor alone as G-CSF, increases neutrophil count and chances of complications. SCD patients, because of repeated vaso-occlusive crises in the marrow and associated fibrosis, could make such patients poor mobilizers, and such patients may need more than one

Table 9.4 Gene therapy and gene editing clinical trials for sickle cell disease till 2021

Goal	Target	Sponsor	Trial ID (NCT)	Expected participant
Elevate HBF	CTX001/BCL11A	Vertex	03745787	45
As above	Plerixafor/ BCL11A	Biorativ	03653247	8
As above	OTQ203/BCL11A HIX 763/BCL11A	Novartis	04443907	30
Repair HbS	Lentiviral AS-3	Calif. Inst	02247843	6
Elevate HBF	ARU-180	Aruvant Sci GmBH	02186418	10
Repair HbS	GLOBE-1	Pub. Hospitaux Paris	03964792	10
As above	Lentivirus BB305	Blue Bird	04293185	35
As above	normal b Globin	Memorial Sloan Kettering	02193197	39
As above	BB305 Lentivirus	Bluebird	02140554	50
Elevate HbF	SiRNA. BCL11A	Boston Child	03282656	15

Recently recognized editing therapy is with CRISPR/Cas9 (Casegevy)

session to have satisfactory yield of HSC (>5 × 10^6/Kg). The collection is then concentrated for CD34-positive cells using a CliniMACS-like system. The collected cells are transduced with an excess amount of the Vector trans gene, and after separating from the excess vector, tested for the number of vector copies per cell and also for integration of the transgene. The product is then infused into the patient who has been conditioned by marrow ablation using one of the chemo protocols, mostly Busulfan conditioning. After this transplantation, the patient is followed up for marrow recovery. Peripheral red cell number, presence of transgene hemoglobin, etc.

9.7 Clinical Trials with Gene Therapy

Several clinical trials have been ongoing or completed as part of gene therapy in SCD or TDT. These trials have been listed in Tables 9.3 and 9.4. These trials have involved gene addition, gene editing, or gene silencing technologies. Some of these gene therapies have been spectacularly successful for both diseases. A recently published phase 3 clinical trial [19] Beticel involving Hb^{T87Q} beta-globin gene addition showed that 21/23 TDT patients were transfusion independent with Hb level more than 9 gms/dl after a median one-year follow-up [20].

In a composite analysis of the trial with the same Beticel therapy involving a phase 1/2/3 trial (Bluebirds Bio, Beticel) on a seven-year follow-up 49/63 patients achieved transfusion independence with minimum hemoglobin levels more than 9Gms/dl. Abdominal pain (18%), thrombocytopenia (14%), and VOD of the liver (11%) were early complications within the first two years of follow-up. Neutrophil recovery and platelet recovery happened within 18 and 45 days post-transplantation. It was found that the final product transplanted (drug product), viral copy number/cell and post-transplantation percentages of transgene hemoglobin after three months were strong predictors of success [20].

Several techniques of autologous modified stem cell therapy using modified beta globin gene as well as BCL11A silencing using shRNA technology were found to be equally successful [21]. Side effects of treatment were consistent with those of autologous stem cell transplantation. A summary of various clinical trials of gene therapy in beta globin haemoglobinopathies, i.e., TDT, severe NTDT, and SCD, is available [22]. Clinical trials for SCD gene therapy are presented separately in Table 9.4.

In 2023, two HSC-targeted gene therapies for SCD were approved by the FDA, including lovotibeglogene autotemcel (Lyfgenia, bluebird bio) and exagamglogene autotemcel (Casgevy, Vertex and CRISPR Therapeutics).

Canter and Falcon have nicely summarized how a patient intending to approach gene therapy for SCD should be evaluated and counseled at the present state of our understanding and development of the process [23]. Basically, a similar approach can be used for TDT and severe NTDT.

9.8 Side Effects of Ex Vivo Gene Therapy in Symptomatic Hemoglobinopathy

Ex vivo gene therapy for symptomatic hemoglobinopathy comes from two procedures: (i) Autologous stem cell transplantation requires conditioning of the marrow to create space for engraftment. Usually, the conditioning regimen involves chemotherapy with Busulphan or its analogs. This can produce MDs/ acute leukemia and solid tumors in the long run. Engraftment of the haemopoietic stem cells and finally production of enough neutrophils and platelets may take time, and during these intervals, various bacterial, viral, and fungal infections can produce some mortality and morbidity. (ii) Transduced hemopoietic stem cells should contain adequate Vector Copy number/cell otherwise the engraftment will not produce desired results. Graft failure and growth of original haemopoietic stem cells will bring back the disease. As lentiviral vectors integrate with the host genome, improper integration close to an oncogene may activate the oncogene and cause leukemogenesis or other malignancy [24, 25]. Trial for SCD was halted temporarily because of the development of MDS and AML in two of the patients. Detailed investigation showed that in one patient, the transduced cell was not involved, but in another patient, the leukemic cells appeared from the gene-modified cells, but integration of the transgene was not near any oncogene. One of the hypotheses is that Sickle cell disease normally has a higher prevalence of leukemia than age matched normal population, hence occasional development of leukemia may be seen as unfolding of that natural history. Chemo induced hematological malignancies have certain cytogenetic features and usually occur 3–5 years after therapy, except for those that happen after Topoisomerase II inhibitor therapy.

Finally, both TDT and SCD cause various organ damage, and this damage is aggravated with higher levels of iron overload in TDT and many vaso-occlusive crises that take place in SCD. Moreover, transfusion-transmitted viral infection can also take its toll.

Table 9.5 Important clinical endpoints for curative genetic therapies for hemoglobinopathy

Clinical efficacy	Clinical laboratory measures	Clinical safety
Transfusion independence	Hemoglobin concentrations	Engraftment
A weighted average	Edited stem cell	Graft failure
Hemoglobin of ≥9 g/dL	Total Hb and HbF levels	Treatment-related
RBC transfusions for ≥12 months	F-cell expression	Mortality/morbidity
	Vector copy number	Long-term organ damage
Reduction of crises	Reversal of vascular path	Mortality/morbidity
Chelation therapy	Ferritin/cardiac	Malignancy
Quality of life	Liver iron (MRI)	
Reduction in pain	Bone marrow	

9.9 Discussion and Future Advances in Gene Therapy for Symptomatic Hemoglobinopathy

Gene therapy in both TDT and SCD has come of age. With a proper gene construct, two broad types of ex vivo gene therapy, i.e., replacement of defective beta-globin gene with wild or more effective recombinant beta-globin gene, i.e., Hb ^{T87Q} is one approach; another approach is activation of fetal Hb (HbF) in the haemopoietic cells, which can be used for both SCD and TDT.

The results of phase 3 trials have demonstrated a near 90% efficiency of transfusion-free (TDT) or crisis-free life (SCD) one year after the procedure. The number of patients responding to the procedure tends to increase with time.

Clinical endpoints in gene therapy in symptomatic haemoglobinopathies and how to do the follow-ups are slowly evolving, as is given in Table 9.5.

However, the procedure is still not applicable to all patients.

Integrative leukemogenesis, though rare, is still a concern and tends to increase as the age of the patient increases. The procedure still requires marrow conditioning using anti-neoplastic drugs that increase the side effects of the procedure.

Hence, there is a need for developing marrow conditioning with non-chemotherapeutic procedures, i.e., using Monoclonal antibodies or recombinant proteins which can home in haemopoietic stem cells to cause apoptosis, that needs to be developed.

Presently, the cost of the procedure is substantial and may not be available for most of the patients who need it!

Allogenic stem cell transplantation is now a well-established procedure. Reduced chemo conditioning with better immunosuppressive therapies have developed, as well as many alternative donors for the procedure, and expertise to carry on the procedure is available more extensively than gene therapy at present. Hence, this procedure for gene therapy should be evaluated first for anyone who needs it. Meanwhile, more and more patients should join clinical trials of gene therapy to make it safe and more extensively available.

Developing a gene therapy protocol similar to hemophilia, i.e., in vivo gene therapy, where injection of a vector containing a transgene directed to haemopoietic stem cells will cut down post-conditioning toxicities as well as future development of secondary leukemia, MDS, and other solid tissue malignancies.

A major problem in developing such therapy is finding the right kind of viral vector directed at haemopoietic stem cells [26].

Newer types of gene correction therapy involving Base deamination (cytidine deaminase /adenine deaminase on the shoulder of CRISPER/ Cas dependent program can be developed. Both types of deaminases are already present in the cells; the need being only to target these enzymes in the right place [27]. Base deamination, unfortunately, cannot replace purine with a pyrimidine base and vice versa.

One of the challenges of present ex vivo gene therapy is over the course of time, transgene or corrected gene-containing stem cells may dwindle, and the disease could come back. One way to prevent this is to harvest a larger number of stem cells

(>5 × 10^6/Kg of CD34 positive cells containing a high copy number of vectors per cell). This may need more than one pheresis for the patient, particularly for sickle cell anemia patients, where stem cell harvest may be poor.

Development of malignancy in gene therapy patients, particularly with sickle cell anemia, mandates that cells which are transfused have been checked for the presence of common AML mutations.

Intrauterine gene therapy for hemoglobinopathy is facing hurdles because the very active fetal marrow has a large number of stem cells in cycle and is competitive. The genetically modified cells are small the engraftment has been poor. However, slow but steady progress in intrauterine gene therapy for alpha thalassemia is being made, as fetal death without gene correction is a real concern [28].

9.10 Conclusion

Gene therapy for hemoglobinopathy is an evolving science. With present technology, several companies are running this trial with high rates of success.

There is little doubt that this mode of therapy will become an important tool to treat symptomatic hemoglobinopathy. The cost of the therapy, like any other new therapy, is a problem, but it may eventually come down when a large number of patients are treated with this therapy and technology becomes simpler.

References

1. Harteveld CL, Achour A, Arkesteijn SJG, Ter Huurne J, Verschuren M, Bhagwandien-Bisoen S, Schaap R, Vijfhuizen L, El Idrissi H, Koopmann TT. The hemoglobinopathies, molecular disease mechanisms and diagnostics. Int J Lab Hematol. 2022;44(S1):28–36.
2. Kohne E. Hemoglobinopathies: clinical manifestations, diagnosis, and treatment. Dtsch Arztebl Int. 2011;108(31-32):532–40.
3. Biswas S, Smrity SZ, Bhuia MS, Sonia FA, Aktar MA, Chowdhury R, Islam T, Islam MT, Gonçalves Alencar G, Paulo CLR, et al. Beta-thalassemia: a pharmacological drug-based treatment. Drugs Drug Candidates. 2024;3:126–47.
4. Jain DL, Apte M, Colah R, et al. Efficacy of fixed low dose hydroxyurea in Indian children with sickle cell anemia: a single centre experience. Indian Pediatr. 2013;50:929–33.
5. Italia KY, Jijina FJ, Merchant R, Panjwani S, Nadkarni AH, Sawant PM, Nair SB, Ghosh K, Colah RB. Response to hydroxyurea in beta thalassemia major and intermedia: experience in western India. Clin Chim Acta. 2009;407(1-2):10–5.
6. Ghosh K, Colah R, Manglani M, Choudhry VP, Verma I, Madan N, Saxena R, Jain D, Marwaha N, Das R, Mohanty D, Choudhary R, Agarwal S, Ghosh M, Ross C. Guidelines for screening, diagnosis and management of hemoglobinopathies. Indian J Hum Genet. 2014;20(2):101–19.
7. Lucarelli G, Galimberti M, Polchi P, Angelucci E, Baronciani D, Giardini C, et al. Bone marrow transplantation in patients with thalassemia. N Engl J Med. 1990;322:417–21.
8. Mathews V, Balasubramaniam P, Abraham A, George B, Srivastava A. Allogeneic stem cell transplantation for thalassemia major in India. J Pediatr Hematol Onco. 2017;2:114–20.

9. Bhalla N, Bhargav A, Yadav SK, Singh AK. Allogeneic hematopoietic stem cell transplantation to cure sickle cell disease: a review. Front Med (Lausanne). 2023;10:1036939. https://doi.org/10.3389/fmed.2023.1036939.
10. Kassim AA, Walters MC, Eapen M, Smith M, Logan BR, Solh M, et al. Haploidentical bone marrow transplantation for sickle cell disease. NEJM Evid. 2025;4(3):EVIDoa2400192. https://doi.org/10.1056/EVIDoa2400192. Epub 2025 Feb 25.
11. Lidonnici MR, Scaramuzza S, Ferrari G. Gene therapy for haemoglobinopathies. Human Gene Therapy. 2023;17–18:793–807.
12. Li C, Wang H, Gil S, Georgakopoulou A, Radtke S, Yannaki E, Papayannopoulou T, Kiem H-P, Lieber A. In vivo HSC gene therapy for hemoglobinopathies: a proof of concept evaluation in rhesus macaques. Blood. 2020;136(Supplement 1):46–7.
13. Cavazzana M, Antoniani C, Miccio A. Gene therapy for β-hemoglobinopathies. Mol Ther. 2017;25:1142–54.
14. McColl B, Vadolas J. Animal models of β-hemoglobinopathies: utility and limitations. J Blood Med. 2016;7:263–74.
15. Moi P, Sadelain M. Towards the genetic treatment of β-thalassemia: new disease models, new vectors, new cells. Haematologica. 2008;93:325–30. https://doi.org/10.3324/haematol.12732.
16. Bulcha JT, Wang Y, Ma H, et al. Viral vector platforms within the gene therapy landscape, vol. 6. Sig Transduct Target Ther; 2021. p. 53. https://doi.org/10.1038/s41392-021-00487-6.
17. Kunz JB, Kulozik AE. Gene therapy of the hemoglobinopathies. Hemasphere. 2020;4(5):e479. https://doi.org/10.1097/HS9.0000000000000479.
18. Park SH, Lee CM, Dever DP, Davis TH, Camarena J, Srifa W, Zhang Y, et al. Highly efficient editing of the β-globin gene in patient-derived hematopoietic stem and progenitor cells to treat sickle cell disease. Nucleic Acids Res. 2019;47:7955–72.
19. Locatelli F, Thompson AA, Kwiatkowski JL, et al. Betibeglogene autotemcel gene therapy for nonbeta(0)/beta(0) genotype beta-thalassemia. N Engl J Med. 2022;386:415–27.
20. Walters MC, Kwiatkowsky JL, Porter JB, et al. Long term outcomes of 63 patients with transfusion-dependent b-thalassemia (TDT) followed up to 7 years post-treatment with betibeglogene autotemcel (beti-cel) gene therapy and exploratory analysis of predictors of successful treatment outcomes in phase 3 trials. Blood. 2022;140:5355–7.
21. Esrick EB, Lehmann LE, Biffi A, et al. Posttranscriptional genetic silencing of BCL11A to treat sickle cell disease. N Engl J Med. 2021;384:205–15.
22. Frangoul H, Altshuler D, Cappellini MD, et al. CRISPRCas9 gene editing for sickle cell disease and βthalassemia. N Engl J Med. 2021;384:252–60.
23. Canter J, Falcon C. Gene therapy for sickle cell disease where we are now? Haematology. 2021:176–80. ASH education programme 2021. https://doi.org/10.1182/hematology.2021000250.
24. Leonard A, Tisdale JF. A pause in gene therapy: reflecting on the unique challenges of sickle cell disease. Mol Ther. 2021;29:1355–6.
25. Goyal S, Tisdale J, Schmidt M, Kanter J, Jaroscak J, Dustin Whitney D, et al. Acute myeloid leukemia case after gene therapy for sickle cell disease. N Engl J Med. 2022;386:138–47. https://doi.org/10.1056/NEJMoa2109167.
26. Li C, Wang H, Gil S, et al. In vivo HSC gene therapy for hemoglobinopathies: a proof of concept evaluation in Rhesus Macaques. Blood. 2020;136(Supplement 1):46–7.
27. Zeng J, Wu Y, Ren C, et al. Therapeutic base editing of human hematopoietic stem cells. Nat Med. 2020;26(4):535–41.
28. Yung NK, Maassel NL, Ullrich SJ, Ricciardi AS, Stitelman DH. A narrative review of in utero gene therapy: advances, challenges, and future considerations. Transl Pediatr. 2021;10:1486–96.

Chapter 10
Role of Flow Cytometry in the Diagnosis of Benign Haematological Disorders

Pankhi Dutta and Shanaz Khodaiji

Abstract Flow cytometry (FCM), with its ability to rapidly analyse multiple parameters on individual cells, is an indispensable tool in haemato-oncology for the rapid diagnosis of various haematological neoplasms. However, FCM is also being increasingly used in the diagnosis of non-neoplastic haematological disorders affecting all three haematopoietic cell lines. Paroxysmal nocturnal haemoglobinuria (PNH) is an acquired stem cell disorder caused by the absence of glycosylphosphatidylinositol (GPI) anchored proteins on cell surfaces and is characterized by haemolysis, increased thromboses and bone marrow failure. Today, demonstration of the absence of GPI-anchored proteins by FCM is the gold standard for the diagnosis of PNH. Osmotic fragility testing using FCM and Eosin 5′ maleimide binding test has shown high sensitivity and specificity in the diagnosis of hereditary spherocytosis. FCM has also found use in the detection of feto-maternal bleeding in the investigation of Rh incompatibility. This technology can be used for the diagnosis of platelet function disorders even in the presence of severe thrombocytopenia, thus overcoming the biggest limitation of light transmission aggregometry, the gold standard in the diagnosis of platelet dysfunction. Primary immune-deficiency disorders are a heterogeneous group of genetic disorders. FCM appears to be a useful modality that provides a rapid diagnosis in many instances and at least guides genetic testing in others. FCM can be used for immunophenotyping or the detection of intracellular proteins as well as for functional assays. International guidelines and well-described protocols for performing FCM in non-neoplastic haematological

P. Dutta (✉)
Consultant Haematopathologist, Haematology Laboratory, Dubai Hospital, Dubai, United Arab Emirates

S. Khodaiji
Consultant Hematology and Transfusion Medicine, P.D. Hinduja Hospital and Medical Research Centre, Mumbai, India

H. P. Pati et al. (eds.), *Clinical Hematology and Hemato-Oncology*,
https://doi.org/10.1007/978-981-92-1167-8_10

disorders are available. This chapter will give an overview of the clinical uses of FCM for the diagnosis of non-neoplastic diseases of haematology, while also reviewing some protocols/guidelines available for performing these assays.

Keywords Flowcytometry · Paroxysmal nocturnal haemoglobinuria · Hereditary spherocytosis · Platelet function defects · Primary immune deficiency disorders

Learning Objectives

- Gain an overview of the applications of flow cytometry in non-malignant haematologic disorders.
- Familiarity with guidelines for performing and reporting flow cytometry for diagnosis of paroxysmal nocturnal haemoglobinuria and platelet function disorders.
- Recognize the utility of flow cytometry in the diagnosis of primary immune deficiency disorders.

10.1 Introduction

Flow cytometry (FCM) is a powerful tool that measures scattered light at different angles from cells passing in a single file and being interrogated by a laser beam in a special flow cell. Cells of different lineages/types have different physical properties and express different antigens. The forward scattered light, i.e., the FSC, reflects the relative size of the cell while the side scattered light, i.e., SSC, reflects the complexity or granularity of the cells. When the cells are exposed to different fluorescent dye-tagged antibodies, the flow cytometer also detects fluorescence emissions, which in turn are dependent on the antibodies' binding to antigens expressed on the cells. Thus, the flow cytometer can characterize cells based on their size, internal complexity, and antigens expressed by them. This technology allows for the rapid multiparametric analysis of individual cells. First introduced around 1970, there have been many advancements over the years and currently, FCM has many applications, both for research as well as for clinical purposes. It is a well-established modality in haemato-oncology and is best known for its application in the diagnosis of haematological neoplasms. However, FCM has many applications in the diagnosis of several benign or non-neoplastic haematological disorders affecting all three types of blood cells, namely, red blood cells, white blood cells as well as platelets.

Clinical Case *A 32-year-old female presented to the emergency department with lower abdominal pain and vomiting. She was initially referred to the obstetrics and gynaecology department with the clinical suspicion of a pelvic infection. Her pelvic ultrasound was normal, and she underwent a computed tomography (CT) scan of the abdomen, which showed infrahepatic, suprarenal IVC thrombosis with IVC wall enhancement. Her haemoglobin, white blood cell (WBC), and platelets were 7.9* *(reference range/RR 12.0 to 15.0 gm), 3900 (RR of 4000 to 11,000/ul), and 51,000 (RR 150,000 to 450,000/ul), respectively. Her unfractionated bilirubin and serum lactate dehydrogenase (LDH) were raised, i.e., LDH was 970 (RR 105-222 U/L) while the serum haptoglobin was low, <0.1 (RR 0.3 to 2.0 gm/L). The Coombs test was negative. There was no history of passing dark urine, but the urine tested positive for haemosiderin, confirming intravascular haemolysis and haemoglobinuria. In view of the thrombosis, pancytopenia, and haemolysis, FCM for Paroxysmal Nocturnal Haemoglobinuria was requested. A diagnosis of PNH was made based on the following FCM report.*

Patient's details—XYZ
Sample: Peripheral blood
Indication for FCM: Thrombosis, pancytopenia, and evidence of haemolysis
PNH clone: Positive in RBCs and WBCs, consistent with a diagnosis of PNH.
PNH clone in the RBCs—31.2%
PNH clone in the neutrophils—77%
PNH clone in the monocytes—89%
Antibodies used: CD45, CD15, CD64, and CD235a for gating and CD59, CD157 as well as fluorescent aerolysin (FLAER) for demonstration of absence of GPI-anchored proteins as well as GPI anchors, respectively.
Red Blood Cells: Type II partial CD59 deficiency:20.39%, Type III complete CD59 deficiency: 10.81%, total clone: 31.2%. (LLOQ: 0.01%)
Neutrophils: FLAER/CD157 deficiency: 77% (LLOQ: 0.1%)
Monocytes: FLAER/CD157 deficiency: 89%

Table 10.1 gives the WBC statistics for the same case. Figure 10.1 shows the WBC (monocytes and granulocytes) plots, Fig. 10.2a–c shows the RBC plots, while Fig. 10.3 shows the RBC histograms, which help to delineate between different types of RBCs based on the degree of loss of GPI-anchored proteins.
The patient underwent a thrombolysis and was put on anticoagulation. Due to financial constraints, the specific therapy for PNH, Eculizumab, was not given.

Table 10.1 WBC statistics

Statistics						
Name	Events	% Parent	% Grandparent	% Total	FSC-A Mean	SSC-A Mean
WBC STAINED:All Events	125,023	***	***	100.00	97,898	103,091
WBC STAINED:Singlets	115,639	92.49	***	92.49	101,412	107,461
WBC STAINED:Viable Cells	97,259	84.11	77.79	77.79	115,668	116,787
WBC STAINED:Neutro+Mono	58,748	60.40	50.80	46.99	144,191	168,368
WBC STAINED:Monos	4,942	5.08	4.27	3.95	133,315	77,477
WBC STAINED:Neutros	50,841	52.27	43.97	40.67	145,692	178,091
WBC STAINED:Abn Mono	4,408	89.19	4.53	3.53	133,764	77,448
WBC STAINED:Abn Neutro	39,451	77.60	40.56	31.55	145,005	177,577

***Not applicable.

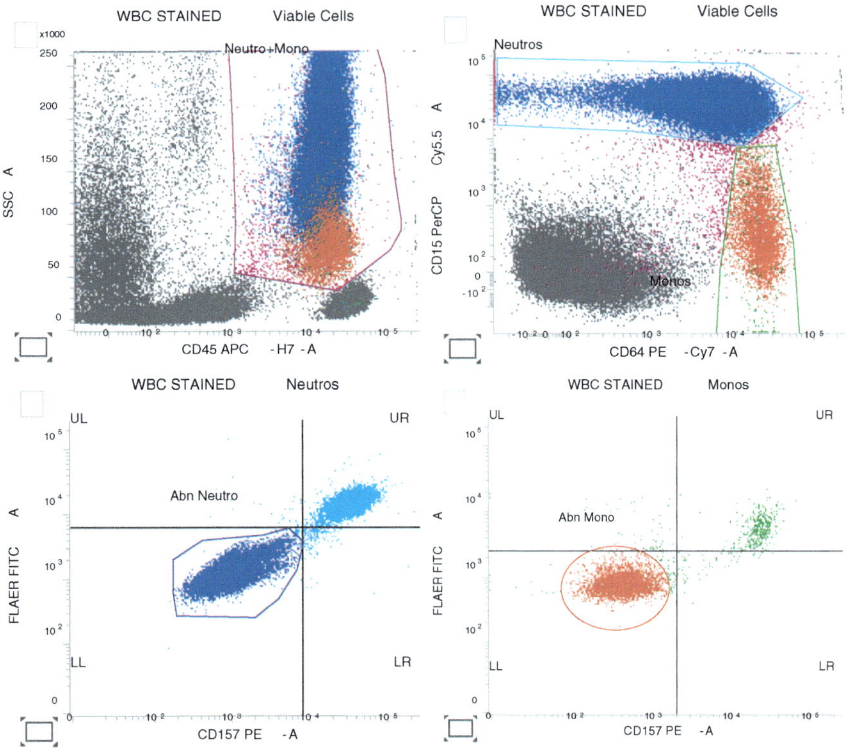

Fig. 10.1 Neutrophils and monocytes stained by antibodies against CD15 and CD64 respectively along with anti CD157 (GPI anchored protein)

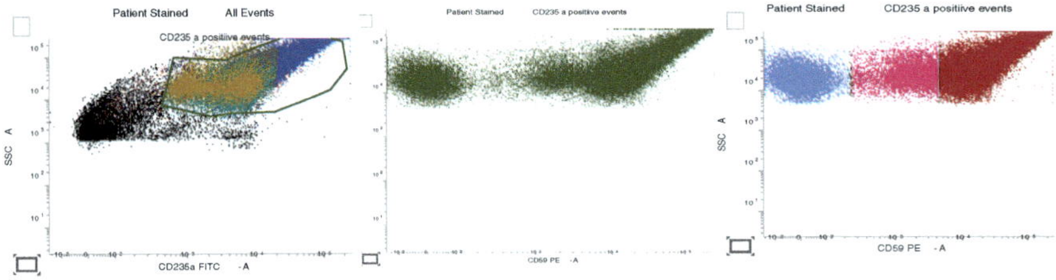

Fig. 10.2 (**a**) RBCs gated by CD235a staining. (**b**, **c**) RBCs showing variable expression of CD59

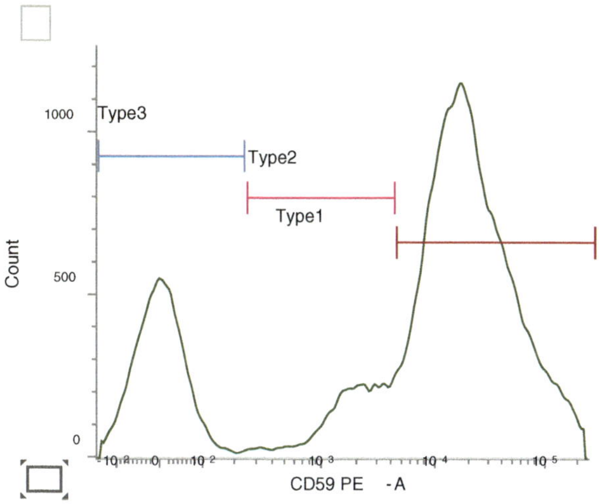

Fig. 10.3 Histogram showing type 1, type 2, and type 3 RBCs. (Flow plots courtesy: Dr.Vidisha Mahajan MD)

10.2 Flow Cytometry and PNH

Paroxysmal nocturnal haemoglobin is an acquired, clonal disorder of the haematopoietic stem cells characterized by impaired synthesis of a cell anchoring protein, i.e., glycosylphosphatidylinositol (GPI), due to an acquired mutation in the PIG-A gene on chromosome X, leading to the absence of numerous GPI-anchored proteins from the surfaces of all haematopoietic cells. Two such proteins recognized earliest and found to have significance are the decay accelerating factor (DAF) or CD55 and membrane inhibitor of reactive lysis (MIRL) or CD59, which regulate complement activity and protect red blood cells (RBCs) from haemolysis. Haemolysis in PNH occurs due to excessive complement activity due to the absence of these complement regulators. Along with haemolysis, PNH is also characterized by thromboses at unusual sites and cytopenias due to bone marrow failure [1].

In the appropriate clinical scenario, the diagnosis of PNH is confirmed by demonstrating lack of GPI anchored proteins on cell surfaces by flow cytometry. First described by van der Schoot CE in 1990 [2], J Schubert et al. showed that flow cytometry was equivalent, if not better than classical Ham's test for diagnosing PNH [3]. Hall and Rosse through a series of 54 patients established optimum conditions for flow cytometric analysis for diagnosis of PNH [4]. They used antibodies against CD55, CD59, and CD16 and found that CD59 was the most useful marker, the demonstration of whose absence on RBCs as well as granulocytes could be standardized for diagnosis. It was also realized that using only CD59 or any single marker was not sufficient for diagnosis, as a single protein deficiency state could represent an isolated inherited defect, and some proteins can have transmembrane forms (besides being GPI-anchored) of expression too. The diagnosis was thus, based on the demonstration of a lack of the GPI-anchored proteins and not on the absence of the anchor itself. Nearly 25 years ago, it was shown that PNH cells are resistant to the cytotoxic effects of a bacterial toxin, aerolysin. It is because the toxin/its inactive precursor, pro-aerolysin, binds to cells via the GPI anchor, and hence, cells lacking this anchor cannot bind the toxin and are resistant to it. Thus, fluorescently labelled pro-aerolysin variant (FLAER, which can bind the GPI anchor but cannot cause cytotoxicity) was introduced to demonstrate the absence of the GPI anchor itself. FLAER assays appeared to be more sensitive and better at differentiating between PNH positive and PNH-negative cells [5]. Almost a decade after the introduction of FLAER, the first comprehensive guidelines on behalf of the International Cell Cytometry Society (ICCS) were published in 2010, which outlined almost all aspects of PNH testing by flow cytometry, including clinical indications for testing, type of samples, pre-analytical issues, choice of monoclonal antibodies with the fluorescent dyes, reporting format, etc. The diagnostic efficiency of PNH tests is much higher when performed under the correct clinical indications [6]. Those guidelines also distinguished between routine PNH assays versus high-sensitivity assays. A paper published after two years outlined protocols and optimum conditions for the high-sensitivity assay [7]. Over the years, with advancements in techniques for rare event analysis (MRD), differentiation between routine and highly sensitive assays has become redundant. Any flow cytometry laboratory wishing to start PNH testing can establish a highly sensitive assay using similar instruments, software, monoclonal antibodies, and efforts. In fact, newer guidelines do not distinguish between the two [8].

FCM for PNH needs to show the absence of the GPI-anchored proteins or of the GPI anchor itself, which can be demonstrated on red blood cells (RBCs), neutrophils, and monocytes. The PNH positive cells can be classified as type III (completely deficient for the GPI-anchored proteins), type II (partial deficiency), type I (normal cells). The percentages of these various types can vary in one patient.

Lymphocytes and platelets have not been found useful for the detection of the defect. Lymphocytes have a long life and also have variable expression of proteins. As protein expressions may vary, it is recommended that both RBCs as well as white blood cells (WBCs) be tested for the PNH defect. For RBCs, CD59 tagged to Phyocerythrin (PE) is the most useful and most efficient to distinguish between type III and type II cells. A logarithmic scale is used to separate the RBCs, and instead of depending on FSC and SSC properties, it is recommended that glycophorin a (CD235a) tagged to FITC be used to identify and gate the red cells [7]. As CD235a is expressed very abundantly on red cells, exposure to the antibody can cause red cell aggregation, and careful titration of the antibody should be performed while validating the assay. CD45, along with CD15 (for neutrophils) and CD64 (for monocytes), is advocated for gating pure populations and avoiding possible contaminants like eosinophils and dendritic cells, respectively. Demonstration of absence of GPI-linked proteins like CD24 (on neutrophils), CD14 (on monocytes), CD157/ADP-ribosyl cyclase 2 (on both neutrophils and monocytes) [9], as well as absence of binding of FLAER, is used for confirming the PNH defect. Because of the advantages of FLAER, it is recommended that FLAER be used when available. FLAER is tagged to Alexa 488 and needs special compensation. It is also more expensive. Additionally, FLAER has not been found to be useful for detecting the defect in RBCs. Assays on granulocytes and monocytes without FLAER (using

CD157, CD24, CD14) have been shown to be equally efficient [10]. A combination of FLAER and CD157 is also equally effective, i.e., without CD24 and CD14 [11].

It is easier to achieve high sensitivity analysis using RBCs as a large number of cells are available for acquisition. Using single marker histograms, it is also easier to differentiate between type I and type II cells. However, the clone size may be misleading due to loss of cells following haemolysis or dilution due to red cell transfusion. These latter situations do not occur with white blood cells. Assaying both neutrophils and monocytes gives more confidence in establishing/ruling out the diagnosis. Table 10.2 summarizes some of the best/current practices and guidelines for PNH flow cytometry.

All testing is performed on peripheral blood samples. Left-shifted samples with the presence of immature cells or bone marrow samples are not suitable, as the expression of antigens on immature cells differs from that of mature cells.

Transfused RBCs may express dim CD59, putting these cells at risk of being detected as type II PNH cells. Use of CD71 to gate reticulocytes and establish PNH defect in them may be helpful in red cell assays in transfused specimens [12].

PNH clones are associated with marrow failure syndrome like aplastic anaemia and myelodysplastic syndromes, and since the presence of such clones has significant therapeutic and prognostic implications, highly sensitive assays able to detect clones as small as 0.01% have become necessary. In such assays, to be confident that abnormal events (for GPI proteins) are real PNH events and not some random, nonspecific ones, the laboratory has to follow guidelines for rare event flow cytometry. One step is to establish the limit of blank (LOB). LOB is the highest reading (from non-specific signals) which might be detected in a normal person's sample who does not have PNH (considered the blank sample). Various studies have shown that these events are generally 2–6/million acquired RBCs and 2–10/million acquired neutrophils.

To be confident that a certain cluster of events is the cells of interest and to quantify the percentage of such a cluster of cells, the size of the cluster has to be large enough, i.e., comprise a certain number of events [13]. A cluster comprising at least 50 events with well-characterized PNH defects is considered a requirement for quantification, as measurements performed on them will have an acceptable standard deviation as per Poisson's distribution statistics (lower limit of quantification, LLOQ). A smaller number of events (i.e., 20 events) might be enough for detection, but not considered enough to quantify the clone (lower limit of detection, LOD). Total number of events to be acquired and analysed will depend upon this number and level of sensitivity desired. To achieve a sensitivity level of 0.01%, at least 500,000 target cell population must be analysed. For RBCs and even neutrophils this is usually possible but difficult in monocytes as they are present in smaller numbers. Generally, acquisition of 100,000 RBCs is enough if no PNH positive cells are seen. The acquisition may be stopped and a negative report issued. If any PNH cells are seen, the acquisition should be increased in order to get a quantifiable cluster as described above [14].

The report should be well standardized and as per guidelines [6]. The report of the patient mentioned at the beginning of this chapter is a good example of one. If

Table 10.2 Summary of current common/best practices and guidelines for PNH flow cytometry

Type of cell	Sample type	Stability	Markers	Processing	Cytometer	Special notes	Advantage/ disadvantage
RBC	Peripheral blood in EDTA, Heparin and ACD acceptable	48 hours from collection	CD235a FITC for gating (PE labelled antibody causes more aggregation), CD59, CD55	Critical racking step before acquisition to dislodge aggregates, washing step	Logarithmic scale for both forward scatter and side scatter, dot plots, single colour histograms	Careful titration of CD235a to prevent RBC aggregates Diluted blood sample used	Large numbers available for analysis for increased sensitivity (up to 0.002%) Easier to distinguish between type II and type III cells Clone size often decreases due to haemolysis or blood transfusion
Neutrophils	Peripheral blood in EDTA Heparin and ACD acceptable	24–48 hours from collection	CD45, CD15 (gating), CD24, CD157, FLAER	Lyse-wash-stain Bulk lysis- clear background	Linear scale	No dilution of blood sample Careful titration of anti-CD15 antibody	Not affected by haemolysis/ transfusion Often challenging to distinguish between type II and type III cells
Monocytes	Peripheral blood in EDTA Heparin and ACD acceptable	24–48 hours from collection	CD45, CD 64 (gating), CD14, CD157, FLAER	Lyse-wash-stain Bulk lysis -clear background	Linear scale		Not affected by haemolysis/ transfusion Reflect clone size better. Due to low numbers, cannot achieve high sensitivity using monocytes

PNH cells are detected but the cluster contains lesser number of events than the lower limit of quantification for the laboratory, the same should be mentioned and a qualitative report may be signed out with advice to follow up.

10.3 Flow Cytometry and Hereditary Spherocytosis (HS)

Hereditary spherocytosis (HS) is the commonest type of inherited haemolytic anaemia, which is characterized by haemolysis, bouts of jaundice, and splenomegaly. HS is a disorder of the red cell membrane characterized by defects in red cell membrane proteins like ankyrin, alpha spectrin, beta spectrin, band 3, and protein 4.2. Due to defective membrane proteins, the RBC membrane becomes less deformable and unstable, leading to loss of membrane, especially when the red cells are subjected to the shear stress of traversing the sinusoids of the spleen. The loss of membrane causes the cells to acquire a spheroidal shape, which can accommodate maximum volume for minimal surface area. Blood film morphology for spherocytes, red cell indices (raised mean corpuscular haemoglobin concentration), demonstration of Coombs negative haemolysis, and family history (as most cases are autosomal dominant) are the mainstays of diagnosis. In many straightforward cases, the diagnosis may not be difficult. However, the blood film morphology may not be helpful in neonates and milder forms. Family history might not help in autosomal recessive cases.

The spheroidal RBCs having no extra membrane are very susceptible to lysis on exposure to hypotonic saline. This was demonstrated by the manual osmotic fragility test wherein red cells are added to varying concentrations of saline solutions, and the amount of haemolysis with decreasing saline strengths is measured by spectrophotometry. This test is cumbersome, time-consuming and lacks specificity for HS and is no longer recommended [15]. Other manual tests to screen for the reduced surface area to volume are the acidified glycerol lysis test (AGLT) and the cryohaemolysis test. However, none of these are sensitive or specific enough to detect all cases of HS. For atypical cases, sodium-dodecyl-sulphate-polyacrylamide gel electrophoresis (SDS–PAGE) of erythrocyte membrane proteins, ektacytometry (technology that actually measures the RBC deformation on exposure to osmotic stress), genetic testing are needed for diagnosis. All the three methodologies are limited by being not easily available.

Though the manual osmotic fragility is no longer recommended as a screening test in any of the current guidelines, osmotic fragility testing using flow cytometer (FC-OFT) appears to have a high sensitivity and specificity for HS. A cost-effective and relatively simple test for performing osmotic fragility by FCM was described in 2009 [16]. Red cells in suspension in isotonic normal saline (NS) are exposed to deionized water (DW) and the red cell count is measured sequentially by FCM in real-time before and after DW spiking. In the time versus FSC plot, eight equal regions are demarcated, and events are measured from left to right (x axis representing time). The RBC saline suspension is acquired immediately after mixing, and the tube is removed after the first region, spiked with DW, and reinstalled at the acquisition site. The acquisition continues, and the result is read as a percentage of residual cells, which is the event count of the last two regions over the counts in the first region (before DW spiking) multiplied by 100. Additionally, the pre-spiking event count is multiplied by a correction factor to correct for the additional dilution caused by the DW after the spiking. A ratio of the residual RBC count of a normal sample to the patient's result appeared to have greater discretionary power. The first authors suggested a value of 23% residual red cell count and a ratio of 3 (normal to patient residual red cell count ratio) to be highly sensitive and specific for HS. Various laboratories have used a similar methodology and found osmotic fragility by flow cytometry to have 97–100% sensitivity and 95.5–98% specificity for HS [17]. Two points are vital: (a) there should be no/minimal time gap between creation of saline suspension and acquisition, (b) ensuring addition of an equal number of RBCs in both patient and control sample tubes (ensured using a formula taking the red cell count of each sample into consideration). The results of FC-OF appear to correlate with clinical severity scores [18], and FC-OF has been found to have high sensitivity for paediatric patients too [19]. It is far less labour and time-consuming and there is no need of an additional test on an incubated sample.

The eosin 5′ maleimide binding test (FC-EMA) is based on the measurement of the binding of EMA, a fluorescent dye to band 3 protein on red cell membrane [20]. Amongst other red cell membrane proteins, band 3 is essential for the stabilization of the cytoskeleton/membrane complex. Loss of band 3 occurs due to gene mutation coding for the protein, and also because of red cell membrane fragmentation caused by the loss of other proteins. Decreased binding of EMA (a measure of the amount of band 3) is reflected by reduced fluorescence as measured by the mean fluorescence or MFI after staining of red cells with EMA. It is a good screening test with the highest specificity for diagnosis of HS, and when compared to SDS–PAGE, it showed a sensitivity of 92.7% and specificity of 99%, respectively [20]. Other authors [21] have reported even higher sensitivity of 96.4% with a specificity of 94.2%, and international guidelines have included it in the list of recommended tests for the diagnosis of HS [22]. The results of FC-EMA have been shown to distinguish between HS and hereditary pyropoikilocytosis (HPP) based on the differences in mean fluorescence intensity (MFI), the MFI for RBC EMA fluorescence being nearly 25% lower in HPP compared to HS [23]. This assay requires a smaller specimen volume compared to traditional OFT, making it ideal for paediatric and neonatal patients. An EDTA sample, which is refrigerated at 4 °C, is stable for testing for up to 72 hours. However, no internationally accepted reference values for MFI of the EMA binding test are available, and assaying normal control samples along with the patient sample is essential. Though there are reports of using fluorescent beads [24] to do away with the use of healthy controls, referral labs mandate shipping a sample from a normal control along with the patient sample.

When FC-OFT and FC-EMA were performed at the same time in children with clinically confirmed disease, a small number tested positive on one method and negative on the other. It is also shown that the EMA binding test is not sensitive to ankyrin defects. Due to the low-specimen volumes needed for both FC-OFT and FC-EMA, and to not miss any case, it may be beneficial to perform both tests concurrently (even in paediatric patients). It is clear that FC-OF and FC-EMA are better than traditional osmotic fragility [25].

10.4 Flow Cytometry and Fetomaternal Haemorrhage

The detection and quantification of feto-maternal haemorrhage is critical in the management of Rh alloimmunization in Rh-positive babies born to Rh-negative mothers. FCM has been used for detecting the presence of foetal RBCs in the peripheral blood of pregnant women in order to establish and quantify feto-maternal haemorrhage [26]. FCM using fluorescent-tagged anti-D antibody is useful only in Rh mismatched cases, but is technically simpler as Rh antigens are present on the surface of RBCs. Antibodies targeting foetal hemoglobin (HbF) can be used to detect feto-maternal bleeding in all situations but is technically more challenging as HbF is intracellular and necessitates intracytoplasmic staining [27]. Moreover, adults also contain small amounts of foetal haemoglobin which might lead to overestimation of the foetal cell counts. To overcome this, an antibody against Carbonic Anhydrase (CA) has been used in combination as CA is expressed by adult red cells only [28]. Detection of foetal cells using FCM has been found to be more accurate and reproducible as compared to the manual Kleihauer Betke test, as a much larger number of cells are analysed rapidly and as it is an automated method. In fact, the FCM method has been recommended in earlier guidelines [29] for confirmation. However, there are disadvantages of flow cytometry like the need for a flow cytometer, trained technologists, increased cost and the need for the testing service to be available round the clock. In light of these, the traditional Kleihauer Betke's method, even with its inaccuracies (as compared to flow cytometry), appears to serve the purpose for which it was intended and hence, flow cytometric detection of FMH has not yet become routine [30].

10.5 Flow Cytometry and Platelet Disorders

Platelets are the blood cells playing the main role in primary haemostasis and thrombosis. They circulate in the blood in an inactivated state but when they come into contact with an area of vascular injury, or are exposed to shear stress, they undergo a number of changes and get activated. At sites of vascular injury, they adhere to Von Willebrand factor and collagen using very specific glycoprotein receptors GPVI and GPIb-IX-V (CD42b/CD42a/CD42d), respectively. This, along with the effect of other agonists released from the site of injury, causes the platelets to get activated and bind fibrinogen and form platelet aggregates (which contribute to the platelet plug) via another set of receptors, GPIIb/IIIa (CD41/CD61) or integrin alpha IIbBeta3 [31]. The activation causes the fibrinogen binding receptor to undergo a conformational change (activated form).

The absence/reduced expression of the glycoprotein receptors leads to bleeding disorders, two of the most well characterized being Glanzmann's Thrombasthenia (reduced/absence of CD41/CD61) and Bernard Soulier Syndrome (reduced/absence of CD42b).

Platelet activation causes the secretion of contents of dense granules and alpha granules, which lead to further activation and aggregation of platelets. Granule release is associated with exposure of the proteins of the membrane of the granules, like CD63 from dense granule membranes and CD62P and TLT-1 [TREM-like transcript-1] from membranes of alpha granules on platelet surface. P-Selectin (CD62P), when exposed to the platelet surface, binds to monocytes and neutrophils and thus, plays a role in inflammation. Strong agonists like thrombin cause platelet phosphatidylserine to be exposed, which is involved in the coagulation cascade. Defects in any of these steps can lead to bleeding disorders.

A procedure for the detection of glycoprotein receptor expression on platelets was first described by Marti et al. [32]. Today, FCM assays using fluorescent-tagged monoclonal antibodies against the main platelet glycoprotein receptors to detect reduced expression of these for the diagnosis of diseases like Glanzman's Thrombasthenia and Bernard Soulier Syndrome are well standardized and relatively straightforward (Figs. 10.4, 10.5, 10.6, and 10.7).

However, platelet function disorders are heterogenous diseases, and there are many conditions that are not well characterized and challenging to diagnose, especially disorders associated with defective activation of platelets. There are assays that utilize monoclonal antibodies against activated receptors (using antibodies that can recognize only activated forms of receptors) as well as monoclonal antibodies

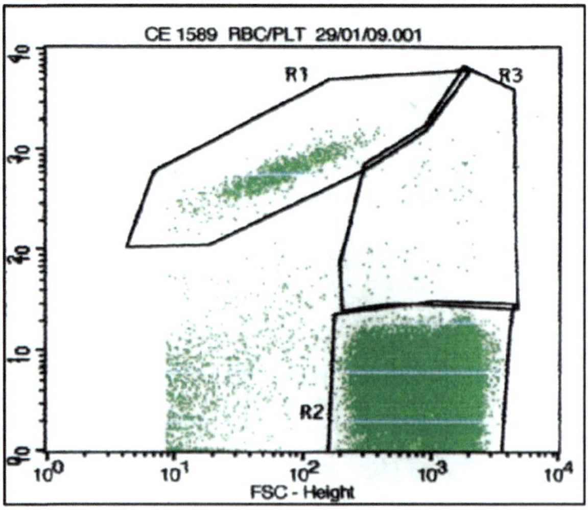

Fig. 10.4 Separation of platelets and RBCs. R1 – platelet events; R2 – RBC events; R3 – Coincidence events

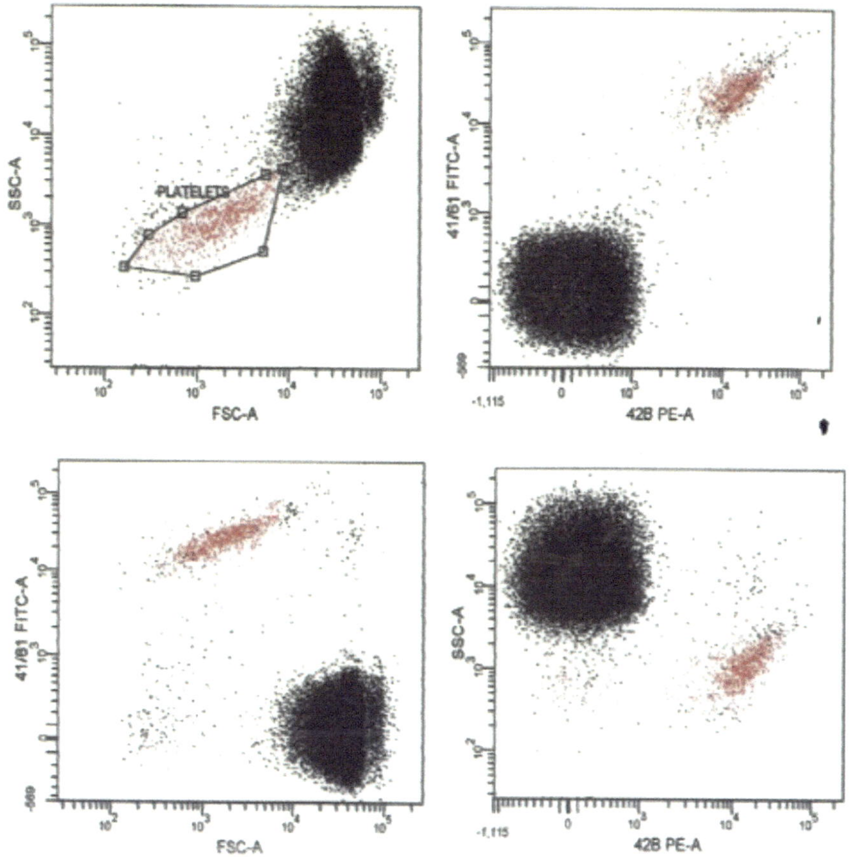

Fig. 10.5 Normal platelets positive for CD41/61 and CD42b

against granule contents (exposed on the surface only after activation by various agonists). FCM methods for the detection of platelet aggregation have also been described [33].

Shattil et al. described a flow cytometric method of detection of activated platelets using PAC-1 antibody, which binds to the activated form of the fibrinogen receptor (GPIIb-IIIa complex) and SI2, which detects an alpha-granule membrane protein that becomes exposed on the platelet surface upon activation. It was also shown that presence of even 0.8% activated platelets could be detected showing that flow cytometry was a sensitive methodology for detecting changes in platelets [34]. Various protocols for both glycoprotein receptor expression as well as detection of platelet activation have been put forward by different laboratories, along with the creation of some reference ranges for various parameters using healthy volunteers [35–37]. In large surveys of laboratories performing platelet functions, including one involving 37 countries over five continents, it was realized that though Light

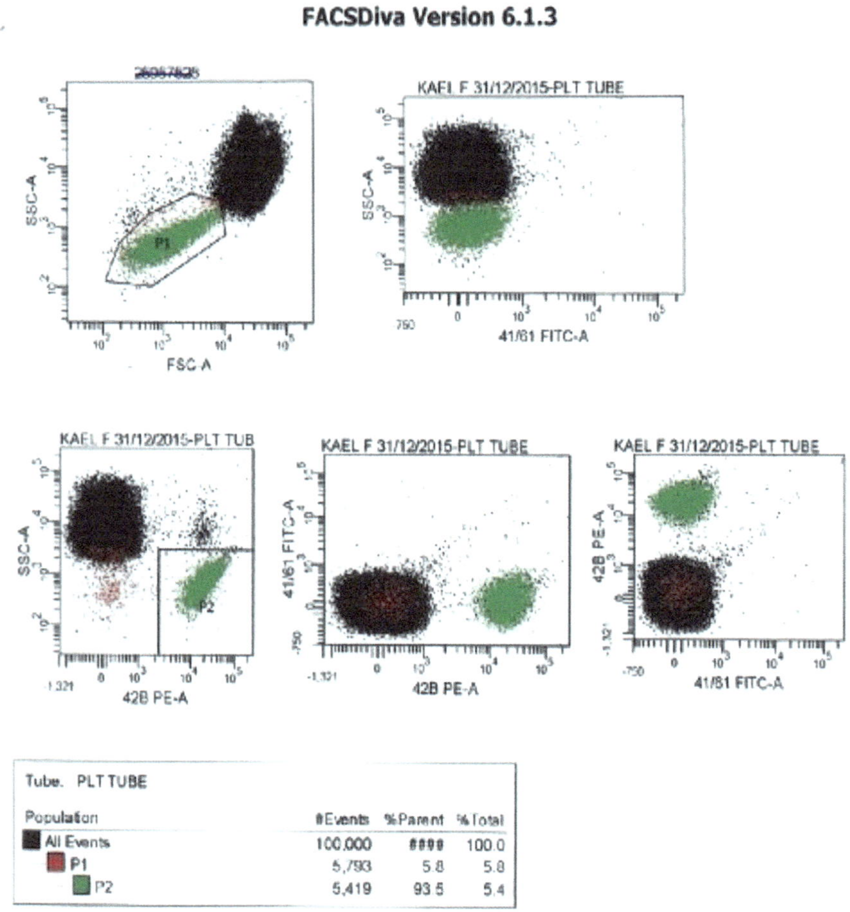

Tube: PLT TUBE

Population	#Events	%Parent	%Total
All Events	100,000	####	100.0
P1	5,793	5.8	5.8
P2	5,419	93.5	5.4

Fig. 10.6 CD41/61 negative and CD42b positive platelets in Glanzman's thrombasthenia

Transmission Aggregometry (LTA) was still the mainstay of diagnosis, FCM for PFD was performed by nearly 70% of the laboratories [38, 39]. It was also realized that there was still a lack of standardization of FCM methods. The subcommittee for platelet physiology for the International Society of Thrombosis and Haemostasis [40] and the International Society of Thrombosis and Haemostasis 2021 consensus recommendation [41], as well as the 2023 consensus report [42] for FCM in thrombocytopenic samples, address a number of issues towards standardization of FCM for the diagnosis of platelet function disorder.

Few pre-analytical variables that need to be considered are the gauge of the needle used for blood collection (19 to 21G), the sample should be kept and transported at ambient room temperature (20–25 °C), it should be hand-carried (no pneumatic chutes), and the time between collection and testing should not exceed 4 hours. The sample is used in a dilution of 1:10 in order to prevent aggregates (dilution can be

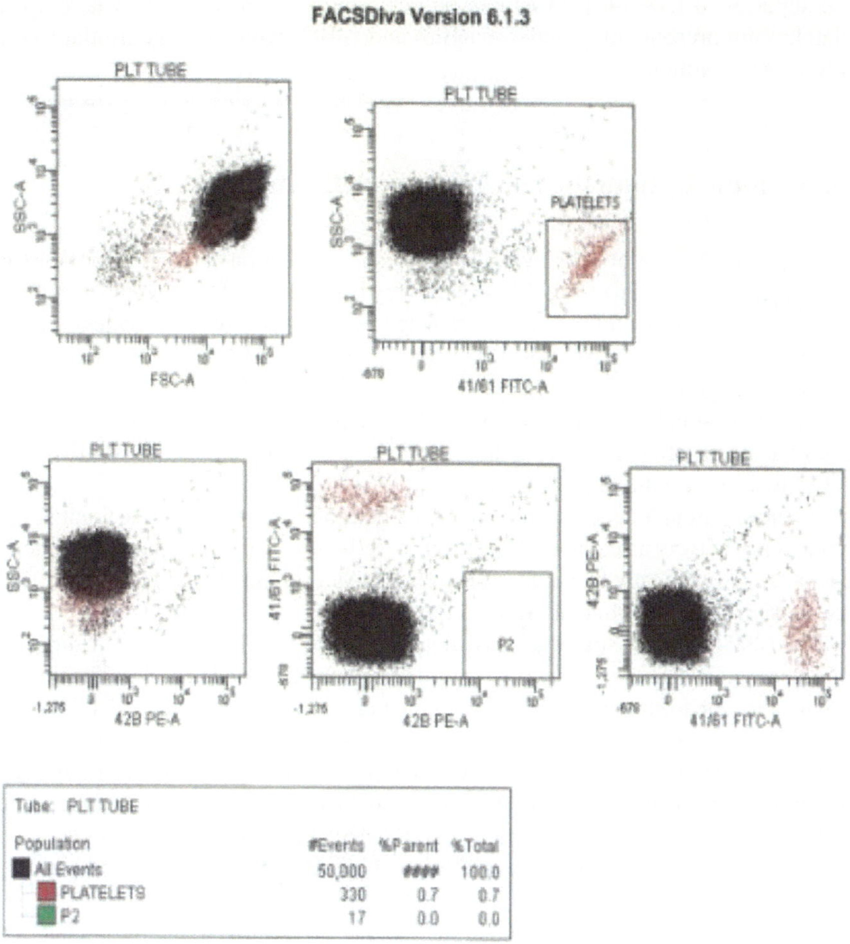

Fig. 10.7 CD41/61 positive and CD42b negative platelets in Bernard Soulier syndrome

reduced in severe thrombocytopenia) [35]. FSC versus SSC, along with a platelet glycoprotein like CD41 on a logarithmic scale, is used to delineate the platelets from RBCs and WBCs. As the sample is usually whole blood, there is usually no need to remove debris. A slower acquisition is recommended, and it is enough to collect 10,000 platelets to analyse them, which is possible even in thrombocytopenic samples.

A major limitation for performing LTA (the mainstay of platelet assays) is the unreliable results with thrombocytopenia. It is well established that low counts associated with platelet function defects are associated with higher bleeding scores. FCM overcomes this and also has the advantage of needing very small amounts (as less as 5 ul) of blood for testing, making it suitable for testing paediatric samples too. Comparisons of FCM with LTA found FCM to be as good if not superior to LTA [43]. FCM can be performed on whole blood wherein the platelets are present along with the RBCs and WBCs which is very similar to the in vivo environment.

10.6 Flow Cytometry and Immunodeficiency Disorders

Immunophenotyping of cells by FCM enables identification/categorisation of cells by antigen expression patterns. Flow cytometry has been used for quantifying CD4+ T cell subsets in the follow-up and management of HIV positive patients. With advances in flow cytometry as well as the availability of a large number of antibodies targeted against surface, intracytoplasmic, and intranuclear antigens, along with a better understanding of immunology, it is now possible to extend the lymphocyte subset analysis into greater detail and to even assess the functional status of various cells involved in immunity [44, 45].

Inherited immunodeficiency disorders are heterogenous diseases due to inherited monogenic defects affecting the function of cells involved in the immune system, characterized clinically by recurrent infections. Autoimmunity, marrow failure, and malignancy are other clinical presentations.

The 2024 Update on the classification from the International Union of Immunological Societies Expert Committee provided an updated classification of Inborn Errors of Immunity (IEI), encompassing a total of 555 IEIs, and 17 phenocopies due to mutations in 504 different genes under 10 classes of disorders.

Genetic testing is most specific, but it can be expensive, with undesirably long turnaround times. Moreover, the phenotype might vary even with the same genetic lesion. It is also important to demonstrate the actual immunological consequences of a genetic defect, and flow cytometry has been found to be very useful in this context.

Severe combined immunodeficiency (SCID) is characterized by severe reduction in T cells (<300/ul), which may be associated with normal or decreased B and NK cells in different combinations [46]. It is genetically heterogenous and immunophenotyping of lymphocytes and subsets is the first step in the diagnosis of SCID. The lymphocyte subset assay by FCM provides the absolute numbers as well as the percentages of the various lymphocytes for preliminary classification of SCID into T-B+NK+ SCID, T-B-NK+ SCID, T-B+NK- SCID, and T-B-NK- SCID. For accurate numerical results, single platform assays using beads are recommended, use of two levels of quality control material, reverse pipetting, and establishing linearity of the assays are other recommendations.

More detailed immunophenotyping, determining the naïve/memory and activation states of T cells using CD45RA, CD45RO, and HLA-DR aids in the diagnosis of Leaky SCID and Omenn syndrome. Most (80–90%) of the T cells in newborns are naïve, while the memory T cells increase with age [47]. More memory cells suggest the possibility of Omenn syndrome (SCID which shows autosomal recessive inheritance, increased immunoglobulin E and eosinophils), a milder form of SCID, like hypo-morphic SCID or engraftment of maternal T-cells. T-cells recently emigrated (RTEs) from the thymus show expression of PECAM-1 (CD-31), and its expression helps identify RTEs to study thymic function in disorders like Di George syndrome, as well as for following haematologic reconstitution following transplantation. Defects in the IL2RG, IL7RA, or JAK3 gene can cause T-B+ SCID. Analysis of specific protein expressions by FCM may serve as a quick method to point out possible genetic defects. Flow cytometric analysis for subsets like CD132 (IL2RG), CD127 (IL7RA), CD3, and CD19 can help classify T-B+ SCID patients into X-Linked SCID or IL7RA-deficient SCID.

Immunophenotyping of B-lymphocyte subsets in peripheral blood is used to diagnose and assess patients with humoral deficiencies such as common variable immunodeficiency (CVID) [48]. CVID is a heterogeneous disease, but often, there is defective differentiation of B cells into memory B cells or antibody-secreting cells. B cells are identified by CD19 expression in the lymphocytes, and B-cell populations can be segregated based on expression of IgD and CD27 [naive (IgD+CD27−), pre-switched (IgD+CD27+), switched memory (IgD−CD27+), and exhausted (IgD−CD27−)] cells. Switched memory cells are absent in abnormal germinal centre function.

T-cell immunophenotyping also helps diagnose autoimmune lymphoproliferative syndrome (ALPS), which is associated with dysregulated lymphocyte proliferation with autoimmune phenomenon, chronic lymphadenopathy, and organomegaly due to defects in the genes controlling lymphocyte apoptosis [49]. Demonstration of elevated double negative-cells (defined as CD3+TCRαβ+CD4-CD8- T cells); either >1.5% of total lymphocytes or >2.5% of CD3+ T-cells in a background of normal or elevated lymphocyte counts is one of the diagnostic criteria. These cells may also express B220. If the double negative (CD4-/CD8-/CD3+) T-cell population is expanded on a routine lymphocyte subset assay, further immunophenotyping with anti-TCRαβ and anti-B220 may be performed. It is essential to consider age-specific reference intervals while issuing the report. This assay is a rapid tool with a positive predictive value of 61% and a negative predictive value of 71% and helps to decide on genetic testing.

Besides immunophenotyping, flow cytometric analysis of the expression of certain intracellular proteins can be performed for the diagnosis of inherited immune diseases. X-linked agammaglobulinemia, characterized by a lack of B-cells and immunoglobulins, is caused by a mutation in the gene for a protein called Bruton's Tyrosine Kinase (BTK) [50]. Peripheral blood lymphocyte subset analysis shows markedly low B-cells, i.e., <1% of all lymphocytes. FCM of monocytes (as B-cell numbers are usually too low in these patients) for intracellular BTK expression will show significantly decreased expression. Carrier females show two types of cell populations (with normal expression as well as decreased expression). FCM analysis of the phosphorylation status of the protein is helpful when the expression is normal, but the protein is non-functional.

Hemophagocytic Lymphohistiocytosis (HLH) is a severe systemic illness due to a hyper inflammatory drive caused by excessive activation of macrophages and T cells, resulting from defective cytotoxicity characterized clinically by fever, cytopenias and hepatosplenomegaly. HLH can either be genetic (familial) or secondary to infections, malignancies, etc. Inherited HLH occurs due to mutations in genes coding for proteins needed for cytotoxic functions of NK cells and cytotoxic lymphocytes. Many flow cytometry assays have been developed to demonstrate the deficient cytotoxic activity of NK cells or cytotoxic lymphocytes (CTL).

Two assays stand out amongst them, i.e., detection of intracellular expression of perforin and surface expression of CD107a [51]. The defective PRF1 gene leads to decreased/absent perforin expression, a protein that is essential for cytotoxicity. Absence of perforin leads to a type of familial HLH (FHL2).

Most other types of FHLs (FHL3, FHL4, FHL5, etc) are due to defects in other genes causing defective degranulation. CD107a is present intracellularly on the lysosomal surface, which is expressed on the cell surface upon activation and release of lysosomal contents. Thus, detection of this protein after activation of NK cells or CTL is a measure of the efficiency of degranulation [44]. Assays have been developed to detect intracellular expression of perforin. In normal individuals, >80% cells express perforin. The expression can be detected in CD56+/CD3- NK cells or CD3+/CD8+ cytotoxic T cells. Though the diagnostic criteria put forward by the Histiocyte Society in 1991 and upgraded in 2007 include demonstration of deficiency of cytotoxicity of NK cells, the perforin assay, as well as the CD107a assay, have been found to be easier, more robust, and equally sensitive and specific for FHL. Experts have found that while investigating for FHL, it is useful to do both these assays simultaneously, as they are seen almost equally, and doing them simultaneously saves time [44].

X-linked lymphoproliferative syndromes (XLP-1 and XLP-2) are rare disorders seen in males wherein the genetic defect (in SH2D1A and BIRCA genes, respectively, leading to absence of SAP and XIAP proteins) leads to HLH. Flow cytometry can detect the absence of expression of SAP as well as XIAP and is recommended in male patients. Functional assays for these disorders have also been described, but only genetic assays for the defective genes are confirmatory.

Immunophenotyping and detection of a CD3+/CD8+/CD38++/HLADR+ subset of cells has also been reported to be useful in differentiating HLH from other inflammatory situations like sepsis [52].

Chronic granulomatous disease (CGD) is a group of disorders characterized by a defective NADPH oxidase system, leading to a defective oxidative burst, which in turn leads to an inability to generate toxic oxygen radicals (superoxide) required to kill bacteria. Typically, patients get recurrent bacterial infections or abscesses. To look for the oxidative burst, neutrophils are loaded with dihydrorhodamine (DHR) dye and then activated with an activator like phorbol-12-myristate-13 acetate (PMA). Normally activated neutrophils produce superoxides that oxidize DHR, resulting in the emission of fluorescence, which in turn is quantified by flow cytometry. Neutrophils from affected patients fail to generate superoxide and, therefore, cannot oxidize the dye, leading to reduced fluorescence. This functional FCM assay assesses the capacity of neutrophils to produce an oxidative burst (Fig. 10.8). Results are expressed as the stimulation index

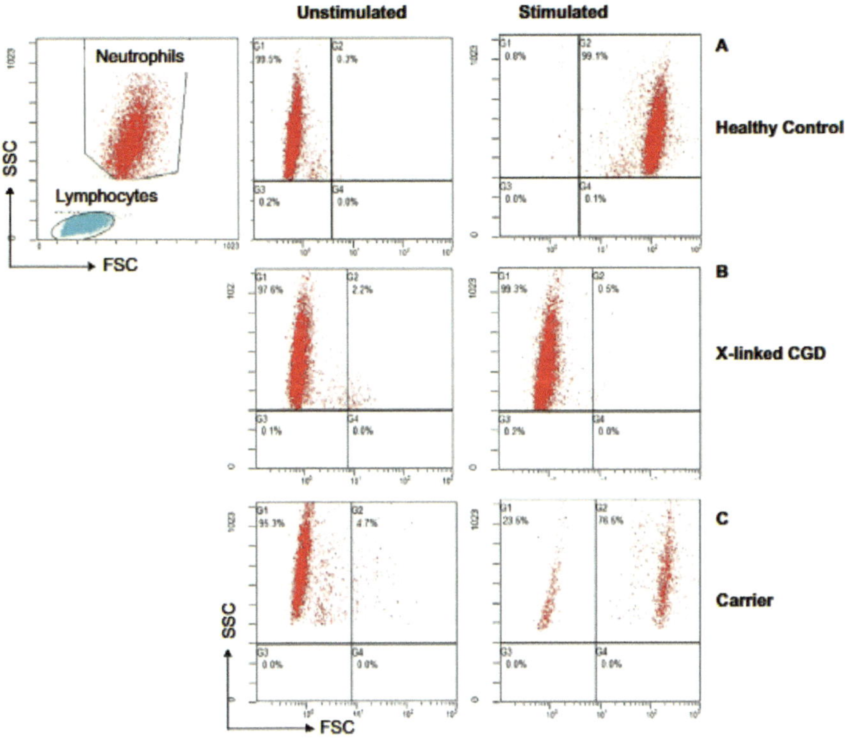

Fig. 10.8 Assessment of oxidative burst in neutrophils

of neutrophils, which is the ratio of peak mean fluorescence of stimulated neutrophils to that of unstimulated neutrophils [53].

The defect occurs due to mutations in one of four known components of the NADPH oxidase system; X-linked form (gp91-phox) is the commonest, along with three autosomal recessive (p22-phox, p47-phox, and p67-phox) ones. It is also possible to study the expression of these component proteins by flow cytometry.

Leukocyte adhesion deficiency Type I (LAD-I) is caused by a decreased expression of CD18. while leukocyte adhesion deficiency Type II (LAD-II) is caused by the decreased expression of CD15 [54].

The hyper IgM syndromes include genetic disorders of immunodeficiency characterized by isotype class-switching defects resulting in decreased immunoglobulins (IgG and IgA), with normal or increased IgM. X-linked hyper IgM syndrome (HIGM), the most common form, is caused by genetic defects in the gene for CD40L or CD154 molecule, expressed primarily on activated CD4+ T-cells. Infections, neutropenia, and liver disease are common. HIGM syndrome can be rapidly diagnosed by flow cytometry for CD40L expression and function on activated CD4+ T-cells [55].

10.7 Summary

FCM is a vital tool for the diagnosis of many non-malignant haematological disorders involving all three haematological cell lines. FCM is the gold standard for the diagnosis of PNH, and guidelines for the same are quite well standardized. For the diagnosis of RBC red cell membrane disorders, FCM offers very sensitive and specific assays like FC-OFT and FC-EMA. Diagnosis of inherited platelet disorders of glycoprotein expression, like BSS and GT, is relatively straightforward. Platelet activation assays are more challenging, but guidelines and protocols are widely available in the literature today. The role of flow cytometry in the diagnosis of immune-deficiency disorders has gone far beyond a B and T-cell lymphocyte subset assay. Even functional assays are being performed, albeit in a limited number of laboratories and FCM appears to be a valuable tool in diagnosis as well as in providing clues towards the type of genetic testing required for confirmation. With more and more experience being reported and shared, it is possible for haematology laboratories who have experience with flow cytometry in leukaemia/lymphoma diagnosis to establish specialized assays for non-malignant haematological disorders. Absence of reference ranges and non-availability of quality control materials are major challenges for accredited clinical laboratories to perform these assays. Added to these are the lack of External Quality Control schemes for many of the assays.

Acknowledgements The authors would like to thank Dr. Vidisha Mahajan for the PNH flow plots and Ms. Anwaar AbdulBaset AlHathrami and Mr. Mohammed Bilal for their help in referencing.

References

1. Hillmen P, Lewis SM, Bessler M, Luzzatto L, Dacie JV. Natural history of paroxysmal nocturnal hemoglobinuria. N Engl J Med [Online]. 1995;333(19):1253–8. Available from: https://doi.org/10.1056/NEJM199511093331904.
2. van der Schoot CE, Huizinga TW, van 't Veer-Korthof, Wijmans R, Pinkster J, von dem Borne AE. Deficiency of glycosyl-phosphatidylinositol-linked membrane glycoproteins of leukocytes in paroxysmal nocturnal hemoglobinuria, description of a new diagnostic cytofluorometric assay. Blood [Online]. 1990;76(9):1853–9. Available from: https://doi.org/10.1182/blood.v76.9.1853.bloodjournal7691853.
3. Schubert J, Alvarado M, Uciechowski P, Zielinska-Skowronek M, Freund M, Vogt H, et al. Diagnosis of paroxysmal nocturnal haemoglobinuria using immunophenotyping of peripheral blood cells. Br J Haematol [Online]. 1991;79(3):487–92. Available from: https://doi.org/10.1111/j.1365-2141.1991.tb08060.x.
4. Hall SE, Rosse WF. The use of monoclonal antibodies and flow cytometry in the diagnosis of paroxysmal nocturnal hemoglobinuria. Blood [Online]. 1996;87(12):5332–40. Available from: https://doi.org/10.1182/blood.v87.12.5332.bloodjournal87125332.
5. Brodsky RA, Mukhina GL, Li S, Nelson KL, Chiurazzi PL, Buckley JT, et al. Improved detection and characterization of paroxysmal nocturnal hemoglobinuria using fluorescent aerolysin. Am J Clin Pathol [Online]. 2000;114(3):459–66. Available from: https://doi.org/10.1093/ajcp/114.3.459.

6. Borowitz MJ, Craig FE, Digiuseppe JA, Illingworth AJ, Rosse W, Sutherland DR, et al. Guidelines for the diagnosis and monitoring of paroxysmal nocturnal hemoglobinuria and related disorders by flow cytometry. Cytometry B Clin Cytom [Online]. 2010;78(4):211–30. Available from: https://doi.org/10.1002/cyto.b.20525.
7. Sutherland DR, Keeney M, Illingworth A. Practical guidelines for the high-sensitivity detection and monitoring of paroxysmal nocturnal hemoglobinuria clones by flow cytometry. Cytometry B Clin Cytom [Online]. 2012;82(4):195–208. Available from: https://doi.org/10.1002/cyto.b.21023.
8. Sutherland DR, Illingworth A, Marinov I, Ortiz F, Andreasen J, Payne D, et al. ICCS/ESCCA consensus guidelines to detect GPI-deficient cells in paroxysmal nocturnal hemoglobinuria (PNH) and related disorders part 2 - reagent selection and assay optimization for high-sensitivity testing. Cytometry B Clin Cytom [Online]. 2018;94(1):23–48. Available from: https://doi.org/10.1002/cyto.b.21610.
9. Sutherland DR, Acton E, Keeney M, Davis BH, Illingworth A. Use of CD157 in FLAER-based assays for high-sensitivity PNH granulocyte and PNH monocyte detection. Cytometry B Clin Cytom [Online]. 2013. Available from: https://doi.org/10.1002/cytob.21111.
10. Marinov I, Illingworth AJ, Benko M, Sutherland DR. Performance characteristics of a non-fluorescent aerolysin-based paroxysmal nocturnal hemoglobinuria (PNH) assay for simultaneous evaluation of PNH neutrophils and PNH monocytes by flow cytometry, following published PNH guidelines: non-flaer-based assay for pnh testing by flow cytometry. Cytometry B Clin Cytom [Online]. 2018;94(2):257–63. Available from: https://doi.org/10.1002/cyto.b.21389.
11. Deka R, Pati HP, Chandra D, Manivannan P, Chauhan R, Tyagi S, et al. CD157 can replace CD24 and CD14 in a single-tube flow-cytometric assay to detect paroxysmal nocturnal hemoglobinuria (PNH) clones on both neutrophils and monocytes: a prospective study from north India. Cureus [Online]. 2022;14(4):e23965. Available from: https://doi.org/10.7759/cureus.23965.
12. Sutherland DR, Richards SJ, Ortiz F, Nayyar R, Benko M, Marinov I, et al. CD71 improves delineation of PNH type III, PNH type II, and normal immature RBCS in patients with paroxysmal nocturnal hemoglobinuria. Cytometry B Clin Cytom [Online]. 2020;98(2):179–92. Available from: https://doi.org/10.1002/cyto.b.21853.
13. Hedley BD, Keeney M. Technical issues: flow cytometry and rare event analysis. Int J Lab Hematol [Online]. 2013;35(3):344–50. Available from: https://doi.org/10.1111/ijlh.12068.
14. Illingworth A, Marinov I, Sutherland DR, Wagner-Ballon O, DelVecchio L. ICCS/ESCCA consensus guidelines to detect GPI-deficient cells in paroxysmal nocturnal hemoglobinuria (PNH) and related disorders part 3 – data analysis, reporting and case studies: ICCS/ESCCA PNH consensus guidelines - part 3. Cytometry B Clin Cytom [Online]. 2018;94(1):49–66. Available from: https://doi.org/10.1002/cyto.b.21609.
15. Bolton-Maggs PHB, Stevens RF, Dodd NJ, Lamont G, Tittensor P, King M-J, et al. Guidelines for the diagnosis and management of hereditary spherocytosis: guideline. Br J Haematol [Online]. 2004;126(4):455–74. Available from: https://doi.org/10.1111/j.1365-2141.2004.05052.x.
16. Won DI, Suh JS. Flow cytometric detection of erythrocyte osmotic fragility. Cytometry B Clin Cytom [Online]. 2009;76(2):135–41. Available from: https://doi.org/10.1002/cyto.b.20448.
17. Pati NK, Sartor MM, Wong S, Nemet A, Bradstock KF. Evaluation of the role of flow cytometry as a diagnostic tool for Hereditary Spherocytosis. Blood [Online]. 2008;112(11):5381–1. Available from: https://doi.org/10.1182/blood.v112.11.5381.5381.
18. Shim YJ, Won D. Flow cytometric osmotic fragility testing does reflect the clinical severity of hereditary spherocytosis: FCM of Test Reflects the Severity of HS. Cytometry B Clin Cytom [Online]. 2014;86(6):436–43. Available from: https://doi.org/10.1002/cyto.b.21143.
19. Ciepiela O, Adamowicz-Salach A, Zgodzińska A, Łazowska M, Kotuła I. Flow cytometric osmotic fragility test: increased assay sensitivity for clinical application in pediatric hematology: Flow Cytometric Osmotic Fragility Test in Children. Cytometry B Clin Cytom [Online]. 2018;94(1):189–95. Available from: https://doi.org/10.1002/cyto.b.21511.

20. King MJ, Behrens J, Rogers C, Flynn C, Greenwood D, Chambers K. Rapid flow cytometric test for the diagnosis of membrane cytoskeleton-associated haemolytic anaemia. Br J Haematol [Online]. 2000;111(3):924–33. Available from: https://doi.org/10.1046/j.1365-2141.2000.02416.x.
21. Kar R, Mishra P, Pati HP. Evaluation of eosin-5-maleimide flow cytometric test in diagnosis of hereditary spherocytosis. Int J Lab Hematol [Online]. 2010;32(1 Pt 2):8–16. Available from: https://doi.org/10.1111/j.1751-553X.2008.01098.x.
22. Bolton-Maggs PHB, Langer JC, Iolascon A, Tittensor P, King M-J, General Haematology Task Force of the British Committee for Standards in Haematology. Guidelines for the diagnosis and management of hereditary spherocytosis – 2011 update: guideline. Br J Haematol [Internet]. 2012;156(1):37–49. Available from: https://doi.org/10.1111/j.1365-2141.2011.08921.x.
23. King M-J, Telfer P, MacKinnon H, Langabeer L, McMahon C, Darbyshire P, et al. Using the eosin-5-maleimide binding test in the differential diagnosis of hereditary spherocytosis and hereditary pyropoikilocytosis. Cytometry B Clin Cytom [Online]. 2008;74(4):244–50. Available from: https://doi.org/10.1002/cyto.b.20413.
24. Glenthøj A, Sharfo A, Brieghel C, Nardo-Marino A, Birgens H, Petersen JB. Improving the EMA binding test by using commercially available fluorescent beads. Front Physiol [Online]. 2020;11:569289. Available from: https://doi.org/10.3389/fphys.2020.569289.
25. Arora RD, Dass J, Maydeo S, Arya V, Radhakrishnan N, Sachdeva A, et al. Flow cytometric osmotic fragility test and eosin-5′-maleimide dye-binding tests are better than conventional osmotic fragility tests for the diagnosis of hereditary spherocytosis. Int J Lab Hematol [Online]. 2018;40(3):335–42. Available from: https://doi.org/10.1111/ijlh.12794.
26. Chen JC, Davis BH, Wood B, Warzynski MJ. Multicenter clinical experience with flow cytometric method for fetomaternal hemorrhage detection. Cytometry [Online]. 2002;50(6):285–90. Available from: https://doi.org/10.1002/cyto.10154.
27. Ward RY. Estimation of fetomaternal haemorrhage using a flow cytometric technique. Int Clin Cytom Soc e-News. 2011;2. Available from: https://www.cytometry.org/newsletters/eICCS-2-2/article3.php.
28. Kumpel BM, MacDonald AP, Bishop DR, Yates AF, Lee E. Quantitation of fetomaternal haemorrhage and F cells in unusual maternal blood samples by flow cytometry using anti-D and anti-HbF: quantitation of FMH by flow cytometry. Transfus Med [Online]. 2013;23(3):175–86. Available from: https://doi.org/10.1111/tme.12030
29. Austin E , Bates S, de Silva M, Howarth D, Lubenko A, Rowley M, et al. Guidelines for the estimation of fetomaternal haemorrhage. Working Party of the British Committee for Standards in Haematology, Transfusion Taskforce. 2009. Available from: https://b-s-h.org.uk/media/15705/transfusion-austin-the-estimation-of-fetomaternal-haemorrhage.pdf.
30. Gereg C, Fung MK. Assessment of flow cytometry and kleihauer-Betke method when calculating fetomaternal hemorrhage and Rh immunoglobulin dose. Arch Pathol Lab Med. 2022;146(3):271. Available from: https://doi.org/10.5858/arpa.2021-0432-LE.
31. Nurden A, Nurden P. Advances in our understanding of the molecular basis of disorders of platelet function: inherited platelet disorders. J Thromb Haemost [Internet]. 2011;9 Suppl 1:76–91. Available from: https://doi.org/10.1111/j.1538-7836.2011.04274.x.
32. Marti GE, Magruder L, Schuette WE, Gralnick HR. Flow cytometric analysis of platelet surface antigens. Cytometry [Online]. 1988;9(5):448–55. Available from: https://doi.org/10.1002/cyto.990090508.
33. Vinholt PJ, Frederiksen H, Hvas A-M, Sprogøe U, Nielsen C. Measurement of platelet aggregation, independently of patient platelet count: a flow-cytometric approach. J Thromb Haemost [Online]. 2017;15(6):1191–202. Available from: https://doi.org/10.1111/jth.13675.
34. ShattilSJ,CunninghamM,HoxieJA.Detectionofactivatedplateletsinwholebloodusingactivation-dependent monoclonal antibodies and flow cytometry. Blood [Online]. 1987;70(1):307–15. Available from: https://doi.org/10.1182/blood.v70.1.307.bloodjournal701307.

35. Spurgeon BEJ, Naseem KM. Platelet flow cytometry: instrument setup, controls, and panel performance: platelet flow cytometry. Cytometry B Clin Cytom [Online]. 2020;98(1):19–27. Available from: https://doi.org/10.1002/cyto.b.21774.
36. Andres O, Henning K, Strauß G, Pflug A, Manukjan G, Schulze H. Diagnosis of platelet function disorders: a standardized, rational, and modular flow cytometric approach. Platelets. 2018;29(4):347–56. Available from: https://doi.org/10.1080/09537104.2017.1386297.
37. Keller Cecconello D, Spagnol F, Alegretti AP, Pilger DA, Farias MG. Flow cytometry immunophenotyping of healthy platelets and hospitalized patients with suspected platelet dysfunction: challenges for establishing a cutoff value. Hematol Transfus Cell Ther [Online]. 2024;46 Suppl 5:S136–42. Available from: https://doi.org/10.1016/j.htct.2023.07.002.
38. Gresele P, Harrison P, Bury L, Falcinelli E, Gachet C, Hayward CP, et al. Diagnosis of suspected inherited platelet function disorders: results of a worldwide survey. J Thromb Haemost [Online]. 2014;12(9):1562–9. Available from: https://doi.org/10.1111/jth.12650.
39. Szanto T, Zetterberg E, Ramström S, Leinøe EB, Holme PA, Antovic JP, et al. Platelet function testing: current practice among clinical centres in Northern Europe. Haemophilia [Online]. 2022;28(4):642–8. Available from: https://doi.org/10.1111/hae.14578.
40. Gresele P. Subcommittee on Platelet Physiology of the International Society on Thrombosis and Hemostasis. Diagnosis of inherited platelet function disorders: guidance from the SSC of the ISTH. J Thromb Haemost [Online]. 2015;13(2):314–22. Available from: https://doi.org/10.1111/jth.12792.
41. Frelinger AL 3rd, Rivera J, Connor DE, Freson K, Greinacher A, Harrison P, et al. Consensus recommendations on flow cytometry for the assessment of inherited and acquired disorders of platelet number and function: communication from the ISTH SSC Subcommittee on Platelet Physiology. J Thromb Haemost [Internet]. 2021;19(12):3193–202. Available from: https://doi.org/10.1111/jth.15526.
42. Jourdi G, Ramström S, Sharma R, Bakchoul T, Lordkipanidzé M, FC-PFT in TP study group. Consensus report on flow cytometry for platelet function testing in thrombocytopenic patients: communication from the SSC of the ISTH. J Thromb Haemost [Online]. 2023;21(10):2941–52. Available from: https://doi.org/10.1016/j.jtha.2023.07.006.
43. Navred K, Martin M, Ekdahl L, Zetterberg E, Andersson NG, Strandberg K, et al. A simplified flow cytometric method for detection of inherited platelet disorders-a comparison to the gold standard light transmission aggregometry. PLoS One [Online]. 2019;14(1):e0211130. Available from: https://doi.org/10.1371/journal.pone.0211130.
44. Madkaikar MR, Shabrish S, Kulkarni M, Aluri J, Dalvi A, Kelkar M, et al. Application of flow cytometry in primary immunodeficiencies: experience from India. Front Immunol [Online]. 2019;10:1248. Available from: https://doi.org/10.3389/fimmu.2019.01248.
45. Martínez-Gallo M, García-Prat M. Flow cytometry applied to the diagnosis of primary immunodeficiencies [Online]. In: Innovations in cell research and therapy. IntechOpen; 2020. Available from: https://doi.org/10.5772/intechopen.89743.
46. Chinn IK, Shearer WT. Severe combined immunodeficiency disorders. Immunol Allergy Clin N Am. 2015;35(4):671–94. Available from: https://doi.org/10.1016/j.iac.2015.07.002.
47. Garcia-Prat M, Álvarez-Sierra D, Aguiló-Cucurull A, Salgado-Perandrés S, Briongos-Sebastian S, Franco-Jarava C, et al. Extended immunophenotyping reference values in a healthy pediatric population: Interpretation of Extended Immunophenotyping Profiles. Cytometry B Clin Cytom. 2019;96(3):223–33. Available from: https://doi.org/10.1002/cyto.b.21728.
48. Warnatz K, Schlesier M. Flowcytometric phenotyping of common variable immunodeficiency. Cytometry B Clin Cytom [Internet]. 2008;74(5):261–71. Available from: https://doi.org/10.1002/cyto.b.20432.
49. Matson DR, Yang DT. Autoimmune lymphoproliferative syndrome: an overview. Arch Pathol Lab Med [Internet]. 2020;144(2):245–51. Available from: https://doi.org/10.5858/arpa.2018-0190-RS.

50. Yadav RM, Desai SS, Gupta M, Dalvi A, Bargir UA, Jodhawat N, et al. Clinical utility of flow-cytometry for diagnosis and genotype phenotype correlation in a cohort of X-linked agammaglobulinemia patients. Indian J Pediatr [Online]. 2024;91(6):638. Available from: https://doi.org/10.1007/s12098-024-05127-9.
51. Rubin TS, Zhang K, Gifford C, Lane A, Choo S, Bleesing JJ, et al. Perforin and CD107a testing is superior to NK cell function testing for screening patients for genetic HLH. Blood [Online]. 2017;129(22):2993–9. Available from: https://doi.org/10.1182/blood-2016-12-753830.
52. Chaturvedi V, Marsh RA, Zoref-Lorenz A, Owsley E, Chaturvedi V, Nguyen TC, et al. T-cell activation profiles distinguish hemophagocytic lymphohistiocytosis and early sepsis. Blood [Online]. 2021;137(17):2337–46. Available from: https://doi.org/10.1182/blood.2020009499.
53. O'Gorman MR, Corrochano V. Rapid whole-blood flow cytometry assay for diagnosis of chronic granulomatous disease. Clin Diagn Lab Immunol [Online]. 1995;2(2):227–32. Available from: https://doi.org/10.1128/cdli.2.2.227-232.1995.
54. Dorfman DM, Karlon WJ, Linden MA. Color atlas of flow cytometry. USA: College of American Pathologists; 2023.
55. Freyer DR, Gowans LK, Warzynski M, Lee W-I. Flow cytometric diagnosis of X-linked hyper-IgM syndrome: application of an accurate and convenient procedure. J Pediatr Hematol Oncol [Internet]. 2004;26(6):363–70. Available from: https://doi.org/10.1097/00043426-200406000-00006.

Chapter 11
Molecular Genetic Tests in Thalassemias and the Hemoglobinopathies: Pros and Cons of Different Techniques

Prashant Sharma and Reena Das

Abstract Thalassemias and hemoglobinopathies are common inherited monogenic disorders, characterized by defects in the quantity and/or quality of globin chain production. Initial diagnostic evaluation typically includes red cell indices and hemoglobin separation techniques such as HPLC or CZE. Molecular genetic testing becomes necessary to resolve diagnostic ambiguities, guiding prenatal diagnosis, elucidating genotype–phenotype correlations, and occasionally, confirming carrier status. This chapter provides a comprehensive overview of molecular diagnostic techniques used in the evaluation of α-, β-, and rarer forms of the thalassemias. For β-thalassemia as well as most hemoglobinopathies, commonly used methods include allele-specific PCRs (especially ARMS-PCR), DNA reverse dot blot hybridization (RDB), Sanger sequencing, and rarely, MLPA and real-time PCR. For α-thalassemia, multiplex gap-PCR and MLPA are used to detect prevalent gene deletions, while sequencing is increasingly preferred over individual end-point PCRs to identify the less common non-deletional variants. The diagnostic yield, cost-effectiveness, throughput, and ability of these techniques to detect known-versus-novel mutations are discussed. Factors influencing the selection of a diagnostic approach include the local mutational spectrum, laboratory capacity, and clinical scenario. Non-transfusion dependent β-thalassemia (NTDT) genotypes often require assessment of secondary and tertiary genetic modifiers, including co-inherited α-globin gene anomalies and polymorphisms influencing fetal hemoglobin production. There is an emerging role of next-generation sequencing (NGS) for comprehensive genotyping and its integration into high-throughput screening platforms. Recent advances in non-invasive prenatal testing (NIPT), including digital PCR and relative haplotype dosage analysis using cell-free fetal DNA, are transforming reproductive counselling in high-risk couples.

P. Sharma (✉) · R. Das
Department of Hematology, Postgraduate Institute of Medical Education and Research (PGIMER), Sector 12, Chandigarh 160012, India

H. P. Pati et al. (eds.), *Clinical Hematology and Hemato-Oncology*,
https://doi.org/10.1007/978-981-92-1167-8_11

Keywords Hemoglobinopathies · Molecular diagnostics · Mutation detection techniques · Next-generation sequencing (NGS) · Non-invasive prenatal testing (NIPT) · Thalassemia

Learning Objectives
- To understand the principles, applications, advantages, and limitations of various molecular techniques used in the diagnosis of thalassemias and hemoglobinopathies, including ARMS-PCR, reverse dot blot, Sanger sequencing, MLPA, and next-generation sequencing (NGS).
- To differentiate between molecular strategies employed for β-thalassemia (primarily point mutations and small indels) and α-thalassemia (predominantly gene deletions), and recognize how mutation type guides the choice of diagnostic technique.
- To identify the clinical scenarios and laboratory findings that warrant molecular genetic testing, including genotype–phenotype discordance, non-transfusion dependent β-thalassemia (NTDT), and prenatal diagnosis in at-risk couples.
- Describe the evolving role of non-invasive prenatal testing (NIPT) and NGS in comprehensive screening, fetal genotyping, and the identification of genetic modifiers of disease severity.

11.1 Introduction

Thalassemias and the hemoglobinopathies represent a diverse group of inherited recessive disorders that comprise the commonest monogenic disorders globally. They arise from quantitative or qualitative defects in the synthesis or structure of globin polypeptide chains. Being among the first genetic diseases to be characterized at the molecular level, they have served as prototypes for the development of molecular techniques. The highly variable clinical manifestations of these disorders necessitate accurate and comprehensive diagnostic approaches. Molecular genetic testing is important for definitive diagnosis of challenging cases, screening of atypical carriers, prenatal diagnosis, and understanding genotype-phenotype correlations [1, 2].

Table 11.1 Salient indications for molecular genetic testing in thalassemia [1, 6]

Clinical indications: Diagnostic dilemmas, genotype-phenotype discorrelations, prenatal diagnosis. Specific instances are
In recently and/or multi-transfused patients, where HPLC/CZE do not reveal a clear picture.
For clinically ambiguous cases, often with a genotype/phenotype mismatch. For e.g.: - Cases of ß-thalassemia intermedia/non-transfusion dependent β-thalassemia (NTDT). - ß-thalassemia trait with disproportionately severe clinical symptoms (testing for α-triplications, unstable hemoglobins, dominant ß-thalassemia with exon 3 mutations). - Patients in whom parental HPLC/CZE testing is not available or not feasible, for e.g. an adopted child.
In couples at risk of carrying a fetus with a significant (i.e., severely symptomatic) hemoglobin disorder. For e.g., ß-thalassemia major/TDT, severe ß-thalassemia intermedia (NTDT), sickle cell anemia, double heterozygosity for sickle/ß^0-thalassemia, sickle/E, sickle/HbD-Punjab etc.)
Infants where both parents are BTT, and a presumptive diagnosis of BTM made on HPLC/CZE needs to be confirmed by genetic studies.
Laboratory indications
Unusual/uncommon hemoglobin variants that remain unexplained even after an independent second-line technique.
Ambiguous HPLC/CZE findings insufficient to distinguish double heterozygous states (for e.g., sickle/ß-thalassemia, HbE/ß-thalassemia) from homozygous states (sickle cell anemia or SS-state, HbE disease or EE-state).
Borderline high HbA2 (typically defined as HbA2% between 3.4% and 3.9%).
Unexplained "thalassemic indices" (i.e., erythrocytosis, microcytosis, hypochromia, normal red cell distribution width) in persons with normal range HbA2% [to exclude α-thalassemia trait/ silent carrier states].
Unexplained elevation of fetal hemoglobin.

11.2 Overview of Diagnostic Strategies

Initial suspicion may stem from hematological parameters indicative of microcytic anemia or the presence of abnormal hemoglobin fraction(s) detected by HPLC/ CZE. Patients may be referred for anemia, jaundice, gallstones, or, less commonly, to look for specific variants (e.g., sickle Hb in thrombosis, high-oxygen affinity variants in polycythemia, methemoglobinemic variants in congenital cyanosis, or to explain pulse oximetric findings, etc.). Screening programs aimed at antenatal women also frequently yield asymptomatic states [1, 3, 4].

HPLC findings are fairly specific for many disorders, especially in conjunction with blood counts or simple tests. ß-thalassemia traits typically exhibit elevated HbA2 levels while HbH disease (α-thalassemia intermedia) shows pre-integration peaks on HPLC and a fast-moving band on alkaline pH hemoglobin electrophoresis. However, these methods provide presumptive diagnoses, and definitive characterization of the underlying genetic defect requires a second technique, and in critical or confusing situations, molecular analysis [1, 2, 4]. Table 11.1 summarizes common diagnostic indications for molecular testing in hemoglobinopathies. Generally, molecular testing targets globin gene mutations, which can be broadly categorized into point mutations, small insertions/deletions, and large deletions or rearrangements affecting the α-globin and β-globin gene clusters [1, 5].

11.3 Molecular Genetic Defects in β-, α-, and δβ-Thalassemias

The thalassemias show remarkable genetic heterogeneity. β-thalassemia is predominantly caused by point mutations and small indels, although larger deletions and insertions also occur. α-thalassemia occurs most often due to deletions. The

Table 11.2 The mutational spectrum of β- and α-thalassemias found in India

Mutation (common name)	HGVS nomenclature	Mutation type	Genetic consequence
β-thalassemias			
IVS-I-5 (G>C)	*HBB*:c.92+5G>C	Substitution at a splice site, β^+ (severe)	nt 147 G > C in *HBB* The G > C mutation at nt 5 of the IVS-I reduces the efficiency of splicing of the normal 5′ splicing site
619 bp deletion	NG_000007.3: g.71609_72227del619	Deletion, β^0	619 nts deleted from (1065 thru 1683) in *HBB* Defective mRNA formation; no normal β-globin is synthesized
IVS-I-1 (G>T)	*HBB*: c.92+1G>T	Substitution at a splice site, β^0	nt 143 G>T in *HBB* A G>T change in the GT dinucleotide that is required for normal splicing abolishes this process; no normal mRNA is formed
Codons 8/9 (+G)	*HBB*: c.27_28insG	Frameshift due to indel, β^0	Insertion of G between codons 8 and 9 of *HBB* Frameshift results in termination of translation at codon 22 (TGA)
Codons 41/42 (-CTTT)	*HBB*: c.126_129delCTTT	Frameshift due to indel, β^0	4 nts deleted between codons 41 and 42 of *HBB* gene This frameshift results in a stop codon at the new codon 59, terminating translation
Codon 15 (G>A) *	*HBB*: c.47G>A	Substitution, stop-gain, β^0	T<u>G</u>G > T<u>A</u>G at codon 15 in the β-globin gene This change of one nucleotide results in the termination of translation at codon 15

(continued)

Table 11.2 (continued)

Mutation (common name)	HGVS nomenclature	Mutation type	Genetic consequence
Codon 16 (-C)*; GGC(Gly)>GG	*HBB*: c.51delC	Frameshift due to indel, β^0	nt C deleted from codon 16 of the β-globin gene Frameshift results in termination of translation at codon 18 (TGA)
CAP +1 (A>C) silent*	*HBB*: c.-50A>C	Substitution at upstream CAP site, β^+	nt 1 A>C in *HBB* Decreased level of mRNA is expected
−88 (C>T)*	*HBB*: c.-138C>T	Substitution at upstream promoter site, β^+	nt −88 C>T in *HBB* Reduced β-globin gene transcription due to decreased binding of transcriptional factors
α-thalassemias			
$-\alpha^{3.7\,kb}$ deletion	*NG_000006.1:g.34164_37967del*	Deletion of 3804 nucleotides from the *HBA2* to *HBA1* genes	Partial deletion of α2 gene and partial deletion of α1 gene resulting in the formation of a fusion α gene (α+ thalassaemia).
$-\alpha^{4.2\,kb}$ deletion	*NG_000006.1:g.16609_20854del*	Deletion of 4246 nucleotides	Deletion of α2 gene, leaving the α1 gene intact (α+).
δβ-thalassemias			
Indian type of deletional $\gamma^G(^A\gamma\delta\beta)^0$ Thalassaemia			Deletion of the $^A\gamma$ and δ as well as β-globin genes; however, an intervening region is preserved but inverted.

In approximate decreasing order of frequencies
Less common mutations are marked with * [1, 6, 12–14]

hemoglobinopathies too, are largely caused by point mutations [1–5, 7–10]. Table 11.2 summarizes the mutational spectrum of thalassemias in India.

11.4 Molecular Genetic Techniques for β-Thalassemia and Hemoglobinopathies

Numerous PCR-based techniques have been developed to detect these mutations, and these are discussed briefly below [1, 2, 5, 11, 12].

- *Amplification Refractory Mutation System (ARMS)-PCR*
  - *Principle:* This technique leverages the principle that single nucleotide mismatches at the critical 3′ end of a primer prevent efficient extension by DNA

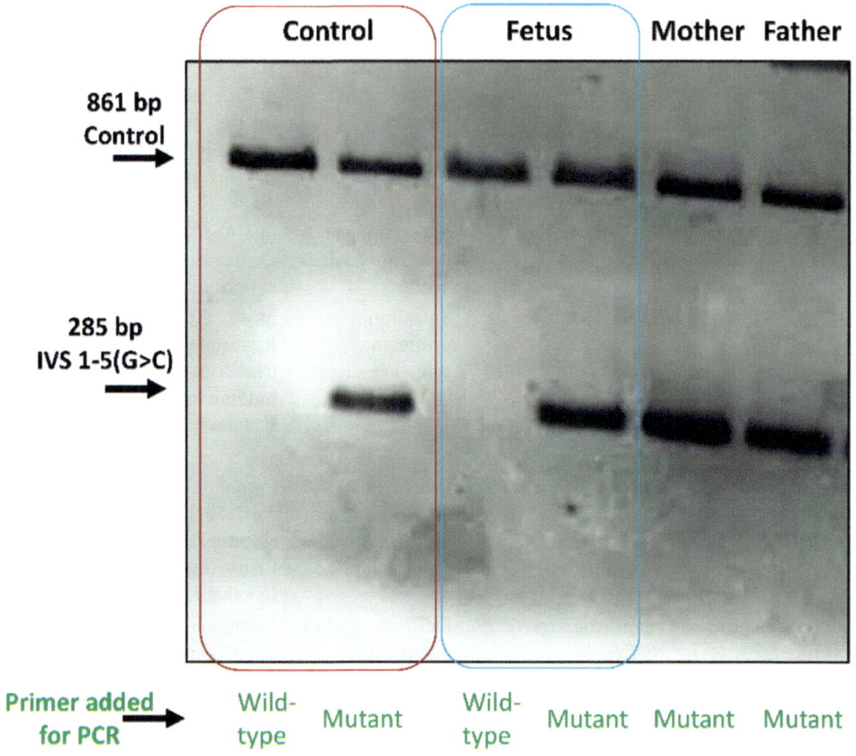

Fig. 11.1 ARMS PCR done for the IVS I-5 mutation. Samples of a thalassemia major control (homozygous IVS I-5), a homozygous fetus, and its parents (both heterozygous for IVS I-5) are shown. Primers used in each tube are written at the bottom

(Taq) polymerase, thus selectively amplifying only the target DNA sequence with the correct base at that position. Typically, a reaction mixture for a single mutation incorporates two amplifications of the same genomic DNA: one using a mutation-specific ARMS primer and the other using a near-identical wild-type-specific primer (with only the 3′ end carrying the nucleotide corresponding to the normal sequence). If the primers are put in separate tubes, then control primers are also added in each, ensuring that the PCR reaction has worked. The presence of a specific PCR product of the expected size indicates the presence or absence of the targeted mutation (Fig. 11.1). Several procedural tweaks and modifications have been designed. ARMS primers ~30 bases long, optimized for a 65 °C annealing temperature, can be easily designed to diagnose over 20 common β-thalassemia mutations, as well as HbS, HbC, and HbE.

Secondary mismatches can also be introduced to increase specificity. For ARMS primers with a weak 3′ terminal mismatch, a strong secondary mismatch is engineered. If the 3′ terminal mismatch is a strong one, only a weak secondary mismatch is required, usually at the second nucleotide. The strength of mismatch pairings is maximum with G-A, C-T, and T-T pairs; C-C is considered strong, while A-A and G-G are medium strength mismatches. C-A and G-T are weak mismatches.

  - *Pros:* ARMS-PCR is a relatively simple, cost-effective, and robust assay. It is widely adopted in many laboratories when screening for a limited number of highly prevalent mutations in a given population (for e.g., the five most common mutations among Indians). The use of internal control primers helps avoid false negative results. ARMS-PCR can be readily applied for prenatal diagnosis to determine the genotype of the fetus when both parents are carriers for a specific mutation each.

  Cons: A particular ARMS-PCR detects its specific mutation only. It requires prior knowledge of the mutations being screened for and necessitates the development of specific primers for each mutation [1, 2, 5, 11, 12].

- *PCR-Restriction Fragment Length Polymorphism (RFLP) Analysis:* RFLP utilizes restriction endonuclease enzymes that cleave DNA at specific recognition sequences. Mutations that create or abolish a restriction site can be detected by changes in the DNA fragment sizes after enzyme digestion and gel electrophoresis. For example, PCR-RFLP has been used for the diagnosis of the Hb Constant Spring mutation using the enzyme *Mse* I. Its pros and cons are largely similar to those of ARMS-PCR. Some mutations do not affect restriction sites [1, 2, 5, 11, 12].
- *Reverse Dot Blot (RDB) Analysis*

  - *Principle:* The region of interest (e.g., the entire β-globin gene exons) of the patient is amplified by PCR. Amplified products are then hybridized to a membrane onto which allele-specific oligonucleotide probes (both wild-type and mutant) are covalently spotted as dots. After hybridization and washing, the presence of a specific mutation is indicated by the binding of the amplified DNA to the corresponding mutant probe. This is visualized through a colorimetric or chemiluminescent detection system. RDB assays simultaneously screen for multiple common mutations (thalassemia as well as hemoglobinopathies) in a given geographical region.
  - *Pros:* Simultaneous detection of multiple known mutations in a single assay make RDB efficient for screening populations with a defined set of common mutations. It is particularly useful for carrier screening and prenatal diagnosis in high-prevalence areas. Commercial line strip assays have been developed that are technically simpler to standardize, for e.g., the Vienna Lab strip assay (21 alpha and 22 beta mutations covered) and BioRad's mDx Gene kits for common Asian and Mediterranean alpha, beta, and variant mutations.

  Cons: Similar to ARMS-PCR, RDB cannot identify novel or uncharacterized mutations. It is limited to the detection of pre-defined mutations for which

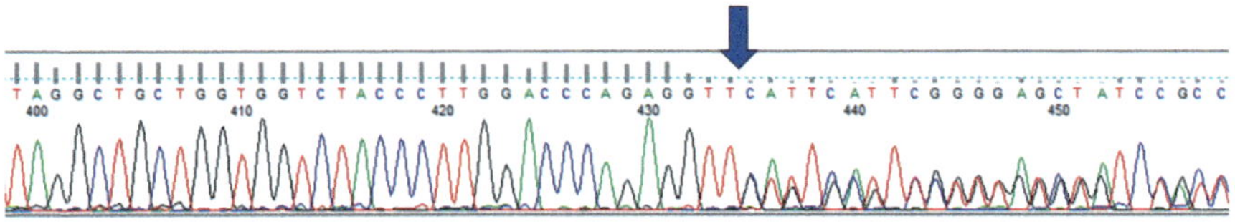

Fig. 11.2 Direct DNA sequencing by Sanger's technique showing the common Indian frameshift 41/42 in a heterozygous state. The sequence electropherogram shows overlapping peaks after the blue arrow due to the deletion of four nucleotides on one allele

probes are included on the membrane. The development, preparation, and storage of the dot blot membranes with specific probes can be technically demanding. There are two elements of quality control in RDB - membrane preparation-related, and patient DNA handling-related, which enhance test complexity [1, 2, 5, 11, 12].

- *Direct DNA Sequencing (Sanger Sequencing)*
  - *Principle:* This involves PCR amplification of the target region (e.g., the exons 1-2 of the β-globin gene) followed by chain termination sequencing using dideoxynucleotides. The resulting fluorescently labelled DNA fragments are then separated by very high-resolution capillary electrophoresis, and the sequence is determined based on the order of the terminating nucleotides (Fig. 11.2). This method allows for the direct determination of the nucleotide sequence of the amplified DNA.
  - *Pros:* Sanger sequencing is considered the gold standard method for identifying unknown mutations in the globin genes and also to confirm mutations detected by other methods. It is a comprehensive technique capable of detecting point mutations and small insertions or deletions..

  Cons: It requires greater capital investment in the form of the capillary electrophoresis instrument. Workflow and analysis can both be time-consuming and labor-intensive, especially when screening for a large number of potential mutations or when analyzing multiple samples. Large deletions and structural abnormalities are missed. Compared to multiplex assays like ARMS-PCR or RDB, it is less efficient for high-throughput screening of known mutations in large populations. Sequencing of the *HBB* gene is less technically complex than for α-globin genes (*HBA1* and *HBA2*) due to the presence of only a single gene and a less GC-rich sequence in the former. Delta globin gene (*HBD*) sequencing, although less commonly required, poses particular challenges due to high sequence homology with HBB [1, 2, 5, 11, 12].

11.5 Less Commonly Used Molecular Methods in ß-Thalassemia and Hemoglobinopathies

- *Real-Time PCR*
  - *Principle:* Real-time PCR integrates microvolume rapid-cycle PCR with fluorometry, enabling the real-time fluorescent monitoring of the amplification reaction. This allows for quantitative PCR and/or characterization of PCR products for rapid genotyping, eliminating the need for post-PCR sample manipulation. Various probe-based chemistries, such as TaqMan probes or melting curve analysis using intercalating dyes, can be employed for mutation detection. For β-globin gene point mutations, allele-specific probes or primers can be used to discriminate between normal and mutant alleles based on fluorescence signal during amplification or differences in melting temperatures of the PCR products. Some assays are designed with probes complementary to the wild-type sequence, potentially allowing for the distinction of any allele with a nucleotide variation under the probe.
  - *Pros:* Real-time PCR offers rapid genotyping capabilities. Melting curve analysis is relatively simple and cost-effective for detecting known mutations and even some unknown variations based on altered melting profiles. It minimizes the risk of contamination associated with post-PCR handling.

  Cons: While melting curve analysis can suggest the presence of a mutation, definitive characterization often requires a second method, such as ARMS-PCR or sequencing. The design and optimization of allele-specific real-time PCR assays can be complex. TaqMan chemistry-based assays are comparatively more expensive than ARMS-PCR or even Sanger sequencing on a per-sample basis [1, 2, 5, 11, 12].

- *Denaturing Gradient Gel Electrophoresis (DGGE) and Conformation-Sensitive Gel Electrophoresis (CSGE)*
  - *Principle:* DGGE separates DNA fragments based on their differential electrophoretic mobility in a polyacrylamide gel containing an increasing gradient of denaturant. DNA fragments with different melting domains will exhibit altered mobility as they reach their specific denaturing concentration. CSGE separates DNA fragments based on subtle differences in their three-dimensional conformation, which can be affected by single-nucleotide changes. PCR products from a heterozygous individual will form heteroduplexes with altered electrophoretic mobility compared to homoduplexes.
  - *Pros:* Before the advent of Sanger sequencing, DGGE and CSGE were used to screen for unknown mutations. They were employed to identify abnormal band patterns vis-à-vis normal controls when ARMS-PCR failed to detect common mutations.

  Cons: These methods were primarily screening techniques and did not directly identify the specific mutation. Abnormal bands needed to be further analyzed

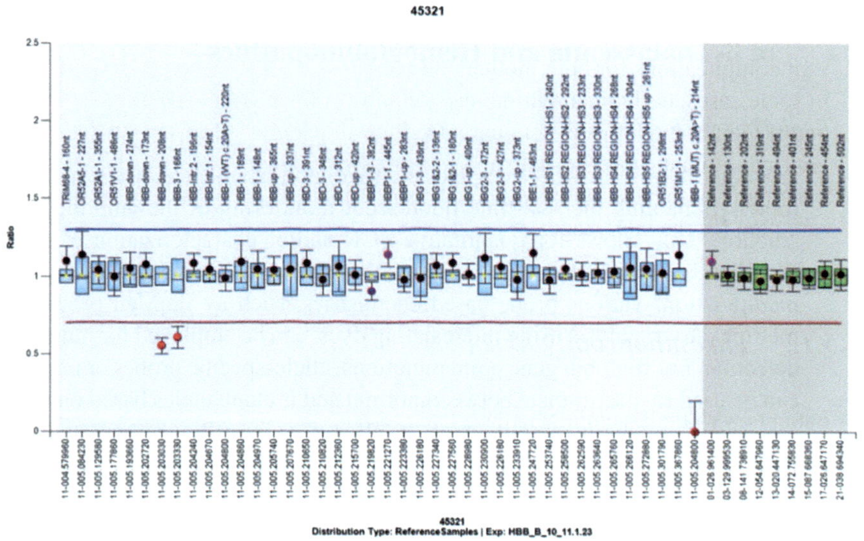

Fig. 11.3 MLPA analysis of the beta globin gene cluster reveals a heterozygous 619-bp deletion in a case of beta thalassemia trait

by sequencing to determine the underlying genetic alteration. They are technically demanding to optimize and to interpret [1, 2, 5, 11, 12].

- *Multiplex Ligation-dependent Probe Amplification (MLPA):*
  - *Principle:* This PCR-based method allows for the detection of copy number variations (CNVs), such as deletions and duplications, as well as the detection of point mutations. It involves the hybridization of multiple probes to their target DNA sequences, followed by a ligation step where only correctly hybridized probes are joined. The ligated probes are then amplified in a single PCR reaction using a common primer pair. The relative amounts of the different amplified products as detected via high-resolution capillary electrophoresis reflect the copy number of the corresponding target sequences in the original DNA sample (Fig. 11.3).
  - *Pros:* MLPA is a relatively simple and robust technique for detection of various deletions and duplications in the β-globin gene cluster, including δβ-thalassemia and HPFH deletions. MLPA is particularly useful for identifying unusual or large deletions that may be missed by standard gap-PCR.

Cons: While MLPA can be used for point mutation detection, other methods like ARMS-PCR or sequencing are generally preferred for this purpose due to their higher sensitivity and specificity for single nucleotide changes. Interpretation of MLPA results requires careful analysis of peak heights to determine copy number variations. Precise breakpoints are usually not revealed by MLPA [1, 2, 5, 11, 12].

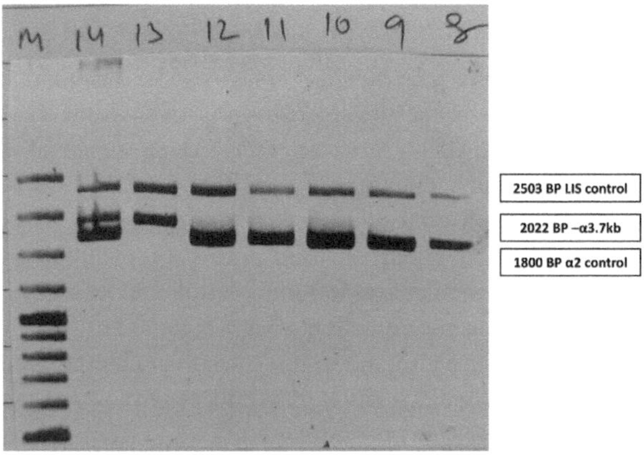

Fig. 11.4 Multiplex gap-PCR for α-globin gene deletions. Lanes labeled 8-12 (toward the right) are normal (both LIS and intact α2 genes are amplified). Lane 13 is homozygous and lane 14 is heterozygous for the common –α3.7 kbp deletion

11.6 Molecular Genetic Techniques for α-Thalassemia and α-Triplications

α-Thalassemias are predominantly caused by deletions of one or more of the four α-globin genes (two α2 and two α1 genes). Non-deletional mutations, such as point mutations affecting gene expression or protein stability, also occur [1, 2, 6, 8, 13–15].

- *Multiplex gap-PCR*
  - *Principle:* Multiplex gap-PCR is a commonly used initial screening method for α-thalassemia deletions. It involves the use of multiple sets of PCR primers that flank the common deletion breakpoints. The presence of a deletion is indicated by the amplification of a specific-sized PCR product that spans the deletion junction. Several comprehensive sets of PCR primers have been described to detect most common *HBA* deletions, such as -α3.7, -α4.2, -SEA, -MED, -SA, αTHAI, αFIL, and -(α)20.5 (Fig. 11.4).
  - *Pros:* Multiplex gap-PCR is a rapid, reliable, and cost-effective method for the initial screening of the most common α-thalassemia deletions. It allows for the simultaneous detection of multiple deletions in a single PCR reaction.

  Cons: Gap-PCR is limited to the detection of known deletions for which the flanking primers are designed. It cannot detect non-deletional mutations or novel deletions with unknown breakpoints.

- *MLPA*

  It is extensively employed in α-thalassemia diagnosis, particularly for the identification of unusual deletions or rearrangements in the α-globin gene cluster that may not be detected by gap-PCR. Pros and cons are the same as discussed for MLPA above.

- *PCR for supernumerary α-genes (also referred to as α-triplications)*
  - *Principle:* Specific PCR assays can be designed to amplify across the junction created by the unequal crossing over event that leads to α-gene triplication (αααanti-3.7 or αααanti-4.2). The presence of a specific PCR product confirms the triplication.
  - *Pros:* Allows for the specific detection of α-gene triplications, which can contribute to silent or mild forms of α-thalassemia and may interact with β-thalassemia. Single-tube multiplex PCR assays have been developed for the simultaneous detection of anti-3.7 and anti-4.2 α-globin gene triplications.

  Cons: This technique cannot resolve heterozygous or homozygous triplication nor yield exact copy numbers [14].

- *α-globin gene sequencing (Sanger sequencing):*
  - *Principle:* Similar to β-globin gene sequencing, but requires specific strategies to overcome the high sequence homology (over 1 kbp including flanking regions, coding sequences, and introns) between the two adult α-globin genes (*HBA1* and *HBA2*) located on chromosome 16. Selective amplification of each gene is necessary, often achieved by using primers designed from sequences at least 1000 base pairs 5′ to the structural genes, combined with a common 3′ primer. The GC-rich nature of the α-globin gene sequences also necessitates optimized PCR conditions. Once amplified, the PCR products are sequenced using standard Sanger methods, and the obtained sequences are compared with databases like HbVar to determine clinical significance. α-gene mutations are more commonly found in the α2 gene compared to the α1 gene.
  - *Pros:* α-globin gene sequencing is essential for identifying non-deletional α-thalassemia mutations, such as point mutations, small insertions, or deletions that affect α-globin chain synthesis or stability. It is the gold standard for characterizing these types of mutations.

  Cons: Sequencing of α-globin genes is technically more challenging than β-globin gene sequencing, and requires careful primer design and optimized PCR conditions. Deletions >500 bp are not reliably detected.

- *Allele-specific PCR and reverse dot blotting:*

  Similar to their applications in β-thalassemia, allele-specific PCR can be used for detecting known non-deletional α-thalassemia mutations prevalent in specific ethnic groups, such as hemoglobin Constant Spring in Southeast Asia. Reverse dot blot assays have also been developed for the simultaneous detection of common α-thalassemia deletions and point mutations. The pros and cons of these techniques are similar to those described for β-thalassemia [1, 2, 5, 8, 11–15].

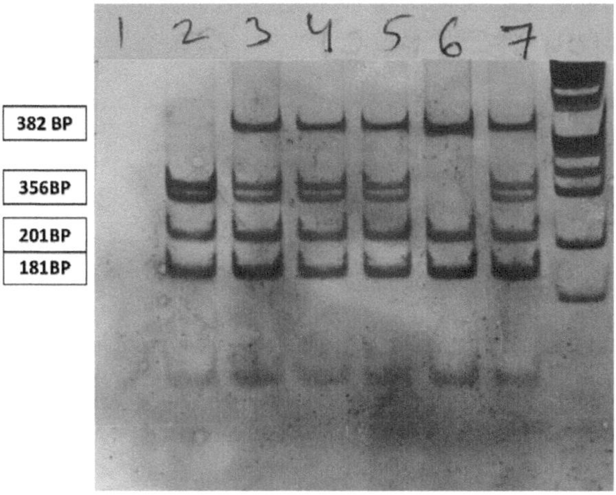

Fig. 11.5 PCR-RFLP for the sickle hemoglobin using the DdeI restriction enzyme. Lane 1 is the no-template control; lane 2 is normal; lanes 3, 4, 5, and 7 are heterozygous, and lane 6 is homozygous for the β^s allele

11.7 Other Molecular Techniques

While PCR-based methods and Sanger sequencing are most widely used, other techniques have also played a role in the molecular diagnosis of hemoglobinopathies [1, 5, 11, 16–19]. These include:

- *Next-Generation Sequencing (NGS)*
  - *Principle:* NGS technologies encompass a variety of high-throughput sequencing methods that allow for the simultaneous sequencing of millions of DNA fragments. They typically involve DNA fragmentation, library preparation with specific adaptors, clonal amplification (or single-molecule amplification), and sequencing-by-synthesis or ligation-based sequencing reactions with fluorescently-labelled nucleotides. The resulting sequence reads are then aligned to a reference genome for variant calling and analysis.
  - *Pros:* High throughput, scalability, and speed, highly efficient for the comprehensive analysis of multiple genes and samples simultaneously. Detects a wide spectrum of genetic variations, including point mutations, small insertions/deletions, large deletions, and even complex structural rearrangements. Particularly valuable for identifying rare or novel mutations that may be missed by targeted assays. Targeted NGS panels covering the α- and β-globin genes, their regulatory regions, and modifier genes are increasingly being used for comprehensive and accurate diagnosis and carrier screening.

  Cons: High cost. Bioinformatic analysis of large datasets requires specialized expertise and infrastructure. Sequencing of the *HBA1 and HBA2* genes presents technical challenges (like low coverage) due to high sequence homology and GC content.

Table 11.3 Summary of molecular tests that may be employed in genetic diagnosis of various thalassemias and hemoglobinopathies [1–4, 9, 10, 13, 14, 18, 20]

Disorder	First-line/commonly used tests	Second-line/less commonly used tests	Older/rarely used tests
Beta thalassemia	ARMS-PCR, reverse dot-blot PCR, Sanger sequencing	PCR-RFLP, NGS, MLPA	Western blot analysis
Alpha thalassemia: deletional variants	Gap-PCR (usually multiplexed for the detection of 4–8 common deletions); MLPA; reverse dot blot analysis	Real-time gap-PCR with HRM curve analysis, denaturing HPLC, NGS	Western blot analysis, mutagenically separated PCR, pyrosequencing, DNA oligonucleotide microarray
Alpha thalassemia: non-deletional variants	Sanger sequencing	ARMS-PCR, NGS	–
Delta-beta thalassemia	MLPA, Gap-PCR followed by Sanger sequencing	NGS	Restriction enzyme mapping using the Southern Blot technique
Hemoglobin Lepore, hemoglobin Kenya	MLPA, Gap-PCR followed by Sanger sequencing	NGS	–
Hereditary persistence of fetal hemoglobin—deletional variants	MLPA, Gap-PCR, and sequencing	NGS	–
Hereditary persistence of fetal hemoglobin—non--deletional variants	Sanger sequencing	NGS	–
Unstable hemoglobins, high- or low-oxygen affinity hemoglobins, methemoglobinemic variants	Sanger sequencing	NGS	–
Clinically important variant hemoglobins	PCR-RFLP [HbS: DdeI; HbE: MnlI; HbD-Punjab and HbO-Arab EcoRI]	Sanger sequencing, ARMS, or another allele-specific PCR	–
Molecular testing of genetic modifiers of clinical phenotype			
Xmn1 $^{G}\gamma$ polymorphism	PCR-RFLP	Sanger sequencing	–
Polymorphic markers in *HBS1L-MYB* intergenic region, *BCL11A*, *KLF1*, etc.	PCR-RFLP, targeted NGS	Real-time PCR (TaqMan arrays or KASP assay)	–
Supernumerary alpha globin genes (e.g., α-triplications)	Gap-PCR, MLPA	–	–

(continued)

Table 11.3 (continued)

Disorder	First-line/commonly used tests	Second-line/less commonly used tests	Older/rarely used tests
Gilbert syndrome	Sanger sequencing of *UGT1A1* promoter	Allele-specific PCR	–
APOE genotyping	PCR-RFLP	Sanger sequencing	–
Vitamin D receptor polymorphisms	PCR-RFLP, other allele-specific PCRs	Real-time PCR (TaqMan arrays or KASP assay)	–
HFE, HAMP, HJV, FPN, and other iron-related gene polymorphisms	PCR-RFLP, Sanger sequencing, targeted NGS.	Allele-specific PCRs	–

- *Pyrosequencing:* A real-time DNA sequencing-by-synthesis method that detects the release of pyrophosphate during nucleotide incorporation. It can be used for short read sequencing and quantification of allelic ratios.
- *Clinically important variant hemoglobins* are commonly diagnosed using ARMS-PCR, PCR-RFLP (Fig. 11.5), Sanger sequencing, and less commonly, by DNA melting curve analysis or loop-mediated isothermal amplification.

Table 11.3 summarizes the molecular genetic techniques used for the diagnosis of β-thalassemia and hemoglobinopathies.

11.8 Factors Influencing the Choice of Molecular Technique

The choice of molecular diagnostic strategy is influenced by several factors, including the technical expertise available within the diagnostic laboratory, the available budget, and the type and spectrum of mutations prevalent in the population being screened [1, 3, 6, 7, 9, 16–18]:

- *Prevalence of Mutations:* In populations with a high prevalence of a limited number of known mutations (e.g., specific β-thalassemia mutations in Mediterranean or Southeast Asian populations), targeted assays like ARMS-PCR or reverse dot blot analysis can be highly efficient and cost-effective for screening purposes.

Table 11.4 Genotypes of NTDT classified based on whether one or both *HBB* alleles are affected

(i) *Homozygous or compound heterozygous* states for β-thalassemia: (a) Inheritance of mild β-thalassemia alleles, β 'silent' and β^{++}, in homozygous or compound heterozygous states. (b) Co-inheritance of α-thalassemia with two β^{0} alleles (c) Increased HbF response due to any of the following: *(a) XmnI*$^{G}\gamma$ polymorphism *(b) HBB* promoter mutations *(c) Trans*-acting quantitative trait loci (QTLs) for HbF on Xp22.2-p22.3, 6q23, 8q, and 2p15
(ii) *Heterozygous* state for β-thalassemia 1. Co-inheritance of additional α-globin genes (ααα/αα, ααα/ααα, αααα/αα, αααα/αααα): This is an important modulator of the severity of βTT or β-NTDT, exacerbating the phenotypic severity of β-thalassemia by causing more globin chain imbalance (Weatherall DJ., 1998; Weatherall DJ., 2001). 2. Dominantly inherited β-thalassemia (hyperunstable β globin chain variants) 3. Somatic deletion of the other β-globin locus—mosaicism
(iii) *Compound heterozygotes* for β-thalassemia and β chain variants e.g., HbE/ β-thalassemia.

- *Spectrum of Mutation Types:* When dealing with populations with a diverse spectrum of known and potentially novel mutations, or when the initial screening fails to identify a common mutation, more comprehensive techniques like Sanger sequencing or NGS become necessary. For α-thalassemia, where deletions are common, gap-PCR is a primary tool, complemented by sequencing for non-deletional forms. For detecting copy number variations, MLPA is a valuable technique.
- *Technical Expertise and Infrastructure:* The availability of skilled personnel and the necessary equipment are crucial considerations. Techniques like ARMS-PCR and gap-PCR are relatively simple to implement, while NGS requires more advanced infrastructure and bioinformatics expertise.
- *Budget:* The cost per sample varies considerably between different techniques. Targeted PCR-based methods are generally less expensive than Sanger sequencing or NGS, making them more suitable for resource-limited settings or large-scale screening programs.
- *Clinical Indication:* The clinical context also dictates the choice of technique. For routine carrier screening for a few common mutations, multiplex PCR assays or RDB are efficient. For diagnosing symptomatic individuals with atypical hematological findings, a more comprehensive approach, like sequencing or NGS, might be warranted to identify rare or novel mutations. NTDT almost always requires molecular testing, and their genotypic bases are summarized in Table 11.4. Prenatal diagnosis often relies on techniques that can rapidly and very accurately identify specific parental mutations in fetal samples. In patients

Table 11.5 Genetic modifiers of phenotypic variability in β-thalassemias

Primary modifiers	Nature of mutations in the β-globin (*HBB*) gene (β^0, β^+, β^{++})
Secondary modifiers	Co-inherited defects in the α-globin (*HBA*) genes (α-thalassemia, α-globin gene triplication or quadruplication)
	Genetic modifiers of fetal hemoglobin (HbF) production: Within the β-globin gene cluster Co-inherited HPFH Co-inherited δβ-thalassemia Xmn1$^{G}\gamma$—158 (C > T) polymorphism Unlinked to the β-globin gene cluster *HBS1L-MYB* intergenic region on chromosome 6q23 *BCL11A* gene polymorphisms on chromosome 2p16 *KLF1* gene variations on chromosome 19p13
Tertiary modifiers	Genes unrelated to hemoglobin production that influence the onset and severity of other complications: Bilirubin metabolism: Polymorphism of the promoter region of bilirubin UDP-glucuronosyl transferase *(UGT1A1)* [TA7/TA7 genotype] Iron metabolism: Homozygous mutation of the *HFE* gene *(C282Y* and *H63D); HAMP* and *HFE2 genes* Bone metabolism: Polymorphisms of the genetic loci of transforming growth factor β1 *(TGFβ1),* vitamin D receptor, estrogen receptor, and *COL1A1* gene Myocardial dysfunction: Apolipoprotein E, ε4 allele; Genes modulating free radical formation (i.e., cytochrome C oxidase), scavenger enzymes (superoxide dismutase, catalase), genes controlling replication of mitochondrial DNA, structural genes involved in the synthesis of membrane lipoproteins, and genes involving DNA repair. Cardiac iron overload: Glutathione S-transferase M1 (*GSTM1*) null (deleted) genotype Response to viral infections: Interleukin-28B (*IFNL3*) gene polymorphisms in relation to HCV infection; Gene polymorphisms of human leucocyte antigen (HLA) haplotypes Coagulation pathways: Factor V Leiden, MTHFR C677T, and prothrombin G20210A mutations

with specific clinical findings or complications, testing for the secondary and tertiary modifiers is indicated (Table 11.5) [1, 6].

- *Need for High-Throughput Analysis:* For large-scale screening programs, techniques that allow for the simultaneous analysis of multiple samples and mutations, such as reverse dot blot assays or NGS, are preferred.
- *Requirement for Novel Mutation Discovery:* When investigating families with uncharacterized hemoglobinopathies, or for research purposes aimed at identifying new disease-causing variants, Sanger sequencing or NGS are essential.

It is recommended that diagnostic laboratories have access to more than one mutation detection method to ensure accurate and reliable results.

11.9 Non-invasive Prenatal Testing (NIPT) Using Cell-Free Fetal DNA (cffDNA) in Maternal Plasma

This advance has significantly reshaped prenatal care for common chromosomal aneuploidies, and substantial progress has also been made in developing NIPT for monogenic diseases like thalassemia. One of the primary challenges in NIPT for monogenic diseases is targeting the low concentration of fetal mutations that differ by only a few nucleotides from the abundant maternal DNA in plasma. Current NIPT strategies for thalassemia involve detecting or excluding paternally inherited fetal mutations absent in the mother's genome. Techniques like allele-specific amplification, the refractory mutation system (ARMS), real-time PCR (RT-PCR), and methods using paternal single-nucleotide polymorphism (SNP) markers have been employed for this purpose. A negative test for paternally inherited ß-thalassemia mutation implies the fetus has not inherited the paternal normal ß-globin allele and is likely unaffected, potentially reducing the need for invasive diagnostic procedures by half.

Assessing maternally inherited mutations or mutations shared by both parents requires highly sensitive DNA quantification techniques. Two powerful approaches to elucidate fetal mutational status in such cases are relative mutation dosage (RMD) and relative haplotype dosage (RHDO).

- The RMD approach examines alterations in the relative proportions of mutant and wild-type alleles using single-molecule counting technologies like droplet digital PCR (ddPCR). ddPCR allows for precise quantification of mutant and wild-type alleles in maternal plasma DNA to determine allelic balance or imbalance, even in populations with lower genetic diversity. This method is particularly useful for targeting previously characterized parental mutations, such as point mutations, small deletions, or insertions, and does not require haplotyping information, making it relatively simple and cost-effective.
- The RHDO approach, on the other hand, utilizes massively parallel sequencing (MPS) or next-generation sequencing (NGS) to obtain a comprehensive mutational profile of the fetus from maternal plasma. RHDO leverages SNP information from parental genomes to deduce paternal and maternal inheritance patterns. For maternal inheritance, SNP markers linked to the mutation (i.e., haplotypes) are interrogated. By assessing the balance or imbalance of maternal haplotypes in the maternal plasma DNA, the fetal mutational status can be inferred. The robustness of RHDO increases by analyzing multiple SNP sites assigned to a haplotype. Targeted sequencing protocols are increasingly used with RHDO to analyze only the genomic region of interest, reducing the need for whole-genome sequencing. RHDO analysis can theoretically detect most types of variants, including large insertions/deletions and copy number variants.

Other recent advancements in NIPT include the exploration of Oxford Nanopore™ sequencing technology combined with RHDO analysis for NIPT of ß-thalassemia. Nanopore sequencing can produce long reads, facilitating direct construction of parental haplotypes, potentially making the process more accurate and less complex, even without a proband sample.

The current focus is on developing cost-effective NIPT approaches that can be integrated into existing conventional prenatal screening protocols. Targeted sequencing protocols coupled with robust RHDO analysis are anticipated to become the preferred method for NIPT of a broad spectrum of monogenic diseases with decreasing sequencing costs. Population-based haplotyping is also being explored as a potentially sensitive, fast, and inexpensive strategy for NIPT of thalassemia, reducing the reliance on family-based haplotyping. Overall, NIPT for thalassemia is rapidly evolving, offering less invasive and potentially more comprehensive diagnostic options for at-risk pregnancies [19–21].

11.10 Future Directions

The field of molecular diagnostics for hemoglobinopathies is continuously evolving. Next-generation sequencing (NGS) is increasingly emerging as a powerful tool for molecular screening and clinical genotyping. Its ability to simultaneously analyze multiple genes and detect a wide range of mutations, including novel variants and structural rearrangements, makes it a promising approach for comprehensive diagnosis and carrier screening. While currently limited by cost, it is anticipated that the cost of NGS technologies will decrease, making them more accessible for routine clinical use, particularly in resource-limited settings where the burden of hemoglobinopathies is highest. The development of user-friendly bioinformatics pipelines and improved strategies for analyzing the complex data generated by NGS will further enhance its clinical utility [16, 17, 19, 21].

11.11 An Illustrative Case

An unusual non-transfusion-dependent thalassemia requiring molecular genetic testing for a definitive diagnosis

- *Presentation:* An 11-year-old girl from Haryana, second-born child of a non-consanguineous marriage, presented with recurrent jaundice and easy fatiguability since approximately 4-5 years of age.
- *Past and family history:* She had required a single blood transfusion 2 years ago. There was a history of neonatal jaundice. There was no family history of jaundice or gallstones. Her older brother was healthy, except for mild jaundice noted rarely by his mother, usually during fever episodes.

- *On examination:* She was mildly icteric with moderate pallor. Her spleen was palpable 4 cm below the left costal margin. No hepatomegaly was noted.
- *Clinical diagnosis:* Chronic mild-to-moderate severity hemolytic anemia or thalassemia intermedia
- *Investigations:*
  - Hemoglobin 6.8 g/dL
  - Corrected reticulocyte count 3.4%
  - Mean corpuscular volume 63.6 fL
  - Red cell distribution width-coefficient of variation (RDW-CV) 31.5%
  - Peripheral smear: Marked anisopoikilocytosis, microcytic hypochromic red cells, teardrop cells, and cells with basophilic stippling. Platelets were adequate. 02 nucleated RBCs per 100 WBCs.
  - Total bilirubin 3.79 mg/dL, conjugated fraction 0.51 mg/dL
  - SGOT, SGPT, and alkaline phosphatase levels were normal
  - Serum iron profile: Ferritin 252 μg/L, iron 100 μg/dL, TIBC 250 μg/dL, %transferrin saturation 40%. Serum vitamin B12 and folate levels were normal
  - High-performance liquid chromatography (HPLC) revealed beta thalassemia trait (HbA2 4.9%) along with mildly elevated HbF (4.5%)
  - Parental HPLCs: Beta-thalassemia trait in the mother (HbA2 5.3%, HbF 0.9%), father's HPLC was normal (HbA2 3.0%, HbF 1.0%)
  - Brother's HPLC was normal (HbA2 2.4%, HbF 0.2%)

  Incubated osmotic fragility, eosin-5′-maleimide (EMA) binding test, and direct Coombs' tests ruled out hereditary spherocytosis and immune hemolysis, respectively. G6PD deficiency screening, urine and plasma hemoglobin, and tests for unstable hemoglobin were all negative

- *Molecular testing*
  - Beta globin gene: ARMS-PCR revealed heterozygous codons 8/9 (+G) frameshift mutation (*HBB*:c.27_28insG) in the child and her mother. Sanger sequencing confirmed that no other *HBB* mutation was present in the child
  - Polymerase chain reaction for supernumerary alpha-globin genes confirmed αααanti-3.7 allele, explaining the non-transfusion-dependent β-thalassemia (NTDT) phenotype
  - No alpha globin gene deletions were found in the index case
  - Sanger sequencing of the *HBB* gene in the father revealed no variants

  Sanger sequencing of the *UGT1A1* gene promoter region in the child identified homozygosity for the (TA)7 variant, confirming the Gilbert syndrome. Her brother also had the Gilbert syndrome

- *Final diagnosis*: Coexisting β-thalassemia trait, alpha-globin gene triplication, and Gilbert syndrome presenting as a non-transfusion dependent β-thalassemia phenotype
- Parental counselling was done, with a suggestion to screen her spouse (in the future) for hemoglobinopathies. As part of cascade screening, HPLCs of all siblings of her mother were advised.

11.12 Conclusion

Molecular genetic testing is an indispensable component of the diagnostic pathway for thalassemias and hemoglobinopathies. A wide array of techniques, each with its own advantages and limitations, is available for the detection of globin gene mutations. The choice of molecular technique is guided by factors such as the prevalence and spectrum of mutations in the population, available resources, technical expertise, and the specific clinical indication. The continued advancements in molecular diagnostic technologies, particularly NGS, promise to further enhance our ability to accurately diagnose, manage, and ultimately prevent these common inherited blood disorders.

11.13 Summary

Thalassemias and hemoglobinopathies are among the most prevalent inherited monogenic disorders worldwide, caused by quantitative or qualitative defects in globin gene expression. Accurate molecular characterization is essential for confirming diagnosis, resolving genotype–phenotype discordances, enabling prenatal diagnosis, and guiding genetic counseling. This chapter presents a comprehensive overview of molecular diagnostic techniques used in the evaluation of α-, β-, and δβ-thalassemias, as well as structural hemoglobin variants.

For β-thalassemia and hemoglobinopathies, where point mutations predominate, commonly employed methods include allele-specific PCR (ARMS-PCR), reverse dot blot (RDB), and Sanger sequencing. α-thalassemias, primarily caused by large gene deletions, are typically evaluated by multiplex gap-PCR and multiplex ligation-dependent probe amplification (MLPA), while sequencing is required for non-deletional variants. Each method's diagnostic yield, throughput, and cost-effectiveness are discussed, with technique selection guided by mutation type, population-specific mutation spectra, laboratory capacity, and clinical context.

The chapter further explores emerging applications of next-generation sequencing (NGS) for comprehensive mutation detection, genetic modifier assessment, and high-throughput screening. The evolving landscape of non-invasive prenatal testing (NIPT) using cell-free fetal DNA is detailed, including relative haplotype dosage (RHDO) and droplet digital PCR (ddPCR) approaches for detecting parental mutations in fetuses.

An understanding of secondary (e.g., α-globin gene alterations, HbF polymorphisms) and tertiary (e.g., bilirubin, iron, bone metabolism genes) modifiers of disease phenotype is emphasized. A tiered, context-specific diagnostic approach incorporating traditional and advanced molecular tools is advocated to enhance diagnostic accuracy and optimize patient care in diverse clinical settings.

References

1. Das R, Sharma P. Molecular genetics of thalassemia syndromes. In: Kumar D, editor. Colloquium series—digital library of genomic and molecular medicine, vol. 5(1). Williston: Morgan and Claypool Publishers. p. 1–57. https://doi.org/10.4199/C00142ED1V01Y201607GMM007.
2. Old J, Harteveld CL, Traeger-Synodinos J, Petrou M, Angastiniotis M, Galanello R. Prevention of thalassaemias and other haemoglobin disorders, vol. 2: Laboratory protocols [Internet]. 2nd ed. Nicosia (Cyprus): Thalassaemia International Federation; 2012. PMID: 24672828.
3. Old JM. Screening and genetic diagnosis of haemoglobinopathies. Scand J Clin Lab Invest. 2007;67(1):71–86. https://doi.org/10.1080/00365510601046466. PMID: 17365985.
4. Shang X, Xu X. Update in the genetics of thalassemia: what clinicians need to know. Best Pract Res Clin Obstet Gynaecol. 2017;39:3–15. https://doi.org/10.1016/j.bpobgyn.2016.10.012. Epub 2016 Oct 26. PMID: 27876354.
5. Tesio N, Bauer DE. Molecular basis and genetic modifiers of thalassemia. Hematol Oncol Clin North Am. 2023;37(2):273–99. https://doi.org/10.1016/j.hoc.2022.12.001. PMID: 36907603; PMCID: PMC10122828.
6. Indian Academy of Pediatrics - Pediatric Hematology Oncology Chapter (IAP-PHO). Guidelines for the diagnosis and management of thalassemia. 2023. Available from: https://www.phoindia.org/cms/thalassemia-guideline-pho-chapter-2023. Last visited May 16, 2025.
7. Mettananda S, Higgs DR. Molecular basis and genetic modifiers of thalassemia. Hematol Oncol Clin North Am. 2018;32(2):177–91. https://doi.org/10.1016/j.hoc.2017.11.003. PMID: 29458725.
8. Farashi S, Harteveld CL. Molecular basis of α-thalassemia. Blood Cells Mol Dis. 2018;70:43–53. https://doi.org/10.1016/j.bcmd.2017.09.004. Epub 2017 Sep 21. PMID: 29032940.
9. Franco E, Karkoska KA, McGann PT. Inherited disorders of hemoglobin: a review of old and new diagnostic methods. Blood Cells Mol Dis. 2024;104:102758. https://doi.org/10.1016/j.bcmd.2023.102758. Epub 2023 May 18. PMID: 37246072.
10. Harteveld CL, Achour A, Arkesteijn SJG, Ter Huurne J, Verschuren M, Bhagwandien-Bisoen S, Schaap R, Vijfhuizen L, El Idrissi H, Koopmann TT. The hemoglobinopathies, molecular disease mechanisms and diagnostics. Int J Lab Hematol. 2022;44 Suppl 1(Suppl 1):28–36. https://doi.org/10.1111/ijlh.13885. PMID: 36074711; PMCID: PMC9542123.
11. Langer AL. Beta-Thalassemia. In: Adam MP, Feldman J, Mirzaa GM, Pagon RA, Wallace SE, Amemiya A, editors. GeneReviews® [Internet]. Seattle: University of Washington, Seattle; 2000. p. 1993–2025. PMID: 20301599.
12. Thein SL. The molecular basis of β-thalassemia. Cold Spring Harb Perspect Med. 2013;3(5):a011700. https://doi.org/10.1101/cshperspect.a011700. PMID: 23637309; PMCID: PMC3633182.
13. Saha D, Chowdhury PK, Panja A, Pal D, Nayek K, Chakraborty G, Sharma P, Das R, Basu S, Chatterjee R, Basu A. Effect of deletions in the α-globin gene on the phenotype severity of β-thalassemia. Hemoglobin. 2022;46(2):118–23.
14. Sundaresan DD, Hira JK, Chhabra S, Trehan A, Khadwal AR, Malhotra P, Sharma P, Das R. Hematological and genetic profiles of persons with co-inherited heterozygous β-thalassemia and supernumerary α-globin genes. Eur J Haematol. 2023;110(5):510–7.
15. Tamary H, Dgany O. Alpha-Thalassemia. 2005 Nov 1 [updated 2024 May 23]. In: Adam MP, Feldman J, Mirzaa GM, Pagon RA, Wallace SE, Amemiya A, editors. GeneReviews® [Internet]. Seattle: University of Washington, Seattle; 1993–2025. PMID: 20301608.
16. Harteveld CL. State of the art and new developments in molecular diagnostics for hemoglobinopathies in multiethnic societies. Int J Lab Hematol. 2014;36(1):1–12. https://doi.org/10.1111/ijlh.12108. Epub 2013 May 31. PMID: 23721114.

17. Rets A, Clayton AL, Christensen RD, Agarwal AM. Molecular diagnostic update in hereditary hemolytic anemia and neonatal hyperbilirubinemia. Int J Lab Hematol. 2019;41 Suppl 1:95–101. https://doi.org/10.1111/ijlh.13014. PMID: 31069991.
18. Sabath DE. Molecular diagnosis of thalassemias and hemoglobinopathies: an ACLPS critical review. Am J Clin Pathol. 2017;148(1):6–15. https://doi.org/10.1093/ajcp/aqx047. PMID: 28605432.
19. Thein SL. Genetic association studies in β-hemoglobinopathies. Hematology Am Soc Hematol Educ Program. 2013;2013:354–61. https://doi.org/10.1182/asheducation-2013.1.354. PMID: 24319204.
20. Lee JS, Cho SI, Park SS, Seong MW. Molecular basis and diagnosis of thalassemia. Blood Res. 2021;56(S1):S39–43. https://doi.org/10.5045/br.2021.2020332. PMID: 33935034; PMCID: PMC8093999.
21. Li DZ, Yang YD. Invasive prenatal diagnosis of fetal thalassemia. Best Pract Res Clin Obstet Gynaecol. 2017;39:41–52. https://doi.org/10.1016/j.bpobgyn.2016.10.011. Epub 2016 Oct 26. PMID: 27889305.

Chapter 12
Prenatal Diagnosis for Hereditary Haematologic Disorders

Bipin Prakash Kulkarni, Prabhakar Kedar, Sharda Shanbhag, Nikesh Kawankar, Pratibha Sawant, and Pallavi Thaker

Abstract Prenatal diagnosis plays a crucial role in the early detection of hereditary haematologic disorders, offering valuable insights for clinical management and genetic counselling. These disorders, which include haemoglobinopathies, haemophilia, inherited platelet disorders, inherited bone marrow failure syndromes, myeloproliferative disorders, and others arise from genetic mutations affecting blood cell production, function, and composition. Advances in molecular genetics, imaging, and diagnostic techniques have significantly improved the accuracy and accessibility of prenatal testing.

Various methodologies are employed in the prenatal diagnosis of hereditary haematologic disorders. Non-invasive prenatal testing (NIPT), which analyses cell-free fetal DNA in maternal blood, provides a safer alternative for identifying specific mutations but has limitations in comprehensiveness. Invasive techniques such as chorionic villus sampling (CVS) and amniocentesis offer high diagnostic accuracy for a broad spectrum of disorders but carry a small risk of pregnancy complications. Furthermore, genetic diagnosis methods for haemophilia, including PCR-based techniques, Sanger sequencing, multiplex ligation-dependent probe amplification (MLPA), and next-generation sequencing (NGS), have enhanced the ability to detect mutations in the F8 and F9 genes. Traditional techniques like Southern blotting and long-range PCR, as well as linkage analysis for indirect genetic testing, also contribute to diagnostic accuracy. Additionally, preimplantation genetic diagnosis (PGD) allows at-risk couples undergoing in vitro fertilization (IVF) to select embryos free from disease-causing mutations.

Despite its benefits, prenatal diagnosis raises ethical concerns, including issues of informed consent, reproductive choices, potential discrimination, and genetic privacy. Proper counselling and ethical considerations must be integrated into clinical

B. P. Kulkarni (✉) · P. Kedar · S. Shanbhag · N. Kawankar · P. Sawant · P. Thaker
ICMR-National Institute for Research on Blood and Immune Disorders (NIRBID) (Formerly ICMR-NIIH), Mumbai, India

H. P. Pati et al. (eds.), *Clinical Hematology and Hemato-Oncology*,
https://doi.org/10.1007/978-981-92-1167-8_12

practice to ensure informed decision-making and mitigate potential psychosocial impacts. As prenatal diagnostic technology continues to evolve, it holds the promise of further improving early detection and intervention strategies for hereditary haematologic disorders, ultimately enhancing patient outcomes and reproductive autonomy.

Keywords Prenatal diagnosis · Hereditary haematologic disorders · Genetic testing · Ethical considerations · Molecular diagnostics

Learning Objectives

- Define prenatal diagnosis and its significance in identifying hereditary haematologic disorders.
- Describe different categories of hereditary haematologic disorders, including haemoglobinopathies, haemophilia, inherited platelet disorders, bone marrow failure syndromes, and others.
- Identify key diagnostic techniques for prenatal testing, including non-invasive prenatal testing (NIPT), chorionic villus sampling (CVS), amniocentesis, and preimplantation genetic diagnosis (PGD).
- Compare molecular genetic diagnostic methods such as PCR, Sanger sequencing, MLPA, NGS, Southern blotting, and linkage analysis in detecting genetic mutations.
- Evaluate the advantages and limitations of each prenatal diagnostic method, considering accuracy, safety, and accessibility.
- Understand the clinical implications of early diagnosis, including its impact on patient management, genetic counselling, and family planning.
- Discuss ethical considerations related to prenatal diagnosis, such as informed consent, reproductive choices, genetic discrimination, and the responsible use of genetic information.
- Explore advancements in genetic testing technologies and their potential role in improving prenatal diagnosis of hereditary haematologic disorders.

12.1 Introduction

Prenatal diagnosis refers to the detection of genetic conditions in a fetus before birth. With the advancements in molecular genetics, imaging, and other diagnostic tools, it has become possible to diagnose a range of hereditary haematologic disorders during pregnancy. Haematologic disorders can affect blood production, function, and composition, and many of them are inherited in an autosomal dominant, autosomal recessive, or X-linked manner. This chapter explores the methods, benefits, challenges, and ethical considerations of prenatal diagnosis for hereditary haematologic disorders.

12.2 Overview of Hereditary Haematologic Disorders

Hereditary haematologic disorders encompass a wide range of blood-related diseases caused by genetic mutations. These disorders can affect red blood cells, white blood cells, platelets, or coagulation factors. Below are the major categories of hereditary haematologic disorders.

12.3 Haemoglobinopathies

Thalassemias Thalassemias are a group of inherited blood disorders caused by mutations in the genes that encode the globin chains of haemoglobin. These mutations result in a reduced or absent production of either the alpha-globin or beta-globin chains, leading to an imbalance in the globin chain synthesis and the formation of abnormal haemoglobin. Beta-thalassemia results from mutations in the HBB gene on chromosome 11 [1]. The severity of thalassemia depends on whether the individual inherits one or two defective alleles of the affected globin gene, with homozygous mutations often leading to more severe disease, such as thalassemia major, characterized by profound anemia and a need for lifelong blood transfusions. The prevalence of beta-thalassemia varies across different population groups, ranging from 1.0% to 17.0%, with an average prevalence of 3.0% to 4.0% nationwide. It is estimated that around 35 to 45 million individuals in India carry the beta-thalassemia trait, and annually 7500 to 12,000 babies are born with a severe form of the disorder [2]. Delta beta (δβ)-thalassemia results from a deletion in both the delta and beta genes on chromosome 11. Because of the large deletions, there is no production of δ- and β-globin chains, leading to $(\delta\beta)^0$ thalassemia. δβ-thalassemia heterozygotes clinically show characteristics of thalassemia minor, but in association with β-thalassemia, it gives rise to a clinical phenotype of thalassemia major [3]. HPFH is a group of conditions characterized by the persistence of fetal haemoglobin synthesis into adult life in the absence of significant haematological manifestations. HPFH occurs due to mutations in the β-globin gene cluster. Co-inheritance of HPFH with β thalassemia or HbE usually leads to severe clinical manifestations similar to those of thalassemia intermedia [4].

Haemoglobin S (HbS) HbS is an abnormal form of haemoglobin caused by a single point mutation that leads to the substitution of amino acid valine for glutamic acid at position 6 of the HBB gene located on chromosome 11 [5]. HbS, when inherited as a single copy, is called sickle cell trait and in the double dose or homozygous form, it is referred to as sickle cell anemia (SCA). It can also be inherited with other haemoglobinopathies like HbD, HbE, or with β-thalassemia. All these conditions are also referred to as sickle cell disease (SCD). Under low oxygen conditions, HbS molecules polymerize, causing red blood cells to adopt a rigid, sickle shape. These sickle-shaped cells are less flexible and prone to haemolysis, leading to chronic anemia, vaso-occlusion, and organ damage. In India, Hb S is primarily found in tribal populations and some socially and economically disadvantaged scheduled caste groups, with the highest carrier prevalence rates of 20.0% to 30.0% in central India (Madhya Pradesh and Chhattisgarh). It is also prevalent in parts of South Gujarat, Maharashtra, Tamil Nadu, and Kerala [2].

Haemoglobin E (HbE) HbE results from a single base substitution of glutamic acid (GAG) with lysine (GAA) at codon 26 of the beta globin chain. The substitution produces unstable haemoglobin when subjected to oxidative stress due to weakening of the bonds between the monomers constituting the tetramers. Hb E disorders may be heterozygous (AE), homozygous (EE), or compound heterozygous with beta-thalassemia and Hb S. Hb E is particularly common in the northeastern regions of India, where some population groups exhibit carrier rates as high as 40.0–50.0%. In West Bengal, the carrier frequency of Hb E is around 4.0–5.0%, reaching 10.0% in some groups [2].

12.4 Haemophilia

Haemophilia A and B Haemophilia A and B are X-linked recessive bleeding disorders caused by mutations in the genes encoding clotting factors. Haemophilia A results from mutations in the F8 gene, which encodes coagulation factor VIII, while Haemophilia B is caused by mutations in the F9 gene, which encodes coagulation factor IX. Both conditions impair the blood's ability to clot properly, leading to prolonged bleeding after injury or surgery, spontaneous joint bleeds, and an increased risk of internal bleeding. The severity of the disease depends on the level of clotting factor activity, with severe forms typically characterized by less than 1% of normal factor activity, moderate forms between 1% and 5%, and mild forms between 5% and 40%. Genetic testing is essential for diagnosing haemophilia, as it enables the identification of specific mutations in the F8 or F9 genes. Techniques such as PCR, inverse PCR, DNA sequencing, and multiplex ligation-dependent probe amplification (MLPA) can detect mutations ranging from point mutations, intron 22 and intron 1 inversions, and small deletions to large gene rearrangements. Early genetic testing allows for effective carrier diagnosis (heterozygous females), who are at risk of passing the disorder to their children, and prenatal diagnosis in the affected families and provides valuable information for family planning and genetic counselling. Genetic testing is also important in differentiating haemophilia from other bleeding disorders. In addition, genetic testing helps in understanding the molecular basis of the disease, which is important for the development of tailored therapies, including gene therapy, and for managing haemophilia more effectively, particularly in the context of emerging treatments like clotting factor replacement and novel haemostatic agents.

12.4.1 Inherited Platelet Disorders

Inherited platelet disorders are a heterogeneous group of genetic conditions that affect platelet function or production, leading to bleeding tendencies. These disorders can result from mutations in genes involved in platelet production, adhesion, aggregation, or secretion. Examples include Bernard-Soulier syndrome, caused by mutations in the GP1BA, GP1BB, or GP9 genes, which impair the platelet glycoprotein complex responsible for adhesion to the vascular subendothelium; Glanzmann thrombasthenia, resulting from mutations in the ITGA2B or ITGB3 genes, which encode the integrin αIIbβ3 complex necessary for platelet aggregation; and other rare platelet disorders, leading to variable bleeding manifestations in the patients. The molecular pathology of these disorders typically involves defective or absent proteins critical for platelet function, leading to either impaired clot formation or a failure to form proper primary haemostasis.

Genetic testing techniques such as next-generation sequencing (NGS) is best suited to identify the pathogenic variants in genes involved in the relevant pathways, enabling precise diagnosis. Early genetic diagnosis is crucial not only for confirming the clinical diagnosis but also for distinguishing between different platelet disorders that may have overlapping symptoms. Moreover, genetic testing is important to identify asymptomatic carriers, especially in autosomal dominant disorders, and to provide genetic counselling to affected families. Understanding the genetic basis of inherited platelet disorders also aids in the development of targeted therapies and enables better management of bleeding risks, including preoperative planning and the use of specific haemostatic agents.

12.4.2 Inherited Bone Marrow Failure Syndromes

Inherited bone marrow failure syndromes (IBMFS) are a group of rare genetic disorders characterized by haematopoietic stem cell failure, leading to bone marrow dysfunction and subsequent haematologic abnormalities such as anemia, neutropenia, and thrombocytopenia. These syndromes, including conditions like Fanconi anemia, dyskeratosis congenita, and Schwachman-Diamond syndrome, often present with multisystem involvement, including growth delays, skeletal anomalies, and increased cancer susceptibility. Molecular pathology plays a crucial role in diagnosing and understanding these disorders, as they are caused by mutations in genes involved in DNA repair, telomere maintenance, or ribosomal function. Genetic testing, including next-generation sequencing (NGS), is essential for accurate diagnosis, as it enables the identification of specific pathogenic variants, informs prognosis, and guides clinical management.

Early genetic diagnosis also facilitates family planning, offers potential therapeutic options, and allows for surveillance of associated malignancies, underscoring the importance of genetic testing in the management of IBMFS.

12.4.3 Polycythemia Vera and Other Myeloproliferative Disorders

Polycythemia vera (PV) and other myeloproliferative disorders (MPDs) are haematologic conditions characterized by the clonal proliferation of haematopoietic stem cells, leading to abnormal blood cell production. Though these conditions are often diagnosed in adulthood, some inherited mutations can predispose individuals to polycythemia and other related myeloproliferative neoplasms. PV is primarily marked by erythrocytosis, while other MPDs, such as essential thrombocythemia and primary myelofibrosis, involve abnormal platelet and megakaryocyte proliferation, respectively. The molecular pathology of these disorders is driven by acquired genetic mutations, most notably the JAK2 V617F mutation, which occurs in approximately 95% of PV cases, and mutations in CALR and MPL genes in other MPDs. These mutations activate the JAK-STAT signaling pathway, promoting uncontrolled cell proliferation. Genetic testing, particularly the detection of JAK2 V617F, CALR, and MPL mutations, is crucial for accurate diagnosis, differentiating PV and other MPDs from reactive conditions and other haematologic malignancies. Furthermore, genetic testing informs prognostic stratification, aids in treatment decisions such as the use of JAK inhibitors, and helps to monitor for disease progression or transformation into acute leukemia. The role of genetic testing in these disorders enhances diagnostic accuracy and personalized management, improving patient outcomes.

12.5 Methods of Prenatal Diagnosis for Hereditary Haematologic Disorders

Prenatal diagnosis for hereditary haematologic disorders involves several techniques, each with specific advantages and limitations. The choice of method depends on factors such as the type of disorder, the risk of maternal or fetal complications, and the stage of pregnancy.

12.5.1 Non-invasive Prenatal Testing (NIPT)

Non-invasive prenatal testing (NIPT) is a rapidly evolving technique that allows for the detection of fetal genetic conditions without the need for invasive procedures. NIPT involves the analysis of cell-free fetal DNA circulating in maternal blood.

Recent studies have reported the application of NIPT in hereditary haematologic disorders [6].

- *Applications*: NIPT is not widely used for detecting haematologic disorders like sickle cell disease or thalassemia, but it can be used to detect specific mutations when a parent is a known carrier of a genetic disorder.
- *Advantages*: Safe for both the mother and the fetus, as it only requires a blood sample from the mother.
- *Limitations*: NIPT is generally not comprehensive for detecting all hereditary haematologic disorders and may be less effective for conditions with complex genetic mutations or variable expression.

12.5.2 Invasive Prenatal Testing

The techniques employed for prenatal diagnosis include chorionic villus sampling (CVS), amniocentesis, and/or cordocentesis. It involves direct sampling of fetal tissue and/or fluid to access the fetus's genotype.

12.5.3 Chorionic Villus Sampling (CVS)

Chorionic villus sampling is an invasive procedure that involves the collection of placental tissue (chorionic villi) for genetic analysis. CVS is typically performed between 10 and 13 weeks of pregnancy.

- *Applications*: CVS biopsy, followed by molecular genetic testing, can detect mutations associated with a variety of hereditary haematologic disorders, including sickle cell disease, thalassemia, haemophilia, and others.
- *Advantages*: High diagnostic accuracy for genetic conditions, including single-gene disorders.
- *Limitations*: Invasive and carries a small risk of miscarriage or other complications. Results may take several days to weeks.

12.5.4 Amniocentesis

Amniocentesis is another invasive procedure where a sample of amniotic fluid is taken in the 2nd trimester of pregnancy, typically between 16 and 18 weeks of gestation. The amniotic fluid contains fetal cells that can be analyzed for genetic disorders.

- *Applications*: Like CVS, amniocentesis can detect a wide range of genetic conditions, including those that cause hereditary haematologic disorders. It is often

used when CVS is not available, the patient reports late or if more time is needed to assess the fetus.
- *Advantages*: Provides a direct sample of fetal cells for analysis, enabling the detection of genetic mutations with high accuracy.
- *Limitations*: Invasive procedure with a small risk of miscarriage or other complications. The procedure is performed later in pregnancy, which may delay decision-making.

12.5.5 Cordocentesis (Fetal Blood Sampling)

It is done between 18th and 20th weeks of gestation for second-trimester prenatal diagnosis of haemoglobinopathies.

- Application: This procedure is only done when couples at risk of having an affected child are identified late or if the diagnosis done during the first trimester is not conclusive. The fetal blood sample can be analyzed by HPLC [7, 8].
- Advantages: The major advantage of cordocentesis is that it allows direct access to the fetus and helps to provide quicker diagnostic results
- Disadvantages: The procedure carries risks such as infection, miscarriage, or fetal injury, and is typically offered when other diagnostic options are not suitable or conclusive.

12.6 Genetic Diagnosis Methods for Haemoglobinopathies

Genetic testing for haemoglobinopathies is crucial for accurate diagnosis, prenatal testing, carrier screening, and newborn screening. It helps identify inherited blood disorders, enabling early detection, better treatment, and prevention of serious health issues. This information supports family planning, informed decisions, and improves health outcomes and public health efforts. Haemoglobinopathies were the first genetic disorders to be characterized at the molecular level. There are many different PCR-based techniques that can be used to diagnose the globin gene mutations, including allele-specific oligonucleotide (ASO) dot blot, reverse dot blot analysis (CRDB), the amplification refractory mutation system (ARMS) gap-PCR, restriction fragment length polymorphisms (PCR-RFLP), Sanger's DNA sequencing, multiple ligation probe amplification assay (MLPA), and real-time PCR.

- Allele-specific oligonucleotide (ASO) dot blot: This method is based on the principle of hybridizing allele-specific oligonucleotides (short DNA probes) to immobilized DNA samples on a membrane. The oligo probes are radioactive labelled. It requires different hybridization and wash temperatures for each probe per mutation and screen many samples for one mutation per membrane [9].

 - Advantages: Technique is widely applicable and reliable.
 Disadvantages: Traditional protocol used radioactively labelled probes. The method is expensive, time consuming and can only screen one mutation at a time.

- Covalent reverse dot blot hybridization (CRDB): CRDB is a non-radioactive method which involves the immobilization of complementary DNA oligonucleotide probes on a nylon membrane and allowing them to anneal with an amplified labelled DNA fragment. Six common Indian mutations, namely IVS 1 nt 5 (G➔C), IVS 1 nt 1 (G➔T), CD 8/9 (+G), CD 41/42 (-CTTT), CD 15 (G➔A), and CD 30 (G➔C), along with two structural variants of haemoglobin, HbS and HbE, are screened for by hybridization with allele-specific oligonucleotide probes followed by color development. Using this method, we can distinguish between heterozygous, homozygous, and compound heterozygous states of β-thalassemia and these abnormal haemoglobins. More than 80% of the β thalassemia carriers and affected cases can be diagnosed using this technique [10].
 - Advantages: CRDB is a simple, rapid, and reliable method that utilizes non-radioactive reagents. It allows for the simultaneous screening of multiple mutations and is relatively cost-effective.
 Disadvantages: This method needs sample controls to standardize the new mutation. It also demands a high level of technical expertise in the laboratory to set up and validate CRDB. Additionally, it can become costly if using a commercial kit.

- Amplification refractory mutation system (ARMS): ARMS is a simple method for detecting any mutation involving single-base changes or small deletions. It is a PCR-based system that discriminates between normal and mutant alleles by selecting primers that have a nucleotide at their 3′ end corresponding to either normal or mutant sequence. This method can be used for screening multiple mutations in one patient but it needs good experience to understand false negatives (Old JM 2001).
 - Advantages: It is a simple, rapid, and inexpensive method that is suitable for technical modification. It can be multiplexed to detect more than one mutation.
 Disadvantages: It requires control DNA to validate the test results every time and for some very rare mutations, a homozygous control is not available. Also, degradation of primers gives non-specific results.

- Gap- PCR: It is a rapid, simple, and non-radioactive method that allows the identification of deletions and gene rearrangements. This method is used to detect α-thalassemia, δβ-thalassemia deletions, and Hb Lepore rearrangements. The limitation of this method is that the deletion endpoints must be known to design the primers [3].
 - Advantages: It is a simple, rapid, and inexpensive method. It can be multiplexed to detect more than one mutation.

Disadvantages: It requires control DNA to validate the test results every time. Useful for only those deletional mutations with known breakpoint sequences. There is a possibility of allele drop-out, and hence one needs to be careful while doing prenatal diagnosis.

- PCR-restriction fragment length polymorphism (PCR-RFLP): A small number of β- globin gene mutations create or abolish a restriction endonuclease recognition site in the globin gene sequence. The PCR fragment is treated with a restriction enzyme that will cut or not cut when the particular point mutation is present. This technique is useful for the diagnosis of the clinically important Hb variants HbS, HbE, and HbD^{Punjab} (Old JM 2001).
  - Advantages: It is a simple, rapid, and reliable method.
    Disadvantages: It is limited to only few mutations. Care must be taken to prevent partial digestion. Frequent cutter enzymes are not useful, and some enzymes are costly.
- Sanger's DNA sequencing: Sanger DNA sequencing is a technique used to identify rare mutations in the β-globin gene that may not be detected by methods like CRDB and ARMS. The entire β-globin gene is sequenced to identify potential mutations. This method involves PCR amplification of the entire β globin gene, followed by dideoxy chain termination sequencing. It is particularly effective in detecting point mutations, including missense, nonsense, and small insertions/deletions (INDELs) [11].
  - Advantages: Use of an automated sequencer makes it more rapid and easier. Mutations are characterized directly.
    Disadvantages: Relatively expensive and PCR products need to be purified before using them for sequencing.
- Multiple Ligation Probe Amplification Assay (MLPA): Multiplex Ligation-dependent Probe Amplification (MLPA) is a technique that involves the ligation of multiple probe pairs hybridized across a specific region of interest. This is followed by quantitative PCR using universal-tag PCR primers for all ligated probe pairs, with fragment analysis conducted afterward. MLPA enables the detection of deletions or duplications across the analyzed locus and serves as a valuable alternative or complementary method to gap-PCR when investigating known or unknown deletions associated with α-, β-, or δβ-thalassemia [12].
  - Advantages: It is a simple and rapid technique that detects all common, rare, and novel deletions and duplications compared to Gap- PCR.
    Disadvantages: It does not provide a definitive diagnosis, the results are typically consistent with an estimated deletion length and the location of breakpoints, which is usually sufficient for diagnostic purposes. Also, it requires an automated DNA sequencer machine.
- Real-time PCR: This technique uses fluorescent probes and dedicated instruments to monitor the accumulation of amplicons produced throughout the prog-

ress of a PCR reaction. Recently, several commercial instruments have been developed, which integrate microvolume rapid cycle PCR with fluorometry, offering real-time fluorescent monitoring of the amplification reaction for quantitative PCR analysis and /or characterization of PCR products for rapid genotyping, precluding any post-PCR sample manipulation.

- Advantages: This technique is quick, and no post-PCR processing is required. Disadvantages: This technique is quite costly per analysis, and the equipment required is also expensive.

For prenatal diagnosis, the genotype of the fetus should be confirmed using two different methods that work on different principles. The final diagnosis should be based on matching the results from both methods to ensure accuracy. This reduces the chance of errors and provides a more reliable diagnosis.

12.7 Checking for Maternal DNA Contamination

Routine examination of short tandem repeats (STRs) or variable number of tandem repeats (VNTRs) in fetal and parental DNA samples by PCR analysis is essential to rule out maternal contamination. It is recommended to check for maternal DNA contamination in every case of prenatal diagnosis, especially when the fetal genotype is the same as the maternal genotype. An informative test is when both parents have two different-sized alleles and the fetus can clearly be seen to have inherited one of the maternal and one of the paternal alleles. If a faint positive signal for the second maternal allele is seen in the fetal DNA, this indicates maternal DNA contamination. In such cases, the fetal genotype cannot be relied upon, and a repeat sample from the fetus should be collected. When a fetal blood sample is collected through cordocentesis, the Kleihauer-Betke (KB) staining method can be used to distinguish fetal cells from maternal cells, which will help to confirm that the sample is not contaminated with maternal blood. The algorithm for prenatal diagnosis of haemoglobinopathies is given in Fig. 12.2.

12.8 Counselling of Couples at Risk of Having a Child with Different Haemoglobinopathies

Not all haemoglobinopathies exhibit clinically severe phenotypes in their homozygous and compound heterozygous forms. Therefore, it is important to provide proper genetic counselling to carrier couples, guiding them in making informed decisions about prenatal diagnosis. Table 12.1 outlines the combinations where prenatal diagnosis is either recommended or not required [4].

Table 12.1 List of the combinations where prenatal diagnosis is required and not required

Prenatal diagnosis required	Prenatal diagnosis is not required
β-thalassemia trait/ β-thalassemia trait	β-thalassemia trait/HbD trait
β-thalassemia trait/δβ-thalassemia trait	β-thalassemia trait/ HbQ India trait
β-thalassemia trait/HPFH trait	HbE trait/ HbE trait
β-thalassemia trait/Hb Lepore trait	Hb D trait/ HbD trait
β-thalassemia trait/ HbS trait	HPFH trait/HPFH trait
β-thalassemia trait/ HbE trait	
β-thalassemia trait/ HbD-β-thalassemia	
HbS trait/HbS trait	
HbS trait/HbD trait	
HbE trait/ Hb Lepore trait	

12.9 Genetic Diagnosis Methods for Haemophilia A and B

Haemophilia A and Haemophilia B are X-linked recessive bleeding disorders caused by mutations in the F8 (Factor VIII) and F9 (Factor IX) genes, respectively. Genetic testing is crucial for confirming a diagnosis, identifying carriers, and facilitating prenatal screening in our country. Various molecular techniques are employed for mutation detection, each differing in sensitivity, specificity, and application. A comprehensive overview of the key methods used for genetic diagnosis of Haemophilia A and Haemophilia B is mentioned below.

PCR-Based Techniques Polymerase chain reaction (PCR) is a fundamental molecular technique used to amplify specific DNA sequences, allowing for the identification of mutations in the F8 and F9 genes. This technique is widely utilized due to its high sensitivity, specificity, and cost-effectiveness. Our algorithm for molecular diagnosis of haemophilia is shown in Fig. 12.1.

12.9.1 Inversion Mutation Analysis for Haemophilia A

12.9.1.1 Intron 22 Inversion

Approximately 45–50% of severe Haemophilia A cases results from intron 22 inversions, where a segment of the F8 gene is inverted due to recombination between the F8 gene and its intronic homologous regions. This results in disruption of normal gene function, leading to Factor VIII deficiency. Specialized PCR-based methods such as inverse-shifting PCR (IS-PCR) and long-range PCR (LR-PCR) are used for detection [13–15]. This test is crucial for the genetic diagnosis of severe Haemophilia A. The accurate identification of intron 22 inversions aids in genetic testing and counselling of the affected families.

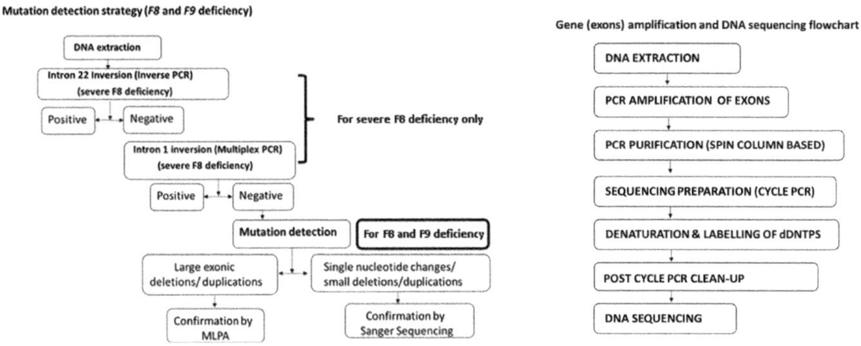

Fig. 12.1 Algorithm for molecular diagnosis of haemophilia

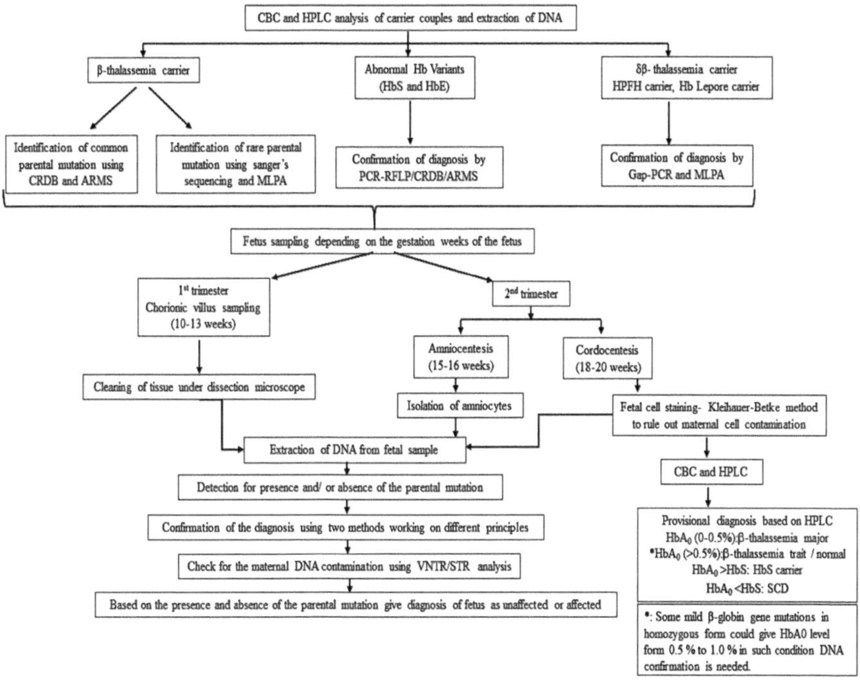

Fig. 12.2 Algorithm for prenatal diagnosis of haemoglobinopathies

12.9.1.2 Intron 1 Inversion

Intron 1 inversions account for 1–5% of severe haemophilia A cases. These inversions occur due to homologous recombination between intronic repeat sequences. PCR-based techniques, including long-range PCR and multiplex PCR, specifically amplify the rearranged regions to identify this mutation [16]. This test is essential for confirming cases of severe Haemophilia A in the absence of intron 22 inversions. Identifying intron 1 inversions ensures precise molecular diagnosis.

12.9.2 Detection of Point Mutations and Small Genetic Variations

12.9.2.1 Sanger Sequencing

Sanger sequencing is considered the gold standard for identifying small mutations within the coding regions of the F8 and F9 genes. This method involves PCR amplification of exonic regions followed by dideoxy chain termination sequencing. It effectively detects point mutations such as missense, nonsense, and small insertions/deletions (INDELs) [11].

Sanger sequencing is useful in the diagnosis of severe and mild to moderate Haemophilia A and B cases, where large deletions or structural variations are absent. It is often employed after ruling out inversion mutations in Haemophilia A patients to identify other causative mutations. Additionally, it plays a crucial role in carrier screening and prenatal diagnosis, enabling precise identification of disease-causing mutations.

12.9.2.2 Multiplex Ligation-Dependent Probe Amplification (MLPA)

MLPA is designed to detect copy number variations (CNVs), such as large deletions or duplications that are not easily identifiable by conventional PCR or Sanger sequencing. This method utilizes hybridization-based probe ligation, followed by PCR amplification and capillary electrophoresis for quantification [17]. MLPA is particularly beneficial when PCR and Sanger sequencing fail to detect mutations. It is an essential tool for diagnosing haemophilia cases caused by exon deletions or duplications, ensuring comprehensive genetic analysis.

12.9.2.3 Next-Generation Sequencing (NGS)

NGS enables high-throughput sequencing of the entire F8 or F9 gene, including exonic and intronic regions. This technique allows for simultaneous detection of multiple mutation types, including single-nucleotide variations (SNVs), insertions/deletions (INDELs), and large structural changes [18]. NGS provides a comprehensive genetic profile. NGS is faster and cost-effective than traditional sequencing for large-scale screening. It is recommended for cases where conventional methods yield inconclusive results.

12.9.2.4 Southern Blotting in Haemophilia Genetic Diagnosis

Genetic diagnosis of Haemophilia A (F8 gene mutations) and Haemophilia B (F9 gene mutations) relies on various molecular techniques. Among these, Southern blotting and long-range PCR (LR-PCR) have been historically used for detecting large-scale mutations, inversions, and structural variations. Below is a detailed evaluation of their advantages and limitations in haemophilia diagnosis.

Southern blotting is a hybridization-based technique that detects large gene deletions, duplications, and rearrangements. It involves DNA digestion, electrophoresis, blotting, and probe hybridization to identify structural mutations in the F8 and F9 genes.

12.9.3 Pros of Southern Blotting in Haemophilia Diagnosis

- Detects Large Structural Variations: Useful for detecting intron 22 inversion in severe Haemophilia A cases.
- Effective for the detection of large deletions and duplications in the F8 or F9 gene.
- Southern blotting is highly specific as it directly detects large genomic rearrangements rather than relying on indirect markers.
- Unlike PCR-based methods, Southern blot does not require specific primer sets, making it useful for cases where sequence variation may prevent proper primer binding.
- Southern blot is not affected by GC-rich sequences or repeat regions, unlike standard PCR, which may struggle with these genomic complexities.

12.9.4 Cons of Southern Blotting in Haemophilia Diagnosis

Time-Consuming and Labor-Intensive: The entire process takes 2–3 days, making it slow compared to modern PCR-based techniques.

Requires multiple steps including DNA digestion, electrophoresis, transfer, and hybridization.

Southern blot needs higher DNA concentrations (10–20 μg), unlike PCR-based methods, which require only nanogram quantity.

Southern blot cannot detect point mutations, small deletions, or single-nucleotide changes, which are common in mild and moderate haemophilia.

Southern blotting involves expensive radioactive or chemiluminescent probes, making it costly compared to PCR-based techniques.

The technique requires high expertise, and results may vary between laboratories due to differences in hybridization conditions and probe specificity.

Long-Range PCR (LR-PCR) in Haemophilia Genetic Diagnosis Long-range PCR is an advanced form of PCR that enables the amplification of large DNA fragments (>10 kb), making it particularly useful for detecting structural rearrangements and large deletions in the F8 and F9 genes.

Pros of Long-Range PCR in Haemophilia Diagnosis

- Long-range PCR detects large mutations (e.g., intron 22 and intron 1 inversions).
- It is highly effective for the detection of intron 22 and intron 1 inversions in the F8 gene, which are major causes of severe Haemophilia A.
- Long-range PCR can also detect large deletions in the F9 gene.
- LR-PCR can provide results within a few hours, compared to 2–3 days for Southern blot.
- Less labor-intensive and requires fewer steps.
- Uses a nanogram quantity of DNA (50–100 ng), unlike Southern blot, which requires microgram quantities.
- LR-PCR is capable of amplifying long genomic regions, making it useful for detecting complex rearrangements that standard PCR cannot amplify.
- LR-PCR is cost-effective and much cheaper than Southern blot, as it does not require radioactive probes or complex blotting procedures.

Cons of Long-Range PCR in Haemophilia Diagnosis

- LR-PCR fails in highly repetitive or GC-rich regions, which may prevent complete amplification of large segments of DNA.
- This method is prone to polymerase errors, secondary structures, and preferential amplification, which can lead to false results.
- While effective for specific known rearrangements, it cannot screen for point mutations or small insertions/deletions, which require sequencing-based methods.
- This method also needs high-fidelity polymerases (e.g., Phusion, LA-Taq) and optimized reaction conditions, which can be technically demanding.

Both Southern blot and long-range PCR are useful for detecting large structural mutations in Haemophilia A and B. However, long-range PCR is the preferred method due to its speed, lower DNA requirements, and cost-effectiveness. Southern blot, though historically significant, is now largely replaced by qPCR, MLPA, and NGS-based approaches, which provide higher sensitivity and broader mutation detection.

12.10 Linkage Analysis (Indirect Genetic Testing)

Linkage analysis is a technique used to track the inheritance of a disease-causing gene within a family. It relies on identifying genetic markers (such as microsatellites or single nucleotide polymorphisms, SNPs) that are closely linked to the F8 gene (Haemophilia A) or F9 gene (Haemophilia B) on the X chromosome. Unlike

Table 12.2 Advantages and limitations of linkage analysis in haemophilia genetic diagnosis

Aspect	Pros	Cons
Mutation knowledge	Works even when the exact mutation is unknown	Cannot directly detect mutations
Carrier detection	Effective for identifying female carriers	Requires multiple family members for accuracy
Prenatal diagnosis	Can be used for early screening in families with a known history	Recombination may lead to incorrect results
Use in sporadic cases	Can sometimes track inheritance patterns if distant relatives are available	Not useful in *de novo* (sporadic) cases with no family history
Reliability	Useful when markers are *informative*	Unreliable if markers are *uninformative* or there is recombination
Cost and accessibility	Less expensive than full sequencing	Requires multiple tests and family member cooperation
Ethical issues	Helps with genetic counselling and reproductive decisions	May uncover non-paternity or unexpected family relationships

direct mutation analysis, linkage analysis does not detect the actual mutation but follows DNA sequences inherited alongside the disease gene.

Linkage analysis remains a valuable tool in carrier detection and prenatal diagnosis of Haemophilia A and B, particularly in families with known haemophilia cases. However, its dependence on family member's samples, risk of recombination errors, and inability to detect new mutations make it less reliable than direct mutation testing (PCR-based sequencing or NGS). We have summarized the advantages and limitations of linkage analysis testing in haemophilia in Table 12.2.

Direct genetic testing (Sanger sequencing, MLPA, or NGS) is preferred due to its accuracy, while linkage analysis is mainly used when direct testing is not feasible.

12.11 Preimplantation Genetic Diagnosis (PGD)

For couples undergoing in vitro fertilization (IVF), preimplantation genetic diagnosis (PGD) offers an option to screen embryos for specific genetic mutations before implantation.

- *Applications*: PGD can be used to screen for mutations associated with hereditary haematologic disorders such as sickle cell disease, thalassemia, or haemophilia. It is an option for couples who are known carriers of such conditions and wish to prevent the transmission of the disorder to their child.
- *Advantages*: Prevents the birth of a child with a hereditary haematologic disorder by selecting embryos free of the mutation.
- *Limitations*: Involves IVF, which can be costly, physically demanding, and may not be accessible to all patients.

12.12 Ethical Considerations in Prenatal Diagnosis

The decision to pursue prenatal diagnosis for hereditary haematologic disorders raises a number of ethical issues. These concerns should be carefully considered by both the parents and the healthcare provider.

12.12.1 Informed Consent

Informed consent is a critical component of prenatal testing. Parents must understand the risks, benefits, and limitations of the diagnostic tests, including the potential outcomes and the implications of a positive or negative result. Additionally, they must be aware of the emotional, psychological, and social consequences of knowing or not knowing about a potential genetic disorder.

12.12.2 Reproductive Choices

Prenatal diagnosis may provide parents with the option to make decisions about the pregnancy, including continuing the pregnancy or considering termination. This raises complex ethical questions about reproductive autonomy, the potential for disability discrimination, and the value placed on individuals with genetic conditions.

12.12.3 Risk of Discrimination and Stigma

There is a risk that individuals diagnosed with hereditary haematologic disorders may face discrimination or stigma. Prenatal diagnosis might inadvertently reinforce societal biases against individuals with genetic conditions, which should be taken into consideration during the counselling process.

12.12.4 Use of Genetic Information

The use of genetic information for reproductive decision-making should be handled with sensitivity, particularly regarding the privacy and potential misuse of genetic data. Genetic testing for non-medical reasons, such as gender selection or social preferences, is also an area of concern.

12.13 Conclusion

Prenatal diagnosis for hereditary haematologic disorders offers significant benefits in terms of early detection and management, as well as providing parents with the opportunity to make informed decisions. Advances in molecular genetics, non-invasive testing methods, and prenatal imaging have expanded the possibilities for diagnosing and managing these conditions. However, the ethical considerations, risks of invasive procedures, and potential for psychological and emotional impact require careful consideration and appropriate counselling. As technology continues to evolve, the landscape of prenatal diagnosis for hereditary haematologic disorders will undoubtedly become more refined, offering new possibilities for prevention and early intervention.

Key Takeaways

- Hereditary haematologic disorders include conditions such as sickle cell disease, thalassemia, haemophilia, inherited platelet disorders, inherited bone marrow failure syndromes, and others.
- Prenatal diagnostic techniques such as NIPT, CVS, amniocentesis, and PGD allow for the detection of these disorders, each with its advantages and limitations.
- Ethical concerns regarding reproductive choices, informed consent, and the potential for discrimination must be carefully addressed in the context of prenatal diagnosis.

12.14 Summary

Prenatal diagnosis of hereditary haematologic disorders has been significantly advanced through molecular genetics and imaging technologies, enabling early detection and informed reproductive decision-making. These disorders, including sickle cell disease, thalassemia, haemophilia, inherited platelet disorders, bone marrow failure syndromes, and others, are caused by genetic mutations affecting genes in the respective pathways.

Diagnostic methods range from non-invasive prenatal testing (NIPT) to invasive procedures like chorionic villus sampling (CVS) and amniocentesis, as well as preimplantation genetic diagnosis (PGD) for embryo selection. Techniques such as PCR, Sanger sequencing, and next-generation sequencing (NGS) facilitate precise mutation detection.

Despite the clinical benefits, ethical considerations, including informed consent, reproductive choices, and potential genetic discrimination, must be addressed. Advances in genetic testing continue to refine prenatal diagnosis, balancing medical possibilities with ethical responsibilities.

Appendix

The cases described below highlight the importance of molecular testing for prenatal diagnosis and carrier detection in haemoglobinopathies and haemophilia.

Case 1 Prenatal diagnosis for δβ-β-thalassemia.

A Couple was referred to us for prenatal diagnosis at 12 weeks of gestation, as they have previous child with β-thalassemia major phenotype. On HPLC the mother was found to be β-thalassemia carrier (HbA_2: 5.4%) and the father was having elevated HbF (19.6%). We performed CRDB to determine the maternal mutation and it was found to be IVS 1-5 (G>C) heterozygous, whereas to determine the paternal genotype we performed Gap-PCR and the mutation was found to be $A\gamma G\gamma(\delta\beta)^0$-thalassemia (Asian Indian inversion) in heterozygous form. The fetal sample was taken out using chorionic villus sampling. The CRDB and Gap-PCR techniques were used to determine the genotype of the fetus. The CRDB showed the presence of maternal mutation IVS 1-5 (G>C) in homozygous form and the Gap-PCR showed the presence of Asian Indian inversion in heterozygous form. This suggested that the fetus was affected and having compound heterozygous condition for β-thalassemia and δβ-thalassemia. The VNTR analysis was done to rule out maternal cell contamination.

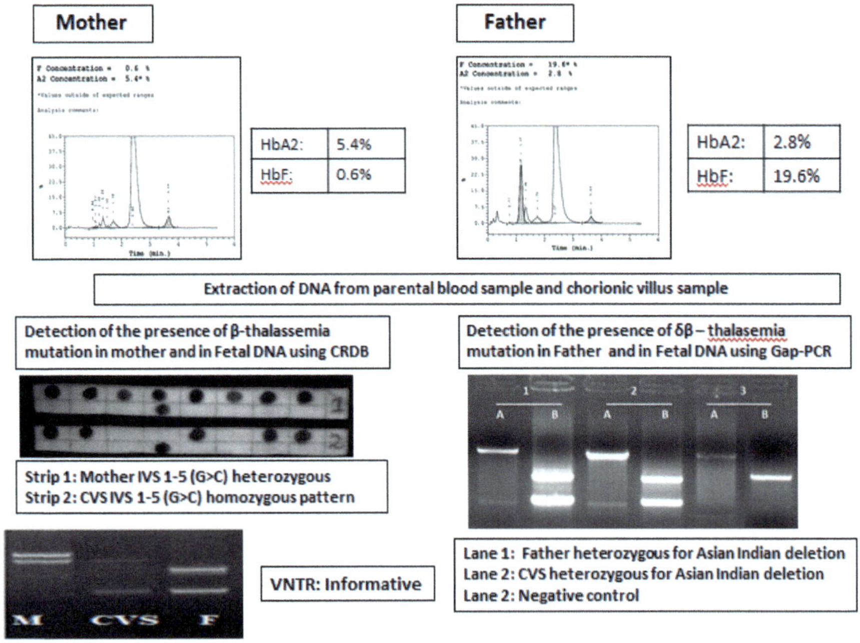

Case 2 Prenatal diagnosis for HbS-β-thalassemia.

A couple referred to us for prenatal diagnosis as the wife was diagnosed as sickle cell carrier (HbS: 38.4%) during the routine ANC screening and on HPLC her husband was found to be β-thalassemia carrier (HbA_2: 4.9%). The wife was 13 weeks pregnant and the fetal sample was obtained by CVS. The presence of HbS in mother and fetus was determined using PCR-RFLP technique. Mother was found to be heterozygous for HbS whereas the HbS was absent in the fetal DNA. The β-globin gene mutation in father and fetal DNA was determined using CRDB technique. Both the father and fetal DNA showed Codon 30 (G>C) mutation in heterozygous form. As the HbS was absent in the fetal DNA the fetus was diagnosed as unaffected (β-thalassemia carrier). VNTR analysis was performed to exclude the possibility of maternal cell contamination.

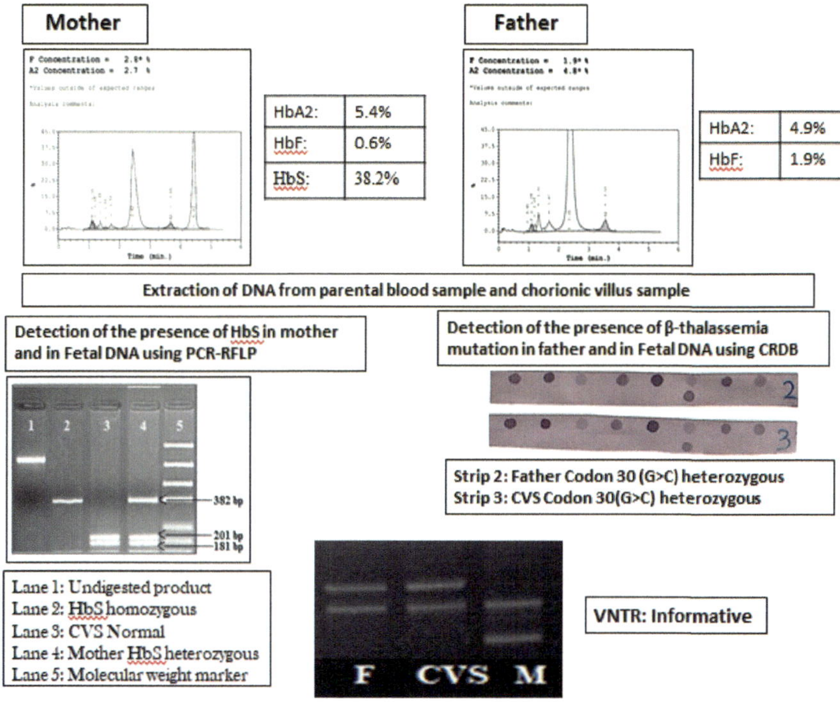

Case 3 Prenatal diagnosis for HbE-β-thalassemia.

A couple referred to us for prenatal diagnosis as they had one affected child with HbE-β-thalassemia and requiring regular blood transfusion. The gestation age of the fetus was 12 weeks hence CVS was done to obtain the fetal sample. On HPLC the wife was found to be β-thalassemia carrier (HbA2: 5.4%) while the husband was HbE trait (HbA2: 26.3%). On CRBD the husband and fetal DNA showed presence of HbE in heterozygous form whereas the five common β-thalassemia mutations were found to be absent in wife. To rule out other rare β-thalassemia mutations, we used the ARMS technique, which revealed that the wife was heterozygous for the FS 16 (-C) mutation, but this mutation was absent in the fetal DNA. Therefore, the fetus was diagnosed as unaffected, with an HbE trait. VNTR analysis was performed to exclude the possibility of maternal cell contamination.

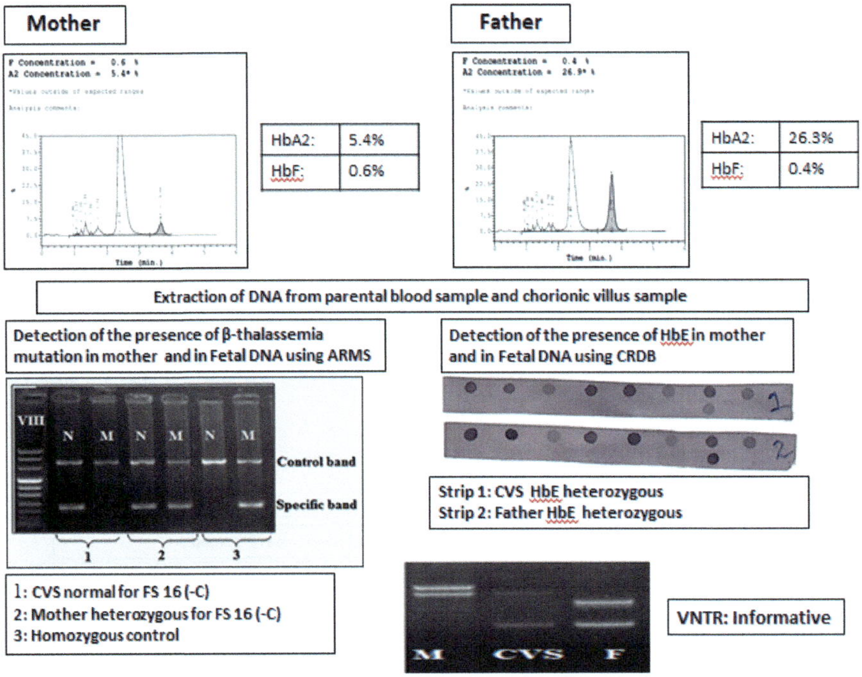

Case 4 Prenatal diagnosis for β-thalassemia.

A β-thalassemia carrier couple was referred to us for prenatal diagnosis. The fetal sample was obtained through CVS. On CRDB wife was found to be having Codon 15 (G>A) mutation in heterozygous form whereas the husband was heterozygous for Codon 30 (G>C) mutation. The fetal DNA showed the presence of both these mutation in compound heterozygous form. Therefore, the fetus was diagnosed as affected (β-thalassemia major). The VNTR analysis was done to rule out maternal cell contamination.

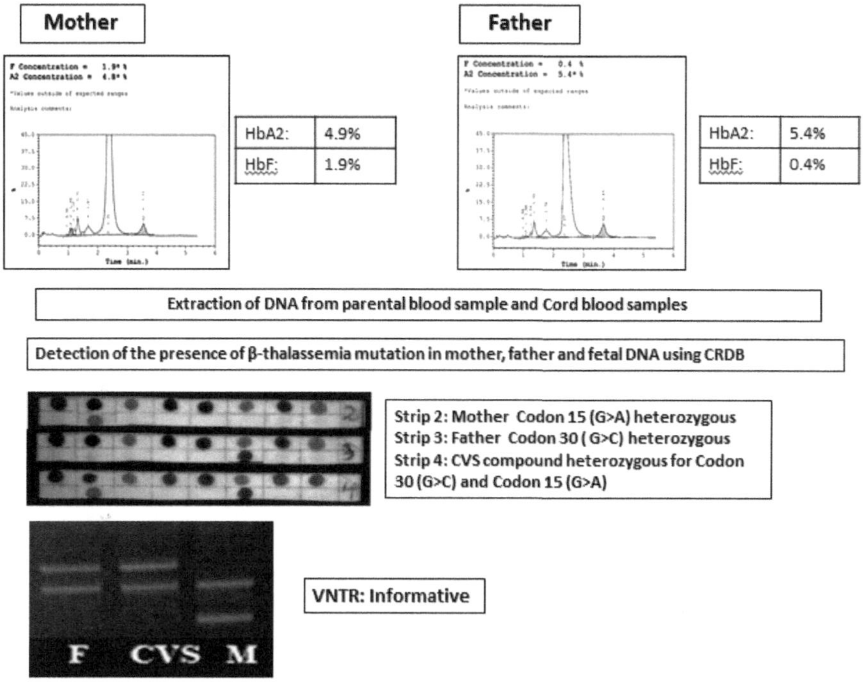

Case 5 Case of severe haemophilia A with *F8* Intron 22 inversion (type 1).

Case 5 demonstrates the results of a complementary and diagnostic tests using 2% agarose gel electrophoresis for identifying different genetic profiles in F8 intron 22 inversion positive severe haemophilia A cases. This electrophoretic analysis effectively differentiates between normal, carrier, and affected individuals based on F8 intron 22 inversion status.

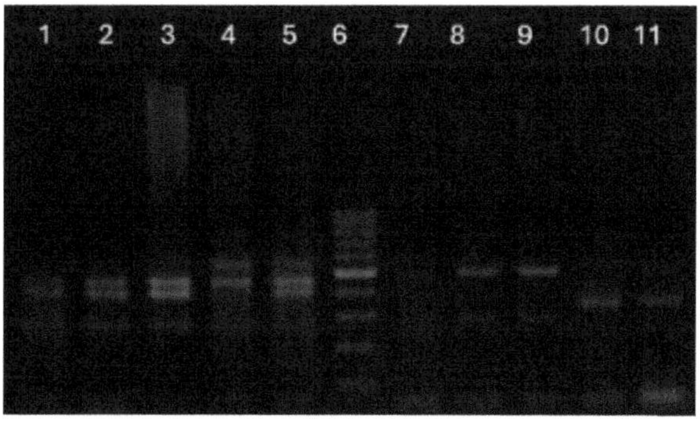

F8 Intron 22 inversion 2% agarose gel image

Complementary test results (lanes 1-5), 100 bp DNA ladder (lane 6), and diagnostic test results (lanes 7–11)

Lanes 1,2 and 3: Normal unaffected fetus/non-carrier sister (405, 457 bp)
Lane 4: Intron 22 inversion type 1 positive index-case (559,457 bp)

In case of Intron 22 inversion type 2 index case will show 559,405 bp bands (not shown in image).

Lane 5: Carrier female (559,457 and 405 bp)
Lane 6: DNA ladder
Lanes 7, 8 and 9: Normal unaffected fetus/non-carrier sister (487 bp)
Lane 10: Intron 22 inversion type 1 positive index-case (333 bp)

In case of Intron 22 inversion type 2 index case will show 385 bp (not shown in image).

Lane 11: Carrier female (333 and 487 bp)

Case 6 Case of severe haemophilia A with *F8* Intron 1 inversion.

Case 6 presents the results of molecular analysis of F8 intron 1 inversion in severe haemophilia A families using multiplex PCR and detection by 2% agarose gel electrophoresis to identify affected individuals and carriers.

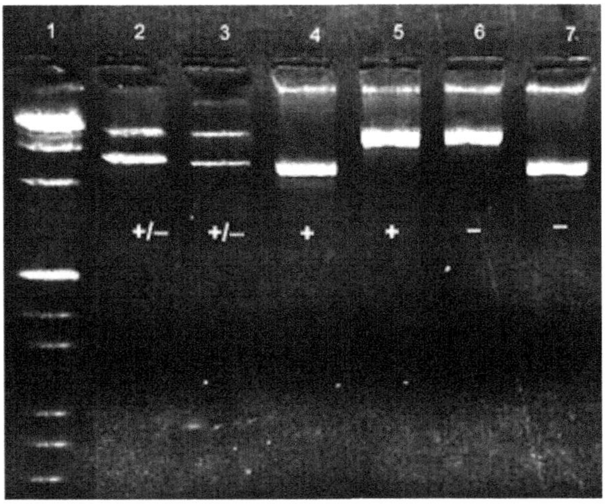

Lanes 1: Molecular marker X
Lane 2 and 3: Carrier mother
Lane 4 and 5: Index case positive for *F8* intron 1 inversion
Lane 6 and 7: Normal unaffected fetus/non-carrier sister

Case 7 Case of severe haemophilia A with single nucleotide variant.

Case 7 represents severe haemophilia A patient presented with recurrent spontaneous bleeding. Genetic analysis identified a missense variant p.Arg2182Cys (c.6544C>T) in exon 23 of the F8 gene, confirmed by electropherogram. This C>T transition at nucleotide 6544 results in an arginine-to-cysteine substitution at position 2182, affecting Factor VIII function. The variant was classified as likely pathogenic due to its impact on protein structure. Family screening confirmed the patient's mother as a heterozygous carrier, and genetic counselling followed by prenatal testing was provided.

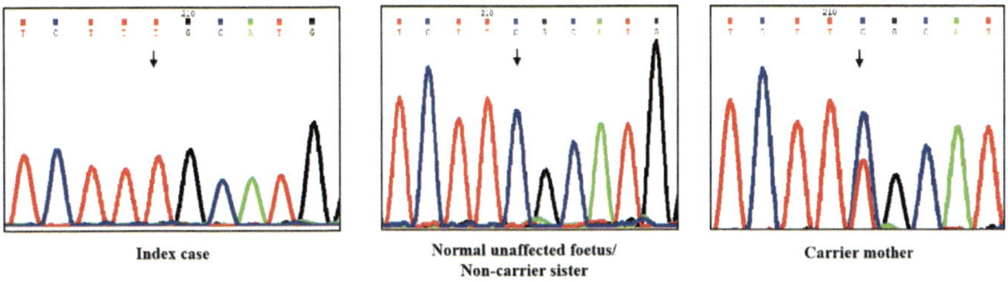

Electropherogram of *F8* missense variant p.Arg2182Cys (c.6544C>T) in exon 23.

Case 8 Case of severe haemophilia A with frameshift variant.

Case 8 represents genetic analysis of a severe haemophilia A family which identified a frameshift (insertion) variant p.Gly469Valfs*18 (c.1405_1406insTTGG) in exon 9 of the F8 gene, confirmed by electropherogram. This TTGG insertion at nucleotide 1405-1406 causes a frameshift, leading to a premature stop codon (*18) and truncation of the Factor VIII protein. The mutation is classified as pathogenic due to its severe impact on protein function. Family testing confirmed the mother as a heterozygous carrier, and genetic counselling was provided.

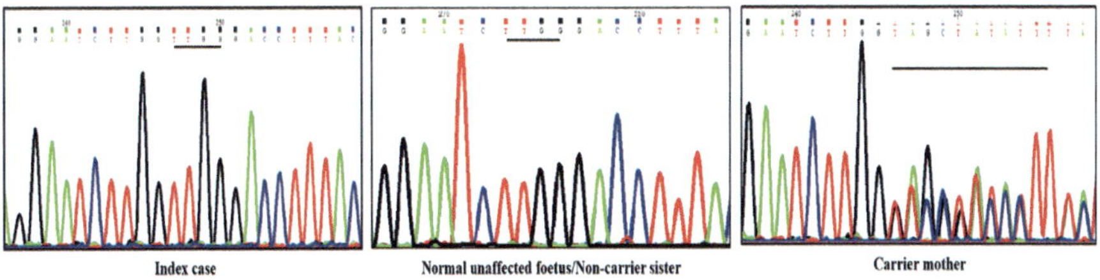

Electropherogram of *F8* frameshift (insertion) variant p.Gly469Valfs*18 (c.1405_1406insTTGG) in exon 9.

Case 9 Case of severe haemophilia A with *F8* exon 1 deletion (*F8* MLPA).

Case 9 is a severe haemophilia A patient identified with a deletion of exon 1 in the F8 gene, confirmed by MLPA. This deletion results in the loss of Factor VIII expression, leading to a severe disease phenotype. Genetic testing confirmed the mother as a heterozygous carrier, while his non-carrier sister showed no deletion. Family counselling was conducted to discuss inheritance patterns and future reproductive options. This case highlights the role of MLPA in detecting large deletions in haemophilia A.

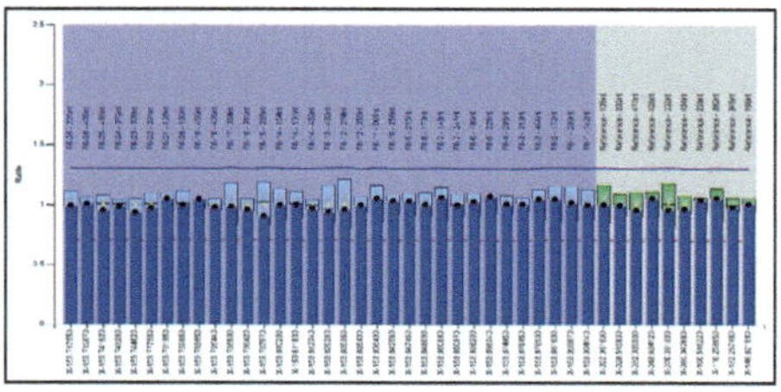

Normal unaffected foetus/non-carrier sister

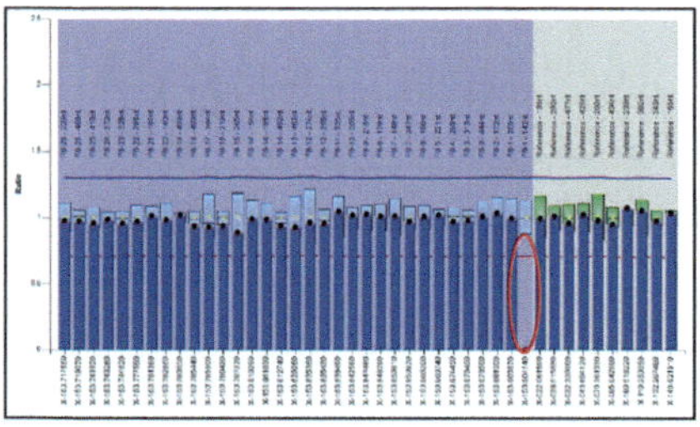

Index case with exon 1 deletion

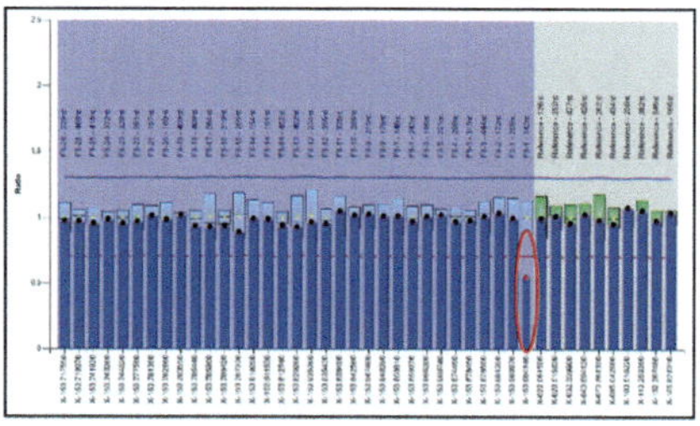

Carrier mother

References

1. Vijian D, Wan Ab Rahman WS, Ponnuraj KT, Zulkafli Z, Bahar R, Yasin N, Hassan S, Esa E. Gene mutation spectrum among alpha-thalassaemia patients in northeast peninsular Malaysia. Diagnostics (Basel). 2023;13(5):894. https://doi.org/10.3390/diagnostics13050894. PMID: 36900038; PMCID: PMC10000533.
2. Colah RB, Nadkarni AH, Gorakshakar AC, Sawant PM, Mehta PR, Gorivale MS, Hariharan P, Mohanty D, Ghosh K. The changing trends in prenatal diagnosis of hemoglobinopathies in India: the quest of a single center to reduce the burden of disease over three decades. Hemoglobin. 2021;45(2):112–8.
3. Nadkarni A, Wadia M, Gorakshkar A, Kimaya R, Colah RB, Mohanty D. Moleculer characterization of delta-beta thalassemia and hereditary persistence of fetal haemoglobin in the Indian population. Hemoglobin. 2008;32:425–33.
4. Weatherall DJ, Clegg JB. The thalassemia syndromes. 4th ed. Blackwell Science; 2001.
5. Inusa BPD, Hsu LL, Kohli N, Patel A, Ominu-Evbota K, Anie KA, Atoyebi W. Sickle cell disease-genetics, pathophysiology, clinical presentation and treatment. Int J Neonatal Screen. 2019;5(2):20. https://doi.org/10.3390/ijns5020020. PMID: 33072979; PMCID: PMC7510211.
6. Alshehri AA, Jackson DE. Non-invasive prenatal fetal blood group genotype and its application in the management of hemolytic disease of fetus and newborn: systematic review and meta-analysis. Transfus Med Rev. 2021;35(2):85–94. https://doi.org/10.1016/j.tmrv.2021.02.001. Epub 2021 Mar 1. PMID: 33781630.

7. Wadia MR, Phanasgaokar SP, Nadkarni AH, Surve RR, Gorakshakar AC, Colah RB, Mohanty D. Usefulness of automated chromatography for rapid fetal blood analysis for second trimester prenatal diagnosis of beta-thalassemia. Prenat Diagn. 2002;22(2):153–7.
8. Rao S, Saxena R, Deka D, Kabra M. Use of HbA estimation by CE-HPLC for prenatal diagnosis of beta-thalassemia; experience from a tertiary care centre in north India: a brief report. Hematology. 2009;14(2):122–4.
9. Old JM, Khan SN, Verma I, Fucharoen S, Kleanthous M, Ioannou P, Kotea N, Fisher C, Riazuddin S, Saxena R, Winichagoon P, Kyriacou K, Al-Quobaili F, Khan B. A multi-center study in order to further define the molecular basis of beta-thalassemia in Thailand, Pakistan, Sri Lanka, Mauritius, Syria, and India, and to develop a simple molecular diagnostic strategy by amplification refractory mutation system-polymerase chain reaction. Hemoglobin. 2001 Nov;25(4):397-407.
10. Colah RB, Goraksahkar AC, Lu CY, Nadkarni AH, Desai SN, Pawar NR, et al.Application of covalent reverse dot blot hybridization for rapid prenatal diagnosis of the common Indian thalassaemia syndromes. Ind J Haematol and Blood Transf 1997; 15:10.
11. Sanger F, Nicklen S, Coulson AR. DNA sequencing with chain-terminating inhibitors. Proc Natl Acad Sci USA. 1977;74(12):5463–7.
12. Old J, Harteveld CL, Traeger-Synodinos J, Petrou M, Angastiniotis M, Galanello R. Prevention of thalassaemias and other haemoglobin disorders: volume 2: laboratory protocols [Internet]. 2nd ed. Nicosia (Cyprus): Thalassaemia International Federation; 2012.
13. Liu Q, Sommer SS. Subcycling-PCR for multiplex long-distance amplification of regions with high and low GC content: application to the inversion hotspot of the factor VIII gene. BioTechniques. 1998;25(6):1022–8.
14. Lakich D, Kazazian HH Jr, Antonarakis SE, Gitschier J. Inversions disrupting the factor VIII gene are a common cause of severe haemophilia A. Nat Genet. 1993;5(3):236–41. PUBMED. NCBI.NLM.NIH.GOV.
15. Rossetti LC, Radic CP, Larripa IB, De Brasi CD. Developing a molecular diagnostic service for haemophilia A: detection of novel and recurrent mutations in the factor VIII gene. Haemophilia. 2005;11(3):292–9.
16. Bagnall RD, Waseem NH, Green PM, Giannelli F. Recurrent inversion breaking intron 1 of the factor VIII gene is a frequent cause of severe haemophilia A. Blood. 2002;99(1):168–74.
17. Schouten JP, McElgunn CJ, Waaijer R, Zwijnenburg D, Diepvens F, Pals G. Relative quantification of 40 nucleic acid sequences by multiplex ligation-dependent probe amplification. Nucleic Acids Res. 2002;30(12):e57.
18. Shen Y, Wan Z, Coarfa C, Drabek R, Chen L, Ostrowski EA, Liu Y, Weinstock GM, Wheeler DA, Milosavljevic A. A SNP discovery method to assess variant allele probability from next-generation resequencing data. Sci Rep. 2016;6:36615.

Chapter 13
NGS for Precision Medicine in Hematologic Disorders

Renu Saxena, Shalini Goel, Ritu Chadha, and Nitin Mathur

Abstract Next-generation sequencing (NGS) has revolutionized hematology by enabling comprehensive analysis of the genetic landscape of hematologic malignancies and inherited blood disorders. It allows high-throughput, simultaneous sequencing of a very large number of genes, providing insights into genetic mutations, structural variations, and epigenetic alterations. In malignancies such as leukemia, lymphoma, and myelodysplastic syndromes, NGS facilitates the identification of diagnostic markers, risk stratification, and detection of minimal residual disease (MRD). This precision guides therapeutic decisions, including targeted therapies, by uncovering actionable mutations like FLT3, NPM1, and IDH1/2. Furthermore, NGS panels allow for the dynamic monitoring of clonal evolution during disease progression and treatment.

In inherited hematologic disorders, such as thalassemia, sickle cell anemia, and hemophilia, NGS enhances diagnostic accuracy by pinpointing causative mutations and identifying carriers. Whole-genome and whole-exome sequencing are particularly valuable for diagnosing complex conditions (such as rare inherited hemolytic disorders, idiopathic bone marrow failure syndromes, inherited, and platelet function disorders, which are not detected by routine tests) and uncovering novel gene variants. Additionally, NGS supports bone marrow transplantation by refining donor selection through high-resolution HLA typing.

Technological advancements, including single-cell sequencing and methylation profiling, have expanded the utility of NGS in hematology, enabling the study of tumor heterogeneity and epigenetic regulation. Despite its transformative impact, challenges remain, including high costs, data interpretation complexity, and the need for robust bioinformatics pipelines. Ethical considerations related to incidental findings and genetic counselling also require attention.

NGS has become an integral tool in hematology, driving precision medicine and advancing our understanding of blood disorders. As technology evolves, its applications are expected to expand, further improving patient outcomes through personalized care.

R. Saxena (✉) · S. Goel · R. Chadha · N. Mathur
Department of Hematopathology, Medanta,The Medicity, Gurugram, Haryana, India

H. P. Pati et al. (eds.), *Clinical Hematology and Hemato-Oncology*,
https://doi.org/10.1007/978-981-92-1167-8_13

Keywords Precision medicine · Next-generation sequencing · AML · CLL · Benign hematology

Learning Objectives
- What is NGS?
- What are its applications in hematology?
- What are its advantages over RT PCR?
- What are its limitations?
- What are future directions in molecular medicine?

13.1 Introduction

Next-generation sequencing (NGS) has emerged as a transformative tool in hematology, enabling comprehensive genomic analysis to better understand, diagnose, and treat blood disorders. By allowing simultaneous sequencing of millions of DNA fragments, NGS offers unparalleled sensitivity, specificity, and depth in genetic investigation. The availability of commercially designed NGS panels, which can provide results within hours to days, has further accelerated the diagnostic process. These panels not only facilitate quicker diagnoses but also assist in selecting targeted therapies, improving treatment precision. Additionally, advancements in treatment have led to deeper responses, necessitating more sensitive tools to evaluate complete remission. Numerous studies have highlighted the importance of NGS-based Minimal Residual disease (MRD) assessment in prognostication and risk stratification, showcasing its potential to influence clinical decision-making and improve patient outcomes. This write-up explores the key applications, benefits, challenges, and future prospects of NGS in hematology.

The fundamental workflow of NGS consists of four steps, including DNA or RNA extraction, library preparation, sequencing, and data analysis. NGS offers various sequencing approaches tailored to specific clinical needs. These include whole-genome sequencing (WGS), which covers the entire genome (~3 billion base pairs) to provide comprehensive genomic insights, whole-exome sequencing (WES) which focuses on coding regions (~30 million base pairs), representing ~1% of the genome but harboring the majority of disease-related mutations and Targeted Mutation Panels which examine specific genes or pathways linked to particular diseases. Mutation panels for hematologic malignancies include mutations for both myeloid and lymphoid malignancies and also for their MRD.

The most common approach for hematologic malignancies is the use of targeted panels for myeloid and lymphoid neoplasia and their MRD. Exome sequencing is often used for the diagnosis of undiagnosed benign hematologic disorders like hemolytic anemia and bleeding disorders, etc. Whole-genome approach is very rarely used as it is expensive. It is used for research or diagnosis of unknown variants, and where exome sequencing fails.

13.2 NGS in Myeloid Neoplasms

NGS has transformed the diagnosis, prognostic assessment, and management of myeloid neoplasms, including acute myeloid leukemia (AML), myelodysplastic syndromes (MDS), myeloproliferative neoplasms (MPNs), and overlapping disorders, such as myelodysplastic syndrome/myeloproliferative neoplasm (MDS/MPN). Below is an overview of the applications, benefits, and challenges of NGS in the context of myeloid neoplasms.

13.2.1 *Applications of NGS in Myeloid Neoplasms*

1. *Diagnostic Utility*

   NGS facilitates the identification of genetic mutations that aid in the diagnosis of myeloid neoplasms:

   (a) *AML*: The World Health Organization classification (2022) [1] and the European Leukemia Net recommendations for AML [2] consider genetic abnormalities as a top priority for diagnosis, prognostication, monitoring of measurable residual disease, and treatment choice [3]. NGS identifies common mutations, which are required for 2022 classification of AML, like FLT3, NPM1, and CEBPA. NGS also identifies less common mutations, such as IDH1/2 and DNMT3A. Recent discoveries highlight the role of premalignant stages in the multistep clonal evolution of AML. Early mutations, such as those in TET2, DNMT3A, and ASXL1, arise at low variant allelic frequencies (VAFs) in individuals without overt hematologic disease. The accumulation of somatic mutations in multipotent stem/progenitor cells of healthy persons is known as clonal hematopoiesis (CH) [4, 5]. WHO 2022 classification of hemato-lymphoid malignancies includes new myeloid precursor lesions, clonal hematopoiesis of indeterminate potential (CHIP), and clonal cytopenia of undetermined significance (CCUS) [4, 5]. CHIP refers to CH harboring somatic mutations of myeloid malignancy-associated genes with a variant allele frequency (VAF) of ≥2% in individuals without a diagnosed hematologic disorder or cytopenia.

   CHIP is referred to as CCUS when it is accompanied by persistent, inexplicable cytopenias. DNMT3A, TET2, ASXL1, JAK2, TP53, SF3B1, PPM1D, SRSF2, ZBTB33, IDH1, IDH2, U2AF1, KRAS, NRAS, CTCF, CBL, GNB1, BRCC3, PTPN11, GNAS, BCOR, and BCORL1 are among the genes that frequently have CH driver mutations. Progression to clinically overt AML occurs with the acquisition of additional mutations.

   NGS has also provided profound insights into the genetic landscape of AML, uncovering novel mutations and refining the understanding of disease heterogeneity [3] (Table 13.1). For instance, in core-binding factor (CBF) AML, mutations in genes such as KIT, FLT3, and N/KRAS are frequently

Table 13.1 Genes and structural variants for clinical testing in leukemia

AML	Required for diagnosis and risk stratification: ASXL1, BCOR, CEBPA, DDX41, EZH2, FLT3-ITD, FLT3-TKD, IDH1, IDH2, NPM1, RUNX1, SF3B1, SRSF2, STAG2, TP53, U2AF1, ZRSR2 Additional recommended: ANKRD26, BCORL1, BRAF, CBL, CSF3R, DNMT3A, ETV6, GATA2, JAK2, KIT, KRAS, NRAS, NF1, PHF6, PPM1D, PTPN11, RAD21, SETBP1, TET2, WT1	BCR::ABL1, CBFB::MYH11, DEK::NUP214, MECOM::R, KMT2A::R, NUP98::R, RUNX1::RUNX1T1, PML::RARA
B-ALL	CREBBP, CRLF2, FLT3, IDH1, IDH2, IKZF1, IL7R, JAK1, JAK2, JAK3, KMT2D, KRAS, NF1, NRAS, PAX5, PTPN11, SETD2, SH2B3, TP53	ABL1::R, ABL2::R, CRLF2::R, CSF1R::R, DUX4::R, EPOR::R, ETV6::R, JAK2::R, KMT2A::R, MEF2D::R, NUTM1::R, PAX5::R, PDGFRA::R, PDGFRB::R, TCF3::R, ZNF384::R
T-ALL	DNMT3A, ETV6, EZH2, FBXW7, FLT3, IDH1, IDH2, IL7R, JAK1, JAK3, KRAS, MSH2, NOTCH1, NRAS, PHF6, PTEN, U2AF1, WT1	BCL11B::R, LMO2::R, MYB::R, NUP::ABL1, NUP214::R, STIL::R, TAL::R, TLX1::R, TLX3::R

observed [6]. Furthermore, Grimwade et al. (2016) demonstrated that mutations in ASXL1 and EZH2 are more common in AML with t(8;21) than in AML with inv(16) [7]. These mutations are associated with poor prognosis, especially in patients with co-occurring tyrosine kinase pathway mutations, such as those in KIT or FLT3. Additionally, a high KIT mutant allele ratio (>35%) correlates with inferior outcomes in t(8;21) AML, emphasizing the importance of genetic profiling for prognosis. ELN guidelines for AML diagnosis recommend conventional cytogenetics and mutational analysis for at least nine key genes, such as NPM1, FLT3, CEBPA, TP53, ASXL1, IDH1, IDH2, RUNX1, and c-KIT. Screening for gene rearrangements, including PML-RARA, CBFB-MYH11, and RUNX1-RUNX1T1, is also recommended to ensure comprehensive risk stratification [2]. The recent WHO classification[2022] has removed the entity "AML with myelodysplasia related changes" and instead introduced cytogenetic and molecular abnormalities under the category AML myelodysplasia related. This entity now includes a set of 8 genes (*ASXL1, BCOR, EZH2, SF3B1, SRSF2, STAG2, U2AF1,* and *ZRSR2*) for AML-MR diagnosis [3].

(b) *MDS*: MDS is a heterogeneous group of disorders and NGS has enabled the identification of an increasing number of genetic abnormalities, including recurrent modifications in the TP53, DNMT3A, NRAS, NPM1, RUNX1, and FLT3 genes. Twenty-one genes were found to have mutations, including ASXL1, TET2, SRSF2, EZH2, CSF3R, NRAS, ETV6, SETBP1, RUNX1, DDX41, U2AF1, JAK2, FLT3ITD, SF3B1, DNAMT3A, PHF6, TP53, CEBPA, CBL, IDH2, and GATA2 (Table 13.2). In nearly half of the cases, the karyotype was normal [8]. Mutations in genes like SF3B1, SRSF2,

Table 13.2 Genes and structural variants for clinical testing in MDS/MPN neoplasms

Indication	Single gene mutations	Structural variants
MDS, MDS/MPN, cytopenia	ASXL1, BCOR, BCORL1, CBL, CEBPA, CSF3R, DDX41, DNMT3A, ETV6, ETNK1, EZH2, FLT3-ITD, FLT3-TKD, GATA2, GNB1, IDH1, IDH2, JAK2, KIT, KRAS, KMT2A-PTD, NF1, NPM1, NRAS, PHF6, PPM1D, PRPF8, PTPN11, RAD21, RUNX1, SAMD9, SAMD9L, SETBP1, SF3B1, SRSF2, STAG2, TET2, TP53, U2AF1, UBA1, WT1, ZRSR2	
MPN and mastocytosis	ASXL1, CALR, CBL, CSF3R, DNMT3A, EZH2, IDH1, IDH2, JAK2, KIT, KRAS, MPL, NRAS, PTPN11, RUNX1, SETBP1, SF3B1, SH2B3, SRSF2, TET2, U2AF1, ZRSR2	BCR::ABL1
Eosinophilia	ASXL1, CBL, DNMT3A, EZH2, KRAS, NRAS, RUNX1, SF3B1, SRSF2, STAT5B, TET2, U2AF1	BCR::ABL1, FGFR1::R, FLT3::R, JAK2::R, PDGFRA::R, PDGFRB::R

TET2, ASXL1, and TP53 are frequently identified. SF3B1 mutations are particularly associated with ring sideroblasts [9].

(c) *MPNs*: Detection of JAK2 V617F, CALR, and MPL mutations is often seen in polycythemia vera (PV), essential thrombocythemia (ET), and primary myelofibrosis (PMF) [10].

Juvenile Myelomonocytic Leukemia (JMML): Around 90% of patients have molecular alterations in one of the five RAS pathway genes (PTPN11, NRAS, KRAS, NF1, or CBL), which define clinically distinct subtypes. In about 50% of the cases, second hits are seen. In 10–15% of cases, the second hit is seen in one of the RAS pathway genes (RAS double mutant cases). It is also seen in SETBP1 mutations (7–9%), PRC2 (EZH2 and ASXL1) mutation in 4–7%, and JAK3 mutations in 3–10% of JMML patients [11].

(d) *MDS/MPN Neoplasms*: While somatic mutations in myeloid-related genes are present in approximately 90% of patients with MDS/MPN, chromosomal abnormalities can be detected in 10–50% of cases using standard cytogenetics. The clinical progression and clinical heterogeneity of these disorders are influenced by these mutations (Table 13.2) [11].

Chronic Myelomonocytic Leukemia (CMML): Since more than 90% of patients with CMML have at least one mutation, which typically affects TET2 (60%), SRSF2 (50%), and ASXL1 (45%), it is the most prevalent and, thus, the best genetically characterized MDS/MPN. RUNX1 (20%), SETBP1 (12%), and EZH2 (8%), which contribute to the myelodysplastic CMML (MD-CMML) phenotype, are recurrent secondary driver hits that contribute to clonal expansion and disease evolution. ASXL1, which is present in both MD and myeloproliferative CMML (MP-CMML), is more common in the latter. Acquisition of RAS pathway mutations or chromosomal abnormalities may cause progression to AML, which is reported in 15–30% of CMML [11].

MDS/MPN Neoplasm with Neutrophilia: This shows initiating mutations in ASXL1 (60–80%), followed by SETBP1 (40%), SRSF2 (40%), TET2 (35%), EZH2 (25%), NRAS (20%), RUNX1 (20%), GATA2 (18%), CBL (15%); 10% for CSF3R, STAG2, and CUX1. The secondary hits (SETBP1, RUNX1, and EZH2) lead to clonal expansion and cytopenia development. Activation of the RAS pathway promotes leukocytosis eventually leading to AML [11].

MDS/MPN with SF3B1 Mutation and Thrombocytosis: This has a normal karyotype in 85% patients. Frequent mutations are seen in SF3B1 (90%), with mutations in JAK2 (40%). CALR mutations are rare. Other recurrent mutations include those associated with clonal hematopoiesis: TET2 (20%), ASXL1 (20%), and DNMT3A (15%); and less frequent mutations in EZH2 (7%), SETBP1 (5%), and SRSF2 (5%) [11].

MDS/MPN Neoplasm-NOS: This is the most heterogeneous group with frequent mutations including ASXL1 (40%), JAK2 (25%), TET2 (25%), SRSF2 (25%), EZH2 (20%), U2AF1 (16%), and RUNX1 (15%). Based on mutations, recently they have been further subcategorized into "CMML-like" (biallelic TET2, TET2/SRSF2 or RUNX1/SRSF2),"aCML-like" (ASXL1/SETBP1, SETBP1/SRSF2, ASXL1/EZH2, RUNX1/EZH2), "MDS/MPN-RT-T-like" (SF3B1, DNMT3A/JAK2), "TP53" and "others" [11].

2. *Prognostic Stratification with NGS:*

   (a) *AML*: NGS-defined mutations help in risk stratification as per the ELN guidelines [2]. The mutations are classified into 3 risk groups.

   - Favorable risk group includes Core Binding Factor AML: *RUNX1-RUNX1T1* (t(8;21)(q22;q22.1)), *CBFB-MYH11* (inv(16)(p13.1q22) or t(16;16)(p13.1;q22)), NPM1-mutated (without FLT3-ITD or with low FLT3-ITD allelic ratio), and Biallelic CEBPA mutations (b ZIP domain mutation)
   - Intermediate risk group includes NPM1-mutated with FLT3-ITD (high allelic ratio), wild-type NPM1 with FLT3-ITD (low allelic ratio), mutations in other genes such as RUNX1, ASXL1, or TP53 (without complex karyotype)
   - Adverse risk includes chromosomal abnormalities (Complex karyotype (≥3 unrelated abnormalities), monosomal karyotype and (9; 22) (q34.1;q11.2) (*BCR-ABL1*) and molecular markers (*FLT3-ITD (high allelic ratio)RUNX1*, *ASXL1*, or *TP53* mutations (regardless of cytogenetics).

   (b) *MDS*: The three most significant genetic predictors of unfavorable outcomes are TP53 multihit, FLT3 mutations, and MLLPTD; the latter two show the strongest tendency to convert into AML. TP53 and ASXL1 mutations indicate poor prognosis, while SF3B1 mutations predict better outcomes. In order to include the somatic mutations and improving the risk stratification, a clinical-molecular prognostic model (IPSS-Molecular [IPSS-M]) has been developed over the previous IPSS R prognostic model. This is based on hematologic parameters, cytogenetic abnormalities, and somatic mutations of 31 genes and identifies patients into six different IPSS-M risk categories with prognostic differences. Compared with the IPSS-R, the IPSS-M improves prognostic discrimination across all clinical endpoints in the patients [12].

The IPSS-M is applicable in primary and secondary/therapy-related MDS. The IPSS-M score is personalized with a virtually unique value per patient, interpretable (a one-unit increase in score results in doubled risk), reproducible (an applicable mathematical formula and an online calculator), and provides a flexible and transparent strategy to account for missing values.

(c) *MPNs*: CALR mutations (type 1/type 2) in ET and PMF are linked to varying thrombosis risks and survival rates.

Juvenile Myelomonocytic Leukemia (JMML): Secondary mutations are often subclonal and may be involved in disease progression rather than initiation of leukemia [11].

(d) *MDS/MPN:*
- *CMML*: The inclusion of molecular markers in CMML-specific prognostic scoring systems has allowed to refine previous models. Now all of these scores contain mutations in ASXL1 since they have been repeatedly linked to negative outcomes. Furthermore, mutations in RUNX1, NRAS, and SETBP1 are included in the molecular CMML-specific prognostic scoring system (CPSS-Mol) as they are linked to a higher probability of AML transformation and a worse OS. Stronger results and a stronger response to treatment are linked to TET2 mutations, particularly when ASXL1 mutations are absent [11] (Table 13.2).
- *MDS/MPN with neutrophilia*: This is the most aggressive of all MDS/MPN overlap syndromes, with a very poor survival and a high transformation rate to AML. The prognostic impact of SETBP1 mutations is controversial, but mutations in TET2, RUNX1, NRAS, and CUX1 are reported to have poor outcome. Mayo Prognostic Model for aCML stratifies patients into two different risk groups based on age, anemia and TET2 mutations, which identifies patients who can benefit from HSCT, the current hallmark of aCML treatment [11].
- *MDS/MPN with SF3B1 mutation and thrombocytosis* usually has a mild course with longer OS when compared to other overlap syndromes and a low rate of transformation to AML. Mutations in ASXL1, SETBP1, and EZH2 have also been associated with adverse outcomes [11].
- *MDS/MPN neoplasm—NOS*: Usually the outcome mimics the corresponding MDS/MPN counterpart, with the "MDS/MPN-RS-T-like" category being associated with the highest median OS and the patients within "TP53" group having the most unfavorable prognosis [11].

3. *Therapeutic Guidance:*

   (a) *AML targeted therapies*: NGS plays a pivotal role in treatment planning for AML by guiding the choice and timing of therapeutic interventions. It identifies actionable mutations for targeted therapies, e.g., FLT3 inhibitors (midostaurin, gilteritinib) and IDH inhibitors (enasidenib, ivosidenib). NGS has also been instrumental in assessing treatment responses in AML. For instance, hypo-methylating agents (HMAs) such as azacytidine and decitabine are often used in patients unfit for intensive chemotherapy. Mutations in TET2 have been associated with improved response to azacytidine in some studies, although the findings are not consistent across all research [13]. Similarly, DNMT3A mutations are linked to better responses to HMAs, whereas IDH mutations are associated with poorer outcomes. Interestingly, Welch et al. observed that AML patients with TP53 mutations responded favorably to decitabine, with a significant reduction in adverse prognostic implications compared to patients with wild-type TP53 [14].

       AML and allogenic transplant: NGS also identifies mutations that predict the likelihood of benefit from allogeneic transplantation, providing critical prognostic insights.

       In a study by Middeke et al., involving 97 patients with AML who were treated with intensive chemotherapy and allogeneic hematopoietic stem cell transplantation (HSCT), a high-risk cytogenetic profile was defined by the presence of complex karyotype, monosomy of chromosome 7, monosomy and/or deletion of the long arm of chromosome 5, or abnormalities of chromosome 17p. The presence of a TP53 mutation at diagnosis was significantly associated with worse outcomes following transplantation. The three-year survival rate was 33% for patients without TP53 mutations compared to only 10% for those with TP53 mutations ($p = 0.002$) [15].

       These findings were corroborated in another study of 113 AML patients treated with intensive chemotherapy and allogeneic transplantation. In this cohort, Quek et al. performed genetic sequencing of 35 genes at diagnosis and relapse (49 patients relapsed) and identified pre-transplant mutations in WT1 ($p = 0.018$), DNMT3A ($p = 0.045$), FLT3 ITD ($p = 0.071$), and TP53 ($p = 0.06$) as predictors of relapse. These results underscore the utility of pre-transplant genetic profiling in predicting outcomes after HSCT [15–17].

   (b) *MDS and CMML*: NGS informs the use of hypo-methylating agents in high-risk patients.

   (c) *MPNs*: Detection of JAK2 mutations guides the use of JAK inhibitors (e.g., ruxolitinib).

4. *Minimal Residual Disease (MRD) Monitoring*

   Serial NGS enables highly sensitive detection of residual disease post-treatment, providing insights into relapse risk and therapy efficacy [13]. NGS-based MRD monitoring has shown high concordance with real-time quantitative PCR (RQ-PCR), emerging as an alternative tool in MRD-based protocols, particularly for pediatric acute lymphoblastic leukemia (ALL). In myeloid malignancies, the focus of NGS-based MRD assays is on tumor-associated somatic mutations. Multiple studies have demonstrated the clinical relevance of NGS-based MRD monitoring in AML patients. The revised ELN guidelines recommend error-corrected NGS with unique molecular identifiers as an MRD technique, achieving a detection limit of 10^{-3} or lower. This guideline also includes a foundational gene panel for AML, which encompasses CALR, CEBPA, DDX41, ETV6, EZH2, FLT3, IDH1, IDH2, JAK2, KIT, KRAS, MPL, NPM1, NRAS, PTPN11, RAD21, RUNX1, SF3B1, SRSF2, STAG2, TP53, U2AF1, and WT1. However, germline mutations and mutations associated with age-related CH (so-called DTA) should be excluded from MRD analysis [3].

5. *Clonal Evolution and Resistance*

   NGS reveals clonal dynamics and resistance mechanisms, such as the emergence of secondary mutations (e.g., FLT3 kinase domain mutations in AML treated with FLT3 inhibitors).

6. *Uncovering Germline Predispositions*

   - NGS can identify germline mutations associated with familial AML syndromes.
   - Recognizing these predispositions is crucial for patient management and family counselling.

13.3 NGS in Lymphoid Neoplasms

NGS has become a pivotal tool in the diagnosis, classification, risk stratification, and management of lymphoid neoplasms, including lymphomas, chronic lymphocytic leukemia (CLL), and plasma cell neoplasms like multiple myeloma.

13.3.1 Diagnosis and Subtyping

NGS enhances the accuracy of diagnosing lymphoid neoplasms by identifying genetic mutations, translocations, and clonal rearrangements. Key genetic alterations are given in Table 13.3.

- *B-ALL*: WHO[2022] [18] introduced *PAX5* mutations as one of the components of a new subtype, "B-acute lymphoblastic leukemia (ALL) with other defined genetic abnormalities" [3].
- *B-cell lymphomas*: Some genetic mutations are being used to support a diagnosis of certain lymphomas. Representative examples include *BRAF* mutations for hairy cell leukemia, *MYD88* or *CXCR4* mutations for lympho-plasmacytic lymphoma, *TCF3* or *ID3* mutations for EBV-negative Burkitt lymphoma ([3]) (Detection of translocations involving MYC, BCL2, and BCL6 in diffuse large B-cell lymphoma (DLBCL) or Burkitt's lymphoma (Table 13.3).

Table 13.3 Key genetic alterations in lymphoid neoplasms

Indication	Key genetic alterations
Diffuse large B-cell lymphoma	MYD88, EZH2, BCL2, BCL6, TP53, CD79A/B
Chronic lymphocytic leukemia	TP53, NOTCH1, SF3B1, ATM, unmutated IGHV
Burkitt lymphoma	MYC translocations (t(8;14), t(8;22), t(2;8)
Follicular lymphoma	BCL2 translocation (t(14;18)), EZH2
Hodgkin lymphoma	PD-L1/PD-L2 amplifications, STAT6 mutations
Multiple myeloma	KRAS, NRAS, TP53, BRAF, t(4;14), t(14;16)
T-cell lymphomas	STAT3, RHOA, DNMT3A, TET2, IDH2

- *T-cell lymphomas*: *STAT3* or *STAT5B* mutations for T-large granular lymphocytic leukaemia [3]. Identification of recurrent mutations in genes like STAT3, DNMT3A, and RHOA.
- *Hodgkin's lymphoma*: Genetic alterations in genes regulating immune evasion, such as PD-L1/PD-L2 amplifications.
- *CLL*: Mutations in TP53, NOTCH1, and SF3B1, along with immunoglobulin heavy chain variable region (IGHV) mutation status, aid in CLL classification. In chronic lymphocytic leukemia (CLL), the genomic landscape revealed by NGS highlights recurrent aberrations, including mutations in ATM, NOTCH1, SF3B1, and TP53, which are observed in more than 10% of cases. Other mutations, affecting less than 1–5% of cases, are linked to signaling pathways like B cell receptor/NF-kB signaling (BIRC3, NFKBIE), NOTCH signaling (NOTCH1, FBXW7), DNA repair (ATM, TP53), and RNA/ribosome processing (RPS15, SF3B1, XPO1). Among these, SF3B1 is notably frequent, occurring in 5–15% of early-stage patients and increasing to 16–28% in relapsed or refractory cases [19].
- *Multiple Myeloma (MM)*: NGS has improved our understanding of MM, but it still needs to be validated in clinical trials and transferred to routine clinical labs. As per current studies, genes which are recurrently mutated,possibly driver mutations in plasma cell myeloma (PCM) include *KRAS, NRAS, IRF4, MAX, HIST1H1E, RB1, EGR1, TP53, TRAF3, FAM46C, DIS3, BRAF, LTB, CYLD,* and *FGFR3* [20, 21]. To accomplish a complete molecular diagnosis in a single essay, a capture-based NGS approach to reliably identify pathogenic mutations (SNVs and indels), genomic alterations (CNVs and chromosomic translocations), and *IGH* rearrangements is being explored [22].

1. *Prognostic Stratification by NGS*

   NGS-derived mutational profiles allow risk stratification in lymphoid neoplasms:

   - *DLBCL*: Genetic subtypes such as MYD88-mutated or EZH2-mutated tumors have distinct prognostic implications.
   - *CLL*: TP53 mutations and unmutated IGHV are associated with poor prognosis, while SF3B1 mutations predict resistance to standard therapies. The current recommendation for TP53 mutation reporting includes pathogenic variants with a variant allele frequency (VAF) above 10%, which corresponds

to the sensitivity of Sanger sequencing. Variants with a VAF between 5% and 10% may be reported with a disclaimer regarding their unclear clinical significance. Additionally, assessing the IGHV gene somatic hypermutation (SHM) status remains important in CLL
- *Mantle cell lymphoma*: SOX11 expression and TP53 mutations are linked to aggressive disease.

2. *Therapeutic Targeting*

   - *Targeted Therapies*: NGS identifies actionable mutations, such as BTK mutations for BTK inhibitors (e.g., ibrutinib) or BCL2 rearrangements for BCL2 inhibitors (e.g., venetoclax).
   - *Immune Checkpoint Inhibitors*: Identification of PD-L1 amplifications guides the use of checkpoint inhibitors in Hodgkin lymphoma and other lymphomas.
   - *CAR-T Cell Therapy*: NGS supports target identification and clonal monitoring post-CAR-T therapy.

3. *Minimal Residual Disease (MRD) Monitoring*

   NGS enables highly sensitive detection of MRD by identifying unique clonal sequences in immunoglobulin or T-cell receptor genes, providing insights into relapse risk and therapy efficacy. It can detect one malignant cell among 1,000,000 normal cells (10^-6). It detects unique clonotypes (IgH, IgK, or TCR gene rearrangements) to track malignant cells over time and simultaneously identifies mutations in multiple genes (e.g., TP53, NOTCH1, SF3B1) in chronic lymphocytic leukemia (CLL) or diffuse large B-cell lymphoma (DLBCL). Its applications in the following lymphoid diseases are

   - *Acute lymphoblastic leukemia (ALL)*: NGS is used for IgH/TCR-based MRD detection with high precision.
   - *Chronic lymphocytic leukemia (CLL)*: Tracks MRD using somatic mutations (e.g., IGHV mutational status).
   - *Multiple myeloma*: Detects clonal rearrangements of Ig genes and mutations in key oncogenes.
   - *Diffuse large B-cell lymphoma (DLBCL)*: Identifies circulating tumor DNA (ctDNA) to monitor disease dynamics.

4. *Clonal Evolution and Resistance Mechanisms*

   - The NGS technique is used to quantify the clonality of IGH and TCR gene rearrangements in lymphoid cancers like PCM or ALL
   - *Monitoring Therapy Resistance*: NGS tracks clonal evolution during treatment, such as secondary mutations in BTK in CLL patients on BTK inhibitors.
   - *Epigenetic Changes*: Identification of mutations in chromatin modifiers like EZH2 or CREBBP that influence treatment response.

13.4 Advantages and Challenges of Next-Generation Sequencing (NGS) in Hematologic Neoplasms

13.4.1 Advantages of NGS

1. *Comprehensive Genomic Profiling*: NGS provides a broad genomic landscape by simultaneously detecting mutations, translocations, copy number variations, and clonal rearrangements. This allows for a more complete understanding of hematologic malignancies.
2. *Personalized Therapy Guidance*: NGS identifies actionable mutations, enabling targeted therapies tailored to individual genetic profiles. For example, FLT3 and IDH inhibitors can be selected based on specific mutations detected in AML.
3. *Clonal Evolution and Resistance Tracking*: Longitudinal NGS monitoring helps track clonal evolution, detect resistance mutations, and monitor MRD, providing insights into disease progression and relapse risk.
4. *Integration into Risk Stratification Systems*: NGS improves prognostic accuracy by integrating molecular data into established risk stratification models, such as:
   - ELN guidelines for AML
   - IPSS-R and IPSS-M for MDS
   - WHO classification for lymphoid neoplasms
5. *Detection of Low-Allele Frequency Mutations*: NGS can detect subclonal populations and mutations at low allele frequencies, crucial for identifying early disease progression and treatment resistance.

13.4.2 Challenges of NGS

1. *Driver* vs. *Passenger Mutations*: Distinguishing driver mutations from passenger mutations or variants of unknown significance (VUS) remains a significant challenge. Misclassification can lead to erroneous clinical decisions.
2. *Limited Functional Data on Novel Mutations*: The functional implications of rare or novel mutations are often unclear, limiting their immediate clinical utility.
3. *High Cost and Infrastructure Requirements*: NGS requires substantial infrastructure and specialized bioinformatics support, making routine clinical implementation difficult in resource-limited settings.
4. *Dynamic Clonal Evolution*: Myeloid neoplasms are inherently heterogeneous and evolve over time. NGS provides only a snapshot of clonal populations at a given point, potentially missing the full complexity of clonal dynamics.
5. *Incidental Germline Findings*: NGS may reveal germline mutations associated with hereditary cancer syndromes, necessitating genetic counselling and raising ethical concerns about disclosure and management.

13.5 NGS in Benign Hematologic Disorders

NGS has significantly advanced the understanding and management of benign hematologic disorders. These include a broad spectrum of inherited and acquired conditions affecting red blood cells, white blood cells, platelets, and the coagulation system. NGS offers a powerful approach to uncover the molecular basis of these disorders, facilitating accurate diagnosis, personalized treatment, and improved patient care.

A. *Diagnosis of Benign Hematologic Disorders*

1. *Inherited Anemias*

   NGS is particularly valuable in diagnosing hereditary red blood cell disorders:

   - *Hemoglobinopathies*: NGS detects mutations in the HBB, HBA1, and HBA2 genes associated with sickle cell anemia, beta-thalassemia, and alpha-thalassemia.
   - *Congenital Dyserythropoietic Anemia (CDA)*: NGS identifies mutations in CDAN1, SEC23B, and other genes.
   - *Hereditary Spherocytosis*: Detects mutations in genes encoding membrane proteins (ANK1, SPTB, SPTA1, EPB42).
   - *Pyruvate Kinase Deficiency*: Mutations in the PKLR gene can be pinpointed using NGS (Table 13.4).

2. *Inherited Bone Marrow Failure Syndromes (IBMFS)*

   - *Fanconi Anemia (FA)*: NGS panels identify mutations in FANCA, FANCC, FANCG, and related genes.
   - *Dyskeratosis Congenita (DC)*: Mutations in telomere-related genes like DKC1, TERT, and TERC are detected by NGS.

Table 13.4 Mutations in benign hematology conditions

Condition	Gene mutations	Remarks
Hereditary hemochromatosis	HFE (C282Y, H63D, S65C), TFR2, HJV, HAMP	HFE C282Y homozygosity most common
Congenital erythrocytosis	EPOR, EGLN1, VHL, HIF2A	VHL-related mutations associated with Chuvash polycythemia
Hereditary spherocytosis	ANK1, SPTA1, SPTB, SLC4A1, EPB42	Most mutations are autosomal dominant
G6PD deficiency	G6PD	X-linked; associated with hemolysis
Congenital neutropenia	ELANE, GFI1, HAX1, CSF3R, WAS, VPS45	ELANE is most frequently mutated
Thrombophilia	F5 (Factor V Leiden), F2 (Prothrombin G20210A)	Increased risk of venous thromboembolism
Hereditary thrombocytopenia	RUNX1, ANKRD26, ETV6, MPL, THPO	Autosomal dominant mutations common

- *Diamond-Blackfan Anemia (DBA)*: Mutations in RPS19, RPL11, and other ribosomal protein genes are identified.

3. *Inherited Platelet Disorders*

   NGS can elucidate genetic causes of thrombocytopenia and platelet dysfunction:

   - *Bernard-Soulier Syndrome*: GP1BA, GP1BB, GP9 mutations.
   - *Glanzmann Thrombasthenia*: ITGA2B and ITGB3 mutations.
   - *MYH9-Related Disorders*: Mutations in MYH9 affecting platelet morphology and function.

4. *Inherited Coagulation Disorders*

   NGS enhances the diagnosis of genetic bleeding disorders by identifying causative mutations:

   - *Hemophilia A and B*: F8 and F9 mutations, respectively.
   - *Von Willebrand's Disease*: Mutations in VWF gene.
   - *Rare Disorders*: Fibrinogen or factor deficiencies (e.g., FGA, FGB, FGG).

5. *Primary Immunodeficiencies (PIDs)*

   - NGS is pivotal in diagnosing PIDs, such as severe combined immunodeficiency (SCID), chronic granulomatous disease (CGD), and others caused by mutations in genes like IL2RG, CYBB, or RAG1/RAG2.

6. *Congenital Neutropenia*

   NGS identifies genetic mutations in ELANE, G6PC3, HAX1, and other genes responsible for severe congenital neutropenia (Table 13.4).
7. *Aplastic Anemia and Paroxysmal Nocturnal Hemoglobinuria (PNH)*

   - While acquired, some cases have genetic predispositions that can be uncovered using NGS.
   - PNH can also involve mutations in PIGA detected through NGS techniques.

8. *Erythrocytosis and Polycythemia*

   - NGS identifies mutations in EPOR, VHL, EGLN1, and HIF2A in cases of hereditary erythrocytosis.

9. *Thrombophilia*

   - NGS facilitates screening for inherited thrombophilic conditions caused by mutations in F5 (Factor V Leiden), F2 (Prothrombin), or deficiencies in antithrombin (SERPINC1), protein C (PROC), and protein S (PROS1) (Table 13.4)

B. *Advantages of NGS in Benign Hematologic Disorders*

- NGS allows for simultaneous analysis of multiple genes, improving diagnostic yield in disorders with overlapping clinical features. This enables early

intervention, particularly in inherited conditions, preventing complications and improving outcomes.
- It identifies mutations that can guide targeted therapies or gene-editing approaches, such as CRISPR-based strategies for haemoglobinopathies.
- Its results facilitate genetic counselling and cascade testing of family members for heritable disorders.
- It also uncovers novel mutations and pathways involved in benign hematologic disorders, expanding the understanding of disease mechanisms.

13.6 Future Directions

13.6.1 Myeloid and Lymphoid Malignancies

- Use of single-cell sequencing, which enables the study of clonal heterogeneity and microenvironment interactions at a single-cell resolution is being explored. NGS is effective in analyzing complex single-gene disorders, such as lymphoid clonality through IGH or TRG/TRB gene rearrangements [23].
- Use of Liquid Biopsies using cell-free DNA (cf DNA) or circulating tumor DNA (ct DNA) for non-invasive disease monitoring is also being explored.
- NGS can help create a holistic understanding of lymphoid/myeloid neoplasm by combining genomic, transcriptomic, and proteomic data.
- It can leverage advanced algorithms by AI for variant interpretation and risk prediction.
- It can also help optimize CART cells by refining CAR-T cell targets and predict patient responses.

13.6.2 Benign Hematology

- NGS-guided therapies like CRISPR-Cas9 are being developed for conditions such as sickle cell disease and beta-thalassemia.
- Efforts are going on for the development of comprehensive panels to cover a wide range of hematologic conditions for improving diagnostic precision.
- Use of cf. DNA and RNA for non-invasive monitoring of disease progression and treatment response is also being studied.

13.7 Conclusion

NGS has revolutionized the approach to benign and malignant hematologic disorders, offering deep insights into their molecular and genetic underpinnings. It facilitates early diagnosis, personalized therapy, and family screening, significantly enhancing patient care. Continued advancements in technology and integration with therapeutic innovations promise to further elevate its role in managing these conditions.

Case Report

A 23-year-old female, known to have beta-thalassemia trait, presented with anemia and thrombocytopenia. Clinical suspicion of MDS prompted further evaluation. Peripheral blood smear revealed ~5% blasts and mild dyspoiesis in the granulocytic lineage (Figs. 13.1 and 13.2) Bone marrow aspirate showed a cellular marrow with

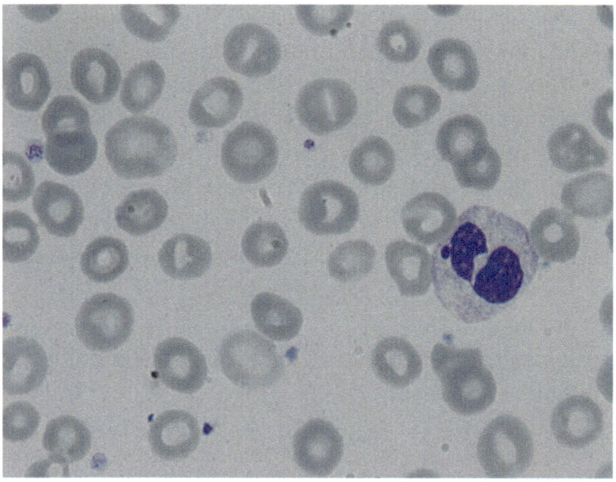

Fig. 13.1 Photomicrograph (Leishman and Giemsa; 100X) of peripheral smear showing pseudo Pelger Huet anomaly

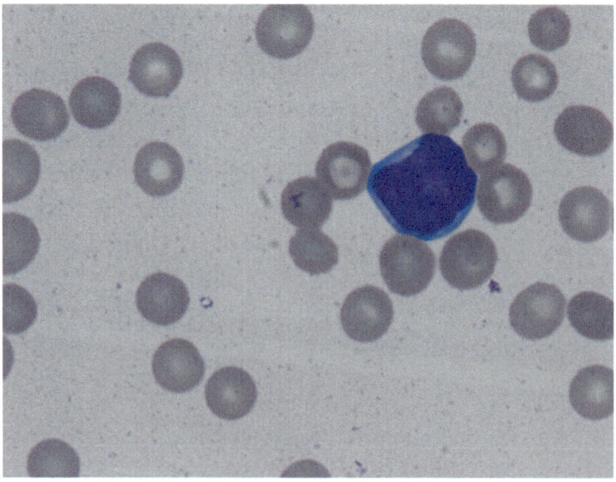

Fig. 13.2 Photomicrograph (Leishman and Giemsa; 100X) of peripheral smear showing a blast

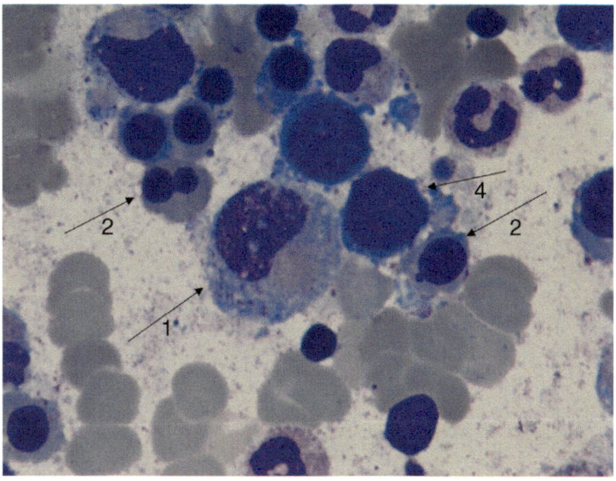

Fig. 13.3 Photomicrograph (Leishman and Giemsa; 100X) of Bone marrow aspirate showing nucleolated myelocyte (dysmyelopoiesis) (1) and dyserythropoiesis in the form of nuclear budding in erythroid cell (2, 3) and megaloblastoid erythroid cell (4)

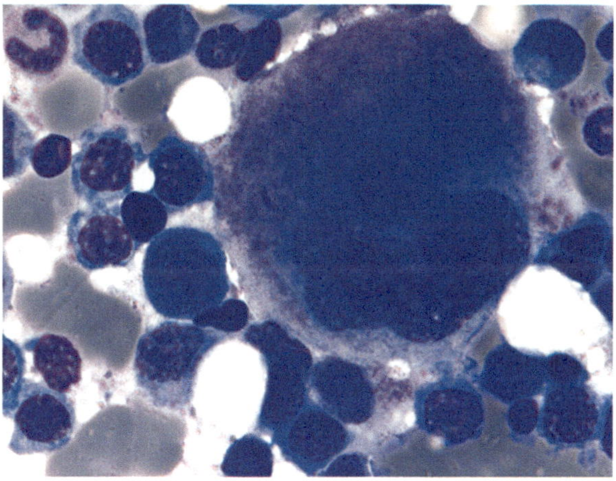

Fig. 13.4 Photomicrograph (Leishman and Giemsa; 100X) of Bone marrow aspirate showing dyspoietic megakaryocyte

trilineage dysplasia (Figs. 13.3 and 13.4) and ~12% blasts, supporting a diagnosis of MDS with Increased Blasts-2 (MDS-IB-2). Bone marrow flow cytometry confirmed ~9% myeloid blasts and significant dyspoiesis in the myeloid lineage. Cytogenetic analysis revealed a karyotype of 47,XX,+8[4]/46,XX[16], indicating trisomy 8 (Fig. 13.5), which is a marker of myeloid disease and is associated with an intermediate prognosis according to the Revised International Prognostic Scoring System (IPSS-R). Molecular testing by next-generation sequencing (NGS) was performed on Ion Gene Studio S5 System from Thermo Fisher Scientific, using Ion Torrent Oncomine Myeloid panel. This gene panel includes 40 key DNA target genes and 29 RNA driver genes (for fusion detection) to cover major myeloid neoplasms. NGS detected presence of mutations in TET2, EZH2, ASXL1, and RUNX1 (Fig. 13.6). These mutations, particularly RUNX1 and ASXL1, are associated with poor prognosis and increased risk of transformation to acute myeloid leukemia (AML). The diagnosis of MDS-IB-2 with high-risk features was established.

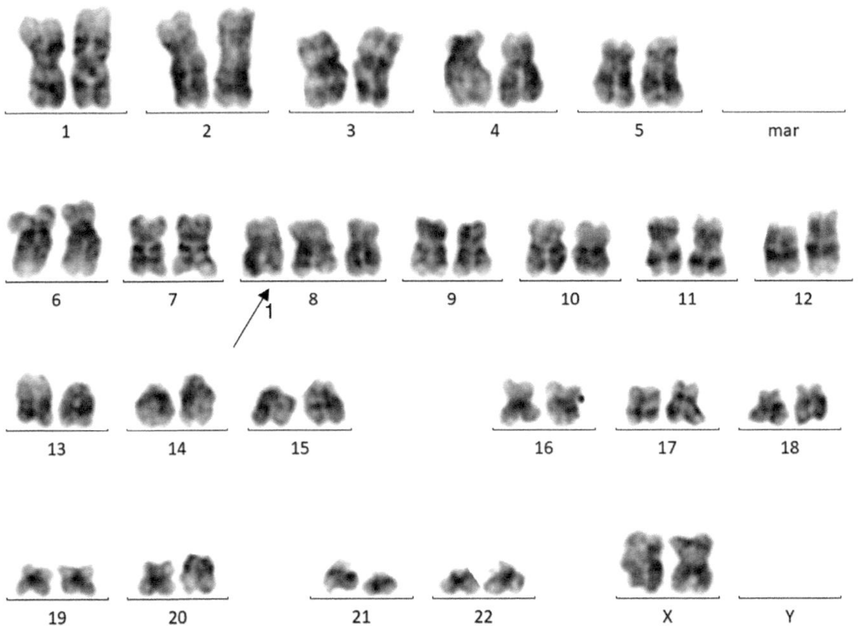

Fig. 13.5 Karyogram showing trisomy 8

Type of Specimen : Bone marrow
Quality of Specimen : Satisfactory
QC Passed : Yes
Equipment and software : Ion PGM System / Ion Reporter
Results

1.Clinically Relevant Mutations Identified.

Genomic Alteration	Function of Gene in Cancer
TET2	Tumor suppressor gene
TET2	Tumor suppressor gene
EZH2	Tumor suppressor and oncogene
ASXL1	Transcriptional activator or corepressor of retinoic acid receptor (RAR) activity
RUNX1	Encodes the alpha subunit of the core binding transcription factor and is involved in determining the lineage fate of HSCs

Variant Details :

Gene	Amino acid change / Exon	Coding	Variant ID	Location	Locus	% Variant Frequency	Transcript	Variant Effect
TET2	p.Arg1452Ter/ 10	c.4354C>T	COSM41706	TET2:exonix:NM_001127208.2, TET2:exonic: NR_126420.1	chr4:106193892	49.21	NM_001127208.2, NR_126420.1	nonsense
TET2	p.Arg1516Ter/ 11	c.4546C>T	COSM43420	TET2:exonix:NM_001127208.2, TET2:exonic: NR_126420.1	chr4:106196213	49.33	NM_001127208.2, NR_126420.1	nonsense
EZH2	p.Arg690His/ 18	c.2069G>A	COSM52980	EZH2:exonic:NM_004456.4	chr7:148506443	44.61	NM_004456.4	missense
ASXL1	p.Arg693Ter/ 12	c.2077C>T	COSM51388	ASXL1:exonic:NM_015338.5	chr20:31022592	54.14	NM_015338.5	nonsense
RUNX1	p.Arg107Cys/	c.319C>T	COSM24736	RUNX1:exonic:NM_001754.4	chr21:36259172	27.59	NM_001754.4	missense

Mean Coverage : 1. TET2: 1782; 2. TET2: 1125; EZH2: 1912; ASXL1: 133; RUNX1: 29
2.Clinically Relevant Gene Fusions : None

Fig. 13.6 NGS report of the patient showing details of clinically relevant mutations found in this patient

The patient and the family were counselled for intensive therapy and hematopoietic stem cell transplantation (HSCT). However, the patient did not take any treatment and was lost to follow-up. Two months later, the patient again presented to OPD with worsening of symptoms, epistaxis and anemia. She was evaluated again with bone marrow aspiration, which showed cellular marrow with significant trilineage dyspoiesis and ~ 24% blasts, consistent with progression to AML. The patient was started on 3 + 7 (Doxorubicin + Cytarabine) therapy, and the Day +14 marrow showed hypocellular marrow with ~2% blasts. The patient is currently on follow-up and the family has been counselled for HSCT post remission.

To conclude, this report provides a comprehensive diagnostic picture of a 23-year-old female suspected to have MDS, diagnosed conclusively as MDS IB2 by bone marrow, cytogenetics, and NGS evaluation. NGS further predicted its prognosis as poor and helped in counselling the patient and treatment decisions.

References

1. Khoury JD, Solary E, Abla O, Akkari Y, Alaggio R, Apperley JF, et al. The 5th edition of the World Health Organization classification of haematolymphoid tumours: myeloid and histiocytic/dendritic neoplasms. Leukemia. 2022;36:1703–19.
2. Arber DA, Orazi A, Hasserjian R, et al. WHO classification of tumours of haematopoietic and lymphoid tissues. 5th ed. Lyon: IARC Press; 2022.
3. Döhner H, Estey E, Grimwade D, et al. Diagnosis and management of AML in adults: 2022 recommendations from an international expert panel. Blood. 2022;139(9):1071–105.
4. Cho YU. The role of next-generation sequencing in hematologic malignancies. Blood Res. 2024;59:11. https://doi.org/10.1007/s44313-024-00010-0.
5. Jaiswal S, Ebert BL. Clonal hematopoiesis in human aging and disease. Science. 2017;355(6332):1316–21.
6. Steensma DP, Bejar R, Jaiswal S, et al. Clonal hematopoiesis of indeterminate potential and its distinction from myelodysplastic syndromes. Blood. 2015;126(1):9–16.
7. Duployez N, Willekens C, Marceau-Renaut A, et al. Prognosis and comprehensive mutational landscape in core-binding factor acute myeloid leukemia. Blood Adv. 2016;128(24):2642–53.
8. Grimwade D, Ivey A, Huntly BJP. Molecular landscape of acute myeloid leukemia. N Engl J Med. 2016;375(2):2005–22.
9. Bülbül H, Kaya ÖÖ, Karadağ FK, Olgun A, Demirci Z, Ceylan C. Prognostic impact of next-generation sequencing on myelodysplastic syndrome: a single-center experience. Medicine (Baltimore). 2024;103(41):e39909. https://doi.org/10.1097/MD.0000000000039909.
10. Papaemmanuil E, Gerstung M, Malcovati L, et al. Clinical and biological implications of driver mutations in myelodysplastic syndromes. Blood. 2013;122(22):3616–27.
11. Vannucchi AM, Lasho TL, Guglielmelli P, et al. Mutations and prognosis in primary myelofibrosis. Leukemia. 2013;27(9):1861.
12. Palomo L, Acha P, Solé F. Genetic aspects of myelodysplastic/myeloproliferative neoplasms. Cancers (Basel). 2021;13(9):2120. https://doi.org/10.3390/cancers13092120.
13. Bernard E, et al. Molecular international prognostic scoring system for myelodysplastic syndromes. NEJM Evid. 2022;1(7):EVIDoa2200008. https://doi.org/10.1056/EVIDoa2200008.
14. Leisch M, Jansko B, Zaborsky N, Greil R, Pleyer L. Next generation sequencing in AML—on the way to becoming a new standard for treatment initiation and/or modulation? Cancers (Basel). 2019;11:252.

15. Welch JS, Petti AA, Miller CA, Fronick CC, O'Laughlin M, Fulton RS, Wilson RK, Baty JD, Duncavage EJ, Tandon B, et al. TP53 and Decitabine in acute myeloid leukemia. Br J Haematol. 2016;172:914–22.
16. Middeke JM, Herold S, Rücker-Braun E, Berdel WE, Stelljes M, Kaufmann M, Schäfer-Eckart K, Baldus CD, Stuhlmann R, Ho AD, et al. TP53 mutation in patients with high-risk acute myeloid leukaemia treated with allogeneic haematopoietic stem cell transplantation. Br J Haematol. 2016;172:914–22.
17. Quek L, Ferguson P, Metzner M, Ahmed I, Kennedy A, Garnett C, Jeffries S, Walter C, Piechocki K, Timbs A, et al. Mutational analysis of disease relapse in patients allografted for acute myeloid leukemia. Blood Adv. 2016;1(3):193–204.
18. Alaggio R, Amador C, Anagnostopoulos I, Attygalle AD, de Oliveira Araujo IB, Berti E, et al. The 5th edition of the World Health Organization classification of haematolymphoid tumours: lymphoid neoplasms. Leukemia. 2022;36:1720–48.
19. Mollstedt J, Mansouri L, Rosenquist R. Precision diagnostics in chronic lymphocytic leukemia: past, present, and future. Front Oncol. 2023;13:1146486. https://doi.org/10.3389/fonc.2023.1146486.
20. Walker BA, Boyle EM, Wardell CP, et al. Mutational spectrum, copy number changes, and outcome: results of a sequencing study of patients with newly diagnosed myeloma. J Clin Oncol. 2015;33:3911–20.
21. Manier S, Salem KZ, Park J, Landau DA, Getz G, Ghobrial IM. Genomic complexity of multiple myeloma and its clinical implications. Nat Rev Clin Oncol. 2017;14:100–13.
22. Rosa-Rosa JM, Cuenca I, Medina A, Vázquez I, Sánchez-delaCruz A, Buenache N, et al. NGS-based molecular karyotyping of multiple myeloma: results from the GEM12 clinical trial. Cancers (Basel). 2022;14(20):5169. https://doi.org/10.3390/cancers14205169.
23. Kwon R, Yeung CCS. Advances in next-generation sequencing and emerging technologies for hematologic malignancies. Haematologica. 2024;109:379–87.

Chapter 14
Cytogenetics and FISH in Hematologic Malignancies

D. S. Udayakumar, Bhawna Jha, Akshay Gore, and Renu Saxena

Abstract Cytogenetics has been there for ages. In 1842, Swiss botanist Karl Nägeli first discovered chromosomes in pollen. From 1960, when the first genetic abnormality, the Philadelphia chromosome, was identified in chronic myeloid leukemia (CML) by Dr. Peter Nowell and Dr. David Hungerford, to the development of FISH in the 1980s, and to the present day, where the classification of tumors incorporates genetic abnormalities as a key component, cytogenetics has stood the test of time. Despite NGS creating the maximum buzz in the world of hematology and solid organ malignancies, this chapter will reiterate, with evidence, that cytogenetics is an essential part of diagnosis, prognostication, and disease follow-up in hematological malignancies.

Keywords Karyotyping · Cytogenetics · FISH · Fluorescent in situ hybridization

Learning Objectives
- What is cytogenetics?
- A brief overview of nomenclature used in cytogenetics.
- How cytogenetics in hematology gave us the significance of genetic abnormalities in malignancies?
- Role of cytogenetics in hematological malignancies (acute leukemia, myeloproliferative neoplasm (MPN), lymphomas, myeloma, and myelodysplastic neoplasms (MDS)).

D. S. Udayakumar (✉)
Department of Hematopathology, Yashoda Hospitals, Hitech City, Hyderabad, India

B. Jha · A. Gore · R. Saxena
Department of Hematopathology, Medanta,The Medicity, Gurugram, Haryana, India

H. P. Pati et al. (eds.), *Clinical Hematology and Hemato-Oncology*,
https://doi.org/10.1007/978-981-92-1167-8_14

14.1 Introduction

Cytogenetics is the study of chromosomes. It is broadly divided into two groups:

1. Conventional cytogenetics: Karyotyping.
2. Molecular cytogenetics: Fluorescent in situ hybridization (FISH), Comparative genomic hybridization (CGH), spectral karyotyping (SKY), whole chromosome painting (WCP).

In a clinical cytogenetics laboratory, karyotyping and FISH are the most commonly used techniques, and they complement each other. Karyotyping and FISH have become central tools in the diagnosis, management, and follow-up of patients with hematological malignancies.

Conventional banding cytogenetics, especially the G-banded karyotype, is crucial in detecting recurrent chromosomal rearrangements of diagnostic significance, prognostic risk stratification, and targeted therapy. G-banding in protease-treated chromosomes results from interactions of both DNA and protein with the thiazine and eosin components of the Giemsa dye.

In a normal human karyotype, 46 chromosomes are arranged in decreasing order of size as 23 matching or homologous pairs in a karyogram, with 22 pairs of autosomes and the sex chromosomes (XX for female, XY for male). An International System for Human Cytogenomic Nomenclature (ISCN 2024) describes a standardized numbering pattern for chromosome identification based on the banding pattern [1].

FISH is a molecular cytogenetic technique that uses fluorescent probes that bind to complementary parts of the chromosome. Most commonly, interphase FISH (iFISH) is performed in hematological malignancies, where the signals of FISH probes are observed on the interphase nuclei of cells. A metaphase FISH (mFISH) is performed in special situations to delineate the chromosomes involved. In mFISH, the individual chromosomes stand out and can be used to locate the abnormality on a particular chromosome.

Two main types of probes are used in FISH to detect chromosomal rearrangements in hematological malignancies: fusion probes and break-apart probes.

Fusion probes detect signals from two genes that are normally separated. In a normal cell, the two probes will hybridize to two separate locations, resulting in two distinct signals. However, in cells with a translocation, the two probes will hybridize to the same location, resulting in a single, fused signal.

Break-apart probes, on the other hand, detect signals from two regions of a single gene that are normally fused. In a normal cell, the two probes will hybridize to two separate locations on the same chromosome, resulting in two distinct signals. However, in cells with a translocation, the two probes will hybridize to two separate locations on different chromosomes, resulting in two distinct signals.

Whole blood, bone marrow aspirate, splenic cells, lymph nodes, and touch preparation from bone marrow or other tissue biopsies are the samples used for FISH and karyotyping. Heparin is the anticoagulant of choice for blood and bone marrow; however, FISH can also be performed with good results from EDTA vacutainers and on unstained bone marrow touch or aspirate smears.

The International System for Human Cytogenomic Nomenclature (ISCN) has standardized and continuously updated symbols and formats for describing numerical and structural chromosomal abnormalities. Common examples include the symbols +, −, t, del, dup, and der, which refer to the gain of a chromosome, loss of a chromosome, translocation, deletion, duplication, and derivative chromosome, respectively [1].

In 1914, Theodor Boveri, in his article "Concerning the Origin of Malignant Tumours (Zur Frage der Entstehung maligner Tumoren)," stated the famous Boveri's hypothesis that chromosome abnormalities are the cellular changes causing the transition from normal to malignant proliferation. In hematology, we more frequently discuss clonal cytogenetic abnormalities; hence, it is important to understand the definition of a clone. According to the ISCN 2020, a clone must have at least two cells with the same chromosomal abnormality in the case of chromosome gain or structural rearrangement. The chromosomal abnormality must be present in at least three cells for chromosome loss. However, two cells with the loss of a chromosome and the same chromosome gain or structural aberration can be clonal. In karyotyping, a minimum of 20 metaphases and in FISH, a minimum of 200 cells must be examined to detect clonal abnormalities.

Only through cytogenetics, the first genetic abnormality associated with cancer, the Philadelphia chromosome, was discovered in 1960 by Dr. Peter Nowell and Dr. David Hungerford in seven patients with chronic myeloid leukemia (CML). In 1973, Dr. Janet Rowley used quinacrine fluorescence and G-banding to document the first recurrent balanced rearrangements in acute myeloid leukemia (AML) patients, a reciprocal translocation between chromosomes 8 and 21, that is, t(8;21)(q22;q22). Dr. Janet Rowley also discovered that the Philadelphia chromosome formed from a specific DNA translocation between chromosomes 9 and 22. The advent of molecular genetic testing in the past few decades has broadened our knowledge and understanding of the mechanisms that are operative in the initiation and progression of malignancies.

In hematological malignancies, karyotyping and FISH have proven roles in diagnosis, prognostication, and disease follow-up.

14.2 Role in Hematological Malignancies

14.2.1 Acute Myeloid Leukemia

Karyotyping and FISH are routinely used to diagnose recurrent genetic abnormalities in AML (Table 14.1) and to risk-stratify patients based on the European LeukemiaNet (ELN) genetic risk classification (Table 14.2). The

Table 14.1 Cytogenetic abnormalities in acute leukemias [3]

Disease group	Specific abnormalities
Acute myeloid leukemia with defining genetic abnormalities	Acute promyelocytic leukaemia with t(15;17)(q24.1;q21.2)/PML::RARA AML with t(8;21)(q22;q22.1)/RUNX1::RUNX1T1 AML with inv.(16)(p13.1q22) or t(16;16)(p13.1;q22)/CBFB::MYH11 AML with t(6;9)(p22.3;q34.1)/DEK::NUP214 AML with RBM15::MRTFA AML with t(9;22)(q34.1;q11.2)/BCR::ABL1 AML with KMT2A rearrangement AML with MECOM rearrangement AML with NUP98 rearrangement
Acute myeloid leukemia, myelodysplasia-related defining cytogenetic abnormalities	Complex karyotype (≥3 abnormalities) 5q deletion or loss of 5q due to unbalanced translocation Monosomy 7, 7q deletion, or loss of 7q due to unbalanced translocation 11q deletion 12p deletion or loss of 12p due to unbalanced translocation Monosomy 13 or 13q deletion 17p deletion or loss of 17p due to unbalanced translocation Isochromosome 17q Idic(X)(q13)
Acute myeloid leukemia with other defined genetic alterations	AML with t(1;3)(p36.3;q21.3)/PRDM16::RPN1 AML with t(1;22)(p13.3;q13.1)/RBM15::MRTFA AML with t(3;5)(q25.3;q35.1)/ NPM1::MLF1 AML with t(5;11)(q35.2;p15.4)/NUP98::NSD1 AML with t(7;12)(q36.3;p13.2)/ETV6::MNX1 AML with t(8;16)(p11.2;p13.3)/KAT6A::CREBBP AML with t(10;11)(p12.3;q14.2)/PICALM::MLLT10 AML with t(16;21)(p11.2;q22.2)/FUS::ERG AML with t(16;21)(q24.3;q22.1)/RUNX1::CBFA2T3 AML with inv.(16)(p13.3q24.3)/CBFA2T3::GLIS2
B-cell acute lymphoblastic leukemia/lymphoma	B—ALL with hyperdiploidy B—ALL with hypodiploidy B—ALL with iAMP21 B—ALL with BCR::ABL rearrangement B—ALL with BCR::ABL like features B—ALL with KMT2A rearrangement B—ALL with ETV6:: RUNX1 rearrangement B—ALL with TCF3::PBX1 rearrangement B—ALL with IGH::IL3 rearrangement B—ALL with TCF3::HLF rearrangement
B-ALL with other defined genetic abnormalities	B—ALL with DUX4 rearrangement B—ALL with MEF2D rearrangement B—ALL with ZNF384 rearrangement B—ALL with NUTM1 rearrangement B—ALL with IG::MYC fusion B—ALL with PAX5
Acute leukemia of ambiguous lineage with defining genetic abnormalities	Mixed-phenotype acute leukemia with BCR::ABL1 fusion Mixed-phenotype acute leukemia with KMT2A rearrangement
Acute leukemia of ambiguous lineage with other defined genetic alterations	Mixed-phenotype acute leukemia with ZNF384 rearrangement Acute leukemia of ambiguous lineage with BCL11B rearrangement

Table 14.2 European Leukemia Net (ELN) risk stratification in AML [4, 5]

	ELN 2022 risk classification for patients treated with intensive chemotherapy	ELN 2024 risk classification for patients treated with less-intensive chemotherapy
Risk category	Genetic abnormality	Genetic abnormality
Favorable	t(8;21)(q22;q22.1)/RUNX1::RUNX1T1 inv.(16)(p13.1q22) or t(16;16)(p13.1;q22)/CBFB::MYH11 Mutated NPM1 without FLT3-ITD bZIP in- frame mutated CEBPA	Mutated NPM1 (FLT3- ITDwt, NRASwt, KRASwt, TP53wt) Mutated IDH2 (FLT3- ITDwt, NRASwt, KRASwt, TP53wt) Mutated IDH1[a] (TP53wt) Mutated DDX41b Other cytogenetic and/or molecular abnormalities (FLT3- ITDwt, NRASwt, KRASwt, TP53wt)
Intermediate	FLT3- ITD (irrespective of allelic ratio or NPM1 mutation) t(9;11)(p21.3;q23.3)/MLLT3::KMT2A Cytogenetic and/or molecular abnormalities not classified as favorable or adverse	Other cytogenetic and/or molecular abnormalities (FLT3- ITDpos and/or NRASmut, and/or KRASmut, TP53wt)
Adverse	t(6;9)(p23;q34.1)/DEK::NUP214 t(v;11q23.3)/KMT2A rearranged (excluding KMT2A- PTD) t(9;22)(q34.1;q11.2)/BCR::ABL1 t(8;16)(p11;p13)/KAT6A::CREBBP inv. (3)(q21.3q26.2) or t(3;3)(q21.3;q26.2)/GATA2, MECOM(EVI1) t(3q26.2;v)/MECOM(EVI1)- rearranged −5 or del(5q) −7 −17/abn(17p) Complex karyotype[b] Monosomal karyotype[c] Mutated ASXL1, BCOR, EZH2, RUNX1, SF3B1, SRSF2, STAG2, U2AF1, or ZRSR2 Mutated TP53 (variant allele frequency ≥ 10%)	Mutated TP53

[a]The favorable risk applies specifically to patients treated with azacitidine+ivosidenib, irrespective of the presence of activating signaling gene mutations

[b]Complex karyotype: ≥ three unrelated chromosome abnormalities in the absence of other class-defining recurring genetic abnormalities; excludes hyperdiploid karyotypes with three or more trisomies (or polysomies) without structural abnormalities

[c]Monosomal karyotype: presence of two or more distinct monosomies (excluding X or Y), or one single autosomal monosomy in combination with at least one structural chromosome abnormality (excluding core- binding factor AML)

genotype-phenotype correlations of most of these recurrent genetic abnormalities are well documented.

14.2.1.1 Diagnosis of AML

The World Health Organization (WHO) classification of hematolymphoid tumors, fifth edition, and the International Consensus Classification (ICC) have recently incorporated additional cytogenetic and molecular findings into AML. In addition, the WHO and ICC have modified the blast percentage cutoff for most AML categories. The WHO has eliminated the 20% blast requirement for all AML types by defining genetic aberrations, with exceptions that include AML with BCR::ABL1 fusion and AML with CEBPA mutation. ICC has reduced the blast cutoff assignment to 10% for nearly all AML types, except for AML with t(9;22)(34.1;q11.2)/BCR::ABL. These changes further emphasize the need for cytogenetic and molecular testing in AML at diagnosis.

One of the categories in AML, myelodysplasia-related AML (AML-MR), requires a 20% blast cutoff, together with specific cytogenetic and gene abnormalities associated with myelodysplastic syndrome (MDS), again reiterating the importance of clonal abnormalities over morphology alone.

FISH plays an important role in the rapid diagnosis of acute promyelocytic leukemia (APL) with PML::RARA. We routinely use a combination of a dual fusion probe and a RARA break-apart probe to detect variant retinoic acid receptor alpha (RARA) translocations. Several variant translocations are known in APL such as ZBTB16::RARA/t(11;17) (q23;q21), NPM1::RARA/ t(5;17)(q35;q21), STAT5B::RARA/der(17), FIP1L1::RARA/ t(4;17)(q12;q21), BCOR::RARA/ t(X;17)(p11;q21), NUMA1::RARA/t(11;17)(q13;q21), PRKAR11::RARA/ t (17;17)(q21;q24), del(17)(q21;q24), NAPB1::RARA/t(2;17)(q32;q21), GTF2I::RARA/t(7;17)(q11;q21), TBLR1::RARA/ t(3;17)(q26;q21), IRF2BP2::RARA/ t(1;17) (q42;q21) [2].

In the WHO classification of hematolymphoid tumors, fifth edition, several retinoic acid receptor gamma (RARG) translocations with acute promyelocytic leukemia-like features have also been included, such as CPSF6::RARG, t(12;12)(q13;q15); NUP98::RARG, t(11;12)(p15;q13); PML::RARG, t(12;15)(q13;q22) and HNRNPC::RARG. A hematopathologist needs to suggest testing for such fusions in cases with morphological and immunophenotypical features of APL, which are negative for RARA fusions, since these rare fusions show resistance to all-trans-retinoic acid (ATRA) based therapy [3].

One of the new genetic abnormalities added in the WHO, fifth edition, is AML with NUP98 fusion, which does not require a blast cut-off of 20%.

Case 1

A 46-year-old male presented with refractory AML after receiving 7 + 3 induction regimen and a high dose of cytarabine treatment. At that time, no previous investigations were available to us. At our hospital, conventional karyotyping was done,

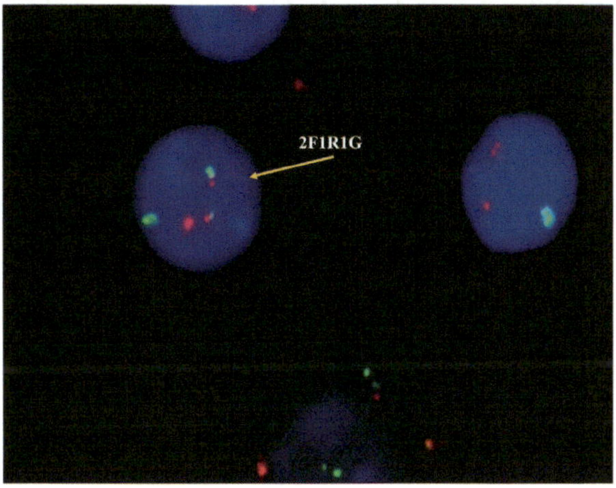

Fig. 14.1 FISH using t(5;11) NSD1/NUP98 Dual Fusion Probe (green-labelled probe for NSD1 gene region at 5q35.2–35.3 and red-labeled probe for NUP98 gene region at 11p15) showing 2Fusion 1Red 1Green (2F1R1G) aberrant signal pattern indicating that t(5;11) is present

which showed a normal male karyotype. Further, FISH testing was performed on interphase cells, which revealed NUP98::NSD1 fusion positivity, indicating that t(5;11) is present, which is a cryptic translocation and cannot be identified by karyotyping alone owing to the terminal location of the NUP98 gene on chromosome 11p15.4 (Fig. 14.1). The patient is treated with azacytidine and venetoclax chemotherapy and is doing well.

14.2.1.2 Risk Stratification of AML

According to ELN genetic classification, cytogenetic abnormalities in AML are also used to prognosticate patients. Originally, ELN genetic classification was developed based on data from younger adults receiving intensive chemotherapy and was not intended for prognostic stratification of older and/or unfit patients receiving less intensive therapeutic options. In general, AML associated with t(8;21), t(15;17) or inv.(16) predicts a favorable outcome. The presence of a complex karyotype, −5, del(5q), −7, or abnormalities of 3q defines a group with a relatively poor prognosis. The remaining group of patients, including those with 11q23 abnormalities, +8, +21, +22, del(9q), del(7q), or other miscellaneous structural or numerical defects not encompassed by the favorable or adverse risk groups, have an intermediate prognosis [4].

Recently, analyses from patients receiving less intensive therapies prompted an ELN genetic risk classification specifically for this patient population. This ELN classification stratifies prognostic outcome in patients receiving hypomethylating agent (HMA)–based regimens alone or in combination with either the B-cell leukemia/lymphoma 2 inhibitor venetoclax (VEN) or azacitidine (AZA) with the IDH1 inhibitor ivosidenib (IVO) for IDH1-mutated acute myeloid leukemia (AML) [5].

14.2.2 Acute Lymphoblastic Leukemia (ALL)

Specific genetic abnormalities are identified in most cases of B-lineage acute lymphoblastic leukemia (B-ALL), either by conventional karyotyping or FISH studies (Table 14.1). Conventional cytogenetics or FISH don't play a significant role in the diagnosis and risk stratification of T-lineage acute lymphoblastic leukemia (T-ALL).

14.2.2.1 Diagnosis and Risk Stratification of B-ALL

Each B-ALL genetic subgroup is important and can be a critical prognostic marker. The decision for early transplantation can be made if BCR::ABL/t(9;22)(q34;q11.2), KMT2A translocations, RUNX1 duplication /amplification (iAMP21) or a hypodiploid clone is identified. In contrast, if the ETV6::RUNX1/ t(12;21)(p13;q22) fusion is detected by FISH or hyperdiploidy is identified by karyotyping, the patient has a favorable prognosis and transplantation is rarely considered. It is important to note that the diagnosis of ETV6::RUNX1 fusion is always done through FISH (fluorescence in situ hybridization) or PCR (polymerase chain reaction) since it is a cryptic translocation and difficult to diagnose only based on conventional karyotyping.

Hypodiploidy is a poor prognostic finding in B-ALL. It is further characterized as near-haploidy (24–31 chromosomes), low hypodiploidy (32–39 chromosomes), and high hypodiploidy (40–43 chromosomes). In some cases, hypodiploid clones undergo endoreduplication, wherein trisomies and tetrasomies of some chromosomes mask the monosomies of several chromosomes and can change the modal number of the karyotype, and can be mischaracterized as hyperdiploidy. These "doubled" hypodiploid clones are termed pseudo-hyperdiploid. Why it is important is true hyperdiploidy is a favorable prognostic finding in B-ALL. In B-ALL, hyperdiploidy is specifically defined as having a chromosome count between 51 and 65 (or 67), and the most common chromosome gains are seen in X, 4, 6, 10, 14, 17, 18, and 21.

It is essential to carefully analyze metaphases with monosomies of some chromosomes and gains of some chromosomes in B-ALL, and care should be taken to delineate pseudo-hyperdiploid cases.

In addition, several new prognostically significant entities detectable by FISH, such as DUX4, MEF2D, ZNF384, NUTM1, and PAX5 rearrangements, have been included in WHO HAEM5 as B-ALL with other defined genetic abnormalities [3].

14.2.2.2 Philadelphia Chromosome (Ph)-like or BCR::ABL1-like ALL

In 2009, Mullighan and colleagues from the Children's Oncology Group (COG) and St. Jude Children's Research Hospital (SJCRH) and Den Boer and colleagues from the Netherlands, described a new subtype of ALL, termed Philadelphia chromosome (Ph)-like or BCR::ABL1–like ALL. This subtype had a gene expression profile highly similar to that of Ph + ALL and a high frequency of deletions of IKZF1, which encodes the lymphoid transcription factor IKAROS.

BCR::ABL1-like ALL is increasingly important due to the poor prognosis in pediatric, adolescent, and young adult ALL. Common features of this entity involve ABL-class fusions (involving ABL1, ABL2, CSF1R, and PDGFRB) that phenocopy BCR-ABL1 and alterations of CRLF2, JAK2, and EPOR that activate JAK/STAT signaling. Additional genomic alterations in Ph-like ALL activate other kinases, including BLNK, DGKH, FGFR1, IL2RB, LYN, NTRK3, PDGFRA, PTK2B, TYK2, and the RAS signaling pathway.

A combination of cytogenetic and FISH testing is currently recommended in all pediatric and adult patients with B-ALL/lymphoblastic lymphoma. A reflex panel of additional FISH testing using a panel of break apart probes for Philadelphia chromosome-like acute lymphoblastic leukemia (ALL) (1q25 rearrangement, ABL2; 5q32 rearrangement, PDGFRB; 9p24.1 rearrangement, JAK2; 9q34 rearrangement, ABL1; 7p-, IKZF1/CEP7; t(Xp22.33;var) or t(Yp11.32;var), CRLF2 rearrangement; t(Xp22.33;var) or t(Yp11.32;var), P2RY8 rearrangement) is recommended in all B-ALL patients without recurrent genetic abnormalities. We routinely test our B-ALL patients with normal karyotype or without recurrent genetic abnormalities with a FISH panel comprising probes for Ph-like ALL.

Most importantly, identifying these Ph-like ALL entities creates new opportunities for precision medicine therapies for this high-risk ALL subtype with ABL class fusions targeted by Imatinib and Dasatinib, JAK/STAT pathway lesions by various JAK inhibitors and RAS/MAPK signaling pathway by MEK inhibitors [6, 7].

Case 2

A 4-year-old male child diagnosed and treated elsewhere as B-ALL with a normal karyotype, presented to our hospital with relapse (15 months from diagnosis). Conventional cytogenetics and RT-PCR for BCR::ABL done in our hospital were found to be normal. Hence, FISH analysis for Ph-like B-ALL was performed, which showed JAK2 gene rearrangement and IKZF1 gene deletion in 90% of cells analyzed each, suggestive of BCR::ABL1-like B-ALL (Ph-like B-ALL) (Fig. 14.2a, b).

14.2.3 Myeloproliferative Neoplasms

14.2.3.1 Chronic Myeloid Leukemia

Bone marrow examination is mandatory in CML at diagnosis, as it can be used for baseline cytogenetic analysis. The Philadelphia chromosome is the shortened chromosome 22, resulting from a translocation between chromosomes 9 and 22. It is the hallmark of chronic myeloid leukemia (CML). It is usually present in 100% of

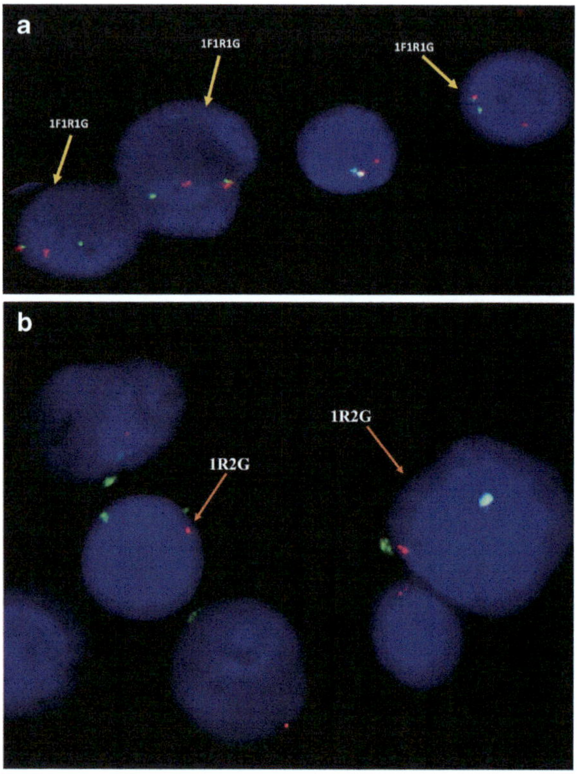

Fig. 14.2 (**a**) FISH using JAK2 break apart probe showing 1Fusion1Red1Green (1F1R1G) aberrant signal pattern indicating JAK2 gene rearrangement. (**b**) FISH using IKZF1/CEN 7 Dual Color Probe (Red for IKZF1 gene region and Green for centromeric region D7Z1 of chromosome 7 showing 1Red 2Green (1R2G) aberrant signal pattern indicating IKZF1 gene deletion

metaphases and often as the sole abnormality. Ten to 15% of CML patients have additional chromosomal abnormalities (ACAs) at diagnosis.

Broadly, the additional chromosomal abnormalities are classified as:

Major route ACAs: These are more frequent and include trisomy 8, isochromosome 17q (i(17q)), trisomy 19, and an additional copy of the Philadelphia chromosome.

Other ACAs: Some abnormalities beyond the major route include trisomy 21, 3q26.2, monosomy 7/7q-, 11q23, and complex karyotypes.

Ninety percentage of patients have a typical t(9;22), and 5% have variant translocations, which can involve chromosome 9 and a chromosome other than chromosome 22; i.e., still an ABL1 translocation, or can be complex involving one or more chromosomes in addition to chromosomes 9 and 22. Less than 5% of patients require molecular testing to detect BCR::ABL translocation, as conventional cytogenetic studies cannot detect the rearrangement.

Baseline cytogenetic analysis is mandatory as per ELN guidelines, as it will allow the detection of ACAs, mainly i(17)(q10)-7/del7q, and 3q26.2 rearrangements, associated with a relatively poor prognosis [8].

14.2.3.2 Utility of Karyotyping in Other Myeloproliferative Neoplasms (MPNs)

Karyotyping abnormalities play an important role in the prognostication of other MPNs. Mutation-enhanced international prognostic system for polycythemia vera (MIPSS-PV) refines treatment approach in polycythemia vera (PV). Karyotyping is an essential component of this prognostic system. MIPSS-PV considers molecular abnormalities, such as SRSF2 mutations (2 points), age > 60 years (2 points), abnormal karyotype (1 point), and leukocytosis $\geq 11 \times 10^9$/l (1 point). Four risk groups are defined with significant differences in median overall survival: Low (0–1 point), Intermediate-1 (2 points), Intermediate-2 (3 points), and High risk (≥4 points) [9].

Although karyotyping does not have a significant role in MIPSS-ET, an abnormal karyotype at diagnosis is seen in <10% of patients with essential thrombocythemia and includes more commonly +9, del 20q, and del 13q [10].

Risk stratification in myelofibrosis includes karyotyping abnormalities as an integral component. Contemporary prognostic systems for myelofibrosis, such as GIPSS (genetically inspired prognostic scoring system) and MIPSS70+ version 2.0 (MIPSSv2; mutation-and karyotype-enhanced international prognostic scoring system), both include karyotyping abnormalities. Very high-risk karyotyping abnormalities included are −7, inv. (3), i(17q), +21, +19, 12p- and 11q-. Favorable risk abnormalities included are normal karyotype or isolated +9, 13q-, 20q-, 1q abnormalities and loss of Y chromosome [11].

Thus, conventional karyotyping is a mandatory test in myelofibrosis and polycythemia vera patients at diagnosis.

14.2.3.3 Eosinophilic Disorders

Hypereosinophilia (HE) workup is incomplete without karyotyping and FISH testing.

Myeloid/lymphoid neoplasms (MLN) with eosinophilia and rearrangements of PDGFRA, PDGFRB, FGFR1, JAK2, ETV6::ABL1, and FLT3 fusions represent a significantly diverse group of hematologic malignancies such as chronic myelomonocytic leukemia (CMML), chronic eosinophilic leukemia (CEL), acute myeloid leukemia (AML), B- ALL and T-ALL, and mixed phenotypic acute leukemias (MPAL). In our laboratory we routinely use a panel of FISH probes comprising 4q12 deletion or rearrangement, FIP1L1, CHIC2, PDGFRA; 4q12 rearrangement, PDGFRA; 5q32 rearrangement, PDGFRB; t(5;12), PDGFRB::ETV6; 8p11.2 rearrangement, FGFR1; 9p24.1 rearrangement, JAK2; 9q34 rearrangement, ABL1; t(9;22), BCR::ABL1 on peripheral blood or bone marrow aspirate specimens in patients with hypereosinophilia.

Identifying PDGFRA, PDGFRB, FGFR1, and JAK2 rearrangements is critical for disease categorization and potential therapeutic intervention. PDGFRA and PDGFRB respond to tyrosine kinase inhibitors such as imatinib mesylate. JAK2 rearrangements have the potential for response to JAK inhibitor therapy. Rearrangements of FGFR1 are typically more aggressive and less responsive to targeted inhibitors [12].

Chronic eosinophilic leukemia (CEL) does not have rearrangements described in MLN with eosinophilia. In the WHO classification of hematolymphoid tumors, fifth edition, three important factors distinguish CEL from hypereosinophilic syndromes (HES): (a) sustained hypereosinophilia for 4 weeks; (b) presence of clonality as indicated by cytogenetic or molecular abnormalities; and (c) bone marrow morphology, such as megakaryocytic or erythroid dysplasia is not required as described in the fourth edition. Evidence of clonality determined by karyotype analysis or molecular testing takes precedence over morphology, and hence identifying the common karyotype abnormalities such as trisomy 8, complex karyotype, del 13q, del 20 q, chromosome 1 abnormalities, and monosomy 7 affirms a diagnosis of CEL [13].

14.2.4 Multiple Myeloma

Multiple myeloma is broadly classified as trisomic/ hyperdiploid multiple myeloma (HDMM) with recurrent trisomies involving odd-numbered chromosomes except for chromosomes 1, 13, and 21, constituting approximately 45% of multiple myeloma, and IgH translocated multiple myeloma with a translocation involving the immunoglobulin heavy chain (IgH) locus on chromosome 14q32, constituting most of the rest. Trisomies and IgH translocations are considered primary cytogenetic abnormalities and occur at the time of establishment of MGUS. Gain(1q), del(1p), del(17p), del(13), and secondary translocations involving MYC are some secondary cytogenetic abnormalities that arise along the disease course. Both primary and secondary cytogenetic abnormalities can influence disease course, response to therapy, and prognosis. Revised International Staging System (RISS) combines elements of tumor burden (ISS) and disease biology (presence of high-risk cytogenetic abnormalities or elevated lactate dehydrogenase level). Due to a lack of availability, only three widely available cytogenetic markers are used in the RISS (high-risk cytogenetics [t(4;14)(p16;q32)/ NSD2, t(14;16)(q32;q23)/ C-MAF, or del(17p)] [14]. The Mayo Clinic mSMART risk stratification (www.msmart.org) provides additional details that are valuable in formulating risk-adapted treatment strategies for multiple myeloma (MM). It has proposed a concept similar to high-grade lymphomas. Presence of any two high-risk factors is considered double-hit myeloma; three or more high-risk factors is triple-hit myeloma [15].

FISH testing also plays a vital role in smoldering multiple myeloma (SMM). t(4;14) involving the fibroblast growth factor 3 (FGFR3) gene on chromosome 4 or del 17p or 1q gain are considered high-risk factors for high-risk smoldering multiple myeloma.

Most importantly, the efficacy of FISH is dependent on the plasma cell enrichment routinely done by CD138—magnetic-activated cell sorting (MACS).

Table 14.3 Diagnostic cytogenetic abnormalities in non-hodgkin lymphomas [3]

B lineage lymphomas	
Mantle cell lymphoma	t(11;14);CCND1::IGH, and IGK/ IGL and CCND2&3 variants
Follicular lymphoma	t(14;18); BCL2::IGH, and IGK/ IGL variants, and less frequently BCL6 rearrangements
Diffuse large B-cell lymphoma (DLBCL)	IGH, BCL6, BCL2, and MYC gene rearrangements
ALK-positive DLBCL	t(2;17)(p23;q23);CLTC::ALK or Other translocations including t(2;5)(p23;q35); NPM1::ALK translocation
Burkitt lymphoma	t(8;14);MYC::IGH, and IGK/IGL Variants, with no additional involvement of BCL2 or BCL6 or complex karyotype
Burkitt-like lymphoma with 11q aberration	Chromosome 11q proximal gains and telomeric losses, and no MYC rearrangement
Extra nodal marginal zone lymphoma of mucosa-associated lymphoid tissue	t(11;18)(q21;q21); BIRC3:: MALT1; t(1;14)(p22;q32);BCL10::IGH; t(14;18)(q32; q21);MALT::IGH and t(3;14)(p14.1;q32);FOXP1::IGH, Trisomy 3 and/or trisomy 18
T lineage lymphomas	
T-cell prolymphocytic leukemia	14q11 (TRA/D) rearrangement in 80–90% T-PLL
Anaplastic large cell lymphoma (ALCL)	ALK gene rearrangement, most frequent t(2;5)(p23;q35);ALK::NPM1
ALK-negative ALCL	DUSP22::IRF4 rearrangement, most commonly a t(6;7)(p25.3;q32.3) or TP63 rearrangements

14.2.5 Non-Hodgkin Lymphoma (NHL)

In lymphomas, FISH testing plays a vital role in diagnosis and risk stratification (Table 14.3).

14.2.5.1 Diagnosis of NHL

FISH testing plays a vital role in the diagnosis of mantle cell lymphoma (CyclinD1), Follicular lymphoma (t(11;14)), high-grade large B-cell lymphomas with MYC, BCL2, and/or BCL6 rearrangements, extranodal marginal zone lymphomas, and for detecting ALK rearrangements [3].

Not all high-grade large B-cell lymphomas will have rearrangements. Some show amplifications in the form of extra copies of BCL2, BCL6, and MYC. These are called extra copy lymphomas or atypical double-hit or triple-hit lymphomas. One study defined atypical double-hit lymphoma cases as tumors with concurrent MYC and BCL2 abnormalities other than coexistent translocations. They further subcategorized them into three groups: (1) MYC translocation coexisting with extra

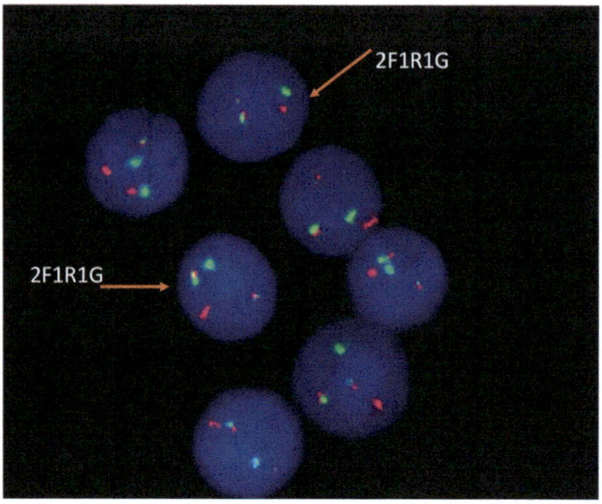

Fig. 14.3 FISH using IGH/CCND1 dual fusion probe (red for 11q13/CCND1 and green for the IGH breakpoint region at 14q32) showing 2Fusion 1Green 1Red (2F1R1G) aberrant signal pattern indicating IGH/CCND1 t(11;14)

copies of BCL2 but lacking evidence of t(14;18)(q32;q21)/IGH::BCL2; (2) t(14;18)(q32;q21)/IGH::BCL2 coexisting with extra copies of MYC, but without evidence of MYC translocation; and (3) extra copies of MYC and BCL2 without translocations involving either gene [16].

Case 3
A 60-year-old male presented with absolute lymphocytosis and cervical and mediastinal lymphadenopathy. Flow cytometric immunophenotyping was suggestive of mantle cell lymphoma. FISH was positive for t(11,14) in 60% of cells, confirming the diagnosis of mantle cell lymphoma (Fig. 14.3).

14.2.5.2 Risk Stratification of CLL

FISH is vital in the prognostication of CLL and therapeutic decision-making. Since CLL cells have a low in vitro proliferation rate, FISH testing on interphase cells is preferred over conventional karyotyping. Based on genetic alterations detected by FISH, Döhner et al. separated CLL patients into five prognostic subgroups, ranging from high to low risk: del(17p) > del(11q) > trisomy 12 > no FISH aberrations (approximately 20% of CLL patients) > isolated del(13q) [17].

14.2.6 Myelodysplastic Neoplasms (MDS)

Karyotyping with or without FISH testing is mandatory for diagnosis and risk stratification of myelodysplastic neoplasms (MDS).

14.2.6.1 Diagnosis of MDS

There are some key differences between the WHO and ICC classification systems in MDS. Pertaining to the role of cytogenetical abnormalities in the diagnosis of MDS, ICC retains the category of MDS-NOS (not otherwise specified), while the WHO fifth edition abandons the morphologic descriptor in favor of MDS with low blasts (MDS-LB). The list of MDS-defining cytogenetic abnormalities is omitted in the WHO, fifth edition. Regardless of these changes, which will surely be revised and updated in upcoming editions, karyotyping remains the center of MDS diagnosis and prognostication along with next-generation sequencing (NGS). Some karyotyping abnormalities, such as MDS with low blasts and isolated 5q deletion (MDS-5q), are diagnostic.

14.2.6.2 Risk Stratification of MDS

The prognosis of patients with MDS can be calculated using scoring systems such as the Revised International Prognostic Scoring System (IPSS-R), which includes analysis of peripheral cytopenias, the percentage of blasts in the bone marrow, and cytogenetic characteristics.

Cytogenetic abnormalities for IPSS-R are classified into five categories, such as

1. Very good: del(11q) or -Y;
2. Good: normal karyotype, del(20q), del(5q), del(12p), or double including del(5q);
3. Intermediate: +8, del(7q), i(17q), +19, or any other single or double independent clone;
4. Poor: −7, inv.(3)/t(3q)/del(3q), double including −7/del(7q), or complex (3 abnormalities)
5. Very poor: complex >3 abnormalities.

IPSS-R, in turn, defines five major prognostic categories (very low, low, intermediate, high, and very high) that are beneficial for predicting the clinical outcomes of untreated MDS patients and aiding the design and analysis of clinical trials in this disease [18].

Case 4

A 63-year-old female presented with persistent transfusion-dependent anemia with normal leucocyte and platelet counts. Bone marrow was hypercellular with prominent dysplasia in megakaryocytic lineage with many hypolobate forms. Blasts were not increased. Conventional karyotype analysis revealed deletion of the long arm of chromosome 5, confirming the diagnosis of MDS with low blasts and 5q deletion (MDS-5q) (Fig. 14.4a, b).

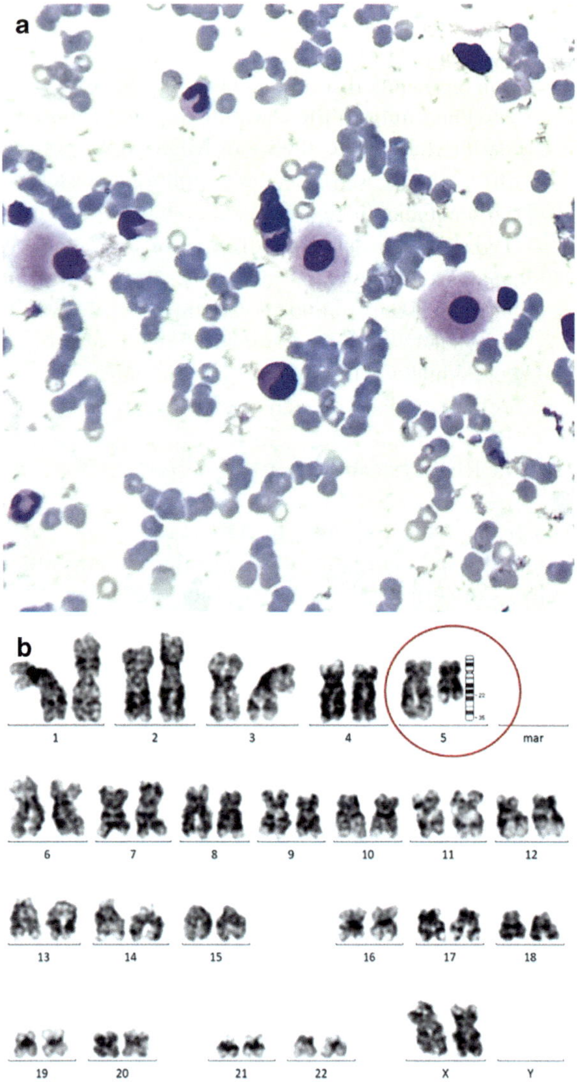

Fig. 14.4 (**a**) Bone marrow aspirate smear showing prominent dysplasia in megakaryocytic lineage with several monolobate forms (Leishman Giemsa, 400x). (**b**) Karyogram showing deletion of the long arm of chromosome 5

14.3 Summary

- Conventional karyotyping and FISH provide immense value in the diagnosis and prognostication of AML, B-ALL, MDS, myeloma, and high-grade and some low-grade lymphomas.
- FISH testing remains the cornerstone for rapid diagnosis of acute promyelocytic leukemia (APL).
- Despite the advances in the field of next-generation sequencing, in hematological malignancies, cytogenetics has a proven role in diagnosis, prognostication, and disease follow-up.

References

1. McGowan-Jordan J, Hastings RJ, Moore S, editors. ISCN 2020: an international system for human Cytogenomic nomenclature. Basel: Karger; 2020.
2. Mannan A, Muhsen IN, Barragán E, Sanz MA, Mohty M, Hashmi SK, Aljurf M. Genotypic and phenotypic characteristics of acute promyelocytic leukemia translocation variants. Hematol Oncol Stem Cell Ther. 2020;13(4):189–201., ISSN 1658-3876,. https://doi.org/10.1016/j.hemonc.2020.05.007.
3. Alaggio R, Amador C, Anagnostopoulos I, et al. The 5th edition of the World Health Organization classification of haematolymphoid tumours: lymphoid neoplasms. Leukemia. 2022;36:1720–48.
4. Döhner H, Wei AH, Appelbaum FR, et al. Diagnosis and management of AML in adults: 2022 recommendations from an international expert panel on behalf of the ELN. Blood. 2022;140(12):1345–77.
5. Döhner H, Dinardo CD, Appelbaum F, et al. Genetic risk classification for adults with AML receiving less- intensive therapies: the 2024 ELN recommendations. Blood. 2024;144(21):2169–73. https://doi.org/10.1182/blood.2024025409.
6. Mullighan CG. The genomic landscape of acute lymphoblastic leukemia in children and young adults. Hematology Am Soc Hematol Educ Program. 2014;2014(1):174–80.
7. Thompson J, Thompson G, White D, Yeung D. Judicious use of precise fluorescence in situ hybridisation panels guided by population prevalence may assist pragmatic detection of clinically targetable Philadelphia chromosome-like acute lymphoblastic leukaemia fusions: a systematic review. Pathology. 2024;56(7):931–41. ISSN 0031-3025.
8. Wang W, Cortes JE, Tang G, et al. Risk stratification of chromosomal abnormalities in chronic myelogenous leukemia in the era of tyrosine kinase inhibitor therapy. Blood. 2016;127(22):2742–50.
9. Pasquer H, Kiladjian J-J, Benajiba L. Current myeloproliferative neoplasm scoring systems for clinical practice. Blood. 2025;145(3):257–76. https://doi.org/10.1182/blood.2024025459.
10. Tefferi A, Vannucchi AM, Barbui T. Essential thrombocythemia: 2024 update on diagnosis, risk stratification, and management. Am J Hematol. 2024;99(4):697–718. https://doi.org/10.1002/ajh.27216.
11. Tefferi A. Primary myelofibrosis: 2023 update on diagnosis, risk-stratification, and management. Am J Hematol. 2023;98(5):801–21. https://doi.org/10.1002/ajh.26857.
12. Metzgeroth G, Steiner L, Naumann N, et al. Myeloid/lymphoid neoplasms with eosinophilia and tyrosine kinase gene fusions: reevaluation of the defining characteristics in a registry-based cohort. Leukemia. 2023;37:1860–7. https://doi.org/10.1038/s41375-023-01958-1.
13. Morsia E, Reichard K, Pardanani A, Tefferi A, Gangat N. WHO defined chronic eosinophilic leukemia, not otherwise specified (CEL, NOS):a contemporary series from the Mayo Clinic. Am J Hematol. 2020;95:E172–4.
14. Palumbo A, Avet-Loiseau H, Oliva S, et al. Revised international staging system for multiple myeloma: a report from international myeloma working group. J Clin Oncol. 2015;33(26):2863–9. https://doi.org/10.1200/JCO.2015.61.2267.
15. Rajkumar SV. Multiple myeloma: 2024 update on diagnosis, risk-stratification, and management. Am J Hematol. 2024;99(9):1802–24. https://doi.org/10.1002/ajh.27422.
16. Li S, Seegmiller A, Lin P, et al. B-cell lymphomas with concurrent MYC and BCL2 abnormalities other than translocations behave similarly to MYC/BCL2 double-hit lymphomas. Mod Pathol. 2015;28:208–17. https://doi.org/10.1038/modpathol.2014.95.
17. Döhner H, Stilgenbauer S, Benner A, Leupolt E, Kröber A, Bullinger L, et al. Genomic aberrations and survival in chronic lymphocytic leukemia. N Engl J Med. 2000;343(26):1910–6. https://doi.org/10.1056/NEJM200012283432602.
18. Greenberg PL, Tuechler H, Schanz J, et al. Revised international prognostic scoring system for myelodysplastic syndromes. Blood. 2012;120(12):2454–65. https://doi.org/10.1182/blood-2012-03-420489.

Chapter 15
Measurable Residual Disease (MRD) in Haematological Malignancies: A Comparative Overview of Flow Cytometry, Molecular, and Next-Generation Sequencing Approaches

Neha Singh and Pradeep Arumugam

Abstract Measurable residual disease (MRD) has emerged as a cornerstone of disease evaluation in haematological malignancies, providing prognostic insight and informing treatment decisions beyond what is achievable through conventional morphological assessment. During morphological remission—defined by less than 5% bone marrow blasts—MRD testing detects persistent leukemic cells at submicroscopic levels, enabling early identification of relapse risk and supporting individualized therapy planning. The principal platforms for MRD assessment include flow cytometry (FCM), molecular diagnostic techniques, and next-generation sequencing (NGS), each offering distinct advantages across different disease contexts. Technological progress has extended detection sensitivity to as low as 10^{-6}—levels unattainable with conventional assays.

Flow cytometry is the most universally applicable method, capable of interrogating leukaemia-specific surface marker profiles across virtually all patients. Instruments range from basic four-colour configurations to next-generation flow cytometry (NGF) platforms employing more than ten markers, permitting the analysis of millions of cells and approaching the sensitivity of molecular methods. However, FCM has notable limitations, including dependence on fresh specimens, significant operator expertise, and susceptibility to immunophenotypic drift that may generate false-positive or false-negative results. On the molecular side, methodologies have progressed from conventional quantitative PCR (qPCR) to sophisticated platforms such as droplet digital PCR (dPCR) and NGS. While NGS offers unparalleled sensitivity and the capacity to identify clonal evolution, its deployment remains confined to specialist centres because of cost and technical complexity.

N. Singh (✉) · P. Arumugam
Tata Memorial Center (HBCH & MPMMCC), Varanasi, India

Homi Bhabha National Institute, Mumbai, India

H. P. Pati et al. (eds.), *Clinical Hematology and Hemato-Oncology*,
https://doi.org/10.1007/978-981-92-1167-8_15

dPCR permits absolute target quantification and surpasses traditional PCR in sensitivity, though standardization remains challenging for genetically heterogeneous targets such as NPM1.

MRD assessment is well-established in B-ALL, T-ALL, AML, MM, and CLL, with each malignancy requiring tailored immunophenotypic and molecular strategies. In CML, serial molecular monitoring by qRT-PCR forms the backbone of response assessment, enabling evaluation of deep molecular remission and informing decisions around treatment-free remission. Liquid biopsy approaches utilizing ctDNA have attracted growing interest in lymphoma, where conventional sampling is less informative. Despite these advances, key challenges persist: the absence of harmonized global standards, biological heterogeneity causing false results, clonal evolution undermining established targets, and restricted access to technologies such as NGS in resource-limited settings.

Keywords Measurable residual disease · Next-generation flow cytometry · Next-generation sequencing · Real-time quantitative PCR · Leukaemia · Lymphoma · Myeloma

Learning Objectives

Conceptual Foundations of MRD

- Understand the definition and clinical relevance of MRD in haematological malignancies.
- Appreciate the principal MRD detection platforms, encompassing flow cytometry, molecular assays, and next-generation sequencing (NGS).

Technical Advances in MRD Detection

- Become familiar with the latest developments in MRD technologies, including droplet digital PCR, error-corrected NGS, and next-generation flow cytometry.
- Identify the principal challenges in MRD detection: biological heterogeneity, clonal evolution, and the ongoing need for global assay standardization.

Disease-Specific Applications

- Examine MRD applications across major malignancy categories, including B-ALL, T-ALL, AML, CLL, MM, and CML.
- Understand how disease-specific immunophenotypic and genetic characteristics inform MRD panel design.

Comparative Assessment of MRD Platforms

- Evaluate the sensitivity, clinical applicability, and practical constraints of FCM, qRT-PCR, dPCR, NGS, and imaging modalities (e.g., PET/CT).

- Compare these platforms with reference to their sensitivity, accessibility, and clinical relevance.

Treatment Personalization
- Grasp how MRD status guides risk-adapted treatment intensification or de-escalation.
- Appreciate the role of MRD surveillance in enabling precision oncology and individualized patient management.

Emerging Directions
- Explore the potential of liquid biopsy, particularly circulating tumour DNA (ctDNA), for non-invasive lymphoma MRD monitoring.
- Discover novel biomarkers and molecular strategies for MRD assessment in multiple myeloma and related conditions.

15.1 Introduction

Measurable residual disease (MRD) is defined as the persistence of detectable malignant cells in the bone marrow or peripheral blood during morphological remission—a state conventionally characterized by fewer than 5% bone marrow blasts on microscopy. Across haematological malignancies, MRD monitoring has gained widespread acceptance as an independent prognostic marker and a guide for risk-stratified therapeutic decision-making. Two complementary analytical frameworks underpin MRD quantification: molecular diagnostics, which characterize tumour-specific genetic abnormalities, and flow cytometric immunophenotyping, which profiles aberrant tumour surface antigens. Both modalities are deployed at the time of diagnosis and repeated during clinical remission phases to achieve consistent and accurate quantification, based on the delineation of case-specific tumour signatures.

Contemporary advances in high-throughput technologies have substantially enhanced the specificity and sensitivity of MRD detection, now achieving levels of 10^{-5} to 10^{-6}. In molecular diagnostics, the field is transitioning away from qualitative PCR and real-time quantitative PCR (RQ-PCR) toward more refined platforms, including droplet digital PCR and next-generation sequencing. In parallel, immunophenotypic methods have undergone substantial evolution—from four-colour flow cytometry through six-to-eight-colour multidimensional platforms to "next-generation flow cytometry" (NGF), which employs more than ten markers and enables rapid acquisition of over 10^7 events, thereby approaching the sensitivity of molecular assays (10^{-6}). Sophisticated software tools for automated gating and

Table 15.1 Comparison of MRD monitoring by different technologies in acute leukaemia

Variables	Next generation multiparametric flow cytometry (MFC)	Real-time quantitative PCR	Next generation sequencing (error-corrected NGS)
Sensitivity	10^{-4} to 10^{-5}	~10^{-5}	~10^{-6}
Availability	Broadly accessible	Broadly accessible	Confined to specialized centres
Applicability	Nearly universal (~100%)	Restricted to cases carrying defined translocations or mutations (e.g., BCR-ABL1, PML-RARA, RUNX1::RUNX1T1, NPM1, JAK2)	Restricted to cases with defined point mutations or indels
Sampling requirements	Viable fresh sample mandatory; analysis within 24–48 hours	Both fresh and archived specimens acceptable	Both fresh and archived specimens acceptable
Baseline sample requirement	Required for LAIP strategy; not needed for DfN approach	Not required, though knowledge of the target genetic aberration is essential	Mandatory
Turnaround time	Results within hours	Typically, within 1 week	Generally, 3–4 weeks
Clonal evolution detection	Feasible	Not feasible	Feasible
Key limitations	Absence of global standardization; considerable technical expertise required; false positives due to phenotypic overlap; immunophenotypic shift may cause false negatives (LAIP approach)	Applicable only in molecularly defined cases; false negatives attributable to clonal evolution	High cost; complex bioinformatics pipeline

maturation pathway analysis have further improved the accuracy and reproducibility of NGF-based MRD (see Table 15.1). Such multiparameter flow cytometry (MFC) monitoring also has the capacity to disclose emerging phenotypic shifts that could serve as therapeutic targets—including antigens addressed by agents such as anti-CD19 blinatumomab and bispecific T-cell engagers (BiTEs). Nevertheless, despite computational and technical progress, reliable MRD evaluation by MFC continues to demand significant specialized expertise, restricting widespread implementation of NGF-MRD analysis to a small number of highly qualified laboratories [1–3].

15.2 MRD Assessment by Flow Cytometry in Acute Leukaemia

Flow cytometric MRD evaluation has been established as a standard component of clinical decision-making in acute leukaemia. Residual disease after induction therapy correlates with elevated relapse risk, and serial monitoring may identify subclinical persistence before clinical relapse becomes evident. Two principal immunophenotypic strategies are employed: the leukaemia-associated immunophenotype (LAIP) approach, which identifies surface marker combinations present on leukaemic cells but absent from normal counterparts, and the "different from normal" (DfN) approach, which characterizes leukaemic blasts by detecting immunophenotypic deviations relative to a defined normal reference population. The foundational principles of sample processing and MRD standardization by flow cytometry are applicable across all acute leukaemia subtypes. An 8-to-10-colour platform is recommended for precise analysis. The first-pull bone marrow aspirate (0.5–1 mL) is the preferred specimen. Samples should be collected in EDTA or heparin anticoagulant, transported at 8 to 20 °C, and processed within 48 to 72 hours of collection. The bulk lysis-staining approach described by the EuroFlow Consortium is the recommended processing method. Acquisition of a minimum of 500,000 CD45-positive events per tube is required, though collecting the highest feasible number of events is strongly encouraged. To maximize assay sensitivity, at least 1 to 2 million cells should be acquired, with a minimum of 100 abnormal blast events required to report a confident MRD-positive result. A minimum of two distinct LAIPs must be identified to assign MRD positivity; otherwise, the result should be reported as suspicious. MRD burden is expressed as the proportion of MRD-positive events relative to total viable cell count.

15.3 B-ALL MRD Strategy

B-ALL MRD detection primarily rests on discriminating B-lymphoblasts from haematogones across their various stages of maturation [4]. A panel incorporating backbone markers—CD19 (for gating), CD10, CD20, CD34, CD38, and CD45—together with more recently validated MRD antigens such as CD123, CD66c, CD58, CD304, CD73, and CD86 should be employed. Haematogones progressively upregulate CD45 and CD20 with maturation while losing CD34, CD10, and CD38 expression through later developmental stages. Beyond haematogones, other immunophenotypic mimickers must be systematically excluded before designating a population as MRD-positive: these include CD34+mature B cells, CD10+mature B cells, CD10+/CD73+mesenchymal stem cells, CD19dim+NK cells in regenerating marrow, and CD123+/CD19+plasmacytoid dendritic cells (Fig. 15.1).

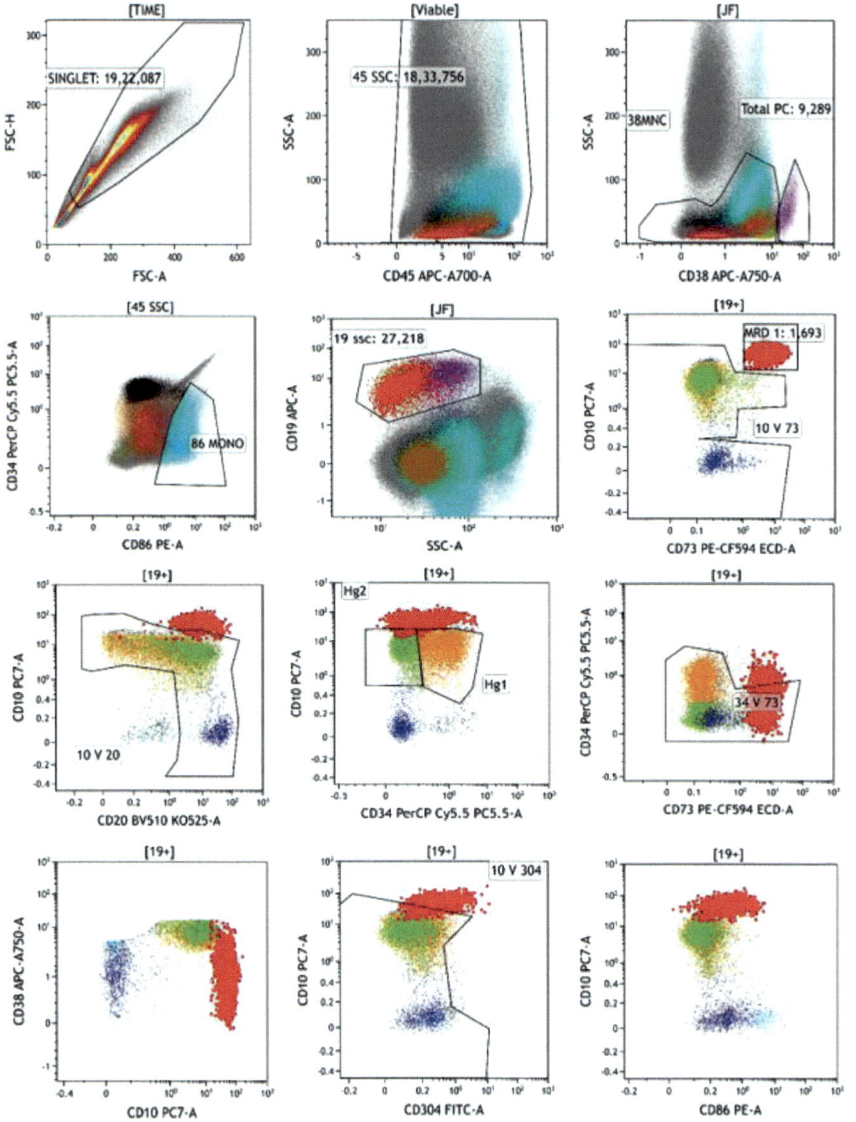

Fig. 15.1 A 9-year-old female diagnosed with B-cell precursor lymphoblastic leukaemia by flow cytometry. NGS identified EBF1-PDGFRB1 fusion by RNA sequencing. The patient was classified as high-risk BCP-ALL and treated with Modified ICiCLe protocol plus Dasatinib. Post-induction MRD positivity of 0.07% was demonstrated by high-sensitivity flow cytometry (10-colour panel); MRD-positive events are highlighted in red

15.4 T-ALL MRD Strategy

In principle, T-ALL MRD detection is more straightforward than B-ALL because normal T-lymphocyte maturation occurs predominantly in the thymus; consequently, the presence of immature T-cell populations in peripheral blood or bone marrow is inherently aberrant. In practice, however, loss of immaturity-associated antigens from blast populations following induction chemotherapy complicates interpretation [5]. T-ALL MRD therefore relies on identifying aberrant expression patterns among T-cell antigens—including CD2, CD3 (cytoplasmic and surface), CD5, CD4, CD8, and CD7—as well as NK-associated markers such as CD16 and CD56, which tend to be relatively stable even when immaturity markers (CD99, TdT, CD34, CD1a) are diminished or absent. The principal diagnostic challenge lies in differentiating T-lymphoblasts from NK cells, surface CD3-negative mature T cells, and myeloblasts with dim CD7 expression (Fig. 15.2). Close follow-up and repeat MRD assessment are advisable in equivocal cases. The clinically relevant threshold for treatment intensification or de-escalation is 0.01%.

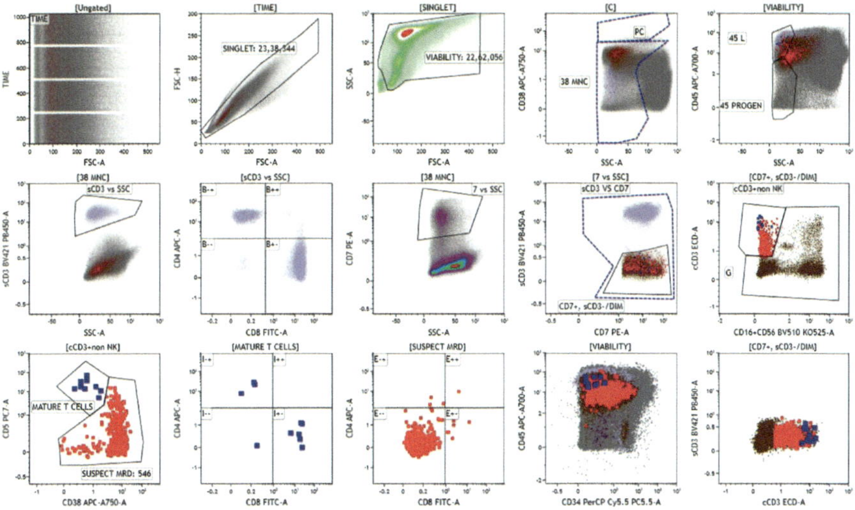

Fig. 15.2 A 15-year-old male presenting with hyperleukocytosis, diagnosed with Early T-precursor acute lymphoblastic leukaemia by flow cytometry. Post-induction bone marrow assessment demonstrates MRD positivity of 0.024% by high-sensitivity flow cytometry using a 10-colour T-MRD panel with the DfN approach; positive events are highlighted in red

15.5 MRD Assessment in AML

AML MRD detection relies on distinguishing normal haematopoietic progenitors from leukaemic cell populations using either the DfN or LAIP approaches [6–9]. Blast-equivalent populations are evaluated across three separate compartments: CD34+/CD117±, CD34−/CD117+, and CD34−/CD117neg. Normal marrow components—including mast cells (bright CD117), basophilic precursors (CD123-bright, HLA-DR-negative), plasmacytoid dendritic cell precursors (CD123-bright, HLA-DR-bright), mesenchymal stem cells (CD13-bright), plasma cells (CD38-bright), erythroid precursors (CD36+/CD117±/CD33-negative), and immature myeloid precursors such as promyelocytes and myelocytes—are systematically segregated. The central interpretive challenge is separating aberrant myeloid blasts or leukaemic stem cells from regenerating normal myeloblasts (CD34+/CD38+) and stem cell progenitors (CD34+/CD38−). This differentiation relies principally on understanding normal progenitor maturation patterns in relation to supplementary markers including CD123, CD117, HLA-DR, TIM-3, CLL-1, CD25, CD32, CD7, CD15, CD19, and CD56 (Fig. 15.3). The universally accepted threshold for clinical decision-making in AML is 0.1% (Table 15.2). Pending clinical validation of emerging NGS-based approaches, molecular MRD monitoring in AML remains feasible only when specific translocations or mutations are present. This leaves MFC-MRD as the sole available method for most AML patients, including the intermediate-risk group characterized by the absence of targetable molecular lesions. It should be noted that MFC may fail to detect mature differentiating myeloid cells harbouring genomic aberrations, such as BCR-ABL1 in CML-chronic phase or NPM1-mutated/PML-RARA-rearranged monocytic and mature myeloid cells [10].

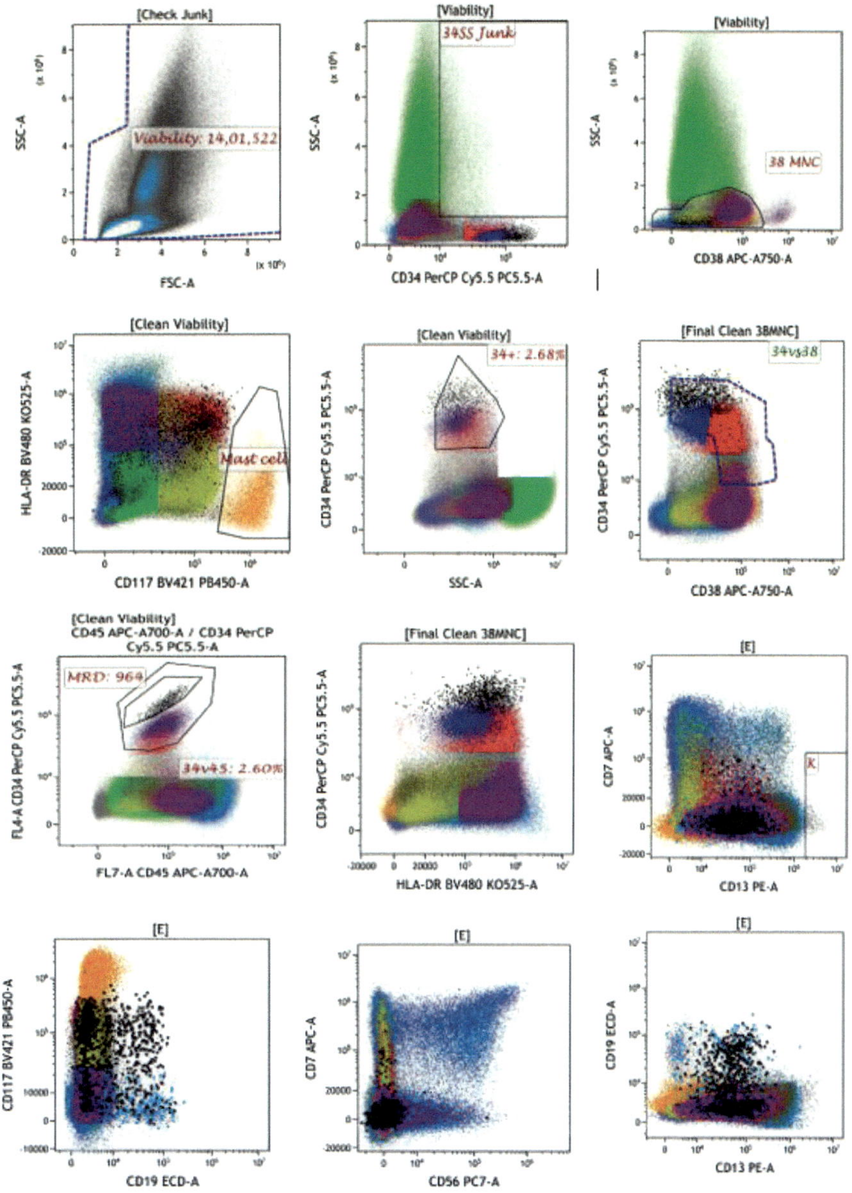

Fig. 15.3 A 45-year-old male diagnosed with AML t(8;21), initiated on 3 + 7 induction. NGS revealed concurrent ASXL1 and ZBTB4 mutations in addition to RUNX1::RUNX1T1. Post-induction bone marrow MRD assessment demonstrates positivity of 0.068% by high-sensitivity flow cytometry; aberrant cells are annotated with black dots

Table 15.2 Key features of MRD monitoring by flow cytometry across haematological malignancies [3]

	AML	B-ALL	T-ALL	CLL	Myeloma
Sensitivity	10^{-3} – 10^{-5}	10^{-4} – 10^{-5}	10^{-4} – 10^{-5}	10^{-4} – 10^{-5}	10^{-5} – 10^{-6}
Sample source	BM	BM	BM, PB	PB, BM	BM
Minimum cell requirement	3×10^6	4×10^6	4×10^6	3×10^6	$5–20 \times 10^6$
Applicability	>97%	>99%	>99%	>95%	>99%
Clinically significant MRD threshold	$\geq 10^{-3}$	$\geq 10^{-4}$	$\geq 10^{-4}$	$\geq 10^{-4}$	$\geq 10^{-5}$
Assessment schedule	Protocol-dependent; typically post-induction and post-consolidation, thereafter every 3–6 months				
Core panel markers	CD34, CD117, CD45, CD13, CD33, CD38	CD34, CD45, CD19, CD38, CD20, CD10	CD3, CD7, CD16, CD56, CD38, CD5, CD4, CD8, CD45, CD34	CD19, CD20, CD5, CD45, CD10, CD23	CD38, CD138, CD45, CD20, CD19, kappa, lambda, CD56, CD81, CD27
Supplementary markers	CD15, CD7, CD14, CD64, HLA-DR, CD123, CD25, CD32, TIM-3, CLL-1, CD56, CD19	CD22, CD73, CD123, CD58, CD66c, CD44, ROR1, CD304, CD81, CD86	TdT, CD10, CD2, CD99, CD1a	CD43, CD79b, CD81, CD200	CD28, CD117, CD200, CD229, CD319, CD33

15.6 MRD Assessment by Quantitative Real-Time PCR and Digital PCR in Acute Leukaemias

qRT-PCR-based MRD monitoring requires identification of a specific target mutation or fusion transcript—such as NPM1, PML-RARA, RUNX1-RUNX1T1, CBF-MYH11, BCR-ABL, TCF3:PBX1, or ETV6:RUNX1. A positive qRT-PCR result is reported when the fluorescent signal crosses a pre-specified threshold after a defined number of amplification cycles. Although conceptually well suited for detecting low-level residual AML, the technique is complicated by tumour heterogeneity and the reliance on relative rather than absolute quantification of target copy numbers. Normalizing the signal against a standardized housekeeping reference gene—such as ABL1 or GUSB—partially addresses this limitation. Nevertheless, the absence of absolute quantification in qRT-PCR hampers assay standardization and precise MRD quantitation [11].

Digital PCR has gained recognition as a technically superior alternative, offering absolute quantification by partitioning the input sample into thousands of individual oil-water emulsion droplets or nanowells. Each partition contains an independent

PCR reaction, and the ratio of positive to negative droplets yields the absolute target count. This methodology minimizes variability in normalized target levels and lends itself to straightforward data interpretation. A significant limitation, however, is that standardization is difficult for genetically heterogeneous targets such as NPM1, which may carry multiple mutation subtypes (types A, B, C, and others).

15.7 MRD Assessment by NGS in Acute Leukaemias

Illustrative Case
A 25-year-old male presented with newly diagnosed acute myeloid leukaemia confirmed by flow cytometry. NGS profiling identified NPM1 Type A mutation together with an IDH2 R140 mutation. He was classified as AML with NPM1 mutation per the revised WHO 2022 classification and assigned to the favourable-risk category per ELN 2022 recommendations. He received 3 + 7 induction chemotherapy followed by three cycles of HiDAC consolidation. After two cycles, flow cytometric MRD was negative, yet persistent unexplained cytopenias prompted an NGS-MRD panel, which revealed residual IDH2 R140 mutation at a VAF of 0.5% alongside an emergent FLT3-ITD clone. Midostaurin was incorporated into the therapeutic regimen, and the patient subsequently underwent allogeneic BMT after achieving pre-transplant NGS-MRD negativity.

In B-cell malignancies, NGS-based MRD primarily exploits the unique rearrangements of the immunoglobulin heavy chain (IGH) gene as a clonal fingerprint; the T-cell receptor (TCR) gene is the equivalent target in T-cell malignancies [12]. In contrast to ALL, where IGH or TCR rearrangements reliably define clonality, the AML genome is more heterogeneous, necessitating a patient-directed multi-mutation testing strategy. For AML, NGS-MRD quantifies the persistence of disease-specific mutations following treatment. Critically, not all mutations identified at diagnosis carry equivalent utility for MRD monitoring—these nuances are summarized in (Table 15.3).

Mutations associated with age-related clonal haematopoiesis—including DNMT3A, TET2, and ASXL1—as well as germline predisposition signatures such as ANKRD26, GATA2, ETV6, CEBPA, RUNX1, DDX41, and TP53 do not necessarily indicate persistent AML and must be interpreted accordingly. Similarly, for therapeutically targetable mutations such as FLT3, KRAS, and KIT, negative MRD results may not fully exclude residual disease.

NGS-MRD requires sufficient read depth to reliably discriminate true signal from PCR-induced background noise—a challenge addressed by error-corrected duplex sequencing. This approach incorporates unique molecular identifiers (UMIs) during library preparation to tag individual DNA molecules with a distinctive fingerprint, enabling in silico removal of PCR amplification and sequencing errors, thereby markedly improving assay specificity [13].

Table 15.3 ELN recommendations for molecular MRD testing in AML [13]

Genetic alteration	ELN AML MRD 2021/ ELN 2022 recommendation	Notes
NPM1	Recommended	Critical for informing post-remission therapy planning
RUNX1-RUNX1T1, CBFB-MYH11, or PML-RARA	Recommended	Fusion transcript quantification by qRT-PCR is highly informative
Other fusions (KMT2A, DEK-NUP214, MECOM)	Not specifically addressed	Supporting evidence is limited but the underlying rationale is valid; KMT2A has over 100 known fusion partners
Signalling pathway genes: FLT3, KIT, RAS	Possibly useful	Informative when positive; however, relapse can occur in test-negative patients
"DTA" genes: DNMT3A, TET2, ASXL1	Specifically recommended against	These may reflect age-related clonal haematopoiesis and must not be conflated with residual AML
Hereditary predisposition genes: ANKRD26, CEBPA, DDX41, ETV6, GATA2, RUNX1, TP53	Not recommended	When present at a variant allele frequency of ~50%, these should be explicitly excluded from MRD consideration
WT1, EVI1	Discouraged	Expression-based assays for these targets are subject to considerable variability

15.8 Minimal Residual Disease Assessment in Multiple Myeloma

With the advent of novel agents and combination regimens, an increasing proportion of MM patients now attain deep remissions. Conventional criteria for complete remission (CR) in MM require negative immunofixation in serum and urine, resolution of soft-tissue plasmacytomas, and fewer than 5% plasma cells in bone marrow aspirates. Despite the fact that more than half of newly diagnosed MM patients fulfil these CR criteria, approximately 68% relapse within 2 years. To address this limitation, the International Myeloma Working Group (IMWG) incorporated MRD assessment as an additional response category in 2016 (Table 15.4). IMWG endorses both intramedullary and extramedullary MRD assessment. For intramedullary evaluation, bone marrow aspirate material is analysed using allele-specific oligonucleotide quantitative PCR (ASO-qPCR), multiparametric flow cytometry (MFC), next-generation flow cytometry (NGF), or NGS (Table 15.5). MFC-based MRD detection in myeloma relies on quantifying and characterizing neoplastic plasma

Table 15.4 IMWG response criteria for MRD in multiple myeloma

Response category	Defining criteria
Sustained MRD-negative	MRD negativity in the marrow (NGF or NGS, or both) and by imaging as defined below, confirmed at minimum 1-year intervals. Subsequent evaluations may further specify the duration of negativity (e.g., MRD-negative at 5 years)
Flow MRD-negative	Absence of phenotypically aberrant clonal plasma cells by NGF‡ on bone marrow aspirates using the EuroFlow standard operation procedure for MRD detection in multiple myeloma (or validated equivalent method) with a minimum sensitivity of 1 in 10^5 nucleated cells or higher
Sequencing MRD-negative	Absence of clonal plasma cells by NGS on bone marrow aspirate, in which the presence of a clone is defined as less than two identical sequencing reads obtained after DNA sequencing of bone marrow aspirates using the Lympho SIGHT platform (or validated equivalent method) with a minimum sensitivity of 1 in 10^5 nucleated cells or higher
Imaging plus MRD-negative	MRD negativity defined by NGF or NGS plus resolution of all areas of increased tracer uptake identified at baseline/preceding PET/CT, or reduction below mediastinal blood pool SUV, or below surrounding normal tissue activity

cells (PCs) relative to their normal counterparts. Normal PCs characteristically express CD38-bright, CD138-bright, CD81-bright, CD45+, CD19+, and CD27+, while lacking CD28, CD20, CD56, and CD117, with polyclonal cytoplasmic kappa/lambda immunoglobulin expression. Neoplastic PCs, by contrast, exhibit one or more aberrancies from the following profile: CD38-dim (weaker than normal PCs), CD45−, CD19−, CD20+, CD27−, CD28+, CD81−, CD117+, CD56+, and monoclonal cytoplasmic kappa or lambda expression (Fig. 15.4). An important caveat is that therapy with anti-CD38 monoclonal antibodies (daratumumab and isatuximab) compromises the utility of CD38 as an MRD marker; alternative markers—including CD200, CD33, CD54, CD229, CD307, CD319, CD150, and VS38—have been proposed as substitutes in post-anti-CD38-therapy MFC panels.

According to IMWG criteria, MRD negativity in myeloma is defined as the absence of detectable cancer cells against a background of at least 10^5 normal cells, as assessed by MFC or NGS technology, in patients achieving CR. Extramedullary MRD monitoring is conducted primarily through imaging modalities, including ^{18}F-fluorodeoxyglucose positron emission tomography with computed tomography (FDG-PET/CT) and magnetic resonance imaging (MRI) [14–17].

Table 15.5 Comparison of MRD monitoring platforms in multiple myeloma

Technique	Sensitivity	Advantages	Disadvantages
MFC — Identification of MM cells by flow cytometry analysis of MM-specific cell surface antigens	10^{-4} (4–6 colour) 10^{-5} (8–10 colour)	(1) Broad applicability (90–100%). (2) Rapid, cost-effective, and efficient. (3) Incorporates built-in sample quality assessment. (4) Not impacted by somatic hypermutation or clonal evolution	(1) Specimen must be processed within 24–48 hours. (2) Data interpretation demands specialized expertise. (3) Complex data visualization. (4) Cannot resolve cytogenetic characteristics
ASO-qPCR — Identification of MM cells by amplifying MM-specific immunoglobulin gene rearrangement	10^{-5}	(1) Broad laboratory applicability. (2) Fully standardized detection protocols. (3) Fresh sample processing is not mandatory	(1) Applicability may decrease (42–75%) with universal primers. (2) Standard curve construction consumes scarce bone marrow DNA. (3) Risk of false-negative results
NGS — Identification of MM cells by sequencing the IGH/IGK/IGL loci	10^{-6}	(1) No immediate sample processing or standard curve required. (2) Captures virtually all Ig gene rearrangements. (3) Consensus primers applicable for clonality detection and MRD follow-up. (4) Adaptive biotechnologies (Seattle, WA) standardization available	(1) Susceptible to somatic hypermutation. (2) No built-in sample quality control. (3) Time-consuming, labour-intensive, expensive, and not universally deployable. (4) Result interpretation demands substantial expertise
FDG-PET/CT — Identification of MM cells by assessing tumour metabolic aberration	Spatial resolution limit ~5 mm	(1) Detects residual active clonal cells in osteolytic lesions. (2) Accurately maps bone and extramedullary disease sites. (3) Complementary to cellular and molecular methods	(1) False-positive results are possible (e.g., recent chemotherapy or growth factor use). (2) False-negative results are possible (e.g., hexokinase deficiency or high-dose steroids). (3) Significant associated cost

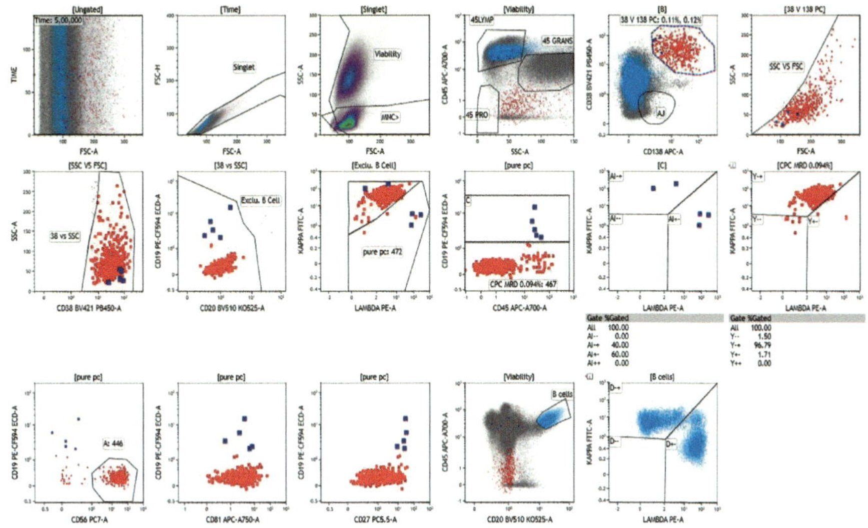

Fig. 15.4 A 52-year-old male with known myeloma, assessed at day +100 post-BMT. Bone marrow aspirate shows trilineage haematopoiesis and 1% plasma cells. Flow cytometric MRD assessment identifies MRD-positive events (highlighted in red), representing residual neoplastic plasma cells

15.9 MRD Assessment in Chronic Lymphocytic Leukaemia

Although most CLL patients are not cured by first-line therapy, meaningful MRD monitoring can be achieved in peripheral blood. Three validated methods meet the established MRD detection threshold of $<10^{-4}$: multicolour flow cytometry (MFC), real-time quantitative polymerase chain reaction (RQ-PCR), and high-throughput sequencing (HTS), each with characteristic strengths and limitations. MFC remains the most widely applied method owing to its broad accessibility, robust standardization, reliability up to the clinically applicable MRD threshold ($<10^{-4}$), and relatively modest cost. MFC-based CLL MRD relies on discriminating residual CLL cells from normal B-cell populations through characteristic differential antigen expression. The co-expression of CD5 and CD23 alongside weaker CD20, CD79b, and CD81 expression compared to normal mature B cells are the hallmark feature of CLL cells (Fig. 15.5). Because contemporary 8-to-10-colour instruments can accommodate the required antibody combinations in a single tube, the ERIC group has developed a standardized core panel comprising six monoclonal antibodies—CD19, CD20, CD5, CD43, CD79b, and CD81—applicable to over 95% of typical CLL cases and feasible in most laboratory settings. Supplementary markers such as CD160, CD200, CD23, and ROR1 provide additional value in atypical presentations or when enhanced sensitivity is required [18].

Treatment strategies with curative intent—including allogeneic stem cell transplantation and, prospectively, CAR T-cell therapy—justify the use of more sensitive

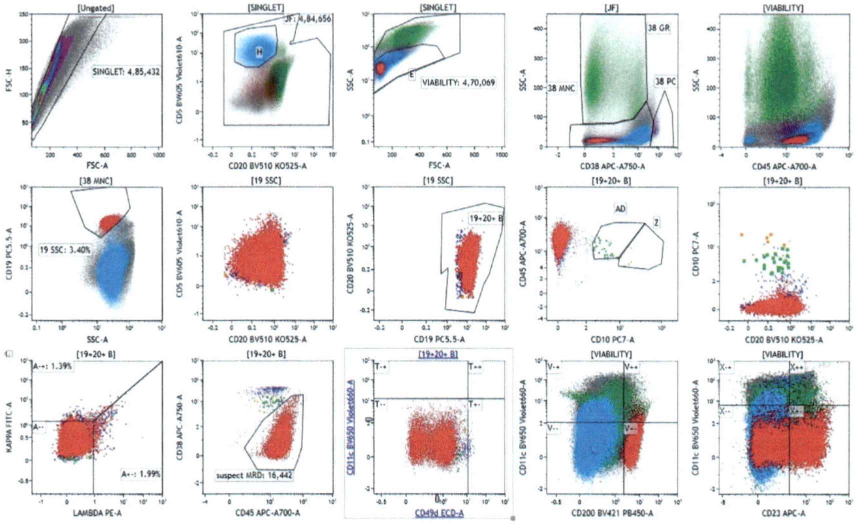

Fig. 15.5 A 66-year-old male diagnosed with CLL by flow cytometry, treated with six cycles of chemotherapy-induced pancytopenia. Flow cytometric MRD analysis of a subsequent bone marrow aspirate demonstrates residual CLL cells; MRD-positive events are highlighted in red

MRD platforms such as HTS. High-throughput IGH sequencing (IGH-HTS) employs consensus primers to amplify all IGH genes, followed by HTS-based quantification of the disease-specific IGH sequence identified in pre-treatment blood samples [19]. This approach has demonstrated MRD detection limits of 10^{-6} (Table 15.6).

15.10 MRD Monitoring in Lymphoma

The application of MRD surveillance in lymphoma is an evolving field, with prospective utility being explored across a widening spectrum of histological subtypes. Liquid biopsy has attracted considerable interest in this context, particularly through the detection of circulating tumour DNA (ctDNA) or cell-free DNA (cfDNA). cfDNA encompasses all DNA shed from cells—whether healthy, inflamed, or malignant—via apoptosis or necrosis, whereas ctDNA represents specifically the tumour-derived fraction of cfDNA, capturing dynamic genetic alterations such as mutations, methylation changes, amplifications, and structural rearrangements.

Table 15.6 Comparison of MRD monitoring platforms in CLL

Techniques	Flow cytometry	RQ-PCR	High-throughput sequencing
Sensitivity/LOD	10^{-4} to 10^{-5}	10^{-5}	10^{-6}
Methodology	Surface antigen profiling via antibody combinations (CD5/CD19/CD20/CD43/CD79b/CD81)	Disease-specific IGHV detection using patient-tailored primers	Disease-specific IGH sequence identification following amplification of all IGH segments with consensus primers
Standardized protocol available?	Yes	Yes	Under development
Fresh sample required?	Yes; sample must be <48 hours old	No; however, DNA extraction is preferred within 48 hours	No; however, DNA extraction is preferred within 48 hours
Advantages	Directly quantitative; widely available; rapid turnaround; highly standardized assay	High sensitivity; viable leucocytes not required	High sensitivity; viable leucocytes not required; multiple mutations detectable in a single assay
Disadvantages	Lower sensitivity than molecular methods; specimens must be fresh	Not directly quantitative; requires a baseline sample; time- and labour-intensive; expensive	Not directly quantitative; baseline sample required; less widely accessible; expensive

While ctDNA constitutes a minor subset of total cfDNA, its identification is indispensable for accurate MRD assessment. Among the various liquid biopsy matrices evaluated in lymphoma, peripheral blood is the most extensively studied and consistently yields detectable ctDNA levels even at early disease stages [20].

Lymphomas are inherently heterogeneous, frequently exhibiting multifocal disease in anatomically distinct sites within a single patient. ctDNA-based liquid biopsy is minimally invasive and captures cell-free DNA shed from diverse tumour foci, providing broader genomic representation than site-specific tissue biopsy. This enables characterization of mutational profiles with prognostic significance, as well as dynamic MRD monitoring throughout treatment. A structured comparison of MRD detection modalities across lymphoma subtypes is presented in (Tables 15.7 and 15.8).

Table 15.7 Comparison of advantages and disadvantages of MRD detection methods in lymphomas.

Methods	FCM-based	PCR-based		NGS-based		
Techniques	MFCM	ASO-RQ-PCR	ddPCR	IgNGS	Panel NGS	LP-WGS
Approximate LOD	4-color:10^{-3} 8-color:10^{-4}	$10^{-4} \sim 10^{-5}$	10^{-5}	10^{-6}	10^{-6}	$10^{-3} \sim 10^{-5}$
Evaluable lesions	Immunophenotype	SNVs Translocations		SNVs, Indels, translocations copy number variants		Copy number variants fragmentation profile
Clonal evolution	Cannot be tracked	Cannot be tracked	Limited by throughout	Can be tracked		Cannot be tracked
Cost	Relatively cheap	Relatively cheap	Relatively expensive	Expensive		
Advantages	Rapid quantification Availability	Low calibration failure Accurate Relatively high sensitivity and reproducibility Fewer technical requirements	Rapid Relatively high sensitivity Absolute quantification	High sensitivity Can detect MRD not identified by MFC or RQ- PCR Patients specific primers unnecessary Commercial availability Analysis is objective and automatically completed by the software	High sensitivity Applicable to all lymphoma subtypes	Relatively high sensitivity Relatively rapid Relatively low cost
Disadvantages	Comparative and insensitive Lack of standardization Require presence of CTCs High professionalism	Primer design necessary Relative quantification Assessment is limited to few genetic lesions	Requires specialized technology not widely accessible Relatively complicated steps Limited capability for multiplexing Application range depends on the panel selected	Relatively complicated steps Requires tumor tissue for clonotype determination	Research laboratories available Sensitivity limited by breadth of genes and sequencing depth Limited detection at low allele frequencies	Sensitivity limited by sequencing depth Assessment is limited by the DNA input

Table 15.8 Comparison of MRD detection methods in some lymphoma subtypes

	HL	DLBCL	FL	MCL
Image methods	Yes	Yes	Yes	Yes
	PET-CT scan or CT scan contrast	PET-CT scan or CT scan contrast	PET-CT scan or CT scan contrast	PET-CT scan or CT scan contrast
Histologic/ pathologic methods	No, unless there is BM involvement at diagnosis	BM biopsy (optional)	BM biopsy (optional)	BM biopsy (optional)
FCM methods	No	No	No	Yes The sensitivity is less than RQPCR
PCR-based methods	No Advanced HL may be detected	Yes, RQPCR ddPCR	Yes ddPCR	Yes, RQPCR ddPCR
NGS methods	NGS liquid biopsy, investigational use	NGS liquid biopsy, investigational use	NGS liquid biopsy, investigational use Relatively low ctDNA concentrations as compared with other lymphoma subtypes	NGS liquid biopsy, investigational use
Low-depth WGS method	Investigational use	Investigational use	Investigational use	Investigational use

15.11 MRD Monitoring in Chronic Myeloid Leukaemia

Illustrative Case

A 35-year-old patient was diagnosed with chronic myeloid leukaemia in chronic phase following confirmation of BCR::ABL1 p210 major transcript by RT-PCR. Imatinib 400 mg was initiated. Six-month molecular assessment by RQ-PCR yielded an IS-normalised copy number (IS-NCN) value of 15%, meeting criteria for TKI failure and prompting kinase domain mutation analysis. Sanger sequencing identified a T315I mutation—known to confer resistance to all approved TKIs except Ponatinib. Following the transition to Ponatinib, the subsequent six-month IS-NCN value was 0.05%.

Molecular monitoring in CML is firmly established in clinical practice and is endorsed by international guidelines as the standard strategy for quantifying treatment response, directing therapeutic adjustments, and triggering BCR::ABL1 kinase domain mutation testing when drug resistance is suspected. Patients achieving a major molecular response (MMR; BCR::ABL1 ratio $\leq$ 0.1% on the International Scale [IS]) face a low probability of disease progression. Deep molecular responses (DMR; BCR::ABL1 ratio $\leq$ 0.01% IS) sustained for 1–2 years constitute a prerequisite for considering TKI discontinuation and pursuing treatment-free remission (TFR). Current guidance from the European LeukemiaNet (ELN) and the National Comprehensive Cancer Network (NCCN) is summarized in Table 15.9.

Table 15.9 ELN 2020 and NCCN V3.2022 treatment response milestones for CML, expressed as BCR::ABL1 on the International Scale

Milestones	ELN 2020 Optimal	NCCN V3.2022 TKI-sensitive	ELN 2020 warning	NCCN V3.2022 possible resistance	ELN 2020 failure	NCCN V3.2022 TKI-resistant
Baseline	NA	NA	High-risk ACA, high-risk ELTS score	NA	NA	NA
3 months	≤10%	≤10%	>10%	>10%	>10% if confirmed within 1–3 months	NA
6 months	≤1%	≤10%	>1–10%	NA	>10%	>10%
12 months	≤0.1%	*≤0.1% or >0.1–1%	>0.1–1%	>1–10%	>1%	>10%
Any time	≤0.1% or ≤0.01% (for patients targeting TFR)	–	>0.1–1%; loss of MMR indicates failure after TFR	–	>1%, resistance mutations and high-risk ACA	–

CML MRD assays should employ ABL1, BCR, or GUSB as internal reference genes to ensure reliability and reproducibility, compensating for differences in BCR::ABL1 transcript levels arising from RNA degradation. RT-qPCR results should be reported on the International Scale for BCR::ABL1 (e13a2/e14a2 transcript type) patients. Continuous internal quality control is required to maintain assay stability over time. The BCR::ABL1 transcript type must be confirmed at diagnosis to guide appropriate monitoring in the approximately 2% of patients who carry atypical fusions; these patients require bespoke RT-qPCR or RT-dPCR assays with results expressed as individual molecular responses normalized to baseline. FISH is generally not recommended because of its substantially lower sensitivity relative to molecular methods, though it may provide utility when molecular testing for atypical fusions is unavailable (Table 15.10).

RT-dPCR represents a valid and potentially superior alternative to conventional RT-qPCR, offering absolute quantification free from the amplification efficiency biases that affect relative quantification. Replicate analysis is feasible using nanofluidic partitioning technology, with workflows and reagents analogous to standard hydrolysis-probe real-time PCR. In the RT-dPCR format, the specimen is partitioned into thousands of water-oil emulsion droplets, each hosting an independent PCR reaction; the proportion of positive droplets is then used to calculate absolute target abundance. The high replication number substantially improves the precision of rare transcript detection. Digital PCR has been shown to achieve greater sensitivity for BCR::ABL1 transcripts than conventional qPCR and has been used to detect residual disease in patients pursuing TFR attempts [21, 22].

Table 15.10 Recommended diagnostic tests for monitoring and investigating CML during treatment

Test	Recommendation and rationale
Interphase FISH	Not recommended as routine. May be considered if quality-controlled RT-qPCR is unavailable, including for atypical BCR::ABL1 fusions. Cannot be used to define MMR or DMR
Qualitative RT-PCR	Not recommended. Offers minimal value for monitoring treatment response
Conventional cytogenetics	Indicated at overt haematological relapse, ELN-defined failure, or suspected/overt disease progression. Also consider in patients in remission with abnormal blood counts. The sole technique capable of detecting prognostically significant ACAs arising during disease course, as well as chromosomal abnormalities in Ph-negative cells
Quantitative RT-qPCR or RT-dPCR	Mandatory for routine molecular monitoring. Currently the only technique(s) capable of quantifying disease across the full response range defined by ELN and other clinical frameworks, including DMR
NGS panel (myeloid/lymphoid genes)	Indicated at overt haematological relapse and in cases of suspected or confirmed disease progression. May help verify progression and identify potential therapeutic targets.
BCR::ABL1 TKD mutation analysis	Strongly recommended when patients fail to achieve defined ELN milestones or experience loss of MMR on TKI therapy. Guides subsequent therapeutic decisions in a substantial proportion of cases.

Summary and Key Take-Home Points

MRD surveillance in haematological malignancies employs immunophenotypic and molecular analysis to detect residual malignant cells in bone marrow and peripheral blood at levels below the threshold of conventional light microscopy. The strong and independent prognostic value of MRD status has established MRD-guided therapy intensification or de-escalation as a cornerstone of modern haematological oncology. The integration of advanced molecular platforms—NGS and ddPCR—with next-generation multiparameter flow cytometry equips clinicians with the tools needed to design truly individualized therapeutic strategies, including the application of precision immunotherapy.

MRD monitoring in B-ALL, T-ALL, AML, and CLL is well-validated by flow cytometry, though NGS and ddPCR are gaining increasing traction, particularly in cases characterized by marked biological heterogeneity. CML monitoring continues to rely principally on conventional qRT-PCR, yet digital PCR for BCR::ABL1 can resolve deeper molecular responses—up to MR5—which is particularly relevant to predicting durable treatment-free remission. In lymphoma, imaging modalities and flow cytometric immunophenotyping remain the primary clinical tools, but cfDNA-based liquid biopsy is emerging as a promising non-invasive adjunct, offering high sensitivity and the capacity to detect clonal evolution through NGS.

Bibliography

1. Radich J. Introduction to the series on measurable residual disease. Haematologica. 2022;107(12):2782. https://doi.org/10.3324/haematol.2022.281079.
2. Riva G, Luppi M, Tagliafico E. From gating to computational flow cytometry: exploiting artificial intelligence for MRD diagnostics. Br J Haematol. 2023;202(4):715–7. https://doi.org/10.1111/bjh.18833.
3. Riva G, Nasillo V, Ottomano AM, et al. Multiparametric flow cytometry for MRD monitoring in hematologic malignancies: clinical applications and new challenges. Cancers (Basel). 2021;13(18):4582.
4. Tembhare PR, Subramanian PG, Ghogale S, et al. A high-sensitivity 10-color flow cytometric minimal residual disease assay in B-lymphoblastic leukemia/lymphoma can easily achieve the sensitivity of 2-in-10^6 and is superior to standard minimal residual disease assay: a study of 622 patients. Cytometry B Clin Cytom. 2020;98(1):57–67.
5. Tembhare PR, Chatterjee G, Khanka T, et al. Eleven-marker 10-color flow cytometric assessment of measurable residual disease for T-cell acute lymphoblastic leukemia using an approach of exclusion. Cytometry B Clin Cytom. 2021;100(4):421–33.
6. Tettero JM, Freeman S, Buecklein V, et al. Technical aspects of flow cytometry-based measurable residual disease quantification in acute myeloid leukemia: experience of the European LeukemiaNet MRD working party. Hema. 2021;6(1):e676.
7. Teixeira A, Carreira L, Abalde-Cela S, et al. Current and emerging techniques for diagnosis and MRD detection in AML: a comprehensive narrative review. Cancer. 2023;15(5):1362.
8. Patkar N, Kakirde C, Shaikh AF, et al. Clinical impact of panel-based error-corrected next generation sequencing versus flow cytometry to detect measurable residual disease (MRD) in acute myeloid leukemia (AML). Leukemia. 2021;35(5):1392–404.
9. Blachly JS, Walter RB, Hourigan CS. The present and future of measurable residual disease testing in acute myeloid leukemia. Haematologica. 2022;107(12):2810–22.
10. Kegyes D, Thiagarajan PS, Ghiaur G. MRD in acute Leukemias: lessons learned from acute Promyelocytic leukemia. Cancers (Basel). 2024;16(18):3208.
11. Chandra DJ, Lachowiez CA, Loghavi S. Practical considerations in clinical application of WHO 5th and ICC classification schemes for acute myeloid leukemia. Blood Rev. 2024;64:101156.
12. Chen H, Gu M, Liang J, et al. Minimal residual disease detection by next-generation sequencing of different immunoglobulin gene rearrangements in pediatric B-ALL. Nat Commun. 2023;14:7468.
13. Heuser M, Freeman SD, Ossenkoppele GJ, et al. 2021 update on MRD in acute myeloid leukemia: a consensus document from the European LeukemiaNet MRD working party. Blood. 2021;138(26):2753–67.
14. Cordone I, Amodeo R, Bellesi S, et al. Consensus for flow cytometry clinical report on multiple myeloma: a multicenter harmonization process merging laboratory experience and clinical needs. Cancers (Basel). 2023;15(7):2060.
15. Medina-Herrera A, Sarasquete ME, Jiménez C, et al. Minimal residual disease in multiple myeloma: past, present, and future. Cancers (Basel). 2023;15(14):3687.
16. Yee AJ, Raje N. Minimal residual disease in multiple myeloma: why, when, where. Hematology Am Soc Hematol Educ Program. 2021;2021(1):37–45.
17. Kumar S, Paiva B, Anderson KC, et al. International myeloma working group consensus criteria for response and minimal residual disease assessment in multiple myeloma. Lancet Oncol. 2016;17(8):e328–46.

18. Wierda WG, Rawstron A, Cymbalista F, et al. Measurable residual disease in chronic lymphocytic leukemia: expert review and consensus recommendations. Leukemia. 2021;35:3059–72.
19. Del Giudice I, Foà R. Measurable residual disease in chronic lymphocytic leukemia. Where do we stand? Leukemia. 2023;37(12):2339–42.
20. Zhang S, Wang X, Yang Z, et al. Minimal residual disease detection in lymphoma: methods, procedures and clinical significance. Front Immunol. 2024;15:1430070.
21. Cross NCP, Ernst T, Branford S, et al. European LeukemiaNet laboratory recommendations for the diagnosis and management of chronic myeloid leukemia. Leukemia. 2023;37:2150–67.
22. Branford S, Apperley JF. Measurable residual disease in chronic myeloid leukemia. Haematologica. 2022;107(12):2794–809.

Part III
Hemostasis & Thrombosis

Chapter 16
Spectrum of Coagulation Factor Deficiencies and the Approach to Diagnosis

Debadrita Ray, Narender Kumar, and Jasmina Ahluwalia

Abstract Coagulation factor deficiencies, which can be inherited or acquired, disrupt the intricate process of hemostasis, leading to bleeding disorders. Inherited deficiencies result from genetic mutations affecting coagulation factor synthesis or function, while acquired deficiencies are more common and arise from factors such as diminished hepatic synthesis, vitamin K deficiency, or increased consumption. In this manuscript, we elaborate on the coagulation pathways, specific factor deficiencies, and the various laboratory tests to detect those entities. Each deficiency is characterized by varying degrees of bleeding severity, specific clinical manifestations, and unique laboratory findings. Effective diagnosis requires a systematic approach, including a detailed clinical history, standardized bleeding assessment tools, and coagulation screening tests such as PT and APTT. Mixing studies and specific factor assays are crucial for differentiating between factor deficiencies and inhibitors. A thorough understanding of these deficiencies is essential for accurate diagnosis and appropriate management.

Keywords Coagulation factors · Bleeding · Laboratory diagnosis · Algorithm

Learning Objectives
- Coagulation factors and their functions.
- History taking and clinical examination in patients with bleeding due to coagulation factor deficiencies.
- Understanding laboratory tests for the diagnosis of bleeding disorders.
- Algorithmic approach to the investigation of bleeding disorders.

D. Ray · N. Kumar · J. Ahluwalia (✉)
Department of Hematology, Postgraduate Institute of Medical Education and Research, Chandigarh, India

H. P. Pati et al. (eds.), *Clinical Hematology and Hemato-Oncology*,
https://doi.org/10.1007/978-981-92-1167-8_16

16.1 Introduction

Hemostasis is a highly regulated physiological process that ensures vascular integrity following injury through the formation of a stable fibrin clot. This dynamic interaction involves endothelial cells, platelets, von Willebrand factor (vWF), and coagulation factors. The coagulation cascade follows a sequential activation of coagulation factors on phospholipid surfaces, primarily platelets or damaged endothelial cells, culminating in covalently cross-linked fibrin to stabilize the platelet plug [1, 2].

16.2 Coagulation Factors

Coagulation factors exist predominantly as inactive zymogens, undergoing proteolytic activation when required, e.g., Factor IX (FIX), Factor II (FII). Cofactors such as tissue factor (TF), Factor V (FV), and Factor VIII (FVIII) facilitate the proteolytic activity of coagulation enzymes on TF-expressing cells, including endothelial cells and platelets. Fibrinogen is the substrate for clot formation, whereas Factor XIII (FXIII) acts as a transglutaminase that enhances fibrin stabilization [1].

The liver is the principal site of coagulation factor synthesis. FII, FV, FVII, FIX, FX, FXI, and FXII are produced in the liver, whereas FVIII is synthesized predominantly by hepatic sinusoidal endothelial cells. Notably, FII, FVII, FIX, and FX undergo post-translational γ-carboxylation, which is vitamin K-dependent and essential for their physiological function [1, 2].

16.3 Classification of Coagulation Factor Deficiencies

Coagulation factor deficiencies can be classified into two broad categories: inherited and acquired.

16.3.1 Acquired Coagulation Factor Deficiencies

Acquired deficiencies are more prevalent than their inherited counterparts and primarily arise due to:

- *Diminished hepatic synthesis*, as observed in liver disease
- *Impaired biosynthesis* secondary to vitamin K deficiency
- *Accelerated consumption or destruction*, seen in conditions such as disseminated intravascular coagulation (DIC) and thrombolytic therapy
- *Autoantibody-mediated neutralization* leading to factor depletion [3]

16.3.2 Inherited Coagulation Factor Deficiencies

Inherited coagulation disorders result from genetic mutations affecting the synthesis or function of specific coagulation factors, leading to an increased propensity for bleeding. The clinical severity varies depending on the degree of factor deficiency.

16.4 Coagulation Pathways

The cell-based model of coagulation is useful to understand the role of cells and cell surfaces, generation, amplification, and propagation of coagulation. However, the traditional coagulation cascade is often resorted to for interpreting lab tests in the workup of bleeding disorders. This is delineated into three interconnected pathways:

1. *Extrinsic pathway*
2. *Intrinsic pathway*
3. *Common pathway*

Thrombin generation is a crucial endpoint in coagulation, where fibrinogen is proteolytically converted to fibrin. FXIII-mediated fibrin cross-linking further stabilizes the fibrin clot.

16.5 Isolated Extrinsic Pathway Defect: FVII Deficiency

Factor VII (FVII) deficiency is probably the commonest among the "rare" inherited bleeding disorders, typically following an autosomal recessive inheritance pattern, though with incomplete penetrance [4]. It forms a common clinical consult in a patient with usually no prior history of bleeding, noticed to have a prolonged Prothrombin Time (PT).

A key characteristic of FVII deficiency is the weak relationship between the measured levels of FVII in the plasma and the observed bleeding tendencies. Clinically, this presents as a wide range of outcomes, where individuals carrying only one affected gene copy (heterozygotes) can experience significant bleeding, while those with two affected copies (homozygotes) and very low FVII levels may show no symptoms. The severity of bleeding in FVII-deficient individuals varies considerably, with roughly 30% reporting no history of bleeding.

Common clinical signs include mucocutaneous bleeding, such as nasal bleeds, easy bruising, gum bleeding, as well as heavy menstrual bleeding in approximately 50–60% of affected women. The pattern of bleeding varies among individuals affected by this deficiency. Notably, mucocutaneous bleeding is more often seen in heterozygotes with mild to moderate FVII deficiency [4, 5].

Women in their reproductive period appear to have a higher likelihood of experiencing bleeding symptoms. These gynecological symptoms include heavy menstrual bleeding (reported in 50–69% of women), bleeding before and after childbirth, and irregular periods. Heavy menstrual bleeding is the initial bleeding symptom in 12% of cases.

Gastrointestinal bleeding and bleeding into deep tissues, including hematomas and joint bleeds, can occur in FVII deficiency and are more frequently observed in individuals with severe forms of the deficiency [5].

The preferred replacement treatment for patients with FVII deficiency who require it is recombinant factor VIIa (rFVIIa) concentrate. However, plasma-derived concentrate can be used if the recombinant form is not available. Fresh frozen plasma is another option if rFVIIa is inaccessible, but its use involves risks such as the transmission of viruses and fluid overload. Prothrombin complex concentrate is a less commonly used alternative treatment.

16.6 Intrinsic Pathway Defects: Contact Activation System

The intrinsic system initiates coagulation via FXII, which undergoes autoactivation upon exposure to anionic surfaces, such as subendothelial collagen. This cascade involves:

- Plasma prekallikrein conversion to kallikrein.
- FXII activation, resulting in FXIIa-mediated cleavage of FXI.
- FXIa activation of FIX, subsequently forming the intrinsic tenase complex with FVIIIa, leading to thrombin generation and clot formation.

The contact activation system is implicated in thrombotic processes but is nonessential for physiological hemostasis. It interacts with inflammatory, fibrinolytic, and complement pathways.

16.7 FXII and Other Contact Factor Deficiencies

Deficiencies in contact factors, including FXII, prekallikrein (Fletcher factor), and high molecular weight kininogen, follow an autosomal recessive inheritance pattern. These deficiencies often result in markedly prolonged activated partial thromboplastin time (aPTT) but do not contribute to haemorrhagic phenotypes [4]. Severe FXII deficiency is rare and typically discovered incidentally during tests for various coagulation parameters.

16.8 Other Intrinsic Pathway Factor Deficiencies

FXI deficiency, previously termed hemophilia C, is characterized by autosomal inheritance with variable penetrance. It is a rare bleeding disorder that presents complexities in patient assessment and bleeding risk management. While generally associated with mild to moderate bleeding symptoms, clinical manifestations are variable, and bleeding tendency does not consistently correlate with FXI plasma levels or genotype.

The prevalence of severe FXI deficiency is estimated to be approximately one in one million. However, it exhibits a higher prevalence in some populations [5].

Severe FXI deficiency is defined by an activity level of less than 20%, most commonly found in homozygotes or compound heterozygotes. Heterozygotes typically demonstrate FXI activity levels of 20–60%. Patients with FXI deficiency typically present with an elevated activated partial thromboplastin time (aPTT). Generally, aPTT prolongation is observed when the FXI activity level is reduced to less than 30%. While a normal aPTT can exclude severe FXI deficiency, it may not detect partial deficiency (FXI activity 20–60%) [6].

However, the bleeding tendency in FXI deficiency is generally mild, even in cases of severe deficiency. Clinical symptoms include bleeding provoked by surgical hemostatic challenge, post-injury bleeding, epistaxis, and heavy menstrual bleeding. Surgical procedures involving areas with high fibrinolytic activity, such as the urogenital tract or the oropharyngeal cavity (tonsillectomy/dental extraction), appear to correlate with the highest bleeding risk (49–67%). In contrast to severe FVIII or FIX deficiency, unprovoked bleeding episodes such as hemarthroses, muscle bleeds, or soft tissue bleeds are not frequently observed in severe FXI deficiency.

Importantly, the bleeding phenotype demonstrates a lack of correlation with the FXI activity level, with bleeding reported in heterozygotes with mild deficiency (FXI levels 20–60%) [5]. This lack of correlation between bleeding risk and FXI activity levels poses a significant therapeutic challenge.

FVIII and FIX Deficiencies

Hemophilia A (HA) and Hemophilia B (HB) are X-linked recessive bleeding disorders resulting from pathogenic variants in the genes encoding FVIII and FIX, respectively. HA exhibits a higher prevalence (approximately 1 in 5000 male live births) compared to HB (approximately 1 in 30,000 male live births) [7].

The clinical severity of hemophilia is classified based on the functional plasma levels of FVIII or FIX. Severe hemophilia is defined by factor activity less than 1%, moderate hemophilia by factor activity between 1% and 5%, and mild hemophilia by factor activity between 5% and 40% [8]. Individuals with severe hemophilia frequently experience spontaneous hemorrhages into joints (hemarthrosis), muscles, or soft tissues, and are at risk for life-threatening bleeding episodes, including intracranial hemorrhage. In contrast, individuals with mild or moderate factor deficiency typically experience bleeding only following trauma or invasive procedures, with spontaneous hemorrhages being infrequent. While residual factor activity generally correlates with the clinical phenotype, inter-individual variability in bleeding manifestations can occur among patients with similar factor levels.

Furthermore, the nature of the genetic variant in the FVIII (HA) and FIX (HB) genes influences residual factor activity and the bleeding diathesis. Generally, larger gene defects are associated with more severe clinical phenotypes. The spectrum of mutations identified in FVIII and FIX includes point mutations, deletions, insertions, rearrangements, or inversions. The relative frequencies of these mutation types differ between HA and HB. Notably, gross genetic abnormalities account for approximately 7% of HB cases, whereas severe HA gene rearrangements, particularly intron 22 inversion, constitute nearly half of the observed defects.

The primary therapeutic strategy for HA and HB involves replacement therapy with FVIII or FIX concentrates, respectively. A significant complication of this treatment is the development of high-affinity neutralizing antibodies (inhibitors) against the infused clotting factor. Inhibitor development against FVIII occurs in approximately 25–30% of patients with severe HA [9], while it is less frequent in HB, occurring in 3–5% of treated patients. Some data suggests that the specific mutation type may also govern the risk of inhibitor development in addition to clinical risk factors like the type and dose of factor replacement [10]. Immune tolerance induction (ITI), nonfactor replacement therapies, and emicizumab remain the approach for inhibitor eradication [11].

16.9 Common Pathway Factor Deficiencies

FII, V, & X deficiencies are uncommon autosomal disorders that present with simultaneous PT and aPTT prolongation.

FII Deficiency

It is a rare inherited coagulation disorder with an estimated prevalence of approximately 1 in 2,000,000 [12, 13]. Two distinct phenotypes are recognized: Type I deficiency (hypoprothrombinemia): This condition is characterized by a concomitant decrease in both the functional activity and antigenic levels of the prothrombin zymogen. Type II deficiency (dysprothrombinemia): In this condition, prothrombin antigen levels are normal or nearly normal. However, it exhibits impaired functional activity [12]. Severe FII deficiency, where plasma levels are less than 5% in homozygous patients, consistently leads to severe bleeding. This includes prolonged bleeding post-injury, mucosal bleeding, and subcutaneous or muscle hematomas. Menorrhagia is a common symptom in homozygous female patients. Heterozygous individuals with FII plasma levels between 30% and 60% are typically asymptomatic. However, excessive bleeding may occur following moderate trauma, tooth extractions, or surgical procedures. Patients with dysprothrombinemia show variable bleeding tendencies, generally less severe than in Type I deficiency. In some dysprothrombinemia, a significant discrepancy exists between coagulation test results and the severity of bleeding. Most FII mutations are missense mutations

(80%), although insertions/deletions (10%), nonsense mutations (6%), and splice site mutations (4%) have also been reported [14].

FV Deficiency

FV is a glycoprotein cofactor essential for hemostasis, participating in both coagulation and anticoagulant pathways. Congenital FV deficiency is a rare bleeding disorder with an incidence of 1 per million live births for the severe homozygous form. However, the incidence is higher in geographical areas with increased consanguinity. Homozygotes or compound heterozygotes typically exhibit FV plasma levels below 10%, whereas heterozygous individuals with mild to moderate FV deficiency usually have plasma levels around 50% [15].

FV deficiency is classified as: Type I (Quantitative): The most common form, characterized by a concordant reduction or absence of both FV antigen and functional plasma levels. Type II (Qualitative): It is characterized by dysfunctional FV with normal or mildly reduced antigen plasma levels and diminished coagulant activity. The clinical presentation of congenital FV deficiency varies widely, ranging from mild to severe hemorrhages. Predominant clinical manifestations include mucosal bleeding, such as epistaxis, oral cavity bleeding, hematemesis, melena, hematuria, and menorrhagia in females. Hemarthroses and deep hematomas are less frequent. Serious internal bleeding, including gastrointestinal and intracranial hemorrhage, is rare.

Laboratory and clinical studies indicate that FV activity levels above 15% to 20% of normal are sufficient for effective hemostasis. Consequently, heterozygotes with FV levels between 25% and 60% are typically asymptomatic. In contrast, homozygotes and compound heterozygotes (FV level less than 10%) may present with a spectrum of bleeding symptoms, from minimal to severe. Notably, there is a weak correlation between residual FV levels and bleeding phenotype; some patients with low FV levels are asymptomatic. This phenomenon appears to correlate with the presence of sufficient hemostatically active platelet FV, which can locally generate enough thrombin to prevent bleeding [15]. Platelet-released FV demonstrates greater resistance to activated protein C (APC) cleavage and higher cofactor activity compared to plasma FV. Furthermore, patients with FV deficiency have reduced levels of tissue factor pathway inhibitor (TFPI), which decreases the FV requirement for thrombin generation.

Assessment of concomitant FVIII activity is recommended to rule out combined FV and FVIII deficiency, a rare inherited disorder resulting from genetic variants in LMAN1 or MCFD2, genes encoding proteins involved in intracellular transport of FV and FVIII [16].

FX Deficiency

FX deficiency is a rare inherited coagulation disorder characterized by autosomal recessive inheritance. The clinical phenotype presents as a variable bleeding tendency. Homozygous FX deficiency has an estimated incidence of 1 in 1,000,000 within the general population [17]. Heterozygous individuals are frequently clinically asymptomatic. Acquired FX deficiency is uncommon and is typically associated with amyloidosis. Individuals with FX deficiency may exhibit a bleeding tendency at any age, with more severely affected individuals demonstrating reduced FX activity.

16.10 FXIII Deficiency

The zymogen FXIII consists of two catalytic A subunits (FXIII-A) and two carrier/protective B subunits (FXIII-B). FXIII-A is produced by cells of bone marrow origin, whereas FXIII-B is synthesized by hepatocytes and forms complexes in the plasma [18].

Inherited FXIII deficiency is a rare autosomal recessive bleeding disorder with an estimated prevalence of one in one to three million individuals. Severe disease is typically observed in homozygotes or compound heterozygotes.

This deficiency also manifests in two primary forms: Type I, a quantitative defect resulting from reduced protein synthesis, and Type II, characterized by a normal or near-normal concentration of a functionally impaired FXIII-A subunit.

Severe congenital FXIII-A deficiency is associated with significant hemorrhagic events, and intracranial hemorrhage is a major cause of mortality. A classic early clinical indicator of this condition is delayed umbilical stump bleeding. Other preferential sites for severe bleeding include muscle and subcutaneous soft tissues. Notably, life-threatening bleeding episodes can occur unexpectedly even after prolonged periods without major bleeding, underscoring the necessity of prophylactic replacement therapy upon confirmation of severe congenital FXIII deficiency, regardless of patient age [19].

Furthermore, FXIII-A deficiency is frequently linked to impaired wound healing and can lead to abortion in pregnant women. Recurrent spontaneous abortions, even with only moderate bleeding symptoms, warrant investigation for underlying FXIII-A deficiency [20]. Severe FXIII-B deficiency is exceedingly rare, with only a few reported cases, and is characterized by milder bleeding symptoms compared to FXIII-A deficiency.

16.11 Fibrinogen Deficiency

Congenital fibrinogen disorders (CFDs) are rare conditions, representing approximately 8% of rare bleeding disorders. These disorders arise from mutations in the FGA, FGB, or FGG genes, resulting in qualitative and/or quantitative defects in fibrinogen [21].

The clinical manifestations of CFDs are heterogeneous, spanning a spectrum from asymptomatic individuals to patients exhibiting bleeding symptoms of varying severity, including easy bruising, menorrhagia, epistaxis, post-partum hemorrhage, post-surgical bleeding, gastrointestinal bleeding, and rarely, intracranial haemorrhage [22, 23].

Notably, patients with CFDs can also present with thrombotic events; both arterial and venous thrombosis have been reported in up to 20% of patients. Several factors are implicated in the pathophysiology of thrombosis in CFDs, including the absence or reduction of antithrombin-like properties of fibrinogen γ' and the production of clots with abnormal fibrin structure.

Due to incomplete penetrance, CFDs may be diagnosed incidentally during routine coagulation assays or during evaluation for a positive family history. It is important to note that even asymptomatic individuals with CFDs, particularly those diagnosed at a young age, may have an increased risk of future bleeding and/or thrombosis, depending on the specific CFD. Global fibrinolysis assays are increasingly utilized in clinical practice; however, their inherent limitations pose a challenge in diagnosing disorders involving clot instability and enhanced fibrinolysis.

Fibrinogen concentrates can be employed to achieve hemostatic control in both congenital and acquired fibrinogen disorders, depending on the clinical context.

16.12 Laboratory Approach to a Patient with a Coagulation Factor Deficiency

An effective and logical approach to evaluating clotting disorders should integrate both laboratory evidence and clinical expertise. This approach must embrace the patient's clinical presentation, their personal and family history of bleeding, and the diagnostic tests available either on-site or at a specialized center. Although standardized testing algorithms are often useful, some cases may need a more tailored evaluation strategy [24].

16.13 Importance of Clinical History

The initial assessment of a patient suspected of having an inherited bleeding disorder should begin with a thorough review of both personal and family bleeding history. The use of standardized bleeding assessment tools (BATs), developed by the International Society on Thrombosis and Haemostasis (ISTH), is fundamental for evaluating the likelihood of a bleeding disorder. The score incorporates the number of bleeding episodes and the degree of medical intervention required to control them. Common reference values for the ISTH-BAT are ≤ 3 in males, ≤ 5 in females, and ≤ 2 in children [25].

The history should help differentiate between spontaneous and provoked bleeding, identify the age at which symptoms first appeared, and note the context of symptom onset, especially if triggered by interventions like surgery. Clinicians should record the location, nature (e.g., oozing vs. profuse), duration, and severity of bleeding episodes, including whether medical interventions like transfusions were necessary. Specific inquiries should include details about easy bruising, recurrent nosebleeds, and abnormal bleeding following minor injuries or surgeries. History of existing co-morbid disorders like liver disease, DIC, use of drugs, especially NSAIDs for rheumatological disorders, prolonged antibiotic use related to vitamin K deficiency in patients, massively transfused trauma patients, coexisting pregnancy or postpartum state, all of which may confound the lab results.

In females, a detailed menstrual history is crucial. Subjective descriptions such as "light" or "heavy" are insufficient. Instead, clinicians should document age at menarche, any excessive bleeding at onset, duration of menstruation, number of sanitary products used on peak flow days, frequency of changing products, and use of combined protection (pads and tampons). A report of needing to change a pad or tampon more often than every 3 h, or using more than 3–5 pads per day for more than 1 day, may indicate an underlying bleeding disorder. Recent evidence suggests that normal ISTH-BAT scores in women may vary with age, and incorporating age-adjusted cut-offs could improve diagnostic accuracy in adult females [26].

A detailed family history should include any known bleeding disorders, along with relevant symptoms. However, clinicians should be cautious when relying on self-reported or family-reported diagnoses such as hemophilia or von Willebrand disease, as these may be inaccurate or misinterpreted. While physical examination can occasionally support the clinical assessment, its utility may be limited in some cases. Structured bleeding assessment tools, which include targeted questions as outlined earlier, can help quantify bleeding symptoms and improve the identification of potential inherited bleeding disorders [27]. Bleeding from a solitary site (epistaxis or uterine bleeding) may be due to an anatomical cause. However, both an anatomical cause and a coagulation factor deficiency may coexist. Caution should be exercised in testing patients who have recently been transfused with plasma, since these may alter the results of coagulation tests. Uncommonly, some coagulation factor deficiencies may predispose to thrombosis, e.g., Factor XII and fibrinogen.

16.14 Initial Coagulation Screening in Coagulation Factor Deficiencies

All patients suspected of having a clotting disorder should undergo initial coagulation screening. Standard practice includes the measurement of prothrombin time (PT) and activated partial thromboplastin time (APTT) to identify coagulation abnormalities and to establish a baseline in anticipation of possible bleeding. PT

Table 16.1 Differential diagnosis of coagulation screening test results in clotting disorders

Coagulation test result	Possible differential diagnoses
↑ PT, normal APTT	Early vitamin K deficiency Liver disease (early/mild)—Factor VII deficiency
↑ APTT, normal PT	Hemophilia A or B (factor VIII or IX deficiency) Factor XI deficiency—Contact factor deficiency (e.g., prekallikrein, HMWK, factor XII—Not associated with bleeding) Von Willebrand disease, especially type 3 and type 2 N VWD
↑ PT and ↑ APTT	Vitamin K deficiency (advanced) Common pathway factor deficiencies (e.g., factor X, V, II, or fibrinogen)
↑ Thrombin time (TT)	Hypofibrinogenemia or dysfibrinogenemia
↓ Fibrinogen	Congenital hypofibrinogenemia
Normal PT and APTT	Factor XIII deficiency Von Willebrand disease Platelet function defect or thrombocytopenia

and APTT assess the extrinsic and intrinsic pathways, respectively, and are typically conducted on citrated, platelet-free plasma using automated analyzers. Among inherited bleeding disorders, APTT is often more informative, as around 98% of these conditions involve deficiencies in factors assessed by the intrinsic pathway. In addition, initial workup should include thrombin time (TT) or Clauss fibrinogen assay to detect abnormalities in fibrinogen. Thrombin time is especially important in samples collected from inpatients, where heparin contamination from an indwelling line may lead to an inhibitor pattern. Although PT and APTT are valuable tools in identifying most coagulation abnormalities, they are not sufficient to detect all disorders. Factor XIII deficiency and von Willebrand disease (VWD) may go unnoticed. Therefore, incorporating a clot solubility test (e.g., in 5 M urea or 2% monochloroacetic acid) for severe FXIII deficiency and VWF assays enhances the sensitivity of the screening and broadens the diagnostic scope [28]. A summary of coagulation defects and corresponding test abnormalities is provided in Table 16.1.

16.15 Mixing Studies and Inhibitor Screening

When coagulation screening tests are prolonged, mixing studies are a key next step in identifying the underlying cause: factor deficiency or inhibitor. In this, patient plasma (PP) is mixed in equal parts (1:1) with normal plasma (NP), and the affected clotting test (either PT or APTT) is repeated on the mixture. If the result is corrected to normal, this suggests a clotting factor deficiency (Figs. 16.1 and 16.2).

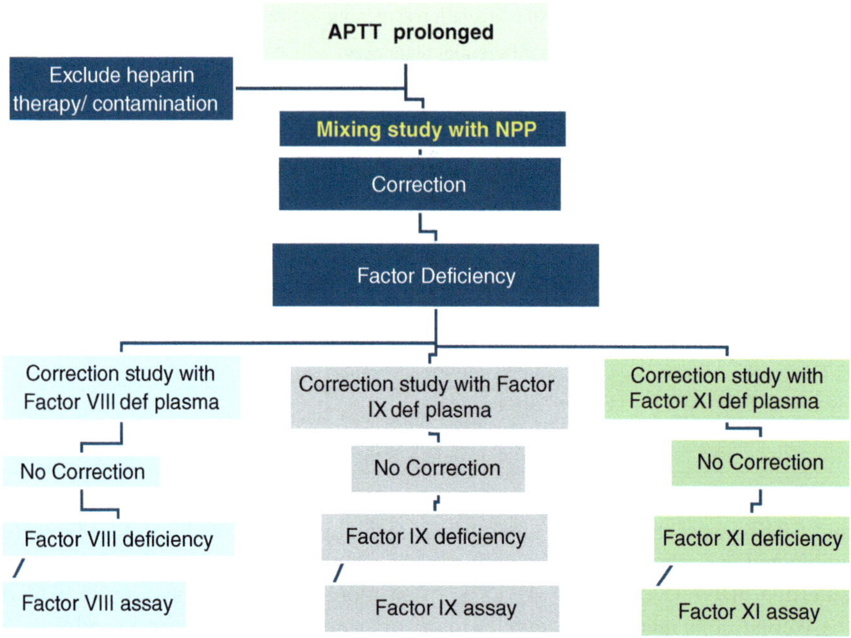

Fig. 16.1 Algorithm for laboratory workup of cases with isolated prolonged aPTT

If it does not correct, an inhibitor is likely to be present. To further pinpoint which factor is deficient, additional mixing can be performed using aged serum or adsorbed plasma, which contain different sets of coagulation factors. However, the use of factor-deficient plasma has become more prevalent in modern practice, as it offers a direct means of identifying specific factor deficiencies. Table 16.2 provides a detailed overview of how various reagents assist in interpreting mixing study results.

In certain cases, the mixing study does not lead to correction of prolonged clotting times, indicating the likely presence of an inhibitor rather than a simple factor deficiency. In such scenarios, further testing is required to distinguish between non-specific inhibitors, such as lupus anticoagulant (LA), and specific inhibitors, like antibodies targeting Factor VIII or IX, which can lead to significant bleeding

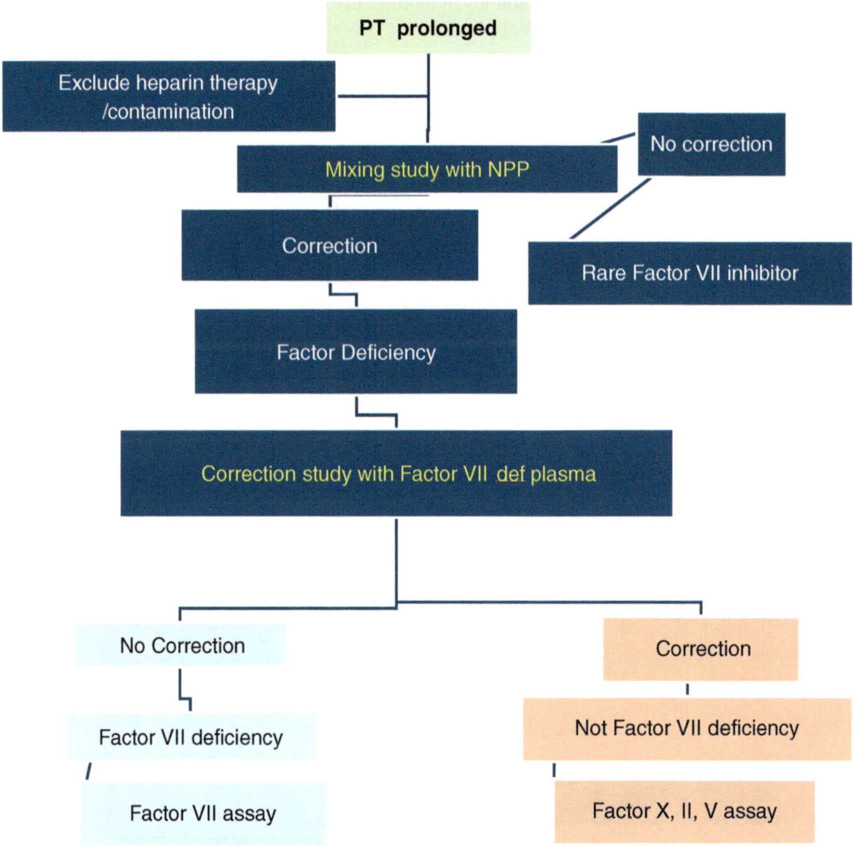

Fig. 16.2 Algorithm for laboratory workup of cases with isolated prolonged PT

episodes. A detailed clinical history, especially concerning previous treatments, can aid in raising suspicion of inhibitor development. For isolated prolongation of APTT, an inhibitor screen is conducted using a 1:1 mixture of patient plasma (PP) and normal pooled plasma (NPP). The APTT is measured immediately (0 h) and after 2 h of incubation at 37 °C. If the clotting time initially corrects but becomes prolonged after incubation, this pattern suggests a time-dependent inhibitor, commonly seen with Factor VIII inhibitors. If prolongation persists at both time points, an immediate-acting inhibitor is likely, such as lupus anticoagulant, Factor IX inhibitors, or high-titer Factor VIII inhibitors [29] (Fig. 16.3).

Table 16.2 Interpretation of mixing studies in clotting disorders using normal plasma, adsorbed plasma, aged serum, and factor-deficient plasmas

Test/material used	Test performed	Corrects deficiency in	Does not correct deficiency in
50:50 mix (normal plasma)	PT, APTT	Most clotting factor deficiencies (except inhibitors)	Time-dependent inhibitors, lupus anticoagulant
Aged serum	PT, APTT	VII, IX, X, XI, XII	V, VIII
Adsorbed plasma	PT, APTT	I (fibrinogen), V, VIII, XI, XII	II, VII, IX, X
Factor VIII-deficient plasma	APTT	Corrects all except factor VIII deficiency	Factor VIII deficiency
Factor IX-deficient plasma	APTT	Corrects all except factor IX deficiency	Factor IX deficiency
Factor XI-deficient plasma	APTT	Corrects all except factor XI deficiency	Factor XI deficiency
Factor V-deficient plasma	PT, APTT	Corrects all except factor V deficiency	Factor V deficiency
Factor X-deficient plasma	PT, APTT	Corrects all except factor X deficiency	Factor X deficiency
Factor II-deficient plasma	PT, APTT	Corrects all except factor II deficiency	Factor II deficiency
Factor VII-deficient plasma	PT	Corrects all except factor VII deficiency	Factor VII deficiency

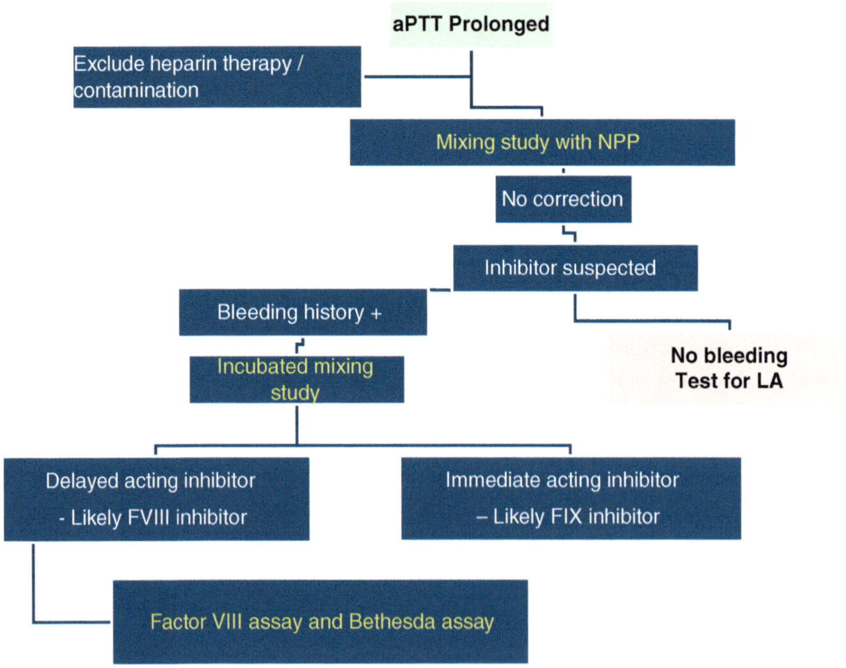

Fig. 16.3 Algorithm for laboratory workup of cases with isolated prolonged aPTT and suspected presence of inhibitor

16.16 Confirmatory Investigations for the Coagulation Factor Deficiencies

Confirmatory tests for clotting disorders typically involve individual clotting factor assays, with the choice of test depending on the results of initial coagulation screening and mixing studies. In many well-funded centers, the mixing study is often bypassed, and direct factor assays are performed.

Clotting factors can be assessed using either functional or antigenic assays. The results are usually reported as percentages of normal activity, with a pooled plasma from healthy individuals being assigned a value of 100%, or as units per milliliter (1 U/mL = 100%). Functional assays are preferred and fall into two categories: clot-based assays, which assess clotting factor activity by measuring clotting time in plasma deficient in the specific factor, and chromogenic assays, which activate the factor to its active enzyme form and mix it with a chromogenic substrate. This substrate, upon cleavage, produces a color change. Antigenic assays, although less commonly requested, are primarily conducted in reference laboratories. However, antigenic assays for von Willebrand factor (vWF) and Factor XIII antigen are commonly performed in many coagulation labs using automated analyzers [30].

16.17 Illustrative Case Studies

16.17.1 Clinical Case 1

A 23-year-old female presented with hematuria of a month's duration. She had no history of any other bleeding episodes. There was no history of recent jaundice, drug intake, or blood transfusions. There was no consanguinity in the parents. She had anemia (Hb 89g/L), and a marginal platelet count -118×10^9/l. The liver function tests and renal function tests were unremarkable. Coagulation tests:

PT 37- s (normal 10–13 s), aPTT -38 s (normal 25–35 s), fibrinogen assay: 3.26 g/l (normal 1.5-4 g/l)

A mixing test was done on PT in a mix of 1:1 PP (patient plasma) and NPP (normal pooled plasma). The results of further testing are shown below.

	PT (seconds)	Interpretation	Remark
Patient plasma (PP)	37	Prolonged	
Normal pooled plasma (NPP)	11		
PP + NPP	13	Shows correction.	Suggests a factor deficiency
PP + FVII-deficient plasma	19	Partial correction	Not factor VII deficiency
PP + FII-deficient plasma	14.6	Partial correction	Not factor II deficiency
PP + FV-deficient plasma	15.2	Partial correction	Not factor V deficiency
PP+ FX-deficient plasma	44.6	No correction	Suggestive of factor X deficiency

Factor assays were done to confirm the results of the mixing studies
Factor X assay—4.1% (normal—77–11%)
Factor VII assay—50% (normal—50–129%)
Factor V assay—116% (normal—62–139%)

Diagnosis: Factor X Deficiency
Mixing tests can be performed on both aPTT and PT, depending on the availability of plasma. Mixing with specific factor-deficient plasmas, like factor II, V, VII, X deficient plasmas, may not show clotting times of the mix within reference ranges; however, most often they do reduce. The likely deficiency is indicated by the deficient plasma with which the clotting time does not shorten or even prolongs (i.e., Factor X in this case). Despite very low levels of Factor X, the patient did not have a history of bleeding in childhood, which is well known in rare bleeding disorders.

16.17.2 Clinical Case 2

An 8-year-old boy presented with a history of recurrent sore throats with fever and was found to have markedly enlarged tonsils. An ENT consultation was sought, and an adenotonsillectomy was advised. At the preanesthetic evaluation, there was no history of a bleeding disorder; however, screening coagulation tests were ordered. The results were

PT -13 s (normal 10–13 s).
aPTT -106 s (normal 25–35 s).
Fibrinogen assay: 3.26 g/l (normal 1.5–4 g/l).

A mixing test was done on aPTT in a mix of 1:1 PP (patient plasma) and NPP (normal pooled plasma).

The results of further testing are shown below.

	aPTT (seconds)	Interpretation	Remark
Patient plasma (PP)	106	Prolonged	
Normal pooled plasma (NPP)	27		
PP + NPP	32	Shows correction	Suggests a factor deficiency
PP + FVIII-deficient plasma	39	Partial correction	Not factor VIII deficiency
PP + FIX-deficient plasma	39	Partial correction	Not factor IX deficiency
PP + XI-deficient plasma	41	Partial correction	Not factor XI deficiency
PP+ FXII-deficient plasma	108	No correction	Suggestive of factor XII deficiency

Factor assays were done to confirm the results of the mixing studies
Factor VIII assay—98% (normal—60–160%), Factor IX assay—60% (normal—55–155%)
Factor XI assay—83% (normal—50–150%), Factor XII assay—9% (normal—50–150%)

Diagnosis: Factor XII Deficiency
Factor XII deficiency is associated with prolonged aPTT but no bleeding risk. This is frequently detected when coagulation testing is done as part of the workup for some other illness. It is more of a nuisance in the laboratory since its deficiency has no clinical relevance related to bleeding. While purchasing aPTT reagents for the lab, it is important to choose one that is insensitive or poorly sensitive to Factor XII deficiency to avoid unnecessary workup, expenditure, delay in treatment, and undue anxiety in patients.

Inherited coagulation factor deficiencies are rare. Laboratory workup is guided by a good bleeding history. Most coagulation factor deficiencies other than Factor XIII and VWF can be detected by simple coagulation screens. Confirmation by a factor assay is mandatory.

16.18 Conclusions

Coagulation factor deficiencies can lead to bleeding disorders. Deficiencies can be inherited, caused by genetic mutations, or acquired, resulting from factors such as liver disease, vitamin K deficiency, or increased consumption. Inherited coagulation factor deficiencies are rare. These deficiencies have a common clinical presentation, which necessitates the use of a systematic diagnostic approach, including clinical history, bleeding assessments, and coagulation tests, to accurately identify and manage these deficiencies.

References

1. Park S, Park JK. Back to basics: the coagulation pathway. Blood Res. 2024;59(1):35. https://doi.org/10.1007/s44313-024-00040-8.
2. Breen P. Basics of coagulation pathways. Int Anesthesiol Clin. 2004;42(3):1–9. https://doi.org/10.1097/00004311-200404230-00003.
3. Ogawa Y. Diagnosis and treatment of autoimmune acquired coagulation factor deficiency. Rinsho Ketsueki. 2023;64(9):1116–23. https://doi.org/10.11406/rinketsu.64.1116.
4. Demidova E, Salomashkina V, Pshenichnikova O, et al. Factor XII deficiency: a clinical and molecular genetic study. Int J Hematol. 2023;117(5):678–83. https://doi.org/10.1007/s12185-023-03535-9.
5. Lewandowska MD, Connors JM. Factor XI Deficiency. Hematol Oncol Clin North Am. 2021;35(6):1157–69. https://doi.org/10.1016/j.hoc.2021.07.012.
6. Bolton-Maggs PH. Factor XI deficiency--resolving the enigma? Hematology Am Soc Hematol Educ Program. 2009;2009:97–105. https://doi.org/10.1182/asheducation-2009.1.97.
7. Bolton-Maggs PH, Pasi KJ. Haemophilias A and B. Lancet. 2003;361(9371):1801–9. https://doi.org/10.1016/s0140-6736(03)13405-8.
8. Müller J, Miesbach W, Prüller F, Siegemund T, Scholz U, Sachs UJ. An update on laboratory diagnostics in Haemophilia A and B. Hamostaseologie. 2022;42(4):248–60. https://doi.org/10.1055/a-1665-6232.
9. Ray D, Kumar N, Hans C, et al. Inhibitor; an uncommon but vexing challenge in North Indian patients with hemophilia A. Indian J Hematol Blood Transfus. 2022;38(4):703–9. https://doi.org/10.1007/s12288-022-01539-9.
10. Ray D, Sharma R, Kumar N, et al. Unearthing the genotype-inhibitor phenotype association in severe haemophilia a: a North Indian cohort study. Haemophilia. 2024;30(2):410–8. https://doi.org/10.1111/hae.14948.
11. Pratt KP, Arruda VR, Lacroix-Desmazes S. Inhibitors-recent insights. Haemophilia. 2021;27(Suppl 3):28–36. https://doi.org/10.1111/hae.14077.
12. Lancellotti S, De Cristofaro R. Congenital prothrombin deficiency. Semin Thromb Hemost. 2009;35(4):367–81. https://doi.org/10.1055/s-0029-1225759.
13. Satyarthi P, Ray D, Kumar V, et al. Prothrombin G20210A mutation is rare but not absent among North Indian patients with thromboembolic events. Indian J Hematol Blood Transfus. 2024;40(3):522–6. https://doi.org/10.1007/s12288-024-01741-x.
14. Meeks SL, Abshire TC. Abnormalities of prothrombin: a review of the pathophysiology, diagnosis, and treatment. Haemophilia. 2008;14(6):1159–63. https://doi.org/10.1111/j.1365-2516.2008.01832.x.
15. Franchini M, Focosi D. Clinical, laboratory, and molecular aspects of factor V deficiency. Semin Thromb Hemost. 2025;51(2):111–5. https://doi.org/10.1055/s-0044-1789021.
16. Zheng C, Zhang B. Combined deficiency of coagulation factors V and VIII: an update. Semin Thromb Hemost. 2013;39(6):613–20. https://doi.org/10.1055/s-0033-1349223.
17. Uprichard J, Perry DJ. Factor X deficiency. Blood Rev. 2002;16(2):97–110. https://doi.org/10.1054/blre.2002.0191.
18. Biswas A, Ivaskevicius V, Thomas A, Oldenburg J. Coagulation factor XIII deficiency. Diagnosis, prevalence and management of inherited and acquired forms. Hamostaseologie. 2014;34(2):160–6. https://doi.org/10.5482/hamo-13-08-0046.

19. Pelcovits A, Schiffman F, Niroula R. Factor XIII deficiency: a review of clinical presentation and management. Hematol Oncol Clin North Am. 2021;35(6):1171–80. https://doi.org/10.1016/j.hoc.2021.07.009.
20. Levy JH, Greenberg C. Biology of factor XIII and clinical manifestations of factor XIII deficiency. Transfusion. 2013;53(5):1120–31. https://doi.org/10.1111/j.1537-2995.2012.03865.x.
21. John MJ, Byreddy P, Modak K, Makkar M. Congenital fibrinogen deficiency in India and role of human fibrinogen concentrate. Acta Haematol. 2021;144(6):595–602. https://doi.org/10.1159/000516339.
22. Casini A, de Moerloose P, Neerman-Arbez M. Clinical features and management of congenital fibrinogen deficiencies. Semin Thromb Hemost. 2016;42(4):366–74. https://doi.org/10.1055/s-0036-1571339.
23. Mohsenian S, Palla R, Menegatti M, et al. Congenital fibrinogen disorders: a retrospective clinical and genetic analysis of the Prospective Rare Bleeding Disorders Database. Blood Adv. 2024;8(6):1392–404. https://doi.org/10.1182/bloodadvances.2023012186.
24. Hayward CPM. How I investigate for bleeding disorders. Int J Lab Hematol. 2018;40(Suppl 1):6–14. https://doi.org/10.1111/ijlh.12822.
25. Rodeghiero F, Tosetto A, Abshire T, et al. ISTH/SSC bleeding assessment tool: a standardized questionnaire and a proposal for a new bleeding score for inherited bleeding disorders. J Thromb Haemost. 2010;8(9):2063–5. https://doi.org/10.1111/j.1538-7836.2010.03975.x.
26. Doherty D, Grabell J, Christopherson PA, et al. Variability in international society on thrombosis and Haemostasis-scientific and standardization committee endorsed bleeding assessment tool (ISTH-BAT) score with normal aging in healthy females: contributory factors and clinical significance. J Thromb Haemost. 2023;21(4):880–6. https://doi.org/10.1016/j.jtha.2022.11.045.
27. Rydz N, James PD. The evolution and value of bleeding assessment tools. J Thromb Haemost. 2012;10(11):2223–9. https://doi.org/10.1111/j.1538-7836.2012.04923.x.
28. Hayward CP, Moffat KA. Laboratory testing for bleeding disorders: strategic uses of high and low-yield tests. Int J Lab Hematol. 2013;35(3):322–33. https://doi.org/10.1111/ijlh.12077.
29. Kumar N, Rajpal S, Ahluwalia J, et al. Acquired hemophilia a: experience of a tertiary care institute from North India. Indian J Hematol Blood Transfus. 2018;34(3):524–9. https://doi.org/10.1007/s12288-017-0873-1.
30. Cheves TA, DeMarinis S, Sweeney JD. Laboratory methods in the assessment of hereditary hemostatic disorders. Hematol Oncol Clin North Am. 2021;35(6):1051–68. https://doi.org/10.1016/j.hoc.2021.07.002.

Chapter 17
Laboratory Monitoring of Newer Anticoagulants and Fondaparinux

Dinesh Chandra, Gurpreet Kaur, and Ankur Ahuja

Abstract Venous thromboembolism (VTE) includes deep vein thrombosis (DVT) and pulmonary embolism (PE). The estimates of incidence are to the tune of ~2 per 1000 first events every year in the West; it is a major cause of morbidity and mortality. The advent of direct oral anticoagulants (DOACs), such as dabigatran, rivaroxaban, apixaban, and edoxaban, has transformed the management of thromboembolic disorders. These newer medications offer several advantages over traditional vitamin K antagonists (VKAs), including predictable pharmacokinetics, fixed dosing, and less need for routine laboratory monitoring. Consequently, DOACs have become the first-line treatment for conditions like atrial fibrillation, deep vein thrombosis, and pulmonary embolism.

Laboratory tests for direct oral anticoagulants (DOACs) are typically unnecessary for regular therapeutic monitoring. However, specific assays can assess their effects: the activated partial thromboplastin time (aPTT) is useful for dabigatran, while anti-Xa assays are preferred for direct factor Xa inhibitors. The thrombin time (TT) can also monitor dabigatran, though it's less common. No single test is universally accepted for DOACS. Fondaparinux, an indirect FXa inhibitor, is monitored by the chromogenic anti-FXa assay.

This chapter explores the clinical applications and mechanisms of Direct Oral Anticoagulants (DOACs) and Fondaparinux, highlighting their significance in patient care. It addresses the necessity of monitoring DOACs, the role of laboratory assessments in managing patients, and the challenges associated with current testing methods. Additionally, it emphasizes recent advancements in DOAC monitoring

D. Chandra (✉)
Department of Hematology, Sanjay Gandhi Post Graduate Institute of Medical Sciences, Lucknow, Uttar Pradesh, India

G. Kaur · A. Ahuja
Department of Pathology, Armed Forces Medical College, Pune, Maharashtra, India

H. P. Pati et al. (eds.), *Clinical Hematology and Hemato-Oncology*,
https://doi.org/10.1007/978-981-92-1167-8_17

aimed at optimizing care, reducing adverse events, and supporting personalized anticoagulation therapy.

Keywords Direct thrombin inhibitors · Factor Xa inhibitors · Liquid chromatography-tandem mass spectrometry (LC-MS/MS) · Chromogenic anti-Xa assays (C-FXa) · Functional assays for quantification of anti-IIa DOACs

Learning Objectives

- *Identify* the key classes of newer anticoagulants, including direct thrombin inhibitors and direct oral anticoagulants (DOACs) and Fondaparinux.
- *Describe* the mechanism of action, pharmacokinetics and pharmacodynamics of newer anticoagulants.
- *List* the common indications for the use of newer anticoagulants in clinical practice.
- *Interpret* laboratory test results to monitor the efficacy and safety of newer anticoagulants.
- Game changer in monitoring of Newer oral anticoagulants.
- *Propose* appropriate strategies for patients with abnormal laboratory values while on newer anticoagulants.

17.1 Introduction

Vitamin K antagonists (VKAs) were introduced in the 1920s and have since become the cornerstone of oral anticoagulation therapy. They are the most widely prescribed oral anticoagulants worldwide. VKAs are primarily used for the prevention and treatment of venous thromboembolic disease (VTE), which includes conditions such as deep vein thrombosis and pulmonary embolism. They also aid in managing thromboembolic complications associated with atrial fibrillation (AF) and mechanical heart valves. However, VKAs are known for causing significant interactions with certain foods and medications. Additionally, their dosing can vary greatly among individuals. As a result, frequent monitoring is necessary to ensure optimal dosing [1].

Vitamin K antagonists (VKAs) exhibit significant variability in their dose–response effects, both among different individuals and within the same individual over time. This variability is influenced by various factors. Endogenous factors include age, gender, body weight, existing health conditions (comorbidities), and genetic makeup. Environmental factors also play a role, such as the presence of other medications and dietary habits. These influences can impact the clearance of VKAs from the body, along with the synthesis or removal of vitamin K–dependent coagulation factors.

Due to this variability and the narrow therapeutic range of VKAs, routine laboratory monitoring is essential. Such monitoring helps assess the anticoagulant effect and allows for appropriate adjustments to the daily dosage [2].

To address the limitations of vitamin K antagonists (VKAs), a new class of anticoagulants known as novel oral anticoagulants (NOACs) or direct oral anticoagulants (DOACs) has emerged. DOACs have become a first-line treatment for various indications, particularly for stroke prevention in patients with atrial fibrillation and for the prevention and treatment of venous thromboembolism (VTE). Five DOACs are approved for clinical use are dabigatran, rivaroxaban, apixaban, edoxaban, and betrixaban [3].

17.2 Mechanism of Action

DOACs, or direct oral anticoagulants, are fast-acting and target-specific anticoagulants that inhibit both free and bound activated serine proteases. Dabigatran directly and reversibly inhibits both free and clot-bound thrombin (Factor IIa). In contrast, rivaroxaban, apixaban, edoxaban, and betrixaban are direct inhibitors of activated Factor X (F Xa) [4]. Fondaparinux is a synthetic analogue of the pentasaccharide. It is an indirect inhibitor of factor Xa, but it does not inhibit thrombin at all (Fig. 17.1).

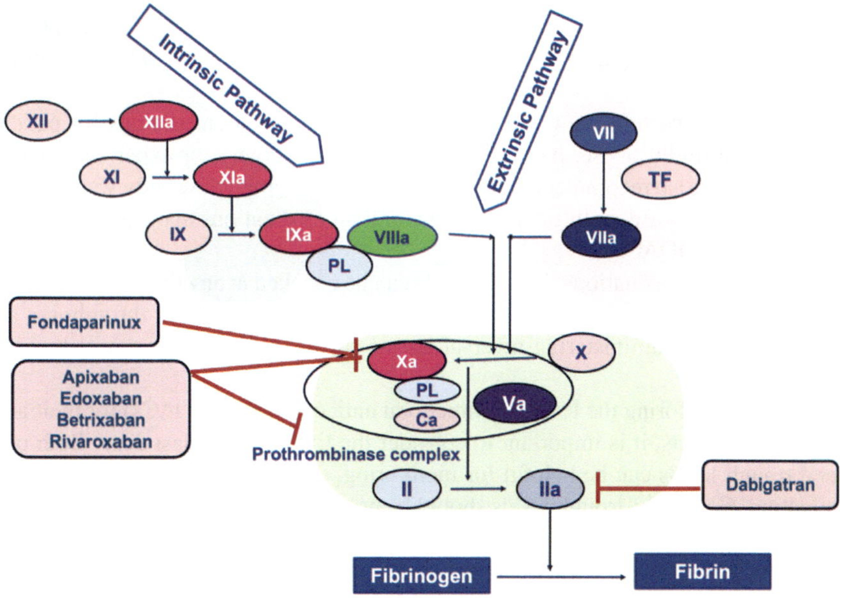

Fig. 17.1 Mechanism of action of various DOACs

Table 17.1 Pharmacological characteristics of DOACs

	Dabigatran	Rivaroxaban	Apixaban	Edoxaban	Betrixaban
Mechanism of Action	Anti-IIa	Anti-Xa	Anti-Xa	Anti-Xa	Anti-Xa
Frequency of intake	Twice daily	Once daily	Twice daily	Once daily	Once daily
T_{max} (h)	1.5–3	2–4	3–4	1–2	3–4
T_{trough} (h)	12	24	12	24	24
Half-life (h)	12–14	5–9	10–14	9–11	35–45
Bioavailability	3–7%	80–100%	50%	62%	34%
Protein binding	35%	92–95%	87%	40–59%	60%
Renal clearance (%)	80%	40%	27%	50%	6–13%

T_{max} time at peak plasma drug concentration, T_{trough} time at trough plasma drug concentration

Most direct oral anticoagulants (DOACs) are metabolized by the liver and excreted by the kidneys. However, dabigatran is primarily eliminated by the kidneys. DOACs typically reach peak plasma levels within about 2 h, and their plasma trough levels are achieved within 12–24 h, depending on how often they are administered [5]. Pharmacological properties of various DOACs are listed in Table 17.1.

17.3 Is There a Need to Monitor DOACs?

Unlike warfarin, routine therapeutic monitoring is not recommended for direct oral anticoagulants (DOACs) due to their predictable pharmacokinetics (PK), pharmacodynamics (PD), and wide therapeutic windows. However, there are several clinical scenarios in which monitoring DOAC levels can be beneficial for treatment decisions.

Laboratory monitoring of DOACs is advised in outpatient settings for patients who are morbidly obese, have undergone bariatric surgery, or experience malabsorption. It is also recommended for patients with extremely low body weight, end--stage kidney disease, or those taking concomitant medications that may enhance the effects of the DOAC.

In emergency situations, DOAC levels can be checked at any time, such as before invasive procedures, during episodes of breakthrough bleeding or thrombosis, and before or after administering reversal agents for patients who have overdosed on DOACs [5].

When monitoring the levels of direct oral anticoagulants (DOACs) for their anticoagulant effects, it is important to consider the timing of the last dose. Both peak and trough levels can be helpful for monitoring, depending on the specific clinical situation. Generally, trough levels should be used to assess clearance, particularly in cases involving elderly patients and those with renal or liver failure. On the other hand, peak levels are best for confirming absorption or evaluating adherence to the

Table 17.2 Timing and expected peak and trough serum concentration of DOACs

Drug	Indication and dose	Peak (hours)	Peak concentration (ng/ml)	Trough (hours)	Trough concentration (ng/ml)
Direct Thrombin Inhibitor					
Dabigatran	Stroke prevention in NVAF treatment of PE or VET (150 mg BID)	1.5–3	175 (117–275)	12	91 (61–143)
Factor Xa Inhibitor					
Apixaban	Stroke prevention in NVAF treatment of PE or VET (5 mg BID)	3–4	171 (91–321)	12	103 (41–230)
Edoxaban	Stroke prevention in NVAF treatment of PE or VET (60 mg daily)	1–2	170 (125–245)	24	36 (19–62)
Rivaroxaban	Stroke prevention in NVAF treatment of PE or VET (20 mg daily)	2–3	249 (184–419)	24	44 (12–137)

BID twice daily, *NVAF* non-valvular atrial fibrillation, *PE* pulmonary embolism, *VTE* venous thromboembolism

medication; however, it is ideal to record the time since the last dose was taken [6]. Characteristics of various DOACs have been mentioned in Table 17.2.

17.4 Laboratory Monitoring of DOACs

When monitoring the levels of direct oral anticoagulants (DOACs) for their anticoagulant effects, it is important to consider the timing of the last dose. Both peak and trough levels can be helpful for monitoring, depending on the specific clinical situation. Generally, trough levels should be used to assess clearance, particularly in cases involving elderly patients, as well as those with renal or liver failure. On the other hand, peak levels are best for confirming absorption or evaluating adherence to the medication; however, it is ideal to record the time since the last dose was taken.

An ideal assay for monitoring direct oral anticoagulants (DOACs) should accurately measure the concentration of these drugs and be sensitive enough to detect the lowest clinically relevant levels. It should also be readily available in laboratories, easy to perform, cost-effective, and able to provide results within a short time frame.

17.5 Sample Requirement for DOACs Assessments [7]

- Platelet-poor plasma prepared with 3.2% sodium citrate can be used for both quantitative and qualitative assays, including clot-based and chromogenic tests.
- Liquid chromatography–mass spectrometry/mass spectrometry (LC–MS/MS) can utilize either serum or plasma samples.
- Citrated whole blood samples should be processed within 4 h of collection.
- For thrombin time testing (specifically for dabigatran), plasma samples remain stable for up to 4 h at room temperature.
- Anti-Xa assays for anti-FXa direct oral anticoagulants (DOACs) should be performed within 8 h of collection. If testing cannot be conducted within this time frame, the samples should be stored at −20 or −70 °C
- Samples can withstand three freeze-thaw cycles without a significant loss of activity.
- Erroneous or unreliable results may arise from causes such as hemolyzed, icteric, or lipemic samples, incorrect timing of sample collection, delays in specimen transportation, or heparin contamination.

17.6 Routine Laboratory Coagulation Tests for Monitoring of DOACs

Routine coagulation tests, such as prothrombin time (PT) and activated partial thromboplastin time (APTT), are not reliable for assessing the effects of direct oral anticoagulants (DOACs). The sensitivity of these tests can vary based on the laboratory and the reagents used. The impact of DOACs on the results of individual coagulation assays like PT, APTT, and thrombin time (TT) depends on their specific mechanism of action. To aid in interpretation, a simplified algorithm is proposed for evaluating screening test results in patients undergoing DOAC therapy (Fig. 17.2).

- Direct thrombin inhibitors, such as dabigatran, primarily impact the thrombin time (TT) and activated partial thromboplastin time (aPTT), while they have a minimal effect on prothrombin time (PT) results.
- In contrast, factor Xa inhibitors like rivaroxaban, edoxaban, and betrixaban significantly affect the PT test, while having a minor or negligible effect on the aPTT test. The TT test is not impacted by these medications at all.
- Apixaban, another factor Xa inhibitor, does not affect the PT, aPTT, or TT.
- The aPTT cannot be used to monitor fondaparinux, although it may become prolonged at therapeutic doses.

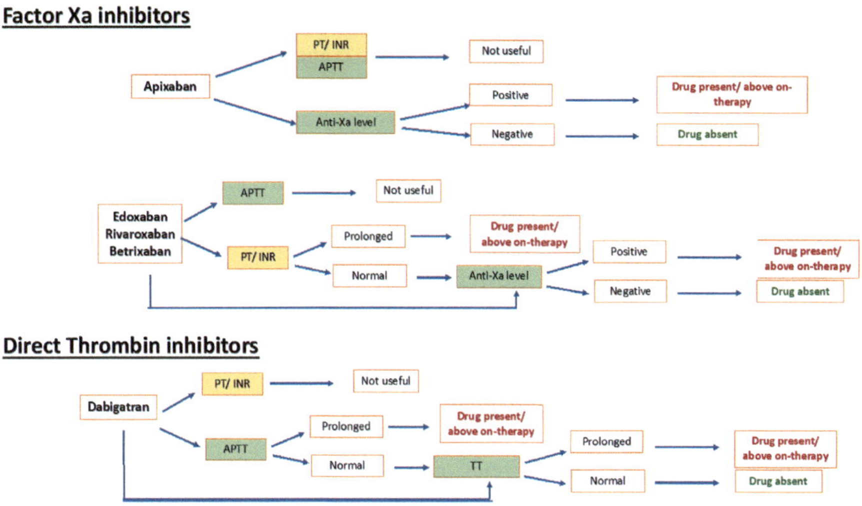

Fig. 17.2 Algorithm for evaluating screening test results in patients undergoing DOAC therapy

17.7 Specific Assays for Quantitative Measurement of DOAC Concentration

Quantitative assessment of DOAC concentration is performed using liquid chromatography–tandem mass spectrometry (LC–MS/MS) or drug-calibrated clot-based methods or chromogenic techniques.

1. *Liquid chromatography–tandem mass spectrometry (LC–MS/MS)*: The gold standard for measuring DOAC levels is liquid chromatography–tandem mass spectrometry (LC–MS/MS); however, this method does not provide the rapid turnaround times required for routine clinical care, making it impractical [8]. The advantages and disadvantages of LC–MS/MS are listed in Table 17.3.

Table 17.3 Advantages and disadvantages of liquid chromatography–tandem mass spectrometry (LC–MS/MS)

Advantages	Disadvantaged
A gold standard method for the measurement of DOACs High degree of specificity, sensitivity, selectivity, and reproducibility The lower limit of detection (LLOD) and quantitation (LLOQ) for DOACs 0.025 and 3 ng/mL Reportable range of quantitation: 5 and 500 ng/mL	Labor-intensive sample preparation steps, the complexity of the technique, and instrument availability Co-elution of other compounds (drugs or xenobiotics), internal standard preparation, and inability to detect drug metabolites Absence of standardization Lack of a universal calibration material or international reference standard

2. *Functional assays for quantification of anti-Xa DOACs*

   Chromogenic anti-Xa assays (C-FXa) are commonly used to assess heparin concentration. These assays are highly sensitive to direct FXa inhibitors. However, C-FXa may not accurately measure drug levels below 30 ng/mL for rivaroxaban, below 15 ng/mL for apixaban, and 10 ng/mL for edoxaban. Specifically, plasma samples with suspected rivaroxaban levels under 30 ng/mL may not provide reliable results.

   For rapid quantitation of anti-Xa direct oral anticoagulants (DOACs), drug-calibrated anti-FXa assays are recommended as the preferred method. It is important to note that antithrombin-supplemented anti-FXa methods should not be used for DOAC assessment, as they tend to overestimate drug concentrations and have not been validated by the manufacturers [5, 9].
3. *Functional assays for quantification of anti-IIa DOACs*

   Various functional assays, such as ecarin clotting time (ECT), chromogenic ecarin assay (ECA), chromogenic anti-FIIa (C-FIIa) assay, dTT, and dilute Russell's viper venom time, are used to quantify direct thrombin inhibitors (DTIs) like dabigatran when appropriately calibrated. Most of these assays are not well standardized in laboratories, except for the Chromogenic anti-FIIa assay (C-FIIa). C-FIIa is the most commonly used assay for measuring dabigatran, as several commercial kits are available. When the drug is calibrated, C-FIIa demonstrates a strong correlation with LC–MS/MS results [5, 9].

17.7.1 Anti-Xa Assays (Factor Xa Inhibitor)

• Anti-Xa assay is a test used to monitor patients on low molecular weight heparins (LMWHs), unfractionated heparin (UFH), and direct oral anticoagulants (DOACs) with anti-Xa activity.

• UFH and LMWHs bind to antithrombin (AT) to form the heparin-antithrombin complex, which enhances its inhibitory activity. LMWHs primarily exhibit anti-Xa activity, while UFH demonstrates both anti-Xa and anti-IIa activity.

Principles

- The test plasma (containing AT and LMWH or UFH or DOAC) is incubated with a known amount of Factor Xa. This results in the formation of an AT-heparin or AT-DOAC complex, which inhibits Factor Xa activity in proportion to their concentration. The residual Factor Xa is then measured using either a clotting-based Factor X assay or, more commonly, a chromogenic substrate specifically designed for Factor Xa.
- A standard curve is created by adding known quantities of LMWH, UFH, or DOACs to plasma, followed by the addition of a fixed amount of Factor Xa.
- The residual FXa activity is inversely proportional to the concentration of heparin or DOAC in the test sample, and it can be quantified using the appropriate calibration curve.

- When used for LMWH/UFH, the results from heparin-specific reference curves are expressed in U/mL. In contrast, when used for DOACs, the results from the reference curve are expressed in ng/mL.

17.7.2 *Anti-IIa Assay (Direct Thrombin Inhibitor Assay)*

- *Principle*: This assay measures the inhibitory effect of direct thrombin inhibitors (like dabigatran) on thrombin (factor IIa). The assay is based on the ability of thrombin to convert fibrinogen to fibrin, which is inhibited in the presence of the drug.
- *Key measurement*: The degree of thrombin inhibition is quantified by measuring the clot formation time or the residual thrombin activity in the sample.

17.7.3 *Fondaparinux (Anti-Xa Inhibitor)*

- In patients treated with fondaparinux, the Xa inhibitory activity of antithrombin is increased. This activity can be measured using either a clot-based assay or, more commonly, a chromogenic assay. In the chromogenic assay, the patient's plasma is mixed with a known amount of Factor Xa, and the degree of Xa inhibition is assessed to determine the residual Xa. This is measured using a chromogenic substrate that is specific for Factor Xa.
- It is important to calibrate the anti-factor Xa activity assay with fondaparinux as a reference standard.
- The results are reported as fondaparinux levels in micrograms per milliliter (mcg/mL). Although a definitive therapeutic range has not been established, typical levels for prophylactic-dose fondaparinux are between 0.39 and 0.5 mcg/mL, while levels for therapeutic-dose fondaparinux range from 0.5 to 1.5 mcg/mL.

17.8 The Game Changer in the Monitoring of DOACs

Global hemostatic tests, such as viscoelastic assays and thrombin generation assays, are utilized to monitor direct oral anticoagulants (DOACs). Point-of-care (POC) tests, like ROTEM (rotational thromboelastometry) and TEG (thromboelastography), analyze whole blood to measure the presence of DOACs. These tests can guide treatment in perioperative and trauma settings. Specifically, the R times in ROTEM and clot formation times (CFT) correlate with dabigatran and rivaroxaban concentrations.

The TEG 6s device employs resonance-frequency viscoelasticity measurements and uses premixed disposable multichannel microfluidic cartridges. Recent data on the use of targeted DOAC cartridges for the TEG 6s platform indicate promising results. The system can accurately recognize and classify DOACs, with sensitivities ranging from 92% to 98% and specificities between 95% and 100%.

The DOAC-specific cartridge contains kaolin in channel 1 (the citrated kaolin [CK] channel), ecarin in channel 2 (the direct thrombin inhibitor [DTI] channel), factor Xa (FXa) in channel 3 (the anti-FXa [AFXa] channel), and kaolin with abciximab in channel 4 (the functional fibrinogen channel) [10, 11].

The ROTEM assay is a rapid and highly sensitive method for detecting apixaban. By using a modified trigger based on factor Xa (FXa), ROTEM can accurately identify apixaban even at low therapeutic levels, surpassing the accuracy of the commercial Ex-tem trigger and those based on Russell's viper venom (RVV). This assay can be performed at the bedside within 20 min, making it much quicker than traditional plasma-based coagulation tests. It is especially valuable in the clinical management of patients who are experiencing acute severe complications while undergoing treatment with apixaban [12].

Global coagulation assays, such as thrombin generation testing using the calibrated automated thrombogram, can evaluate direct oral anticoagulants (DOACs) by measuring total thrombin formation, which is the final product of the coagulation pathway. Factor Xa inhibitors, like rivaroxaban and apixaban, significantly affect the thrombin peak compared to the endogenous thrombin potential (ETP). The anticoagulant effects of various agents, including vitamin K antagonists (VKAs), low molecular weight heparin (LMWH), factor Xa inhibitors, and direct thrombin inhibitors, can all be assessed through thrombin generation assays; however, the responses may vary among these different drugs [13].

In emergency situations, point-of-care (POC) coagulometer instruments may offer advantages over conventional clotting assays for detecting direct oral anticoagulants (DOACs). Depending on the specific DOAC, between 30% and 80% of these medications are excreted in urine by the kidneys.

The DOAC Dipstick is a diagnostic tool that contains a matrix with specific enzymes and substrates designed to detect direct oral factor Xa and thrombin inhibitors. This certified in vitro diagnostic (IVD) medical device, developed by DOASENSE GmbH, operates on the principle that DOACs can be excreted into urine and are detectable there.

The test provides qualitative results indicating the presence or absence of DOACs in a patient's urine sample for both direct oral factor Xa inhibitors and oral thrombin inhibitors. It is a single-use assay with a turnaround time of just 10 min, and the results can be visually identified by observing color changes without the need for additional equipment [14].

DOAC quantification can be conducted using dried blood spots (DBS) for blood collection, followed by the highly sensitive technique of ultra-performance liquid chromatography/tandem mass spectrometry (UPLC/MS/MS). All DOACs remain stable in DBS for up to 52 days at room temperature, provided the DBS are protected from light and humidity. There is a strong correlation between the drug concentration in samples taken from DBS and blood plasma. Patients can easily collect

DBS samples at home and send them to the laboratory for drug concentration measurement [15].

The impact of direct oral anticoagulants (DOACs) on laboratory assays used for thrombophilia testing—such as antithrombin, protein S, protein C, lupus anticoagulant, and activated protein C resistance (APC-R)—is a well-documented issue that can lead to false-positive and false-negative results. The DOAC-Stop® adsorbent procedure, which utilizes adsorbent tablets (DOAC-Stop®; Haematex Research, Hornsby, Australia), offers an effective and straightforward method to mitigate the interference of DOACs in coagulation tests. It is important to interpret thrombophilia screening tests in patients taking DOACs carefully and consider the use of the DOAC-Stop® treatment in clinical practice to avoid potential misclassifications and their associated clinical consequences [16].

17.9 Interference of DOAC on Coagulation Assays

Most assays used to diagnose bleeding disorders or inherited thrombophilia are functional routine tests that rely on a coagulation endpoint or a chromogenic endpoint involving factor Xa or IIa. Direct Oral Anticoagulants (DOACs) can interfere with these tests, leading to inaccurate results. Specifically, rivaroxaban and edoxaban tend to prolong the Prothrombin Time/International Normalized Ratio (PT/INR) more significantly than the Activated Partial Thromboplastin Time (APTT) [17].

- Most clot-based assays, such as those measuring the activities of factors II, V, VII, VIII, IX, X, XI, and XII, as well as protein C and protein S, along with activated protein C resistance (APC), tend to overestimate results in the presence of either rivaroxaban or apixaban. An antithrombin activity assay based on factor Xa will also be overestimated when anti-Xa DOACs (direct oral anticoagulants) are present, but assays based on factor IIa are not affected.
- Moreover, DOACs can significantly and falsely decrease the chromogenic activity of factor VIII. They may also lead to false positive results for lupus anticoagulant (LA) even when the activated partial thromboplastin time (APTT) is normal, although they do not impact ELISA-based antiphospholipid antibody assays.
- Other testing platforms, including selected chromogenic or latex immunoassays such as plasminogen activity, quantitative D-dimer, free protein S antigen, chromogenic protein C activity, von Willebrand factor antigen, and von Willebrand factor activity, remain unaffected by the presence of anti-Xa DOACs [18, 19]. The effects and interferences of DOACs on other coagulation factor testing are summarized in Table 17.4.

In many clinical situations, understanding whether abnormal laboratory test results are solely due to the effect of direct oral anticoagulants (DOACs) or if there are additional underlying abnormalities can be crucial in the decision-making process. To address this, in vitro techniques have been developed to either remove or

Table 17.4 Effect of DOACs on various coagulation assays

Coagulation test	Test endpoint	Anti-Xa inhibitors	Anti-IIa inhibitors
PT/INR	Coagulation	Yes	Yes
APTT	Coagulation	Yes	Yes
Thrombin time	Coagulation	No	Yes
Fibrinogen	Coagulation	No	Yes
Factor II, V, VII, VIII, IX, X, XI, XII	Coagulation	Yes	Yes
Factor VIII chromogenic	Chromogenic	Yes	Yes
Protein C activity	Chromogenic	No	No
Protein S activity	Coagulation	Yes	Yes
Antithrombin activity	Chromogenic	Yes	Yes
Protein S antigen	Immunoassay	No	No
Protein C antigen	Immunoassay	No	No
Antithrombin antigen	Immunoassay	No	No
APC-resistance	Coagulation	Yes	Yes
Lupus anticoagulant	Coagulation	Yes	Yes
D-Dimer	Immunoassay	No	No

block DOACs from patient samples, allowing other coagulation assays to be performed without interference.

Activated charcoal or carbon, marketed as DOAC Remove® and DOAC Stop®, has been utilized both in clinical settings for hemoperfusion and in laboratory tests for eliminating DOACs. The application of these agents to mitigate the effects of DOACs will facilitate accurate diagnosis of various hemostatic conditions and help confirm or rule out the presence of lupus anticoagulants and inherited thrombophilia's [16].

17.10 Summary

Newer anticoagulants, including direct thrombin inhibitors (e.g., dabigatran) and direct factor Xa inhibitors (e.g., rivaroxaban, apixaban, edoxaban), offer significant advantages over traditional agents like warfarin, including predictable pharmacokinetics, fewer dietary restrictions, and reduced need for routine monitoring. However, laboratory monitoring remains important in specific clinical situations, such as bleeding, overdose, or when rapid reversal is necessary. The chromogenic anti-factor Xa assay is currently the gold standard for monitoring LMWH and fondaparinux therapy. Anti-IIa and anti-Xa assays are the primary tests used to assess drug levels and guide management. Drug-specific calibrated anti-Xa assays, as well as the diluted thrombin time (dTT), ecarin clotting assay (ECA), ecarin chromogenic test (ECT), and anti-factor IIa chromogenic assays, can estimate the concentration of DOACs. These methods are comparable to liquid chromatography-tandem mass spectrometry (LC–MS/MS) for measuring DOAC levels. Emerging techniques such as DOAC stop, urine DOAC dipsticks, rotational thromboelastometry (ROTEM), thrombin generation assays, and TEG 6s NOAC assays are game changers in the monitoring of DOACs. While these newer agents reduce the burden of monitoring, understanding their pharmacodynamics, potential drug interactions, and proper use of laboratory tests is essential for ensuring safe and effective patient care.

References

1. Ansell J, Hirsh J, Hylek E, Jacobson A, Crowther M, Palareti G. Pharmacology and management of the vitamin K antagonists: American College of Chest Physicians Evidence-Based Clinical Practice Guidelines (8th Edition). Chest. 2008;133:160S–98S.
2. Ageno W, Gallus AS, Wittkowsky A, Crowther M, Hylek EM, Palareti G, American College of Chest Physicians. Oral anticoagulant therapy: antithrombotic therapy and prevention of thrombosis, 9th ed: American College of Chest Physicians Evidence-Based Clinical Practice Guidelines. Chest. 2012;141(2 Suppl):e44S–88S.
3. Conway SE, Hwang AY, Ponte CD, Gums JG. Laboratory and clinical monitoring of direct acting oral anticoagulants: what clinicians need to know. Pharmacotherapy. 2017;37(2):236–48. https://doi.org/10.1002/phar.1884.
4. Dale BJ, Chan NC, Eikelboom JW. Laboratory measurement of the direct oral anticoagulants. Br J Haematol. 2016;172(03):315–36.
5. Gosselin RC, Adcock DM, Bates SM, et al. International Council for Standardization in Haematology (ICSH) recommendations for laboratory measurement of direct oral anticoagulants. Thromb Haemost. 2018;118(03):437–50.
6. Douxfils J, Ageno W, Samama CM, et al. Laboratory testing in patients treated with direct oral anticoagulants: a practical guide for clinicians. J Thromb Haemost. 2018;16(2):209–19.
7. McGrail R, Revsholm J, Nissen PH, Grove EL, Hvas AM. Stability of direct oral anticoagulants in whole blood and plasma from patients in steady state treatment. Thromb Res. 2016;148:107–10.
8. Rohde G. Determination of rivaroxaban–a novel, oral, direct Factor Xa inhibitor–in human plasma by high-performance liquid chromatography-tandem mass spectrometry. J Chromatogr B Analyt Technol Biomed Life Sci. 2008;872(1–2):43–50.
9. Cuker A, Siegal DM, Crowther MA, et al. Laboratory measurement of the anticoagulant activity of the non vitamin K oral anticoagulants. J Am Coll Cardiol. 2014;64:1128–39.
10. Bliden KP, Chaudhary R, Mohammed N, et al. Determination of non-Vitamin K oral anticoagulant (NOAC) effects using a new-generation thrombelastography TEG 6s system. J Thromb Thrombolysis. 2017;43(4):437–45.
11. Dias JD, Lopez-Espina CG, Ippolito J, et al. Rapid point-of-care detection and classification of direct-acting oral anticoagulants with the TEG 6s: implications for trauma and acute care surgery. J Trauma Acute Care Surg. 2019;87(2):364–70.
12. Taune V, Skeppholm M, Agren A, Wikman A, Hillarp A, Wallén H. Rapid detection of Apixaban by a ROTEM-based approach and reversibility with Andexanet Alfa or DOAC-stop. TH Open. 2022;6(3):e238–47.
13. Pfrepper C, Metze M, Siegemund A, Kl¨oter T, Siegemund T, Petros S. Direct oral anticoagulant plasma levels and thrombin generation on ST Genesia system. Res Pract Thromb Haemost. 2020;4(4):619–27.
14. Harenberg J, Schreiner R, Hetjens S, Weiss C. Detecting anti-IIa and anti-Xa direct oral anticoagulant (DOAC) agents in urine using a DOAC dipstick. Semin Thromb Hemost. 2019;4(3):275–84.

15. Foerster KI, Huppertz A, Meid AD, Müller OJ, Rizos T, Tilemann L. Dried-blood-spot technique to monitor direct oral anticoagulants: clinical validation of a UPLC-MS/MS-based assay. Anal Chem. 2018;90(15):9395–402.
16. Favresse J, Lardinois B, Sabor L, Devalet B, Vandepapeliere J, Braibant M. Evaluation of the DOAC-stop® procedure to overcome the effect of DOACs on several thrombophilia screening tests. TH Open. 2018;2(2):e202–9. https://doi.org/10.1055/s-0038-1657785.
17. Tsakiris DA. Direct oral anticoagulants–interference with laboratory tests and mechanism of action. Semin Hematol. 2014;51(2):98–101.
18. Samuelson BT, Cuker A, Siegal DM, et al. Labora tory assessment of the anticoagulant activity of direct oral anticoagulants: a systematic review. Chest. 2017;151:127–38.
19. Helin TA, Pakkanen A, Lassila R, Joutsi-Korhonen L. Effects of apixaban on prothrombin time, activated partial thromboplastin time and anti-Xa assays: a European survey. Clin Chem Lab Med. 2017;55(8):e178–80.

Chapter 18
Management of ITP: Including Approach in Refractory Patients in Children and Adults

Pravas Mishra, Saphalta Baghmar, and Prashant Mehta

Abstract Immune thrombocytopenia (ITP) is characterized by immune-mediated platelet destruction. While first-line treatment options such as corticosteroids and IVIG are effective initially, relapse and chronicity affect most adults. This review evaluates current studies in the management of chronic ITP, both paediatric and adult, with a focus on refractory cases. Second-line therapies, including splenectomy, rituximab, thrombopoietin receptor agonists (TPO-RAs), fostamatinib, and other immunosuppressives, are reviewed.

Keywords Immune thrombocytopenia · Splenectomy · Rituximab · TPO-RA · Fostamatinib · Refractory ITP

Learning Objectives
- First-line therapies in adults and children.
- Understand the outcome data for various interventions beyond the first line.
- Learn to make evidence-based decisions on treatment selection, keeping patient perspectives in mind.

18.1 Introduction

Immune thrombocytopenia (ITP) is an immune-mediated accelerated platelet destruction, along with, in some cases, suppressed platelet production. The aetiology is mostly idiopathic (primary ITP) and is a diagnosis of exclusion. Secondary

P. Mishra (✉) · S. Baghmar · P. Mehta
Department of Hematology, Medical Oncology and BMT, Amrita Institute of Medical Sciences, Faridabad, India
e-mail: pravasmishra@fbd.amrita.edu

H. P. Pati et al. (eds.), *Clinical Hematology and Hemato-Oncology*,
https://doi.org/10.1007/978-981-92-1167-8_18

ITP is diagnosed in systemic lupus erythematosus, HIV, Hepatitis C, antiphospholipid antibody syndrome, drugs and haematological, typically lymphoid malignancies. This review is focussed on idiopathic ITP. We will understand the outcomes of various interventions in ITP with a more extensive coverage of relapsed, refractory ITP.

18.2 Acute ITP

Case 1: A 9-year-old girl presented with a history of easy bruising for 10 days. She had no preceding fever, and the general examination was normal. Her haemoglobin was 13.5 g/dL, WBC count was 7 × 10^9/l and platelet count was 20 × 10^9/l. Her peripheral smear showed few macrocytic and microcytic erythrocytes with thrombocytopenia, giant platelets, and no atypical cells. Per institutional policy, a marrow examination was not done

Case 2: A 65-year-old male presented with a history of black coloured stools preceded by bruises for 15 days. As in case 1, the systemic examination was normal. His haemoglobin was 5 g/dL, WBC count was 12 × 10^9/l and platelet count was 2 × 10^9/l. His peripheral smear showed few microcytic erythrocytes with thrombocytopenia and no atypical cells. An endoscopy outside had shown bleeding mucosa in the stomach and jejunum. In view of age and anaemia, a bone marrow examination was done which confirmed megakaryocytic thrombocytopenia

Case 1 does not ideally require any immediate treatment as 75–80% of paediatric cases would resolve on their own whatever the line of therapy, including observation. However, 75% of adults will not recover or have a lingering course [1]. A Buchanan and Adix bleeding score of 3 or more, denoting mucosal bleeding, is an indication for treatment in a paediatric presentation. Other patients with lower scores might not require therapy in the paediatric cohort. However, guidelines provide significant leeway in deciding the need for therapy even in lower scores. Therefore, in the author's opinion, many cases with lower scores, in the real world, might be treated if they present to the hospital. The AIEOP guidelines recommend IVIG as first-line therapy in children based on data that suggests that IVIG exposure at the outset reduces the risk of chronic ITP, an assertion not borne out by randomized data [2]. The ASH guidelines do not recommend IVIG except perhaps in situations that demand a rapid recovery [3], as in case 2. Dexamethasone may be preferred over prednisolone if a faster response is required. Case 1 received a short course of prednisolone, rapidly tapered over 6 weeks. Case 2 received high-dose dexamethasone. Adults with less threatening bleeds receive oral prednisolone, again tapered over 6 weeks. Table 18.1 (paediatric) and Table 18.2 (adult) tabulate the approved first-line therapy in ITP.

Table 18.1 Paediatric ITP: first-line therapeutic options

Therapy	Dose	Response rate	Time to response	Duration of response
Prednisone	1–2 mg/kg/day orally for 15 days	60–80% overall, 30–50% sustained	Within 1–3 days	30–50% sustain after stopping
Dexamethasone	0.6 mg/kg/day for 4 days	Similar to prednisone, faster onset	1–2 days	Similar to prednisone
IVIG	0.8–1 g/kg single dose (or 0.4–0.5 g/kg for 4–5 days)	80% response	Within 48 h	Short (1–4 weeks)
IV Methylprednisolone	5–10 mg/kg/day IV for 3 days	Comparable to prednisone	1–3 days	Similar to prednisone
IVIG + methylprednisolone	IVIG 0.4 g/kg/day (day 1–2) + methylpred 20 mg/kg/day (day 1–3)	Used in uncontrolled bleeding; rapid response	Within 1–2 days	Not defined

Table 18.2 Adult ITP: first-line therapeutic options

Therapy	Dose	Response rate	Time to response	Duration of response
Prednisone	0.5–2 mg/kg/day orally (typical ~1 mg/kg)	60–80% initial response	Within days (1–3)	30–50% sustain after stopping
Dexa-methasone	40 mg/day orally for 4 days (sometimes repeated courses)	Faster initial response than prednisone; higher sustained remission in some studies	1–2 days	Variable; may be higher than prednisone with repeated courses
IVIG	1–2 g/kg single dose or divided over 2–5 days	~70–80% response	Within 1–2 days	Short (1–4 weeks)
IV Methylprednisolone	High dose (e.g., 30 mg/kg IV for 3 days in emergencies)	Used in emergency bleeding situations	Rapid (within days)	Not clearly defined
Combination therapies	Corticosteroids + recombinant human TPO or others	Some trials show improved response rates compared to steroids alone	Faster than steroids alone	Not well defined
Anti-D (Rh-positive pts)	50–75 μg/kg IV single dose	~60% response	Within 2–3 days	Short (weeks) Note *: No longer being marketed owing to safety concerns

18.3 Second Line Therapy in ITP

The various drugs currently approved or most widely studied in relapsed refractory ITP lasting ≥3 months, with their mechanism of action are summarized in Table 18.3. Subsequent sections will discuss their efficacy in this setting.

Table 18.3 Second line drugs and their mechanism of action

Drug/class	Mechanism of action
Splenectomy	Removes the primary site of platelet destruction and autoantibody production; reduces phagocytosis of antibody-coated platelets
Rituximab	Anti-CD20 monoclonal antibody that depletes B cells, reducing autoantibody production against platelets
TPO receptor agonists (Romiplostim, Eltrombopag, Avatrombopag)	Stimulate thrombopoietin receptor (c-MPL) to increase megakaryocyte proliferation and platelet production via JAK/STAT, PI3K/AKT, MAPK pathways. Avatrombopag has no relation to food intake and binds to different sites on c-MPL receptor than eltrombopag. Romiplostim, a peptide/peptibody, binds to the extracellular domain of the TPO receptor while the small molecules bind to the transmembrane section of the receptor
Fostamatinib	Syk inhibitor that blocks Fc receptor signalling in macrophages, reducing phagocytosis of platelets
Rilzabrutinib (Ongoing LUNA III study)	Reversible Bruton tyrosine kinase inhibitor (BTKi): Inhibits B cell antibody formation and antibody coated platelet phagocytosis via FcR in spleen and liver. No bleeding or cardiac side-effects seen with non-selective irreversible BTKi
Mycophenolate mofetil (MMF)	Inhibits inosine monophosphate dehydrogenase, impairing lymphocyte proliferation and antibody production
Cyclosporine	Calcineurin inhibitor that suppresses T-cell activation and cytokine production
Azathioprine	Purine analogue, inhibits lymphocyte proliferation and reduces autoantibody production
Dapsone	Unclear; thought to act via oxidative stress on immune cells and modulation of macrophage activity
IVIG	Saturates Fc receptors on splenic macrophages, blocking destruction of antibody-coated platelets
Sirolimus	mTOR inhibitor that blocks T-cell activation and reduces cytokine production
Danazol	Attenuates immune response by suppressing gonadotropins and possibly T-cell function
Tacrolimus	Calcineurin inhibitor similar to cyclosporine; inhibits T-cell activation and cytokine production

18.4 Splenectomy in Immune Thrombocytopenia (ITP)

The spleen is a major site of platelet clearance in immune thrombocytopenia (ITP). Platelets coated with autoantibodies are removed by macrophages in the spleen. Fcγ receptors (FcγR) on splenic macrophages attach to antibody-coated platelets. These platelets are phagocytosed in the spleen via spleen tyrosine kinase (syk) signalling pathways [4]. Our spleen is an important site of autoantibody production. The splenic antigen-presenting cells activate $CD4^+$ T cells, which in turn stimulate B cell differentiation into long-lived antiplatelet autoantibody-producing plasma cells through CD40-CD40L interactions [4]. These contribute to the development of chronic ITP. Therefore, splenectomy potentially provided a curative option in ITP. Table 18.4 includes outcomes from global and national studies. Complete response (CR) rates range from 58% to 90%, with speedy responses within a week, both paediatric and adult. Long-term event-free survival ranges between 70% and 90%.

Table 18.4 Splenectomy in ITP

Study (year)	Study period	Origin	*n*	Median age (yrs)	CR Rate	Time to response	Reported long-term outcomes
Ahmed et al., 2016 [5]	1995–2009	India	254 total	24 (4–65)	90.2%	1 day	10-yr EFS: 71% Infections 16% Deaths 1.57%
Pediatric subset—Ahmed et al., 2016 [5]	1995–2009	India	87	10 (4–14)	93.1%	1 day	10-yr EFS: 70%
Chaturvedi et al., 2018 [4]	1973–2016	Various international series	>2000 cases	Not specified	50–70%	Days	Relapses in first 2 yrs.: 20–30%
Mishra et al., 2021 [10]	2001–2020	India	45	38 (19–56)	61.8% at day 30 48.8% at 1 year	<30 days	5-yr RFS: 57.4%, OS: 92.6%
ICIS—Avila et al., 2020 [6]	1997–2017	International paediatric study	239	11.7 (7.9–15.3)	93% (CR + R)	7 days (median peak)	Clinically relevant non-major bleeding 8.7%, sepsis 2.7%
French Study—Ducassou et al., 2020 [7]	1990–2014	France	108	12 (3.5–18.9)	84% received no further therapy	Not reported	Not specifically mentioned for splenectomy

Table 18.4 (continued)

Study (year)	Study period	Origin	*n*	Median age (yrs)	CR Rate	Time to response	Reported long-term outcomes
Japanese Study—Isshiki et al., 2023 [9]	1985–2018	Japan	23	10 (5–22)	74% CR 83% PR	<4 weeks	91% drug-free at FU
Mendoza et al., 2024 [8]	2012–2020	Spain	51	Mean 32 years	78.4% at 3 years	3 days	72.5% sustained CR at 6 years
Zoletto et al., 2025 [11]	2012–2022	Italy	47	32 years	93%	≤1 week	Loss of response in 24%; 10-yr RFS: 70.3%

18.5 Complications of Splenectomy

The complication rates after splenectomy are generally low, particularly in children. Adult studies report perioperative mortality between 0.2% and 1.0%, and thrombosis, including portal vein thrombosis and venous thromboembolism (approximately 4% [4]), as well as early bacterial infections, remain the primary risks. Vaccination and antibiotic prophylaxis (e.g., amoxicillin or erythromycin) are essential to reduce post-splenectomy infection. In paediatric cohorts, no mortality or serious infections were reported, highlighting the safety of splenectomy with proper supportive care. The early infection rate is 5.6% [4], and the reported annual incidence rate of overwhelming post-splenectomy infection (OPSI) of approximately 0.13 per 100 person-years [12].

18.6 Predictors of Favourable Response to Splenectomy

Younger age in adults and older in children corresponds to the teenager/young adult population, steroid responsiveness prior to splenectomy, female sex, and splenic sequestration patterns (Table 18.5), identifying those more likely to respond. Age > 40, autoimmunity, steroids ≥37.5 mg/day, low T follicular helper cell density predicted those less likely to respond [11]. Vaccination and antibiotic prophylaxis are key to ensuring infection-free survival (Tables 18.6 and 18.7) along with appropriate post splenectomy surveillance (Table 18.7).

Table 18.5 Predictors of response to splenectomy from various studies

Study	Age group	Predictors of response
Ahmed et al., 2016 [5]	Combined adult and children	Female sex, steroid sensitivity, higher pre-splenectomy platelet count
Mendoza et al., 2024 [8]	Adults	Splenic sequestration pattern on 111In scan; OR 36.8, $p = 0.001$
Zoletto et al., 2025 [11]	Adults	Age < 30 at diagnosis of ITP, no autoimmune comorbidity, lower steroid requirement, higher Tfh density
Chaturvedi et al., 2018 [4]	Adults	Younger age, early platelet rise post-op; inconsistent predictors across studies
ICIS—Avila et al., 2020 [6]	Children	Older age in children and higher early platelet response post-splenectomy

Table 18.6 Vaccination guidelines post splenectomy

Pathogen	Vaccine type	Schedule	Notes
S. pneumoniae	PCV15/20 + PPSV23	Initial + PPSV23 after 8 wks	Revaccinate PPSV23 q5y
H. influenzae type b	Hib conjugate	Single dose	Even if vaccinated in childhood
Neisseria meningitidis	MenACWY + MenB	MenACWY q5y; MenB 2 doses	Age < 25, endemic areas
Influenza	IIV	Annually	Reduces bacterial superinfection
COVID-19	Per national guidelines	Prior to splenectomy	Strongly recommended

Table 18.7 Post-splenectomy surveillance, prophylaxis, and fever management

Strategy	Recommendation	Details/notes
Antibiotic prophylaxis children	Amoxicillin 250 mg orally twice daily (age < 5 or high risk) or erythromycin 250 mg BID if allergic	Continue for ≥2 years post-op and until age 5
Antibiotic prophylaxis adults	Consider amoxicillin 500 mg BID or erythromycin 500 mg BID for 3–6 months post-op	Extend if immunocompromised, elderly, or vaccine non-responders
Fever management	Educate patients to seek urgent care for fever ≥38 °C; initiate empiric antibiotics promptly	Cover for *S. pneumoniae*, *H. influenzae*, and *N. meningitidis*
Travel precautions	Avoid malaria-endemic areas or take full antimalarial prophylaxis; screen for babesiosis if febrile	Due to increased risk of parasitic infections (malaria, babesiosis) in asplenic individuals
Patient education	Carry splenectomy alert card; wear medical alert bracelet; awareness of sepsis risk	Improves emergency management and outcomes
Lifelong follow-up	Continue annual influenza, 5-year PPSV23 boosters, and monitor for late VTE or infections	Emphasize coordinated primary and haematology care

18.7 Splenic Embolization

Notably, while generally safe, splenectomy has declined in recent years [7, 10], due to the availability of thrombopoietin receptor agonists and rituximab, though it possibly remains the most curative approach. Nevertheless, it could be a challenge for elderly individuals and those with significant comorbidities. In such cases, splenic artery embolization (SE) could be considered. In a collected analysis of 228 patients across several published series, SE was associated with CR rates of 50.1% and 74.4% overall response, 46% sustained response at 10 years, which compares well with splenectomy [13]. It would perhaps be necessary to target >60% embolization to achieve the desired results with easily manageable post embolization syndrome (abdominal pain, fever). Splenic abscess was seen in 1.3% cases, with one death in the entire analysis. A second embolization helped only those who had relapsed or had a partial response to the first SE procedure [13].

18.8 Rituximab in ITP

Rituximab has shown overall response rates of approximately 50–80% across studies (Table 18.8). Interestingly, the RITP randomized placebo-controlled study failed to show any significant benefit compared to placebo, albeit with a longer response interval. The low-dose rituximab studies showed results like standard dose schedules. Smaller studies with combination therapy appeared to show better response rates (Table 18.9) in the short term, with no long-term benefit (Table 18.10).

Table 18.8 Rituximab monotherapy in ITP

Study	*N*	Dose	ORR (%)	CR (%)	Median time to relapse	Notes
Mishra et al., India 2021 [20]	81	375 mg/m²/week ×4	51.7% at day 30	16.7% 37.8% PR	28 days 30% at 1 year	Median follow-up 789 days
RITP trial—Rituximab arm [14]	55	375 mg/m²/week ×4	81%	58%	Relapse-free 36 weeks	Relapse 68%
RITP trial—Placebo arm [14]	54	Placebo	73%	50%		Relapse 78%
Lucchini et al. 2019 Review [15]	313	375 mg/m²/week ×4	52–73%	20–54%	Median duration of response: 10.5 months	Systematic review
Kapoor et al., India 2017 [17]	21	100 mg/week ×4	47.6%	33.3%	Median time to CR 75 days; and PR 105 days	RFS 78% at 13 months
Zaja et al. 2010 [21]	48	100 mg × 4	60.5%	39.5%	–	55% relapse by 24 mo

Table 18.9 Rituximab in combination therapies

Study	Combination	*N*	ORR (%)	CR (%)	Notes
Chu et al., Vietnam 2024 [16]	Eltrombopag + low-dose RTX	4	100%	50%	All responded; no AEs
Zhou et al. [18]	rhTPO + RTX (100 mg × 4)	77	79.2%	45.4%	Time to response 7 d (median 7–28) vs 28 d (median 4–90): No long-term benefit
Gomez Almaguer 2017 [19]	Eltrombopag + Dex + RTX	13	100%	92%	High CR; 5/13 received additional high-dose dexamethasone

Splenectomy has better response rates and durability as compared to rituximab (Table 18.10)

Table 18.10 Rituximab vs. splenectomy—comparative efficacy

Study	N (RTX/Splx)	Response 3 mo	Response 12 mo	CR 3 mo	CR 12 mo	5 yr. Sustained	Median duration of response
Shamoon et al., Iraq 2024 [23]	27/47	NA	NA	44.4/83.0%	NA	52/74%	Not stated
Moulis et al., France 2014 [22]	43/62	69.8/91.4%	59.0/87.9%	39.5/82.8%	35.9/81.0%	NA	20.1 mo (RTX); 81.0 mo (Splx)

RTX Rituximab, *Splx* Splenectomy, *NA* not available

6 months, bleeding history, or anticoagulant use [44]. It is appropriate to taper in all others with normal/ above normal platelet counts irrespective of duration of therapy or time to response. The taper schedule is generally similar to those experienced with a steroid taper. There is no definite guidance on how to monitor platelet counts after taper [44]. For eltrombopag and avatrombopag, tapering involves dose reduction followed by interval prolongation. For romiplostim, only dose reduction is appropriate. Patients should be monitored for 1–2 weeks post-discontinuation. Restarting therapy is advised if platelets fall <30 × 10^9/L with bleeding. Tables 18.13 and 18.14 summarize the STOPAGO and TAPER study protocol and outcomes, respectively. The TAPER studied patients on eltrombopag who were steroid relapsed-refractory [43].

18.12 Fostamatinib

Fostamatinib is an oral spleen tyrosine kinase (SYK) inhibitor. It has a dual mechanism whereby it blocks Fcγ receptor-mediated phagocytosis of antibody-coated platelets. It also impairs B-cell receptor signalling, thus reducing autoantibody

18.9 Rituximab in Children

The two studies from India included children with the youngest being 2.5 years in Mishra et al. [20]. A retrospective cohort study of 64 patients (24 children <18 years and 40 adults ≥18 years) treated with rituximab for ITP showed no significant difference in complete response (CR) between children (58%) and adults (55%). The median age at first rituximab dose was 12.1 years for children and 52.6 years for adults. Fifteen responders required additional therapy more than 6 months after rituximab [24]. In another systematic review and meta-analysis of prospective clinical trials comparing thrombopoietin receptor agonists (TPO-RAs) with rituximab (RTX) in children with ITP, both therapies showed similar rates of achieving platelet response (71% for TPO-RAs vs. 68% for RTX) [25]. However, TPO-RAs, particularly romiplostim, had superior sustainability of platelet response in this meta-analysis. The mean time to response was 6.75 weeks for rituximab, compared to 4.75 weeks with TPO-RAs. Patients on rituximab were more likely to require rescue therapy [25]. The long-term immunosuppressive effects of Rituximab are a concern, but hypogammaglobulinaemia was noted in one RTX study by Wang et al. in 3 out of 24 patients (12.5%) without subsequent serious infections or need for IVIG replacement [26].

There have been variable data on potential predictors of response to rituximab, and hence no meaningful conclusion can be made with regard to rituximab versus TPO agonists in children [25].

18.10 Thrombopoietin Receptor Agonists (TPO-RA) in Immune Thrombocytopenia (ITP)

Thrombopoietin receptor agonists (TPO-RAs) are second-line agents in immune thrombocytopenia (ITP), acting through stimulation of the thrombopoietin receptor (c-MPL) to promote megakaryocyte proliferation and platelet production. Romiplostim is a peptibody that competitively binds to the extracellular domain of c-MPL, mimicking endogenous TPO and primarily stimulating mature megakaryocyte precursors [27]. The small molecule agents (eltrombopag and avatrombopag) activate key intracellular signalling pathways—namely JAK2/STAT5, PI3K/AKT, and MAPK/ERK—that lead to megakaryocyte maturation and increased thrombopoiesis. Unlike Romiplostim, their binding to the TPO receptor is noncompetitive. These agents may have immunomodulatory effects by enhancing regulatory T-cell activity and modulating antigen presentation, suggesting a role beyond thrombopoiesis [28]. TPO receptor agonists have similarities in structure to iron chelators and have been described to cause iron deficiency anaemia [29] with a potential effect on the antiproliferative effects of malignant cells due to antiproliferative effects and reduced intracellular iron. Table 18.11 summarizes the key TPO agonists, indications besides ITP, and their features.

Table 18.11 Comparison of various TPO agonists

Drug name [27]	Indications	Dosing regimen (for ITP)	Common adverse effects	Food/cation restrictions
Romiplostim: Adults and children	Chronic ITP, refractory ITP, severe aplastic anaemia (EU)	1 μg/kg SC weekly, titrated	Arthralgia, myalgia, headache	None
Eltrombopag: Adults and children	Chronic ITP, SAA, HCV-associated thrombocytopenia	50 mg daily, adjust to a lower dose for Asians/ children	Transaminitis, cataracts	Avoid food, Ca^{2+}, Fe^{2+}, Mg^{2+}
Avatrombopag: Adults only	Chronic ITP, chronic liver disease-related thrombocytopenia	20 mg daily, max 40 mg	Headache, URTI Minimal hepatotoxicity	Take with food
Lusutrombopag	Chronic liver disease-related thrombocytopenia	3 mg daily × 7 days	Headache, nausea	None

Table 18.12 summarizes the published data on the TPO receptor agonists. They induce platelet responses in 60–90% of patients with ITP with similar efficacy and safety in both adult and paediatric populations, while avatrombopag has shown high initial response rates and favourable safety in adults. Real-world data support switching between agents for intolerance or suboptimal efficacy. Avatrombopag has been effective in patients with prior exposure and resistance/ intolerance to TPO receptor agonists. Patients who have undergone splenectomy have also responded to avatrombopag [40]. The TPO receptor agonists are generally well tolerated with no long-term side effects on bone marrow fibrosis, cataract or other adverse effects. 6.2% of 961 patients on follow-up developed antibodies to romiplostim at a median follow-up of 14 weeks without any effect on platelet counts [39].

18.11 Tapering of TPO-RAs

Only up to a third of patients with ITP who respond to TPO-RAs may safely discontinue therapy [28] and less than 10% have sustained responses off drug. In a paediatric analysis of romiplostim in 262 patients across clinical trials, 7% patients were able to hold all therapy, including romiplostim for more than 6 months [37]. Tapering TPO-RAs is considered in patients with stable platelet counts $\geq 150 \times 10^9/L$, no recent bleeding, no anticoagulants, and low trauma risk. In a prospective multicentric trial (STOPAGO), with most patients on eltrombopag, 27 of 48 achieved SROT (sustained response off treatment), 15 of 48 achieved SCROT (sustained complete remission off treatment) at Week 24; 25 of 48 achieved SROT, and 14 of 48 achieved SCROT at week 52 [35]. Patients who had increased expression of CD69 on CD8 T cells at the time of taper were less likely to benefit [35]. These responses were sustained in the majority at 4 year followup [42]. Tapering is inappropriate with platelet counts $<30–50 \times 10^9/L$, recent therapy intensification within

Table 18.12 Summary of published response outcomes with thrombopoietin-receptor agonists

Study (year)/design/ population	TPO-RA dose/ regimen	Overall platelet response	Complete response	Median time to response	Durable/sustained response	Notes
PETIT–Phase-1/2 DB-RCT, paediatric persistent/chronic ITP ($n = 67$) [30]	Eltrombopag (weight-adjusted): 45 Placebo 22	62%	–	–	36% sustained (wks 2–6)	Included a dose-finding arm
PETIT-2 (2015)—Phase-3 DB-RCT, paediatric persistent/chronic ITP ($n = 92$) [31]	Eltrombopag 63 Placebo 29	40%	–	N-	41% sustained (weeks 5–12)	
Zhang et al. 2018—Meta-analysis of 5 paediatric RCTs = 261 [32]	Eltrombopag vs Romiplostim	Similar (RR 0.57; CI 0.21–1.56)	NR	–	Similar (RR 2.48; CI 0.31–19.97)	
Neunert et al. 2016—ICON ($n = 87$) [33]	TPO agonist in children (Romiplostim 51 Eltrombopag 36	86–89% %	N	6.4–7 weeks	40% sustained responses at consistent doses	67% had a bone marrow examination: 17% of which had increased reticulin No cataract
Mishra et al. 2020—Indian cohort ($n = 53$ adults) [34]	Eltrombopag (50–75 mg)	81.1% at 3 months	34%	35 days	Relapse: 25.3% at 3 years and 47.7.% at 5 years	Hepatobiliary adverse effects in 17% and anaemia in 47%
Tomasello et al. 2023—Norwegian registry ($n = 16$) [36]	Romiplostim	70%	61%	7 days	Durable 52%; SROT 9%	
Tomasello et al. 2023—Norwegian registry ($n = 35$) [36]	Eltrombopag	68%	56%	10 days	Durable 74%; SROT 6%	

Tomasello et al. 2023—Norwegian registry (*n* = 14) [36]	Avatrombopag	100%	100%	7 days	Durable 64%; SROT 0%	
Romiplostim pooled paediatric data (*n* = 262) [37]	Romiplostim	88–90%	NR	5–6 weeks		7% cases could come off all therapy
UK ITP Registry 2019 (*n* = 118 adults) [38]	Romiplostim	Mean increase from 38 to 103×10^9/L	Not reported	4 weeks	Responses maintained 3 yrs	
Jurczak et al. 2018—Phase III RCT (*n* = 49) [40]	Avatrombopag (20–40 mg/day)	65.6%	28.1%	8 days	34.4% durable (6/8 wks)	
Pascual-Izquierdo et al. 2025—AVAMAD study (*n* = 66) [41]	Avatrombopag (20–40 mg/day)	86.36%	72.7%	2 weeks (IQR 1.3–4.3)	74.2% no rescue; in 56,% reduced concomitant meds	

SROT Sustained Response Off Treatment

production. Table 18.15 summarizes the available data on fastamatinib. The table shows data from pivotal FIT1/ FIT2 trials, comparing them with the results of a meta-analysis.

Fostamatinib and TPO agonists could potentially complement each other's mechanism of action. In a retrospective real-world study on 113 patients receiving various combinations, the platelet counts were maintained at more than ≥50,000/μL in ≥50% readings, 60% of the time [47]. The common side-effects were Diarrhoea (23%), hypertension (18%), bleeding (12%), fatigue (8%), headache (5%), thrombosis (4%).

Table 18.13 STOPAGO and TAPER studies

Study	Drug	Tapering step	Interval	Discontinuation criteria
STOPAGO [35, 42]	Eltrombopag	↓ 25 mg every 2 weeks	Every 2 weeks	≥30 × 10^9/L, stopped by week 10
	Romiplostim	↓ 1 μg/kg every 2 weeks	Every week	≥30 × 10^9/L, stopped by week 10
TAPER [43]	Eltrombopag	↓ 25 mg every 2 weeks	Every 2 weeks	Stable counts, no bleeding/ rescue use

↓ = dose reduction; q2w = every 2 weeks

Table 18.14 Outcomes of STOPAGO and TAPER studies on TPO-RA discontinuation

Study	Population	Median TPO exposure	TPO agent	SROT / SCROT at 48 months	SROT at 24 months	Relapse after discontinuation
STOPAGO [35, 42]	48 adults with chronic ITP	2.1 years	Eltrombopag and Romiplostim; Eltrombopag 92%	SROT 52.1%, SCROT 29.2%	SROT 47.9% ≥30 × 10^9/L SCROT 39.6% complete response ≥100 × 10^9/L	2 (1 regained CR on reinitiation)
TAPER [43]	105 adults, relapsed/ refractory ITP	5.6 months	Eltrombopag	30.5%	Not reported	12 relapsed; 7/8 responded to restart. Median duration of SROT: 22 months at month 24 of follow-up

SROT Sustained Response Off Treatment, SCROT Sustained complete response off treatment, *CR* Complete Response, *NR* Not Reported

Table 18.15 Fostamatinib trial data

Outcome	FIT1/FIT2 trials [45]	Meta-analysis (2024) [46]
Stable response (platelets ≥50,000/μL at ≥4/6 visits, weeks 14–24)	18% (18/101) vs. 2% placebo (p = 0.0003)	ORR 0.80 (95% CI: 0.72–0.88), NNT = 10
Overall response (≥1 platelet count ≥50,000/μL within 12 weeks)	43% vs. 14% placebo (p = 0.0006)	ORR at week 12 = 0.80 (95% CI: 0.72–0.90); at week 24 = 0.82
Patients with baseline <15,000/μL achieving ≥30,000 and ≥ 20,000 rise	21% at week 12; 15% at week 24	ORR 0.81 at week 12; 0.82 at week 24
Median time to response	15 days	Consistent with trial data
Dose	100 mg twice daily	100–150 mg twice daily
Adverse effects	Diarrhoea 31%, hypertension 28%, raised ALT 11%	Increased risk of diarrhoea, hypertension, and raised liver enzymes

18.13 Other Immunosuppressive Drugs

Recent studies on various immunosuppressive and immunomodulating therapies in refractory immune thrombocytopenia (ITP) are highlighted in Table 18.16. Dapsone is popular because it is a cheap alternative and has shown some activity with variable results from Indian studies. A large French study failed to show any benefit with frequent discontinuations [54]. The AIIMS Delhi study on cyclosporine reported a 36% complete response rate [49]. Another commonly available drug, Danazol, was studied in Nepal and had response rates of 65%, albeit with liver side effects [50]. The other drugs, mycophenolate, azathioprine, and sirolimus have been used with similar response rates ranging between 30–40%, with a small case series showing 57% response for daratumumab. In a randomized study on Mycophenopate glucocorticoid combination compared to glucocorticoid alone, the combination showed greater efficacy and lesser failures over time [55]. The response rates, time to response, duration of response, and other outcome measures are too varied, and without randomized comparative data, it is not possible to make any recommendations on the choice of therapy beyond TPO agonists, rituximab, and splenectomy.

18.14 Which Intervention is Best Used as Second Line?

Table 18.17 summarizes data from selected trials discussed in this review. Splenectomy is still considered a reasonable option in terms of response rates and durability of response. In experienced centres with vaccination and good post-splenectomy prophylaxis, morbidity and mortality rates are minimal. However, this might not be an option in children <5 years of age and patients with comorbidities

Table 18.16 Other immunosuppressives in ITP

Drug	Study and design (Country, Year)	Number of patients	Median age (range)	Complete remission†	Overall response†	Time to response	Duration of response	Adverse events‡	Dose used
Aza-thioprine	Mishra et al., Retrospective (India, 2021) [48]	63	28 (15–68)	1 patient	38.1% @ 90d	95 days	FU 870d; relapse 21% at 5y	41% (≥Grade 3: 4.7%): Leukopenia, anaemia, 1 death due to sepsis	1–2 mg/kg/day
Cyclo-sporine A	Choudhary et al., Prospective Single-Centre (India, 2008) [49]	25	12 (4–73)	36% (9/25)	44% (CR + PR)	Not reported	Mean follow-up 7.3 ± 2.1 mo; 3 relapsed	Gingival hyperplasia (8%); no HTN/hirsutism	5 mg/kg/day ×1 wk. → 3 mg/kg/day (target level 200–400 ng/mL)
Danazol	Shah et al., Meta-analysis (Nepal 2024) [50]	901	Range 16–86 (median NR)	≈46%	61%	~3 months	ORR 65% at 12 mo	12–21% (LFT↑, wt gain)	200–800 mg/day
Daratu-mumab	Strüßmann et al., case series (Germany, 2024) [51]	7	59 (22–87)	57% (4/7)	57%	1–10 weeks	Sustained 9–36 mo	None ≥Grade 3	1800 mg SC weekly (4–17 doses)
Dapsone	Karthika et al., prospective (India, 2021) [52]	50: 36 female	20 (3–60)	4.1%	20.8% @ 12 mo	2–6 months	Assessed to 12 mo	46% mild-mod; 4% severe	2 mg/kg/day
Dapsone	Khera et al., Paediatric Case Series (India, 2020) [53]	29	9.8 (3–14)	24%	72%	2.9 months	FU 28 mo; relapse 21%	MetHb 3%, ulcers 7%	1–2 mg/kg/day

Dapsone	Larue et al., RCT + Observational (France, 2025) [54]	93 (RCT) 46 (Obs)	48.5 (RCT), 50.7 (Obs)	–	ORR 21.7% (RCT)/13.6% (Obs)	Median 4.6 weeks	Follow-up 52 weeks	78% early d/c; 67% SAE	100 mg/day
MMF first line	Bradbury et al., RCT (UK, 2021) [55]	59 MMF plus steroid	Mean 54 (17–87)	91.5%	91.5%	38 days (6–65)	Sustained for 2 years	No ↑ severe AEs	0.5–1 g BID
		61 steroid alone		63.9%	63.9%	46 days (6–58)			
MMF	Abdelwahab et al., Meta-analysis (Egypt, 2023) [56]	411	Mostly adults 17–87	32%	50–62%	4–6 weeks	Not pooled	12% (GI commonest)	0.5–1 g BID
Sirolimus	Feng et al., Prospective Single-Arm (China, 2020) [57]	86	40 (5–85)	40% (3 mo); 41% (6 mo)	85% (3 mo); 70% (6 mo)	Median 19 days	ORR 65% at 12 mo	Dyslipidaemia 12%, ulcers 7%, rash 5%, Gr3 pneumonia 1%	2–4 mg/day (target 5–15 ng/ml)

MMF Mycophenolate Mofetyl, *NR* Not reported, *FU* follow-up, *d/c* discontinued

[a]CR: Platelets >100 × 10^9/L. PR: ≥30 × 10^9/L & ≥2× baseline.

[b]Percent of patients with any AE; most common or serious types in parentheses.

that preclude splenectomy. TPO agonists would be preferred over rituximab in adults and over rituximab and splenectomy in children who did not respond to first line therapy [58]. The responses with TPO agonists appear comparable, but the drug has to be continued indefinitely in the majority of cases. Fostamatinib data comes from heavily pre-treated individuals and could perhaps be combined with TPO agonists to achieve synergistic action.

18.15 Thrombotic Risk in ITP

Splenectomy has been associated with a 4% risk of thrombosis [4]. Laparoscopic surgeries are likely associated with lesser risk [59]. In a retrospective analysis of 220 patients by Goncalves et al., 26 experienced thrombosis events, which included 29 venous thromboembolism (VTE) cases and 8 arterial thromboembolism (ATE) cases, giving an incidence rate of 2.71 thrombosis events per 100 person-years [59]. The risk factors associated with thrombosis in ITP were older age, pre-existing prothrombotic states, prior thromboembolic episodes, TPO agonists (HR 1.82, $P = 0.16$), secondary ITP (SLE) [59, 60]. One needs to be aware of pre-existing prothrombotic states and manage those accordingly, as ITP itself and its treatment modalities, like splenectomy and TPO RA, would add to the risk.

Table 18.17 Summary of data across different interventions for relapsed/refractory ITP

Therapy	Overall rate (%)	Complete response rate (%)	Sustained response at 1 Year (%)	Sustained response at 5 Years (%)	Median time to response	References
Splenectomy	88–89%	61.8–88%	~65%	54–57%	Immediate (~1 month)	Zoletto et al. 2025 [11], Mishra et al. 2021 [10]
Rituximab	54.5%	16.7%	~69%	~43%	28 days	Mishra et al. 2021 [20]
Romiplostim	92.3%	84.6%	~50% at 1 year	Not reported	7 days	Tomasello et al. [36]
Eltrombopag	81.1%	34%	93.4%	~52%	35 days	Mishra et al. 2020 [34]
Fostamatinib	43%	18% stable response	54%	Not reported	15 days	Bussel et al. FIT1/FIT2 trials [45]
Dapsone	22%	4.1%	20.8% @ 12 mo	Not reported	Not reported 72.9% at 2 months	Karthika et al. 2021 [52]
Azathioprine	38.1%	1.8%	~79%	78.8%	95 days	Mishra et al. 2021 [48]
Cyclosporine	50–60%	~20%	~30%	Not reported	1–3 months	Choudhary et al. 2008 [49]

18.16 Patient and Physician Perspectives on ITP

So how do patients and physicians perceive ITP? The I-Wish study from India provided some interesting insights [61]. While both physicians and patients agreed that quality of life is important, treatments should target once-daily oral treatments with minimal toxicity wherever possible. However, patients wanted their physicians to address fatigue, while physicians felt that ensuring bleed-free periods alone would perhaps improve a patient's quality of life. More importantly, physicians self-assessed that they provided all information, whereas patients actually felt otherwise, highlighting the need for empowering patients with more communication regarding their disease.

18.17 Summary

Initial therapy in ITP is guided by bleeding severity. Paediatric cases often resolve spontaneously or respond to IVIG or steroids, while adult cases are more prone to chronicity.

For relapsed or refractory ITP, treatment options have been expanding beyond splenectomy. Splenectomy remains efficacious, but despite being safe might not be feasible in certain situations and is associated with thrombotic and infectious risks. Thrombopoietin receptor agonists (romiplostim, eltrombopag, and avatrombopag) offer comparable and durable response rates and are increasingly used as second-line or adjunct therapies. Fostamatinib has shown efficacy combined with TPO – RAs. Along with Fosatmatinib, other selective, short-acting, and reversible BTKi could become additional treatment options in chronic ITP. Immunosuppressants like azathioprine, MMF, cyclosporine, sirolimus, and danazol provide additional, though perhaps less effective options. Finally, patient and physician perspectives need to be aligned, and this is critical for shared decision-making in chronic disease.

References

1. Mititelu A, Onisâi M-C, Rosca A, Vlădăreanu AM. Current understanding of immune thrombocytopenia: a review of pathogenesis and treatment options. Int J Mol Sci. 2024;25(4):2163.
2. Russo G, Parodi E, Farruggia P, Notarangelo LD et al. Recommendations for the management of acute immune thrombocytopenia in children. A Consensus Conference from the Italian Association of Pediatric Hematology and Oncology. Blood Transfus. 2024;22:253–65.
3. Neunert C, Terrell DR, Arnold DM, Buchanan G, Cines DB, Cooper N, et al. American Society of Hematology 2019 guidelines for immune thrombocytopenia. Blood Adv. 2019;3(23):3829–66.
4. Chaturvedi S, Arnold DM, McCrae KR. Splenectomy for immune thrombocytopenia: down but not out. Blood. 2018;131(11):1172–82.
5. Ahmed R, Devasia AJ, Viswabandya A, et al. Long-term outcome following splenectomy for chronic and persistent immune thrombocytopenia (ITP) in adults and children. Ann Hematol. 2016;95(9):1429–34.

6. Avila ML, Amiri N, Pullenayegum E, et al. Long-term outcomes after splenectomy in children with immune thrombocytopenia: an update on the registry data from the Intercontinental Cooperative ITP Study Group. Haematologica. 2020;105(11):2682–5.
7. Ducassou S, Gourdonneau A, Fernandes H, et al. Second-line treatment trends and long-term outcomes of 392 children with chronic immune thrombocytopenic purpura: the French experience over the past 25 years. Br J Haematol. 2020;189(5):931–42.
8. Mendoza A, Álvarez-Román MT, Monzón-Manzano E, et al. Study of platelet kinetics in immune thrombocytopenia to predict splenectomy response. Br J Haematol. 2024;204(1):315–23.
9. Isshiki K, Mori M, Irikura T, et al. Long-term efficacy and safety profile of splenectomy for pediatric chronic immune thrombocytopenia. Int J Hematol. 2023;117(5):774–80.
10. Mishra K, Kumar S, Sandal R, Jandial A, et al. Safety and efficacy of splenectomy in immune thrombocytopenia. Am J Blood Res. 2021;11(4):361–72.
11. Zoletto S, Pizzi M, De Crescenzo A, et al. Predictors of splenectomy response in immune thrombocytopenia: a multicentric Italian study. J Clin Med. 2025;14(1):30.
12. Goshua G, Sinha P, Kunst N, Pischel L, Lee AI, Cuker A. Cost-effectiveness of second-line therapies in adults with chronic immune thrombocytopenia. Am J Hematol. 2023;98:122–30.
13. Egbaria A, Touma E, Cohen-Abadi M, Bisharat N. The use of splenic embolization in immune thrombocytopenia: a systematic review and meta-analysis. Br J Haematol. 2024;204:1966–76.
14. Ghanima W, Khelif A, Waage A, et al. Rituximab as second-line treatment for adult immune thrombocytopenia (the RITP trial): a multicentre, randomised, double-blind, placebo-controlled trial. Lancet. 2015;385:1653–61.
15. Lucchini E, Zaja F, Bussel J. Rituximab in the treatment of immune thrombocytopenia: what is the role of this agent in 2019? Haematologica. 2019;104(6):1124–35.
16. Chu TH, Huynh TN, Trinh-Le QV, et al. Refractory immune thrombocytopenia responding to combination therapy of eltrombopag and low-dose rituximab: a case series. Hematol Transfus Cell Ther. 2024;46(S5):S299–304.
17. Kapoor R, Kumar R, Mahapatra M, Pati HP, Pramanik SK. Low dose rituximab in chronic ITP: still an option in resource limited settings. Indian J Hematol Blood Transfus. 2017;33(4):568–73.
18. Zhou H, Xu M, Qin P, et al. A multicenter randomized open-label study of rituximab plus rhTPO vs rituximab in corticosteroid-resistant or relapsed ITP. Blood. 2015;125(10):1541–7.
19. Gómez-Almaguer D, Colunga-Pedraza PR, Gómez-De León A, Gutiérrez-Aguirre CH, Cantú-Rodríguez OG, Jaime-Pérez JC. Eltrombopag, low-dose rituximab, and dexamethasone combination as frontline treatment of newly diagnosed immune thrombocytopaenia. Br J Haematol. 2019;184(2):288–90.
20. Mishra K, Kumar S, Jandial A, et al. Real-world experience of rituximab in immune thrombocytopenia. Indian J Hematol Blood Transfus. 2021;37(3):404–13.
21. Zaja F, Vianelli N, Volpetti S, et al. Low-dose rituximab in adult patients with primary immune thrombocytopenia. Eur J Haematol. 2010;85(4):329–34.
22. Moulis G, Sailler L, Sommet A, et al. Rituximab versus splenectomy in persistent or chronic adult primary immune thrombocytopenia: an adjusted comparison of mortality and morbidity. Am J Hematol. 2014;89(1):41–6.
23. Shamoon RP, Yassin AK, Alnuaimy SL. Rituximab versus splenectomy in chronic primary ITP: experience of a single hematology clinic. Mediterr J Hematol Infect Dis. 2024;16(1):e2024019.
24. Harris EM, Hillier K, Al-Samkari H, Berbert L, Grace RF. Response to rituximab in children and adults with immune thrombocytopenia (ITP). Res Pract Thromb Haemost. 2021;5:e12587.
25. Ayad N, Grace RF, Al-Samkari H. Thrombopoietin receptor agonists and rituximab for treatment of pediatric immune thrombocytopenia: a systematic review and meta-analysis of prospective clinical trials. Pediatr Blood Cancer. 2022;69(3):e29447.
26. Wang J, Wiley JM, Luddy R, Greenberg J, Feuerstein MA, Bussel JB. Chronic immune thrombocytopenic purpura in children: assessment of rituximab treatment. J Pediatr. 2005;146(2):217–21.
27. Gilreath JA, Lo M, Bubalo J. Thrombopoietin Receptor Agonists (TPORAs): drug class considerations for pharmacists. Drugs. 2021;81(11):1285–1305.

28. Ghanima W, Cooper N, Rodeghiero F, Godeau B, Bussel JB. Thrombopoietin receptor agonists: ten years later. Haematologica. 2019;104(6):1112–23.
29. Lambert MP, Witmer CM, Kwiatkowski JL. Therapy induced iron deficiency in children treated with eltrombopag for immune thrombocytopenia. Am J Hematol. 2017;92(6):E88–91.
30. Bussel JB, de Miguel PG, Despotovic JM, et al. Eltrombopag for the treatment of children with persistent and chronic immune thrombocytopenia (PETIT): a randomised, multicentre, placebo-controlled study. Lancet Haematol. 2015;2(8):e315–25.
31. Grainger JD, Locatelli F, Chotsampancharoen T, et al. Eltrombopag for children with chronic immune thrombocytopenia (PETIT2). Lancet. 2015;386(10004):1649–58.
32. Zhang J, Liang Y, Ai Y, et al. Eltrombopag versus romiplostim in treatment of children with persistent or chronic immune thrombocytopenia: a systematic review incorporating an indirect-comparison meta-analysis. Sci Rep. 2018;8(1):576.
33. Neunert C, Despotovic J, Haley K, et al. Thrombopoietin receptor agonist use in children: data from the pediatric ITP consortium of North America ICON2 study. Pediatr Blood Cancer. 2016;63(8):1407–13.
34. Mishra K, Pramanik S, Jandial A, et al. Real-world experience of eltrombopag in immune thrombocytopenia. Am J Blood Res. 2020;10(5):240–51.
35. Guillet S, Crickx E, Azzaoui I, et al. Prolonged response after TPO-RA discontinuation in primary ITP: results of a prospective multicenter study. Blood. 2023;141(23):2867–77.
36. Tomasello R, Garabet L, Pettersen H, et al. Real-world use, effectiveness and safety of romiplostim, eltrombopag and avatrombopag in immune thrombocytopenia: data from the Norwegian ITP registry. Blood. 2023;142(Suppl 1):3952.
37. Tarantino MD, Despotovic J, Roy J, et al. Romiplostim treatment for children with immune thrombocytopenia: Results of an integrated database of five clinical trials. Pediatr Blood Cancer. 2020;67(11):e28630.
38. Doobaree IU, Newland A, McDonald V, et al. Primary immune thrombocytopenia (ITP) treated with romiplostim in routine clinical practice: retrospective study from the United Kingdom ITP registry. Eur J Haematol. 2019;102(5):416–23.
39. Mytych DT, Park JK, Kim J, Barger TE, Boshier A, Jawa V, Kuter DJ. Assessment of romiplostim immunogenicity in adult patients in clinical trials and in a global postmarketing registry. Br J Haematol. 2020;190(6):923–32.
40. Jurczak W, Chojnowski K, Mayer J, Krawczyk K, Jamieson BD, Tian W, Allen LF. Phase 3 randomised study of avatrombopag, a novel thrombopoietin receptor agonist for the treatment of chronic immune thrombocytopenia. Br J Haematol. 2018;183(3):479–90.
41. Pascual-Izquierdo C, Llacer-Ferrandis MJ, de-la-Iglesia A, Monsalvo-Saornil S, et al. Avatrombopag in adults with immune thrombocytopenia: a multicentre real-life observational study in Madrid, Spain (AVAMAD study). Br J Haematol. 2025;206(2):652–6.
42. Cottu A, Guillet S, Viallard JF, et al. Long-term follow-up of the STOPAGO study. Blood. 2025;145(2):244–7.
43. Cooper N, Ghanima W, Vianelli N, et al. Sustained response off-treatment in eltrombopag-treated adult patients with ITP who are refractory or relapsed after first-line steroids: primary, final, and ad-hoc analyses of the phase II TAPER trial. Am J Hematol. 2024;99(1):57–67.
44. Cuker A, Despotovic JM, Grace RF, et al. Tapering thrombopoietin receptor agonists in primary immune thrombocytopenia: RAND/UCLA Delphi panel. Res Pract Thromb Haemost. 2020;5(1):69–80.
45. Bussel J, Arnold DM, Grossbard E, Mayer J, et al. Fostamatinib for the treatment of adult persistent and chronic immune thrombocytopenia. Am J Hematol. 2018;93(7):921–30.
46. Tungjitviboonkun S, Bumrungratanayos N, Jitwimungsanon J, Kheamakulvanich T, Siramongkholkarn S. Efficacy and safety of fostamatinib in refractory immune thrombocytopenia: a meta-analysis from randomized controlled trials. Ann Hematol. 2024;103:3357–68.
47. Bowhay-Carnes E, Kreychman Y, Buxman L, Todd L. Real-world experience with combination therapy of fostamatinib and thrombopoetin receptor agonists (TPO-RAs) for treatment of immune thrombocytopenia (ITP): patient-reported outcomes. Blood. 2024;144(Supplement 1):5080.
48. Mishra K, Pramanik SK, Sandal R, et al. Safety and efficacy of azathioprine in immune thrombocytopenia. Am J Blood Res. 2021;11(3):217–26.

49. Choudhary DR, Naithani R, Mahapatra M, Mishra P, Saxena R. Efficacy of cyclosporine as a single agent therapy in chronic idiopathic thrombocytopenic purpura. Haematologica. 2008;93:e61-2.
50. Shah S, Yadav R, Bhattarai A, et al. Safety and efficacy of danazol in immune thrombocytopenia: a systematic review. Res Pract Thromb Haemost. 2024;8(4):e102444.
51. Strüßmann T, Heinz J, Wäsch R, et al. Long-term complete remissions of refractory severe idiopathic immune thrombocytopenia treated with daratumumab: A case series. Br J Haematol. 2024;205(4):1618–21.
52. Karthika S, Mandal PK, Baul S, Dolai TK. A Study from Eastern India on the Role of Dapsone Therapy in Patients of Persistent and Chronic Immune Thrombocytopenia; Where Do We Stand ? J Indian Med Assoc. 2021;119(6):16–21.
53. Khera S, Pramanik SK, Yanamandra U, et al. Dapsone: an old but effective therapy in paediatric refractory immune thrombocytopenia. Indian J Hematol Blood Transfus. 2020;36:690–4.
54. Larue M, Moulis G, Rueter M, et al. Efficacy and safety of dapsone in adult primary immune thrombocytopenia. Blood Adv. 2025;9(8):1976–83.
55. Bradbury CA, Pell J, Hill Q, et al. Mycophenolate mofetil for first-line treatment of immune thrombocytopenia. N Engl J Med. 2021;385 (10):885–95.
56. Abdelwahab OA, Mechi A, Gahlan S, et al. Efficacy and safety of mycophenolate mofetil in immune thrombocytopenic purpura: a systematic review and meta-analysis. Clin Rheumatol. 2024;43:621–32.
57. Feng Y, Xiao Y, Yan H, et al. Sirolimus as Rescue Therapy for Refractory/Relapsed Immune Thrombocytopenia: Results of a Single-Center, Prospective, Single-Arm Study. Front Med (Lausanne). 2020;7:110.
58. Neunert CE, Arnold DM, Grace RF, Kuhne T, McCrae KR, Terrell DR. The 2022 review of the 2019 American Society of Hematology Guidelines on immune thrombocytopenia. Blood Adv. 2024;8(13):3578–82.
59. Goncalves I, Lewis C, Grainger B, Dring R, Lee N, Pasricha S-R, et al. Thrombosis in patients with immune thrombocytopenia: incidence, risk, and clinical outcomes. Res Pract Thromb Haemost. 2024;8(1):102342.
60. Tjepkema M, Amini S, Schipperus M. Risk of thrombosis with thrombopoietin receptor agonists for ITP patients: a systematic review and meta-analysis. Crit Rev Oncol Hematol. 2022;171:103581.
61. Chakrabarti P, George B, Shanmukhaiah C, et al. How do patients and physicians perceive immune thrombocytopenia (ITP) as a disease? Results from Indian analysis of ITP World Impact Survey (I-WISh). J Patient Rep Outcomes. 2022;6(1):24.

Chapter 19
Comprehensive Management of Hemophilia, Including Recent Therapeutic Advances

Prantar Chakrabarti and Archit S. Pandharipande

Abstract Hemophilia remains one of the most challenging inherited bleeding disorders, especially in low- and middle-income countries (LMICs) where late diagnosis, suboptimal factor availability, and limited access to novel therapies hinder optimal outcomes. This chapter presents an integrated approach to the management of Hemophilia A and B, encompassing pathophysiology, classification, and clinical manifestations across different age groups. Using a real-life illustrative case, the narrative explores the evolution of treatment strategies—from plasma-derived concentrates to recombinant factor replacement and novel non-factor therapies. The role of low-dose prophylaxis, the importance of early joint protection, and LMIC-specific implementation barriers are emphasized.

Particular attention is paid to the advent of emicizumab and other non-factor therapies, which has transformed prophylaxis in both inhibitor and non-inhibitor patients, with insights from the HAVEN trials and Indian low-dose data. Gene therapy's promise is critically evaluated, including limitations related to cost, vector immunity, and durability of response. A cost-effectiveness comparison between conventional therapy, emicizumab, and gene therapy is presented. The chapter also outlines current international treatment guidelines (WFH, ISTH) and how they can be contextualized for resource-constrained settings.

This chapter aims to equip clinicians, researchers, and policymakers with a comprehensive yet practical understanding of hemophilia management tailored to regional needs and emerging global standards.

Keywords Hemophilia A · Emicizumab · Low-dose prophylaxis · Gene therapy · Inhibitor management · LMIC health policy · Recombinant factor replacement · WFH guidelines

---

P. Chakrabarti (✉)
Chief Medical Director, Sugah HealthCorp OPC Pvt Ltd, Chennai, India

Ex HOD, Department of Hematology, NRS Medical College, Kolkata, India

A. S. Pandharipande
Department of Clinical Hematology, All India Institute of Medical Sciences, Nagpur, India

H. P. Pati et al. (eds.), *Clinical Hematology and Hemato-Oncology*,
https://doi.org/10.1007/978-981-92-1167-8_19

Learning Objectives

By the end of this chapter, the reader will be able to:

- Understand the pathophysiology and clinical spectrum of Hemophilia A and B, including the role of clotting factor deficiencies.
- Describe the epidemiology and socioeconomic burden of hemophilia, particularly in low- and middle-income countries (LMICs).
- Recognize early signs and formulate a diagnostic approach, including laboratory and genetic investigations, for the timely identification of hemophilia and its complications.
- Evaluate the evolution of hemophilia treatment, from plasma-derived factors to recombinant products and cutting-edge gene therapies.
- Differentiate between primary, secondary, and tertiary prophylaxis strategies and assess their application in both HIC and LMIC settings.
- Understand the management of inhibitors, including immune tolerance induction and bypassing agents.
- Appreciate the critical role of physiotherapy and rehabilitation in preventing long-term joint damage and disability.
- Analyze the clinical efficacy and cost-effectiveness of novel therapies such as emicizumab, fitusiran, and concizumab.
- Interpret key data from landmark clinical trials and international guidelines (WFH/ISTH) that shape current hemophilia care.
- Explore the potential and limitations of gene therapy, including the latest developments in lentiviral and AAV-based approaches.
- Formulate context-specific strategies for LMICs, focusing on affordability, accessibility, and sustainable implementation of care.

19.1 Introduction

Hemophilia is a rare yet significant hereditary bleeding disorder resulting from a deficiency of clotting factors VIII (Hemophilia A) or IX (Hemophilia B). The disorder follows an X-linked recessive pattern of inheritance, making it primarily affect males, while females are typically carriers with variable clinical expression. Severe hemophilia, characterized by clotting factor levels below 1% of normal, leads to spontaneous bleeding, particularly in joints (hemarthrosis) and muscles, significantly impairing quality of life if left untreated.

The evolution of hemophilia management over the past century has been remarkable, transitioning from plasma-derived factor concentrates to recombinant products and now advanced therapies like rebalancing agents and gene therapy [1, 2]. Despite these advances, challenges persist, particularly in low- and middle-income countries (LMICs), where limited access to clotting factor replacement therapy leads to suboptimal care, increased morbidity, and early mortality. Even in high-income settings, the emergence of inhibitors—neutralizing antibodies that render factor therapy ineffective—continues to pose a formidable challenge. This chapter presents an overview of Hemophilia A, illustrating key issues in diagnosis and management.

19.1.1 Epidemiology and Burden of Disease

The global prevalence of hemophilia is estimated at 1 in 5000 male births for Hemophilia A and 1 in 30,000 for Hemophilia B [3]. There is significant underreporting of hemophilia diagnosis, especially in LMICs (low-middle-income countries). According to the WFH Annual Global Survey, only 30% of people with hemophilia worldwide receive adequate treatment, highlighting the disparity between high-income and resource-limited settings [4].

Hemophilia imposes a significant socioeconomic burden, and patients often experience high out-of-pocket expenses, loss of productivity due to disability, and limited access to comprehensive care, thus necessitating a planned approach to diagnosis, management, rehabilitation, and prevention.

19.1.1.1 Advancements in Hemophilia Care

The treatment landscape for hemophilia has shifted dramatically over the past few decades [1, 2]:

1. *Early Era (Pre-1950s)*: Whole blood transfusions were used with limited efficacy.
2. *1960s–1980s*: The development of plasma-derived factor concentrates significantly improved outcomes but introduced infectious risks (e.g., HIV, hepatitis B, and C).
3. *1990s–2010s*: Recombinant factor VIII/IX products became the standard of care, minimizing viral transmission risks. The standard half-life factors (SHLs) were modified to prolong their half-lives (EHLs), leading to fewer injections and consistent blood levels.
4. *2010s–Present*: The era of non-factor therapies (e.g., emicizumab), rebalancing agents (e.g., fitusiran, concizumab), and gene therapy (e.g., etranacogene dezaparvovec, valoctocogene roxaparvovec) is changing the treatment paradigm.

19.1.1.2 Illustrative Case Presentation

Patient Profile: 15-year-old Male, a diagnosed case of Severe Hemophilia A (Factor VIII <1%)

19.1.2 Early Childhood: Missed Diagnosis (Ages 0–10)

He was born to non-consanguineous parents with no known family history of hemophilia. His parents noticed frequent bruising, particularly after minor falls. At 18 months, he developed oral mucosal bleeding while teething, which was treated with home remedies. By the age of 3 years, he began experiencing painful joint swelling, particularly in his knees and ankles, often following minor trauma. He was prescribed analgesics without further hematologic evaluation. Episodes of prolonged

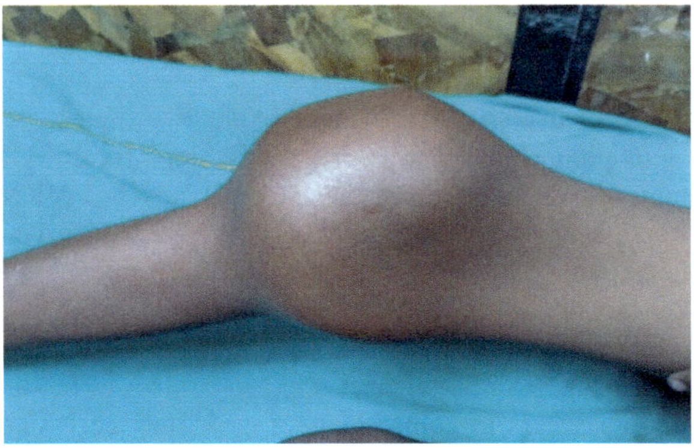

Fig. 19.1 Worsening of the target right knee joint with wasting of muscles

bleeding post-injections were treated at home with cold compressions with ice. At the age of 5 years, after a dental extraction, he experienced prolonged oozing for 24 h, which was treated with local measures. By the age of 10 years, the child had severe, recurrent joint bleeds (hemarthrosis), resulting in progressive joint deformities and reduced mobility. He was evaluated later at a tertiary hospital, where a diagnosis of severe Hemophilia A (Factor VIII <1%) was made.

19.1.3 Initiation of Secondary Prophylaxis and Inhibitor Development (Ages 10–13)

After diagnosis, he was initiated on on-demand therapy with recombinant Factor VIII (rFVIII) at 20–30 IU/kg thrice weekly. His parents were counseled on the need for keeping up with on-demand treatment and regular follow-up. Within a span of 18 months, he developed inhibitors, presenting with persistent joint bleeds (Fig. 19.1) despite adequate dosing of factor VIII, suggestive of suboptimal response to factor therapy. Mixing studies were positive for inhibitor and a Bethesda assay showed high-titer inhibitors (>5 BU/mL). Immune tolerance induction (ITI) was not feasible due to high costs and healthcare infrastructure limitations. Due to inhibitor development, his treatment was shifted to bypassing agents with limited access on a demand basis with FEIBA & recombinant factor VIIa.

19.1.4 Physiotherapy Non-adherence and Progressive Arthropathy (Ages 13–15)

There was a progressive deterioration in joint health due to

- Limited access to physiotherapy
- Socioeconomic constraints
- Pain and psychological distress

By age 15, he had severe hemophilic arthropathy (Fig. 19.1):

- *Fixed knee flexion contractures*, restricting mobility
- *Chronic pain*
- *Dependency on crutches* significantly affecting the quality of life.

His parents began exploring alternative medicine, further complicating his care. These issues affect the life of a person living with hemophilia.

19.2 Diagnosis and Challenges in Hemophilia

19.2.1 Laboratory Diagnosis of Hemophilia

Diagnosing hemophilia requires a combination of clinical suspicion, laboratory investigations, and genetic testing.

Stepwise Approach to Diagnosis: Assessment of bleeding risk and severity with bleeding assessment tools (BAT–ISTH)

1. *Screening Tests*
   - *Prothrombin Time (PT)*: Normal (indicating intact extrinsic pathway).
   - *Activated Partial Thromboplastin Time (aPTT)*: Prolonged (suggesting intrinsic pathway deficiency).
   - *Platelet Count and Bleeding Time*: Normal (rules out platelet disorders).
2. *Confirmatory Factor Assays*
   - *Factor VIII Activity*: <1% (consistent with severe Hemophilia A).
   - *Factor IX Activity*: Normal (excludes Hemophilia B).
3. *Bethesda Assay for Inhibitors*
   - Used to detect *factor-neutralizing antibodies.*
   - Titer result: *High-titer inhibitors (>5 Bethesda Units [BU]/mL)*, indicating *poor response to standard factor replacement therapy.*
4. *Genetic Testing (Optional but informative)*
   - Genetic testing can confirm causative molecular changes responsible for the phenotype.
   - Useful for *prenatal diagnosis* and *carrier screening* in affected families.

19.2.2 Challenges in Diagnosis

Despite established diagnostic pathways, several barriers exist, especially in LMICs, leading to delayed or missed diagnoses:

19.2.2.1 Developmental Hemostasis and Diagnostic Pitfalls

- *Neonatal Diagnosis Challenges[5]*:
  - Factor VIII levels are physiologically low at birth and rise within the first 6 months, leading to false negatives in newborns, especially with factor IX deficiency.
- *Misinterpretation of Early Symptoms*:
  - *Bruising and oral bleeds* in infants are often mistaken for nutritional deficiencies (e.g., vitamin C or iron deficiency anemia).
    Late umbilical stump bleeding is often under-recognized as a potential red flag.
- *Limited Awareness Among Physicians*:
  - Primary care doctors in rural settings may not suspect hemophilia early due to its rarity.
  - *Arthropathy and joint swelling* may be misdiagnosed as juvenile arthritis, leading to unnecessary interventions, delayed referral, and subsequent diagnosis.

19.2.2.2 Challenges in Identifying Inhibitors

- Patients on on-demand therapy (vs. prophylaxis) often develop inhibitors unnoticed until multiple bleeding episodes fail to respond to factor replacement.
- *Regular inhibitor screening* is recommended in high-income settings but is infrequently performed in LMICs due to cost constraints and logistical issues.
- Inhibitor testing should be done:
  - Before starting prophylaxis (especially secondary and tertiary)
  - After the first 50 factor exposure days
  - Before surgeries or major interventions

19.2.3 Diagnostic Recommendations in LMIC Settings

To improve early diagnosis and inhibitor detection in resource-limited settings, the following strategies can be adopted:

- *Expand access to basic coagulation tests* in regional hospitals.
- *Increase awareness* among primary care physicians for early symptom recognition.

19.3 Management Strategies in Hemophilia [3, 6]

Effective hemophilia management revolves around prophylaxis, inhibitor treatment, and physiotherapy, with significant variations between countries globally.

19.3.1 Prophylaxis: The Gold Standard of Hemophilia Management

Prophylaxis with clotting factor replacement has been the gold standard in preventing spontaneous bleeds and promoting joint health and kinetics.

19.3.1.1 Types of Prophylaxis

Type	Description	Recommended for
Primary prophylaxis	Factor replacement started before the first joint bleed, typically before age 3 years	Ideal for HICs, reduces joint disease progression
Secondary prophylaxis	Started after the first joint bleed but before significant arthropathy develops	Common in LMICs due to resource constraints
Tertiary prophylaxis	Started after arthropathy has developed to prevent further damage	Limited impact on joint disease; often used in older children/adults
Intermittent prophylaxis	Short-term prophylaxis (e.g., perioperative, post-injury)	Cost-effective alternative for LMICs

19.3.1.2 Prophylaxis Guidelines (WFH Versus LMIC Reality)

Aspect	WFH guidelines	LMIC Challenges
Factor dosing	Standard dosing: 25–40 IU/kg, 2–3 times per week	High cost limits availability
Product choice	Recombinant factor concentrates are preferred over plasma-derived products	Plasma-derived factors are more accessible in LMICs
Home therapy	Encouraged for early intervention	Infrequent in LMICs due to a lack of awareness and education
Long-acting factors	Extended half-life (EHL) products) reduce infusion frequency, especially in hemophilia B	Limited access due to increased costs

- *LMIC STRATEGY*: Low-dose prophylaxis (10–15 IU/kg twice weekly) in Hemophilia A can promote joint health and allow for optimal resource utilization.

19.3.2 Inhibitor Management: Overcoming Treatment Resistance

Approximately 30% of severe Hemophilia A and 5% of Hemophilia B [3] patients develop inhibitors, rendering standard factor therapy ineffective, thereby necessitating the use of bypassing agents, escalating costs, and visits for care.

19.3.2.1 Immune Tolerance Induction (ITI)

- *Goal*: Suppress inhibitor production by administering high-dose factor VIII (FVIII).
- *Success Rate*: ~70% in Hemophilia A but lower in Hemophilia B (risk of anaphylaxis and nephropathy).
- *WFH Protocol*: Daily FVIII at 50–200 IU/kg for several months.
- *Limitations in LMICs*: Cost-prohibitive (~$100,000–$300,000 per year), requires continuous monitoring.

Alternative Approaches in LMICs:

- *Modified ITI*: Lower-dose FVIII with intermittent escalation.
- *Delayed ITI*: Initiation when inhibitors naturally decline (<10 BU).

19.3.2.2 Bypassing Agents

When ITI fails or is infeasible, bypassing agents like recombinant factor VIIa (rFVIIa) and activated Prothrombin complex concentrate (aPCC) are used.

Bypassing agent	Mechanism	Dose	Challenges
rFVIIa (e.g., NovoSeven)	Enhances thrombin generation independent of FVIII/IX	90 mcg/kg IV every 2–3 hrs during bleeds	Expensive, short half-life, frequent dosing
aPCC (e.g., FEIBA)	Provides activated clotting factors to bypass FVIII function	50–100 IU/kg every 8–12 hrs	Risk of thrombosis with repeated use

Cost-Effective Strategy for LMICs:
- *On-demand rFVIIa therapy*, though expensive, reduces the need for ITI.
- *Plasma-derived aPCC (if available) offers a cheaper alternative.*

19.3.3 Physiotherapy: Preserving Joint Health

Musculoskeletal issues contribute to reduced mobility, dependence, and disability in hemophilia. Therefore, physiotherapy remains the cornerstone for rehabilitation.

19.3.3.1 Role of Physiotherapy in Hemophilia

Objective	Intervention
Prevent hemarthrosis	Strengthen muscles around joints to reduce bleeding risk
Minimize joint damage	Stretching and range-of-motion exercises
Improve mobility	Functional training

19.3.3.2 Barriers to Physiotherapy in LMICs

1. *Limited availability* of rehabilitation centers.
2. *Financial burden*—families prioritize clotting factor therapy over physiotherapy.
3. *Lack of trained physiotherapists* familiar with bleeding disorder-specific rehabilitation.

Proposed Solutions:

- *Home-based physiotherapy regimens* with caregiver involvement.
- *Low-cost assistive devices* to reduce joint strain.
- *Patient education initiatives* to emphasize the role of exercise.
- *Digital health initiatives* through remote audiovisual interactions.

19.3.4 Future Directions: The Shift Toward Non-factor Therapies

In recent years, non-factor therapies have transformed hemophilia care, providing alternative means to allow people with hemophilia to achieve their full potential

19.3.4.1 Emicizumab: The Game-Changer in Hemophilia A with Inhibitors

- *Mechanism*: A bispecific antibody that mimics FVIII function. Approved in most countries.

19.3.4.2 Rebalancing Agents: The Next Frontier

Drug	Mechanism	Status
Fitusiran	siRNA that reduces antithrombin levels to enhance thrombin generation	Phase 3 trials
Concizumab	An anti-TFPI monoclonal antibody to restore the clotting balance	Phase 3 trials

Implications for LMICs:

- *Fewer injections* → Increased patient adherence.
- *Potentially lower long-term costs* once biosimilar versions become available.

Strategy	HIC standard	LMIC alternative
Prophylaxis	High-dose recombinant factors	Low-dose prophylaxis, intermittent dosing
Inhibitor management	ITI + bypassing agents	Selective ITI, on-demand bypassing agents
Physiotherapy	Comprehensive rehab programs	Home-based exercise regimens
Novel therapies	Emicizumab, gene therapy	Pending regulatory approval

19.3.5 Novel Therapies: Emicizumab, Fitusiran, and Concizumab

In recent years, non-factor therapies have significantly transformed hemophilia management by providing long-acting, subcutaneous alternatives to traditional intravenous clotting factor infusions. Among them, emicizumab, fitusiran, and concizumab represent major breakthroughs, particularly in inhibitor-positive patients and resource-limited settings where conventional clotting factor therapy is expensive and difficult to administer.

19.3.5.1 Emicizumab: A Paradigm Shift in Hemophilia Care [7–11]

1. Mechanism of Action

   Emicizumab is a bispecific monoclonal antibody that bridges activated Factor IX (FIXa) and Factor X (FX), mimicking the cofactor function of Factor VIII. Unlike conventional FVIII replacement therapy, emicizumab does not require functional FVIII, making it particularly beneficial for patients with inhibitors to factor VIII.
2. Advantages of Emicizumab

   - *Subcutaneous administration* (weekly, biweekly, or monthly) instead of frequent IV infusions.
   - *Effective in both inhibitor-positive and inhibitor-negative Hemophilia A.*
   - *Lower risk of spontaneous bleeds compared to factor-based prophylaxis.*
   - *Does not induce inhibitors*, making it useful for newly diagnosed patients.
   - *Lower overall treatment costs (~50% cheaper than bypassing agents in some studies).*

     – Low-dose emicizumab efficacy published from multiple HTCs from India.
     – Potentially reduces cost in the long term.

3. Clinical Trial Data Supporting Emicizumab [11–14]
   Multiple pivotal trials have substantiated the efficacy of emicizumab in reducing bleeding episodes and improving life quality in patients with Hemophilia A.

Trial name	Target population	Annualized bleed rate (ABR) reduction	Key findings
HAVEN 1	Adults with inhibitor-positive Hemophilia A	87% reduction in ABR	An effective alternative to bypassing agents
HAVEN 2	Children with Hemophilia A inhibitors	99% of children had zero treated bleeds	Strong safety and efficacy profile in young patients
HAVEN 3	Adults with inhibitor-negative Hemophilia A	68% lower ABR vs. FVIII prophylaxis	Comparable or superior to standard FVIII therapy
HAVEN 4	Extended dosing (once per month)	Similar efficacy to weekly dosing	Monthly regimen feasible

These findings have reshaped prophylactic strategies, particularly for patients with inhibitors and those seeking less frequent administration schedules.

4. Low-Dose Emicizumab: Cost-Effective Use in LMICs [9, 15].
   Low-dose emicizumab, which retains efficacy while *reducing costs.*

   - *Standard dose*: 3 mg/kg weekly x 4 weeks (loading), followed by 1.5 mg/kg weekly or 3 mg/kg every 2 weeks.
   - *Low-dose alternative dosing* maintains hemostasis in many patients with reduced cost, as demonstrated.
   - *Limitations*: Some patients with high physical activity or severe joint disease may still require higher dosing.

Implications for LMICs:

- *Less frequent administration* reduces healthcare burden.
- *Lower drug consumption reduces overall treatment costs.*
- *More equitable access to prophylaxis* in resource-limited settings.

19.3.5.2 Fitusiran: The Rebalancing Agent Targeting Antithrombin

1. Mechanism of Action
   Fitusiran is an RNA interference (siRNA) therapy that inhibits antithrombin (AT), thereby enhancing thrombin generation and restoring hemostasis in both Hemophilia A and B.
2. Advantages of Fitusiran

   - Subcutaneous injection (monthly) instead of frequent IV infusions.
   - Works in both inhibitor-positive and inhibitor-negative patients.
   - Applicable to both Hemophilia A and Hemophilia B.
   - Potential for reduced treatment costs due to the long-acting nature.

3. Clinical Trials Supporting Fitusiran [16, 17]

Trial name	Population	Annualized bleed rate (ABR) reduction	Key findings
ATLAS-INH	Inhibitor-positive Hemophilia A/B	89% reduction in ABR	An effective alternative to bypassing agents
ATLAS--A/B	Inhibitor-negative Hemophilia A/B	61% reduction in ABR	Effective across all hemophilia types
ATLAS-PPX	Previously on prophylaxis	79% reduction in ABR vs. standard therapy	Comparable to FVIII/FIX prophylaxis

4. Limitations and Safety Concerns
    - *Increased risk of thrombosis* if combined with high doses of FVIII or bypassing agents.
    - Requires strict monitoring of D-dimer and thrombotic markers.
    - *Long-acting nature* reduces the need for frequent medical visits.
    - *Applicable to both Hemophilia A and B*, making it a versatile alternative.

19.3.5.3 Concizumab: The Anti-TFPI Antibody

1. Mechanism of Action
   Concizumab is a monoclonal antibody targeting tissue factor pathway inhibitor (TFPI), enhancing thrombin generation to reduce the anti-clotting hemostasis.
2. Advantages of Concizumab
    - First treatment option that works for both Hemophilia A and Hemophilia B with inhibitors.
    - Subcutaneous dosing (daily or every few days) instead of IV infusions.
    - Potentially lower risk of thrombosis compared to fitusiran.
    - Daily subcutaneous administration makes it feasible for home therapy.
    - More affordable than gene therapy, making it a realistic alternative.
3. Clinical Trial Data [18]

Trial name	Population	Annualized bleed rate (ABR) reduction	Key findings
Explorer 4	Hemophilia A/B with inhibitors	86% reduction in ABR	Reduced breakthrough bleeds
Explorer 5	Hemophilia A/B without inhibitors	76% reduction in ABR	Suitable for broader patient groups

19.3.5.4 Future Role of Non-Factor Therapies

These novel therapies are redefining hemophilia management, particularly in settings where:

1. Intravenous access is challenging (e.g., children poor venous access).
2. Conventional factor replacement is unavailable or too expensive.
3. Inhibitor development limits standard therapies.

Therapy	Administration	Target population	Key advantage
Emicizumab	Subcutaneous (weekly/monthly)	Hemophilia A (inhibitor+ and inhibitor-)	Eliminates the need for FVIII infusions
Fitusiran	Subcutaneous (monthly)	Hemophilia A and B (inhibitor+ and inhibitor-)	Universal hemophilia treatment
Concizumab	Subcutaneous (daily/every few days)	Hemophilia A and B (inhibitor+ and inhibitor-)	Alternative to fitusiran

With continued research and cost-optimization strategies, these agents hold great promise for improving hemophilia care in LMICs.

19.4 Recent Advances and Cost-Effectiveness in Hemophilia Management

Despite remarkable advancements in hemophilia treatment, cost remains a major barrier, particularly in low- and middle-income countries (LMICs).

19.4.1 Gene Therapy: A Potential One-Time Cure? [19–21]

Gene therapy represents the most revolutionary approach in hemophilia treatment, offering the potential for a single-dose, long-term correction of clotting factor deficiency. Currently, two gene therapy products have been approved in high-income countries, with multiple others in clinical trials.

19.4.1.1 Mechanism of Gene Therapy

- Uses viral vectors (Adeno-Associated Virus, AAV) to deliver functional Factor VIII (F8) or Factor IX (F9) genes to liver cells.
- Allows hepatocytes to produce endogenous clotting factors that were missing, reducing or eliminating the need for prophylactic therapy.
- This strategy aims to restore baseline hemostasis and reduce or eliminate the need for regular prophylactic infusions.

19.4.1.2 Approved Gene Therapy Products

Product	Target	Vector used	Trial results
Valoctocogene roxaparvovec (Roctavian®)	Hemophilia A	AAV5-F8	Sustained FVIII levels for ~3 years in most patients
Etranacogene dezaparvovec (Hemgenix®)	Hemophilia B	AAV5-F9	Factor IX levels increased >40%, reducing bleeding episodes by 90%

Long-Term Outcomes:
- Some patients remain off prophylaxis for 5+ years.
- Bleeding rates drop significantly, improving the quality of life.

Limitations and Challenges:
- Not all patients respond equally—some show declining factor levels over time.
- AAV-based therapies require pre-screening for pre-existing antibodies, which may exclude 20–30% of candidates.
- Extremely high cost (~$2–3.5 million per dose) limits accessibility.
- Up to 80–90% of Hemophilia A patients require corticosteroids at some point post-gene therapy to manage ALT elevations or hepatic immune responses.
- Approximately 20–40% of patients require long-term corticosteroid use, defined as use beyond 12–20 weeks, sometimes up to 6–12 months.

19.4.2 Lentiviral Gene Therapy for Hemophilia A Using CD34+ Hematopoietic Cells [21]

19.4.2.1 Mechanism

A gene therapy approach for severe hemophilia A by utilizing autologous CD34+ hematopoietic stem cells (HSCs) transduced with a lentiviral vector (CD68-ET3-LV) carrying a novel F8 transgene (ET3) under the control of a myeloid-specific CD68 promoter. Following myeloablative conditioning, these modified HSCs were infused back into patients, aiming to achieve sustained endogenous production of factor VIII (FVIII) through differentiation into myeloid lineage cells.

19.4.2.2 Opportunities

The therapy demonstrated promising results in a single-center study involving five participants aged 22–41 years with severe Hemophilia A. Notably, the annualized bleeding rate was zero for all participants over a cumulative follow-up of 81 months. Participants who received transduction enhancers exhibited higher peripheral blood vector copy numbers (3.2–4.8 copies per cell) and correspondingly elevated FVIII activity levels (19.3–39.9 IU/dL), indicating a dose-response relationship. These findings suggest that lentiviral gene therapy can achieve stable and clinically meaningful FVIII expression.

19.4.2.3 Challenges

Despite the encouraging outcomes, several challenges remain. The procedure requires myeloablative conditioning, which carries risks such as severe neutropenia and thrombocytopenia, observed to last between 7 and 11 days and 1 and 7 days, respectively. Additionally, the variability in FVIII expression among participants underscores the need for optimization of transduction protocols and vector design. Long-term safety concerns, including the potential for insertional mutagenesis and clonal expansion, necessitate extended follow-up studies. Furthermore, the complexity and cost of the therapy may limit its accessibility, highlighting the need for scalable and cost-effective solutions.

In conclusion, lentiviral gene therapy using CD34+ HSCs presents a viable and potentially transformative treatment for Hemophilia A, offering sustained FVIII expression and bleeding control. It is necessary to address the associated risks, optimize efficacy, and ensuring accessibility remain critical for its broader clinical application.

19.4.3 Cost of Hemophilia Treatments: The Global Divide

Hemophilia treatment remains one of the most expensive chronic disease therapies worldwide. The annual cost of clotting factor therapy varies dramatically between high-income countries (HICs) and LMICs.

19.4.3.1 Estimated Costs of Treatment (Per Patient, Per Year)

Therapy	Estimated annual cost (HIC) (USD)	Estimated annual cost (LMIC) (USD)	Notes
Recombinant factor VIII	$200,000–300,000	$30,000–50,000	LMICs rely more on plasma-derived factors
Plasma-derived factor VIII	$30,000–50,000	$5000–15,000	Still expensive but more accessible
Emicizumab (standard dose)	$450,000 (first year), then $250,000/year	$30,000–100,000	LMIC costs vary based on procurement
Gene therapy (one-time cost)	$2–3.5 million	Not available	Cost is prohibitive in LMICs

- HICs predominantly use recombinant factor concentrates due to higher safety and purity.
- LMICs rely on plasma-derived factors due to affordability, but supply chain issues limit access.
- Emicizumab and rebalancing agents offer potential cost savings by reducing bleeding-related complications.
- Gene therapy remains out of reach for LMICs due to upfront costs and infrastructure challenges.

19.4.4 Cost-Effectiveness of Novel Therapies

While non-factor therapies like emicizumab, fitusiran, and concizumab have high upfront costs, their long-term benefits, including fewer bleeding events and reduced hospital visits, make them a cost-effective option in many scenarios.

19.4.4.1 Emicizumab Versus Factor VIII: Which is More Cost-Effective?

A cost-effectiveness analysis comparing emicizumab vs. standard FVIII prophylaxis found:

- Emicizumab reduced total lifetime treatment costs by 50% due to fewer bleeding-related hospitalizations and lower infusion frequency.
- In LMIC settings, low-dose emicizumab regimens (0.6 mg/kg/month) can provide comparable bleed prevention at a fraction of the cost.
- Emicizumab requires fewer medical visits, reducing transportation costs for rural patients.

Conclusion Emicizumab-based regimens are more cost-effective than FVIII prophylaxis in the long run.

19.4.4.2 Rebalancing Agents: A Cost-Effective Alternative?

Therapy	Annual cost (USD)	Potential savings
Fitusiran	$200,000–250,000	Reduces annual infusions from 150+ to ~12 (monthly dosing).
Concizumab	$150,000–180,000	Cheaper than frequent bypassing agents for inhibitor patients.

Conclusion Both fitusiran and concizumab reduce treatment burden, and once biosimilar versions emerge, their costs are expected to drop significantly.

19.4.5 Strategies to Improve Affordability in LMICs

Given cost constraints, several strategies can improve access to hemophilia treatment in resource-limited settings:

19.4.5.1 Government and International Procurement Programs

- Bulk purchasing through the WHO and the WFH Humanitarian Aid Programs reduces costs.
- The WFH Global Alliance for Progress (GAP) initiative has improved access to clotting factor therapy in 60+ LMICs.

19.4.5.2 Local Production of Plasma-Derived Products

- Countries like India, China, and Brazil have developed national plasma fractionation programs, increasing domestic supply.
- Plasma-derived FVIII remains a cost-effective alternative to recombinant products.

19.4.5.3 Low-Dose Prophylaxis Strategies

- "Dose-sparing" approaches (e.g., 10–15 IU/kg FVIII once or twice weekly) provide partial bleed prevention at a fraction of standard prophylaxis costs.
- Low-dose emicizumab regimens offer sustained protection with fewer injections.

19.4.5.4 Expanding Access to Home Therapy

- Training caregivers in home-based infusion therapy reduces hospital dependency.
- Subcutaneous therapies (emicizumab, fitusiran, concizumab) improve adherence due to ease of administration.

19.4.6 Future Perspectives: What's Next?

As research continues, several future developments could further reduce costs and improve access:

- Biosimilar recombinant factors: Generic versions of FVIII and FIX concentrates expected to enter the market within the next 5 years.

- Cheaper AAV-free gene therapy platforms: Efforts are underway to develop non-viral gene therapy delivery, which could significantly lower costs.
- Universal screening & early diagnosis programs: Earlier identification of hemophilia in newborns and carriers will enable timely intervention and better outcomes.

19.5 Guidelines and Clinical Trials in Hemophilia Management

The management of hemophilia is largely guided by international consensus documents, particularly from the World Federation of Hemophilia (WFH) and the International Society on Thrombosis and Haemostasis (ISTH). These guidelines ensure standardized care, emphasizing prophylaxis, inhibitor management, and comprehensive hemophilia treatment centers (HTCs). Additionally, recent clinical trials have been pivotal in shaping treatment paradigms, particularly for non-factor therapies and gene therapy.

19.5.1 WFH and ISTH Guidelines for Hemophilia Management

The WFH and ISTH guidelines provide evidence-based recommendations for the diagnosis and management of hemophilia across different healthcare settings.

19.5.1.1 Prophylaxis Recommendations

Guideline	Recommended prophylaxis	Target factor levels
WFH 2020	Factor replacement prophylaxis is the standard of care for severe hemophilia	Maintain >3–5% trough FVIII/FIX levels to prevent spontaneous bleeds
ISTH 2022	Personalized prophylaxis based on bleeding phenotype and lifestyle	Encourages use of non-factor therapies (e.g., emicizumab) as an alternative to FVIII prophylaxis

LMIC Considerations:

- WFH supports lower-dose prophylaxis (10–15 IU/kg twice weekly) in LMICs where full-dose regimens are not feasible.
- Encourages use of alternative therapies like emicizumab, which may offer cost savings in long-term care.

19.5.1.2 Inhibitor Management

Guideline	Management approach
WFH 2020	Immune tolerance induction (ITI) is first-line for high-titer inhibitors.
ISTH 2022	Supports use of bypassing agents (rFVIIa, aPCC) for inhibitor patients.
Latest update	Encourages non-factor therapies (e.g., emicizumab) as first-line for inhibitor-positive patients, especially in LMICs where ITI is not feasible.

Emicizumab is now recommended over ITI in many patients due to lower cost and better adherence.

19.5.1.3 Hemophilia Treatment Centers (HTCs)

Both WFH and ISTH recommend the establishment of HTCs for multidisciplinary care, integrating:

- Hematologists
- Physiotherapists
- Orthopedic specialists
- Psychosocial support teams

19.5.2 Key Clinical Trials Shaping Hemophilia Care

Over the past decade, landmark clinical trials have led to paradigm shifts in hemophilia management. The introduction of extended half-life factors, non-factor therapies, and gene therapy has significantly altered treatment approaches.

19.5.2.1 Clinical Trials Supporting Emicizumab

Trial name	Population	Key findings
HAVEN 1	Inhibitor-positive adults	87% reduction in annualized bleed rate (ABR) vs. bypassing agents
HAVEN 2	Inhibitor-positive children	99% had zero treated bleeds with emicizumab
HAVEN 3	Inhibitor-negative adults	68% lower ABR compared to FVIII prophylaxis
HAVEN 4	Once-monthly dosing	Monthly dosing was as effective as weekly/biweekly regimens

Implications
- Emicizumab is now the preferred prophylactic agent for inhibitor-positive patients.
- Low-dose regimens (0.6 mg/kg monthly) are being explored to improve cost-effectiveness in LMICs.

19.5.2.2 Fitusiran and Concizumab Trials

Trial name	Therapy	Key findings
ATLAS-INH	Fitusiran (RNAi therapy)	89% reduction in ABR in inhibitor patients
ATLAS-PPX	Fitusiran	Comparable efficacy to FVIII prophylaxis, with significantly fewer injections
EXPLORER 4	Concizumab (anti-TFPI)	86% ABR reduction, providing an alternative for both Hemophilia A and B

Implications:
- Fitusiran offers a universal hemophilia treatment, covering both Hemophilia A and B.
- Concizumab may be an alternative to emicizumab for patients with Hemophilia B.

19.5.2.3 Gene Therapy Trials

Trial name	Therapy	Target	Key findings
HOPE-B	Etranacogene dezaparvovec	Hemophilia B	Factor IX levels increased to 40%+, reducing bleed rates by 90%
GENEr8–1	Valoctocogene roxaparvovec	Hemophilia A	Factor VIII production is maintained in most patients for 3+ years

Implications:
- Gene therapy provides long-term factor expression, reducing the need for regular infusions.
- Extremely high costs (~$2–3.5 million per dose) remain a major challenge.

19.5.3 Global Disparities: LMIC Versus HIC Treatment Strategies

Despite strong clinical trial data and new guidelines, the real-world implementation of these therapies remains highly unequal.

Aspect	High-income countries (HICs)	Low- and middle-income countries (LMICs)
Access to recombinant factor VIII	Standard of care	Limited; plasma-derived products are still widely used
Inhibitor treatment	ITI + emicizumab	ITI is often unaffordable; bypassing agents are used sparingly
Prophylaxis approach	Full-dose FVIII, extended half-life factors	Low-dose or intermittent prophylaxis
Gene therapy availability	Available in some centers	Not yet accessible
Comprehensive care centers	Widespread	Largely unavailable

Potential Solutions for LMICs:

- Lower-cost prophylaxis regimens (e.g., low-dose FVIII, dose-sparing emicizumab).
- Humanitarian aid & bulk procurement programs (e.g., WFH GAP Initiative).
- Subcutaneous alternatives (e.g., fitusiran, concizumab) to improve adherence.

19.5.4 Future Directions in Hemophilia Research

Emerging areas of research in hemophilia include:

1. Next-generation gene therapy platforms to improve the durability of factor expression.
2. Biosimilar development to reduce the cost of recombinant clotting factors.
3. Oral or subcutaneous therapies that eliminate the need for frequent injections.

19.5.5 Conclusion: Integrating Guidelines and Trial Data into Practice

Hemophilia management has undergone a paradigm shift, moving beyond factor replacement therapy to long-acting subcutaneous alternatives and gene therapy.

By integrating evidence-based guidelines with real-world constraints, we can ensure that all individuals with hemophilia receive optimal care, regardless of geographical and economic barriers.

19.6 Summary

19.6.1 Summary of Key Points

Hemophilia management has evolved from episodic clotting factor infusions to continuous prophylaxis and now to non-factor therapies and gene therapy. Despite significant advancements, accessibility and cost remain major concerns, particularly in low- and middle-income countries (LMICs). This chapter provided a case-based approach to highlight challenges such as delayed diagnosis, inhibitor development, and physiotherapy non-adherence, while exploring WFH/ISTH guidelines and landmark clinical trials that define modern hemophilia care.

19.6.1.1 Evolution of Hemophilia Treatment

Era	Treatment approach	Limitations
Pre–1960s	Whole blood & plasma transfusions	Ineffective, short-lived clotting factor levels
1970s–1980s	Plasma-derived factor concentrates	Risk of viral infections (HIV, hepatitis C)
1990s–2010s	Recombinant factor products (standard half-life and extended half-life)	High cost, frequent IV infusions needed
2010s–present	Non-factor therapies (emicizumab, rebalancing agents)	High cost but improved convenience and efficacy
Future	Gene therapy	Potential cure, but prohibitively expensive

19.6.1.2 Major Challenges and Proposed Solutions

Challenge	HIC approach	LMIC-appropriate solution
Delayed diagnosis	Neonatal screening, genetic testing	Physician training, early aPTT screening in high-risk infants
Cost of factor therapy	Recombinant FVIII standard	Plasma-derived FVIII, dose-sparing strategies
Inhibitors	ITI + Emicizumab	Selective ITI, bypassing agents on demand
Prophylaxis access	Standard high-dose prophylaxis	Low-dose prophylaxis (10–15 IU/kg twice weekly)
Gene therapy	Available but expensive	Not yet a viable option; research on alternative platforms ongoing

19.6.2 The Future of Hemophilia Treatment

As we look forward, several groundbreaking developments could further transform hemophilia care, particularly in making therapies more accessible and cost-effective worldwide.

19.6.2.1 Long-Term Gene Therapy Solutions

- Next-generation viral vectors (LentiVirus, CRISPR-based approaches) may provide more durable gene expression with lower immune response risk.
- Oral or subcutaneous gene therapy formulations are being explored, which may reduce costs.

19.6.2.2 Biosimilars and Cost-Reduction Strategies

- Biosimilar recombinant FVIII and FIX products will enter the market in the next few years, potentially reducing factor costs by 30–50%.
- Manufacturing non-factor therapies (e.g., emicizumab, fitusiran) in LMICs could significantly reduce import costs.

19.6.2.3 Improving Global Hemophilia Care Equity

- WFH humanitarian aid programs continue to expand access to clotting factors in LMICs.
- Training programs for healthcare workers to improve early diagnosis and multidisciplinary care.

19.6.3 Final Thoughts: Bridging Innovation and Accessibility

The future of hemophilia management is promising, but equitable access remains the biggest challenge. While high-income countries have rapidly adopted gene therapy and non-factor therapies, LMICs must prioritize practical solutions such as low-dose prophylaxis, cost-effective inhibitors, and subcutaneous therapies.

Key Points

- Personalized treatment approaches, integrating both factor and non-factor therapies, will define modern hemophilia care.
- Gene therapy is a game-changer, but affordability must be addressed before widespread implementation.
- Cost-effective solutions such as low-dose prophylaxis, biosimilars, and government procurement programs can improve access in LMICs.
- Multidisciplinary care, including physiotherapy and psychosocial support, is critical for optimizing long-term outcomes.

By balancing scientific advancements with real-world accessibility, the goal of providing optimal hemophilia care to all patients, regardless of geography or socioeconomic status, can become a reality.

References

1. Mannucci PM. Hemophilia treatment innovation: 50 years of progress and more to come. J Thromb Haemost. 2023;21(3):403–12. https://doi.org/10.1016/j.jtha.2022.12.029.
2. Seth T. The last 50 years of hemophilia care: a golden era. Indian Pediatr. 2024;61:489–93. https://doi.org/10.1007/s13312-024-3140-1.
3. Srivastava A, Santagostino E, Dougall A, Kitchen S, Sutherland M, Pipe SW, Carcao M, Mahlangu J, Ragni MV, Windyga J, Llinás A, Goddard NJ, Mohan R, Poonnoose PM, Feldman BM, Lewis SZ, van den Berg HM, Pierce GF, WFH Guidelines for the Management of Hemophilia panelists and co-authors. WFH Guidelines for the Management of Hemophilia, 3rd edition. Haemophilia. 2020;26(Suppl 6):1–158. https://doi.org/10.1111/hae.14046. Epub 2020 Aug 3. Erratum in: Haemophilia. 2021;27(4):699. doi:10.1111/hae.14308.
4. WFH Global Survey on Access to Hemophilia Treatment. World Federation of Hemophilia. Annual Global Survey Report. 2023. Available from: https://www.wfh.org.
5. Monagle P, Barnes C, Ignjatovic V, Furmedge J, Newall F, Chan A, De Rosa L, Hamilton S, Ragg P, Robinson S, Auldist A, Crock C, Roy N, Rowlands S. Developmental haemostasis. Impact for clinical haemostasis laboratories. Thromb Haemost. 2006;95(2):362–72. https://doi.org/10.1160/TH05-01-0047.
6. International Society on Thrombosis and Haemostasis (ISTH) Guidelines. ISTH 2022 recommendations for hemophilia management. J Thromb Haemost. 2022;20(3):403–15. https://doi.org/10.1111/jth.15789.
7. Patil R, Shanmukhaiah C, Gogtay NJ, Pandey P, Patil K, Jijina F, Madkaikar M. Low-dose emicizumab prophylaxis in patients with severe Hemophilia A: a retrospective study bringing new hope for our patients. J Thromb Haemost. 2024;22(4):1024–30. https://doi.org/10.1016/j.jtha.2023.12.023. Epub 2023 Dec 30
8. Radhakrishnan N, Pandharipande A, Singh S, Verma S, Baby EP, Pandey A. Freedom from bleeds with low-dose emicizumab prophylaxis in inhibitor-positive Hemophilia A. J Hematol. 2024;13(5):186–91. https://doi.org/10.14740/jh1346. Epub 2024 Oct 21. PMID: 39493600; PMCID: PMC11526584.
9. Seth T, John MJ, Chakrabarti P, Shanmukhaiah C, Verma SP, Radhakrishnan N, Dolai TK. Cost-effectiveness analysis of emicizumab prophylaxis in patients with haemophilia A in India. Haemophilia. 2024;30(2):426–36. https://doi.org/10.1111/hae.14921. Epub 2023.
10. Verma SP, Dutta TK, Mahadevan S, Nalini P, Basu D, Biswal N, Ramesh A, Charles D, Vinod KV, Harichandra Kumar KT. A randomized study of very low-dose factor VIII prophy-

laxis in severe haemophilia – a success story from a resource limited country. Haemophilia. 2016;22(3):342–8. https://doi.org/10.1111/hae.12838. Epub 2016
11. Oldenburg J, Mahlangu JN, Kim B, et al. Emicizumab prophylaxis in Hemophilia A with inhibitors. N Engl J Med. 2017;377(9):809–18. https://doi.org/10.1056/NEJMoa1703068.
12. Young G, Liesner R, Sidonio RF, et al. Emicizumab prophylaxis in pediatric Hemophilia A with inhibitors. Blood. 2019;134(24):2127–36. https://doi.org/10.1182/blood.2019002018.
13. Mahlangu J, Oldenburg J, Paz-Priel I, et al. Emicizumab prophylaxis for patients who have Hemophilia a without inhibitors. N Engl J Med. 2018;379(9):811–22. https://doi.org/10.1056/NEJMoa1803550.
14. Callaghan MU, Negrier C, Paz-Priel I, et al. Long-term efficacy and safety of monthly subcutaneous Emicizumab prophylaxis for Hemophilia A. Blood Adv. 2021;5(7):2137–45. https://doi.org/10.1182/bloodadvances.2020004190.
15. Cost Analysis of Hemophilia Therapy, Srivastava A, Brewer A, Mauser-Bunschoten EP, et al. Cost of hemophilia treatment: a global perspective. Haemophilia. 2021;27(Suppl 1):110–8. https://doi.org/10.1111/hae.14321.
16. Pasi KJ, Georgiev P, Mant T, et al. Fitusiran, an siRNA therapeutic targeting antithrombin for Hemophilia A and B. N Engl J Med. 2021;385(10):885–95. https://doi.org/10.1056/NEJMoa2106990.
17. Pasi KJ, Rangarajan S, Georgiev P, et al. Efficacy and safety of fitusiran prophylaxis for patients with hemophilia. Blood. 2022;140(10):1107–16. https://doi.org/10.1182/blood.2022015601.
18. Shapiro A, Khair K, Liesner R, et al. Concizumab prophylaxis in Hemophilia A and B with inhibitors. Lancet Haematol. 2023;10(1):e45–54. https://doi.org/10.1016/S2352-3026(22)00443-0.
19. Mannucci PM, Chowdary P, Pipe SW, et al. Etranacogene Dezaparvovec gene therapy for hemophilia B. Lancet. 2022;400(10359):603–15. https://doi.org/10.1016/S0140-6736(22)01331-9.
20. Rangarajan S, Walsh L, Lester W, et al. AAV5-factor VIII gene therapy in severe Hemophilia A. N Engl J Med. 2020;382(1):29–40. https://doi.org/10.1056/NEJMoa1908490.
21. Srivastava A, Abraham A, Aboobacker F, Singh G, Geevar T, Kulkarni U, Selvarajan S, Korula A, Dave RG, Shankar M, Singh AS, Jeba A, Kumaar N, Benjamin C, Lakshmi KM, Srivastava VM, Shaji RV, Nair SC, Brown HC, Denning G, Lollar P, Doering CB, Spencer T. Lentiviral gene therapy with CD34+ hematopoietic Cells for Hemophilia A. N Engl J Med. 2025;392(5):450–7. https://doi.org/10.1056/NEJMoa2410597. Epub 2024. PMID: 39655790; PMCID: PMC11875532.

Chapter 20
Point-of-Care Testing in Diagnosis and Management of Haemostatic Disorders

Rucha Patil and Sayli Rasal

Abstract Point-of-care testing (POCT) refers to diagnostic tests performed at or near the site of patient care, offering rapid and accurate results that support timely clinical decision-making. These tests, ranging from simple dipsticks to sophisticated automated devices, are designed to satisfy the REASSURED criteria outlined by the World Health Organization (WHO). This is particularly crucial in the management of haemostatic disorders, which involve abnormalities in blood clotting and include conditions like Haemophilia, thrombophilia, Disseminated Intravascular Coagulation (DIC), and liver disease.

In this chapter, we highlight the role of key POCTs in diagnosing and managing haemostatic disorders, specifically using Thromboelastography (TEG) and Rotational Thromboelastometry (ROTEM). These viscoelastic assays assess real-time clot formation, stability, and dissolution, helping to guide treatment decisions in conditions like Haemophilia A, trauma-induced coagulopathy, and liver disease. Furthermore, POCT devices for Prothrombin Time (PT)/INR and D-dimer are emphasized for their utility in monitoring anticoagulation therapy, thrombotic risk, and bleeding. The chapter includes clinical cases demonstrating the application of ROTEM–NATEM in monitoring haemophilia patients on different doses of Emicizumab prophylaxis. Despite their high cost and the need for trained personnel, these technologies provide real-time, dynamic evaluations of clot formation, stability, and dissolution, assisting in the management of conditions like Haemophilia, trauma-induced coagulopathy, liver disease, and obstetric bleeding disorders. Additionally, the chapter explores the application of these devices in perioperative settings, highlighting their role in guiding transfusions and adjusting therapies in a personalized manner. Ultimately, this chapter underscores the importance of POCT

R. Patil (✉) · S. Rasal
Department of Haemostasis and Thrombosis, ICMR-National Institute of Immunohaematology, Mumbai, India

H. P. Pati et al. (eds.), *Clinical Hematology and Hemato-Oncology*,
https://doi.org/10.1007/978-981-92-1167-8_20

in improving the diagnosis, monitoring, and management of haemostatic disorders, ultimately leading to more personalized and timely interventions.

Keywords Thromboelastography (TEG) · Rotational thromboelastometry (ROTEM) · Point-of-care tests (POCT) · Haemophilia · Bleeding states

Learning Objectives
- Understand the importance of point-of-care testing (POCT)
- Evaluate the role of POCT in the diagnosis and management of haemostatic disorders
- Interpret the results of thromboelastography (TEG) and rotational thromboelastometry (ROTEM) in the context of haemostatic disorders
- Explore the clinical applications of TEG and ROTEM in various bleeding states

"Point-of-care test (POCT)" is defined as a laboratory test that takes place at or near the site where the patient is located. This can range from simple dipsticks to sophisticated automated tests on portable analyzers and imaging systems. POCTs are to satisfy the REASSURED criteria, which is a set of standards for diagnostic tests developed by the World health Organization (WHO), with the main aim being to improve access to diagnostic tests [1, 2]. REASSURED stands for:

- Real-time connectivity
- Ease of specimen collection
- Affordable
- Sensitive
- Specific
- User-friendly
- Rapid and robust
- Equipment-free or simple
- Deliverable to end-users

Haemostatic disorders are conditions that affect the blood's ability to form clots properly, either causing excessive bleeding (haemorrhage) or inappropriate clotting (thrombosis). These disorders can arise due to issues with the blood vessels, platelets, coagulation factors, or fibrinolysis (the breakdown of clots). Haemostatic disorders can be inherited or acquired and require careful diagnosis and management to prevent severe complications such as bleeding or thrombosis.

In bleeding disorders, the manifestation can be mild, moderate or severe, and the cause can be congenital or acquired [3]. Some common bleeding disorders include:

- Haemophilia A and Haemophilia B are inherited bleeding disorders which result due to the deficiency in factor VIII and Factor IX, respectively.
- Von Willebrand disease, a genetic disorder wherein the von Willebrand factor is affected and mainly of three types (Types 1, 2, and 3); type 3 being the most severe.
- Vitamin K deficiency, which results in reduced clotting factors.
- Platelet disorders like thrombocytopenia or qualitative platelet defects.
- Disseminated intravascular coagulation (DIC) is a condition wherein abnormal blood clotting occurs, leading to both clot formation and bleeding.
- Liver disease.
- Acquired coagulation disorders, which may develop due to other conditions like autoimmune disease or malignancies.

Thrombophilia refers to conditions that increase the risk of abnormal blood clot formation, leading to thrombosis (e.g., deep vein thrombosis, pulmonary embolism, stroke). These disorders may be inherited or acquired and include:

- Factor V Leiden Mutation
- Antithrombin III Deficiency
- Protein C and Protein S Deficiency
- Antiphospholipid Syndrome (APS)

20.1 Point-of-Care Testing in Haemostatic Disorders

Point-of-care testing (POCT) plays a crucial role in the diagnosis, monitoring, and management of haemostatic disorders by providing quick and accurate results at the site of patient care, which leads to not only personalised treatment but also effective management, especially where the conditions are unstable.

The common POC tests used for haemostatic disorders are:

1. Thromboelastography (TEG)
2. Rotational thromboelastometry (ROTEM)
3. POC device for D-dimer, prothrombin time (PT)/international normalized ratio (INR), Haemophilia A and von Willebrand disease

This chapter aims to highlight the use and the interpretation of the results obtained from the above equipment and tests in different haemostatic disorders.

20.2 Point-of-Care Tests and Equipment Used in the Diagnosis and Management of Different Haemostatic Disorders

20.2.1 *Thromboelastography (TEG) and Rotational Thromboelastometry (ROTEM)*

These are viscoelastic haemostasis assays used to assess the coagulation status of a patient in real time and provide dynamic information on the clot formation, stability and dissolution, making them valuable point-of-care tests helping in guiding diagnosis, transfusion therapy, and monitoring different treatments.

Thromboelastography (TEG) measures clot formation in whole blood by detecting viscoelastic properties, whereas Rotational thromboelastometry (ROTEM) is similar to TEG but is optimised for automation, uses a rotating pin, has multiple assays for clot assessment, and provides faster results [4].

Both TEG and ROTEM have different parameters and clinical significance (Tables 20.1 and 20.2).

Using the parameters above, TEG and ROTEM help:

Haemophilia A

- Assess the severity (Fig. 20.1), perioperative haemostatic ability, in monitoring low doses of emicizumab (Fig. 20.2) and monitoring the effect of drugs like tranexamic acid in combination with FVIII in haemophilia patients.
- Monitor Factor IX prophylaxis in Haemophilia B.
- Distinguish between lobar and deep intracranial haemorrhage (ICH), assess anticoagulation reversal and prognosis of hypercoagulation state in ICH.
- Guided treatment during surgical procedures and the effect of recombinant FVII (rFVII) in Glanzmann's thrombasthenia.
- For guided transfusion and impromptu status of different parameters in women with bleeding in obstetrics, like post-partum haemorrhage (PPH).
- Predicting bleeding events and guided transfusion in liver disease.

Table 20.1 Definition and clinical significance of TEG parameters

Parameters	Definition	Clinical significance
R-time (reaction time)	Time to initial fibrin formation (min)	Prolonged in coagulation factor deficiency (e.g. warfarin, liver disease, DIC)
K-time (kinetics time)	Time to reach 20-mm clot strength (min)	Prolonged in fibrinogen deficiency
α-angle	Rate of fibrin cross-linking (degrees)	Decrease in hypofibrinogenemia or platelet dysfunction
MA (maximum amplitude)	Maximum clot strength (mm)	Low in thrombocytopenia or platelet dysfunction
LY30 (lysis at 30 min)	% Clot lysis at 30 min	High in hyperfibrinolysis (e.g. trauma, tissue plasminogen activator (tPA) overdose)

Table 20.2 Definition and clinical significance of ROTEM parameters

Parameters	Definition	Clinical significance
CT (clotting time)	Time until initial fibrin formation (sec) i.e. until an amplitude of 2 mm is reached	Prolonged in factor deficiencies
CFT (clot formation time)	Time to reach 20-mm clot firmness (sec)	Prolonged in hypofibrinogenemia
Alpha angle	Clot formation rate: Angle between the baseline and a tangent to a clotting curve through the 2-mm point	Decrease in fibrinogen abnormalities
MCF (maximum clot firmness)	Maximum clot strength, i.e. the maximum amplitude reached during the test	Reduced in thrombocytopenia, fibrinogen deficiency
ML (Maximum Lysis)	Percentage of clot breakdown	Increase in hyperfibrinolysis
MaxVel (maximum velocity of clot formation)	Rate of clot formation	Lower values associated with blood loss during surgeries
MaxVel-T (maximum velocity of clot formation-time taken)	Time taken by the clot formation to reach maximum velocity	Shorter MaxVel-T indicates rapid clot formation Prolonged MaxVel-T may indicate delayed clotting
MCE (Maximum Clot Elasticity)	Overall strength and stability of the blood clot	Low MCE is associated with higher risk of bleeding, and elevated MCE may indicate an increased risk of thrombosis
A5, A10, and A20 (Amplitude at 5 min, 10 min and 20 min)	Amplitude of clot firmness at 5, 10, and 20 min after clotting begins	A5 indicates early clot firmness Low A10 is indicative of hypo-fibrinogenemia or platelet dysfunction A20 represents the maximum clot strength

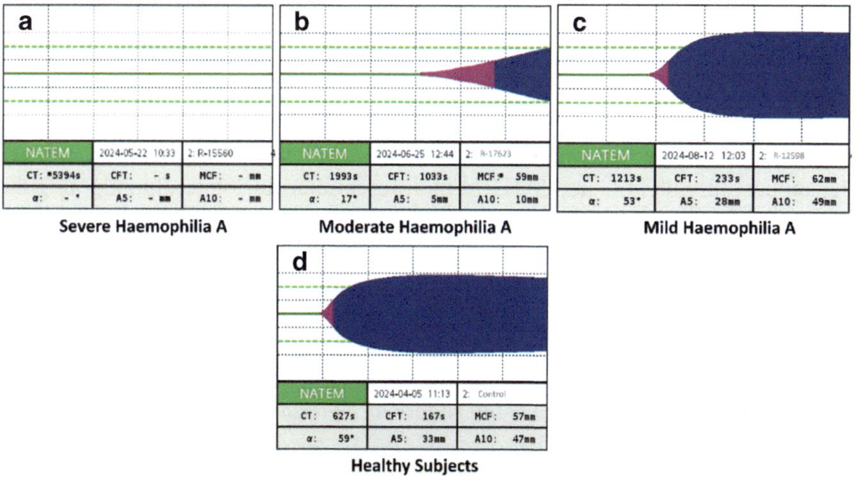

Fig. 20.1 ROTEM–NATEM Clotting Graph in different severities of haemophilia A. The clotting time (CT) and clot formation time (CFT) show how ROTEM-NATEM can help in assessing severity and differentiating between severe, mild, and moderate haemophilia A patients.

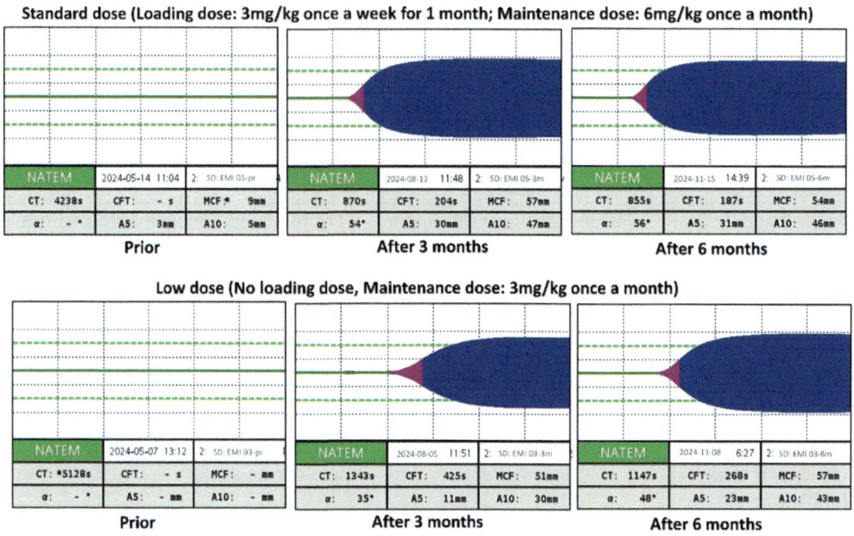

Fig. 20.2 Monitoring of haemophilia patients on different doses of Emicizumab prophylaxis using ROTEM–NATEM. Using ROTEM–NATEM, patients on low dose emicizumab are monitored by evaluating the clotting time (CT) and clot formation time (CFT). Patients on standard dose immediately obtain a clotting profile similar to that of a moderate haemophilia patient; where as those on low dose obtain this profile after a period of time.

- Predicting mortality and guided transfusion in trauma-induced coagulopathy.
- Detection of DIC.
- Detection of hypofibrinogenemia and anticoagulation therapy monitoring in cardiac surgery.
- Coagulation monitoring and prediction of transfusion in orthopaedic and renal surgery.

Limitations of these two tests are that they require trained personnel, the tests are expensive, and some variability is observed between the two tests. Table 20.3 shows the applicability of TEG and ROTEM in different bleeding states, highlighting the different parameters that can be used and how the results can be interpreted.

20.2.2 *Point-of-Care Device*

For Prothrombin Time (PT) and International Normalized Ratio (INR): Point-of-Care (POC) Testing

These are crucial coagulation tests used to assess the extrinsic and common pathways of coagulation. This device uses capillary or venous whole blood, and results are typically available within 1–2 min. The INR test, typically performed via POCT

Table 20.3 Application of TEG and ROTEM in bleeding states

Sr	Bleeding state	Specific utility	Test used	Interpretation	Ref
1	Haemophilia A	To assess severity and differentiate between patients with and without FVIII inhibitor	ROTEM–INTEM, NATEM	Highly prolonged CT, CFT and MaxVel-T and shortened alpha angle and MaxVel in severe haemophilia A patients	[5]
		Perioperative haemostatic ability	ROTEM–Startem	Shortened CT and CFT in patients infused with FVIII and a bypassing agent	[6]
		Emicizumab Monitoring	ROTEM–INTEM, EXTEM, Startem, and NATEM	In Startem CT and CT + CFT are sensitive enough for different concentrations of Emicizumab, unlike INTEM and EXTEM Using NATEM, prolonged CT, and CFT before administration and shortened values after administration of emicizumab based on the dose	[7, 8]
		Low-dose FVIII prophylaxis monitoring	ROTEM–NATEM	Using NATEM, CT, and CFT of patients on low-dose FVIII prophylaxis remains in the range of that of moderate haemophilia	Unpublished data
		Monitoring the effect of Tranexamic acid (TXA) combined with Factor VIII (FVIII) concentrate	TEG: Innovin (Tissue Factor), t-PA, $CaCl_2$	Only TXA normalises the CT, CFT, Alpha angle, MCF and LY30 and shows improvement when spiked with FVIII	[9]

(continued)

Table 20.3 (continued)

Sr	Bleeding state	Specific utility	Test used	Interpretation	Ref
2	Haemophilia B	Factor IX (FIX) prophylaxis	ROTEM–INTEM	Prior prophylaxis, INTEM CT and CFT are prolonged, the alpha angle is shortened and MCF is normalised. Post FIX infusion, CT and CFT are reduced and the alpha angle is increased	[10]
3	Intracranial haemorrhage (ICH)	To distinguish between lobar and deep ICH	ROTEM–INTEM, EXTEM, FIBTEM	EXTEM CT is prolonged for deep ICH as compared to lobar ICH. Whereas, EXTEM MCF and ML values are found to be similar in both the groups. INTEM CT is found to be reduced and INTEM MCF is found to be elevated in deep ICH as compared to lobar ICH. FIBTEM MCF is slightly elevated in Lobar ICH when compared to deep ICH	[11]
		Anticoagulation reversal in patient with ventricular assist device with intracranial haemorrhage	ROTEM–INTEM, EXTEM, FIBTEM	CT, CFT, MCF and alpha angle show normal values in INTEM, EXTEM and FIBTEM. Only A10 and MCF are found to be slightly elevated in EXTEM; suggestive of a hypercoagulable state	[12]
		Prognosis of Hypercoagulation state for Spontaneous Subarachnoid Haemorrhage	ROTEM–INTEM, EXTEM, FIBTEM	Elevated MCF and MCE in INTEM, EXTEM and FIBTEM	[13]
4	Glanzmann's thrombasthenia	Guided treatment during surgical procedures	ROTEM–EXTEM	Reduced MCF is seen with a decline in donor platelet count, indicating further transfusion	[14, 15]
		Effect of Recombinant Factor VII (rFVII)	ROTEM–EXTEM	Increase in CT across different concentrations of rFVII, Increase in CFT post-FVII transfusion, but CFT remains same for different concentrations. MCF remains same for Pre and Post dosing	[16]

5	Bleeding in obstetrics like postpartum haemorrhage (PPH)	Point of care testing and guided transfusion	TEG (Kaolin and Fibrinogen) ROTEM (INTEM or FIBTEM)	MA and MCF in Fibrinogen activated TEG/ROTEM FIBTEM is higher in pregnant women. However, women with PPH found to have low MA and lower A5, A10, and A20 correlated with a high risk of bleeding A5 is a crucial parameter for rapid prediction of hypofibrinogenaemia in women with PPH. Significant decrease in A5, A15 and MCF in third trimester is seen in PPH Low fibrinogen levels detected by FIBTEM A5 are a predictor marker for the progression to severe PPH (>2500 mL of blood loss) Low MA and alpha angle in Kaolin-activated TEG and low MA fibrinogen-activated TEG are predictive markers for severe PPH (>2500 mL), which requires >4 U of RBCs and FFP transfusion	[17–20]
		Fibrinolysis in PPH	TEG (Kaolin)	Monitoring of Hyperfibrinolysis by elevated LY30 (≥3%)	[21]
6	Liver disease and coagulopathy	Predicting bleeding events in liver cirrhosis and liver transplant	ROTEM–EXTEM and INTEM	Significant reduction in MCF in both INTEM and EXTEM, however, prolonged CT in INTEM. MCF in EXTEM is a significant risk predictor for bleeding. Low MaxVel and higher t-MaxVel are seen in bleeders	[22, 23]
		Guided transfusion in liver cirrhosis or liver transplantation	ROTEM–FIBTEM	FIBTEM MCF is strongly associated with intraoperative blood loss and postoperative transfusions	[24]

(continued)

Table 20.3 (continued)

Sr	Bleeding state	Specific utility	Test used	Interpretation	Ref
7	Trauma-induced coagulopathy	Fibrinogen supplementation	ROTEM–FIBTEM	A5 in FIBTEM is a better parameter than A10 for early guidance for transfusion of fibrinogen, as it is an early detection parameter	[25, 26]
		Guided transfusion	ROTEM–EXTEM, INTEM, FIBTEM	Suggested plasma replacement if EXTEM CT > 100 s and/or INTEM CT > 230 s; cryoprecipitate (fibrinogen preparation) and/or plasma administration if FIBTEM MCF < 8 mm; administration of platelet concentrates suggested if EXTEM MCF < 45 mm and FIBTEM MCF > 10 mm. Administration of fibrinolytic agents such as tranexamic acid is suggested if EXTEM ML > 15%	[29]
		Predictor for mortality	ROTEM–APTEM	Low alpha angle, elevated CFT and high CT predict mortality	[27]
		Fibrinolysis	ROTEM–INTEM, EXTEM	CT and CFT are significantly prolonged, and MCF is reduced due to hyperfibrinolysis	[28, 29]
8	DIC	Detection and diagnosis	ROTEM–INTEM, EXTEM, FIBTEM	Elevated CT, reduced MCF, A10, A20, A30, LY30, ML, alpha angle	[30, 31]
9	Cardiac surgery	Detection of hypofibrinogenemia	ROTEM–FIBTEM	FIBTEM A10 for early detection of hypofibrinogenemia and correlation with fibrinogen levels	[32]
		Monitoring anticoagulation therapy	ROTEM–INTEM, EXTEM, FIBTEM, HEPTEM, and APTEM	EXTEM and INTEM CT prolongation reflects coagulation factor deficiency, with INTEM CT specifically reflecting the effect on anticoagulants such as heparin. A low MCF indicates a weak clot and severe bleeding risk as a result of decreased fibrinogen or platelet concentration/ function. Shorter CT in HEPTEM than INTEM is indicative of protamine administration. APTEM assay is utilised for monitoring antifibrinolytic therapy	[33–35]

10	Orthopaedic surgery	Coagulation monitoring and prediction of transfusion	ROTEM–FIBTEM, EXTEM	FIBTEM MCF has high predictive ability for determining excessive bleeding and transfusion requirement. Improvement in CT and A10 is seen after transfusion. Prolonged CT and decreased CT, along with increased MCF, indicate requirement for FFP transfusion and prophylactic anticoagulation, respectively. Decreased alpha angle and MCF indicate cryoprecipitate and fibrinogen concentrate requirement and platelet requirement in case of decreased MCF. Elevated LY30 indicates the need for tranexamic acid	[36–39]
11	Renal surgery	Monitoring coagulation status in chronic kidney disease	ROTEM–INTEM, EXTEM	INTEM and EXTEM CFT are significantly shorter and alpha angle, A5, A10, A20, and MCF are significantly elevated in patients with CKD ML shows significant difference in CKD and healthy control and is the parameter to determine hypercoagulability state in patients with CKD	[40]

Table 20.4 PT/INR values for warfarin monitoring at the point of care

PT–INR value	Interpretation	Recommended action
<1.5	Sub-therapeutic	Increase warfarin dose to achieve the target range
1.5–1.9	Low-therapeutic range	Consider increasing warfarin dose, depending on clinical indication
2.0–3.0	Therapeutic range (standard for most indications)	Goal range for most patients on warfarin
2.5–3.5	Therapeutic range (for some conditions)	Target range for patients with certain conditions, like mechanical heart valves
>3.5	High INR (increased risk of bleeding)	Decrease warfarin dose. Monitor for signs of bleeding. Consider reversal agents if clinically necessary
>5.0	Very high INR (significant risk of bleeding)	Immediate reduction of warfarin dose. Consider vitamin K administration if INR > 9 or in the presence of bleeding
>9.0	Critical high INR	Urgent intervention needed. Vitamin K administration and close monitoring are required

devices, is used to monitor warfarin therapy, ensuring patients stay within the therapeutic range. This is especially important for preventing bleeding or thrombosis in conditions like atrial fibrillation or venous thromboembolism.

Table 20.4 shows, in general, the PT/INR values for warfarin monitoring at the point of care. The Key considerations include:

- *Therapeutic Range*: For most indications (e.g. atrial fibrillation, venous thromboembolism), the target INR range is 2.0–3.0. For patients with mechanical heart valves or other high-risk conditions, the target INR may be slightly higher (2.5–3.5).
- *Monitoring Frequency*: Initially, patients on warfarin therapy are monitored more frequently (e.g. weekly or bi-weekly), and the frequency of testing is reduced once the INR stabilizes within the target range (e.g. every 4–6 weeks).

PT/INRPOCT is also used in:

- Liver disease and cirrhosis to assess if there is a need for fresh frozen plasma (FFP) or vitamin K
- Disseminated Intravascular coagulation (DIC) to help guide blood product transfusion
- Perioperative screening to help decide on perioperative anticoagulation

A few common POC PT/INR devices used are CoaguChek by Roche, i-STAT by Abbott, Hemochron Signature Elite and ProTime Microcoagulation System, etc.

The limitations of this POCT are that it is costly, there exists variability between devices and lab-based INR results, limited accuracy in severe coagulopathy (INR > 4.0), and it is not reliable in certain conditions like antiphospholipid syndrome [41–43].

- *For D-Dimer Testing*

D-dimer is a fibrin degradation product released during clot breakdown and is a crucial biomarker for thrombosis and fibrinolysis. This D-dimer POC device allows immediate risk stratification and clinical decision-making in emergency and critical care settings. It is a semi-quantitative or quantitative immunoassay standardized to detect D-dimer levels in whole blood or plasma within 5–15 min.

A few common POC devices are Cobas h 232 by Roche, Afinion D-Dimer by Abbott, HemosIL D-Dimer HS 500, etc.

The main limitation of the test is that D-Dimer is elevated in many conditions like pregnancy, infection, cancer and leads to false positivity [44, 45].

- *For Diagnosis of Haemophilia and von Willebrand Disease*

The Indian Council of Medical Research–National Institute of Immunohaematology (ICMR–NIIH) in Mumbai has developed a cost-effective point-of-care (POC) rapid diagnostic test for the detection of severe Haemophilia A and von Willebrand Disease (VWD). This innovative test is the first of its kind globally, designed for the specific diagnosis of these common bleeding disorders.

The 2 POCs have a detection limit of 5%, which means all patients having Factor VIII or vWF Antigen levels >5% will be detected. The results are obtained in 10–15 min and are a cost-effective test when compared to the gold standard test. This POC test is particularly beneficial in resource-limited settings, including primary healthcare centres, as it does not require specialized equipment or expertise. Its affordability and ease of use make it a valuable tool for early detection and management of bleeding disorders, potentially improving patient outcomes in underserved populations [46].

- *For Heparin Monitoring*

Patients treated with unfractionated heparin (UFH) are typically monitored using the APTT (Activated Partial Thromboplastin Time) method in the laboratory, which uses ellagic acid as an activator. This method, while effective, can be time-consuming, leading to delays in dose adjustment. In contrast, point-of-care testing (POCT) devices offer a quicker alternative by providing electrochemical measurements of PT (Prothrombin Time) and APTT following activation of the coagulation cascade [47].

The Activated Coagulation Time–Low Range (ACT–LR) is commonly used to measure plasma levels of Non–Vitamin K Antagonist Oral Anticoagulants (NOACs), such as dabigatran, using the portable Hemochron Signature Elite (Werfen). This simple, single-use, cartridge-based technology measures fibrin clot formation. Additionally, the Coaguchek XS Pro (Roche) is used to assess International Normalized Ratio (INR) levels, which are useful for measuring rivaroxaban and apixaban levels, as well as Warfarin levels, especially in cases of antiphospholipid syndrome. Furthermore, the CoaguChek®-INR (CC–INR) (Roche) is utilized for the reversal of direct oral anticoagulants (DOACs) in stroke patients, guiding thrombolysis therapy [48–50].

Paper-based microfluidics is an emerging field in diagnostic devices, particularly for point-of-care (POC) testing. It combines the simplicity, low cost, and portability of paper with microfluidic techniques, enabling the rapid and efficient analysis of biological samples such as blood or serum. The ability to monitor heparin levels, a critical anticoagulant used in the treatment of thrombosis and other clotting disorders, in real time and at the point of care has significant potential for improving patient outcomes.

Paper-based microfluidic devices for heparin monitoring offer a promising solution for point-of-care testing in thrombosis management. They can provide affordable, portable, and rapid monitoring of heparin levels, potentially improving patient outcomes by enabling better management of anticoagulation therapy. Despite challenges in sensitivity, accuracy, and regulatory approval, ongoing research and innovation in this field could make paper-based heparin monitoring a viable tool for clinical practice in the near future [51].

Case Presentations

I. *We present the ROTEM clotting profiles of three haemophilia patients with varying severities of the condition* (Fig. 20.1).

Laboratory test results of the three cases are mentioned in Table 20.5, and Bleeding details were as follows:

Case 1A: spontaneous bleeds from the age of 4 years, joint bleeds, prolonged bleed after injury, multiple transfusions

Case 1B: Bleeding on trauma, occasional spontaneous bleeds from a young age

Case 1C: Bleeding after dental surgery at the age of 27 years

II. *We present a case involving two patients with haemophilia, each receiving different doses of Emicizumab for prophylaxis. The patients' haemostatic status was closely monitored using ROTEM–NATEM* (Fig. 20.2)

Patients 1 and 2 are known cases of severe Haemophilia A, one is on standard dose emicizumab prophylaxis, i.e. loading dose of 3 mg/kg/week followed by a maintenance dose of 6 mg/kg/month, and the other is on low dose emicizumab prophylaxis, i.e. no loading dose and maintenance dose of 3 mg/kg/month. ROTEM NATEM Clotting profile of two patients is shown in Table 20.6.

Table 20.5 Laboratory test results of three haemophilia patients with varying severities of the condition

Sr	Tests	Result			
		Patient 1A	Patient 1B	Patient 1C	Healthy control
1	Prothrombin time (PT) (secs)	Control: 12.5 Patient: 13.4	Control: 12.5 Patient: 12.9	Control: 12.5 Patient: 14.1	Control: 12.5 Patient: 13.1
2	Activated partial Thromboplastin time (APTT) (secs)	Control: 29.9 Patient: 69.8 Mixing (with NPP): 30.7	Control: 29.9 Patient: 49.2 Mixing (with NPP): 30.7	Control: 29.9 Patient: 38.2 Mixing (with NPP): 30.7	Control: 29.9 Patient: 28.2
3	One stage FVIII levels (IU/dL)	<1	3.8	33	121
4	One stage FIX levels (IU/dL)	110	98	125	95
5	Von Willebrand factor antigen levels (IU/dL)	98	121	105	101
6	Impression	Severe Haemophilia A	Moderate Haemophilia A	Mild Haemophilia A	–
7	ROTEM NATEM CT (secs)	5394	1993	1213	627
8	ROTEM NATEM CFT (secs)	Not detected	1033	233	167

Table 20.6 ROTEM–NATEM clotting profile of two patients with haemophilia on standard and low-dose Emicizumab prophylaxis

	ROTEM–NATEM clotting profile		
Timeline	Prior	3 months	6 months
Patient on standard dose emicizumab prophylaxis	CT: 4238 sec CFT: Not detected	CT: 870 sec CFT: 204 sec	CT: 855 sec CFT: 187 sec
Patient on low dose emicizumab prophylaxis	CT: 5128 sec CFT: Not detected	CT: 1343 sec CFT: 425 sec	CT: 1147 sec CFT: 268 sec

20.3 Summary

Point-of-care testing (POCT) refers to diagnostic tests performed near the patient, offering rapid results to guide treatment. POCTs are essential in managing haemostatic disorders, which involve impaired blood clotting, such as Haemophilia, thrombophilia, DIC, and liver disease. Key tests include Thromboelastography (TEG) and Rotational Thromboelastometry (ROTEM), which assess clot formation and breakdown, helping diagnose and manage conditions like Haemophilia and trauma-induced coagulopathy. POCT devices for Prothrombin Time (PT)/INR and D-dimer are also used for monitoring anticoagulation, thrombotic risk, and bleeding. These tests are crucial in emergency and resource-limited settings, despite their cost and need for trained personnel.

References

1. Larkins MC, Thombare A. Point-of-Care Testing. Treasure Island (FL): StatPearls Publishing; 2023. Available from: https://www.ncbi.nlm.nih.gov/books/NBK592387/.
2. Land KJ, Boeras DI, Chen XS, Ramsay AR, Peeling RW. REASSURED diagnostics to inform disease control strategies, strengthen health systems and improve patient outcomes. Nat Microbiol. 2019;4(1):46–54.
3. Doherty TM, Kelley A. Bleeding Disorders. StatPearls Publishing; 2023. Available from: https://www.ncbi.nlm.nih.gov/books/NBK541050/.
4. Veigas PV, Callum J, Rizoli S, Nascimento B, da Luz LT. A systematic review on the rotational thrombelastometry (ROTEM®) values for the diagnosis of coagulopathy, prediction and guidance of blood transfusion and prediction of mortality in trauma patients. Scand J Trauma Resusc Emerg Med. 2016;24(1):114.
5. Gupta D, Arya V, Dass J, Gupta N, Kalra M, Sachdeva A, et al. Assessment of the phenotypic severity of haemophilia A: using rotational thromboelastometry (ROTEM) and APTT-clot waveform analysis. Blood Res. 2024;59(1):19.
6. Yagyuu T, Furukawa S, Zaizen M, Yata S, Imada M, Nogami K, et al. Peri-operative hemostatic management of tooth extraction in patients with hemophilia A, with and without inhibitors, receiving emicizumab prophylaxis. Haemophilia. 2022;29:172.

7. Barg AA, Avishai E, Budnik I, Levy-Mendelovich S, Barazani TB, Kenet G, et al. Emicizumab prophylaxis among infants and toddlers with severe hemophilia A and inhibitors—a single-center cohort. Pediatr Blood Cancer. 2019;66(11):e27886.
8. Yada K, Nogami K, Ogiwara K, Shida Y, Furukawa S, Yaoi H, et al. Global coagulation function assessed by rotational thromboelastometry predicts coagulation-steady state in individual hemophilia A patients receiving emicizumab prophylaxis. Int J Hematol. 2019;110(4):419–30.
9. Janbain M, Enjolras N, Bordet JC, Bolbos R, Brevet M, Leissinger C, et al. Hemostatic effect of tranexamic acid combined with factor VIII concentrate in prophylactic setting in severe hemophilia A: a preclinical study. J Thromb Haemost. 2019;18(3):584–92.
10. Nummi V, Jouppila A, Lassila R. Monitoring once-weekly recombinant factor IX prophylaxis in hemophilia B with thrombin generation assay and factor IX activity. Int J Lab Hematol. 2017;39(4):359–68. Available from: https://pubmed.ncbi.nlm.nih.gov/28406575/.
11. Roh D, Chang T, Zammit C, Wagener G, Reynolds AS, Yoh N, et al. Functional coagulation differences between lobar and deep intracerebral hemorrhage detected by rotational thromboelastometry: a pilot study. Neurocrit Care. 2019;31(1):81–7. Available from: https://pubmed.ncbi.nlm.nih.gov/30693412/.
12. Bonderski VA, Portillo J, Sharp L, Rech MA. Thromboelastometry-guided anti-coagulation reversal in a patient with ventricular assist device with intra-cranial hemorrhage. Am J Emerg Med. 2020;41:265.e5–8. Available from: https://www.sciencedirect.com/science/article/abs/pii/S0735675720307488.
13. Lauridsen SV, Hvas CL, Sandgaard E, Gyldenholm T, Mikkelsen R, Obbekjær T, et al. Thromboelastometry shows early hypercoagulation in patients with spontaneous subarachnoid hemorrhage. World Neurosurg. 2019;130:e140–9.
14. Grassetto A, Fullin G, Lazzari F, Panizzo F, Polese F, Gessoni G, et al. Perioperative ROTEM and ROTEMplatelet monitoring in a case of Glanzmann's thrombasthenia. Blood Coagul Fibrinolysis. 2017;28(1):96–9. Available from: https://pubmed.ncbi.nlm.nih.gov/26825624/.
15. Barg AA, Hauschner H, Misgav M, Lubetsky A, Levy-Mendelowitz S, Livnat T, et al. A novel approach using ancillary tests to guide treatment of Glanzmann thrombasthenia patients undergoing surgical procedures. Blood Cell Mol Dis. 2018;72:44–8. Available from: https://www.sciencedirect.com/science/article/pii/S107997961830247X.
16. Lak M, Scharling B, Blemings A, Sharifian R, Maleki Z, Daraee A, et al. Evaluation of rFVIIa (NovoSeven) in Glanzmann patients with thromboelastogram. Haemophilia. 2007;14(1):103–10.
17. Antony K, Mansouri R, Arndt M, Hui SKR, Jariwala P, Mcmullen V, et al. Establishing thromboelastography with platelet-function analyzer reference ranges and other measures in healthy term pregnant women. Am J Perinatol. 2015;32(06):545–54.
18. Gillissen A, Thomas, Caram-Deelder C, Dacia, Kitty, Eikenboom J, et al. Comparison of thromboelastometry by ROTEM® Delta and ROTEM® Sigma in women with postpartum haemorrhage. Scand J Clin Lab Investig. 2019;79(1–2):32–8.
19. Butwick AJ. Postpartum hemorrhage: wherefore art thou, hyperfibrinolysis? Anesth Analg. 2020;131(5):1370–2.
20. Dias JD, Butwick AJ, Hartmann J, Waters JH. Viscoelastic haemostatic point-of-care assays in the management of postpartum haemorrhage: a narrative review. Anaesthesia. 2022;77:700.
21. Agarwal S, Laycock HC. The debate ROTEMs on – the utility of point-of-care testing and fibrinogen concentrate in postpartum haemorrhage. Anaesthesia. 2020;75(9):1247–51. (previous 38).
22. Janko N, Majeed A, Commins I, Gow P, Kemp W, Roberts SK. Rotational thromboelastometry predicts future bleeding events in patients with cirrhosis. Scand J Gastroenterol. 2024;59(9):1062–8. Available from: https://pubmed.ncbi.nlm.nih.gov/39010734/.
23. Tafur LA, Taura P, Blasi A, Beltran J, Martinez-Palli G, Balust J, et al. Rotation thromboelastometry velocity curve predicts blood loss during liver transplantation. Br J Anaesth. 2016;117(6):741–8. Available from: https://pubmed.ncbi.nlm.nih.gov/27956672/.

24. Carrier FM, Denault AY, Nozza A, Rioux-Massé B, Roy A, Massicotte L. Association between intraoperative rotational thromboelastometry or conventional coagulation tests and bleeding in liver transplantation: an observational exploratory study. Anaesth Crit Care Pain Med. 2020;39(6):765–70. Available from: https://pubmed.ncbi.nlm.nih.gov/33011332/.
25. Blayney A, McCullough J, Wake E, Walters K, Campbell D, Ho D, et al. Substitution of ROTEM FIBTEM A5 for A10 in trauma: an observational study building a case for more rapid analysis of coagulopathy. Eur J Trauma Emerg Surg. 2021;48:1077.
26. Campbell D, Wake E, Walters K, Ho D, Keijzers G, Wullschleger M, et al. Implementation of point-of-care ROTEM ® into a trauma major haemorrhage protocol: a before and after study. Emerg Med Australas. 2020;33:457.
27. Smith AR, Karim SA, Reif RR, Beck WC, Taylor JR, Davis BL, et al. ROTEM as a predictor of mortality in patients with severe trauma. J Surg Res. 2020;251:107–11.
28. Kim JS, Wang IJ, Yeom SR, Cho SJ, Kim JH, Seok JP, et al. Usefulness of rotational thromboelastometry as a mortality predictor of hyperfibrinolysis in patients with severe trauma. Acute Crit Care. 2018;33(3):162–9. Available from: https://pubmed.ncbi.nlm.nih.gov/31723880/.
29. Sakamoto Y, Koami H, Miike T. Monitoring the coagulation status of trauma patients with viscoelastic devices. J Intensive Care. 2017;5(1):7.
30. Koami H, Sakamoto Y, Hirota Y, Sasaki A, Ogawa H, Furukawa Y, et al. Effect of hypofibrinolysis on clinical outcomes of patients with septic disseminated intravascular coagulation. Thromb Res. 2024;245:109235.
31. Koami H, Sakamoto Y, Yamada KC, Matsuda T, Nishi J, Nakayama K, et al. What factor within the Japanese Association for Acute Medicine (JAAM) disseminated intravascular coagulation (DIC) criteria is most strongly correlated with trauma induced DIC? A retrospective study using thromboelastometry in a single center in Japan. Eur J Trauma Emerg Surg. 2017;43(4):431–8.
32. Fernández Suárez FE, Fernández Del Valle D, González Alvarez A, Pérez-Lozano B. Intraoperative care for aortic surgery using circulatory arrest. J Thorac Dis. 2017;9(S6):S508–20.
33. Reinhöfer M, Brauer M, Franke U, Barz D, Marx G, Lösche W. The value of rotation thromboelastometry to monitor disturbed perioperative haemostasis and bleeding risk in patients with cardiopulmonary bypass. Blood Coagul Fibrinolysis. 2008;19(3):212–9.
34. Görlinger K, Dirkmann D, Hanke AA, Kamler M, Kottenberg E, Thielmann M, et al. First-line therapy with coagulation factor concentrates combined with point-of-care coagulation testing is associated with decreased allogeneic blood transfusion in cardiovascular surgery. Anesthesiology. 2011;115(6):1179–91.
35. Vasques F, Spiezia L, Manfrini A, Tarzia V, Fichera D, Simioni P, et al. Thromboelastometry guided fibrinogen replacement therapy in cardiac surgery: a retrospective observational study. J Anesth. 2017;31(2):286–90.
36. Tsantes AG, Papadopoulos DV, Roustemis AG, Trikoupis IG, Piovani D, Tsante KA, et al. Rotational thromboelastometry predicts transfusion requirements in total joint arthroplasties. Semin Thromb Hemost. 2023;49(2):134–44.
37. Hanke AA, Bartlau J, Flöricke F, Przemeck M, Horstmann H, Weber-Spickschen TS, et al. Coagulation monitoring and transfusion in major non-emergency orthopaedic surgery: an observational study. J Orthop. 2020;22:22–8. Available from: https://pubmed.ncbi.nlm.nih.gov/32280164/.
38. Mamczak CN, Speybroeck J, Stillson JE, Dynako J, Piscoya AS, Peck EE, et al. Viscoelastic hemostatic assays for orthopedic trauma and elective procedures. J Clin Med. 2022;11(14):4029.
39. Gonzalez E, Moore EE, Moore HB, Chapman MP, Chin TL, Ghasabyan A, et al. Goal-directed hemostatic resuscitation of trauma-induced coagulopathy. Ann Surg. 2016;263(6):1051–9.
40. Abdelmaguid A, Roberts LN, Tugores L, Joslin JR, Hunt BJ, Parmar K, et al. Evaluation of novel coagulation and platelet function assays in patients with chronic kidney disease. J Thromb Haemost. 2022;20(4):845–56.

41. Wool GD. Benefits and pitfalls of point-of-care coagulation testing for anticoagulation management. Am J Clin Pathol. 2018;151(1):1–17.
42. Vazquez SR, Fleming RP, Johnson SA. Comparison of two point-of-care international normalized ratio devices and laboratory method. Blood Coagul Fibrinolysis. 2017;28(7):534–9.
43. Arline K, Rodriguez C, Sanchez K. Reliability of point-of-care international normalized ratio measurements in various patient populations. Point of Care: J Near-Patient Test Technol. 2020;19(1):12–8.
44. Heerink JS, Oudega R, Gemen E, Hopstaken R, Koffijberg H, Kusters R. Are the latest point-of-care D-dimer devices ready for use in general practice? A prospective clinical evaluation of five test systems with a capillary blood feature for suspected venous thromboembolism. Thromb Res. 2023;232:113–22.
45. Tan M, Huisman MV. Point-of-care D-dimer tests can contribute to patient management in outpatients with suspected venous thromboembolism, particularly those at low risk. Evid Based Med. 2010;15:28.
46. (ICMR IN NEWS) (Syed Adil Shamim Andrabi) Information Interface Officer. 2019. [cited 2025 Feb 17]. Available from: https://www.icmr.gov.in/icmrobject/custom_data/1702965413_icmr_news_2.pdf?.
47. Lardinois B, Hardy M, Michaux I, Horlait G, Rotens T, Jacqmin H, et al. Monitoring of unfractionated heparin therapy in the intensive care unit using a point-of-care aPTT: a comparative, longitudinal observational study with laboratory-based aPTT and anti-Xa activity measurement. J Clin Med. 2022;11(5):1338. Available from: https://www.mdpi.com/2077-0383/11/5/1338/htm.
48. Padayattil Jose S, Banzato A, Carraro P, Haleh A, Rossi K, Nante G, et al. Point of Care Testing (POCT) to assess drug concentration in patients treated with non-vitamin K antagonist oral anticoagulants (NOACs). Thromb Res. 2018;163:100–4. Available from: https://pubmed.ncbi.nlm.nih.gov/29407620/.
49. Jepsen SY, Larsen JB, Christensen TD, Grove EL, Maegaard M, Hvas AM. Warfarin monitoring and interference by lupus anticoagulant in patients with antiphospholipid syndrome. Thromb Res. 2022;211:127–32.
50. Härtig F, Birschmann I, Peter A, Hörber S, Ebner M, Sonnleitner M, et al. Point-of-care testing of coagulation in patients treated with edoxaban. J Thromb Thrombolysis. 2020;50(3):632–9. Available from: https://pubmed.ncbi.nlm.nih.gov/32436010/.
51. Zhou J. The development of the heparin monitoring system based on microfluidics technology. J Biomater Nanobiotechnol. 2020;11:195–213. https://doi.org/10.4236/jbnb.2020.113013.

Chapter 21
Advances in the Diagnosis of DIC and Fibrinolysis

Sonal Jain

Abstract Disseminated intravascular coagulation (DIC) represents a critical clinical syndrome characterized by systemic activation of coagulation pathways and concurrent dysregulation of fibrinolysis. It commonly arises as a complication of severe infections, trauma, malignancies, or obstetric emergencies. Fibrinolysis, the physiological mechanism responsible for clot breakdown, is often impaired in DIC, exacerbating the risk of microvascular thrombosis and organ dysfunction. Over the past decade, significant strides have been made in the early recognition and diagnosis of DIC and its fibrinolytic disturbances. Modern scoring systems—such as those by ISTH and JAAM—integrate laboratory and clinical variables to guide diagnosis with improved specificity and sensitivity. Concurrently, biomarker discovery, including D-dimer, thrombin-antithrombin complexes, and histone-DNA complexes, has enriched diagnostic precision. Technological innovations like thromboelastography (TEG), rotational thromboelastometry (ROTEM), and clot waveform analysis (CWA) offer dynamic, bedside insights into coagulation and fibrinolysis. Moreover, the role of molecular triggers such as DAMPs, PAMPs, and NETs in modulating coagulation is being increasingly appreciated. Imaging modalities like Doppler ultrasound and CT angiography have also augmented diagnostic capabilities by identifying microvascular thrombi. This review outlines these advances, with emphasis on integrating biomarkers, point-of-care technologies, and scoring systems to optimize the diagnosis and management of DIC and fibrinolysis abnormalities.

Disseminated intravascular coagulation (DIC) is a complex and life-threatening disorder characterized by widespread activation of coagulation and fibrinolytic pathways, leading to excessive consumption of clotting factors and platelets, as well as microvascular thrombosis and organ dysfunction. In recent years, there have been significant advances in the diagnosis of DIC, allowing for earlier recognition and improved management of patients with this condition.

Key recent advances include refined scoring systems, the identification of novel biomarkers, and the exploration of advanced imaging techniques.

S. Jain (✉)
Modern Diagnostics and Research Center, Gurgaon, India

Art of Healing Cancer, Gurgaon, India

H. P. Pati et al. (eds.), *Clinical Hematology and Hemato-Oncology*,
https://doi.org/10.1007/978-981-92-1167-8_21

Keywords Disseminated intravascular coagulation · Fibrinolysis · D-dimer · Diagnostic biomarkers · Thromboelastography

Learning Objectives

- Understand the Pathophysiology of DIC
  Explain the mechanisms underlying the development of DIC, including the interplay between coagulation, fibrinolysis, and inflammatory pathways.
- Compare Diagnostic Scoring Systems for DIC
  Identify and contrast the major DIC diagnostic scoring systems, including those by ISTH, JMHW, JAAM, BCSH, and SISET, and understand their clinical applications.
- Recognize the Role of Novel Biomarkers in DIC Diagnosis
  Describe emerging biomarkers such as TAT, F1 + 2, soluble fibrin, MP-TF, and PAP, and evaluate their diagnostic and prognostic significance in various clinical contexts.
- Evaluate Point-of-Care Technologies in DIC Assessment
  Assess the utility of thromboelastography (TEG), rotational thromboelastometry (ROTEM), and clot waveform analysis in the real-time monitoring and management of DIC.
- Appreciate the Clinical Relevance of Molecular Triggers in DIC
  Discuss the role of molecular mediators like DAMPs, PAMPs, NETs, and histones in the pathogenesis of DIC and explore their potential as diagnostic and therapeutic targets.

21.1 Introduction

Disseminated intravascular coagulation (DIC) is a multifactorial and life-threatening disorder involving widespread activation of both coagulation and fibrinolytic pathways. This pathological imbalance results in simultaneous thrombus formation and hemorrhagic complications, predominantly seen in critically ill patients. The fibrinolytic system, which normally serves to dissolve clots and maintain vascular patency, is often dysregulated in DIC, further complicating clinical outcomes. Recent advancements in diagnostic techniques have provided a clearer understanding of DIC's complex pathogenesis, particularly with regard to the interplay between coagulation and fibrinolysis.

Notably, diagnostic scoring systems have become more refined, incorporating a combination of clinical features and laboratory findings. Additionally, biomarkers such as D-dimer, thrombin-antithrombin complexes, and histone–DNA complexes are emerging as key indicators for early detection and risk stratification. Advanced imaging techniques and point-of-care coagulation monitoring tools, including thromboelastography (TEG) and rotational thromboelastometry (ROTEM), have also revolutionized bedside diagnostics. This chapter reviews the current diagnostic strategies and technological innovations that are shaping the early recognition and effective management of DIC and associated fibrinolytic disorders.

21.2 Background

Disseminated intravascular coagulation (DIC) is a complex, acquired syndrome characterized by widespread activation of the coagulation cascade and dysregulation of fibrinolysis. It arises as a secondary complication of numerous conditions, including severe infections, trauma, malignancies, and obstetric complications. The underlying pathophysiology involves excessive thrombin generation, leading to microvascular thrombosis and multiorgan dysfunction, alongside consumption of platelets and coagulation factors that increase bleeding risk. DIC is not a disease in itself but a manifestation of a systemic insult, making diagnosis particularly challenging due to its variable clinical presentation and overlap with other coagulopathies.

Timely diagnosis is essential to guide appropriate therapeutic interventions. Over recent decades, several diagnostic scoring systems and biomarkers have been developed to enhance clinical accuracy and prognostic stratification. Traditional diagnostic criteria often rely on static laboratory parameters such as platelet count, prothrombin time, fibrinogen, and fibrin degradation products. However, growing insight into the molecular drivers of DIC has prompted the integration of novel biomarkers, dynamic clotting assays, and point-of-care diagnostics into clinical algorithms. These advancements reflect a shift toward early recognition, individualized assessment, and dynamic monitoring of coagulopathy in critically ill patients. This review highlights these emerging diagnostic tools and their relevance to contemporary DIC evaluation and management.

21.3 Refined Scoring Systems

One of the key recent advances in the diagnosis of DIC has been the development of scoring systems that use a combination of clinical and laboratory parameters to assess the likelihood of DIC in a given patient. Today, there are five different diagnostic scoring systems for DIC established by the ISTH, the Japanese Ministry of Health and Welfare (JMHW), the Japanese Association for Acute Medicine (JAAM), the British Committee for Standards in Hematology (BCSH), and the Italian Society of Thrombosis and Hemostasis (SISET) [1–5].

The International Society on Thrombosis and Haemostasis (ISTH) scoring system is the most widely used and validated tool. It incorporates platelet count, fibrin-related markers (e.g., D-dimer), prothrombin time, and fibrinogen level. A cumulative score ≥ 5 suggests overt DIC.

The Japanese Ministry of Health and Welfare (JMHW) score evaluates platelet count, fibrin degradation products (FDP), prothrombin time, and clinical symptoms (e.g., bleeding or organ failure). It was among the earliest scoring systems and is widely used in Japan, particularly in sepsis and leukemia.

The Japanese Association for Acute Medicine (JAAM) system is tailored for acute DIC, especially in sepsis. It includes systemic inflammatory response syndrome (SIRS) criteria along with platelet count, prothrombin time ratio, and FDP/D-dimer levels. It is more sensitive for early DIC diagnosis.

The British Committee for Standards in Haematology (BCSH) guidelines recommend a more qualitative approach based on clinical suspicion and supportive laboratory tests rather than a formal scoring system, emphasizing exclusion of alternative diagnoses.

The Italian Society for Thrombosis and Hemostasis (SISET) adapted ISTH criteria, stressing serial monitoring and integrating clinical context for dynamic DIC evaluation (Table 21.1).

Table 21.1 Here is a comparative table of the five major DIC diagnostic scoring systems

Scoring system	Origin	Key components	Scoring threshold	Main use/features
ISTH (International Society on Thrombosis and Haemostasis)	International	Platelet count, prolonged PT, fibrin-related markers (e.g., D-dimer), fibrinogen	≥5 indicates overt DIC	Most validated system, standard for research and general clinical use
JMHW (Japanese Ministry of Health and Welfare)	Japan	Platelet count, FDP, PT prolongation, clinical symptoms	≥7 indicates DIC	Older system, includes clinical features, used in hematologic and septic conditions
JAAM (Japanese Association for Acute Medicine)	Japan	SIRS criteria, platelet count, PT ratio, FDP/D-dimer	≥4 indicates DIC	Sensitive to early DIC, especially in sepsis and ICU settings
BCSH (British Committee for Standards in Haematology)	UK	Clinical judgment, platelet count, PT, fibrinogen, D-dimer	No formal score	Emphasizes clinical context and exclusion of other causes; less structured
SISET (Italian Society for Thrombosis and Hemostasis)	Italy	Adapted ISTH criteria; serial lab monitoring and clinical evaluation	Based on ISTH thresholds	Emphasizes repeated testing and dynamic assessment in a clinical context

21.4 Biomarkers

Recent advances in laboratory diagnostics have identified several novel biomarkers that enhance the early detection and accuracy of Disseminated Intravascular Coagulation (DIC) diagnosis, beyond conventional markers such as platelet count, D-dimer, and fibrinogen.

Thrombin–Antithrombin Complexes (TAT) are sensitive indicators of thrombin generation. Elevated TAT levels reflect ongoing coagulation activation and correlate with DIC severity, especially in sepsis-related cases [6]. Similarly, Prothrombin Fragment 1 + 2 (F1 + 2) is released during prothrombin activation and is a specific marker for thrombin generation, offering early insight into coagulation imbalance [7].

Soluble Fibrin (SF) levels indicate fibrin monomer presence before the formation of cross-linked fibrin, making it a promising early marker for hypercoagulability. Elevated SF often precedes increases in D-dimer, potentially identifying DIC at a preclinical stage [8].

Microparticle-Associated Tissue Factor (MP-TF), derived from activated monocytes and endothelial cells, plays a role in initiating coagulation. Increased levels of MP-TF have been associated with poor prognosis in DIC and may serve both diagnostic and prognostic functions [9].

Plasmin–α2-antiplasmin Complex (PAP) is a marker of fibrinolytic activity, useful in distinguishing DIC with enhanced fibrinolysis, such as in acute promyelocytic leukemia [10].

Emerging omics-based approaches, including proteomics and metabolomics, have also identified novel protein and metabolite signatures associated with early DIC stages. These methods may offer personalized insights and risk stratification in the future [11] .

While these new biomarkers show promise, their clinical utility is still being evaluated. Many are limited by cost, assay standardization, or availability. However, in combination with established scoring systems, they may improve early detection, allow better differentiation of DIC subtypes, and guide targeted therapies.

Levels of endogenous anticoagulants, including AT, PC, and TM, are among the most promising candidates as biomarkers for use in sepsis and DIC [12]. In a large cohort of patients with sepsis and suspected DIC, reduced AT and PC levels were predictive of mortality, regardless of whether the patient met the ISTH criteria for overt DIC [13]. Other studies have focused on markers of endothelial activation, on markers of inflammation, or on novel markers, including extracellular nucleosomes and histones.

In a recent study including 20 patients with sepsis, researchers performed a peptidome analysis using a new target plate, BLOTCHIP, that enables 1-step direct electric transfer of analytes from the 1-dimensional polyacrylamide gel electrophoresis (PAGE) gel to the target plate. In this study, 8 peptides were successfully identified as marker peptides for DIC in patients with sepsis. The peptides were fragments of serum amyloid A-2 protein, a2-HS-glycoprotein, fibrinogen a chain, fibrinogen b chain, serum albumin, collagen a1 (I) chain, collagen a1 (III) chain, and coagulation factor XIII A chain [14].

21.5 Molecular Markers

Extracellular histones and neutrophil extracellular traps. Extracellular histones may be found in the circulation (either free or complexed with DNA 'nucleosomes') or localized (and modified) as part of the extracellular traps released upon damage or activation of nucleated cells, primarily neutrophils. The various roles of neutrophils as key modulators of the complex interaction between innate immunity, inflammation, and coagulation (also known as "immunothrombosis") are increasingly recognized.

NETs were first described in 2004 as a neutrophil-derived amalgam of elastases, histones, and DNA that collectively trap and kill bacteria. Like histones, NETs have important physiological but potentially pathological manifestations. Their uncontrolled or inappropriate release by neutrophils can contribute to the pathogenesis of sepsis, micro- and macro-vascular thrombosis, and multiple organ injury. Consequences of NETs are typically site-specific, but breakdown products, such as cell-free DNA (cfDNA) or DNA-myeloperoxidase (DNA-MPO) complexes, can be found in the circulation.

Histones can arise from endothelial cells following damage or from an exaggerated inflammatory response and, in turn, can mediate further significant damage to vascular endothelial cells. Directly and indirectly, histones can cause pro-inflammatory cytokine release and contribute to "inflammation gone amok," as described in the ISTH communication. With the bi-directional relationship between histones and NETs, along with their functional consequences, histones can be considered mediators of distant organ injury, with NETs being the effectors of multi-organ failure.

There are a number of studies showing histone–DNA complexes as important prognosticators in patients with DIC, and their levels correlate with increasing DIC scores. As such, there appears to be potential in using these molecules as biomarkers in early DIC before full decompensation occurs. This could be a major advancement in the diagnosis and management of critically ill patients at risk of DIC.

There is no simple, rapid test for quantifying histones that could be suitable for the acute hospital setting. Furthermore, there is controversy regarding the level of circulating histones; some papers quote levels in the microgram-per-milliliter range using Western blotting quantification, whereas others suggest that levels are in the nanogram-per-milliliter or picogram-per-milliliter range using enzyme-linked immunosorbent assay (ELISA). Most studies rely on measuring cfDNA, histone-DNA, and DNA-MPO complexes as surrogate markers of NET formation. Recent studies have illustrated promising potential for the use of neutrophil side fluorescence as a marker of neutrophil chromatin decondensation (hence NETosis) in predicting DIC development in patients with septic shock. This new marker correlated significantly (yet with a weak correlation coefficient) with circulating nucleosomes and DNA-MPO complexes in patients with DIC. Standardization for histone and NET measurements using accurate high-output techniques is therefore a pressing need.

21.6 DAMPs

These are endogenous molecules released from damaged or stressed cells, acting as "danger signals" that can trigger inflammation. Examples include high-mobility group box 1 (HMGB1), uric acid, and ATP. Damage-associated molecular patterns (DAMPs) play a crucial role in the pathogenesis of Disseminated Intravascular Coagulation (DIC) and are increasingly recognized as important diagnostic and therapeutic targets. DAMPs, released from damaged or dead cells, can trigger systemic inflammation, activate the coagulation cascade, and impair fibrinolysis, leading to the hallmark features of DIC, including thrombus formation and bleeding [15].

21.6.1 DAMPs and DIC Pathogenesis (Fig. 21.1)

DAMPs, such as histones, extracellular DNA, and other molecules, are released during tissue injury, trauma, sepsis, or other conditions. These DAMPs can activate pattern recognition receptors (PRRs) on immune cells, leading to the release of pro-inflammatory cytokines and the activation of the coagulation system.

DAMPs can directly activate the coagulation cascade through various mechanisms. DAMPs can induce the expression of TF on monocytes and endothelial cells, which is a crucial factor for initiating coagulation. Some DAMPs, like extracellular nucleic acids, can directly activate factor XII (FXII), initiating the intrinsic coagulation pathway. DAMPs can contribute to impaired fibrinolysis by activating enzymes that inhibit fibrinolysis, such as plasminogen activator inhibitor-1 (PAI-1) [16].

21.6.2 Diagnostic and Therapeutic Implications

While DAMPs themselves are not typically used in direct DIC diagnosis, their presence and the inflammatory response they trigger are important considerations in evaluating patients with suspected DIC, particularly in conditions like sepsis or trauma. Modulating the inflammatory response and DAMP-mediated coagulation activation is a potential therapeutic strategy for DIC. For example, targeting DAMPs

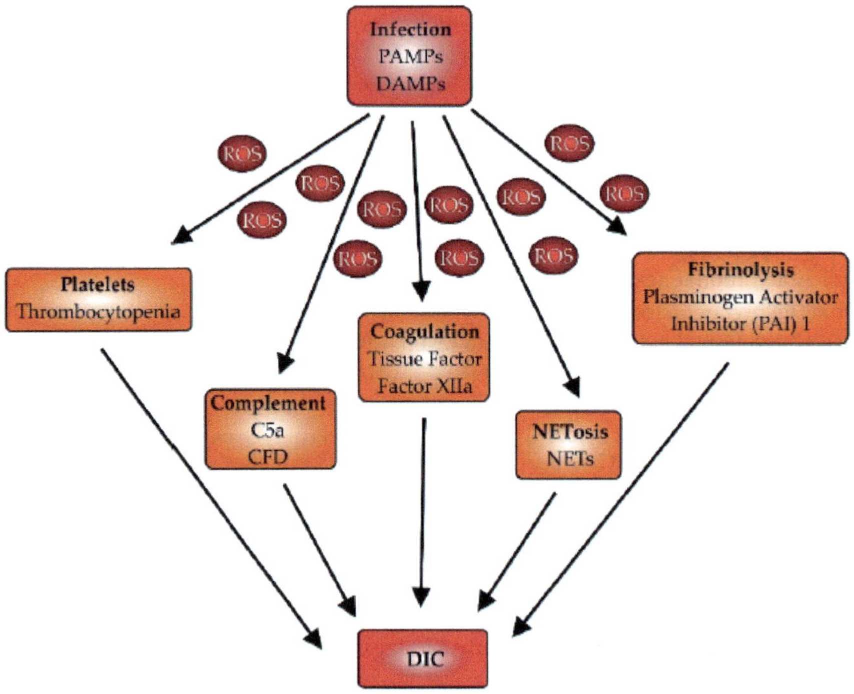

Fig. 21.1 Disseminated intravascular coagulation (DIC). Infectious pathogens via their associated PAMPs release resultant DAMPs, following cell activation or damage, leading to ROS production. These proinflammatory mediators contribute to the activation of platelets, leading to thrombocytopenia [175]; attract immune cells due to the liberation of the chemotactic complement factor C5a [89]; induce tissue factor (TF) production by endothelial cells [169]; and increase coagulation factor FXIIa [166] and plasminogen activator inhibitor (PAI) I, reducing fibrinolysis [17]

like histones or using anticoagulants to control thrombin generation might be beneficial in managing DIC, according to a study in Frontiers.

21.7 Pathogen-Associated Molecular Patterns (PAMPs)

These are conserved molecular structures derived from pathogens (bacteria, viruses, fungi, etc.) that are recognized by the innate immune system. Examples include lipopolysaccharide (LPS), lipoteichoic acid (LTA), and various microbial DNA/RNA. PAMPs (Pathogen-Associated Molecular Patterns) play a crucial role in the development of Disseminated Intravascular Coagulation (DIC), a condition characterized by widespread clotting and bleeding. PAMPs, along with DAMPs (Damage-Associated Molecular Patterns), trigger tissue factor expression and the release of NETs (Neutrophil Extracellular Traps), leading to a cascade of events that can result in immunothrombosis and, ultimately, DIC.

21.7.1 PAMPs and DIC Pathogenesis (Fig. 21.1)

When the body encounters PAMPs from pathogens or DAMPs from damaged cells, it initiates an inflammatory response. This response involves the activation of cells like monocytes and neutrophils. Monocytes, upon detecting PAMPs, express tissue factor, a potent activator of coagulation. Neutrophils, another type of immune cell, can release NETs, which are complex networks of DNA, proteins, and antimicrobial peptides. NETs can activate coagulation, inactivate anticoagulant proteins, and provide a scaffold for platelet aggregation, further promoting clot formation. The inflammatory response, including the release of NETs, can also cause damage to the endothelium (the lining of blood vessels), further disrupting coagulation. These events can lead to a systemic activation of coagulation, resulting in widespread thrombus formation (DIC with a thrombotic phenotype) or, in some cases, hyperfibrinolysis leading to severe bleeding (DIC with a fibrinolytic phenotype).

21.8 Measuring PAMPs and DAMPs

Measuring Pathogen-Associated Molecular Patterns (PAMPs) and Damage-Associated Molecular Patterns (DAMPs) involves detecting these molecules and their effects on the immune system, often through assays that measure receptor activation or downstream signaling. These molecules are recognized by Pattern Recognition Receptors (PRRs), and their detection triggers a variety of physiological responses, including inflammation.

Here's a more detailed breakdown of how PAMPs and DAMPs are measured:

21.8.1 Identifying PAMPs and DAMPs

In Vitro Assays

(a) *Enzyme-Linked Immunosorbent Assay (ELISA):* This method can be used to measure the levels of specific PAMPs or DAMPs in biological samples, such as serum or tissue extracts.
(b) *Flow cytometry:* This technique allows for the analysis of cell populations and can be used to detect the expression of PRRs or the release of DAMPs from cells.
(c) *TLR reporter cell assays:* These assays use cells that express a specific PRR (like a Toll-like receptor) and a reporter gene that is activated when the PRR binds to its ligand (PAMP or DAMP). The reporter gene activity can be measured to assess the strength of the signaling pathway.

In Vivo Approaches

(a) *Measuring cytokine levels:* PAMPs and DAMPs can trigger the release of cytokines, which are signaling molecules involved in inflammation. Measuring cytokine levels in blood or tissue samples can provide insight into the immune response to PAMPs and DAMPs.
(b) *Observing cellular activation and recruitment:* PAMPs and DAMPs can also cause the activation and recruitment of immune cells to the site of infection or injury. Flow cytometry and microscopy can be used to track these changes.

21.8.2 Measuring Receptor Activation

Measuring downstream signaling: When PRRs recognize PAMPs or DAMPs, they trigger a cascade of signaling events that lead to changes in gene expression, cell activation, and the release of cytokines.

Assessing cell surface marker expression: Changes in cell surface marker expression can indicate the activation of PRRs or downstream signaling pathways.

Measuring phosphorylation status: Changes in the phosphorylation status of proteins involved in signaling pathways can also indicate PRR activation.

21.8.3 Challenges

Specificity: Some PRRs can recognize multiple PAMPs and DAMPs, making it challenging to determine the specific molecule that is triggering the response.

Context-dependence: The immune response to PAMPs and DAMPs can be influenced by the context of the immune environment, such as the presence of other signals or the type of cells involved.

In summary, measuring PAMPs and DAMPs involves a combination of techniques to detect these molecules, their effects on receptor activation, and downstream signaling pathways. These measurements provide valuable insights into the innate immune system's response to pathogens and tissue damage, which can help in understanding disease mechanisms and developing new therapeutic strategies.

21.9 Point of Care Devices

Another important advance in the diagnosis of DIC has been the use of point-of-care testing devices that allow for rapid assessment of coagulation parameters at the bedside. These devices, such as thromboelastography, rotational thromboelastometry, and clot waveform analysis, can provide valuable information on the dynamic changes in coagulation and fibrinolysis that occur in DIC, helping to guide management decisions in real time.

21.9.1 Thromboelastography (TEG)

Thromboelastography (TEG) can be a valuable tool for predicting disseminated intravascular coagulation (DIC) early on, especially in patients with septic shock. TEG assesses the entire coagulation process, offering a comprehensive view that traditional coagulation tests may miss. While TEG may initially show hypercoagulability (e.g., shorter R-time), it can later shift to hypocoagulability as DIC progresses, particularly in severe cases.

TEG can be used to assess the overall balance of coagulation, potentially identifying early changes related to DIC before they are fully evident in standard tests. Studies have shown that TEG parameters, such as the maximum amplitude (MA), can be different between patients who develop DIC and those who do not.

Longping et al. [18] carried out a retrospective, single-center study of 67 patients with heatstroke admitted to an intensive care unit (ICU) at a comprehensive hospital between July 2016 and August 2021. Conventional coagulation tests (CCTs) and TEG were performed within 2-h of admission to the ICU. Patients were diagnosed with DIC based on International Society of Thrombosis and Hemostasis criteria, and those with or without DIC were compared in terms of CCTs and TEG findings. The ability of individual parameters to predict DIC was assessed based on logistic regression and the area under receiver operating characteristic curves (AUC).

Of the 67 patients, 19 (28.4%) were diagnosed with DIC. Compared to patients without DIC, those with DIC had significantly longer reaction time [14.5(10.6–26.0) vs. 6.2(5.1–10.1) min] ($p < 0.001$) and kinetic time [10.9(5.9–25.0) vs. 2.7(2.2–4.7) min] ($p < 0.001$). Conversely, those with DIC had significantly lower alpha angle [22(9.1–43.3) vs. 55.0(44.8–61.7)°] ($p < 0.001$), maximum amplitude (MA) [(26.9(17.7–41.4) vs. 52.2(45.8–58.1) mm)] ($p < 0.001$) and coagulation index [−17.3(−39 to −7.9) vs. −2.4(−6.2 to −0.6)] ($p < 0.001$). MA at a cutoff value of 45.4 mm gave an AUC of 0.9 for predicting DIC, with a sensitivity of 77.1%, specificity of 89.5%, positive predictive value of 10.5%, and negative predictive value of 22.9%. Multifactorial logistic regression identified MA < 45.4 mm as an independent predictor of DIC (odds ratio 9, 95% confidence interval 1.2–69.2, $p = 0.035$). MA decreased significantly as DIC score increased and was significantly lower in the non-survivors on admission. The maximum amplitude (MA) value of TEG decreased significantly with the increase of DIC score. MA < 45.4 mm was first demonstrated to be an independent predictor of heatstroke-induced DIC.

Kim et al. conducted TEG prospectively in 1294 patients [19] with septic shock at the emergency department (ED) between January 2016 and December 2019. After exclusion of 405 patients with "do not attempt resuscitation" orders, those refusing enrollment, and those developing septic shock after ED presentation, 889 patients were included. DIC was defined as an International Society on Thrombosis and Hemostasis score ≥ 5 points within 24 h. Of the 889 patients with septic shock (mean age 65.6 ± 12.7 years, 58.6% male), 158 (17.8%) developed DIC. TEG values, except for lysis after 30 min, were significantly different between the DIC and non-DIC groups. Among the TEG values, the maximal amplitude (MA) had the highest discriminating power for DIC, with an area under the curve of 0.814. An MA < 60 indicated DIC with 79% sensitivity, 73% specificity, and 94% negative predictive value. Based on multivariable analysis, MA < 60 was an independent predictor of DIC (odds ratio 5.616 (95% confidence interval: 3.213–9.818)). In patients with septic shock, the MA value in TEG could be a valuable tool for early prediction of DIC. The authors concluded that early diagnosis of coagulopathy and initiation of treatment are crucial for patients with sepsis. Considering that TEG results are rapidly available at bedsides, MA < 60 could be a valuable tool for DIC prediction in patients with septic shock.

TEG can reveal changes in coagulation over time, allowing for monitoring of disease progression and potential interventions. TEG may help guide decisions about managing DIC, particularly in situations like septic shock, where early diagnosis and intervention are crucial.

While TEG is a valuable tool, it's important to consider that it reflects the overall coagulation process and may not be a perfect predictor of DIC in all situations. It should be used in conjunction with other diagnostic tests, such as the International Society on Thrombosis and Hemostasis (ISTH) score and D-dimer, for a more comprehensive assessment of DIC risk.

21.9.2 Clot Waveform Analysis and ROTEM

Clot waveform analysis (CWA) involves an analysis of the activated partial thromboplastin time (CWA-APTT), diluted prothrombin time (CWA-dPT), and a small amount of thrombin time (CWA-sTT), and clot fibrinolysis waveform analysis (CFWA). CWA exhibits an abnormal waveform, as well as peak times and heights in its derivative curves. Traditionally, clotting times, such as activated partial thromboplastin time (APTT),1 prothrombin time (PT),2 and thrombin time (TT),3 have been measured manually (Fig. 21.2). After the development of automatic optical coagulation analyzers, it became possible to visualize the clot reaction curves using different clotting time techniques [20].

The routinely measured APTT reflects the status of the "cascade system in plasma" but does not sufficiently reflect the "thrombin burst" or "enhancement of clotting activation by PLs. In contrast, the automatic optical end-point coagulation analyzers have the ability to show the clot reaction curve of the PT and APTT and to reflect the "thrombin burst" and "enhancement of clotting activation by PLs"; this is referred to as, a clot waveform analysis (CWA).

The MDA system (Organon Teknika, Cambridge, United Kingdom) (Fig. 21.2) was first able to visualize clot formation to detect biphasic waveforms in disseminated intravascular coagulation (DIC). The visual inspection of APTT clot reaction curves, and abnormal biphasic clot reaction curves have been reported to be associated with the early detection of DIC [21, 22]. The biphasic clot reaction curve was reported to be caused by a complex with C-reactive protein, very low-density lipoprotein, and calcium ion [23].

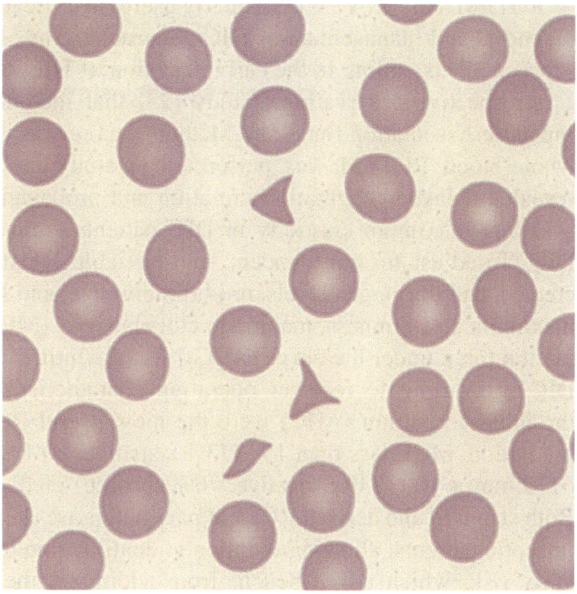

Fig. 21.2 Peripheral smear showing schistocytes

Additionally, the clot reaction curves with an abnormal biphasic pattern have been linked to morbidity and mortality in patients with DIC.

Automatic optical coagulation analyzers that contain software programs for CWA include the ACL TOP series, CN-Series analyzers, STACIA (PHC Corporation, Tokyo, Japan), and S-400CF (Sekisui Corporation, Tokyo, Japan). This software can display clot reaction curves as well as associated first- and second-derivative plots. These derivative plots were automatically calculated from the absorbance data and were reflected in the first and second derivative curves. The first and second derivative curves are called velocity and acceleration, respectively. The first derivative curve reflects coagulation ability, and the second derivative curve reflects FVIII activity or its interaction with phospholipids.

Waveform analysis, particularly clot waveform analysis (CWA), is increasingly used alongside ROTEM in the diagnosis and management of Disseminated Intravascular Coagulation (DIC). ROTEM provides a comprehensive assessment of coagulation and fibrinolysis, while CWA, obtained from conventional clotting tests like APTT, offers insights into the dynamics of clot formation and fibrinolysis [24].

Serial ROTEM and CWA can be used to monitor the progression of DIC and guide treatment strategies. ROTEM measures the mechanical properties of blood clots, providing a whole-blood perspective on coagulation and fibrinolysis. It assesses parameters like Clotting Time (CT), Maximum Clot Firmness (MCF), and Maximum Lysis (MLEX). CWA analyzes the optical waveform generated during conventional clotting tests (APTT, PT). It assesses parameters like Clot Formation Time (CFT) and Maximum Coagulation Velocity.

ROTEM and CWA are particularly useful in critically ill patients where prompt diagnosis and management of DIC are crucial. They can help identify and stage sepsis patients, aiding in the early detection of DIC. Scarlatescu et al. conducted a retrospective observational study [25] that included 97 septic patients. The Japanese Association for Acute Medicine score was used for DIC diagnosis and whole-blood ROTEM was performed at study inclusion. Univariate analysis revealed delayed coagulation initiation and propagation, and reduced clot firmness and maximum elasticity in DIC patients compared with patients without DIC. To adjust for confounders, multivariable logistic regression models were created, and fibrinogen levels, prothrombin time, and ROTEM parameters such as maximum clot firmness, maximum clot elasticity (MCE), and total thrombus formation [area under the curve (AUC)] were identified as significant predictors of DIC. According to receiver operating characteristic analysis, MCE and total thrombus formation (AUC) were the most useful ROTEM parameters for DIC prediction. MCE less than 158 (73% sensitive, 80% specific) and AUC less than 6175 mm × 100 (73% sensitive, 76% specific) predicted DIC in septic patients. Both standard and derived ROTEM parameters are useful for rapid DIC prediction in septic patients, allowing the timely identification of patients with higher mortality risk, which might benefit from additional therapies. Further studies are needed to assess the clinical relevance of these findings.

Muller et al. conducted a study [26] to detect the diagnostic ability of thromboelastometry to detect DIC. A predefined subgroup analysis of a clinical trial in critically ill patients with a coagulopathy was done. ROTEM and markers of coagulation and levels of natural anticoagulants were measured in patients with and without DIC. Twenty-three patients were included; 13 fulfilled criteria for overt DIC. Patients with DIC had lower platelet count, lower levels of fibrinogen, factors II, VII, and VIII compared with those without DIC. Antithrombin, protein C, and S were also reduced in DIC patients. Receiver operator characteristic analyses showed that EXTEM CFT, alpha angle, and MCF were capable of discriminating between patients with and without DIC. A combination of ROTEM values with protein C or antithrombin further improved discriminatory ability. In patients with DIC, thromboelastometry profiles were more hypocoagulable compared with those without DIC. ROTEM correlates well with ISTH DIC score; the diagnostic strength improves when ROTEM values are combined with antithrombin or protein C levels. Thereby, ROTEM may be a useful tool in diagnosing DIC in the critically ill.

ROTEM and aPTT-CWA were found to be valuable diagnostic tools in critically ill children who might require point-of-care tests. Min2 showed significant clinical implications for predicting bleeding events in this population [27].

In summary, waveform analysis, particularly CWA, complements ROTEM by providing a more detailed and dynamic view of clot formation and fibrinolysis. This enhanced information is invaluable in the diagnosis, staging, and management of DIC, especially in critical care settings.

21.10 Imaging Technology

Finally, advances in imaging technology have also played a role in the diagnosis of DIC, particularly in cases where there is suspicion of microvascular thrombosis. Techniques such as Doppler ultrasound and contrast-enhanced computed tomography can help to identify thrombotic occlusions in small vessels, providing valuable information on the extent of organ damage and guiding treatment decisions.

21.11 Clinical Case Scenario

Patient Profile**:** A 58-year-old male presented with a 3-day history of fever, confusion, and progressive shortness of breath.

Vital Signs: BP 85/50 mmHg, HR 120 bpm, Temp 38.9 °C. Physical Examination showed purpura on the lower limbs, bleeding from venipuncture sites.

21.11.1 Laboratory Findings

Test	Result	Normal range	Interpretation
Platelet count	38 × 10^9/L	150–400 × 10^9/L	↓ Thrombocytopenia
Prothrombin time (PT)	22 s	11–15 s	↑ Prolonged
aPTT	45 s	25–35 s	↑ Prolonged
Fibrinogen	0.8 g/L	2.0–4.0 g/L	↓ Hypofibrinogenemia
D-dimer	>20.0 µg/mL	<0.5 µg/mL	↑↑ Elevated fibrinolysis
Peripheral blood smear (Fig. 21.2)	Schistocytes present	–	Microangiopathic hemolysis

Blood Cultures: Positive for *Escherichia coli*

21.11.2 Diagnosis

The patient meets the ISTH DIC scoring system criteria with a score of 6, indicating overt DIC. JAAM criteria also support the diagnosis of DIC, consistent with early-stage coagulopathy.

21.11.3 Advanced Diagnostic Tools

- Thromboelastography (TEG): Prolonged R-time, decreased maximum amplitude (MA), indicating hypocoagulability
- Biomarkers: Elevated levels of thrombin–antithrombin complexes and soluble fibrin

21.11.4 Treatment Plan

- Underlying Cause Management: Initiation of broad-spectrum antibiotics targeting *E. coli*
- Supportive Care: Admission to ICU for organ support and hemostatic monitoring
- Blood Component Therapy: Administration of platelet concentrates and fresh frozen plasma (FFP) to address thrombocytopenia and coagulopathy
- Anticoagulation: Heparin therapy is considered due to the predominance of thrombosis; however, bleeding risk is assessed before initiation
- Monitoring: Serial TEG and ROTEM assessments to guide ongoing management. Over 72 h, the patient's DIC scores and coagulation parameters improved with the above interventions.

21.12 Conclusion

The evolving understanding of disseminated intravascular coagulation and the complexities of associated fibrinolytic dysfunction have led to marked improvements in diagnostic capabilities. Enhanced scoring systems, a growing panel of biomarkers, and sophisticated point-of-care tools such as TEG and ROTEM allow for more timely and accurate diagnosis. Furthermore, the identification of molecular contributors like NETs, DAMPs, and PAMPs has provided deeper insights into the immunothrombotic nature of DIC. As technological advancements continue to refine diagnostic methodologies, integrating these tools into clinical practice will be essential for optimizing patient outcomes in this challenging and high-risk condition.

21.13 Summary

Disseminated intravascular coagulation (DIC) is a critical, acquired condition marked by systemic activation of coagulation pathways and impaired fibrinolysis, often resulting in widespread microvascular thrombosis, bleeding, and organ dysfunction. It arises as a complication of conditions such as sepsis, trauma, malignancy, or obstetric emergencies. Due to its variable presentation, timely diagnosis is essential yet challenging.

Several diagnostic scoring systems have been established to improve recognition of DIC. The most widely adopted is the ISTH scoring system, while others—such as those developed by JMHW, JAAM, BCSH, and SISET—are tailored to specific clinical contexts and offer varying levels of sensitivity and specificity.

Beyond traditional tests, emerging biomarkers like thrombin–antithrombin complexes, prothrombin fragment 1 + 2, soluble fibrin, microparticle-associated tissue factor, and plasmin–α2-antiplasmin complex provide earlier and more accurate diagnostic information. Additionally, molecular triggers such as DAMPs, PAMPs, histones, and neutrophil extracellular traps (NETs) have advanced understanding of DIC pathogenesis.

Technologies like thromboelastography (TEG), rotational thromboelastometry (ROTEM), and clot waveform analysis (CWA) offer real-time coagulation monitoring at the bedside. These tools, along with imaging modalities such as Doppler ultrasound and CT angiography, enhance early detection and clinical decision-making.

Together, these advances support more precise, timely, and individualized approaches to DIC diagnosis and management.

References

1. Iba T, Levy JH, Maier CL, Helms J, Umemura Y, Moore H, Othman M, Thachil J, Connors JM, Levi M, Scarlatescu E. Updated definition and scoring of disseminated intravascular coagulation in 2025: communication from the ISTH SSC subcommittee on disseminated intravascular coagulation. J Thromb Haemost. 2025;23:2356.
2. Helms J, Severac F, Merdji H, Clere-Jehl R, François B, Mercier E, Quenot JP, Meziani F, CRICS TRIGGERSEP group (clinical research in intensive care and sepsis trial Group for Global Evaluation and Research in sepsis). Performances of disseminated intravascular coagulation scoring systems in septic shock patients. Ann Intensive Care. 2020;10(1):92. https://doi.org/10.1186/s13613-020-00704-5. PMID: 32651674; PMCID: PMC7352012
3. Iba T, Di Nisio M, Thachil J, Wada H, Asakura H, Sato K, et al. A proposal of the modification of Japanese society on thrombosis and hemostasis (JSTH) disseminated intravascular coagulation (DIC) diagnostic criteria for sepsis-associated DIC. Clin Appl Thromb Hemost. 2018;24:439–45. https://doi.org/10.1177/1076029617720069.
4. Levi M, Toh CH, Thachil J, Watson HG. Guidelines for the diagnosis and management of disseminated intravascular coagulation. British committee for standards in haematology. Br J Haematol. 2009;145(1):24–33. https://doi.org/10.1111/j.1365-2141.2009.07600.x.
5. Di Nisio M, Baudo F, Cosmi B, D'Angelo A, De Gasperi A, Malato A, Schiavoni M, Squizzato A, Italian Society for Thrombosis and Haemostasis. Diagnosis and treatment of disseminated intravascular coagulation: guidelines of the Italian Society for Haemostasis and Thrombosis (SISET). Thromb Res. 2012;129(5):e177–84. https://doi.org/10.1016/j.thromres.2011.08.028.
6. Levi M, Scully M. How I treat disseminated intravascular coagulation. Blood. 2018;131(8):845–54.
7. Wada H, Thachil J, Di Nisio M, et al. Guidance for diagnosis and treatment of DIC from harmonization of the recommendations from three guidelines. J Thromb Haemost. 2013;11(4):761–7.

8. Iba T, Nisio MD, Levy JH, Kitamura N, Thachil J. New criteria for sepsis-induced coagulopathy (SIC) following the revised sepsis definition: a retrospective analysis of a nationwide survey. BMJ Open. 2017;7(9):e017046.
9. van der Meijden PEJ, Heemskerk JWM. Platelet biology and functions: new concepts and clinical perspectives. Nat Rev Cardiol. 2019;16(3):166–79.
10. Okamoto K, Tamura T, Sawatsubashi Y. Sepsis and disseminated intravascular coagulation. J Intensive Care. 2016;4:23.
11. Park J, Kim D, Kim K, et al. Proteomic analysis of plasma for early diagnosis of DIC in sepsis. Clin Proteomics. 2021;18:12.
12. Iba T, Ito T, Maruyama I, et al. Potential diagnostic markers for disseminated intravascular coagulation of sepsis. Blood Rev. 2016;30(2):149–55.
13. Hjorleifsson E, Sigurdsson MI, Gudmundsdottir BR, Sigurdsson GH, Onundarson PT. Prediction of survival in patients suspected of disseminated intravascular coagulation. Acta Anaesthesiolog Scand. 2015;59(7):870–80.
14. Wakabayashi I, Mambo N, Ueda T, Nonaka D, Lee LJ, Tanaka K, et al. New biomarkers for prediction of disseminated intravascular coagulation in patients with sepsis. Clin Appl Thromb Hemost. 2018;24(9S):223S–9S. https://doi.org/10.1177/1076029618804078.
15. Popescu NI, Lupu C, Lupu F. Disseminated intravascular coagulation and its immune mechanisms. Blood. 2021;138(1):103–24.
16. Gando S, Levi M, Toh CH. Trauma-induced innate immune activation and disseminated intravascular coagulation. J Thromb Haemost. 2024;22:337–51. https://doi.org/10.1016/j.jtha.2023.09.028.
17. von Knethen A, Heinicke U, Laux V, Parnham MJ, Steinbicker AU, Zacharowski K. Antioxidants as therapeutic agents in acute respiratory distress syndrome (ARDS) treatment—from mice to men. Biomedicines. 2022;10:98.
18. He L, Lin Q, Zhong L, Zeng Q, Song J. Thromboelastography maximum amplitude as an early predictor of disseminated intravascular coagulation in patients with heatstroke. Int J Hyperth. 2022;39(1):605–10. https://doi.org/10.1080/02656736.2022.2066206.
19. Kim SM, Kim SI, Yu G, Kim JS, Hong SI, Chae B, Shin YS, Kim YJ, Jang S, Kim WY. Role of thromboelastography as an early predictor of disseminated intravascular coagulation in patients with septic shock. J Clin Med. 2020;9(12):3883. https://doi.org/10.3390/jcm9123883. PMID: 33260354; PMCID: PMC7760761
20. Wada H, Shiraki K, Ichikawa Y, Matsumoto T, Shimpo H, Shimaoka M. Clinical application of clot waveform analysis. Clin Appl Thromb Hemost. 2025;31:10760296251331606. https://doi.org/10.1177/10760296251331606. Epub 2025 Apr 1. PMID: 40170405; PMCID: PMC11963788
21. Toh CH, Giles AR. Waveform analysis of clotting test optical profiles in the diagnosis and management of disseminated intravascular coagulation (DIC). Clin Lab Haematol. 2002;24(6):321–7.
22. Matsumoto T, Wada H, Nishioka Y, Nishio M, Abe Y, Nishioka J, Kamikura Y, Sase T, Kaneko T, Houdijk WP, Nobori T. Frequency of abnormal biphasic aPTT clot waveforms in patients with underlying disorders associated with disseminated intravascular coagulation. Clin Appl Thromb Hemost. 2006;12(2):185–92.
23. Toh CH, Samis J, Downey C, Walker J, Becker L, Brufatto N, Tejidor L, Jones G, Houdijk W, Giles A, Koschinsky M. Biphasic transmittance waveform in the APTT coagulation assay is due to the formation of a ca++-dependent complex of C-reactive protein with very-low–density lipoprotein and is a novel marker of impending disseminated intravascular coagulation. Blood. 2002;100(7):2522–9.
24. Matsumoto T, Wada H, Nishioka Y, Nishio M, Abe Y, Nishioka J, Kamikura Y, Sase T, Kaneko T, Houdijk W, Nobori T, Shiku H. Frequency of abnormal biphasic aPTT clot waveforms in patients with underlying disorders associated with disseminated intravascular coagulation. Clin Appl Thromb Hemost. 2006;12:185–92. https://doi.org/10.1177/107602960601200206.

25. Ecaterinaa S, White NJ, Tomescu DR. Standard and derived rotational thromboelastometry parameters for prediction of disseminated intravascular coagulation in septic patients. Blood Coagul Fibrinolysis. 2020;31(5):317–23. https://doi.org/10.1097/MBC.0000000000000919.
26. Müller MCA, Meijers JC, van Meenen DM, Thachil J, Juffermans NP. Thromboelastometry in critically ill patients with disseminated intravascular coagulation. Blood Coagul Fibrinolysis. 2019;30(5):181–7. https://doi.org/10.1097/MBC.0000000000000808.
27. Chanthong S, Choed-Amphai C, Manowong S, Tuntivate P, Tansriratanawong S, Makonkawkeyoon K, Natesirinilkul R. Rotational thromboelastometry and clot waveform analysis as point-of-care tests for diagnosis of disseminated intravascular coagulation in critically ill children in Thailand. Pediatr Crit Care Med. 2024;25(5):e221–31. https://doi.org/10.1097/PCC.0000000000003452. Epub 2024 Feb 1

Chapter 22
Thrombophilia: Their Relevance in Arterial and Venous Thrombosis

Ankur Ahuja, Gurpreet Kaur, and Dinesh Chandra

Abstract Thrombophilia refers to a group of inherited or acquired disorders that predispose individuals to excessive blood clot formation, either in the veins (venous thrombosis) or arteries (arterial thrombosis). This chapter explores the relevance of thrombophilia in the pathogenesis, diagnosis, and management of both arterial and venous thrombotic events. The key genetic mutations, such as Factor V Leiden, Prothrombin gene mutation, and deficiencies in natural anticoagulants like Protein C, Protein S, and Antithrombin, are discussed in the context of their role in increasing thrombogenicity. The chapter also discusses antiphospholipid syndrome. The relationship between thrombophilia and thrombotic events such as deep vein thrombosis, pulmonary embolism, and arterial events like myocardial infarction and stroke is examined, with a focus on how these conditions influence treatment strategies, including anticoagulation therapy and lifestyle modifications. Overall, this chapter provides a comprehensive overview of thrombophilia, emphasising its importance in both venous and arterial thrombotic disorders and the need for personalised approaches in their management.

Keywords Antiphospholipid syndrome · Arterial thrombosis · Venous thrombosis · Prevalence of thrombosis in an Indian population · Oral contraceptives and thrombosis

---

A. Ahuja (✉) · G. Kaur
Department of Pathology, Armed Forces Medical College, Pune, Maharashtra, India

D. Chandra
Department of Hematology, Sanjay Gandhi Post Graduate Institute of Medical Sciences, Lucknow, Uttar Pradesh, India

H. P. Pati et al. (eds.), *Clinical Hematology and Hemato-Oncology*,
https://doi.org/10.1007/978-981-92-1167-8_22

Learning Objectives

- *Understanding of the definition and types of thrombophilia:*
  - Define *thrombophilia* and differentiate between *inherited* and *acquired* thrombophilic disorders.
    Key genetic mutations associated with inherited thrombophilias (e.g., *Factor V Leiden, Prothrombin G20210A, Protein C* and *S deficiencies, Antithrombin deficiency*).
- *Pathophysiology of thrombosis.*
- *Discussion of the role of thrombophilia in arterial thrombosis.*
- *Evaluation of the clinical relevance of thrombophilia testing.*
  - Discuss indications for *thrombophilia testing* in patients with venous or arterial thrombosis.
    Assess the limitations and potential risks of routine thrombophilia testing, especially in unprovoked thrombosis or recurrent VTE cases.
- *Correlate thrombophilia with risk stratification in venous and arterial thrombosis.*

  Explain the *provoked vs unprovoked thrombosis* concept and its impact on the duration of anticoagulation therapy.
- *Discussion in brief regarding the treatment strategies in patients with thrombophilia and thrombosis.*
  - Reviewing the management of *venous thrombosis* in patients with thrombophilia.
    Explore the role of *direct oral anticoagulants (DOACs), vitamin K antagonists (VKAs),* and other therapeutic agents in patients with thrombophilia.

22.1 Introduction

Thrombophilia, as the name suggests, is characterised by the tendency to develop thrombosis or predisposition to develop thromboembolism because of inherited or acquired factors. At times, there are no identifiable events/risk factors (unprovoked), sometimes there are identifiable risk factors (Provoked) which are caused by an established known factor. These factors may be transient, whereas the risk factors are reversible, which are further subcategorised into major risk factors favouring limited duration of anticoagulation. These major risk factors may be the major surgery of more than 30 min duration or hospitalisation confined to the bed for ≥3 days due to acute illness, oestrogen therapy, pregnancy and puerperium. The other subcategory in the transient risk factors includes minor risk factors, wherein anticoagulation is continued. These minor risk factors include minor surgery of less than

30 min duration, hospitalisation of less than 3 days, and reduced mobilisation of ≥3 days at home due to an acute illness. The other category of risk factors is persistent risk factors wherein the risk factors persist for a prolonged duration or persist forever, like active malignancy, autoimmune diseases, nephrotic syndrome, continued hormonal therapy and obesity.

The aetiology and the risk factors vary from inherited to acquired and have been tabulated in Table 22.1. Most of them have been validated to have moderate to high risk for thrombophilia. Methylenetetrahydrofolate reductase (MTHFR) polymorphism, previously hypothesised to link with thrombophilia, has been downgraded to be the cause of thrombophilia by numerous meta-analyses.

In various studies, the relative prevalences and risk factors have been incorporated in detail (Table 22.2).

Table 22.1 Aetiology/risk factors of thrombophilia (hereditary and acquired) [1]

Hereditary thrombophilia	Acquired/Risk factors (overall risk (OR))
Factor V Leiden	*Strong risk factors with an overall risk of >10* Fracture of lower limb/Major trauma/Spinal cord injury Hip or knee replacement/Major vascular/neuro/onco/pelvi surgeries Hospitalisation for Myocardial infarction/heart failure/atrial fibrillation/flutter (within the previous 3 months) Previous VTE Haemato-onco Myeloproliferative neoplasms—Essential thrombocythemia; Polycythemia vera
Protein C deficiency[a]	*Moderate risk factors with an overall risk of 2–9* In vitro fertilisation (IVF) Postpartum, especially within 6 weeks Arthroscopic knee surgery Congestive heart failure (CHF) Respiratory failure Infection (pneumonia, urinary tract infection (UTI), HIV) Autoimmune disease/Inflammatory bowel disease Paralytic stroke Superficial vein thrombosis Malignancy Drugs: hormone replacement therapy (HRT); oral contraceptives (OCs); heparin; COVID-19 vaccines; tranexamic acid; certain cancer therapies (e.g., tamoxifen, thalidomide, lenalidomide, bevacizumab, asparaginase); erythropoiesis-stimulating agents (ESA) Central venous catheter Blood transfusion
Protein S deficiency[b]	*Weak risk factors with an overall risk of <2* Old age (>65 yrs) Obesity Pregnancy Laparoscope surgery Immobilisation/rest >3 days Diabetes mellitus Hypertension Varicose veins

(continued)

Table 22.1 (continued)

Hereditary thrombophilia	Acquired/Risk factors (overall risk (OR)
Antithrombin deficiency[c]	
Prothrombin G20210A	*Other risk factors* Benign haematology disorders; (HIIT) heparin-induced thrombocytopenia; (VITT) vaccine-induced immune thrombotic thrombocytopenia; hyperviscosity syndrome (hypergammaglobulinemia, hyperfibrinogenaemia, hyperleukocytosis, sickle cell disease)
Heparin cofactor II deficiency	
Dysfibrinogenemia	

[a]*Acquired Protein C deficiency*: Neonates; liver disease; DIC; vitamin K deficiency; chemotherapy (cyclophosphamide, methotrexate, and 5-fluorouracil); inflammatory conditions; patients on warfarin or L-asparaginase
[b]*Acquired protein S deficiency*: Neonates; pregnancy; liver disease; DIC; vitamin K deficiency; patients on warfarin, L-asparaginase, oestrogens
[c]*Acquired AT deficiency*: Neonates; pregnancy; liver disease; nephrotic syndrome; DIC; major surgery; acute thrombosis; patient on L-asparaginase, heparin, oestrogens

Table 22.2 Prevalences in the overall and Indian population [2]

Hereditary thrombophilia	General prevalence	Relative risk of the first episode of VTE	Relative risk of recurrent episode of VTE
Factor V Leiden	2–5% *0.6–1.5% in Indians*	10–20% *2–6% in Indians*	15–25% *4–12% in Indians*
Prothrombin G20210A	1–3% *0–1% in Indians*	0% to <1%	6–8%
Protein C deficiency	0.2–0.5% *<0.2–0.4% in Indians*	3–5% *1–3% in Indians*	4–6% *3–5% in Indians*
Protein S deficiency	0.03–0.13% *0.1–0.3% in Indians*	2–6% *1–4% in Indians*	4–7% *3–5% in Indians*
AT deficiency	0.02–0.2% *0.05–0.2% in Indians*	1–3% *1–2% in Indians*	4–8% *2–4% in Indians*

22.2 Pathophysiology [3]

The pathophysiology of thrombosis has been explicated by Virchow's triad, which embraces venous stasis, hypercoagulability, and endothelial injury in the blood vessels. However, with years, the advancements in molecular techniques, including whole-genome sequencing, have widened the pathophysiology of thrombotic.

(a) *Venous Stasis*

The salient reasons for venous stasis include factors leading to immobilisation, atrial fibrillation, akinetic/infarcted/necrotic myocardium, and external obstruction in the blood outflow. The stasis leads to a lower shear rate of blood below the physiological level and causes the interaction of leukocytes, platelets and erythrocytes, especially with endothelial cells, which is mediated by intercellular adhesion molecule-4 (ICAM-4). This further leads to slowing of blood flow and increased haematocrit, thus leading to the risk of endothelial injury.

(b) *Hypoxia*

The mechanism of hypoxia leading to thrombus formation is through activation of Protein Kinase alpha and beta protein in the cytosol, which leads to activation of the RAS/RAF-1/ERK1/ERK2 pathway, which further leads to extracellular growth response-1 induction. The latter leads to increased transcription of the tissue factor, which is responsible for the thrombus formation.

Besides hypoxia, it also leads to the stabilisation of hypoxia inducible factor-1, which further upregulates plasminogen activation inhibitor 1, which suppresses fibrinolysis and thus promotes thrombosis.

(c) *Genetic Components*

The role of Protein C, Protein S and antithrombin in balancing the coagulation cascade is a well-known fact where these anticoagulants play an important role. Thrombin-thrombomodulin complex interacts with the endothelial cells and activates Protein C with the Protein S as a cofactor. The activated protein C leads to the inactivation of the factor Va and VIIIa, thus inhibiting prothrombin formation. This pathway is an important checkpoint for the inhibition of thrombus. However, any causes inherited or acquired leading to their deficiencies will lead to a predisposition to thrombosis.

Similarly, the FV Leiden mutation leads to resistance to become inactivated by Protein C and hence leads to thrombosis.

Antithrombin inhibits thrombin along with FIXa and FXa, similarly, because of inherited or acquired causes, which can lead to thrombosis.

G20210 A mutation leading to hyperprothrombinemia is also a leading cause of thrombosis, especially in Western countries.

Recently studied gene is STAB2, whose corresponding protein, Stabilin-2, acts as a receptor on the endothelial surface when mutated, it leads to impaired intracellular transport, which results in the elevation of the von Willebrand factor, thus leading to thrombosis.

(d) *Interplay Between Platelets, Coagulation Factors and the Endothelium*

The factors which are prone to cause thrombosis, like inflammation, direct or indirect injuries leading to exposure of the endothelial cell lining, can lead to the release of endothelin, a potent vasoconstrictor; increased von Willebrand factor release, forming a plug with the platelets; expression of P-selectin and collagen, which also forms a platform for the platelets; and recruitment of neutrophils. Besides platelets, when activated, they release protein disulphide isomerase, which further alters the tissue factor, thus proning to thrombosis.

Inflammation, as discussed, carries a high risk for thrombosis and has also been evident by COVID-19 infection. The cytokines and the factors that lead to thrombosis are

(i) Interleukins—IL1β. IL6, IL18, IL9 and IL17A. These interleukins can cause thrombosis due to varied reasons, from increased platelet aggregation rate, the expression of P-selectin, to increased FVIII.

(ii) Activated neutrophils-

(a) Release of neutrophil extracellular traps (NETs):

(i) Histones in NETs have cytotoxic effects on the endothelium, including vacuolation of the endothelium.
(ii) NETs entrapped platelets release Poly P, which activates the intrinsic pathway.

(b) Leukocyte elastase cleaves tissue factor pathway inhibitor, thus keeping tissue factor in an activated mode.

(e) *Cancer-Associated Thrombosis*—Many factors lead to thrombosis in patients with cancer. Some salient ones have been summarised as below

(i) Patient-related risk factors: immobilisation, old age.
(ii) Treatment-related risk factors.

(a) Catheter vein associated.
(b) Anthracyclines: endothelial injury.
(c) Immunomodulators: platelet activation, increased FVIII.
(d) Tamoxifen: increased calcium, FVIII, and reduction of inhibition of coagulation.
(e) Platinum agents: release of extracellular vesicles, exposure of CD 62P, Activation of FXa.
(f) L-Asparaginase: reduction of the inhibition of coagulation.
(g) Second-generation tyrosine kinase inhibitors (Ponatinib): increased expression of Von Willebrand factor, platelet adhesion, microvascular angiopathy.

(iii) Cancer-related risk factor.

(a) Mucins interact with the binding sites for selectins (P-selectins and L-selectins), leading to platelet aggregation & thrombin generation.
(b) Cancer procoagulant (CP), which is a cysteine proteinase, is present in malignant tissues and directly activate F X to Xa.
(c) Tissue factor (TF) is expressed highly in many cancers. These TF are shed from the tumour cells in the form of the extracellular vesicles and get assembled on a negatively charged phospholipid surface. This, as we know, leads to the initiation of thrombin formation.

22.3 Lab Investigations [4–6]

Testing is advised in thrombophilia whenever there is a likelihood of alteration of management in it or in the family members (Table 22.3) or in certain unusual situations, as mentioned in Tables 22.4 and 22.5.

There is an algorithm approach for the deep vein thrombosis (DVT) or pulmonary embolism (PE), Table 22.3.

Table 22.3 Recommended tests

Conditions	Provoked first-time episode of DVT/PE	Unprovoked time DVT/ PTE[a]	Provoked recurrent DVT/PE
Tests indicated	No testing is required	10% risk of recurrence in the first year and 50% in 10 yrs	1. FV Leiden mutation 2. Prothrombin mutation (May be omitted in Indian settings) 3. Antiphospholipid antibodies

[a]Unprovoked first PTE/DVT diagnosis not required, as management of indefinite anticoagulation will not get altered [4]

Table 22.4 Indications for workup

Thrombosis at a young age
Weakly provoked/unprovoked event
Positive family history (first-degree relative having the event at a young age)
Recurrent events
Unusual sites (cerebral veins/splanchnic veins)
Recurrent pregnancy loss

Besides prevention of the risk factors aforementioned, thrombophilia is being managed by anticoagulation therapy which is being administered immediately following its diagnosis (Initial anticoagulation), followed by its administration for the finite period of time frequently for 3 months period or extended anticoagulation wherein the anticoagulation therapy is being administered beyond the 3 months but with a scheduled stop date which is around 6–12 months or may be for the indefinite period which is defined as administration of the anticoagulation beyond typical of 3 months but without any scheduled stoppage date.

Management of thrombosis is based upon the existing co-morbidities and certain conditions, as tabulated below. Anticoagulation therapy is continued for at least 3 months. The choice depends upon the conditions/co-morbidities as tabulated in Table 22.6 [6].

The diagnostic aspects and the monitoring of thrombosis are known to have interference with the known anticoagulants and episodes, and they need to be kept in mind. These have been summarised in Table 22.7. The initiation of the management of thrombosis becomes essential as fast as possible to prevent mortality and morbidity. However, the decision to investigate is hampered by the acute episodes and anticoagulants. It is therefore very important to have an understanding of this aspect. There are a few advanced labs that can perform testing by using a reagent to inactivate or remove the anticoagulant (heparinase for heparin, activated charcoal for DOACs). Some functional assays for protein C, protein S, and AT deficiency are not subject to interference by DOACs.

Though in the acute episodes of thrombosis or in an emergency, anticoagulants have been started, then some tests like Protein C, etc., are not advisable to be done as the chances of reductions in the levels are there, if performed and the plasma levels are still in the normal range, then it rules out their deficiency.

Table 22.5 Elaborated specific recommendations

Patient	Recommendation (Conditional)	Explanation
Symptomatic VTE/VTE provoked by the surgical process	Thrombophilia work-up not required	Indefinite anticoagulation is required, so no change in management Risk of recurrent bleeding if anticoagulation is stopped for the test
VTE provoked by a major non-surgical but transient risk Factors/pregnancy/ post-partum/OCs	Thrombophilia work-up required	Test for thrombophilia, if positive, then indefinite anticoagulant treatment is required
VTE in unusual sites (CVT, Splanchnic veins)	1. Thrombophilia work-up required 2. Thrombophilia workup not required	1. When anticoagulation is discontinued, a thrombophilia workup is required, and if it comes positive, then lifelong anticoagulation is done 2. When lifetime anticoagulation is required
Asymptomatic person/ patients with VTE with mild transient risk factor with Positive family history of VTE & thrombophilia in first-degree relatives	1. *Heterozygous FVL or heterozygous Prothrombin gene mutation (PGM)*—Thrombophilia workup not required 2. *Protein C, S, or antithrombin deficiency*—Thrombophilia workup required, which is known in the family, and if present, thromboprophylaxis is given	1. Firstly, there are only heritable causes, and we need not rule out acquired factors Secondly, they have low penetrance in the family 2. Firstly, there are acquired Protein C & S deficiency conditions that need to be ruled out Secondly, they have high penetrance in the family
Women from the general population considering to start HRT/OCs	Do not test for thrombophilia	
Women with a family history of VTE but unknown thrombophilia in the family, considering to start HRT/ OCs	Do not test for thrombophilia	
Women with a family history of VTE and thrombophilia considering to start HRT/ OCs	*1. Heterozygous FVL or heterozygous Prothrombin gene mutation (PGM)*—Thrombophilia workup not required 2. *Protein C, S, or antithrombin deficiency*—Thrombophilia workup required & avoid giving HRT/OCs in women with thrombophilia	

Table 22.6 Conditions influencing anticoagulant selection [6]

Conditions/Co-morbidities	Preferable anticoagulant	Remarks
Liver disease and coagulopathy	LMWH	DOACs are contraindicated in patients with raised INR VKA are difficult to control
Cancer	LMWH, factor Xa inhibitors	Indicated in neoplasia, especially when newly diagnosed, having extensive VTE, metastatic deposits, or when on chemotherapy
Renal disease and creatinine clearance	VKA	LMWH & DOACs are contraindicated in renal impairment
Dyspepsia or history of GI bleeding	VKA, Apixaban	Other DOACs are associated with dyspepsia/ GI bleeding
Coronary artery disease 9CAD)	VKA, Rivaroxaban, Apixaban, Edoxaban	Dabigatran is not safe in CAD
Poor compliance	VKA	VKA can be monitored with INR, and hence, poor compliance can be ruled out
Pregnancy	LMWH	Other anticoagulants are unsafe in pregnancy
High risk of bleeding, but not having massive deep vein thrombosis	Inferior vena cava (IVC) filter	
High risk of bleeding, but having massive deep vein thrombosis	Surgical thrombectomy followed by an IVC filter	

DOACs direct oral anticoagulants, *INR* international normalised ratio, *GI* gastrointestinal, *LMWH* low molecular weight heparin, *VTE* venous thromboembolism, *VKA* vitamin K-dependent antagonist (i.e., warfarin), *UFH* unfractionated heparin

Table 22.7 Interfering factors with commonly available tests

Thrombophilic state	Acute episode of thrombosis	Warfarin	Heparin	DOACs
Protein C deficiency	Yes	No	Yes	Yes, with some functional assays
Protein S deficiency	No	No	Yes	Yes, with some functional assays
Antithrombin deficiency	No	Yes	No	Yes, with some functional assays
Molecular tests (Factor V Leiden; Prothrombin G20210A)	Yes	Yes	Yes	Yes
Antiphospholipid antibodies (anti-Beta GPI, anti-cardiolipin)	Yes	Yes	Yes	Yes
Lupus anticoagulant	Yes	No	No	No

22.4 Clinical Case 1

A 24-year-old female, a medical graduate, requested a review before starting an oral contraceptive (OCs) because of her strong history of thrombophilia in her family, as her mother died of pulmonary thromboembolism after a brief history of fever and her brother suffered from deep vein thrombosis at his younger age while participating in one of the Marathon. Though she never had any relevant history of thrombosis, she, with a knowledge of thrombophilia, wanted to exclude any hereditary thrombophilia. She negated any history of smoking, medicines, or any chronic illnesses. Her Protein C levels were found to be reduced with Activated protein C resistance (APCR) and Factor V Leiden (FVL) mutation.

22.4.1 Analysis and Learning Points from Case 1

How is family history important in the case of thrombosis?
How are OCs connected to thrombosis development?
What investigations are required to be done, especially in this case?

Thrombosis is a deadly disease if not managed in time. It can arise due to provoked and unprovoked causes. It can be a cause of concern, especially when there is a strong family history like in this case we dealt with. The medical graduate was correct in her approach to have a detailed evaluation of the thrombophilia workup before starting OCs in the background of a strong family history. It's very important to know the hereditary and acquired causes, provoked factors, causing thrombosis.

In this case, we had a strong family history, which suggested the existence of inherited thrombophilia due to a genetic mutation. On many a times, we may not get a direct family history; hence, in those cases, it is very important to ask the indirect history from the patients as below:

A. *Thrombosis in Family Members*

- History of venous thromboembolism (VTE), including DVT, PE, or unusual clots (cerebral vein thrombosis, splanchnic vein thrombosis) in any *first-degree relatives* (parents, siblings, children) or *second-degree relatives* (grandparents, aunts, uncles, cousins).

B. *Age at Onset of Thrombosis*

- Thrombosis at a *young age* (typically <50 years) in family members.
- Recurrence of thrombotic events at a young age in multiple family members.

C. *Thrombotic Events in Unusual Sites*

- Unusual sites involvement such as cerebral veins, portal veins, or renal veins.

D. *Known Inherited Thrombophilia*

- If family members have been diagnosed with specific *genetic thrombophilias* (e.g., *Factor V Leiden mutation, Prothrombin 20210A mutation, Protein C/S deficiency, antithrombin deficiency*).

E. *Cardiovascular Disease and Stroke History*

- A family history of *early cardiovascular disease*, myocardial infarctions, or stroke can also be relevant, as some prothrombotic disorders may contribute to arterial thrombosis.

F. *Pregnancy-Related Thrombosis in Female Relatives*

- *Pregnancy-related complications* like *recurrent miscarriages*, *preeclampsia*, or *thrombosis* during pregnancy or postpartum are often linked to conditions like *antiphospholipid syndrome* or *inherited thrombophilia.*

It is not recommended to go for the regular screening of inherited thrombophilia preceding the commencement of OCs; however, testing can be pursued in patients with a known family history of thrombophilia. Those patients can be counselled for the commencement of the low-risk OCs.

This medical graduate had concerns because she was starting the OCs. She has the right concern because of support by the statistics, particularly the association with the venous thromboembolism (VTE), which includes *deep vein thrombosis (DVT)* and *pulmonary embolism (PE).*

Risk of Thrombosis with Oral Contraceptives: Statistics

- In *healthy women*, the risk of VTE is about *1–5 per 10,000 women per year.*
- With the *OC use*, the risk increases to *3–9 per 10,000 women per year.*
- The risk is higher with *inherited thrombophilias* or *other risk factors.*
- The risk is highest in the initial first 6–12 months of OC initiation.
- The risk of the FV Leiden mutation correlating with OCs is tabulated in Table 22.8.

Mechanism of Thrombosis Development with Oral Contraceptives

- Increased Coagulation Factor Production:
  - Oestrogen in OCs leads to an *increase in clotting coagulation factors* (Fibrinogen, Factors II (Prothrombin), VII, VIII, and X.
- Decrease in anticoagulant proteins.
- Reduced Fibrinolysis.

Table 22.8 Association of OCs with the FV Leiden mutation

OCs	FV Leiden heterozygous mutation	Risk compared to no OCs and no heterozygous FV Leiden mutations
Yes	No	Four-fold increase
No	Yes	Seven-fold increase
Yes	Yes	35-fold increase

- Venous Stasis:
  - OCs may promote *venous stasis* in certain situations, such as prolonged immobilisation.

Risk of Thrombosis with Different Types of Oral Contraceptives

Combined Oral Contraceptives (COCs)

- *COCs* contain both *estrogen* and *progestin*. The risk of thrombosis is mainly accredited to the *estrogen* component, mainly *ethinyl estradiol*.
- The risk of VTE increases with the *dose of estrogen*. Older COCs with higher estrogen doses (*50 mcg or more*) had a significantly higher risk of thrombosis. Modern COCs typically contain lower estrogen doses (*20–35 mcg*) and have a lower but still present risk.
- *Progestins* (synthetic progesterone) can also affect clotting risk. *Third- and fourth-generation progestins* (such as desogestrel, gestodene, and drospirenone) have been associated with a slightly *higher risk* of thrombosis compared to earlier generations (levonorgestrel and norethindrone).

Progestin-only Pills (POPs)

- *Progestin-only contraceptives* (also called "mini-pills") generally have *minimal or no increased risk* of thrombosis compared to combined pills, as they do not contain oestrogen. They are considered safer for women at higher risk of clotting.
- Second-generation OCs, having low-dose oestrogen and progestins, e.g., levonorgestrel, are very safe in comparison to other OCs.

22.5 Clinical Case 2

A 26-year-old woman was referred for the workup of recurrent early trimester abortions. The obstetric workup negated any anatomical or physiological issues. There was no relevant past or family history. The woman was a non-smoker and had never taken any alcohol. She had been taking oral contraceptives in her first 2 years of marriage with no thrombotic episodes during the period. Her screening coagulogram showed borderline increase in activated partial thromboplastin time (APTT) (APTT test being 39 s against the control of 32 s). A mixing study was performed, which revealed no correction. Her antiphospholipid lupus anticoagulant (APLA) workup was initiated, which revealed dilute Russel viper venom (dRVVT) positive, which persisted to be positive after 12 weeks. Besides her antiβ2 GPI and anticardiolipin, she also came out to be positive at the time of presentation and on repetition after 12 weeks.

22.5.1 Analysis and Learning Points from Case 3

What are the updated diagnostic criteria of APLA, and why is there a need to update them?s
What does triple positivity mean, and what is its relevance?
What are the recent understandings of pathophysiology in APLA?
How are these cases to be managed?

Till lately, the APS was being diagnosed based on the Sapporo criteria, which were published in 1991 and were revised in 2006. There has been some development in pathophysiology and clinical features, which include some non-thrombotic ones and involvement of some more systemic diseases and risk stratification. Besides, the Sapporo criteria didn't incorporate the evidence-based definitions, which resulted in confusion and heterogeneity; hence, there was a need for a classification that incorporates the lacunae in the previous classification.

Recently, in 2023, the American College of Rheumatology (ACR) and EULAR [2] have proposed a classification system for the APS (Tables 22.9 and 22.10). In this classification many parameters have been added, making the diagnosis of APS more specific overall and improved sensitivity in some patients, such as those

Table 22.9 2023 ACR/EULAR antiphospholipid syndrome (APS) classification clinical criteria

Domian 1—Macrovascular (Venous thromboembolism)
Unexplained. Confirmed by appropriate test.
Macrovascular (Arterial thrombosis)
Unexplained. Confirmed by appropriate test.
Microvascular
Suspected aetiology Livedo racemosa (Physical examn)—Non uniform, irreversible, broken and assymetric persistent discolouration are the ones only which are scored. Antiphospholipid antibody nephropathy[a] (Physical examn or lab test). *Established aetiology* Livedoid vasculopathy confirmed by pathology. Histopathology(HPE) confirmed microthrombosis/ endothelial cell proliferation. Histopathology confirmed aPl nephropathy. Cytopathology/ HPE confirmed pulmonary haemorrhage. Imaging/ HPE confirmed otherwise unexplained myocardial disease. Imaging/ HPE confirmed otherwise unexplained Adrenal hemorrhage or microthrombosis.
Domain 4—Obsetrics
Prefoetal death[b] Foetal death[c] Pre-eclampsia with severe featurers[d] Placental insufficiency with severe features[e]
Domain 5—Cardiac
Unexplained valve thickening[f] Unexplained valve vegetaion.
Domain 6—Haematology
Unexplained thrombocytopenia.

(continued)

Table 22.9 (continued)

Adapted from Reference [8]

(a) Antiphospholipid antibody (aPl) nephropathy
  (i) Hypertension: New onset/deterioration of previous hypertension;
  (ii) Protein ≥0.5 gm in 24-h urine specimen or protein: creatinine ratio ≥0.5 mg/mg (50 mg/mmoles)
  (iii) Increased serum creatinine levels above normal)
  (iv) Glomerular microscopic haematuria. Pulmonary haemorrhage; unexplained respiratory symptoms
(b) Pre-foetal death (pre-embryonic or embryonic loss)—Pregnancy loss before 10 weeks
(c) Foetal death—Pregnancy loss between 10 weeks and 34 weeks
(d) Pre-eclampsia
  (a) Systolic BP ≥140 mm Hg or diastolic blood pressure ≥90 mm Hg on 2 occasions at least 4 h apart after 20 weeks of gestation with new onset of one or more of the following: (i) proteinuria ≥0.3 mg/mg (30 mg/mmoles) (ii) dipstick protein ≥2+
  (b) Severe features are defined as
    (i) Severe blood pressure elevation: Systolic blood pressure ≥160 mm Hg or diastolic blood pressure ≥110 mm Hg on 2 occasions at least 4 h apart while the patient is on bed rest
    (ii) Central nervous system dysfunction
    (iii) Visual disturbances
    (iv) Pulmonary oedema
    (v) Impaired liver function
    (vi) Renal dysfunction: Serum creatinine concentration >1.1 mg/dL or a doubling of the serum creatinine concentration in the absence of other renal disease.
    (vii) Thrombocytopenia: platelet count of <1 lac/microL
(e) Placental insufficiency with severe features:
  (a) Intrauterine foetal growth restriction: Unexplained foetal weight of <10th percentile for gestational age or postnatal birth weight <10th percentile for gestational age
  (b) Severe features
    (i) Abnormal foetal surveillance tests suggestive of foetal hypoxemia
    (ii) Abnormal Doppler flow velocimetry waveform analysis suggestive of foetal hypoxemia
    (iii) Severe intrauterine foetal growth restriction-- foetal or postnatal birth weight of <3rd percentile for the gestational age
    (iv) Oligohydramnios: Amniotic fluid index of ≤5 cm, or deepest vertical pocket of <2 cm
  (c) Poorly perfused maternal vasculature, though not specific for APS
(f) Valve thickening: Mitral valve of >4 mm between ages 20 and 39 years, and >5 mm for those older than age 40 years, and >3 mm for other valves for any age

Table 22.10 2023 ACR/EULAR antiphospholipid syndrome (APS) classification laboratory criteria

Domain 7—aPL test by the coagulation based functional assay
Lupus anticoagulant (lAC) assay 3- step (screening—mixing study—confirmation) with 2 screening test systems[a] Positive if at least 1 test systems yields a positive result following all 3 steps.
Domain 8—aPl test by solid phase based assay
Anticardiolipin antibody (aCl) and anti–β2- glycoprotein I antibody (anti-β2 GPI). Cut-off—moderate (40–79 units) and high (>80 units). Only ELISA methodology.

Adapted from Reference [8]

[a]Diluted Russell's viper venom time (dRVVT) and Lupus sensitive activated partial thromboplastin time (APTT) [low phospholipids and silica as activator]

having thrombocytopenia, microvascular manifestations, SLE and cardiac valvular disease, in comparison to the 2006 criteria [7].

The pathophysiology of APLA-induced thrombosis is primarily because of the presence of anti-beta2GPI, as shown in Fig. 22.1.

While the role of tissue factor is well defined in the activation of the extrinsic pathway of the coagulation, the NETs, which are comprised of chromatin (histones) from the neutrophils and microbicidal proteins. NETs have a role in the activation of the complement pathway (thus reducing complement C3 & C4), platelets and endothelial cells, thus inducing thrombosis in both arterial and venous vessels. It has been seen that both NETs and anti-NET antibodies are raised in patients with antiphospholipid syndrome (APS). Patients in whom IgG against NETs is present are prone to have increased complications like lupus nephritis because of poor degradation of NETs. While IgM NET antibodies target the DNA component of the NETs, IgG targets the histones [9].

The management of APLA is to give warfarin followed by low molecular weight heparin [LMWH], which is preferred over the direct oral anticoagulant (DOAC). Heparins are mostly reserved for certain situations, such as in pregnancy (LMWH) or during an initial treatment of acute venous thromboembolism.

In patients of APS having an unprovoked thrombotic event, it is recommended to have lifelong anticoagulation. The rationale behind it is, firstly, the high recurrence rate without anticoagulation and secondly, possibly life-endangering recurrent thromboembolic events, especially when it is arterial thrombosis.

The secondary prophylaxis management of APLA with a history of thrombosis is based upon the triple positivity or non-triple positivity. Triple positive for APS antibodies is defined as positivity for all three tests: APTT-LA, β2GP1, and aCL. If the patient has a history of thrombosis and APLA tests come positive, then secondary prophylaxis is required, which is managed as below

1. Venous thrombosis.
    (a) Triple positive.
        (i) Vitamin K anticoagulants (VKA) (Warfarin) with standard intensity, i.e., aiming INR of 2.0–3.0.
        (ii) Heparin/LMWH.

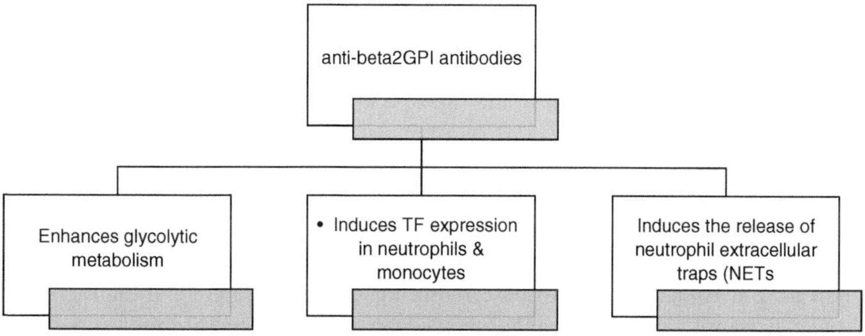

Fig. 22.1 Role of anti-beta2GPI antibodies over neutrophils to induce thrombosis. TF Tissue factor

(b) Non-triple positive.

(i) Vitamin K anticoagulants (Warfarin)/Heparin/LMWH.
(ii) Serious allergy/adverse event with VKA/Low adherence to VKA/No facility for Lab monitoring—Direct oral anticoagulants (DOACs).

(c) Recurrent venous thrombotic events.

(i) Add low-dose aspirin or.
(ii) Aim for the high INR target of 3–4 or.
(iii) Transition to LMWH.

2. Arterial thrombosis.

(a) Low risk/non recurrent.

(i) Vitamin K anticoagulants (VKA) (Warfarin) with standard intensity, i.e., aiming INR of 2.0–3.0 plus low-dose Aspirin.
(ii) Heparin/LMWH.

(b) High risk/recurrent.

(i) Vitamin K anticoagulants (VKA) (Warfarin) with high intensity, i.e., aiming for an INR of 3.0–4.0.

3. In cases of refractory APS, the recently updated management is Chimeric antigen receptor (CAR) T-cell therapy.
4. TNF-α blockers (adalimumab, certolizumab) role in aPL-positive women with a history of recurrent pregnancy complications despite routine therapy.
5. Two medications with anti-neutrophil functions against Neutrophil extracellular traps (NETs) (defibrotide and dipyridamole).
6. Daratumumab—Reset the humoral immunity in patients with APS patient having refractory thromboembolic episodes.

22.6 Clinical Case 3

A 62-year-old presented with a sudden episode of intermittent claudication for past 10 days. Patient complained of leg pain, especially when he walked some steps. Patient was a known case of Type 2 diabetes mellitus, a deranged lipid profile and hypertension. On examination, the arterial pulse was felt over the right common femoral artery but was absent in the right popliteal artery. Further, investigations revealed hemoglobin of 14.2 g/dl (normal range of 14–16 g/dl), TLC count of 8900/cumm (normal range of 4000–11,000/cumm), Platelets—2,34,000/cumm (normal range of 1,50,000-4,00,000/cumm); Haemoglobin A1c (Hba1c)—7.2% (normal range of 4.9–6.0%) with D-dimer of 0.70 IU/L (normal range of 0.0–1.0 μg/mL). The right ankle brachial index (ABI) was 0.40 (normal range of 1.0–1.4), indicating peripheral artery disease requiring ultrasonography and angiography. Lower extremity ultrasonography showed an occlusion in the right superficial femoral artery (SFA). The popliteal artery is shown to have perfusion via collateral channels from the deep femoral artery, thus signifying the atherosclerotic lesion.

Questions Arising from Case 3

Q1. What are the incidences of peripheral arterial occlusion?

Q2. Enumerate the causes of arterial thrombosis.

Q3. What is the lab approach to arterial thrombosis?

Analysis of Answers [10]

- Ans 1. Peripheral arterial occlusion incidence is approximately 1.5 cases per 10,000 persons per year.

Ans 2. The causes are enumerated in Table 22.11.

Ans 3. Approach to arterial thrombosis.

A brief approach is defined in Fig 22.2.

Table 22.11 Causes of arterial thrombosis

Local factors	Systemic factors
Fluid dynamics 1. Reduced flow—shear stress/tensile stress	*Thrombophilia* 1. Neoplasms—solid/haematological (myeloproliferative neoplasms) 2. APLA 3. Hyperhomocystinaemia 4. Paroxysmal nocturnal haemoglobinuria (PNH)
Internal 1. Atherosclerotic plaques 2. Thrombosis of an aneurysm 3. Dissection of the artery 4. Local inflammation	*Emboli* 1. *Source from artery*—Atherosclerotic plaque/aneurysm 2. *Source from cardiac*—Myocardial infarction/atrial fibrillation/endocarditis/valvular disease/prosthetic valves
External 1. Compression of the artery 2. Entrapment of the artery	*Thrombocytopenic* 1. Heparin-induced thrombocytopenia 2. Disseminated intravascular coagulation
Intervention/Injury 1. Bypass graft 2. Angioplasty site/stent 3. Iatrogenic injury	*Infections* 1.COVID-19 infection 2. Systemic infections
	Metabolic 1. Diabetes mellitus 2. Hypertension 3. Deranged lipid profile
	Drugs/Agents 1.Smoking/cocaine/marijuana/cannabis 2. Platinum-based drugs (e.g., cisplatin) 3. Vascular endothelial growth factor inhibitors—Bevacizumab, Sunitinib, and Sorafenib. 4. Tyrosine kinase inhibitors—dasatinib, nilotinib, and ponatinib 5. Thalidomide 6. L-Asparaginase 7. OCs/HRTs/anabolic steroids 8. IV immunoglobulins 9. Erythropoietic stimulating agents

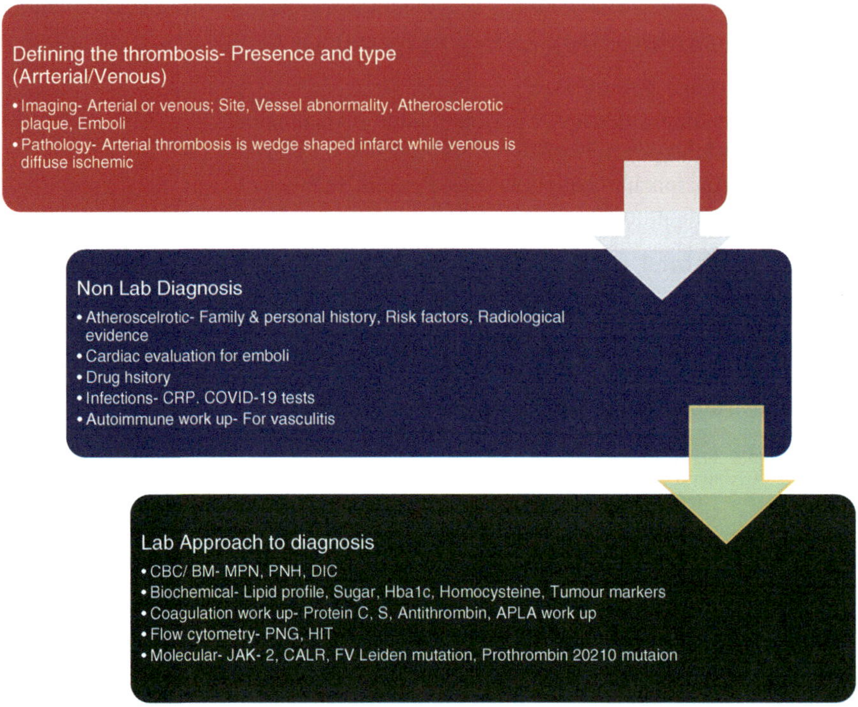

Fig. 22.2 A comprehensive approach to thrombophilia [4, 5]

22.7 Summary

This chapter on thrombophilia explores the significance of inherited and acquired conditions that increase the risk of abnormal blood clot formation, leading to arterial and venous thrombosis. It covers the primary genetic factors, including mutations such as Factor V Leiden, Prothrombin gene mutation, and deficiencies in natural anticoagulants like Protein C, Protein S, and Antithrombin, which contribute to an elevated tendency for clot formation. The chapter also discusses acquired conditions, such as antiphospholipid syndrome, which further predispose individuals to thrombosis.

The relationship between thrombophilia and common thrombotic events, including deep vein thrombosis (DVT), pulmonary embolism (PE), and arterial events like stroke and myocardial infarction, is thoroughly examined. The chapter highlights how these conditions impact diagnosis, risk assessment, and treatment options, focusing on anticoagulation therapy as a primary treatment strategy.

In addition, the chapter underscores the importance of a personalised approach to managing thrombophilia, taking into account the type of thrombophilic disorder, the individual's thrombotic history, and other contributing factors such as lifestyle.

Overall, this chapter provides a comprehensive understanding of thrombophilia and its crucial role in both venous and arterial thrombotic diseases.

References

1. Dicks AB, Moussallem E, Stanbro M, Walls J, Gandhi S, Gray BH. A comprehensive review of risk factors and thrombophilia evaluation in venous thromboembolism. J Clin Med. 2024;13:362.
2. Report of Task Force on Venous Thrombo Embolism by National Academy of Medical Sciences (India) Directorate General of Health Services Ministry of Health & Family Welfare Government of India 2022, p. 58–60.
3. Schulman S, Makatsariya A, Khizroeva J, Bitsadze V, Kapanadze D. The basic principles of pathophysiology of venous thrombosis. Int J Mol Sci. 2024;25(21):11447.
4. Middeldorp S, Nieuwlaat R, Baumann Kreuziger L, Coppens M, Houghton D, James AH, Lang E, Moll S, Myers T, Bhatt M, et al. American Society of Hematology 2023 guidelines for management of venous thromboembolism: thrombophilia testing. Blood Adv. 2023;7:7101–38.
5. Arachchillage DJ, Mackillop L, Chandratheva A, et al. Thrombophilia testing: a British Society for Haematology guideline. Br J Haematol. 2022;198:443.
6. Kearon C, Akl EA, Ornelas J, et al. Antithrombotic therapy for VTE disease: CHEST guideline and expert panel report. Chest. 2016;149:315.
7. Barbhaiya M, Zuily S, Naden R, on Behalf of the ACR/EULAR APS Classification Criteria Collaborators, et al. 2023 ACR/EULAR antiphospholipid syndrome classification criteria. Ann Rheum Dis. 2023;82:1258–70.
8. Zhao Y, Huang C, Zhou Y, Qi W, et al. Performance validation of the 2023 American College of Rheumatology/European League Against Rheumatism antiphospholipid syndrome classification criteria in an antiphospholipid syndrome cohort. J Thromb Haemost. 2024;22:1660–74.
9. Tambralli A, Harbaugh A, Naveen Kumar SK, et al. Neutrophil glucose flux as a therapeutic target in antiphospholipid syndrome. J Clin Invest. 2024;134(15):e169893.
10. May JE, Moll S. Unexplained arterial thrombosis: approach to diagnosis and treatment. Hematology Am Soc Hematol Educ Program. 2021;2021(1):76–84.

Chapter 23
Diagnosis of Antiphospholipid Syndrome and Role in Different Clinical Conditions

Eveeta Baruah, Tejasvi Sharma, and Abhishek Purohit

Abstract *Antiphospholipid Syndrome (APS)*, also referred to as *Antiphospholipid Antibody Syndrome (APLA)*, is an autoimmune prothrombotic condition characterized by a sustained presence of antiphospholipid antibodies (aPL). These autoantibodies target proteins that bind to phospholipids on cell membranes and promote a prothrombotic or hypercoagulable state. As a result, affected individuals are at increased risk for both arterial and venous thrombotic events, in addition to pregnancy-related complications. APS may present as a primary condition or develop secondary to other autoimmune diseases, most commonly in association with systemic lupus erythematosus (SLE). The underlying pathogenesis involves antibody-mediated disruption of normal endothelial and anticoagulant mechanisms, resulting in enhanced thrombin generation and vascular thrombosis.

Clinically, APS demonstrates considerable heterogeneity. Patients may present with recurrent pregnancy loss, deep vein thrombosis, pulmonary embolism, ischemic stroke, or other thrombotic manifestations affecting various vascular beds. Diagnosis is established based on validated classification systems, most notably the Sydney criteria. These criteria mandate the coexistence of at least one clinical event (vascular thrombosis or defined pregnancy morbidity) and persistent laboratory evidence of antiphospholipid antibodies, including anticardiolipin antibodies, lupus anticoagulant, and/or anti–β2 glycoprotein I antibodies.

Management primarily focuses on the prevention of recurrent thrombotic episodes through long-term anticoagulation therapy, typically using warfarin or heparin. In pregnant patients, a combination of low-dose aspirin and heparin is commonly administered to reduce the risk of miscarriage and other obstetric complications such as preeclampsia. Therapeutic decisions require careful balancing of thrombotic risk against potential bleeding complications, necessitating regular monitoring.

The prognosis of APS depends on the extent and recurrence of thrombotic events, along with the presence of associated autoimmune conditions. Long-term care aims to minimize recurrent thrombosis, manage coexisting systemic diseases, and

E. Baruah · T. Sharma · A. Purohit (✉)
Department of Pathology and Lab Medicine, All India Institute of Medical Sciences, Jodhpur, Rajasthan, India

H. P. Pati et al. (eds.), *Clinical Hematology and Hemato-Oncology*,
https://doi.org/10.1007/978-981-92-1167-8_23

improve maternal and fetal outcomes. Owing to its multifaceted presentation and potential complications, APS requires coordinated multidisciplinary management and comprehensive patient education.

Keywords Anti-phospholipid antibody · Anticardiolipin · Anti-beta2 glycoprotein1 · Thromboembolism · Preeclampsia

Learning Objectives
- To be able to define APS—autoimmune disorder with pathogenic aPL (lupus anticoagulant, anti-cardiolipin/β2GPI).
- To know about the underlying mechanisms—aPL causes thrombosis via endothelial activation, platelet aggregation, and complement dysregulation.
- To develop an understanding of the key clinical manifestations, including venous and arterial thrombotic events, recurrent pregnancy morbidity, livedo reticularis, and thrombocytopenia.
- To know how to reach the diagnosis—Sydney criteria: clinical event + lab-confirmed aPL (repeat testing required).
- To understand the approach to management—warfarin/DOACs for thrombosis; heparin + aspirin for pregnancy; triple therapy for CAPS.

23.1 Introduction

23.1.1 Definition

Antiphospholipid syndrome (APS), also referred to as Hughes syndrome, is a systemic autoimmune condition characterized by the sustained presence of circulating antiphospholipid antibodies (aPL) and an increased predisposition to thrombotic events, including deep vein thrombosis (DVT), pulmonary embolism (PE), and cerebrovascular accidents, as well as pregnancy-related complications such as recurrent miscarriage and stillbirth [1]. First recognized in the 1980s, APS is characterized by the presence of defined clinical features and laboratory criteria.

23.1.2 History

In 1906, Wassermann introduced the first serological test for the diagnosis of syphilis. This assay was based on the interaction between nonspecific antibodies (reagins) present in syphilis and a reaction antigen, later identified as cardiolipin, a phospholipid component of the inner mitochondrial membrane [2]. When the test began to be applied widely for population screening, it became apparent that certain individuals with positive results did not have syphilis. These cases were termed biologically false-positive serologic tests for syphilis (BFP–STS). Persistent BFP–STS reactions were subsequently observed in patients diagnosed with systemic lupus erythematosus (SLE).

In 1952, Conley and Hartmann described two patients with SLE who exhibited a circulating anticoagulant associated with hemorrhagic manifestations, attributed to prolonged prothrombin–thrombin conversion [3]. During the 1970s, this anticoagulant activity was shown to result from an acquired immunoglobulin (IgG or IgM) that could be partially neutralized by the addition of phospholipids or platelets. It was subsequently termed "lupus anticoagulant" (LA), as it was initially believed to contribute to bleeding tendencies in patients with SLE [2]. However, the designation proved to be somewhat misleading, since LA was more frequently associated with thrombotic complications than with hemorrhage. Further observations linked LA to recurrent pregnancy loss and intrauterine fetal demise.

The development of a solid-phase anticardiolipin immunoassay by the Graham Hughes group in London enabled direct detection of anticardiolipin antibodies (aCL). A strong association was identified between the IgG isotype of aCL antibodies and clinical thrombotic events. Subsequent research also demonstrated a relationship between aCL antibodies and the presence of LA [3].

These cumulative findings culminated in the description of a distinct clinical entity by G.R.V. Hughes in 1983, in his British Medical Journal publication titled "Thrombosis, abortion, cerebral disease, and the lupus anticoagulant." [4] Hughes was the first to comprehensively define the syndrome, highlighting its multisystem nature and its association not only with lupus anticoagulant but also with anticardiolipin antibodies.

23.1.3 Criteria for Diagnosis of APS

For the classification and diagnosis of APS, clinicians have relied on the Sapporo criteria formulated in 1999, which incorporate defined clinical and laboratory parameters. These criteria were subsequently updated during the Sydney International Antiphospholipid Antibodies Congress in 2006 and are now known as the revised Sapporo or Sydney criteria. To establish a diagnosis of APS, the presence of at least one clinical criterion and one laboratory criterion is required [5].

Clinical Criteria

1. One or more episodes of vascular thrombosis involving arterial, venous, or small-vessel (microvascular) circulation.
2. Pregnancy-related morbidity attributed to placental dysfunction, including:

   A. Three or more consecutive unexplained spontaneous abortions occurring before 10 weeks of gestation.
   B. One or more unexplained fetal deaths beyond the tenth week of gestation.

C. Stillbirth.
D. Unexplained obstetric complications such as pre-eclampsia, preterm delivery, placental abruption, intrauterine growth restriction (IUGR), or oligohydramnios.

Laboratory Criteria

1. Detection of medium- to high-titer anticardiolipin antibodies or anti–β2 glycoprotein I (IgG and/or IgM) antibodies on two or more occasions at least 12 weeks apart, measured by ELISA.
2. Presence of lupus anticoagulant on two separate occasions at least 12 weeks apart.

Despite their widespread use, these criteria have certain limitations. They do not clearly differentiate the clinical significance of IgG versus IgM isotypes—IgG antibodies being more strongly associated with thrombotic manifestations and IgM more commonly linked to obstetric presentations. Additionally, they do not adequately distinguish between early and late pregnancy complications, fail to sufficiently account for small-vessel thrombosis, and do not incorporate other supportive laboratory or imaging findings relevant to APS.

23.1.4 ACR/EULAR Criteria

In 2023, the American College of Rheumatology (ACR) and the European Alliance of Associations for Rheumatology (EULAR) introduced updated classification criteria for APS. These revised guidelines are designed to better evaluate the relative weight of different clinical and laboratory features, while also incorporating relevant aspects of a patient's medical history. Importantly, they assign value to biopsy-proven microvascular thrombosis in the absence of alternative causes. The updated framework gives greater importance to well-defined late pregnancy complications and comparatively less weight to early pregnancy losses. It also incorporates additional clinical features such as cardiac valvular abnormalities and thrombocytopenia to improve diagnostic recognition. Furthermore, diffuse alveolar hemorrhage, a rare but recognized manifestation of APS, has been included. Reduced emphasis is placed on isolated IgM antibody positivity [6].

The ACR/EULAR criteria require an entry condition of at least one documented positive antiphospholipid antibody test within 3 years of a clinical event suggestive of APS. Following this, a set of weighted criteria—ranging from 1 to 7 points—is applied across six clinical domains and two laboratory domains. A diagnosis of APS is classified when a patient achieves a minimum of 3 points in both the clinical and laboratory categories.

23.1.4.1 Clinical Criteria

Domain 1: Macrovascular (Venous Thromboembolism)
- Documented venous thromboembolism that is otherwise unexplained and confirmed by appropriate diagnostic methods.
- This encompasses, but is not restricted to, pulmonary embolism, deep vein thrombosis involving the upper or lower extremities, thrombosis of the splanchnic veins, renal vein thrombosis, cerebral venous sinus thrombosis, and retinal vein thrombosis or occlusion.

Domain 2: Macrovascular (Arterial Thrombosis)
- Confirmed arterial thrombosis without an alternative explanation, established through suitable investigations.
- Examples include myocardial infarction due to coronary artery thrombosis, thrombosis of peripheral, splanchnic, or retinal arteries, ischemic stroke, and infarctions of organs such as the kidney, liver, or spleen, even when a thrombus is not directly visualized.

Domain 3: Microvascular

Suspected Involvement:

- Livedo racemosa identified on clinical examination.
- Cutaneous lesions consistent with livedoid vasculopathy on physical examination.
- Antiphospholipid antibody (aPL)–associated nephropathy suggested by clinical or laboratory findings.
- Pulmonary hemorrhage indicated by symptoms and supportive imaging.

Established Involvement:

- Livedoid vasculopathy confirmed histopathologically.
- aPL nephropathy verified by biopsy.
- Pulmonary hemorrhage demonstrated by bronchoalveolar lavage (BAL) findings or tissue pathology.
- Myocardial involvement documented through imaging or histological examination.
- Adrenal hemorrhage or microthrombotic changes confirmed by imaging studies or pathology.

Domain 4: Obstetric
- Prefetal loss (pre-embryonic or embryonic): unexplained pregnancy loss occurring before 10 weeks 0 days of gestation.
- Fetal loss: unexplained pregnancy loss between 10 weeks 0 days and 15 weeks 6 days (early fetal death), or between 16 weeks 0 days and 34 weeks 0 days of gestation.
- Severe preeclampsia.
- Severe placental insufficiency.

Domain 5: Cardiac Valve

- Thickening of cardiac valves.
- Presence of valvular vegetations.

Domain 6: Hematologic

- Thrombocytopenia is defined as an otherwise unexplained nadir platelet count between 20 and 130 × 10^9/L, confirmed by peripheral smear evaluation and repeat testing.

23.1.4.2 Laboratory Criteria

Domain 7: Antiphospholipid Antibody Testing by Coagulation-Based Functional Assay (Lupus Anticoagulant, LAC)

- Detection of lupus anticoagulant is performed using a three-step approach consisting of screening, mixing study, and confirmatory testing. Two screening assays are required: the diluted Russell's viper venom time (dRVVT) and a lupus-sensitive activated partial thromboplastin time (aPTT) that employs low phospholipid concentration with silica as an activator.
- The LAC result is interpreted as positive when at least one of the two screening systems demonstrates positivity after completion of all three stages, including confirmation of phospholipid-dependent correction of the initially prolonged clotting time.

Domain 8: Antiphospholipid Antibody Testing by Solid-Phase Immunoassay

- Anticardiolipin (aCL) antibodies and anti–β2-glycoprotein I (anti-β2GPI) antibodies are measured using solid-phase assays.
- Moderate titer: 40–79 units.
- High titer: ≥80 units.

The recently introduced criteria adopt a structured, evidence-based methodology intended to enhance diagnostic precision and ultimately improve patient outcomes [6, 7]. They also seek to identify distinct APS subgroups, which may be particularly relevant for future research applications. Compared with the revised Sapporo criteria, the 2023 ACR/EULAR classification system exhibits greater specificity but reduced sensitivity. This variation is largely due to more stringent definitions related to thrombotic risk stratification, obstetric manifestations, and laboratory parameters. Current evidence indicates that the ACR/EULAR criteria are better suited for research purposes because of their higher specificity and ability to define more uniform APS populations, whereas the Sapporo criteria continue to hold importance in routine clinical practice owing to their superior sensitivity [7].

23.1.5 Epidemiology

The classification criteria for APS have undergone revisions largely because of the absence of standardized methods for detecting antiphospholipid antibodies (aPL). In addition, challenges such as confirming persistent aPL positivity at least 12 weeks after the initial test have made it difficult to determine the true prevalence of APS. According to population studies, the estimated incidence and prevalence ranged between 1 and 2 cases per 100,000 and 40 and 50 cases per 100,000 respectively [8]. The prevalence of antiphospholipid antibodies was 10% in patients with deep vein thrombosis (DVT) and 14% in patients with stroke, while in cases of obstetric morbidity, it ranged from 6% to 9% [9]. Around 50% of individuals diagnosed with antiphospholipid syndrome (APS) have "primary APS," while the remaining 50% of patients have "secondary APS" due to a concomitant systemic autoimmune disorder, more commonly as a consequence of SLE [10]. The core clinical features of APS—namely, arterial or venous thrombosis and pregnancy-related morbidity—generally remain consistent, regardless of whether the condition occurs as a primary disorder or in association with an underlying connective tissue disease.

23.2 Pathophysiology of APS

The pathogenesis of Antiphospholipid Syndrome (APS) involves a complex interaction among immune mechanisms, the vascular endothelium, and the coagulation system. In APS, B lymphocytes generate antiphospholipid antibodies (aPLs) that primarily target phospholipid-binding proteins, including β2-glycoprotein I (β2GPI), prothrombin, and annexin, among others [11]. Of these, anti-β2GPI antibodies are considered the most clinically significant. β2GPI is a 326–amino acid plasma protein synthesized predominantly in the liver and has the ability to bind to multiple cell types implicated in APS pathogenesis, such as endothelial cells, monocytes, platelets, trophoblasts, neurons, and neutrophils. Structurally, β2GPI is composed of five domains (DI–DV). The fifth domain contains 14 lysine residues that facilitate attachment to negatively charged phospholipids. Upon binding to these phospholipids, β2GPI undergoes a structural transformation into an open "J-shaped" configuration, which exposes cryptic epitopes within Domain I. This conformational shift enhances the binding of pathogenic aPLs and promotes prothrombotic and proinflammatory processes characteristic of APS [12].

Thrombosis in APS mediated by β2GPI-dependent aPLs is thought to occur through three principal mechanisms: (1) interference with natural anticoagulant pathways in the fluid phase, including disruption of protein C, antithrombin, annexin A5, and fibrinolytic activity; (2) direct effects on cellular elements of hemostasis via interactions with endothelial cells, monocytes, neutrophils, and platelets, thereby amplifying coagulation; and (3) activation of the complement cascade. Notably, the presence of circulating antibodies alone is often insufficient to precipitate thrombosis, and an additional triggering factor—commonly referred to as a "second hit," such as infection or systemic inflammation—is typically necessary for the manifestation of clinical thrombotic events [13].

Antiphospholipid antibodies (aPLs) interfere with the protein C anticoagulant system by impairing the formation and activation of the protein C complex, thereby facilitating thrombin generation [14]. Anti-β2GPI antibodies and β2GPI-dependent lupus anticoagulant (LA) further contribute to a hypercoagulable state by promoting resistance to activated protein C (APC), which increases the risk of venous thromboembolism in APS [15]. Binding of aPLs to β2GPI expressed on cellular surfaces enhances tissue factor expression, a pivotal initiator of the extrinsic coagulation pathway. In endothelial cells, this interaction results in upregulation of adhesion molecules such as E-selectin, decreased activity of endothelial nitric oxide synthase (eNOS), and downregulation of tissue factor pathway inhibitor (TFPI), collectively favoring thrombosis [16]. Moreover, aPLs stimulate neutrophil activation and the release of neutrophil extracellular traps (NETs), which significantly amplify thrombus formation [17]. Thrombocytopenia, frequently observed in APS, is attributed to platelet activation mediated by the anti-β2GPI/β2GPI complex through its interaction with apolipoprotein E receptor 2 (ApoER2) and glycoprotein Ibα [18].

Activation of the complement cascade is another central mechanism in aPL-associated thrombosis and endothelial dysfunction. aPLs initiate cleavage of complement components C3 and C5, leading to the generation of C5a, a potent chemoattractant that recruits and activates neutrophils and enhances tissue factor expression [19]. Decreased levels of complement factor H (FH), an important regulatory protein, may further intensify complement activation in APS [20]. Complement activation has also been implicated in obstetric complications, particularly early pregnancy loss, with elevated levels of Bb and sC5b-9 during early gestation being associated with adverse outcomes in aPL-positive women [21]. Experimental evidence indicates that inhibition of C3 convertase or blockade of C5a receptor signaling can attenuate these pathogenic effects. In addition to their anticoagulant properties, heparins may contribute to improved pregnancy outcomes in APS by modulating complement activation [22].

Two-Hit Hypothesis

The "two-hit hypothesis" (Fig. 23.1) proposes that thrombotic events in APS develop as a consequence of two consecutive processes. The first hit consists of the sustained presence of antiphospholipid antibodies (aPLs), which establish an underlying prothrombotic milieu. The second hit involves an additional precipitating factor—such as infection, trauma, or surgical intervention—that perturbs the hemostatic equilibrium and precipitates thrombosis. Infectious or inflammatory stimuli may activate Toll-like receptors (TLRs), leading to enhanced expression of aPL-related epitopes and thereby amplifying thrombotic risk. In cases of obstetric APS, pregnancy itself may function as this secondary trigger [23]. Although this conceptual framework provides insight into disease mechanisms, it does not universally apply to all patients with APS.

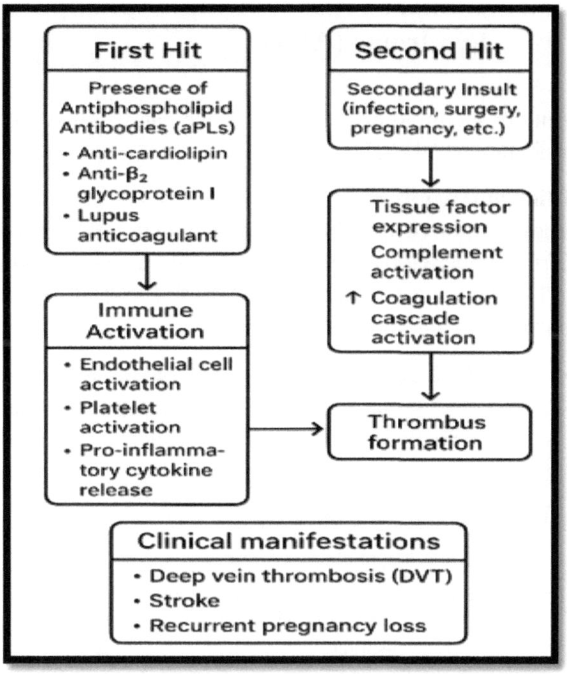

Fig. 23.1 Two-hit hypothesis for the development of antiphospholipid antibody syndrome

Obstetric and Vascular APS

Both obstetric and thrombotic forms of APS are fundamentally driven by β2-glycoprotein I (β2GPI) and β2GPI-dependent antiphospholipid antibodies (aPL). Nevertheless, accumulating data indicate that the biological behavior of aPL may differ between these clinical phenotypes. For example, IgG isolated from patients with isolated obstetric APS has been demonstrated to impair trophoblast invasion and modulate monocyte gene expression in a manner distinct from IgG derived from patients with vascular APS [24]. This suggests that even when antibody specificity is similar, their downstream cellular effects may vary according to the clinical presentation.

β2GPI is constitutively expressed on trophoblasts and decidual cells, where it plays a physiological role in placental development [25]. The binding of β2GPI through its Domain V results in a high-density, J-shaped configuration that promotes enhanced recognition by autoantibodies. In contrast to vascular APS—where β2GPI expression on endothelial cells often requires prior endothelial injury—its baseline expression within placental tissues may account for why an additional triggering factor is not invariably required in obstetric APS [26].

Conversely, vascular APS and its most severe manifestation, catastrophic APS (CAPS), generally conform to the two-hit paradigm. CAPS is characterized by markedly increased levels of proinflammatory cytokines and ferritin, leading to widespread activation of endothelial cells, monocytes, platelets, and neutrophils. This extensive and simultaneous cellular activation across multiple organs underlies the diffuse thrombotic involvement observed in CAPS.

23.3 Clinical Types of Antiphospholipid Antibody Syndrome (APS)

Antiphospholipid antibody syndrome can be clinically classified into four categories (Table 23.1) [27].

Clinical Phenotypes

The detection of aPL alone is insufficient to establish a diagnosis of APS. Diagnostic certainty increases when there is a clear temporal and clinical association between aPL positivity and characteristic clinical events, as well as when distinct clinical phenotypes are identified.

- *Thrombotic APS*: When other risk factors for venous thromboembolism (VTE) or cardiovascular disease (CVD) are present at the time of a thrombotic event, the diagnostic specificity may be reduced.

Table 23.1 Clinical subtypes of APS

Type	Definition	Key feature	Associated condition
Primary APS	APS occurring without any underlying autoimmune disorder	Arterial/venous thrombosis Pregnancy morbidity Positive aPL antibodies	None (isolated APS)
Secondary APS	APS occurring in association with another autoimmune disease	Similar clinical features to the primary Often more severe	Most common: Systemic Lupus Erythematosus (SLE) Others: RA, Sjögren's syndrome
Seronegative APS	APS-like clinical manifestations without detectable aPL antibodies	Clinical features of APS Negative standard lab tests May have non-criteria antibodies	Diagnosis remains clinical; controversial subtype
Catastrophic APS[a] (CAPS)	A rare, acute, life-threatening form of APS with widespread thrombosis	Rapid multiorgan failure Small vessel thrombosis Requires ICU care	Often triggered by infection, surgery, trauma

[a]Catastrophic APS

Catastrophic APS (CAPS) is recognized as a severe, potentially fatal condition characterized by: (i) rapid onset of involvement of multiple organs—typically three or more—within a short duration; (ii) histological confirmation of widespread small-vessel thrombosis; and (iii) the presence of antiphospholipid antibodies, often at high titers [27]

- *Microvascular APS*: Characterized by involvement of small vessels, affecting organs such as the lungs (e.g., diffuse alveolar hemorrhage), kidneys (aPL-associated nephropathy), and skin (livedoid vasculopathy).
- *Catastrophic APS (CAPS)*: Manifests as systemic thrombotic microangiopathy (TMA), often accompanied by hemolytic anemia with schistocytes, thrombocytopenia, and multiorgan dysfunction. The presence of overlapping conditions such as sepsis, heparin-induced thrombocytopenia (HIT), or complement-mediated TMA may make diagnosis more challenging.
- *Obstetric APS*: The diagnosis is strengthened by the occurrence of otherwise unexplained late pregnancy loss, especially when accompanied by evidence of placental vascular abnormalities, while early pregnancy losses are comparatively less specific.
- *Non-thrombotic Manifestations of aPL*: These include unexplained autoimmune thrombocytopenia, hemolytic anemia, and valvular heart disease [27].

23.4 Clinical Manifestations of APS

Because APS is fundamentally a vascular disorder, its clinical manifestations are varied and may involve multiple organ systems. These can be categorized as criteria and non-criteria manifestations:

23.4.1 Criteria Manifestations

23.4.1.1 Systemic Vascular Thrombosis

Thrombosis represents the central clinical feature of APS. The syndrome is capable of producing thrombotic events in vessels of all calibers, involving arterial, venous, and microvascular circulations. Among these, venous thromboembolism is the most common presentation. Deep vein thrombosis of the lower extremities is the predominant site, occurring in approximately 20–30% of individuals with APS [28].

Within the arterial system, ischemic stroke and transient ischemic attacks (TIAs) are the most frequently observed manifestations associated with APS [29]. Notably, APS is responsible for up to 20% of stroke cases in individuals younger than 45 years [30]. Therefore, in younger patients presenting with ischemic stroke in the absence of conventional cerebrovascular risk factors, evaluation for APS should be strongly considered.

In addition to typical sites, APS may present with thrombosis in less common vascular territories, including the portal, renal, and mesenteric veins, as well as cerebral venous sinuses [31]. Other reported complications include avascular osteonecrosis, mesenteric arterial occlusion, and adrenal infarction. Importantly, recurrent thrombotic episodes may occur even in patients receiving appropriate therapeutic anticoagulation.

23.4.1.2 Obstetric APS

The association between recurrent spontaneous pregnancy loss and lupus anticoagulant (LA) was initially reported by Nilson et al., while in 1984, Graham Hughes described the link between anticardiolipin (aCL) antibodies and recurrent miscarriages [32]. Obstetric APS (OAPS) is now recognized as one of the leading identifiable causes of recurrent pregnancy loss and late gestational complications resulting from placental dysfunction. Data from the APS ACTION group indicate that approximately 6% of women with significant pregnancy morbidity test positive for antiphospholipid antibodies [33].

The presence of antiphospholipid antibodies has been linked to various obstetric complications, such as intrauterine growth restriction, preeclampsia, chorea gravidarum, and recurrent spontaneous pregnancy loss. Although the precise mechanisms underlying pregnancy-related morbidity in APS remain incompletely elucidated, proposed contributors include inflammatory pathways, activation of the complement system, and placental thrombosis, all of which are believed to play a role in the development of OAPS [34].

23.4.1.3 Non-criteria Manifestations

1. Cardiovascular Manifestations

   Cardiac involvement in APS most frequently affects the heart valves, presenting as valvular thickening, nodular lesions, or sterile vegetations consistent with Libman–Sacks endocarditis. The mitral valve is most commonly involved, followed by the aortic valve [35]. Patients with APS are at a higher risk of ischemic heart disease than the general population. Myocardial infarction can result from coronary thrombosis without significant underlying atherosclerosis, from accelerated atherosclerotic changes causing atherothrombosis, or from involvement of the coronary microvasculature. Registry data indicate that myocardial infarction occurs in approximately 5.5% of individuals with APS [36].
2. Neurological Manifestations

   Cerebrovascular involvement represents the leading cause of neurological symptoms in APS and includes acute ischemic stroke, transient ischemic attack (TIA), and cerebral venous thrombosis (CVT). Additional neurological features may include Sneddon syndrome, cognitive impairment, multiple sclerosis–like presentations, Guillain–Barré syndrome, transverse myelopathy or myelitis, seizures, psychosis, and chorea [37].
3. Cutaneous Manifestations

   Skin findings may serve as the initial indicator of APS. Livedo reticularis, characterized by a violaceous, net-like rash commonly seen on the extremities, trunk, and buttocks, is the most frequent dermatologic manifestation. It results from altered blood flow within cutaneous vessels and has been linked to recurrent thrombosis and stroke [38]. The prevalence of livedo reticularis is approximately 25% in primary APS and up to 70% in APS associated with systemic lupus erythematosus (SLE). Other dermatologic features include livedo racemosa (a more irregular and broken reticular pattern), digital gangrene, splinter hemorrhages, skin necrosis, ulcerations, and lesions resembling pyoderma gangrenosum.

4. Pulmonary Manifestations

   Pulmonary involvement in APS may arise from vascular or parenchymal pathology. Pulmonary embolism (PE) is the most common pulmonary complication, reported in up to 14% of patients [36]. Less frequently observed manifestations include pulmonary hypertension, acute respiratory distress syndrome (ARDS), and intra-alveolar hemorrhage [39].

5. Renal and Adrenal Manifestations

   APS is associated with a wide range of renal abnormalities, including systemic hypertension, large-vessel involvement (such as renal artery stenosis, thrombosis, infarction, and renal vein thrombosis), intrarenal vascular lesions collectively termed APS nephropathy, and glomerular disease. The true frequency of renal involvement remains uncertain due to limitations related to biopsy feasibility, histopathological evaluation, and overlap with SLE-associated disease [40].

6. Ocular Manifestations

   Although previously considered uncommon, ocular involvement has been reported in up to 37% of patients in recent studies. Clinical features may include conjunctivitis sicca, conjunctival telangiectasia and microaneurysms, punctate epithelial keratopathy, limbal keratitis, blurred vision, amaurosis fugax, and transient visual field defects such as scotoma [41].

7. Hematological Manifestations

   Thrombocytopenia in APS is generally attributed to peripheral platelet consumption and/or immune-mediated destruction following platelet activation by antiphospholipid antibodies. It is typically mild in severity and infrequently necessitates specific therapy [42].

23.5 Assays for APS

Since the clinical manifestations of APS are not pathognomonic and may overlap with other conditions driven by different underlying mechanisms, laboratory identification of antiphospholipid antibodies (aPL) plays a critical role in ensuring accurate diagnosis and preventing both underdiagnosis and overdiagnosis. Given that aPL comprises a diverse and heterogeneous group of autoantibodies, their evaluation includes both established classification (criteria) assays and additional non-criteria tests for comprehensive.

23.5.1 Criteria Assays

According to the established classification criteria, the laboratory parameters include lupus anticoagulant (LA), anti–β2-glycoprotein I antibodies (aβ2GPI), and anticardiolipin (aCL) antibodies of the IgG or IgM isotype [43]. Detection of at least one of these antibodies—LA, aCL, or aβ2GPI—is essential for confirming a diagnosis of APS. Beyond their diagnostic value, these antibodies also play a role in risk assessment. The specific antibody profile, whether single, double, or triple positivity, along with the titers of aCL and aβ2GPI, has prognostic significance for both thrombotic and obstetric outcomes [44]. Laboratory evaluation of aPL involves two principal methodologies: coagulation-based functional assays and immunologic assays.

23.5.1.1 Lupus Anticoagulant Detection

As per the recommendations of the Scientific and Standardization Committee (SCC) of the International Society on Thrombosis and Haemostasis (ISTH), lupus anticoagulant (LA) can be identified using several assay systems, including:

1. Diluted Russell's viper venom time (dRVVT).
2. Kaolin clotting time.
3. Activated partial thromboplastin time (aPTT) employing both LA-sensitive and LA-insensitive reagents.
4. Dilute prothrombin time.
5. Hexagonal phase phospholipid neutralization assay.
6. Ecarin/taipan clotting time.

For proper assessment, two tests employing distinct methodological approaches should be performed at the outset. The first-line test is dRVVT, while the second is an aPTT assay using a reagent validated for LA sensitivity.

LA is suggested when a phospholipid-dependent clotting assay is prolonged, and this prolongation corrects upon addition of excess phospholipid during the confirmatory phase, but fails to correct in mixing studies with normal plasma. If the prolongation does not normalize during the confirmatory step, the findings do not support the presence of LA, and other potential causes of clotting time prolongation should be investigated. In certain cases, mixing with normal plasma may paradoxically result in further prolongation, possibly due to the contribution of a deficient or absent LA cofactor from the added plasma. In such scenarios—particularly when a strong LA is suspected—interpretation may benefit from combining mixing studies with confirmatory testing.

A person is classified as LA-positive if at least one of the two tests produces a positive result. An isolated prolongation of aPTT in an otherwise healthy individual without a history of bleeding may be attributable to the presence of lupus anticoagulant [45].

Patient Selection for Lupus Anticoagulant Testing

1. <50 years with unprovoked venous thromboembolism
2. <50 years with ischemic stroke, transient ischemic attack
3. <50 years with arterial thrombosis
4. Venous thromboembolism at unusual sites.
5. Microvascular thrombosis.
6. Recurrent venous thromboembolism unexplained.
7. Pregnancy morbidities.
8. Systemic lupus erythematosus.

False results are seen when patients are tested during an acute attack or when they are on anticoagulation [45].

23.5.1.2 Anticardiolipin and Anti Beta2GP 1 Antibodies

Anticardiolipin (aCL) and anti–β2-glycoprotein I (aβ2GPI) antibodies have traditionally been measured using ELISA techniques; however, variability in reagents and analytical systems has led to inter-method differences. The growing adoption of fully automated platforms has improved standardization, ensuring more uniform protocol implementation and minimizing variability between laboratories. It is recommended that aCL and aβ2GPI antibodies be assessed using the same solid-phase assay platform to maintain consistency [46].

Certain factors, including rheumatoid factor, intravenous immunoglobulin (IVIG) therapy, and heterophile antibodies, may interfere with testing and produce false-positive results [47].

IgG isotypes show a more robust association with thrombotic manifestations, whereas IgM antibodies are more frequently linked to obstetric complications. Simultaneous testing for both IgG and IgM enhances assessment of the likelihood of APS. Notably, triple positivity—defined as the presence of lupus anticoagulant (LA) together with aCL (IgG and/or IgM) and aβ2GPI (IgG and/or IgM)—shows the strongest association with both thrombotic events and pregnancy morbidity. To confirm persistence, repeat antibody testing after an interval of at least 12 weeks is recommended [48].

23.5.2 Non-criteria Assays

Non-criteria antibodies include Ig A anticardiolipin/anti-beta2-glycoprotein1 antibodies, antiphosphatidyl serine or antiprothrombin antibodies, anti-annexin A2 antibodies, anti-domain1 beta2 GP1 antibodies, etc. While standard aPL testing remains essential for APS diagnosis, non-criteria antibodies show promise in improving diagnostic sensitivity, especially in seronegative APS. Some of them (e.g., aPS/PT, anti-DI β2GPI) correlate with higher thrombotic risk. Hence, these have a potential role in risk stratification by identifying high-risk APS patients.

However, there is a lack of standardization for non-criteria aPL assays [49].

23.5.3 *Others*

23.5.3.1 Genomic and Biomarker Testing

Recently, Genome-Wide Association Study (GWAS) has identified 16 key genes linked to thrombotic and autoimmune pathways in primary APS, which include PF 4 variant 1, Selectin P, TLR2, TLR4, SERPINE1, TFPI, VEGFA, FLT1, TNF alpha, etc. [45, 49]

23.5.3.2 Proteomic Testing

Proteomic testing aids in the identification of dysregulated proteins in APS, offering insights into thrombotic and autoimmune mechanisms. Key proteins include annexin A1, A2, rhoA, HSP60 etc. [45, 49]

23.5.3.3 Biomarker Assay

A key pathogenic mechanism in APS is dysregulated complement activation, which contributes to rapid disease progression. Complement inhibition shows promise. Current fluid-phase complement biomarkers (e.g., C3, C4) are limited because they primarily reflect immune complex activity rather than cell-surface complement regulation (e.g., CD46, CD55, CD59). More informative assays, like the modified Ham test, detect cell-bound complement activation (e.g., C4d), offering better insights into pathogenic complement activity. However, these tests remain largely confined to research settings [46].

23.6 Management of APS

The prevailing management strategy for patients with APS largely follows a uniform "one-size-fits-all" approach. Antithrombotic therapy remains the cornerstone of treatment; however, it is often inadequate for addressing microvascular involvement and non-thrombotic manifestations associated with antiphospholipid antibodies. With advancing insight into the underlying mechanisms of aPL-driven clinical manifestations, there has been a growing trend toward incorporating immunosuppressive therapies in selected aPL-positive patients [50, 51].

23.6.1 Primary Thrombosis Prevention

In individuals without clinical manifestations, antiphospholipid antibodies are often detected incidentally, raising the question of whether primary thromboprophylaxis is warranted. Current guidelines from the British Society for Hematology advise against routine use of anticoagulant or antiplatelet therapy for primary prevention in asymptomatic aPL carriers, including those with triple positivity, with the exception of high-risk circumstances, such as the postoperative period. In contrast, European recommendations support the use of low-dose aspirin for asymptomatic individuals with triple-positive aPL profiles [52].

Non-pharmacological measures, including maintenance of a healthy diet, regular physical activity, and smoking cessation, are strongly encouraged. Estrogen-containing therapies should be avoided due to their prothrombotic potential. Appropriate control of coexisting systemic autoimmune disorders is essential, and hydroxychloroquine is recommended in patients with lupus or lupus-like conditions.

23.6.2 Secondary Thrombosis Prevention

Addressing modifiable risk factors and ensuring optimal treatment of coexisting systemic autoimmune conditions are important components of management. Anticoagulation with vitamin K antagonists is recommended, targeting an international normalized ratio (INR) of 2.0–3.0. In patients with prior arterial thrombotic events and/or additional cardiovascular risk factors, low-dose aspirin may be added to the regimen [50, 51].

23.6.3 Microvascular Antiphospholipid Syndrome

A standardized treatment strategy is challenging due to the variable and multisystem nature of organ involvement in APS. The response to anticoagulation alone may be inadequate, particularly in cases with certain organ manifestations. In such situations, additional therapies—including glucocorticoids, immunosuppressive agents such as azathioprine, mycophenolate mofetil, cyclophosphamide, or sirolimus, as well as biologic agents like rituximab—may be incorporated into the treatment regimen [50, 51].

23.6.4 Catastrophic Antiphospholipid Syndrome

For individuals with suspected or confirmed catastrophic antiphospholipid syndrome (CAPS), a combination regimen consisting of heparin, glucocorticoids, and either plasmapheresis or intravenous immunoglobulin is recommended. In cases characterized by significant microvascular involvement and/or marked thrombocytopenia, rituximab may be considered as an adjunctive therapy. Additionally, in patients exhibiting pronounced systemic thrombotic microangiopathy (TMA), targeted complement inhibition is advised as part of the therapeutic approach [50, 51].

23.6.5 Obstetric APS

A regimen combining low-dose aspirin (LDA) with low-molecular-weight heparin (LMWH) is advised for the majority of patients with a prior history of pregnancy-related morbidity. In contrast, for individuals without previous obstetric complications, low-dose aspirin alone is generally recommended [50, 51].

23.6.6 Non-Thrombotic aPL Manifestations

In cases of moderate to severe thrombocytopenia, treatment options include glucocorticoids, intravenous immunoglobulin, and/or rituximab. For hemolytic anemia, glucocorticoids may be administered in combination with rituximab, azathioprine, or mycophenolate mofetil. In patients presenting with significant systemic thrombotic microangiopathy (TMA), consideration should be given to complement inhibitory therapy [50, 51].

23.6.7 Ongoing Trials for the Management of APS

Approximately seven ongoing clinical trials in APS are currently targeting B cells or plasma cells, evaluating therapeutic agents such as B lymphocyte stimulator (BLyS) inhibitors, the Bruton tyrosine kinase inhibitor zanubrutinib, and the proliferation-inducing ligand (APRIL) antagonist telitacicept.

It has been proposed that selective depletion of CD38-expressing plasmablasts and plasma cells may yield greater therapeutic benefit compared with broader modulation of other B cell subsets. Consequently, therapies under investigation include the anti-BLyS monoclonal antibody belimumab, novel anti-CD38 monoclonal antibodies, and the anti-CD38 agent daratumumab [50, 51].

23.7 An Illustrative Case Scenario

A 32-year-old woman was hospitalized in the medical ward with progressive shortness of breath, worsening on exertion and physical activity, along with a productive cough for the past 2 months. Her obstetric history was significant for a single pregnancy loss at 6 months of gestation.

On examination, she was noted to be pale, with blackish discoloration over the right lower limb. Her vital parameters were stable, except for tachypnea with a respiratory rate of 32 breaths per minute.

Laboratory evaluation showed significant anemia (hemoglobin 6.5 g/dL), thrombocytopenia (65,000 cells/cumm), and an elevated reticulocyte count of 11%. Computed tomography (CT) of the chest demonstrated multiple thrombi within the right lobar pulmonary arteries. Lupus anticoagulant testing was negative. Her anticardiolipin antibody levels were 30 units/mL (IgM) and 35 units/mL (IgG), while anti-β2 glycoprotein I antibody levels were 32 units/mL (IgM) and 40 units/mL (IgG).

Considering the clinical features, laboratory results, and imaging findings, the patient was diagnosed with APS with pulmonary embolism secondary to DVT and thrombocytopenia.

The patient was treated with aspirin (75 mg orally once daily) and rivaroxaban (20 mg orally once daily) for anticoagulation and prevention of blood clots, and a cough syrup for symptomatic relief. She was counseled on the need for long-term anticoagulation, follow-up, and pregnancy planning.

23.8 Summary

Antiphospholipid syndrome (APS) is a systemic autoimmune condition defined by the persistent presence of antiphospholipid antibodies (aPL), which predispose affected individuals to thrombotic events and adverse pregnancy outcomes. The 2023 ACR/EULAR classification criteria have provided a more structured framework for the classification of APS; however, these criteria are primarily intended for research purposes. Despite well-established diagnostic standards, APS continues to demonstrate marked heterogeneity in its clinical presentation and prognosis.

In clinical practice, excessive reliance on laboratory detection of aPL without adequate correlation with the clinical scenario or detailed antibody profiling may result in overdiagnosis, underdiagnosis, or delayed recognition of the disease. This is particularly relevant in so-called "non-criteria" APS manifestations, including microvascular involvement and non-thrombotic organ damage. Appropriate risk stratification is therefore essential, as not all individuals with positive aPL require intensive therapeutic intervention. Although anticoagulation remains the cornerstone of management, it does not uniformly prevent disease progression, and a subset of patients develops refractory manifestations. These challenges underscore the need for well-designed randomized controlled trials to assess emerging therapeutic options.

Future directions should emphasize the development of comprehensive guidelines that integrate clinical features with molecular and genetic data to better define APS endotypes. Such an approach would facilitate personalized, mechanism-driven treatment strategies, ultimately moving beyond the traditional uniform management model and improving overall patient outcomes.

References

1. Lim W. Antiphospholipid antibody syndrome. Hematology Am Soc Hematol Educ Program. 2009;2009(1):233–9.
2. Tincani A, Fontana G, Mackworth-Young C. The history of antiphospholipid syndrome. Reumatismo. 2023;74:144–50.
3. Ortel TL. Antiphospholipid syndrome: laboratory testing and diagnostic strategies. Am J Hematol. 2012;87(Suppl. S1):S75–81.
4. Hughes GR. Thrombosis, abortion, cerebral disease, and the lupus anticoagulant. Br Med J (Clin Res Ed). 1983;287:1088–9.
5. Miyakis S, Lockshin MD, Atsumi T, Branch DW, Brey RL, Cervera R, Derksen RH, de Groot PG, Koike T, Meroni PL, et al. International consensus statement on an update of the classification criteria for definite antiphospholipid syndrome (APS). J Thromb Haemost. 2006;4:295–306.
6. Barbhaiya M, Zuily S, Naden R, Hendry A, Manneville F, Amigo MC, Amoura Z, Andrade D, Andreoli L, Artim-Esen B, et al. The 2023 ACR/EULAR antiphospholipid syndrome classification criteria. Arthritis Rheumatol. 2023;75:1687–1702S.
7. Usta A, Yayla ME, Uslu E, Sezer S, Us E, Ate¸s A, Turgay M. The performance of 2023 American College of Rheumatology (ACR)/European Alliance of Associations for Rheumatology (EULAR) antiphospholipid syndrome classification criteria in a real-world rheumatology department. Mediterr J Hematol Infect Dis. 2024;16:e2024074.
8. Dabit JY, Valenzuela-Almada MO, Vallejo-Ramos S, Duarte-García A. Epidemiology of antiphospholipid syndrome in the general population. Curr Rheumatol Rep. 2022;23:85.
9. Andreoli L, Chighizola CB, Banzato A, Pons-Estel GJ, Ramire de Jesus G, Erkan D. Estimated frequency of antiphospholipid antibodies in patients with pregnancy morbidity, stroke, myocardial infarction, and deep vein thrombosis: a critical reviewof the literature. Arthritis Care Res. 2013;65:1869–73.
10. Cervera R, Serrano R, Pons-Estel GJ, Ceberio-Hualde L, Shoenfeld Y, de Ram6n E, Buonaiuto V, Jacobsen S, Zeher MM, Tarr T, et al. Morbidity and mortality in the antiphospholipid syndrome during a 10-year period: a multicentre prospectivestudy of 1000 patients. Ann Rheum Dis. 2015;74:1011–8.
11. Bo Ic B. Pathogenesis of antiphospholipid syndrome. EJIFCC. 2004;15:54–7.
12. De Groot PG, Meijers JC. β(2)-glycoprotein I: evolution, structure and function. J Thromb Haemost. 2011;9:1275–84.
13. Garcia D, Erkan D. Diagnosis and management of the antiphospholipid syndrome. N Engl J Med. 2018;378:2010–21. https://doi.org/10.1056/NEJMra1705454.
14. De Groot PG, Horbach DA, Derksen RH. Protein C and other cofactors involved in the binding of antiphospholipid antibodies: relation to the pathogenesis of thrombosis. Lupus. 1996;5:488–93. https://doi.org/10.1177/096120339600500532.
15. Nojima J, Kuratsune H, Suehisa E, Iwatani Y, Kanakura Y. Acquired activated protein C resistance associated with IgG antibodies against beta2-glycoprotein I and prothrom-

bin as a strong risk factor for venous thromboembolism. Clin Chem. 2005;51:545–52. https://doi.org/10.1373/clinchem.2004.043414.
16. Ramesh S, Morrell CN, Tarango C, Thomas GD, Yuhanna IS, Girardi G, Herz J, Urbanus RT, de Groot PG, Thorpe PE, et al. Antiphospholipid antibodies promote leukocyte-endothelial cell adhesion and thrombosis in mice by antagonizing eNOS via β2GPI and apoER2. J Clin Invest. 2011;121:120–31.
17. Sule G, Kelley WJ, Gockman K, Yalavarthi S, Vreede AP, Banka AL, et al. Increased adhesive potential of antiphospholipid syndrome neutrophils mediated by b2 integrin mac1. Arthritis Rheumatol. 2020;72:114–24. https://doi.org/10.1002/art.41057.
18. Nayak L, Sweet DR, Thomas A, Lapping SD, Kalikasingh K, Madera A, et al. A targetable pathway in neutrophils mitigates both arterial and venous thrombosis. Sci Transl Med. 2022;14:eabj7465. https://doi.org/10.1126/scitranslmed.abj7465.
19. Ritis K, Doumas M, Mastellos D, Micheli A, Giaglis S, Magotti P, et al. A novel C5a receptor-tissue factor cross-talk in neutrophils links innate immunity to coagulation pathways. J Immunol. 2006;177:4794–802. https://doi.org/10.4049/jimmunol.177.7.4794.
20. Nakamura H, Oku K, Ogata Y, Ohmura K, Yoshida Y, Kitano E, et al. Alternative pathway activation due to low level of complement factor H in primary antiphospholipid syndrome. Thromb Res. 2018;164:63–8. https://doi.org/10.1016/j.thromres.2018.02.142.
21. Kim MY, Guerra MM, Kaplowitz E, Laskin CA, Petri M, Branch DW, et al. Complement activation predicts adverse pregnancy outcome in patients with systemic lupus erythematosus and/or antiphospholipid antibodies. Ann Rheum Dis. 2018;77:549–55. https://doi.org/10.1136/annrheumdis-2017-212224.
22. Chaturvedi S, Braunstein EM, Yuan X, Yu J, Alexander A, Chen H, et al. Complement activity and complement regulatory gene mutations are associated with thrombosis in APS and CAPS. Blood. 2020;135:239–51. https://doi.org/10.1182/blood.2019003863.
23. Pierangeli SS, Liu XW, Barker JH, Anderson G, Harris EN. Induction of thrombosis in a mouse model by IgG, IgM and IgA immunoglobulins from patients with the antiphospholipid syndrome. Thromb Haemost. 1995;74:1361–7.
24. Poulton K, Ripoll VM, Pericleous C, et al. Purified IgG from patients with obstetric but not IgG from non-obstetric antiphospholipid syndrome inhibit trophoblast invasion. Am J Reprod Immunol. 2015;73:390–401.
25. Beltagy A, Trespidi L, Gerosa M, et al. Anti-phospholipid antibodies and reproductive failures. Am J Reprod Immunol. 2021;85:e13258.
26. Meroni PL, Macor P, Durigutto P, et al. Complement activation in antiphospholipid syndrome and its inhibition to prevent rethrombosis after arterial surgery. Blood. 2016;127:365–7.
27. Cervera R, Rodrıguez-Pinto´ I, Espinosa G. The diagnosis and clinical management of the catastrophic antiphospholipid syndrome: a comprehensive review. J Autoimmun. 2018;92:1–11.
28. Cervera R, Khamashta MA, Shoenfeld Y, Camps MT, Jacobsen S, Kiss E, Zeher MM, Tincani A, Kontopoulou-Griva I, Galeazzi M, et al. Morbidity and mortality in the antiphospholipid syndrome during a 5-year period: a multicentre prospective study of 1000 patients. Ann Rheum Dis. 2009;68:1428–32.
29. Mezhov V, Segan JD, Tran H, Cicuttini FM. Antiphospholipid syndrome: a clinical review. Med J Aust. 2019;211:184–8.
30. Berkman SA, Song SS. Ischemic stroke in the young. Clin Appl Thromb Hemost. 2021;27:10760296211002274.
31. Sayar Z, Moll R, Isenberg D, Cohen H. Thrombotic antiphospholipid syndrome: a practical guide to diagnosis and management. Thromb Res. 2021;198:213–21.
32. Nilsson IM, Astedt B, Hedner U, Berezin D. Intrauterine death and circulating anticoagulant ("antithromboplastin"). Acta Med Scand. 1975;197:153–9.
33. Martinez-Zamora MA, Peralta S, Creus M, Tassies D, Reverter JC, Espinosa G, Cervera R, Carmona F, Balasch J. Risk of thromboembolic events after recurrent spontaneous abortion in antiphospholipid syndrome: a case-control study. Ann Rheum Dis. 2012;71:61–6.

34. Antovic A, Sennström M, Bremme K, Svenungsson E. Obstetric antiphospholipid syndrome. Lupus Sci Med. 2018;5:e000197.
35. Bernardi M, Spadafora L, Andaloro S, Piscitelli A, Fornaci G, Intonti C, Fratta AE, Hsu CE, Kaziròd-Wolski K, Metsovitis T, et al. Management of cardiovascular complications in antiphospholipid syndrome: a narrative review with a focus on older adults. J Clin Med. 2024;13:3064.
36. Cervera R, Serrano R, Pons-Estel GJ, Ceberio-Hualde L, Shoenfeld Y, de Ramón E, Buonaiuto V, Jacobsen S, Zeher MM, Tarr T, et al. Morbidity and mortality in the antiphospholipid syndrome during a 10-year period: a multicentre prospective study of 1000 patients. Ann Rheum Dis. 2015;74:1011–8.
37. Leal Rato M, Bandeira M, Romão VC, Aguiar de Sousa D. Neurologic manifestations of the antiphospholipid syndrome—an update. Curr Neurol Neurosci Rep. 2021;21:41.
38. Toubi E, Krause I, Fraser A, Lev S, Stojanovich L, Rovensky J, Blank M, Shoenfeld Y. Livedo reticularis is a marker for predicting multi-system thrombosis in antiphospholipid syndrome. Clin Exp Rheumatol. 2005;23:499–504.
39. Parthvi R, Sikachi RR, Agrawal A, Adial A, Vulisha A, Khanijo S, Talwar A. Pulmonary hypertension associated with antiphospholipid antibody: call for a screening tool? Intractable Rare Dis Res. 2017;6:163–71.
40. Turrent-Carriles A, Herrera-Félix JP, Amigo MC. Renal involvement in antiphospholipid syndrome. Front Immunol. 2018;9:1008.
41. Uludag G, Onghanseng N, Tran ANT, Hassan M, Halim MS, Sepah YJ, Do DV, Nguyen QD. Current concepts in the diagnosis and management of antiphospholipid syndrome and ocular manifestations. J Ophthalmic Inflamm Infect. 2021;11:11.
42. Moulinet T, Dufrost V, Clerc-Urmès I, Wahl D, Zuily S. Risk of thrombosis, pregnancy morbidity or death in antiphospholipid antibodies positive patients with or without thrombocytopenia. Eur J Intern Med. 2021;84:101–3.
43. Barbhaiya M, Zuily S, Naden R, et al. 2023 ACR/EULAR antiphospholipid syndrome classification criteria. Ann Rheum Dis. 2023;82(10):1258–70.
44. Vandevelde A, Chayoua W, de Laat B, et al. Semiquantitative interpretation of anticardiolipin and antibeta2glycoprotein I antibodies measured with various analytical platforms: communication from the ISTH SSC subcommittee on lupus anticoagulant/antiphospholipid antibodies. J Thromb Haemost. 2022;20(2):508–24.
45. Devreese KMJ, de Groot PG, de Laat B, et al. Guidance from the Scientific and Standardization Committee for lupus anticoagulant/antiphospholipid antibodies of the International Society on Thrombosis and Haemostasis: update of the guidelines for lupus anticoagulant detection and interpretation. J Thromb Haemost. 2020;18(11):2828–39.
46. Devreese KMJ, Ortel TL, Pengo V, de Laat B. Laboratory criteria for antiphospholipid syndrome: communication from the SSC of the ISTH. J Thromb Haemost. 2018;16(4):809–13.
47. Devreese KM, Pierangeli SS, de Laat B, Tripodi A, Atsumi T, Ortel TL. Testing for antiphospholipid antibodies with solid phase assays: guidance from the SSC of the ISTH. J Thromb Haemost. 2014;12(5):792–5.
48. Pengo V, Ruffatti A, Legnani C, Gresele P, Barcellona D, Erba N, et al. Clinical course of high-risk patients diagnosed with antiphospholipid syndrome. J Thromb Haemost. 2010;8(2):237–42.
49. Devreese KMJ. Noncriteria antiphospholipid antibodies in antiphospholipid syndrome. Int J Lab Hematol. 2024;46(S1):34–42.
50. Manning JE, Arachchillage DJ, et al. Dilemmas in the diagnosis and management of antiphospholipid syndrome. J Thromb Haemost. 2024;22:2156–70.
51. Knight JS, Erkan D. Rethinking antiphospholipid syndrome to guide future management and research. Nat Rev Rheumatol. 2023;19(5):273–83.
52. Keeling D, Mackie I, Moore GW, Greer IA, Greaves M, British Committee for Standards in Haematology. Guidelines on the investigation and management of antiphospholipid syndrome. Br J Haematol. 2012;157:47–58.

Chapter 24
Diagnosis of Thrombotic Thrombocytopenic Purpura and Current Management

Prattipati Lumen Agarkar, Prabhu Manivannan, and Rajan Kapoor

Abstract Thrombotic thrombocytopenic purpura (TTP) is a rare and life-threatening condition that is characterized by microangiopathic hemolytic anemia (MAHA), severe thrombocytopenia, and organ ischemia. A severe deficiency of ADAMTS13 (<10%) is the most specific biological marker of TTP and has recently been added to its definition. The estimated annual incidence of both immune thrombotic thrombocytopenic purpura (iTTP) and congenital thrombotic thrombocytopenic purpura together (cTTP) combined is two to six cases per million.

There are two types of TTP, namely, congenital and acquired. cTTP is extremely rare, inherited in an autosomal pattern, and occurs due to either homozygous or compound heterozygous mutations of the ADAMTS13 gene (located on chromosome 9q34). This results in a deficiency of von Willebrand factor-cleaving metalloprotease, a disintegrin and metalloproteinase with a thrombospondin type 1 motif, member 13 (ADAMTS13).

Immune TTP (iTTP) occurs due to autoantibodies (Abs) formed against ADAMTS13, resulting in a deficiency of ADAMTS13 (<10%). Over the years, understanding of TTP has evolved alongside advancements in diagnostic modalities and treatment strategies, which provide the basis for updates at various time points.

This chapter on TTP provides an overview of its current definitions, pathogenesis, types, current diagnostic modalities, and treatment strategies. Newer treatment modalities like caplacizumab, rituximab, and plasma-cell-directed therapies have significantly improved the management of TTP by improving treatment outcomes and reducing morbidity. Consequently, we describe current guidelines and recommendations in detail, which would help in the prompt diagnosis and effective treatment of TTP.

P. L. Agarkar · P. Manivannan
Department of Pathology, JIPMER, Puducherry, India

R. Kapoor (✉)
Hematology and Bone Marrow Transplant, Army Hospital RR, New Delhi, India

H. P. Pati et al. (eds.), *Clinical Hematology and Hemato-Oncology*,
https://doi.org/10.1007/978-981-92-1167-8_24

Keywords Thrombotic thrombocytopenic purpura · ADAMTS13 · Caplacizumab · Plasma exchange therapy · Rituximab

Learning Objectives
- To know the updated definition and learn about its types, pathogenesis and the laboratory diagnosis of thrombotic thrombocytopenic purpura.
- To understand the different modalities of treatment options available and the recent advances in its management.

24.1 Introduction

In 1924, nearly a century ago, Eli Moschcowitz first described thrombotic thrombocytopenic purpura (TTP) in a 16-year-old girl as a fatal thrombotic microangiopathy (TMA) presenting with weakness, fever, neurological symptoms, microangiopathic hemolytic anemia (MAHA), and thrombocytopenia, linked to systemic visceral microthrombosis [1]. This showed very fatal outcomes in nearly 90% cases, and its etiology was not known until the 1980s to 1990s.

Subsequently, the introduction of therapeutic plasma exchange (TPE) has drastically improved outcomes, with almost 85% improved survival [2]. It remains both a rare and life-threatening condition, characterized by MAHA, severe thrombocytopenia, and organ ischemia [3]. The estimated annual incidence of both immune thrombotic thrombocytopenic purpura (iTTP) and congenital thrombotic thrombocytopenic purpura together (cTTP) combined is two to six cases per million [4].

24.2 Definition

The definition of TTP has changed over the years. Earlier, it was defined by the presence of pentad, which includes MAHA, thrombocytopenia, fever, and ischemic symptoms affecting the brain and kidneys. Currently, a severe deficiency of ADAMTS13 activity (<10%) is considered as the most specific biological marker and has been added to the updated definition [5]. Accordingly, there are two types of TTP, namely congenital TTP (cTTP) and acquired TTP (aTTP) [6].

24.3 Pathogenesis and Types of TTP

TTP belongs to a group of disorders characterized by MAHA, thrombocytopenia, and occlusive disease affecting small and large vessels. TTP, a rare and fatal medical emergency, arises due to a deficiency of a metalloproteinase known as ADAMTS13 synthesized by the liver. ADAMTS13 has 14 domains and cleaves von Willebrand factor at the Tyr1605-Met1606 site in the A2 domain.

24.3.1 Congenital TTP (cTTP)

cTTP is also called as Upshaw–Schulman syndrome and is defined by the following criteria: (1) Reduced ADAMTS13 activity (<10 IU/dL), (2) Absence of anti-ADAMTS13 autoantibodies, and (3) Confirmatory variants in the ADAMTS13 gene. cTTP is extremely rare, inherited in an autosomal pattern, and occurs due to either homozygous or compound heterozygous mutations in the ADAMTS13 gene (located on chromosome 9q34). This results in a deficiency of von Willebrand factor (VWF)-cleaving metalloprotease, a disintegrin and metalloproteinase with a thrombospondin type 1 motif, member 13 (ADAMTS13) [7]. Absence of ADAMTS13 causes an increase in ultra-large VWF multimers, which subsequently causes the formation of platelet-rich microthrombi. The current estimated prevalence of cTTP cases is 0.5–2.0 per million [7]. These cases manifest immediately after birth or during childhood and present with severe neonatal jaundice and thrombocytopenia accompanied by schistocytes in peripheral smear. However, in some cases, the disease manifests later in adulthood [6].

To date, 758 pathogenic variants of ADAMTS13 have been identified, including 140 reported and 618 novel variants [7]. Seidizadeh et al. conducted a population-based genetic epidemiology analysis, which showed that the estimated prevalence of cTTP is actually 20–40 times higher than previously estimated. Their study emphasizes the importance of suspecting cTTP in cases presenting with MAHA and thrombocytopenia, and it concludes that many cTTP patients remain undiagnosed and would have died during the neonatal period [7].

Nearly 150 mutations of ADAMTS13 have been described in the literature, most of which are spread over the N-terminal region of the gene [3]. The majority of the mutations are missense mutations (~70%), while the remaining ~30% are truncating mutations, including nonsense, frame shift, and splicing mutations [3, 6]. cTTP has a wide spectrum of clinical presentation as evidenced by some of these individuals experiencing disease onset during the neonatal period, followed by multiple recurrent episodes resulting in progressive organ failure. On the other hand, others may have only one episode directly in adulthood, which often responds well to plasma infusion.

24.3.2 Acquired TTP

Immune TTP (iTTP) occurs due to autoantibodies formed against ADAMTS13, resulting in a deficiency of ADAMTS13 (<10%). These autoantibodies can be either neutralizing or non-neutralizing. Neutralizing antibodies inhibit the proteolytic activity of ADAMTS13 by binding to its N-terminal domain and are picked up by functional assays in vitro, while non-neutralizing antibodies accelerate the clearance of ADAMTS13 through opsonization and are picked up in vitro only by enzyme-linked immunosorbent assay (ELISA) [8]. However, both these mechanisms lead to an increase in large VWF multimers in plasma, resulting in the formation of microthrombi.

Autoantibodies formed against ADAMTS13 are polyclonal, with the majority of them belonging to the IgG4 subtype, followed by IgG1. Several studies have demonstrated that the most common site for binding of autoantibodies is the cysteine-rich/Spacer domain (CS domain) [9]. Under normal physiological conditions, ADAMTS13 circulates in a folded configuration. However, allosteric activation of ADAMTS13 by autoantibodies causes loss of folded structure, resulting in an open configuration, which is the most characteristic feature of iTTP [9]. A European multicenter study and a Japanese cohort study have described autoantibodies against the CS domain (anti-CS autoantibodies) as the major and most consistent immunoprofile. Other minor immune profiles have also been described, including anti-CUB1–2, anti-Dys, anti-T2-T5, and anti-T6-T8 Abs [10, 11].

24.4 Basic Laboratory Tests and Differential Diagnosis

TTP is a life-threatening condition and must be identified as early as possible. Due to the broad spectrum of clinical presentation of TTP, not all cases of TTP will present with the classic pentad of symptoms. Thus, it is very important to diagnose TTP with the help of laboratory parameters.

Most TTP cases during acute presentation demonstrate anemia and thrombocytopenia, resulting from platelet consumption in forming platelet-rich microthrombi. In addition, features of hemolysis, such as reticulocytosis, elevated LDH, and decreased haptoglobin, can be seen [12]. A peripheral smear of TTP cases typically shows >1% schistocytes; however, one should keep in mind that the percentage of schistocytes is never considered an indicator for determining the severity of hemolysis, and it is strictly advised not to use this percentage for monitoring therapy response [13].

Knowing the heterogeneity of TTP, which can have both typical and atypical presentations, assessment of renal function (serum creatinine and urea) and cardiac enzyme (troponins) should be done in all suspected cases [14]. Patients with elevated cardiac troponin have a six-fold higher risk of mortality compared to those with normal-range troponin, suggesting that evaluating cardiac troponin helps in identifying patients with high-risk TTP [4]. Organs such as the liver or lungs are not typically involved in TTP due to minimal circulatory shear force. Hence, liver function tests do not show any elevated liver enzymes, which helps to differentiate TTP from other TMAs like HELLP (hemolysis, elevated liver enzymes, and low platelets) syndrome [15].

Microthrombi in TTP are predominantly composed of platelets with a minimal fibrin component, suggesting limited activation of coagulation. In contrast, other TMAs, such as disseminated intravascular coagulation (DIC) or hemolytic uremic syndrome (HUS), show fibrin-rich thrombi with significant activation of coagulation. For this reason, basic coagulation profile—including PT, APTT, TT, fibrinogen, and fibrin-degraded products (FDPs)—is typically normal in TTP but abnormal in other TMAs such as DIC or HUS [12].

Solid organ malignancies, such as mucin-producing tumors of the gastrointestinal tract, ovary, pancreas, and breast, as well as hematological malignancies like acute promyelocytic leukemia, tend to induce DIC. In addition, some of the cancer therapy drugs can cause drug-induced thrombotic microangiopathy (DI–TMA). However, none of these cancer-associated TMAs show a severe reduction in ADAMTS13 levels; therefore, it is recommended not to use TPE in this group of patients [3].

Very rarely, TTP can be mimicked by autoimmune hemolytic anemia with thrombocytopenia (Evans syndrome) [16]. In all hemolytic anemias with worsening anemia and thrombocytopenia despite giving intravenous immunoglobulin and prednisolone, the differential diagnosis of TTP should be kept in mind. Although TTP classically presents as Coombs-negative hemolytic anemia, it can occasionally show Coombs positivity, especially in systemic lupus erythematosus [17]. Failure to promptly recognize TTP masquerading as Evans syndrome can lead to fatal outcomes.

Paroxysmal nocturnal hemoglobinuria (PNH) presents with diverse manifestations, including hemolysis, bone marrow failure, and thrombosis. In 25–30% of cases, hemoglobinuria is the presenting symptom. Cola-colored urine, presence of urine hemosiderin, and evidence of intravascular hemolysis can aid in suspecting these cases. On the other end of the spectrum, thrombotic PNH presents with thrombosis in unusual sites, including the microvasculature in the brain and kidneys [18].

Differentiating TTP from catastrophic antiphospholipid syndrome (CAPS) can be clinically difficult, as both conditions can present with anemia, thrombocytopenia, and recurrent thrombosis. Therefore, measuring ADAMTS13 activity is very crucial in such circumstances [19]. Moreover, literature mentions that antiphospholipid syndrome (APS) itself can cause anti-ADAMTS13 antibodies, resulting in TTP. While APS and TTP are individually treatable conditions, their simultaneous occurrence is associated with poor outcomes despite following good treatment strategies [19, 20].

A baseline pretreatment screening for viral markers is essential to exclude human immunodeficiency virus (HIV) and hepatitis virus before plasma exposure [3].

24.5 Laboratory Investigations for ADAMTS13

With advances in technology, various tests are now available for assaying ADAMTS13, including first-generation and second-generation assays.

24.5.1 First-Generation Assays

In 1982, Moake et al. evaluated ultra-large VWF multimers using immunoelectrophoresis with uncleaved VWF as a substrate obtained from endothelial cell culture, and their study shed light for the first time on laboratory measurement of ADAMTS13 [21]. Although this assay served as the gold standard for detecting ADAMTS13 activity, it was cumbersome and time-consuming, with a turnaround time of 2–3 days—a significant limitation given that TTP is a clinical emergency.

To overcome this limitation, two additional first-generation assays, namely, VWF collagen-binding assay (VWF:CB) [22] and ristocetin-cofactor (Rco)-based VWF cleaving protease (VWFcp) activity assay, were developed [23]. VWF:CB assay, described in 1999, is based on the preferential binding of high-molecular-weight VWF multimer to collagen. The Rco-based VWFcp activity assay, described in 2002, is based on the positive correlation between VWF multimer size and Rco activity [22, 23]. The invention of synthetic VWF peptides with a cleavage site for ADAMTS13 paved the way for the development of second-generation assays [24].

24.5.2 Second-Generation Assays

A second-generation assay known as surface-enhanced laser desorption/ionization time-of-flight mass spectrometry (SELDI–TOF–MS) was introduced based on its ability to provide rapid protein and peptide analysis. It is a highly sensitive assay that can detect ADAMTS13 as low as 2.5% activity and is the only second-generation assay that does not depend on measuring light signals. However, still its application is limited due to longer turnaround time and the requirement for good expertise in the technique [25].

Kato et al. developed mouse monoclonal antibodies directed against the VWF cleavage site for ADAMTS13, which led to the development of TECHNOZYM® (Technoclone, Vienna, Austria), an enzyme-linked immunosorbent assay (ELISA) [26]. In this assay, VWF peptides are initially tagged with glutathione S-transferase (GST) and captured onto an anti-GST-coated plate. The captured GST-tagged VWF peptides are then incubated with patient plasma, during which the peptides are cleaved by the enzyme, and the amount of cleavage depends on the activity of ADAMTS13.

Next, the mixture is further incubated with horseradish peroxidase (HRP)-conjugated antibody, which binds to the cleaved peptides, followed by the addition of a chromogenic substrate. The absorbance measured corresponds to the number of cleaved peptides and reflects ADAMTS13 activity [12, 26]. The major advantage is its high sensitivity, as it can detect as low as 0.5% activity of the normal control levels. Other advantages of this assay include its sensitivity in detecting ADAMTS13 inhibitors, which is essential for diagnosing acquired TTP. The detection limit for this ELISA-based assay is 0.1 BU/mL [26].

Fluorescence resonance energy transfer (FRET) is another second-generation assay that uses a synthetically prepared 73-amino-acid peptide known as FRETS–VWF73 [27]. This peptide is modified such that the fluorophore is attached to one side of the cleavage site and a quencher to the other side. The quencher, being in proximity, blocks the emission of the fluorophore.

Upon incubation of this peptide with patient plasma, ADAMTS13 cleaves the peptide. The cleaved peptides move far away from the quencher and start emitting fluorescence. The measured fluorescence corresponds to the amount of ADAMTS13 activity in the patient's plasma [12, 27]. Several studies have been done comparing FRET with other second-generation assays and have shown good correlation [28, 29]. However, one of the main disadvantages of FRET is that it is affected by hyperbilirubinemia. Bilirubin in the plasma quenches the fluorescence signal, resulting in falsely low ADAMTS13 levels, which can lead to misdiagnosis of TTP [30].

The HemosIL AcuStar®, a fully automated and rapid assay with a run time of just 33 min, is a two-step immunoassay. In the first step, magnetic particles coated with VWF73 peptide with a cleavage site for ADAMTS13 are incubated with patient plasma. The cleavage of the VWF73 peptide occurs in proportion to the extent of ADAMTS13 activity. The second step includes washing and incubation of contents with isoluminol-labeled monoclonal antibodies that bind to the cleavage sites. Chemiluminescence is then measured as relative light units, which are proportional to ADAMTS13 activity. This assay shows a lower limit of quantification of 0.3% with good precision (CV <5.2%) [31]. Figure 24.1 highlights the different second-generation functional assays for measuring ADAMTS13 activity.

24.6 ADAMTS13 Antigen (Ag) Assay

Several assays are currently available to quantitatively measure VWF protein. Some of the methods include ELISA, latex-enhanced immunoassay (LIA), chemiluminescent immunoassay, and flow cytometry, with ELISA and LIA being the most widely used assays [32]. However, these tests vary in their ability to differentiate between full-length, truncated, and mutant forms of ADAMTS13.

ADAMTS13 Ag is consistently reduced in cTTP. However, it shows greater variability in iTTP, with some cases showing normal ADAMTS13 Ag levels due to immune complex formation, while others show reduced levels due to accelerated clearance. Consequently, this assay may not be helpful without ADAMTS13 activity assays. Because of this limited diagnostic utility, this assay is not currently recommended in the routine workup of TTP, except in cTTP cases where ADAMTS13 Ag levels are very low [33].

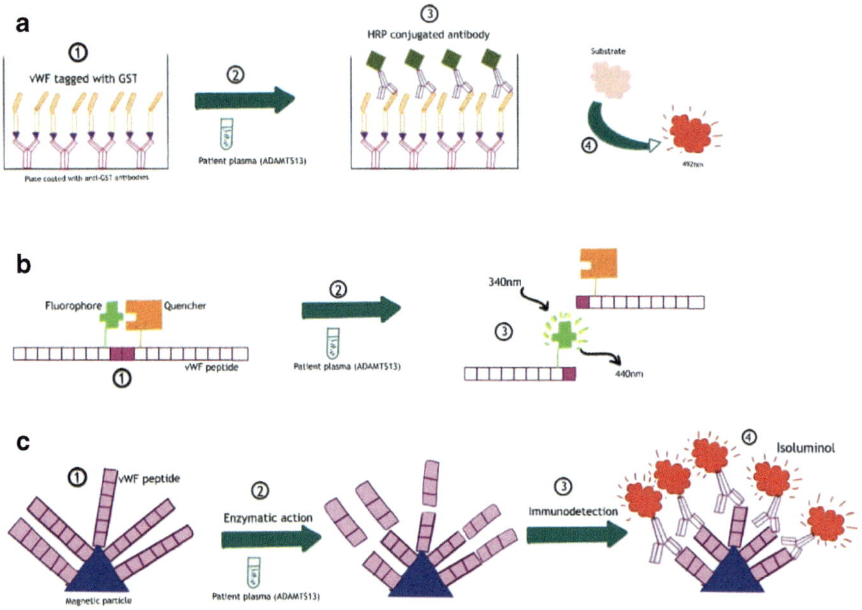

Fig. 24.1 Different second-generation functional assays for measuring ADAMTS13 activity. (**a**) ELISA based TECHNOZYM® showing: (1) Capturing of glutathione S-transferase (GST) tagged VWF. (2) Incubation with patient plasma. (3) Incubation with horseradish peroxidase (HRP) conjugated antibody. (4) Amount of HRP is measured using colorimetric substrate reaction as it corresponds to ADAMTS13 activity; (**b**) FRET assay showing: (1) VWF peptide with a fluorophore and a quencher. (2) Incubation with patient plasma. (3) Measuring fluorescence from fluorophore which corresponds to ADAMTS13 enzymatic activity. (**c**) HemosIL® chemiluminescent assay: (1) Capturing of VWF peptide on magnetic particle. (2) Incubation with patient plasma. (3) Incubation with isoluminol-conjugated antibodies. (4) Measurement of chemiluminescence

24.7 French Score and PLASMIC Score

The French score is a two-component predictive diagnostic score that predicts severe ADAMTS13 deficiency based on platelet count and serum creatinine [34]. PLASMIC score is a seven-component predictive tool that stratifies the risk of having severe ADAMTS13 deficiency in TMA cases. It includes platelet count $<30 \times 10^9/\mu L$, MCV <90 fL, PT-international normalized ratio (INR) <1.5, serum creatinine <2.0 mg/dL, no active cancer, no history of solid-organ or stem cell transplant, and hemolysis biomarkers [35]. This score helps in differentiating TTP from other TMAs, such as HUS, which closely mimics TTP. A PLASMIC score of 0–4, 5, and 6–7 is considered low, intermediate, and high risk, respectively. Studies have shown that the PLASMIC score is superior to the French score, as it accurately categorizes a greater number of non-TTP cases as low risk [35].

24.8 Revised Definitions of Outcomes for iTTP

Clinical Response There should be sustained platelet counts of $\geq 150 \times 10^9/L$, reduced LDH (<1.5 times the upper limit of normal) without any evidence of new or ongoing ischemic organ damage [36]. The current definition for clinical response lacks ADAMTS13 activity, as the primary aim of TPE is to attain clinical response rather than rapid recovery of ADAMTS13 activity [36].

Clinical Exacerbation A decrease in platelet count (to $<150 \times 10^9/L$) after achieving clinical response but prior to clinical remission, with or without evidence of new or ongoing ischemic organ damage for 30 days period after discontinuation of TPE or anti-VWF therapy [36].

Clinical Remission Sustained clinical response in either of the two following conditions:

1. In the absence of TPE or anti-VWF therapy for the last 30 days
2. By attaining ADAMTS13 remission, either partial or complete [36]

Partial ADAMTS13 Remission It is defined as ≥20% ADAMTS13 activity but less than the lower limit of normal (LLN) [36].

Complete ADAMTS13 Remission It is defined as ADAMTS13 activity of ≥LLN [36].

In view of the biological variability of ADAMTS13 activity and variability in ADAMTS13 laboratory measurement, it is recommended to repeat ADAMTS13 activity testing before confirming ADAMTS13 remission. Moreover, it is advised to focus on trends of ADAMTS13 activity rather than emphasizing a single specific value [36, 37].

These revised remission definitions sharply demarcate the difference between clinical remission and ADAMTS13 remission (partial or complete) [36]. It is further highlighted that some of the patients may attain clinical remission even before attaining ADAMTS13 remission, putting them at risk of clinical relapse [38]. In such scenarios, intervention with immunosuppressive therapy using rituximab, to achieve ADAMTS13 remission, can help prevent clinical relapse [39, 40].

Clinical Relapse It is defined as a decline in platelet count to $<150 \times 10^9/L$ after achieving clinical remission, with or without evidence of new-onset ischemic damage. It should be noted that other causes of thrombocytopenia must be ruled out, and severe ADAMTS13 deficiency (i.e., <10% ADAMTS13 activity) should be documented to confirm the relapse [36].

ADAMTS13 Relapse It is defined as a reduction in ADAMTS13 activity to <20% following ADAMTS13 remission (either partial or complete) [36].

In contrast to older definitions, these revised definitions have distinguished clinical relapse from ADAMTS13 relapse and have highlighted that ADAMTS13 relapse can occur in a patient without any clinical relapse [36]. Since a decline in ADAMTS13 activity to <20% (i.e., ADAMTS13 relapse) is well known to predict clinical relapse, intervention with immunosuppressive therapy such as prophylactic rituximab during ADAMTS13 relapse is recommended to prevent clinical relapse [39].

24.9 Treatment Strategies

TTP is a life-threatening condition, and all suspected cases require immediate referral and rapid transfer to a center with better facilities. It is very important to consider a pretransfer review by a skilled medical team to ensure safe transfer, especially if intubation is required in the acute phase of TTP [3]. Irrespective of the time of day at presentation, TPE must be commenced ideally within 4 h of presentation and within 8 h to reduce mortality risk [3].

24.10 Therapeutic Plasma Exchange (TPE) Therapy

The introduction of TPE in the management of TTP has significantly reduced the mortality from 90% to 10–20%, and proved to be superior to plasma infusion, which is now restricted to inevitable emergencies. Since human serum albumins lack ADAMTS13, they are not recommended in TTP management [2, 3]. TPE is carried out once daily with fresh frozen plasma (FFP) with a volume of 1.5 times the circulating plasma volume of the patient, calculated using the following equation:

$$\begin{aligned}\text{Circulating plasma volume}(\text{mL}) = {} & \text{Body weight}(\text{kg}) \times 70(\text{mL}/\text{Kg}) \\ & \times \left(1 - \text{hematocrit value}(\%)/100\right)\end{aligned}$$

According to earlier recommendations, TPE was continued for 2 days after the platelet count returned to normal. However, caplacizumab enables us to stop TPE upon normalization of the platelet count [3]. TPE can be done twice daily in refractory cases, especially those with new-onset neurological and cardiac symptoms [36]. It replenishes functional ADAMTS13 while simultaneously removing autoantibodies and ultra-large VWF multimers [3].

24.10.1 Steroid Therapy

Although corticosteroid usage is presumed to reduce the formation of autoantibodies against ADAMTS13, there has not been sufficient data to demonstrate its efficacy in TTP. In 2017, Cataland et al. demonstrated the efficacy of prednisolone and cyclosporine as adjuvants to TPE in TTP management. They concluded that prednisolone is superior to cyclosporine in suppressing ADAMTS13 autoantibody production. In their study, prednisolone-treated patients showed quicker suppression of autoantibodies, whereas cyclosporine-treated patients took a longer time [3, 41]. However, cyclosporine is not an ineffective drug for immunosuppression, as there are a good number of reports that describe its efficacy in refractory TTP or as prophylactic therapy to prevent relapse [42, 43].

In a randomized multicentric study done by Balduini et al., high-dose methylprednisolone (10 mg/kg/day for 3 days followed by 2.5 mg/kg/day) achieved quicker hematological response and higher remission rates with respect to standard dose (1 mg/kg/day) [44].

24.10.2 Rituximab and Obinutuzumab

Rituximab is a humanized monoclonal antibody targeted against CD20 on B-lymphocytes and has been used in the treatment of iTTP for the past two decades. Initially, its usage was restricted to patients refractory to frontline treatment. Nowadays, the following are the indications of rituximab in iTTP treatment: (1) as an early adjunct to standard treatment, (2) in cases refractory to standard treatment, and (3) as a prophylactic treatment for iTTP patients in clinical remission with reduced ADAMTS13 activity [45].

Early administration of rituximab, ideally within 3 days of admission, along with standard treatment, reduces inpatient stay, relapse rates, and mortality [46, 47]. A dose of 375 mg/m^2 rituximab is recommended with a minimum of four infusions; however, it can be further continued if the ADAMTS13 activity fails to normalize. During TPE therapy, rituximab should be infused once every 3–4 days, as TPE affects the pharmacokinetics of rituximab and clears it from circulation [48].

Obinutuzumab is an effective alternative treatment option for patients who are refractory or experience anaphylaxis with rituximab. It comes with an acceptable safety profile and has been proven to partially overcome rituximab refractoriness in heavily pretreated patients [49].

24.10.3 Caplacizumab

Caplacizumab is a humanized, bivalent, variable domain-only immunoglobulin fragment. It is directed against the A1 fragment of VWF and prevents its interaction with the platelet glycoprotein Ib-IX-V receptor [50]. Caplacizumab marks a milestone in the treatment of aTTP, being the first approved targeted therapy [51]. Scully et al. in their double-blinded clinical trial stated that the time taken for normalization of platelet count was shorter among individuals treated with caplacizumab than the individuals who were given a placebo, indicating that caplacizumab prevents the formation of microthrombi and reduces platelet consumption. They mentioned that patients treated with caplacizumab showed a lower incidence of TTP-related deaths, recurrence, and major thromboembolic events during the trial period [50]. However, one should understand that caplacizumab prevents the fall in platelet counts but does not change the underlying immune disease process.

Upon confirmation of TTP, a 10-mg dose of caplacizumab should be administered intravenously 15 min prior to TPE, followed by a 10-mg dose given subcutaneously after completion of TPE. After completing TPE, a daily 10-mg subcutaneous dose should be continued for 30 days, with subsequent assessment of ADAMTS13 activity. Caplacizumab can be discontinued if the ADAMTS13 activity is >10%; otherwise, it is advised to continue for an additional 28 days. Although caplacizumab should be started based on suspicion of TTP, it should be discontinued once TTP is ruled out [3, 52].

Caplacizumab reduces VWF activity and can cause mild bleeding events, such as epistaxis or gingival bleeding, which resolve with minimal intervention. Rarely, severe bleeding events occur requiring VWF concentrates for intervention [50].

Initially, caplacizumab was approved for only adults (>18 years); later, the Bergstrand et al. study came up with recommendations for pediatric patients aged between 2 and 18 years. A 5-mg dose is recommended for those weighing <40 kg, and a 10-mg dose for those >40 kg [53].

24.10.4 Plasma Cell-Directed Therapy

In patients who are refractory to standard treatment, corticosteroids and rituximab, plasma cell-directed therapy such as daratumumab (an anti-CD38 antibody) and bortezomib (a proteasome inhibitor) are viable options. Both drugs are well-tolerated with acceptable safety profiles. Lee et al. suggest the use of bortezomib in specific scenarios: (1) where caplacizumab is unaffordable or unavailable, (2) in patients who attain clinical remission but without normalization of ADAMTS13 activity, and (3) in relapsed patients where caplacizumab and rituximab have failed [54]. Additionally, Berg et al. mention that daratumumab rapidly normalizes ADAMTS13 activity by targeting autoantibody-producing plasma cells, making it a valuable option in refractory or relapsed iTTP cases [55]. The treatment approach for iTTP is summarized in Fig. 24.2.

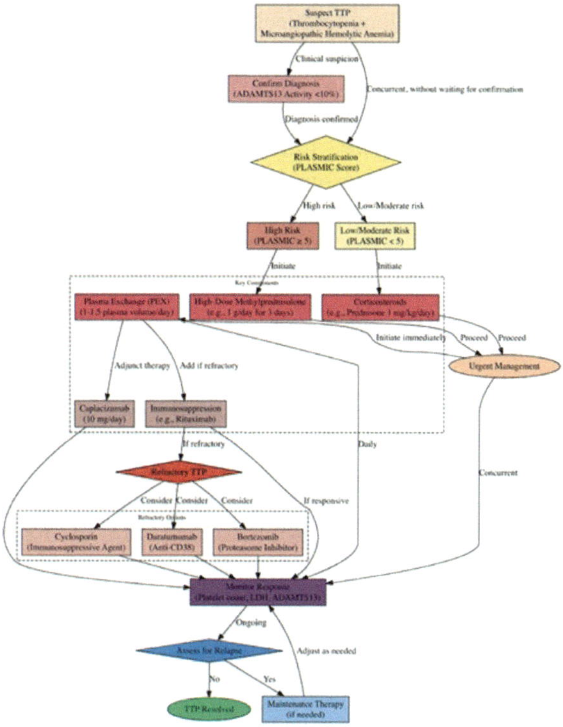

Fig. 24.2 The treatment approach for iTTP

24.11 Treatment for cTTP

ADAMTS13 replacement can be done through either FFP infusion or intermediate purity factor VIII (FVIII) concentrates, such as BPL 8Y/Koate-DVI®. Scully M et al. have confirmed the therapeutic response of BPL 8Y, resulting in rapid normalization of platelet count, reduced number of inpatient days, and can be easily administered on an outpatient basis for treatment [56].

Plasma infusion is preferred over BPL 8Y as there is no clear evidence to support the superiority of using FVIII concentrates. Moreover, plasma infusion has demonstrated better posttreatment ADAMTS13 activity than FVIII concentrates [56, 57]. In addition, there has been much variability in ADAMTS13 concentrations among various FVIII products [58]. However, FVIII products like BPL 8Y can be considered in acute episodes of cTTP.

Peyvandi et al. used Koate–DVI®, a plasma-derived VWF-FVIII concentrate, for off-label treatment in both acute episodes and prophylaxis of cTTP in a limited number of cases. It has a higher functional ADAMTS13 content compared to the other VWF-FVIII concentrates. However, the data on post-infusion recovery is limited, and further studies are needed to establish its role in cTTP treatment [57].

The International Society on Thrombosis and Hemostasis (ISTH) recommends 10–15 mL/kg of FFP once every 1–3 weeks [58]. The regimens vary, with some patients needing long-term periodic FFP transfusions, while other cases may require only episodic transfusions during disease exacerbations [52].

Recombinant ADAMTS13 is a novel treatment option that avoids many risks associated with products derived from plasma. However, it is currently in phase 3 clinical trials; its phase 1 clinical trial proved safety and efficacy without antibody production against recombinant ADAMTS13, even after repeated administration [59, 60].

24.12 TTP in Pregnancy

TTP association with pregnancy is well known, primarily resulting from hemostatic and immune changes that occur during pregnancy. Physiologically, pregnancy itself is a hypercoagulable state, which gets exaggerated during the last trimester to reduce blood loss during childbirth. VWF concentration gradually increases, reaching the peak in the last trimester, while ADAMTS13 activity gradually reduces and reaches as low as 25–30%. Nevertheless, ADAMTS13 level typically normalizes within 1–3 weeks postpartum [61].

The treatment of TTP in pregnancy is essentially similar to that of a non-pregnant woman, with additional cautious measures for drug toxicity to the fetus and decisions regarding delivery. Women who present with TTP for the first time during pregnancy are advised to be treated as iTTP cases with daily TPE and steroids. They should be further investigated, whether they fit in iTTP or are the first manifestation of cTTP during pregnancy [3, 61].

Once cTTP is proven, they are treated with solvent/detergent FFP infusion (SD–FFP) or TPE regularly at a dose of 10–15 ml/kg daily until clinical remission and platelet recovery, followed by maintenance infusions twice every month throughout pregnancy and postpartum period [61]. For refractory iTTP cases in pregnancy, additional immunosuppressive drugs such as corticosteroids (oral prednisolone 1 mg/kg recommended), with other options including cyclosporine, azathioprine, and rituximab. For all women with iTTP, normalization of ADAMTS13 is recommended prior to pregnancy [3].

Caplacizumab administration in pregnancy is currently not recommended, as it is a nanobody that can cross the placental barrier, imposing a risk of bleeding as it reduces VWF activity markedly [3]. However, there are some case reports that suggest caplacizumab as an effective option in the treatment of iTTP cases refractory to TPE and corticosteroids [34, 62]. Notably, Coppo et al. mentioned that there were no adverse events noted in mother or neonate following caplacizumab therapy [34].

In all women with acute TTP episodes, once platelet count crosses over $50 \times 10^9/\mu L$, it is advised to start low-dose aspirin and/or prophylactic low-molecular-weight heparin to reduce the risk of placental vascular damage [3, 61].

24.13 Prognostic Factors

The following factors were considered as predictors of mortality in TTP, which include elderly age (especially >60 years), renal failure, neurological involvement, arterial thrombosis, and platelet transfusion [63]. Jin et al. demonstrated that younger age has been associated with a higher risk of relapse when ADAMTS13 activity is reduced [38]. Ethnicity can play a role in the outcomes, with Black ethnicity showing better survival over Whites, even with similar disease severity [64].

24.14 Follow-Up of TTP

Once platelet normalization is consistently attained, the patient can be discharged and reviewed on an outpatient basis. It is recommended to review once every week till the completion of immunosuppressive therapy, with monitoring of ADAMTS13 activity [3]. Caplacizumab may be continued or reordered if the ADAMTS13 activity remains low. Patient, family members, and relatives should be educated and trained in the administration of caplacizumab. Moreover, they must also be informed regarding TTP and its expected adverse events, which may occur at any time [3].

TTP requires long-term follow-up to deal with both physical and psychological complications. Patients should also be monitored regularly for ADAMTS13 activity to prevent clinical relapses. Various organ damage can be assessed by checking renal function tests, echocardiogram, magnetic resonance imaging of the brain, blood pressure checks, and urine protein-to-creatinine ratio. Assessment of memory, particularly short-term memory, is crucial and can be done with the help of questionnaires. Whenever possible, assessment of neurocognition is advised [3]. In addition, psychological assessment pertaining to depression and anxiety should be made, as nearly 60% of patients have shown these symptoms following an acute episode of iTTP [65].

24.15 A Case History with Details

A 30-year-old female developed acute onset of seizure on the second day of the postpartum period. On examination, she is found to have pallor, mild icterus, febrile with a temperature of 102 °F, and petechial rashes all over the body. Her baseline investigation revealed hemoglobin of 50 g/L, total white blood cell count of 25×10^9/L, platelet count of 15×10^9/L, corrected reticulocyte count of 7%, total bilirubin (5 mg%) with direct fraction of 0.2 mg%, serum creatinine (4 mg%), serum lactate dehydrogenase (LDH) (2000 units), activated partial thromboplastin time (APTT): 22 s (test)/30 s (control), prothrombin time (PT): 12 s (test)/12 s

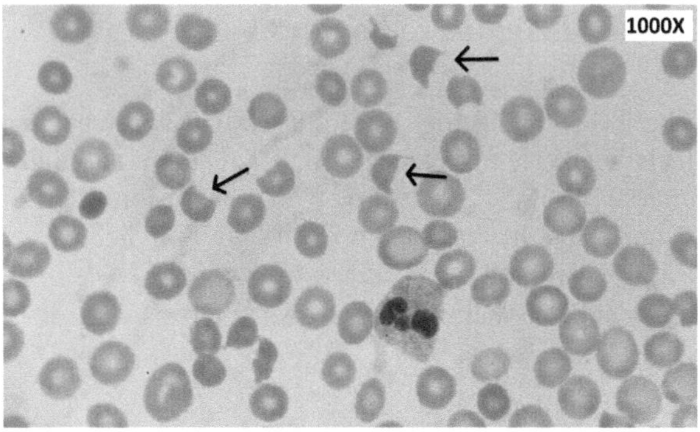

Fig. 24.3 Peripheral smear picture (1000X) showing schistocytes marked with black arrow (←) and thrombocytopenia

(control), thrombin time (TT): 15 s (test)/15 s (control), fibrinogen—300 s (test)/400 s (control), and negative D-dimer. What is your diagnosis, and how will you diagnose and confirm this entity?

Along with neurological and renal dysfunction, our case demonstrated laboratory evidence of MAHA and thrombocytopenia in the peripheral smear (Fig. 24.3), with a normal baseline coagulation profile, which helped us to effectively rule out other differential diagnoses, such as HELLP syndrome/atypical HELLP syndrome, and narrowed down the diagnosis toward TTP. Viral markers, dengue, and malaria work-up turned out to be negative. Coombs test was negative, following which ADAMTS13 activity testing was ordered. Meanwhile, PLASMIC score assessment was performed to evaluate the risk of severe ADAMTS13 deficiency, which turned out to be six (i.e., high risk).

With a high suspicion of TTP based on clinical grounds and laboratory parameters, the patient was shifted to the intensive care unit and started on high-dose methylprednisolone and TPE while awaiting ADAMTS13 test results. The results revealed severe ADAMTS13 deficiency (5%) with the presence of anti-ADAMTS13 antibodies, thereby confirming the diagnosis of iTTP.

The patient received high-dose methylprednisolone and TPE for 5 days, resulting in normalization of platelets by the fifth day. Steroid therapy was then tapered, and TPE was continued for two additional days. She was discharged on tenth day with weekly follow-up planned until the completion of steroid therapy. Family members were educated about potential adverse events, and the patient remained in clinical and complete ADAMTS13 remission at the last follow-up.

References

1. Moschcowitz E. An acute febrile pleiochromic anemia with hyaline thrombosis of the terminal arterioles and capillaries; an undescribed disease. Am J Med. 1952;13(5):567–9.
2. Rock GA, Shumak KH, Buskard NA, Blanchette VS, Kelton JG, Nair RC, et al. Comparison of plasma exchange with plasma infusion in the treatment of thrombotic thrombocytopenic purpura. Canadian Apheresis Study Group. N Engl J Med. 1991;325(6):393–7.

3. Scully M, Rayment R, Clark A, Westwood JP, Cranfield T, Gooding R, et al. A British Society for Haematology Guideline: diagnosis and management of thrombotic thrombocytopenic purpura and thrombotic microangiopathies. Br J Haematol. 2023;203(4):546–63.
4. Alwan F, Vendramin C, Vanhoorelbeke K, Langley K, McDonald V, Austin S, et al. Presenting ADAMTS13 antibody and antigen levels predict prognosis in immune-mediated thrombotic thrombocytopenic purpura. Blood. 2017;130(4):466–71.
5. Joly BS, Coppo P, Veyradier A. Thrombotic thrombocytopenic purpura. Blood. 2017;129(21):2836–46.
6. Bain BJ, Hoffbrand AV, Steensma DP. Hoffbrand's essential haematology. 8th ed. Oxford: Wiley Blackwell; 2020. Br J Haematol 2020;191(1):130–130.
7. Seidizadeh O, Cairo A, Mancini I, George JN, Peyvandi F. Global prevalence of hereditary thrombotic thrombocytopenic purpura determined by genetic analysis. Blood Adv. 2024;8(16):4386–96.
8. Ferrari S, Mudde GC, Rieger M, Veyradier A, Kremer Hovinga JA, Scheiflinger F. IgG subclass distribution of anti-ADAMTS13 antibodies in patients with acquired thrombotic thrombocytopenic purpura. J Thromb Haemost. 2009;7(10):1703–10.
9. Dainese C, Valeri F, Bruno B, Borchiellini A. Anti-ADAMTS13 autoantibodies: from pathophysiology to prognostic impact—a review for clinicians. J Clin Med. 2023;12(17):5630.
10. Kangro K, Roose E, Joly BS, Sinkovits G, Falter T, von Auer C, et al. Anti-ADAMTS13 autoantibody profiling in patients with immune-mediated thrombotic thrombocytopenic purpura. Blood Adv. 2021;5(17):3427–35.
11. Sakai K, Matsumoto M, De Waele L, Dekimpe C, Hamada E, Kubo M, et al. ADAMTS13 conformation and immunoprofiles in Japanese patients with immune-mediated thrombotic thrombocytopenic purpura. Blood Adv. 2023;7(1):131–40.
12. Dimopoulos K, Tripodi A, Goetze JP. Laboratory investigation and diagnosis of thrombotic thrombocytopenic purpura. Crit Rev Clin Lab Sci. 2023;60(8):625–39.
13. Egan JA, Hay SN, Brecher ME. Frequency and significance of schistocytes in TTP/HUS patients at the discontinuation of plasma exchange therapy. J Clin Apher. 2004;19(4):165–7.
14. Imanirad I, Rajasekhar A, Zumberg M. A case series of atypical presentations of thrombotic thrombocytopenic purpura. J Clin Apher. 2012;27(4):221–6.
15. Martin JN, Rinehart BK, May WL, Magann EF, Terrone DA, Blake PG. The spectrum of severe preeclampsia: comparative analysis by HELLP (hemolysis, elevated liver enzyme levels, and low platelet count) syndrome classification. Am J Obstet Gynecol. 1999;180(6):1373–84.
16. Mudra SE, Ardoin K, Aggarwal V, Diltz G, Alcedo Andrade PE, Broome CM. Thrombotic thrombocytopenic purpura masquerading as Evans syndrome. Am J Hematol. 2024;99(12):2381–5.
17. Aleem A, Al-Sugair S. Thrombotic thrombocytopenic purpura associated with systemic lupus erythematosus. Acta Haematol. 2006;115(1–2):68–73.
18. Manivannan P, Ahuja A, Pati HP. Diagnosis of paroxysmal nocturnal hemoglobinuria: recent advances. Indian J Hematol Blood Transfus. 2017;33:453–62.
19. Viner M, Murakhovskaya I. A rare combination of thrombotic thrombocytopenic purpura and antiphospholipid syndrome. Blood Coagul Fibrinolysis. 2017;28(5):411–5.
20. Dolin HH, Dziuba M, Pappada SM, Papadimos TJ. Presumed antiphospholipid syndrome and thrombotic thrombocytopenic purpura: an infrequent association. Clin Case Reports. 2019;7(10):1984–8.
21. Moake JL, Rudy CK, Troll JH, Weinstein MJ, Colannino NM, Azocar J, et al. Unusually large plasma factor VIII: von Willebrand factor multimers in chronic relapsing thrombotic thrombocytopenic purpura. N Engl J Med. 1982;307(23):1432–5.
22. Gerritsen HE, Turecek PL, Schwarz HP, Lämmle B, Furlan M. Assay of von Willebrand factor (vWF)-cleaving protease based on decreased collagen binding affinity of degraded vWF: a tool for the diagnosis of thrombotic thrombocytopenic purpura (TTP). Thromb Haemost. 1999;82(5):1386–9.

23. Böhm M, Vigh T, Scharrer I. Evaluation and clinical application of a new method for measuring activity of von Willebrand factor-cleaving metalloprotease (ADAMTS13). Ann Hematol. 2002;81(8):430–5.
24. Cruz MA, Whitelock J, Dong JF. Evaluation of ADAMTS-13 activity in plasma using recombinant von Willebrand factor A2 domain polypeptide as substrate. Thromb Haemost. 2003;90(6):1204–9.
25. Jin M, Cataland S, Bissell M, Wu HM. A rapid test for the diagnosis of thrombotic thrombocytopenic purpura using surface enhanced laser desorption/ionization time-of-flight (SELDI-TOF)-mass spectrometry. J Thromb Haemost JTH. 2006;4(2):333–8.
26. Kato S, Matsumoto M, Matsuyama T, Isonishi A, Hiura H, Fujimura Y. Novel monoclonal antibody-based enzyme immunoassay for determining plasma levels of ADAMTS13 activity. Transfusion (Paris). 2006;46(8):1444–52.
27. Kokame K, Nobe Y, Kokubo Y, Okayama A, Miyata T. FRETS-VWF73, a first fluorogenic substrate for ADAMTS13 assay. Br J Haematol. 2005;129(1):93–100.
28. Crist RA, Rodgers GM. A comparison of two commercial ADAMTS13 activity assays with a reference laboratory method. Lab Med. 2009;40(4):232–5.
29. Palla R, Valsecchi C, Bajetta M, Spreafico M, De Cristofaro R, Peyvandi F. Evaluation of assay methods to measure plasma ADAMTS13 activity in thrombotic microangiopathies. Thromb Haemost. 2011;105(2):381–5.
30. Meyer SC, Sulzer I, Lämmle B, Kremer Hovinga JA. Hyperbilirubinemia interferes with ADAMTS-13 activity measurement by FRETS-VWF73 assay: diagnostic relevance in patients suffering from acute thrombotic microangiopathies. J Thromb Haemost. 2007;5(4):866–7.
31. Posters from congress ISTH2017 [Internet]. ES: DRAFT EDITORS S.L.; 2017 [cited 2025 Feb 11]. Available from: https://doi.org/10.3252/pso.eu.ISTH2017.2017.
32. Favaloro EJ, Mohammed S, Patzke J. Laboratory testing for von Willebrand Factor Antigen (VWF:Ag). Methods Mol Biol. 2017;1646:403–16.
33. Peyvandi F, Palla R, Lotta LA, Mackie I, Scully MA, Machin SJ. ADAMTS-13 assays in thrombotic thrombocytopenic purpura. J Thromb Haemost. 2010;8(4):631–40.
34. Coppo P, Schwarzinger M, Buffet M, Wynckel A, Clabault K, Presne C, et al. Predictive features of severe acquired ADAMTS13 deficiency in idiopathic thrombotic microangiopathies: the French TMA reference center experience. PLoS ONE. 2010;5(4):e10208.
35. Bendapudi PK, Hurwitz S, Fry A, Marques MB, Waldo SW, Li A, et al. Derivation and external validation of the PLASMIC score for rapid assessment of adults with thrombotic microangiopathies: a cohort study. Lancet Haematol. 2017;4(4):e157–64.
36. Cuker A, Cataland SR, Coppo P, De La Rubia J, Friedman KD, George JN, et al. Redefining outcomes in immune TTP: an international working group consensus report. Blood. 2021;137(14):1855–61.
37. Page EE, Kremer Hovinga JA, Terrell DR, Vesely SK, George JN. Thrombotic thrombocytopenic purpura: diagnostic criteria, clinical features, and long-term outcomes from 1995 through 2015. Blood Adv. 2017;1(10):590–600.
38. Jin M, Casper TC, Cataland SR, Kennedy MS, Lin S, Li YJ, et al. Relationship between ADAMTS13 activity in clinical remission and the risk of TTP relapse. Br J Haematol. 2008;141(5):651–8.
39. Westwood JP, Thomas M, Alwan F, McDonald V, Benjamin S, Lester WA, et al. Rituximab prophylaxis to prevent thrombotic thrombocytopenic purpura relapse: outcome and evaluation of dosing regimens. Blood Adv. 2017;1(15):1159–66.
40. Jestin M, Benhamou Y, Schelpe AS, Roose E, Provôt F, Galicier L, et al. Preemptive rituximab prevents long-term relapses in immune-mediated thrombotic thrombocytopenic purpura. Blood. 2018;132(20):2143–53.
41. Cataland SR, Kourlas PJ, Yang S, Geyer S, Witkoff L, Wu H, et al. Cyclosporine or steroids as an adjunct to plasma exchange in the treatment of immune-mediated thrombotic thrombocytopenic purpura. Blood Adv. 2017;1(23):2075–82.

42. Nosari A, Redaelli R, Caimi TM, Mostarda G, Morra E. Cyclosporine therapy in refractory/relapsed patients with thrombotic thrombocytopenic purpura. Am J Hematol. 2009;84(5):313–4.
43. Yilmaz M, Eskazan AE, Unsal A, Taninmis H, Kara E, Cetiner M, et al. Cyclosporin a therapy on idiopathic thrombotic thrombocytopenic purpura in the relapse setting: two case reports and a review of the literature. Transfusion (Paris). 2013;53(7):1586–93.
44. Balduini CL, Gugliotta L, Luppi M, Laurenti L, Klersy C, Pieresca C, et al. High versus standard dose methylprednisolone in the acute phase of idiopathic thrombotic thrombocytopenic purpura: a randomized study. Ann Hematol. 2010;89(6):591–6.
45. Özpolat HT, Stolla M. Rituximab in the treatment of immune-mediated thrombotic thrombocytopenic purpura. Blood Transfus. 2023;21(5):369–74.
46. Westwood JP, Webster H, McGuckin S, McDonald V, Machin SJ, Scully M. Rituximab for thrombotic thrombocytopenic purpura: benefit of early administration during acute episodes and use of prophylaxis to prevent relapse. J Thromb Haemost. 2013;11(3):481–90.
47. Scully M, McDonald V, Cavenagh J, Hunt BJ, Longair I, Cohen H, et al. A phase 2 study of the safety and efficacy of rituximab with plasma exchange in acute acquired thrombotic thrombocytopenic purpura. Blood. 2011;118(7):1746–53.
48. Mcdonald V, Manns K, Mackie IJ, Machin SJ, Scully MA. Rituximab pharmacokinetics during the management of acute idiopathic thrombotic thrombocytopenic purpura. J Thromb Haemost. 2010;8(6):1201–8.
49. Weisinger J, Fadlallah J, Barbet C, Provot F, Poullin P, Neel A, et al. Obinutuzumab in rituximab refractory or intolerant immune-mediated thrombotic thrombocytopenic purpura. Blood. 2024;144(Supplement 1):139.
50. Scully M, Cataland SR, Peyvandi F, Coppo P, Knöbl P, Kremer Hovinga JA, et al. Caplacizumab treatment for acquired thrombotic thrombocytopenic purpura. N Engl J Med. 2019;380(4):335–46.
51. Gavriilaki E, Koravou E, Dimou-Mpesikli S, Nikolousis E, Banti A, Pontikoglou C, et al. Caplacizumab for acquired thrombotic thrombocytopenic purpura: real-world multicenter data on re-administration and plasma exchange free treatment. Blood. 2022;140(Supplement 1):8503–4.
52. Matsumoto M, Miyakawa Y, Kokame K, Ueda Y, Wada H, Higasa S, et al. Diagnostic and treatment guidelines for thrombotic thrombocytopenic purpura (TTP) in Japan 2023. Int J Hematol. 2023;118(5):529–46.
53. Bergstrand M, Hansson E, Delaey B, Callewaert F, De Passos SR, Sargentini-Maier ML. Caplacizumab model-based dosing recommendations in pediatric patients with acquired thrombotic thrombocytopenic purpura. J Clin Pharmacol. 2022;62(3):409–21.
54. Lee NCJ, Yates S, Rambally S, Sarode R, Ibrahim IF, Shen Y, et al. Bortezomib in relapsed/refractory immune thrombotic thrombocytopenic purpura: a single-centre retrospective cohort and systematic literature review. Br J Haematol. 2024;204(2):638–43.
55. van den Berg J, Kremer Hovinga JA, Pflеger C, Hegemann I, Stehle G, Holbro A, et al. Daratumumab for immune thrombotic thrombocytopenic purpura. Blood Adv. 2022;6(3):993–7.
56. Scully M, Gattens M, Khair K, Liesner R. The use of intermediate purity factor VIII concentrate BPL 8Y as prophylaxis and treatment in congenital thrombotic thrombocytopenic purpura. Br J Haematol. 2006;135(1):101–4.
57. Peyvandi F, Mannucci PM, Valsecchi C, Pontiggia S, Farina C, Retzios AD. ADAMTS13 content in plasma-derived factor VIII/von Willebrand factor concentrates. Am J Hematol. 2013;88(10):895–8.
58. Zheng XL, Vesely SK, Cataland SR, Coppo P, Geldziler B, Iorio A, et al. ISTH guidelines for treatment of thrombotic thrombocytopenic purpura. J Thromb Haemost. 2020;18(10):2496–502.
59. Stubbs MJ, Kendall G, Scully M. Recombinant ADAMTS13 in severe neonatal thrombotic thrombocytopenic purpura. N Engl J Med. 2022;387(25):2391–2.

60. Scully M, Knöbl P, Kentouche K, Rice L, Windyga J, Schneppenheim R, et al. Recombinant ADAMTS-13: first-in-human pharmacokinetics and safety in congenital thrombotic thrombocytopenic purpura. Blood. 2017;130(19):2055–63.
61. Ferrari B, Peyvandi F. How I treat thrombotic thrombocytopenic purpura in pregnancy. Blood. 2020;136(19):2125–32.
62. Odetola O, Martin KA, Dreyer M, Rajan P, Zakarija A, Stein BL. A safe and effective use of caplacizumab in pregnancy-related acquired thrombotic thrombocytopenic purpura. Br J Haematol. 2023;202(4):879–82.
63. Goel R, King KE, Takemoto CM, Ness PM, Tobian AAR. Prognostic risk-stratified score for predicting mortality in hospitalized patients with thrombotic thrombocytopenic purpura: nationally representative data from 2007 to 2012. Transfusion (Paris). 2016;56(6):1451–8.
64. Martino S, Jamme M, Deligny C, Busson M, Loiseau P, Azoulay E, et al. Thrombotic thrombocytopenic purpura in black people: impact of ethnicity on survival and genetic risk factors. PLoS One. 2016;11(7):e0156679.
65. Falter T, Alber KJ, Scharrer I. Long term outcome and sequelae in patients after acute thrombotic thrombocytopenic purpura episodes. Hamostaseologie. 2013;33(2):113–20.

Part IV
Myeloma & Lymphoid Malignancies

Chapter 25
Liquid/Fluid Biopsy and Its Role in Lymphomas

Dheeraj Gautam and Rashi Sharma

Abstract Circulating tumor DNA (ctDNA) has emerged as a powerful biomarker for the detection, monitoring, and genotyping of hematopoietic malignancies, particularly lymphoid cancers. This chapter explores the characterization of ctDNA in lymphoid malignancies, highlighting its applications in diagnosis, treatment response assessment, and minimal residual disease (MRD) detection. Early studies focused on immunoglobulin heavy chain (IgH) rearrangements, while advancements in next-generation sequencing (NGS) techniques, such as Immunoglobulin High-Throughput Sequencing (IgHTS) and Cancer Personalized Profiling by Deep Sequencing (CAPP-seq), have significantly improved sensitivity and accuracy.

We discuss large-scale studies that validate the clinical utility of ctDNA, including comparisons with traditional imaging methods like PET-CT. While extensive research has been conducted on B-cell lymphomas, there remains a gap in T-cell lymphoma ctDNA profiling, necessitating further investigations. Additionally, we examine the role of ctDNA genotyping in detecting single-nucleotide variations (SNVs), insertions/deletions (Indels), copy number variations (CNVs), and fusion events, with an emphasis on its integration into clinical decision-making.

Emerging evidence underscores the significance of DNA methylation analysis as a biomarker for tumor suppressor gene silencing in lymphomas. Furthermore, ctDNA quantification has been linked to risk stratification, with studies demonstrating its predictive value in treatment outcomes. However, challenges persist, including the lower sensitivity of plasma ctDNA detection in central nervous system (CNS) lymphomas and the potential for false positives due to clonal hematopoiesis.

Finally, the chapter explores the role of liquid biopsies in MRD detection, emphasizing their advantages over invasive tissue biopsies. Despite the absence of

D. Gautam (✉) · R. Sharma
Medanta, The Medicity, Gurgaon, India
e-mail: Dheeraj.Gautam@Medanta.org

H. P. Pati et al. (eds.), *Clinical Hematology and Hemato-Oncology*,
https://doi.org/10.1007/978-981-92-1167-8_25

standardized protocols, liquid biopsies show promise in guiding therapeutic decisions, reducing reliance on invasive procedures, and improving patient outcomes. Future advancements in ultra-deep sequencing, tumor-informed approaches, and optimized sample processing will be critical in refining ctDNA-based diagnostics for lymphoid malignancies.

Keywords Liquid biopsy · Circulating tumor DNA · Cell-free DNA · Circulating tumor cells · Minimal residual disease · Next-generation sequencing · Droplet digital PCR · MicroRNAs

Learning Objectives

- Explain the concept and significance of liquid biopsy in medical diagnostics.
- Identify the limitations of traditional tissue biopsies.
- Recognize different tumor-derived substances (e.g., ctDNA, cfDNA, CTCs, microRNAs).
- Clinical applications of liquid biopsy.
- Identify and explain circulating tumor DNA (ctDNA) markers, circulating tumor cells (CTCs), and extracellular vesicles.
- Understand liquid biopsy technologies and techniques.
- Discuss the role of ctDNA in diagnosing and monitoring lymphoma.
- Summarize key studies on ctDNA in lymphoma, including IgH and TCR rearrangement analysis.
- ctDNA quantification and risk stratification in lymphoma,
- Evaluate the role of ctDNA levels in predicting lymphoma prognosis.
- Future Directions in cfDNA and ctDNA research.

25.1 Introduction

The term "biopsy" originated from Besnier in France during the late 1800s while he was engaged in dermatological studies. It stems from the Greek words (bio), meaning life, and (opsis), meaning to see.

Today, a biopsy is understood as the process of extracting cells or tissues for further examination by a pathologist. Traditional tissue biopsies face several challenges, including common complications such as pain and bleeding at the site of the procedure. Moreover, these methods are not very effective in detecting early-stage tumors or residual lesions, and their use for assessing treatment response and prognosis is limited. Additionally, capturing the molecular diversity of metastatic tumors can be challenging, as the evolving nature of cancer genomes often cannot be fully represented by a single localized biopsy [1].

Table 25.1 Components and sources of liquid biopsy

Fluids biopsied	Materials isolated/evaluated
Blood	ctDNA/cfDNA, CTCs, proteins, RNA, DNA, methylation, extracellular vesicles
Urine	ctDNA/cfDNA, proteins, RNA
Ascites fluid	ctDNA/cfDNA
Pleural fluid	ctDNA/cfDNA
Cerebrospinal fluid (CSF)	ctDNA/cfDNA

Table 25.2 Clinical applications of liquid biopsy

Application category	Purpose
Tumor heterogeneity	Understand genetic diversity within tumors
Predicting immune checkpoint response	Evaluate the likelihood of immunotherapy success
Prognostic tool	Forecast disease outcome or progression
Potentially actionable alterations	Identify mutations with therapeutic potential
Evaluating response/resistance	Monitor treatment response and drug resistance
Assessing residual disease	Detect remaining cancer post-treatment
Early cancer detection	Identify cancer at an initial stage
Assessing difficult-to-biopsy tumors	Analyze cancers where tissue biopsy is hard or risky

The phrase "liquid biopsy" was introduced by Pantel and colleagues in their 2010 assessment of circulating tumor cells (CTCs), highlighting the clinical value of analyzing peripheral blood samples [2]. Broadly, liquid biopsy encompasses the extraction and examination of tumor-derived substances, such as DNA, RNA, or intact cells, from blood or various body fluids. Sources for liquid biopsies can include plasma, serum, urine, saliva, stool, and cerebrospinal fluid (Table 25.1). However, some experts argue that cerebrospinal fluid should not be considered a suitable specimen for liquid biopsy due to the invasive procedure required for its collection.

Liquid biopsies are increasingly recognized as a valuable tool for diagnosing hematological malignancies, assessing prognosis, and monitoring treatment [3] (Table 25.2). Instead of performing invasive lymph node biopsies, we can evaluate circulating tumor DNA (ctDNA) or other biomarkers present in the bloodstream.

The primary functions of liquid biopsies in hematological malignancies include:

- Early Detection and Diagnosis: Liquid biopsies can identify genetic mutations and tumor loads associated with lymphoma, sometimes prior to the manifestation of symptoms.
- Risk Stratification and Prognosis: Levels of ctDNA often correlate with the severity of the disease, facilitating predictive assessments of outcomes [4].

- Treatment Monitoring: They offer an immediate assessment of the effectiveness of therapies (such as CAR T-cell therapy), which allows for timely intervention if treatment resistance arises [5].
- Detection of Minimal Residual Disease (MRD): Following treatment, even small quantities of lymphoma can be detected in the blood, aiding in decisions regarding further therapeutic approaches. Liquid biopsies, although still in development, hold the potential to transform the management of lymphoma, ensuring monitoring is less invasive and more accurate [6].

Liquid biopsies primarily depend on the analysis of circulating tumor DNA (ctDNA), but researchers are also exploring other markers, including circulating tumor cells (CTCs), microRNAs, and extracellular vesicles.

The key markers utilized in liquid biopsies for hematological malignancies are

1. Circulating Tumor DNA (ctDNA) Markers.
    - Clonal Immunoglobulin (Ig) Gene Rearrangements: Employed to identify specific B-cell clones linked to lymphoma, aiding in diagnosis and monitoring disease progression.
    - Mutations such as TP53, MYD88, EZH2, and CARD11: Commonly observed in aggressive B-cell lymphomas like DLBCL and mantle cell lymphoma [7].
    - BCL2, BCL6, and MYC Rearrangements: Significant in the context of double-hit and triple-hit lymphomas, impacting treatment strategies.
2. Tracking Minimal Residual Disease (MRD).
    - ctDNA Clearance: Patients demonstrating rapid clearance of ctDNA post-treatment typically exhibit more favorable outcomes [6].
    - Pre-treatment ctDNA Levels: Elevated levels of ctDNA before treatment are associated with a poorer prognosis.
3. Circulating Tumor Cells (CTCs).
    - Detected in peripheral blood, offering insights into the advancement of disease [8].
    - Although less researched compared to ctDNA, it shows potential for non-Hodgkin lymphomas (NHL).
4. Cell-Free RNA (cfRNA) and MicroRNAs (miRNAs).
    - Profiles of miRNAs assist in distinguishing between various lymphoma types [9].
    - Specific miRNAs are linked to resistance to treatment and the likelihood of relapse.
5. Extracellular Vesicles and Exosomes.
    - Transport RNA and proteins specific to lymphoma.
    - Might shed light on the tumor microenvironment and the immune system's response [10].

25.1.1 Liquid Biopsy: Innovative Technologies and Clinical Uses

Various techniques have been developed for isolating and analyzing circulating tumor DNA (ctDNA) and cell-free DNA (cfDNA). These methods include droplet digital polymerase chain reaction, BEAMing (beads, emulsion, amplification, magnetics), tagged-amplicon deep sequencing (TAm-Seq), cancer personalized profiling by deep sequencing (CAPP-Seq), whole genome bisulfite sequencing (WGBS-Seq), whole exome sequencing (WES), and whole genome sequencing (WGS).

Circulating tumor cells (CTCs) are captured using biomarker-driven cell capture methods and can undergo either positive or negative enrichment based on their biophysical characteristics and other properties. Blood biopsies present a less invasive alternative to traditional tissue biopsies, allowing for easier serial samples that yield essential molecular insights in real time. cfDNA consists of DNA fragments that circulate freely in the bloodstream; these fragments may originate from tumors or from normal cellular processes. In contrast, ctDNA specifically refers to DNA that comes from tumor cells. CTCs are cells that are released from tumors into the bloodstream, and although they generally exist in the circulation for a short period (about 1 to 2.5 h) before being eliminated by the immune system, a small portion can persist and contribute to metastatic spread. Both ctDNA/cfDNA and CTCs can be analyzed through next-generation sequencing (NGS) (Fig. 25.1).

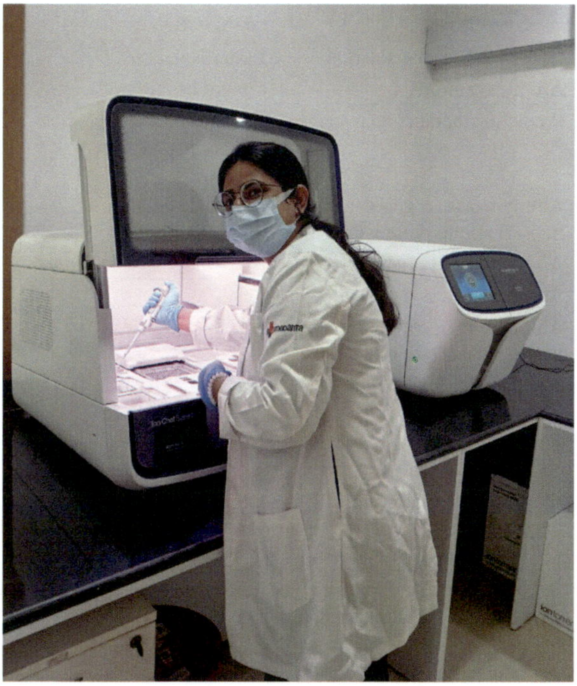

Fig. 25.1 NGS laboratory with the Ion Genestudio S5 System

25.2 Methods for Detecting ctDNA/cfDNA

DdPCR is capable of detecting genomic material at concentrations as low as 0.01–1.0%, making it useful for identifying rare mutations and assessing copy number variants. However, it is limited to analyzing known genomic sequences [3] (Table 25.3).

Similarly, BEAMing is an economical and sensitive technique for identifying known mutations, integrating PCR with flow cytometry to detect changes as low as 0.01%, demonstrating strong agreement with tissue testing results [3].

CAPP-Seq specializes in observing changes in ctDNA and cfDNA by constructing extensive genomic libraries tailored to individual patients.

TAm-Seq offers highly specific and sensitive detection, achieving an accuracy of around 97% and capable of identifying DNA levels down to 2% by using primers for tagging and recognizing genomic sequences [3]. This method is noteworthy for its high sequencing capacity, reduced processing time and costs, as well as the ability to sequence millions of DNA molecules concurrently.

Whole exome sequencing endeavors to thoroughly characterize all tumor mutations present, thereby identifying potential oncogenes and tumor suppressor genes. Yet, its sensitivity might be compromised compared to other techniques due to its focus on exomic variations. Nonetheless, it is appreciated for its cost-effectiveness and high output.

Table 25.3 Comparison of ctNDA/cfDNA and CTCs

	ctDNA/cfDNA	CTCs
Ease of collection/isolation	Easier isolation	More difficult to isolate
Ability to culture	Cannot be cultured	Can be cultured
Predicting therapeutic response	Changes in levels predict response/resistance/relapse	Changes in levels can predict response/resistance/relapse
Ability to assess genomic/transcriptomic/protein data	Can analyze DNA	Can analyze DNA, RNA, and protein
Ability to assess functional data	No	Yes
Ability to assess methylation	Yes	Yes
Ability to perform fluorescent in situ hybridization analysis	No	Yes
Ability to perform single cell analysis	No	Yes
Ability to perform chromosomal analysis	No	Yes
Challenges in collection/interpretation	Cell death under therapy can modify ctDNA levels	Small quantities of ctDNA in circulation can be confounded by CHIP

CHIP clonal hematopoiesis of indeterminate potential, *cfDNA* cell-free DNA, *ctDNA* circulating tumor DNA, *CTC* circulating tumor cells

WGBS-Seq is recognized as the benchmark for analyzing DNA methylation. It delivers precise measurements at the cytosine level and boasts exceptional accuracy. Although it can identify partially methylated regions in tumor cells, the presence of DNA in different states of degradation can lead to decreased sensitivity in this approach. Cells are collected through specific biomarkers present on their surface, which adhere to a device or magnetic material. Nonetheless, there is no all-encompassing CTC antigen, as CTCs express an array of surface markers.

25.3 Technologies for CTC Detection

The following methods have been used to isolate CTCs: immunogenicity, positive enrichment, negative enrichment, and enrichment based on biophysical properties (i.e., size, density). CTC enrichment by immunogenicity is one of the most widely used techniques for isolating CTCs [11].

There are various approaches to achieving positive enrichment of circulating tumor cells (CTCs). The Adna Test employs antibody-coated beads designed for specific cancer types, followed by real-time polymerase chain reaction to analyze the expression patterns in the cells. Another technique, magnetic-activated cell sorting (MACS), utilizes magnetic nanoparticles.

1. CTC Enrichment Techniques

CTC enrichment is necessary due to their low concentration in blood. The main methods fall under two categories

A. Immunogenicity-Based Enrichment

These methods use antibodies to isolate or deplete specific cell types based on surface markers and include

(i) Positive Enrichment (Capturing CTCs) Techniques

- ADNA Test: Uses antibody-coated beads specific to cancer types; followed by real-time PCR for gene expression analysis.
- Magnetic-Activated Cell Sorting (MACS): Magnetic nanoparticles linked to antibodies capture CTCs.
- MagSweeper: Automated system with a robotic magnetic rod and antibody-coated beads for precise CTC capture [12].

(ii) Negative Enrichment (Removing Non-CTCs) Techniques

- EasySep System: Targets and removes CD45+ white blood cells using magnetic particles and antibodies.
- Quadrupole Magnetic Separator: Functions as a magnetic flow cytometer to deplete labeled unwanted cells.
- Any of the above methods can be used.

B. Biophysical Property-Based Enrichment

This relies on physical differences between CTCs and normal blood cells and includes

- Size-based filtration.
- Density-gradient centrifugation.

These approaches are marker-independent but may be less specific.

2. Molecular Analysis of Isolated CTCs

Once enriched, CTCs can be analyzed at the molecular level to detect abnormalities. The following analysis can be done

A. DNA Analysis

This includes

- DNA Amplification: To detect mutations or copy number variations.
- Fluorescence In Situ Hybridization (FISH): To identify gene amplifications or translocations.

B. RNA/Transcriptome Analysis

This includes

- RNA Sequencing: For comprehensive gene expression profiling.
- In Situ Hybridization: To visualize RNA expression within individual cells.

3. Use of cfDNA.

CAR-T therapy is used for treating hematologic cancers with high success. However, new tools are needed for monitoring treatment response beyond imaging or biopsies.
cfDNA and Genomic Instability Number (GIN) in CAR-T therapy response

- cfDNA is a non-invasive biomarker obtained from blood,
- In a pilot study with 12 patients receiving CAR-T for aggressive B-cell lymphoma [13]
  - Patients with a complete response had GIN <170.
    Those with relapse showed GIN elevation before imaging confirmation.
- cfDNA can potentially predict relapse earlier and monitor therapy effectiveness over time,

4. Clinical Significance of CTCs

CTCs originate from cancer stem cells undergoing epithelial–mesenchymal transition (EMT)—A key process in metastasis [14].

Clinical applications

- Early cancer detection.
- Metastasis analysis.
- Prognosis prediction.
- Treatment response monitoring.
- Understanding therapy resistance.

5. Extracellular Vesicles (EVs) and Their Role in Lymphoma.

   A. History and Types.

      - Discovered in 1983; named exosomes in 1987 [9].
      - Now collectively referred to as extracellular vesicles (EVs), which include.

        - Exosomes.
        - Microvesicles.
        - Shedding vesicles.
          Ectosomes.

   B. Contents and Functions.

      - Carry proteins, RNAs (including miRNAs), lipids, and metabolites.
      - Enable intercellular communication.
      - miRNAs in EVs are especially linked to tumor progression and drug resistance.

25.4 Cell-Free DNA and Circulating Tumor DNA

Cell-free DNA, abbreviated as cfDNA, encompasses all DNA fragments that circulate in the bloodstream and are not enclosed within cells. In individuals with no health issues, cfDNA concentration typically ranges between 0 and 100 ng/mL, with an average around 30 ng/mL, primarily deriving from cells that have undergone apoptosis or necrosis. In the context of cancer, the portion of cfDNA that originates from tumors is referred to as ctDNA [4]. This ctDNA can provide valuable information about mutations, methylation patterns, fragment sizes, transcriptomic data, and viral loads. Research conducted by Dennis Lo and colleagues has indicated that the average half-life of circulating fetal DNA post-delivery is approximately 16.3 min, hinting at the possibility of quick clearance for tumor-associated DNA as well.

For the collection of cfDNA, plasma obtained from centrifuged whole blood or specialized blood collection tubes designed for cfDNA sampling is typically employed. Common extraction techniques include the phenol-chloroform method, sodium iodide method, magnetic bead method, and various commercial kits for DNA isolation (Table 25.4).

Table 25.4 Methods of circulating tumor DNA (ctDNA) detection in peripheral blood

Method	Sensitivity	Advantages	Limitations
qPCR	0.01%	High reproducibility of data, and many facilities available for implementation	Time-consuming, laborious
Digital PCR (ddPCR)	0.001%	Easy to perform, standard curve not needed	Lack of standardization data analysis, expensive
Targeted sequence (panel)	0.01%	Available on a commercial basis	Low sensitivity
Whole genome sequence	1%	Detect rare mutations	Suitable for tumor-rich samples

25.5 Characterization of ctDNA in Lymphoid Malignancies

- Research on ctDNA in hematopoietic tumors primarily focuses on lymphoid malignancies, possibly due to the higher prevalence of lymphoma compared to other blood cancers [15]. Early studies focused on immunoglobulin heavy chain (IgH) rearrangements. Key Historical Studies in ctDNA Detection for Lymphoid Cancers997 (Frickhofen et al.): Used PCR to detect rearranged IgH DNA in plasma from NHL and B-precursor ALL patients [32]. 2011 (He et al.): Used IgCap technology to isolate and sequence rearranged IgH DNA fragments in plasma [33].NGS Advances: High-throughput deep sequencing (IgHTS) of B-cell receptor (BCR) genes using multiplex PCR is now widely used.

25.6 ctDNA in Lymphoma Diagnosis and Monitoring

A. Use of ctDNA in large-scale studies.

- Armand et al.: Used Sequenta LymphoSIGHT to detect IgH and IgK reconstitution in DLBCL and MLBCL [16].).
- Kurtz et al.: Compared IgHTS-based ctDNA analysis with PET-CT in 75 cases of DLBCL [15].
- Roschewski et al.: Five-year follow-up of 126 DLBCL patients confirmed the utility of ctDNA monitoring post-treatment [17].
- Sarkozy et al.: Used IgHTS to analyze tumor vs. plasma ctDNA in follicular lymphoma (FL) [18].
- Wagner-Johnston et al. & Kumar et al.: Investigated HIV-related B cell lymphoma and mantle cell lymphoma (MCL) using IgHTS [19].

B. Limited Research on T-cell Lymphomas.

- Zhang et al. (2021): Detected T cell receptor (TCR) rearrangements in 78% of T-cell lymphoma cases via HTS, highlighting the need for more research [20].

25.7 ctDNA Genotyping and Advanced Sequencing Techniques

A. Early studies on ctDNA Mutations 2009 (Hosny et al.): Used direct sequencing to detect TP53 mutations in NHL patients [21].

   - However, early methods were restricted to a few target genes.

B. Introduction of Advanced Sequencing Methods.

   - CAPP-seq (2014, Newman et al.) [22].
     - Hybrid-capture-based targeted sequencing.
     - Detects SNVs, Indels, copy number variations (CNVs), and fusion regions in cell-free tumor DNA.
       Applied to NHL ctDNA, demonstrating improved sensitivity compared to IgHTS.
   - Low-Pass Whole-Genome Sequencing (WGS).
     - Identifies fusion events, copy number variations (CNVs), and mutations.
       Agarwal et al. used it to refine ibrutinib + venetoclax therapy.

C. ctDNA Genotyping in Clinical Applications,

   - Botzen et al.: First detected SNVs/Indels in lymphoid malignancies via ctDNA [23].
   - Rushton et al.: Used a 63-gene panel for ctDNA genotyping in 135 DLBCL cases [19].
   - Camus et al.: Conducted the first prospective ctDNA genotyping after chemotherapy in cHL, showing better MRD detection than PET-CT [24].
   - Rossi et al. & Spina et al.: Applied CAPP-seq to DLBCL and cHL [25].

D. Challenges and Considerations.

   - Plasma ctDNA detection is less sensitive in CNS lymphomas, raising concerns about feasibility.
   - cfDNA from cerebrospinal fluid (CSF) may be more reliable in CNS lymphoma cases,

25.8 DNA Methylation and Tumor Suppressor Gene Analysis

Methylation as a Cancer Biomarker: CpG island methylation in gene promoter regions silences tumor suppressor genes. It has been heavily studied in leukemia and lymphoma.

Key Studies in ctDNA Methylation are given below

- 2003 (Deligezer et al.): Found methylated tumor suppressor gene 16 in cfDNA of lymphoma patients [26].
- 2007 (Shi et al.)
  - Developed a CpG island DNA microarray for methylation profiling [27].
  - Detected DLC-1 gene methylation in NHL plasma ctDNA.
    DLC-1 methylation disappeared after successful chemotherapy, as confirmed by quantitative methylation-specific PCR.

Clinical Applications

- DNA methylation analysis is now integral for genetic assessment and treatment monitoring in lymphoid malignancies.

25.9 ctDNA Quantification and Risk Stratification in Lymphoma

A. ctDNA Quantification Studies done by Delfau-Larue et al. Used ddPCR to measure ctDNA [28] and found a correlation between pre-treatment ctDNA levels and total metabolic tumor volume (PET-CT) in FL. Kurtz et al. developed the Continuous Individualized Risk Index (CIRI) for DLBCL [29] and used pre-treatment ctDNA levels to classify high- and low-risk groups.

Challenge in Clinical Implementation is the need to define how to integrate ctDNA data with PET-CT and other lab results for lymphoma monitoring.

25.10 Techniques for ctDNA and cfDNA Detection in Lymphomas

A. Methods for cfDNA evaluation include the detection of gene mutations or the identification of immunoglobulin heavy chain (IGHV) rearrangement.
B. Additionally, cfDNA analysis is used when a tissue biopsy is not possible and also for.
   - disease monitoring without repeated biopsies.
C. ctDNA genotyping using ultra-deep NGS is used for cancer personalized profiling by deep sequencing (CAPP-seq) and detects point mutations, indels, rearrangements, and CNVs,
D. The Oncomine cell-free total nucleic acid research assay is used for detecting cfDNA in NSCLC patients. It uses Tag sequencing for barcoded library generation.

Assay Workflow

Reverse transcribe cell-free total nucleic acid.

↓

Amplify targets in a 96-well plate.

↓

Target amplicons.

↓

Amplify target amplicons with barcoded primers.

↓

Purify the barcoded library.

↓

Size-select the barcoded library.

25.11 Quantify the Library by qPCR

Dilute the library, and if the library read length is 200 base pairs, then an optimal concentration of 50pM is achieved. Then, polyclonality and low-quality filter results from a sequencing run performed with ion sphere particles (ISPs), and the concentration is properly titrated. Combine libraries, and finally, the analysis is done.[8]

All the B-cell lymphomas have a unique IGHV rearrangement that can be detected on CT DNA using PCR or an NGS-based assay. However, to confirm the tumor origin of the IGHV rearrangement, initial identification of IGHV has to be done on tissue biopsy. So we can use NGS-based methods like coloSeQ, which is an FDA-approved assay for minimal residual disease (MRD) detection in patients with chronic lymphocytic leukemia(CLL), B cell acute lymphoblastic leukemia(B ALL), using IGHV and ctDNA MRD monitoring in lymphoma patients [30]. The drawback of these kinds of assay used for IGHV rearrangement is that they fail to detect clonal V(D)J rearrangements in 20% of lymphomas. The tumor agonist approach poses a lot of challenges because the cfDNA data is not compared with the tissue biopsy data in these cases, which can result in false-positive variants. The tumor-informed approach is better suited for the MRD monitoring and detection of new variants; however, genetic variants associated with clonal hematopoiesis(CH) still remain the source of false positive results.

25.12 The Role of Liquid Biopsies in Detecting Minimal Residual Disease in Lymphoma

Evaluating treatment response in hematological malignancies is crucial for optimizing patient care. Generally, achieving a deeper level of response has been associated with improved outcomes, and methods for assessing minimal residual disease

(MRD) have become more refined. The implementation of liquid biopsies, which involves analyzing genetic alterations in nucleic acids from peripheral blood or other body fluids, is being explored and developed through advanced molecular techniques like next-generation sequencing (NGS) for MRD monitoring. This approach often reduces the need for more invasive testing across various hematological malignancies. Although there is currently no standardized protocol for MRD monitoring via liquid biopsies, accumulating evidence supports its correlation with other response measurement techniques and patient prognosis.

Hematological cancers arise from changes at the molecular level that affect genes responsible for regulating cell growth and proliferation. In cases such as lymphomas, only a small sample of the tumor may be analyzed to determine its molecular characteristics, which can result in incomplete information due to the tumor's heterogeneity or the existence of multiple tumor sites. Additionally, acquiring an adequate sample for analysis can be challenging, often requiring invasive techniques that heighten patient risk. Therefore, follow-up monitoring through repeat biopsies is typically impractical.

Minimal or measurable residual disease (MRD) refers to the existence of a limited number of cancerous cells remaining after the initial treatment, which go undetected by standard morphologic or conventional screening techniques. The methodologies employed in clinical practice to assess treatment response for various hematological cancers [31].

In lymphoid diseases, MRD-guided methods relying on the monitoring of clonal rearrangements of immunoglobulins or T-cell receptors (TCRs) have also become an important therapeutic approach for acute lymphoblastic leukemia (ALL) and multiple myeloma (MM). Yet, the existing MRD strategies have not yet been integrated into the clinical management of other lymphoid malignancies, where imaging techniques continue to be the preferred choice for evaluating treatment responses.

Liquid biopsies offer several benefits compared to bone marrow aspirates for MRD detection: they are less invasive, provide a broader molecular picture of tumor diversity, and allow for easier collection of multiple blood samples over time to monitor treatment response dynamics. Numerous studies indicate that the detection of circulating tumor DNA (ctDNA) has a satisfactory positive predictive value, as its presence correlates with a decrease in disease-free survival rates. However, several challenges keep the negative predictive value of this method relatively low. These issues include inadequate sensitivity in detection methods for very low levels of ctDNA, the potential emergence of new clones not detected by the current techniques, and suboptimal timing of post-treatment sample collection. Additionally, in the case of cell-free DNA (cfDNA), the logistics surrounding sample processing are vital to prevent white blood cell lysis and subsequent genomic DNA contamination. To mitigate this risk, samples should be processed within four hours post-collection or gathered in tubes containing a stabilizing agent for cells.

25.13 Summary

Liquid biopsy has emerged as a promising tool for monitoring treatment responses in onco-hematological disorders, offering rapid implementation either alone or in combination with imaging techniques. While early studies and small-scale trials have shown encouraging results, challenges remain. These include optimizing sample collection methods to ensure sufficient cfDNA yield, enhancing the sensitivity of next-generation sequencing (NGS) techniques, and conducting larger clinical trials to validate findings. Standardization of protocols is essential for liquid biopsy to become a widely accepted diagnostic and monitoring tool in clinical practice.

References

1. Alieva M, van Rheenen J, Broekman ML. Potential impact of invasive surgical procedures on primary tumor growth and metastasis. Clin Exp Metastasis. 2018;35:319–31.
2. Armakolas A, Kotsari M, Koskinas J. Liquid biopsies, novel approaches and future directions. Cancer. 2023;15(5):1579.
3. Bankó P, Lee SY, Nagygyörgy V, Zrínyi M, Chae CH, Cho DH, Telekes A. Technologies for circulating tumor cell separation from whole blood. J Hematol Oncol. 2019;12:1–20.
4. Tivey A, Church M, Rothwell D, Dive C, Cook N. Circulating tumour DNA—looking beyond the blood. Nat Rev Clin Oncol. 2022;19(9):600–12.
5. De Rubis G, Rajeev Krishnan S, Bebawy M. Liquid biopsies in cancer diagnosis, monitoring, and prognosis. Trends Pharmacol Sci. 2019;40:172–86.
6. Jongen-Lavrencic M, Grob T, Hanekamp D, Kavelaars FG, al Hinai A, Zeilemaker A, Erpelinck-Verschueren CAJ, Gradowska PL, Meijer R, Cloos J, et al. Molecular Minimal Residual Disease in Acute Myeloid Leukemia. N Engl J Med. 2018;378:1189–99.
7. Roschewski M, Dunleavy K, Pittaluga S, Moorhead M, Pepin F, Kong K, Shovlin M, Jaffe ES, Staudt LM, Lai C, Steinberg SM. Circulating tumour DNA and CT monitoring in patients with untreated diffuse large B-cell lymphoma: a correlative biomarker study. Lancet Oncol. 2015;16(5):541–9.
8. Adashek JJ, Janku F, Kurzrock R. Signed in blood: circulating tumor DNA in cancer diagnosis, treatment and screening. Cancer. 2021;13(14):3600.
9. Jahromi FN, Dowran R, Jafari R. Recent advances in the roles of exosomal microRNAs (exomiRs) in hematologic neoplasms: pathogenesis, diagnosis, and treatment. Cell Commun Signal. 2023;21(1):88.
10. Musi A, Bongiovanni L. Extracellular vesicles in cancer drug resistance: implications on melanoma therapy. Cancer. 2023;15(4):1074.
11. Ferreira MM, Ramani VC, Jeffrey SS. Circulating tumor cell technologies. Mol Oncol. 2016;10(3):374–94.
12. Deng Z, Wu S, Wang Y, Shi D. Circulating tumor cell isolation for cancer diagnosis and prognosis. EBioMedicine. 2022;1:83.
13. Kedmi M, Shouval R, Fried S, Bomze D, Fein J, Cohen Z, Danilesko I, Shem-Tov N, Yerushalmi R, Jacoby E, Besser M. Point-of-care anti-CD19 CAR T-cells for treatment of relapsed and refractory aggressive B-cell lymphoma. Transpl Cell Therap. 2022;28(5):251–7.
14. Keller L, Belloum Y, Wikman H, Pantel K. Clinical relevance of blood-based ctDNA analysis: mutation detection and beyond. Br J Cancer. 2021;124(2):345–58.

15. Kurtz DM, Green MR, Bratman SV, Scherer F, Liu CL, Kunder CA, Takahashi K, Glover C, Keane C, Kihira S, Visser B. Noninvasive monitoring of diffuse large B-cell lymphoma by immunoglobulin high-throughput sequencing. Blood. 2015;125(24):3679–87.
16. Soscia R. Non-invasive minimal residual disease (MRD) analysis in diffuse large B-cell lymphoma (DLBCL).
17. Cuzzo B, Lipsky A, Cherng HJ. Measurable residual disease monitoring in lymphoma. Curr Hematol Malig Rep. 2023;18(6):292–304.
18. Sarkozy C, Huet S, Carlton VE, Fabiani B, Delmer A, Jardin F, Delfau-Larue MH, Hacini M, Ribrag V, Guidez S, Faham M. The prognostic value of clonal heterogeneity and quantitative assessment of plasma circulating clonal IG-VDJ sequences at diagnosis in patients with follicular lymphoma. Oncotarget. 2017;8(5):8765.
19. Ogawa M, Yokoyama K, Imoto S, Tojo A. Role of circulating tumor DNA in hematological malignancy. Cancer. 2021;13(9):2078.
20. Huang Z, Fu Y, Yang H, Zhou Y, Shi M, Li Q, Liu W, Liang J, Zhu L, Qin S, Hong H. Liquid biopsy in T-cell lymphoma: biomarker detection techniques and clinical application. Mol Cancer. 2024;23(1):36.
21. Hosny G, Farahat N, Hainaut P. TP53 mutations in circulating free DNA from Egyptian patients with non-Hodgkin's lymphoma. Cancer Lett. 2009;275(2):234–9.
22. Bratman SV, Newman AM, Alizadeh AA, Diehn M. Potential clinical utility of ultrasensitive circulating tumor DNA detection with CAPP-Seq. Expert Rev Mol Diagn. 2015;15(6):715–9.
23. Desch AK, Hartung K, Botzen A, Brobeil A, Rummel M, Kurch L, Georgi T, Jox T, Bielack S, Burdach S, Classen CF. Genotyping circulating tumor DNA of pediatric Hodgkin lymphoma. Leukemia. 2020;34(1):151–66.
24. Ferreira TM. Innovations and new approaches regarding the detection of measurable residual disease in lymphomas-a systematic review. PQDT-Global. 2023;
25. Rossi D, Spina V, Bruscaggin A, Gaidano G. Liquid biopsy in lymphoma. Haematologica. 2019;104(4):648.
26. Elshimali YI, Khaddour H, Sarkissyan M, Wu Y, Vadgama JV. The clinical utilization of circulating cell free DNA (CCFDNA) in blood of cancer patients. Int J Mol Sci. 2013;14(9):18925–58.
27. Estécio MR, Yan PS, Ibrahim AE, Tellez CS, Shen L, Huang TH, Issa JP. High-throughput methylation profiling by MCA coupled to CpG Island microarray. Genome Res. 2007;17(10):1529–36.
28. Delfau-Larue MH, van Der Gucht A, Dupuis J, Jais JP, Nel I, Beldi-Ferchiou A, Hamdane S, Benmaad I, Laboure G, Verret B, Haioun C. Total metabolic tumor volume, circulating tumor cells, cell-free DNA: distinct prognostic value in follicular lymphoma. Blood Adv. 2018;2(7):807–16.
29. Kurtz DM, Scherer F, Jin M, Soo J, Craig A, Esfahani MS, Chabon JJ, Stehr H, Liu CL, Tibshirani R, Maeda LS. Development of a dynamic model for personalized risk assessment in large B-cell lymphoma.
30. Gao YJ, He YJ, Yang ZL, Shao HY, Zuo Y, Bai Y, Chen H, Chen XC, Qin FX, Tan S, Wang J. Increased integrity of circulating cell-free DNA in plasma of patients with acute leukemia. Clin Chem Lab Med. 2010;48(11):1651–6.
31. Rivas-Delgado A, Nadeu F, Enjuanes A, Casanueva-Eliceiry S, Mozas P, Magnano L, Castrejón de Anta N, Rovira J, Dlouhy I, Martín S, Osuna M. Mutational landscape and tumor burden assessed by cell-free DNA in diffuse large B-cell lymphoma in a population-based study. Clin Cancer Res. 2021;27(2):513–21.
32. Frickhofen N, Muller E, Sandherr M, Binder T, Bangerter M, Wiest C, Enz M, Heimpel H. Rearranged Ig heavy chain DNA is detectable in cell-free blood samples of patients with B-cell neoplasia. Blood. 1997;90(12):4953–60.
33. Bo J, Sun L, Wang W, Ma C, Li H, Zhao Y. Novel diagnostic biomarker for patients with non-Hodgkin's lymphoma by IgH gene rearrangement. J Cancer Res Ther. 2016;12(2):903–8.

Chapter 26
Flow Cytometric Diagnostic Approach to Low-Grade Lymphomas

Tathagat Chatterjee, Gurpreet Kaur, and Ankur Ahuja

Abstract Chronic lymphoproliferative disorders (CLPD) are heterogenous clonal disorders in their presentation, morphology and immunophenotyping. Flowcytometric immunophenotyping (FCM) is a valuable and indispensable tool in the diagnosis of CLPDS. FCM has many advantages, being multiparamteric it helps analyze several antigens simultaneously on the same cell of interest both in a quantitative and a qualitative manner. It provides us a quick diagnosis and helps us take on other ancillary testing such as cytogenetics and molecular studies.

In this review, the aim to provide common and practical approaches in utlizing FCM in the diagnostic workup of low-grade lymphomas.

Keywords Low-grade lymphomas · Flowcytometry · Chronic lymphoproliferative disorders

Learning Objectives
- A rational and methodical step wise approach to low-grade lymphomas.
- Choosing molecular methods judiciously while diagnosing low-grade lymphomas by integrating clinical history, imaging, lab parameters and flowcytometry.

T. Chatterjee (✉)
Department of Pathology and Haemtology, ESIC Medical College Hospital, NIT3, Faridabad, India

G. Kaur
Department of Pathology, Command Hospital, Kolkata, India

A. Ahuja
Department of Pathology, Command Hospital, Kolkata, India

Department of Pathology, Armed Forces Medical College, Pune, India

H. P. Pati et al. (eds.), *Clinical Hematology and Hemato-Oncology*,
https://doi.org/10.1007/978-981-92-1167-8_26

26.1 Introduction

Chronic lymphoproliferative disorders are characterized by clonal proliferation of B, T, or NK-T lymphocytes in the blood, bone marrow, lymph nodes, and in extra-nodal sites. They account for 2.8% of all diagnosed malignancies and 2.6% of malignancy-associated mortality worldwide. NHL burden in India is high accounting for an incidence rate of 0.22 per million and a mortality rate of 0.15 per million. The mature small B-cell lymphomas comprise more than 30% of the non-Hodgkin lymphomas, Follicular lymphoma (FL) grades I & II, 16%, extra nodal marginal zone lymphoma (ENMZL) 8%, small lymphocytic lymphoma/chronic lymphocytic lymphoma(CLL/SLL) 7%, mantle cell lymphoma (MCL) 6%, nodal marginal zone lymphoma (NMZL) 2%, lymphoplasmacytic lymphoma (LPL) 1%. Based on their clinical course, lymphomas are further classified as either indolent or aggressive [1, 2].

Evaluation of a CLPD involves adequate clinical history examination, radiological evaluation, laboratory investigations including complete blood count (CBC), peripheral smear (PS), lactate dehydrogenase (LDH), beta 2 microglobulin, immunophenotyping for diagnosis, subtyping and prognosis, cytogenetics, and lastly molecular studies [3].

26.2 General Approaches for Analyzing Mature B Cells

The review of the CBC and PS tells us the stage of maturation, whether these are mature cells or immature cells or blasts. Morphological features vary by subtype and give a diagnostic clue. FCM helps us delineate the full immunophenotypic profile of the cells, including the patterns and intensity of staining, whether the staining is surface or cytoplasmic. FCM helps us confirm the lineage and stage of maturation and assess for specific markers or and combinations of antigens that are being expressed. Genotyping followed by the FCM diagnosis helps in assessing recurrent cytogenetic abnormalities and the molecular assessment for gene mutations provides important diagnostic and prognostic information for specific CLPD subtypes and patterns.

The samples for FCM are fresh specimens, which include peripheral blood, bone marrow aspirate, fine needle aspirate, body fluids, and cell suspensions of fresh tissues. For running FCM on tissue specimens, samples are gently cut into tiny pieces (1–2 mm) in Roswell Park Memorial Institute (RPMI) media using scissors, scalpels, or a razor blade to increase surface area for digestion. Following RBC lysis, the resulting suspension is filtered through a 70 μm or 100 μm cell strainer to remove debris to ensure a single-cell suspension is formed and then this sample is processed [4].

Normal B-cells express for B-cell markers CD19, CD20, CD22, and CD79a and are negative for T-cell markers cCD3, CD4, and CD8, and similarly normal T-cells are positive for T markers, i.e. CD3, CD4, CD8, and are negative for B-cell markers as mentioned; however, a minor population of benign B-cells may be CD5+. CD5+ cells comprise 15–25% of the B-cell population in adult secondary lymphoid organs and are rare in peripheral blood. Normal mature B-cells consist of one population expressing kappa (κ) and the other expressing lambda (λ) light chains. The κ to λ ratio ranges from 0.5 to 3.0:1 in the peripheral blood and bone marrow and 1.2–2.7:1 in lymph nodes. Mature B-cell neoplasms most often show a single clone of cells and are either kappa or lambda-restricted. B CLPDS have bright CD45, are HLA-DR positive and have moderate to bright expression of B-cell markers such as CD19, CD20, CD22, and CD79a. A B-cell population that has dim to negative CD20, bright CD10, and is negative for surface light chain immunoglobulins raises the possibility of a B-ALL (B acute lymphoblastic leukemia) and requires additional immaturity markers such as TdT and CD34. B-lymphoblasts are dim or negative CD45 and are positive for CD34, TdT, CD19, CD22, and CD79a, they are negative or dim for CD20. CD10 (CALLA antigen) may be positive or negative. Hematogones, similar to B-ALL, have absent surface light chain expression as these are immature cells, and are partially positive for CD34 and TdT. They have a variable heterogeneous expression for CD10 and CD20. A characteristic waterfall pattern on the CD 20 vs CD10 plot. Initial stage I Hematogones are CD10 positive and they slowly lose this expression and gain CD20 in stage III [3]. We now discuss each of the individual low-grade B-cell lymphomas.

Table 26.1 delineates morphology and immunophenotypic profiles of B CLPDS.

Table 26.1 Morphology and immunophenotypic abnormalities in common low-grade B CLPD

Lymphoma	Morphology	Immunophenotyping	FISH and cytogenetics	Remarks
CLL/SLL	Small lymphocytes, soccer ball chromatin, round nuclei, diffuse infiltrate, pseudo follicles	Weak CD20, CD5=, CD23+, Bcl2 +, CD43+, CD200+, LEF1+, TCL1+	11, 12q, 13q,17p, probes	BCl2 +ve, causes misdiagnosis of FL
MCL	Small--intermediate sized lymphoid cells (blastoid, pleomorphic variants also)	Cyclin D1+, bright CD20+, FMC7+, CD5+, CD23-ve, SOX11 + LEF1-, CD200-, Bcl6 -ve in classical type	IgH/CCND1 fusion probe	Leukemic blood picture common may be SOX11-, CD200 +ve, and CD5-ve
MZL	Monocytoid B-cells, clear cytoplasm, mildly irregular nuclei, and inconspicuous nucleoli	CD5-ve, CD23--ve,variable BCL2 +ve,CIg +ve,lacks distinctive IP	API2/MALT1 fusion, Del (7q) common	MYD88 detected in the subset

(continued)

Table 26.1 (continued)

Lymphoma	Morphology	Immunophenotyping	FISH and cytogenetics	Remarks
LPL	Small lymphocytes, plasmacytoid lymphocytes, and plasma cells, with mast cells admixed	CD5-ve, CD23-ve, CIg +ve, plasma cells monoclonal	t(9;14) (p13;q3)	Associated with hepatitis C, cryoglobulinemia, and amyloid deposition
HCL	Medium in size with moderately abundant pale blue cytoplasm, reniform nuclei, open chromatin, absent nucleoli, and a characteristic serrated cytoplasmic border	CD19+, CD20bright+, CD200 +ve, CD25+, CD103+, CD123+, CD11c+, CD305(LAIR)+, CD5-ve, CD23-ve, CD10-ve AnnexinA1 +ve, DBA-44 +ve	Del7q and 13q and gains chromosome 5	Pancytopenia, monocytopenia, splenomegaly BRAF V600E mutation in >95% of cases
SBLPN	intermediate--sized blastic/ convoluted nuclei, prominent nucleoli, circumferential shaggy contours	CD19+, CD20+, CD22+ (variable), CD11c (bright), CD103 (variable), FMC7 (variable), CD5-ve, CD10-ve, CD25-ve, CD123-ve	Gains on chromosome 5 and losses on 7q and 17p	Negative BRAF V600 mutation MAP2K1 (15q22.31) mutations common
FL	Neoplastic cells are small to intermediate in size, with highly indented nuclei, known as buttock cells	CD19+, CD20+, CD22+ CD79a+,CD5-ve, CD23-ve, CD43-ve, CD10+, BCL6+, HGAL+, LMO2+, Grade 3B can be more commonly negative	t(14;18) (q32;q21) IGH/BCL2: 85% of follicular lymphomas	MYC rearrangement/ activation of MYC is rare <5%, associated with transformation to DLBCL

26.3 Monoclonal B-Cell Lymphocytosis (MBL)

Incidentally detected low numbers <5 × 10^9/cumm of circulating monoclonal B-cells in a healthy person with no evidence of CLL/other lymphoproliferation, with no lymphadenopathy or organomegaly is defined as monoclonal B-cell lymphocytosis (MBL). MBL is postulated to arise from chronic antigenic stimulation leading to the development of an oligoclonal and subsequently monoclonal B cells. 75% of all MBLs express markers that are similar to CLL/SLL with dim CD20 and dim surface immunoglobulins and a co-expression of CD5 and CD23. These are known as CLL-like MBLs. The remaining MBLs may be atypical CLL (CD5+/

CD23 – CD20bright+) and or may be CD5 negative. MBL may be a low count MBL with a monoclonal circulating population of atypical lymphocytes <0.5 × 10^9/cumm or a high count MBL with >0.5 × 10^9/cumm atypical cells. The high count MBL shows progression to CLL at about 1–2% per year, while low count MBL rarely progresses to CLL. The overall incidence of MBL increases with age, with a frequency of >20% in persons >60 years and also shows a familial predisposition. Rawstron et al. reported minute MBL populations <3.5 × 10^9/cumm with a CLL phenotype in 05% of healthy individuals who were older than 60 years of age. The differentials of an MBL may include reactive lymphoid proliferations, SLL with minimal peripheral blood involvement, in which case physical examination and lymph node biopsy is most important. In peripheral blood involvement in an MCL, MBL with atypical CLL phenotype needs to be excluded, and the presence of t(11;14) may help distinguish these two. The majority of CLL-like MBL cases have mutated IGHV genes in up to 90% cases. Genetic abnormalities identified in CLL, such as deletion of 13q, deletion of 11q, deletion of 17p, and the presence of trisomy 12, are also seen in MBL [5].

26.4 Chronic Lymphocytic Leukemia (CLL)

CLL is a low-grade lymphoproliferative disorder of mature peripheral lymphoid B cells characterized by lymphocytosis, CD5/CD23 co-expression, and involvement of blood, bone marrow, spleen, and lymph nodes. The diagnosis of CLL requires ≥5 × 10^9/cumm monoclonal lymphocytes with a CLL phenotype for more than 3 months. A level below this threshold is considered an MBL, as brought out before. In 1994, Matutes et al. devised a scoring system for the diagnosis of CLL based on its common immunological profile CD5+, CD23+, FMC7-, and weak expression (+/–) of surface immunoglobulin (SmIg) and CD22. Each of these five markers scored as 0 or 1; CLL cases scored 5 or 4; however, for most other B cell leukemias/lymphomas the score was 0 or 1. Additional FCM markers are CD43, CD79b, CD81, CD200, CD10, and ROR1. Rarely two clones are detected. Transformation of CLL to a more aggressive disease, which is known as Richter syndrome, occurs in 2% to 12% cases. CLL cases with NOTCH1 mutation have a higher risk of Richter transformation and need close monitoring. Immunoglobulin heavy chain variable region (IgH) mutation status and expression of ZAP-70 and CD38 are important in prognosticating CLL. ZAP-70 and CD38 expression correlate with the unmutated IgH and can be studied by immunohistochemistry or FCM. CD38 expression >30%, ZAP 70 expression >20%, CD49d > 30% positivity in CLL cells has been associated with poor outcomes [6]. Although CD38 expression is associated with mutated CLL, recent reports suggest that a combination of CD38 and IGVH mutational status had greater prognostic power than either marker alone. In the WHO-HAEM5, the term "prolymphocytic progression of CLL" has been introduced [1]. Those CLL/SLL cases that have ≥15% prolymphocytes are now called prolymphocytic progression of CLL; those with <15% prolymphocytes continue to be classified as CLL/SLL in WHO-HAEM5. Cases with >55% prolymphocytes are now renamed as "splenic B-cell lymphoma/leukemia with prominent nucleoli (SBLPN)". SBLPN includes hairy cell leukemia variant (HCLv) and cases of splenic marginal zone lymphoma with similar morphological features. The ultimate goal here was to delineate biologically defined entities and improve therapy, as these are overlapping clinical diseases [1]. The clinical staging is done using the Rai and Binet systems, beta-2 microglobulin: high levels associated with high tumor burden and adverse prognosis. The TP53 mutation/17p deletion is linked with poor response to chemotherapeutic regimens. Complex karyotype with 3 or more unrelated abnormalities is seen in 10–15% cases and is also a bad prognostic marker. 13q deletion is favorable, 11q deletion is unfavorable, whereas trisomy 12 is associated with an intermediate prognosis [7].

26.5 Mantle Cell Lymphoma (MCL)

MCL is a CD5 + CLPD of small- to medium-sized lymphocytes with irregular (indented) nuclei characterized t(11;14)(q13;q32) or IGH/CCND1 and cyclin D1 overexpression. 70% of all MCLs have stage IV disease at presentation. There are two subtypes: an aggressive variant with SOX11+ and nodal presentation and a more indolent form with SOX11- and leukemic presentation with no nodal involvement. Morphologically, MCL most commonly presents with a diffuse or vaguely nodular pattern, effacing the lymph node architecture. The blastoid variant of MCL may mimic an acute lymphoblastic leukemia/lymphoma. On FCM there is CD5+, CD19+, CD20+, CD22+, CD79b+, FMC7+. It is CD10-, CD11c+/−, CD23-, CD43+/−, CD200−/+. Some rare cases may have an atypical immunophenotype with CD5- or CD10+, CD200+, or CD23+. CD23 + ve MCL has better outcomes when compared to the CD23−ve MCL. Both FL and MCL may present with leukemic blood involvement. FCM and FISH studies (CCND1, BCL2) are helpful in differential diagnosis [8]. The translocation (11;14) (q13;q32) is most often detected on FISH and is convenient because it can be performed on fixed tissue sections. Conventional cytogenetics may be carried out if fresh material is available. PCR assays may also be used. Cyclin D2 rearrangements by FISH can be detected in some of the cyclin D1 negative cases [9].

Table 26.2 delineates the major immunophenotypic abnormalities in CLPDs.

Table 26.2 Delineates the major immunophenotypic abnormalities in CLPDs

	CD5	CD10	B CL2	BCL6	CD23	CD20	CD 38	CD 200	CD 43	IgM	IgD	79a	CCND1	Surface light chain	IRTA*#	MNDA	LEF 1
LPL	--/+	--/+	+/-	-	-/+	++	+/-	+	-/+	+	-	+	-	++	-	+	-
EN MZL	--/+	--	-	-	-/+	++		-/+	+	+	+	+	-		++	++	-
N MZL			+	-				-/+	+			+	-		++	+	-
SMZL	-	-	+	-	-	++	-	+	-	+	+	+	-	++	-	+	-
CLL	+	-	+	-	+	+	+/-	++	+	+/-	+/-	+	-	+/-	-	+	+
FL	-	+	+	+		++		-/+	-	+	+/-	+	-		-	-	-
MCL	+	-	+	-	-/+	++		-	+	++	++	+	+	++	-	+	-

IRTA: Immunoglobulin Superfamily receptor translocation associated protein 1
MNDA: Myeloid cell nuclear differentiation antigen
LEF 1 Lymphocyte Enhancer factor 1

26.6 Lymphoplasmacytic Lymphoma (LPL)

Lymphoplasmacytic lymphoma (LPL) is an indolent neoplasm comprising small B lymphocytes, plasmacytoid cells, and plasma cells. LPLs may have a familial predisposition. Cold agglutinin or cryoglobulins may be present sometimes and 15–30% of patients with Waldenström macroglobulinemia (discussed later) have hyperviscosity particularly when the IgM level reaches ≥6 g/dL. Bone marrow infiltration, cryoprecipitation, autoimmune or nonautoimmune antibody activity may lead to cytopenias, cold agglutinin hemolytic anemia and also peripheral neuropathy. Hepatitis C association is common in LPLs. LPL is diagnosed when clonal lymphoplasmacytic aggregates represent≥10% of BM cellularity in biopsies. WHO-HAEM5 recognizes two subtypes of LPL: (1) Waldenström Macroglobulinemia (WM) or IgM-LPL (comprising 95% of cases). (2) Non-WM type LPL (comprising about 5% of cases), which includes those with IgG or IgA monoclonal component, the non-secretory LPL, and IgM-LPL without BM involvement [1].

LPL is a diagnosis of exclusion when features do not match other small B-cell neoplasms. Differential diagnoses include MZL, CLL/SLL, FL, and DLBCL. FCM commonly shows two clonal populations (B cells and plasma cells), with B cells positive for CD19, CD20, CD22, and CD79a, negative for CD5, CD10, and CD103, and showing moderate-to-bright surface Ig. The population of plasma cells expresses CD19 and CD45, which helps distinguish LPL from other plasma cell dyscrasias that usually lack these markers. Over 90% of LPLs harbor MYD88 L265P mutations; CXCR4 mutations occur in a subset (40%) and may be associated with hyperviscosity and predict response to ibrutinib. Testing for MYD88 L265P can be helpful but sensitivity depends on sample type and method. Plasma cell myeloma (PCM) with t(11;14) can mimic LPL but is usually CD19− and lacks PAX5 and CD138 co-expression seen in LPL; cyclin D1 IHC can assist in these cases being positive in PCM with t(11;14). LPL/WM may be difficult to separate from MZL since both disorders show a non-specific phenotype which is CD5−ve, CD10−ve. A high level of serum IgM protein favors LPL. It is important to note that lymphadenopathy is reported in ~15% of LPL. Presence of MYD88 L265P mutation favors LPL/WM over MZL. Plasmacytoid differentiation with Dutcher bodies is less frequently seen in MZL than in LPL. Deletion of 6q21–q25 is a common copy number abnormality in LPL seen in up to 40% cases [10–12].

26.7 Follicular Lymphoma (FL)

Follicular lymphoma is a B-cell neoplasm of follicle center cell origin. Most cases of FL have stage IV disease with BM and blood involvement and it follows a chronic relapsing course. PS shows atypical lymphocytes, centrocytes with irregular nuclei with prominent nuclear cleaving and scanty cytoplasm. Larger lymphocytes, centroblasts, may be seen in various proportions, depending on stage and grade. Immunophenotypically, follicular lymphomas are CD20 bright+, CD19 dim+, CD10+, CD5-, cyclin D1-. On IHC, the expression of BCL2 is usually dimmer than in residual benign small T-cells. Subsets of FL may be negative for either CD10 and/or BCL2. In many cases, FCM reveals two B-cell populations: neoplastic B-cells, a subpopulation of residual benign polyclonal B-cells, and sometimes an increased number of reactive T-cells. The dim expression of CD19 and co-expression of CD10 usually confirms a neoplastic process in these cases [1].

CD10 expression by atypical B-cells may be positive, but down-regulated in the BM. Similarly, there may be a discrepancy in morphologic features between the nodal morphology and BM disease observed, and the phenotype may also differ between primary and secondary sites. FL is characterized by t(14;18)(q32;q21) by cytogenetics/FISH. FISH is more sensitive than PCR-based approaches because of variation in breakpoint regions. Juxtaposition of the Ig light chain promoters to BCL2 leads to t(2;18) and t(18;22) translocations as well. 3q27 BCL6 rearrangement or amplification is seen commonly in follicular lymphoma 3B. Loss of 1p36, which contains TNFRSF14, is common. MAP 2 K1 mutations favor a diagnosis of pediatric-type FL. Detection of EZH2 mutations is important when therapy with an EZH2 inhibitor is considered [13, 14].

26.8 Marginal Zone Lymphoma (MZL)

Marginal zone lymphoma may present with localized or generalized nodal disease; marrow involvement is seen in <50%, peripheral blood involvement is less common, and systemic symptoms are infrequent. EMZL (MALT) arises in tissues that acquire lymphoid aggregates after chronic inflammation, e.g., H. pylori gastritis, Chlamydia psittaci ocular infection, and autoimmune disorders. Characteristic monocytoid B cells of MZL have clear cytoplasm and mildly irregular nuclei.

Splenic and nodal presentations differ by site involvement. The classical immunophenotype is CD19+, CD20+, CD22+, CD79a+, typically negative for cyclin D1, CD5, CD10, CD23, and CD103; some MZLs may be CD5+. Surface Ig and CD20 expression are generally moderate. Based on the expression of CD5, MCL has to be differentiated from other CD5+ B-cell lymphoproliferations, B-CLL/SLL, especially the atypical variants of B-CLL/SLL, which are negative for CD23 expression and have moderate CD20 expression with surface light immunoglobulins, de novo CD5+ DLBCL, and other B-cell lymphoproliferations with aberrant expression of CD5, i.e., MZL, LPL/WM. Monotypic plasma cells are frequent and can support nodal MZL diagnosis. Genetic alterations include mutations in KMT2D, PTPRD, NOTCH2, KLF2, and occasionally MYD88; cytogenetic changes include gains of chromosomes 3 and 18 and 6q loss [1, 15, 16].

26.9 Hairy Cell Leukemia (HCL)

Hairy cell leukemia is an uncommon indolent B-cell neoplasm presenting with cytopenia's, splenomegaly, and few circulating cells with hair-like projections. Classical HCL must be differentiated from SBLPN (formerly HCL-variant). Massive splenomegaly is a hallmark but less frequent with earlier detection these days. Lymphadenopathy is uncommon. Annexin A1 IHC is specific for classical HCL but should be interpreted with B-cell marker correlation. TRAP staining and DBA-44 are less used now, but they help support the diagnosis. Three flow--cytometry clues that need to be kept in mind while diagnosing HCL are: slightly larger cells with higher forward scatter and increased side scatter often in monocyte position, markedly bright CD11c/CD22/CD200 expression, and relative monocytopenia. These findings should prompt a panel including CD25 and CD103; CD305 (LAIR1) is a relatively new supportive marker. HCL immunophenotype includes CD19+, bright CD20+, CD200+, CD25+, CD103+, CD123+, CD11c+, CD305+, CD5−, CD23−, CD10−; annexin A1 positive by IHC. 10% HCL cases may however show CD10 positivity. Reticulin is increased due to the presence of fibrosis. BRAF V600E mutation is characteristic of classical HCL (>95%) but absent in SBLPN (formerly HCL-v), which often shows CD103+/CD11c bright but is CD25−, CD123−, CD200−, and BRAF V600E–negative. Bright CD200 expression among CD5−/CD10− B-cell neoplasms supports HCL. Rare cases that are BRAF V600E mutation negative will be positive for IGHV4–34 [17, 18].

26.9.1 CD5-Positive Mature B-Cell Neoplasms

CD5-positive mature B-cell neoplasms: mainly CLL/SLL and MCL; usually distinguishable, but occasional overlap exists.

26.9.2 CD10-Positive Mature B-Cell Neoplasms

CD10 is a germinal center B-cell (GCB) marker. CD10-positive neoplasms: mostly Follicular Lymphoms (FL), Burkitt lymphoma, "Germinal centre type" DLBCL (GCB-type DLBCLs).

26.9.3 CD5-Positive and CD10-Positive Mature B-Cell Neoplasm

Coexpression of CD5 and CD10 occurs very rarely. The most common neoplasms coexpressing CD5 and CD10 are large B-cell lymphoma, followed by FL, MCL, and CLL/SLL.

26.9.4 CD5-Negative, CD23-Negative, CD10-Negative Mature B-Cell Neoplasm

CD5-negative, CD10-negative low-grade B-cell lymphoproliferative disorders are a fascinating group of indolent, neoplastic, mature B-cell proliferations. These include HCL, SBLPN, LPL, and MZL.

Splenomegaly is prominent with involvement of PB and bone marrow but no involvement of lymph nodes. HCLv which was a provisional entity which in WHO-HAEM4 and ICC in WHO-HAEM5 is classified as SBLPN because it is biologically different from classic HCL [19, 20]. This disease behaves more aggressively than HCL and is resistant to cladribine alone. SMZL is one of the prototypic, best studied, and most frequently encountered CD5-CD10-LPD of the spleen that preferentially involves the white pulp. In contrast, HCL involves red pulp. The characteristic features of HCL, SBLPN are tabulated in Table 26.1.

26.10 Selected Marker Patterns CD200, CD148, and CD180

CLL typically shows weak CD148 and CD180 with strong CD200; MCL exhibits strong CD148 with weak to negative CD180 and CD200; SMZL shows weak CD148 and CD200 with strong CD180. expression [21, 22].

26.11 Summary

This review presents a concise, practical algorithm for routine diagnostic workup of common mature B-cell lymphomas/leukemias. Accurate classification depends on integrating histology, immunophenotype, and ancillary tests. And it is the combination of diagnostic modalities that provides the most reliable assessments when coupled with history and examination findings.

Case 1

A 78-year-old female presented with a history of increasing fatigue of 2 months duration. She also complained of yellowish discoloration of the eyes. She was a known case of diabetes mellitus type II, had a hysterectomy and cholecystectomy done along with macular degeneration of left eye. On examination, she was pale with jaundice. There was no lymphadenopathy or organomegaly. USG Abdomen & MRCP revealed a liver span of 13 cm and normal findings. On being sent for a CBC initial report by an outside laboratory was given as a clotted sample. Repeat testing in our lab showed a clotted sample as well. Mean corpuscular volume (MCV), mean corpuscular hemoglobin (MCH), mean corpuscular hemoglobin concentration (MCHC), platelet (PLT) count, and mean platelet volume (MPV) could not be measured. Overt agglutination was observed when the patient's test tubes with EDTA were seen under the light microscope. Total leucocyte count was 11, 600 cumm, N 48 L 42 M4 E5 B1, atypical lymphocytes seen, ALC: 4872 cumm. These values improved after the sample was warmed to 37 °C, which showed her Hb as 11.7 gm/dl, MCV—37.2, MCHC- 33.

Her biochemical values were normal except indirect bilirubin −6.42 mg/dl. The viral markers were all negative. Investigations done to rule out infection with EBV and Parvovirus, IgG and IgM indices were negative. Tumor markers CA125, CA 19.9, CEA, and AFP were done, all of which were negative, along with CECT abdomen, which revealed a normal study, ruling out malignancy.

Based on her agglutinin on peripheral smear and clinical findings, a direct antiglobulin test (DAT) was advised. DAT was positive for anti-IgG and C3d. Indirect antiglobulin test was also positive for anti-IgG and C3d. The titer by CTT (at 4 Celsius): 1: 1024. Indicating autoantibodies of the IgM type, having a wide thermal amplitude. Indirect antiglobulin test was also positive for anti-IgG and C3d.

In view of the raised lymphocyte count, a flow cytometry on peripheral blood was carried. The CD 45 vs SCC reveals 18.29% lymphocytes, 41.33% granulocytes, 3.73% monocytes. Of these lymphocytes, 10.04% were CD19-positive B cells. These cells express CD19, CD5, CD23 dim kappa, and CD200. they were negative for CD20, FMC7, and CD103. Based on the characteristic immunophenotypic findings and an absolute count of less than 5000/cumm this was diagnosed as monoclonal B-cell lymphocytosis leading to CAD.

Case 2

A 78-year-old female presented with a history of increasing fatigue of 2 months duration. She also complained of yellowish discoloration of the eyes. She was a known case of diabetes mellitus type II, had a hysterectomy and cholecystectomy done along with macular degeneration of left eye. On examination, she was pale with jaundice. There was no lymphadenopathy or organomegaly. On being sent for a CBC, an initial report by an outside laboratory was given as clotted sample. Repeat testing in our lab showed a clotted sample as well as hemoglobin (Hb) 8.6gm% was. Mean corpuscular volume (MCV) was 120 fl, mean corpuscular hemoglobin (MCH), and mean corpuscular hemoglobin concentration (MCHC), could not be measured and were represented as +++, implying these were out of the measurable ranges for the counter. Overt agglutination was observed on the peripheral smear with polychromasia, anisocytosis, and poikilocytosis as shown in Fig. 26.1a. Keeping the possibility of cold agglutination, the warm chain was maintained, and these counter values showed the following: Hb 8.6gm%, total leucocyte count (TLC) 11, 600 cumm, N 48 L 42 M4 E5 B1, absolute lymphocyte count (ALC) was 4872 cumm, MCV 97.2 fl, MCH 31.2 pg, and MCHC33 g/dL. A few smudge cells were also seen (Fig. 26.1b).

Her biochemical parameters revealed a total bilirubin of 7.8 mg/dl with indirect bilirubin of 6.42 mg/dl. The urea/creatinine was 27/0.9 mg/dl. Lactate dehydrogenase (LDH) was raised as per institutional cutoffs at 490 IU/ml. The viral markers were all negative, including those for EBV and parvovirus. Tumor markers CA125, CA 19.9, CEA, and AFP were done, all of which were negative, along with CECT abdomen, which revealed a normal study, ruling out malignancy.

Based on her agglutinin on peripheral smear and clinical findings, a Direct antiglobulin test (DAT) was advised. The direct antiglobulin test was positive for C3d.

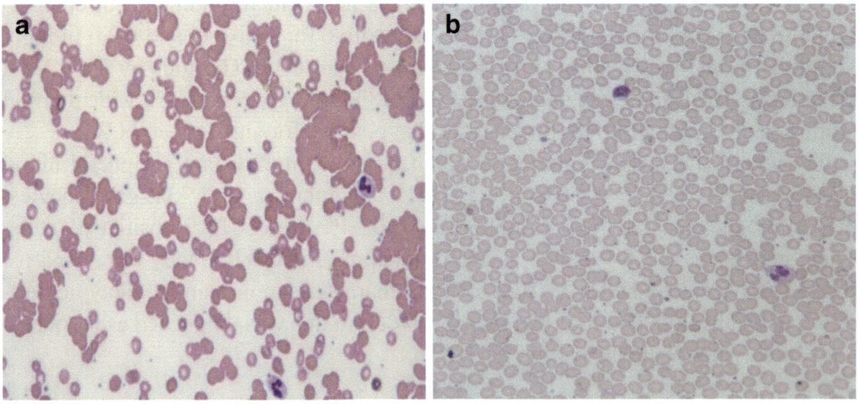

Fig. 26.1 Agglutination seen on peripheral smear on a prewarmed sample. Post warming, the agglutination reduced, and a predominant population of small mature lymphocytes with "soccer ball chromatin" and few smudge cells was seen

The titer by cold agglutinin Titer (CAT) (at 4 Celsius) was 1:1024, indicating autoantibodies of the IgM type, having high thermal amplitude >30 Celsius.

In view of the raised lymphocyte count, a flow cytometry on peripheral blood was carried. The CD 45 vs SCC in flow cytometry reveals 18.29% lymphocytes, 41.33% granulocytes, 3.73% monocytes. Of these lymphocytes, 10.04% were CD19-positive B cells and these expressed CD19, CD5, CD23 dim kappa, and CD200 as shown in Fig. 26.2. They were negative for CD10, CD20, FMC7,CD 123, and CD103. Based on the characteristic immunophenotypic findings and an absolute count of less than 5000/cumm this was diagnosed as monoclonal B-cell lymphocytosis leading to CAD. The patient responded to the Bendamustine Rituximab regimen.

Case 2

A 56-year-old female, post-menopausal, diabetic with a history of bleeding tendencies x 06 months which were primarily mucosal bleeding per vaginum, epistaxis, and melena. Clinically, she had pallor generalized lymphadenopathy and no hepatosplenomegaly. There was no history of drugs, previous bleeding episodes, or history of menorrhagia or postpartum bleeding. There was a relevant family history of bleeding tendencies. Her Hb was 6.1gm%, HCT was 21.0%, MCV was 85.4 fL, RDW 16.9%, total TLC was 9680/mm^3 with differential count being N37, L54, M6, E3 platelets 4.5lac/mm^3. Peripheral smear showed normocytic normochromic anemia with rouleaux formation and plasmacytoid lymphocytes. Figure 26.3a On screening coagulogram, she had isolated deranged aPTT not correcting on a mixing study, thereby implying inhibitors. Her total protein/albumin/globulins (mg/dl) were 15/2/13 gm/dl, revealing an AG reversal. Lactate dehydrogenase (LDH) was 488 IU/ml, which was on the higher side. Her viral markers were negative. A serum protein electrophoresis (SPEP) and immunofixation electrophoresis (IFE) were carried out, which revealed an M spike of 9.2 g/dL of Ig M Kappa subtype. Imaging was essentially normal. Her renal function and liver function were within normal limits. A bone marrow was performed, which showed a predominance of lymphocytes and lymphoplasmacytic cells along with plasma cells (71%). Bone marrow biopsy and aspirate showed the marrow was hypercellular (90% cellularity) with increased small lymphocytes and plasma cells (Fig. 26.3b, c) positive for CD19, kappa, and negative for CD5, and CD10 and lambda. Scattered CD138-positive plasma cells positive for CD56 were seen (aberrant plasma cells) as seen in Fig. 26.4. Flow cytometric analysis revealed that most B cells (49% of the CD45+ events) were positive for CD19, CD20, CD22, and CD23, negative for CD5, CD10, CD34, CD38, CD103, and CD11c, as shown in these B cells showed expression of kappa (Fig. 26.5). Molecular studies showed a positive MYD88 L265P mutation (c.794 T > C). No other mutations, translocations (including CCND1 and IgH), and chromosomal abnormalities were identified. This was therefore diagnosed as a case of IgM lymphoplasmacytic lymphoma or Waldenstorm's macroglobulinemia presenting as bleeding diathesis.

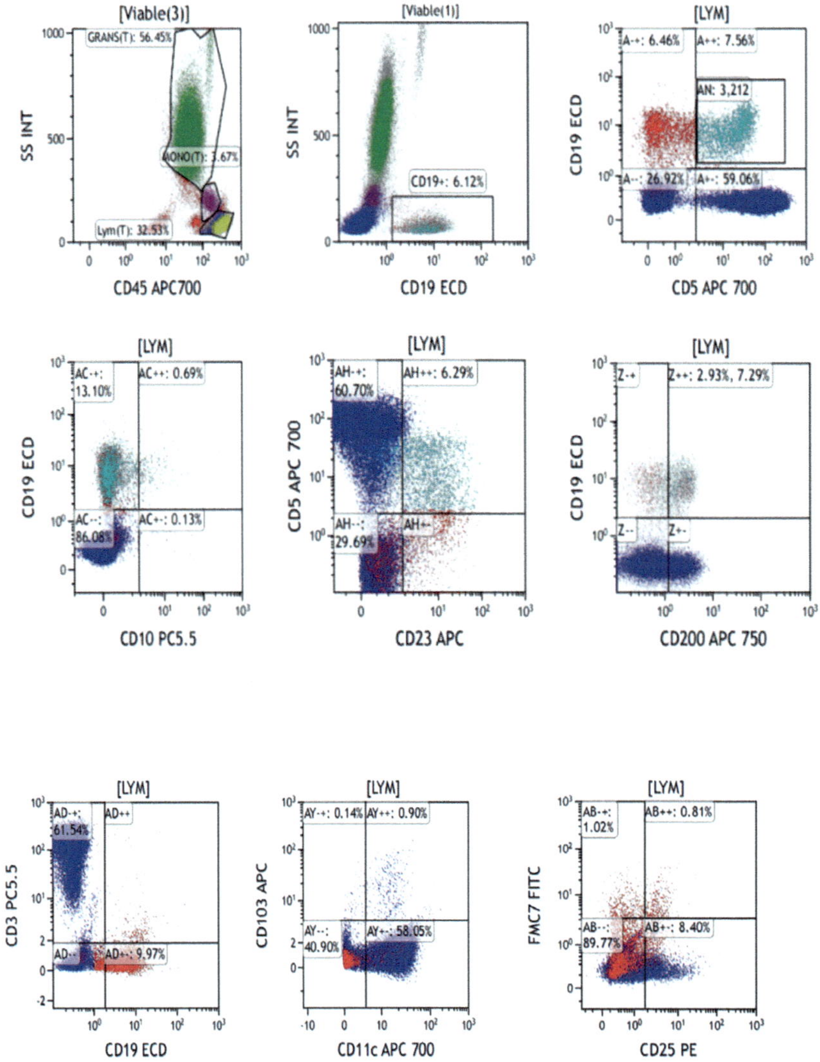

Fig. 26.2 Multiparametric flowcytometry plots showing an aqua blue colored populating which identified CD19 positive B cells, which also expressed CD5, CD23, CD200, and were negative for FMC7, CD10, CD103, CD11c, and CD123. These amounted to a total of 3212/cumm, and hence the diagnosis of monoclonal B-cell lymphocytosis was given

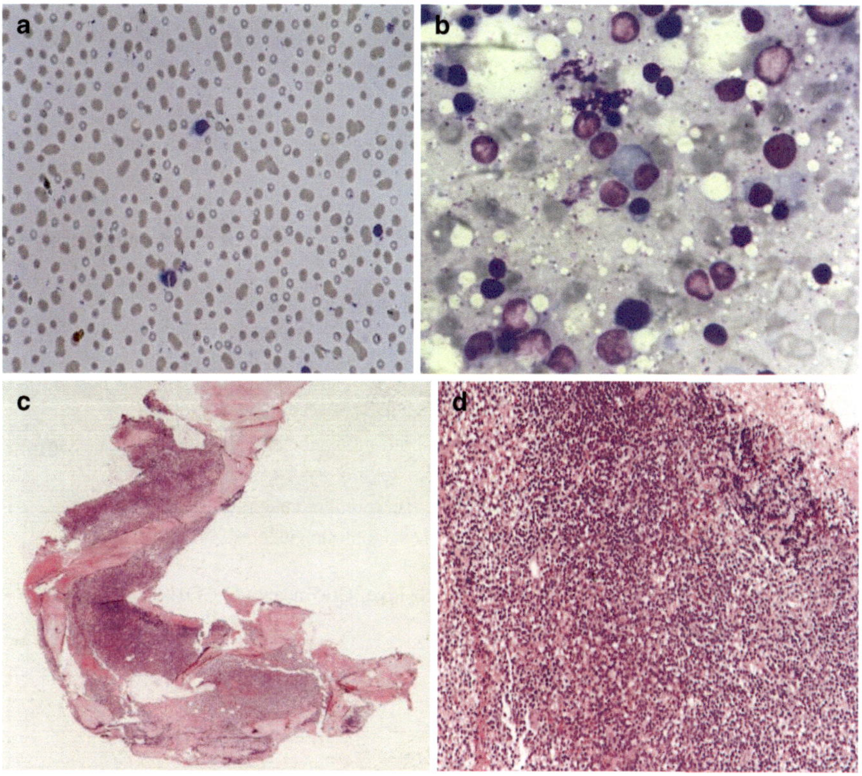

Fig. 26.3 (**a**) Peripheral smear with marked rouleaux formation and a bluish tinge indicating increased paraproteins. The bone marrow aspirate (**b**) reveals a mixture of lymphocytes, plasma cells, and lymphoplasmacytoid lymphocytes. (**c**, **d**) Bone marrow biopsy is hypercellular with a diffuse infiltrate of lymphocytes, plasma cells, and lymphoplasmacytoid lymphocytes

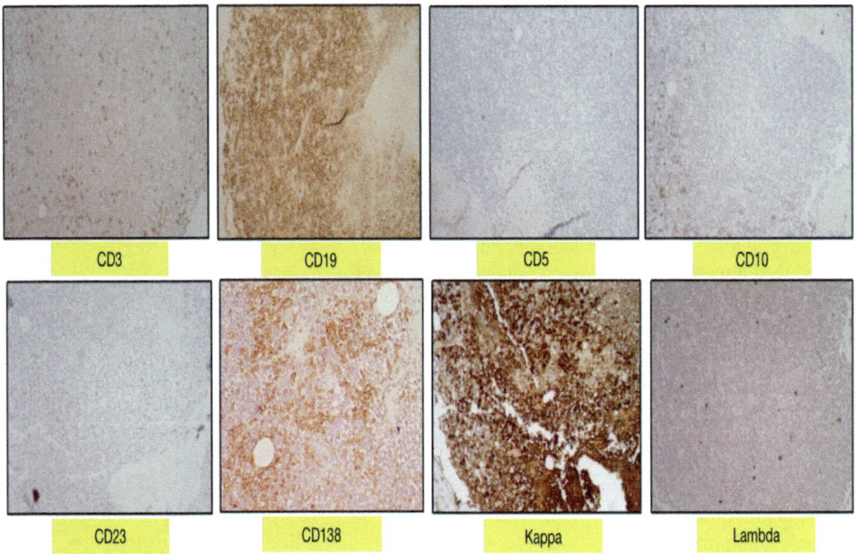

Fig. 26.4 IHC on the marrow shows a CD19-positive, CD5-negative, CD10-negative, CD23--negative, and kappa-restricted infiltrate

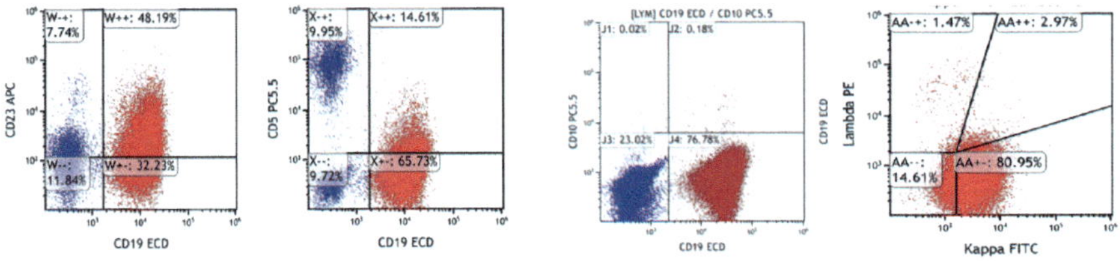

Fig. 26.5 Peripheral blood flow cytometry reveals CD19 positive, CD5 negative, CD23 heterogenous positive, CD10 negative, and a kappa-restricted population of atypical cells

Caveats

1. False-negative flow cytometric evaluation may occur, which may be due to cell loss during processing, especially for large cells and plasma cells. For this, compare smears from a fresh sample with the cytospin. Sometimes there may be paucity of neoplastic cells and hence require more events.
2. CD20-negative B cells post rituximab may be there therefore use flow markers/ IHCs for multiple lineage representative Ag.
3. Small proportion of CD5+ B cells, in the absence of a previously established lymphoma diagnosis, have to be evaluated with caution, especially in autoimmune conditions.
4. 5% of LPL and SMZL are CD5 + .
5. Follicular lymphoma has relatively weak CD19 and is CD10 –ve in bone marrow infiltration settings.

6. Although the presence of a clonal B-cell population is usually associated with malignancy, several studies demonstrated clonal B-cell populations in reactive conditions, especially in antigen-driven proliferation of mucosa-associated lymphoid tissue (MALT) in the stomach, thyroid, orbit, and salivary gland. This has to be kept in mind.
7. B-cell lymphoproliferations may also have non-detectable surface light chain immunoglobulins when analyzed by FC, most likely due to the very low density of antigens on the cells' surfaces. The most common type of lymphoma with a lack of surface κ and surface λ expression by FC is follicular lymphoma, followed by diffuse large B-cell lymphoma (DLBCL) and CLL/SLL. Plasma cells and primary mediastinal large B-cell lymphoma also usually lack surface immunoglobulin expression by FC.
8. FCM analysis of lymph nodes, blood, and bone marrow from patients with HIV often shows B-cells with strong κ and λ expression and poor resolution between κ+/κ and λ+/λ− cells, giving the false impression of dual κ and λ positivity

References

1. Campo E, Jaffe ES, Cook JR, Quintanilla-Martinez L, Swerdlow SH, Anderson KC, et al. The International Consensus Classification of mature lymphoid neoplasms: a report from the Clinical Advisory Committee. Blood. 2022;140:1229–53.
2. Naresh KN, Srinivas V, Soman CS. Distribution of various subtypes of non-Hodgkin's lymphoma in India: a study of 2773 lymphomas using R.E.A.L. and WHO classifications. Ann Oncol. 2000;11(Suppl 1):63–7.
3. Alaggio R, Amador C, Anagnostopoulos I, Attygalle AD, Araujo IBO, Berti E, et al. The 5th edition of the World Health Organization Classification of haematolymphoid tumours: lymphoid neoplasms. Leukemia. 2022;36:1720–48.
4. Bain BJ. Bone marrow trephine biopsy. J Clin Pathol. 2001;54(10):737–42.
5. Gujral S, Subramanian PG, Patkar N, et al. Report of proceedings of the national meeting on "Guidelines for Immunophenotyping of Hematolymphoid Neoplasms by Flow Cytometry". Indian J Pathol Microbiol. 2008;51(2):161–6.
6. Rawstron AC, et al. Monoclonal B-cell lymphocytosis and chronic lymphocytic leukemia. N Engl J Med. 2008;359(6):575–83.
7. Hallek M, Cheson BD, Catovsky D, Caligaris-Cappio F, Dighiero G, Dohner H, et al. iwCLL guidelines for diagnosis, indications for treatment, response assessment, and supportive management of CLL. Blood. 2018;131:2745–60.
8. Hallek M, Al-Sawaf O. Chronic lymphocytic leukemia: 2022 update on diagnostic and therapeutic procedures. Am J Hematol. 2021;96:1679–705.
9. Armitage JO, Longo DL. Mantle-cell lymphoma. N Engl J Med. 2022;386:2495–506.
10. Tam CS, Anderson MA, Pott C, Agarwal R, Handunnetti S, Hicks RJ, et al. Ibrutinib plus venetoclax for the treatment of mantle-cell lymphoma. N Engl J Med. 2018;378:1211–23.
11. Jimenez C, Sebastian E, Chillon MC, Giraldo P, Mariano Hernandez J, Escalante F, et al. MYD88 L265P is a marker highly characteristic of, but not restricted to, Waldenstrom's macroglobulinemia. Leukemia. 2013;27:1722–1728.
12. Treon SP, Gustine J, Xu L, Manning RJ, Tsakmaklis N, Demos M, et al. MYD88wild-type Waldenstrom macroglobulinaemia: differential diagnosis, risk of histological transformation, and overall survival. Br J Haematol. 2018;180:374–80.

13. Hunter ZR, Xu L, Tsakmaklis N, Demos MG, Kofifides A, Jimenez C, et al. Insights into the genomic landscape of MYD88 wild-type Waldenstrom macroglobulinemia. Blood Adv. 2018;2:2937–46.
14. Xing KH, et al. Outcomes in splenic marginal zone lymphoma: analysis of 107 patients treated in British Columbia. Br J Haematol. 2015;169(4):520–7.
15. Laurent C, Adelaide J, Guille A, Tesson B, Gat E, Evrard S, et al. High-grade follicular lymphomas exhibit clinicopathologic, cytogenetic, and molecular diversity extending beyond grades 3A and 3B. Am J Surg Pathol. 2021;45:1324–36.
16. Campo E. Genetic and molecular genetic studies in the diagnosis of B-cell lymphomas I: mantle cell lymphoma, follicular lymphoma, and Burkitt's lymphoma. Hum Pathol. 2003;34(4):330–5.
17. Rossi D, Bertoni F, Zucca E. Marginal-zone lymphomas. N Engl J Med. 2022;386:568–81.
18. Clipson A, Wang M, de Leval L, Ashton-Key M, Wotherspoon A, Vassiliou G, et al. KLF2 mutation is the most frequent somatic change in splenic marginal zone lymphoma and identifies a subset with distinct genotype. Leukemia. 2015;29:1177–85.
19. Angelova EA, Medeiros LJ, Wang W, Muzzafar T, Lu X, Khoury JD, et al. Clinicopathologic and molecular features in hairy cell leukemia-variant: single institutional experience. Mod Pathol. 2018;31:1717–32.
20. Falini B, De Carolis L, Tiacci E. How I treat refractory/relapsed hairy cell leukemia with BRAF inhibitors. Blood. 2022;139:2294–305.
21. Miguet L, Mayeur-Rousse C, Eischen A, et al. The contribution of CD148, CD180 and CD200 combination in the diagnosis of chronic B-cell lymphoproliferative disorders. Blood. 2021;138(Supplement 1):3520. https://doi.org/10.1182/blood-2021-150810.
22. Gautam A, Sreedharanunni S, Sachdeva MUS, et al. The relative expression levels of CD148 and CD180 on clonal B cells and CD148/CD180 median fluorescence intensity ratios are useful in the characterization of mature B cell lymphoid neoplasms infiltrating blood and bone marrow—results from a single centre pilot study. Int J Lab Hematol. 2021;43:1123–31. https://doi.org/10.1111/ijlh.13467.

Chapter 27
Risk Stratification and Advances in CLL Management. How to Choose Best BTK Inhibitor for CLL Patient?

Maitreyee Bhattacharyya

Abstract The treatment landscape of chronic lymphocytic leukemia (CLL) has changed significantly with the introduction of targeted therapies like Bruton tyrosine kinase inhibitor (BTKi) and BCL-2 inhibitor (venetoclax). At diagnosis, patients are stratified into four groups according to CLL-IPI. Targeted therapy has been proven to be more effective than chemoimmunotherapy even in high-risk group patients defined by unmutated IGHV, deletion 17p (17p-), and mutation TP53. While monotherapy with BTKi is an excellent option for many patients, combination therapies can induce deep and durable remissions. There are several doublet therapies that are currently in clinical use. These include combinations of BTKi with BCL2 inhibitors (venetoclax). Triplets combine BTKi with venetoclax and CD20 inhibitors. Selecting proper treatment depends on the patient's co-morbidities, concomitant use of other drugs, cost, and the patient's preference.

Keywords Chronic lymphocytic leukemia (CLL) · Bruton tyrosine kinase inhibitor (BTKi) · Venetoclax · Chemoimmunotherapy (CIT) · Progression-free survival (PFS) · Minimal residual disease (MRD)

Learning Objectives
- Review the risk stratification factors for CLL
- Evaluate the current treatment options for CLL
- Evaluate the safety and efficacy of available BTKi
- Compare various combinations (targeted) therapies
- To decide how to select the right drug for the right patient

---

M. Bhattacharyya (✉)
Institute of Haematology & Transfusion Medicine (IHTM), Medical College, Kolkata, West Bengal, India

H. P. Pati et al. (eds.), *Clinical Hematology and Hemato-Oncology*,
https://doi.org/10.1007/978-981-92-1167-8_27

27.1 Introduction

CLL is the most common adult leukemia in the Western world. This is a disease of Elderly. There have been significant changes in the treatment approach of CLL over the last decade. Even a decade back, the mainstay of treatment was chemoimmunotherapy (CIT), consisting of various chemotherapeutic agents with CD20 antibodies. With a better understanding of the disease biology, therapy has been shifted towards targeted therapy with either continuous Bruton tyrosine kinase inhibitors (BTKi) or a fixed duration BCL 2 inhibitor (Venetoclax), and CD20 antibodies. Despite these advances, many unresolved issues remain, like

(i) Which BTKi should be used?
(ii) Whether BTKi needs to be combined with the CD20 antibody
(iii) What should be the preferred therapy—continuous BTKi or fixed dose Venetoclax

This article will try to find out answer of these by reviewing available literature.

27.2 Clinical Case

A 74-year-old patient presents with cervical lymphadenopathy with comorbidities like hypertension, high cholesterol, and benign prostatic hypertrophy (BPH). Extensive bulky nodes in the neck, axilla, and groin; WBC—88,000 (90% lymphocytes), Hb—9.1 g/dl, PLT—104,000. Flow cytometry confirms CLL diagnosis, IGHV unmutated, beta 2 micro-globulin 5.8 ug/ml. Marrow is 70% replaced with CLL. CT scan reveals widespread adenopathy with the largest nodes 12 cm in the mesentery and 8 cm in the retroperitoneum. FISH testing reveals del(11q), TP53 not detected. His creatinine clearance is 42 ml/min. ECG and echocardiography are normal.

The patient is /hypertensive/dyslipidemic/ underwent PTCA 2 years back. Current medication includes aspirin, bisoprolol, candesartan, and atorvastatin

27.3 Risk Stratification in CL

All patients should undergo risk stratification at diagnosis as per the CLL International Prognostic Index (CLL-IPI) [1]. CLL-IPI includes age > 65 years, Rai stage I-IV, serum beta-2 microglobulin >3.5 mg/L, unmutated immunoglobulin heavy chain (IGHV) genes, and del17p by fluorescence in situ hybridization (FISH) or TP53 mutation by sequencing. Four risk groups (low, intermediate, high, and very-high risk) with different 5-year OS (93%, 79%, 63%, and 23%, respectively) were identified (Table 27.1). This prognostic stratification was associated with

Table 27.1 CLL International Prognostic Index

Prognostic factors	Points
Del 17p on FISH or TP53 mutation	4
Unmutated IGHV	2
Serum beta 2 microglobulin >3.5	2
Rai stage I-IV	1
Age > 65 yrs	1

Table 27.2 Time to first therapy

CLL-IPI	Median years	5 years TTFT Estimated risk	10 years TTFT Estimated risk
Low (0–1)	Not reached	23%	40%
Intermediate (2, 3)	3.7	58%	74%
High (4–6)	2.1	77%	83%
Very high (7–10)	0.7	87%	Not estimable

overall survival (OS) in the past. However, in the era of novel targeted agents, this cannot be used for the prediction of OS. However, it is a very strong predictor of time to first therapy (TTFT) in patients with previously untreated CLL (Table 27.2).

In addition to this ß2-MG, TK, CD38, CD49, ZAP-70, telomere length, metaphase chromosome karyotype, and specific gene mutations (e.g., *NOTCH1*, *SF3B1*, *ATM*, *NFKBIE*, *BIRC3*) have been found to be of prognostic significance, but their role in the era of targeted therapy is less well established and not used in clinical practice. Complex karyotype is also not used currently due to unclear cut points (3 or 5 aberrations), less consistent associations with outcome [2], MRD, though found to have prognostic value, is not considered, as there was no advantage of MRD-directed therapy over fixed-duration therapy.

27.4 Clinical Case (Continued)

CLL—IPI score of our patient was 6, so the patient was in the high-risk group. Whatever the risk score of the patients, asymptomatic patients are kept under watch & wait (Fig. 27.1) when the iwCLL criteria for "active disease" are met [3] (Fig. 27.1).

27.5 Advances in Management

Preferred treatment options are targeted therapy with Bruton tyrosine kinase inhibitor (BTKi) either as monotherapy or in combination. The BTK gene was the 17th identified gene in 1980 [4]. This enzyme, Bruton's tyrosine kinase, a member of the

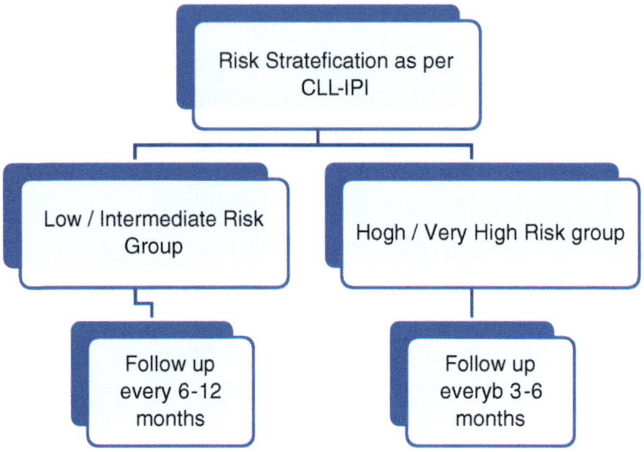

Fig. 27.1 Approach to management of newly diagnosed CLL

Tec kinase family, is vital for B-cell signaling, development, and differentiation, and is a prerequisite for B-cell survival and proliferation. Studies found that inhibition of this pathway was likely to provide clinical benefit in B-cell malignancies. All three bind covalently and irreversibly to the C481 receptor of BTK. blocking its ability to phosphorylate its substrates and subsequently suppressing downstream signaling (Fig. 27.2). The first was ibrutinib, then came acalabrutinib and Zanubrutinib. Acalabrutinib and Zanubrutinib are more selective with less off target effects [5]. Currently, newer BTK-inhibitor pirtobrutinib, which is a non-covalent, reversible binding at functions primarily through the blockage of ATP-binding sites, has alternative sites to the traditional C481 [6]. B-cell leukemia/lymphoma-2 (BCL2) protein is overexpressed in CLL patients. Venetoclax is a highly selective, second-generation BCL2 inhibitor. In the phase I clinical trial, 116 high-risk R/R CLL patients received venetoclax; the overall response rate (ORR) was 79%, and 20% patients achieved complete remission (CR) [7]. Venetoclax has also undergone study in combination with CD20 inhibitors and BTKI treatment of CLL, initially started with mechlorethamine in 1949. Important landmarks of therapy are chlorambucil in 1957, FCR 2000, bendamustine in 2008, Ibrutinib in 2014, venetoclax in 2017, acalabrutinib in 2019, and zanubrutinib in 2023 [8]. The treatment paradigm has shifted from chemoimmunotherapy (CIT) to BTKi. We have many BTKi for the treatment of CLL. So the physicians are faced with the challenges of selecting appropriate BTKi considering efficacy, safety, and comorbidity of the patient. BTKi needs continuous therapy and prolongs PFS only, but venetoclax is of fixed duration and MRD directed (Table 27.3).

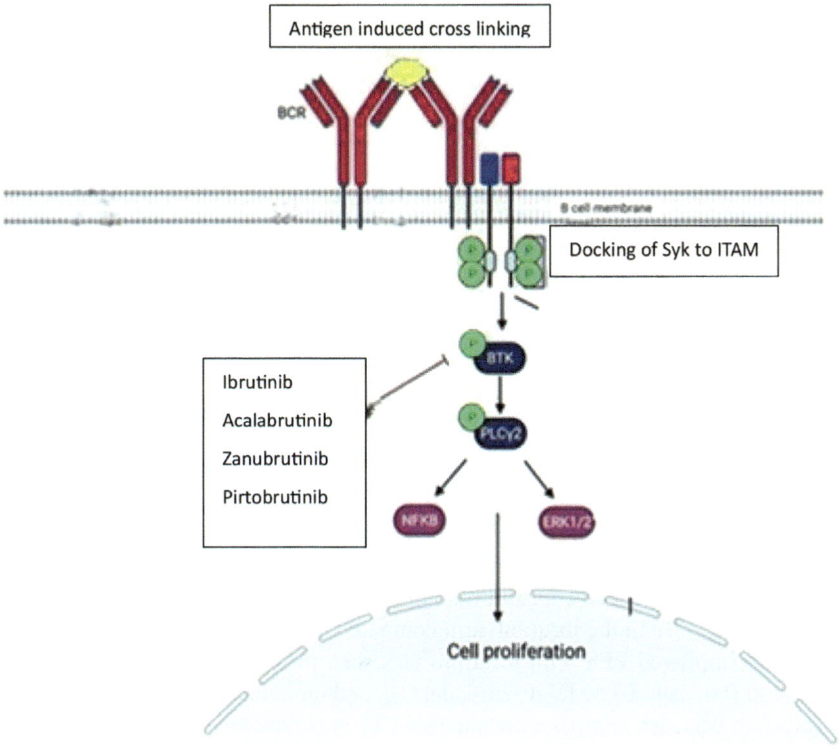

Fig. 27.2 Mechanism of action of BTKi

Table 27.3 Modern goal of therapy

Continuous therapy	Goal of therapy
Ibrutinib Acalabrutinib Zanubrutinib Pirtobrutinib	Disease control Prolonged PFS
Fixed duration therapy	
Venetoclax	Disease eradication

27.5.1 Ibrutinib

Ibrutinib was approved by the FDA for use in CLL in 2014. In the RESONATE study, Ibrutinib was evaluated in relapse/refractory CLL patients against ofatumumab. About 400 patients were recruited and randomized. High-risk cytogenetics were present in about 50% patients in both groups. After a median follow-up of 44 months, PFS had not been reached in the ibrutinib arm, whereas it was 8.1 months with ofatumumab ($p < 0.001$). Overall survival at 1 year was also much better with

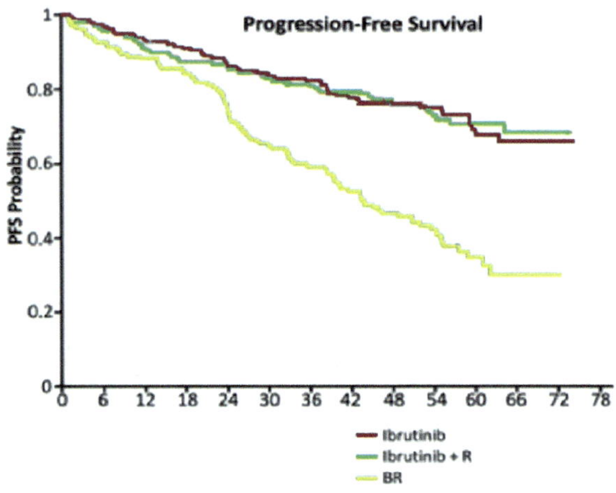

Fig. 27.3 Ibrutinib ± rituximab vs. BR in untreated elderly CLL patients

Ibrutinib 90% vs 81% in ofatumumab (p + 0.005). The 3-year PFS was 59% with ibrutinib, whereas it was only 3% with ofatumumab [9, 10].

In the RESONATE 2 study, newly diagnosed patients who were 65 years of age were randomized to receive ibrutinib or chlorambucil. Five-year PFS and OS rates were 70% and 83% in the ibrutinib arm compared to 12% and 68% in the chlorambucil arm. Improved PFS with ibrutinib was seen in high-risk subgroups such as those with Rai stage III or IV disease, del11q, and unmutated *IGHV* status [11, 12]

Ibrutinib was also compared to standard CIT bendamustine + rituximab (BR) in Alliance A041202 trial, either alone or in combination with rituximab. The 2-year PFS were 74% with BR, 87% with ibrutinib ($p < 0.001$), and 88% with ibrutinib plus rituximab ($p < 0.001$), ORRs were higher in the ibrutinib-containing arms compared with the BR arm; however, complete response (CR) rates and rates of minimal residual disease (MRD) negativity were numerically higher with BR [13, 14] (Fig. 27.3).

Ibrutinib in combination with rituximab was compared with another CIT—FCR in patients aged 70 yrs. or younger. Three-year PFS were 89% with ibrutinib plus rituximab and 73% with FCR (HR = 0.35, $p < 0.001$). Three-year OS rates were 99% and 92% for ibrutinib plus rituximab compared with FCR (HR = 0.17, $p < 0.001$) [15].

27.5.2 Acalabrutinib

It is a second-generation BTKi that binds covalently and irreversibly to C481 of BTK [16]. Less off-target effects on other kinases such as TEC, EGFR, and ITK [17]. Two landmark trials of acalabrutinib in CLL are ASCEND and ELEVATE-TN. In the ASCEND trial, relapse-refractory CLL patients were randomized to receive acalabrutinib, idelalisib plus rituximab, or BR.

The median age was 67 years (range, 32–90). Sixteen percent had del17p; 42% had Rai stage III/IV. The 12-month PFS was much better with acalabrutinib compared to the other two protocols (88% in the acalabrutinib arm vs 68% in the IdR and BR arm), OS with acalabrutinib was 94% compared to 91% with the other two regimens [18].

In the ELEVATE-TN study, treatment-naïve CLL patients were randomized to receive acalabrutinib/acalabrutinib with obinutuzumab/obinutuzumab with chlorambucil. Median age of the patients was 70 years. As per the CLL International Prognostic Index score, 69% patients were high risk and 12% very high risk. Chlorambucil plus obinutuzumab had a PFS of 22.6 months; PFS has not been reached for acalabrutinib and acalabrutinib plus obinutuzumab ($p < 0.001$). The ORR for acalabrutinib plus obinutuzumab was 94%, for acalabrutinib was 85%, and for obinutuzumab plus chlorambucil was 79% [19]. 4-year estimated PFS rates were 87%, 78%, and 25% for obinutuzumab plus acalabrutinib, acalabrutinib monotherapy, and obinutuzumab plus chlorambucil, respectively [20].

In the ELEVATE-RR clinical trial, acalabrutinib and ibrutinib were compared in relapsed/refractory CLL patients; acalabrutinib was found to be non-inferior in terms of PFS (38.6 months) compared to ibrutinib (38.4 months PFS). Acalabrutinib had a better safety profile compared to ibrutinib [21], Fig. 27.4.

Patients intolerant to ibrutinib received acalabrutinib [22]. Patients experienced persistent grade 3 or 4 adverse events or had persistent or recurrent grade 2 adverse events despite dose modification and interruption. The 36-month estimated PFS was 58%. The ORR was 73. The results of this study demonstrate that acalabrutinib is a safe and effective option for patients with relapsed/refractory CLL who are not able to tolerate ibrutinib

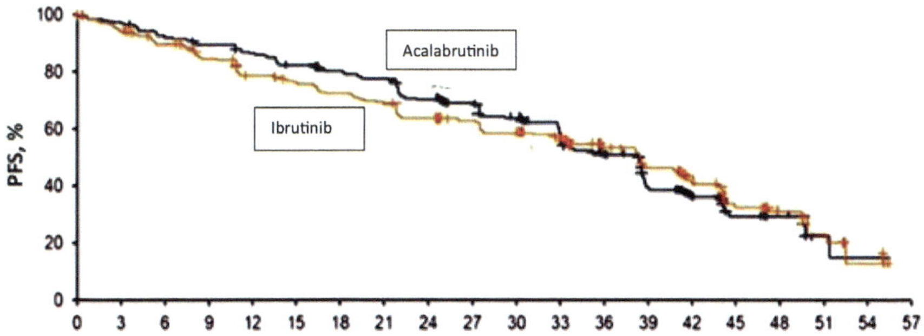

	Events,n(%)	Medilan (95% CI)
Acalabrutinib	143 (53.4)	38.4 (33.0-38.6)
Ibrutinib	136 (51.3)	38.4 (33.0-41.6)

Fig. 27.4 ELEVATE-RR trial showing non-inferiority of acalabrutinib compared to Ibrutinib (PFS)

27.5.3 Zanubrutinib

Zanubrutinib is a second-generation BTKi, approved for CLL. This is also a selective inhibitor with less off target effects. This drug was compared to Imatinib in relapse/refractory CLL patients in the ALPINE trial. The ORR after a median of 15 months was 78% with zanubrutinib compared to 63% with Ibrutinib ($p = 0.0006$). At 24 months, PFS were 78.4% in the zanubrutinib group and 65% in the Ibrutinib group. Response with zanubrutinib was better in patients [23].

In the SEQUOIA trial, zanubrutinib was compared to bendamustine plus rituximab (BR) in treatment-naive patients with chronic lymphocytic leukemia/small lymphocytic. At a median follow-up of 61.2 months, median PFS was not reached in the zanubrutinib group; median PFS was 44.1 months in the BR-groups (hazard ratio [HR], 0.29; one-sided P 5.0001). Prolonged PFS was seen in patients with mutated immunoglobulin heavy-chain variable region (IGHV) genes (HR, 0.40; one-sided P 5 0.0003) and unmutated IGHV genes (HR, 0.21 [95%CI, 0.14 to 0.33]; one-sided $P < 0.0001$). Median overall survival (OS) was not reached in either treatment arm; estimated 60-month OS rates were 85.8% and 85.0% in zanubrutinib- and BR-treated patients, respectively [24] (Fig. 27.5).

27.5.4 Pirtobrutinib

Pirtobrutinib is a non-covalent, reversible BTK inhibitor, which is effective in C481-mutated disease, a common mechanism of resistance to covalent BTK inhibitors in CLL [25]. The BRUIN trial evaluated pirtobrutinib in the BRUIN trial in

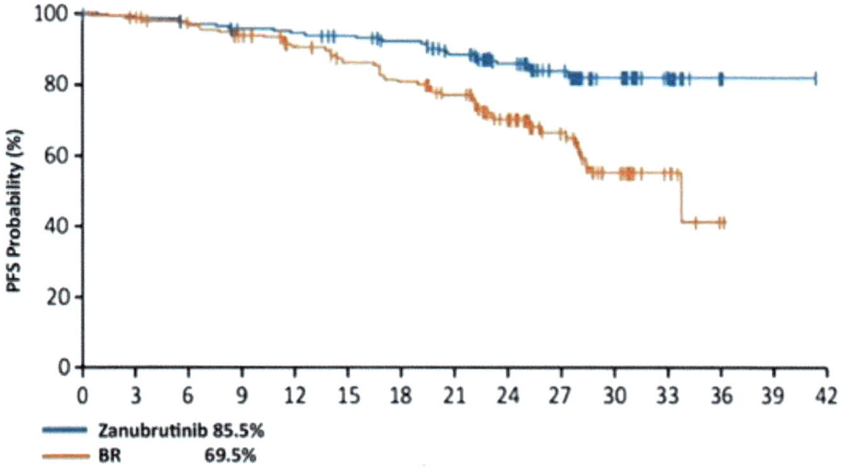

Fig. 27.5 SEQUIOA Trial: PFS with zanubrutinib vs BR

Table 27.4 Superiority of BTKi over CIT

Study	Alliance	ELEVATE-TN	SEQUOIA
Drugs	Ibrutinib ± rituximab Vs BR	Acalabrutinib ± G vs G + Clb	Zanubrutinib vs BR
Duration of follow-up	4.5 years	5 years	26 months
Efficacy	48 months PFS 76% for ibrutinib, 47% for BR	60 months PFS 84% and 72% A + G, acalabrutinib vs 21% for G + Clb	24 months PFS 86% for zanubrutinib vs 70% for BR

relapsed refractory B-cell malignancies, including CLL, SLL, and MCL.38. The 86% of CLL or SLL patients who had received prior BTKi, the ORR with pirtobrutinib was 62%. And 52% in previous BTKi inhibitor-resistant cases. In patients with the C481 mutation, ORR was 71% [26].

BTKi monotherapy is preferred over chemoimmunotherapy (CIT) due to superior efficacy and better tolerability (Table 27.4). However, BTKi needs continuous therapy and is not MRD-directed.

27.6 Combination Therapy with BTKi

In the HELLOS trial, BR was combined with ibrutinib in one arm and a placebo in the other. Patients in both groups had received a median of two prior lines of therapy and the most common prior therapy was FCR. ORR was significantly higher in the ibrutinib arm than in the placebo plus BR arm (83% versus 68%). MRD negativity was also higher in the Ibrutinib pls BR arm [27]. After 5 years of follow-up, PFS was 65.1 months in the ibrutinib plus BR arm compared to 14.3 months in the placebo plus BR arm 42. The CR/CRi was 40.8% at 5 years. OS benefit was also noted in the Ibrutinib arm [28]. Ibrutinib was added to fludarabine, cyclophosphamide, and obinutuzumab (iFCG), for a definitive duration of Ibrutinib [29]. Patients received three cycles of iFCG. Obinutuzumab 3 more cycles and 9 more cycles of ibrutinib given to patients who achieved MRD negativity. Nine additional cycles of obinutuzumab plus ibrutinib were given to the rest of the patients. Patients who achieved MRD negativity at the end of 12 cycles discontinued all treatment,

MRD-positive patients continued ibrutinib. 41. At 12 months, 98% of patients had achieved MRD negativity. Three-year PFS and OS rates were 98% and 98%, respectively.

Fixed-duration ibrutinib was also studied along with venetoclax. In this study, high-risk CLL patients received ibrutinib monotherapy for three cycles [29]. Venetoclax was added from 4th cycle, and combined therapy was given for 24 cycles. After 12 cycles, 88% of previously untreated patients achieved CR/CRi, and 61% achieved MRD negativity. Estimated 3-year PFS and OS rates were 93% and 96%, respectively.

In another study (CAPTIVATE trial,) newly diagnosed CLL patients were given 3 cycles of ibrutinib followed by 12 cycles of ibrutinib plus venetoclax [30].

Patients who were MRD (uMRD) negative were randomized to receive a placebo or ibrutinib until MRD relapse or disease progression. Patients with detectable MRD detectable disease (uMRD) received Ibrutinib or ibrutinib plus venetoclax zanubrutinib has also been combined with venetoclax, a combination given for 12–24 months. If the pt's uMRD $<10^{-4}$, it's stopped early. ORR was 97% [31].

The most recent combination is venetoclax plus ibrutinib plus Obinutuzumab. Acalabrutinib and zanubrutinib have also been studied in a triplet. The rate of uMRD after 24 months was more than 80% with both the drugs [32–34].

27.7 Safety

Major concern for selecting a drug is its toxicity, patients' characteristics, comorbidities, and concomitant use of other drugs. BTKi has many off-target effects, which lead to various adverse effects like skin rash, diarrhea, bleeding manifestations, hypertension, and arrhythmia [35].

As BTK is a regulator of innate immunity, BTK inhibition leads to opportunistic infections. Invasive fungal infections have also been documented [36].

In addition, in CLL patients who were on treatment with BTKi, the seroconversion rate to various vaccines—hepatitis B, influenza, COVID 19 was very poor [37–39].

Incidence of bleeding is very high with Ibrutinib; in one study, it was reported that bleeding of any kind occurred in 50.6% cases [40].

Being a member of the Tec kinase family, BTK functions to signal downstream of various platelet transmembrane receptors, which is inhibited by BTKi [41].

Inhibition of CSK by BTKi leads to cardiac arrhythmia, the most common of which is atrial fibrillation. Ventricular arrhythmia leading to sudden cardiac death has also been reported [42, 43]. In the ELEVATE-RR study, the rate of atrial fibrillation was 9.4% with acalabrutinib compared to 16% with ibrutinib [44]. Atrial fibrillation was only 2.5% with zanubrutinib [45]. Another important cardiovascular effect is hypertension, new or worsened, reported as 78.3 and 17.7%, respectively [46] (Fig. 27.6). Therapy discontinuation rate due to ibrutinib intolerance is around 41% [47].

The most frequent adverse events with acalabrutinib were diarrhea (53%), headache (42%), contusion (40%), dizziness (33%), upper respiratory tract infection (33%), and cough (30%). Acalabrutinib discontinuation was because of adverse events only in 17% cases.

BTK inhibition leads to situations where it is actually difficult to take therapeutic decision. Increased bleeding risk, along with the need for anticoagulation in atrial fibrillation are really difficult situation.

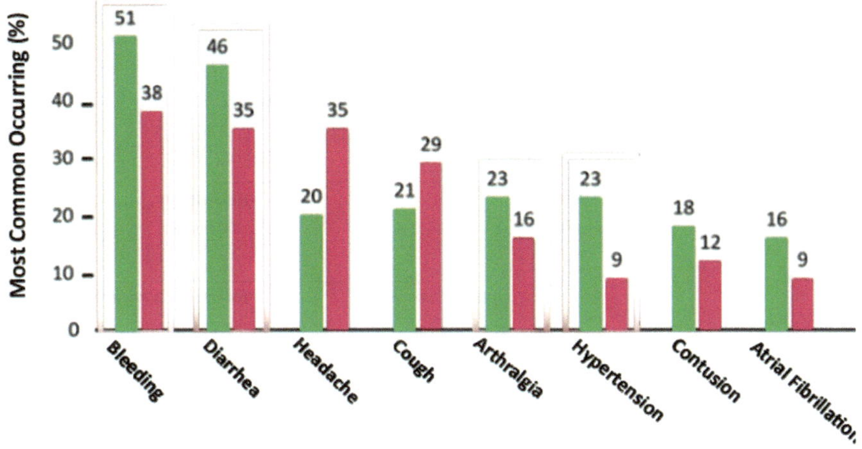

Fig. 27.6 Adverse effects of acalabrutinib vs ibrutinib

27.8 Selecting BTKi

Selecting a BTKi out of the available three depends on consideration of the adverse effects of the drug, co-morbidities of the patient, and concomitant drugs used by patients.

Ibrutinib is the least selective BTKi and leads to many side effects, especially cardiovascular side effects. Zanubrutinib and acalabrutinib are more selective inhibitors and have less cardiovascular side effects. So these two drugs, instead of Ibrutinib to be considered in patients with pre-existing cardiovascular diseases. Most of the trials with acalabrutinib and zanubrutinib have not included patients on anti-coagulation; however, the SEQUOIA trial demonstrated the safety of zanubrutinib in this group of patients [48].

BTKi are metabolized in the liver through CYP3A4 [49–51]. It is recommended to avoid acalabrutinib and reduce the dose of ibrutinib and zanubrutinib with concomitant use of strong CYP3A inhibitors. Solubility of acalabrutinib decreases with an increase of gastric ph, so it should be avoided in patients on proton pump inhibitors and should be given 2 hours prior to any H2 blocker. However, ibrutinib and zanubrutinib can be given in these situations. Ibrutinib and zanubrutinib can be given once daily; however, acalabrutinib needs twice daily doses

BTKi monotherapy gives only better PFS and needs to continue till disease progression, if MRD-directed and fixed duration therapy is preferred, then a combination of BTKi with venetoclax should be given [30, 31]. So, a combination of BTKi either with CD20 antibody or with venetoclax is the preferred treatment of choice for newly diagnosed CLL (Fig. 27.7).

In case of CLL with Tp53 mutation, zanubrutinib has shown superiority over Ibrutinib.

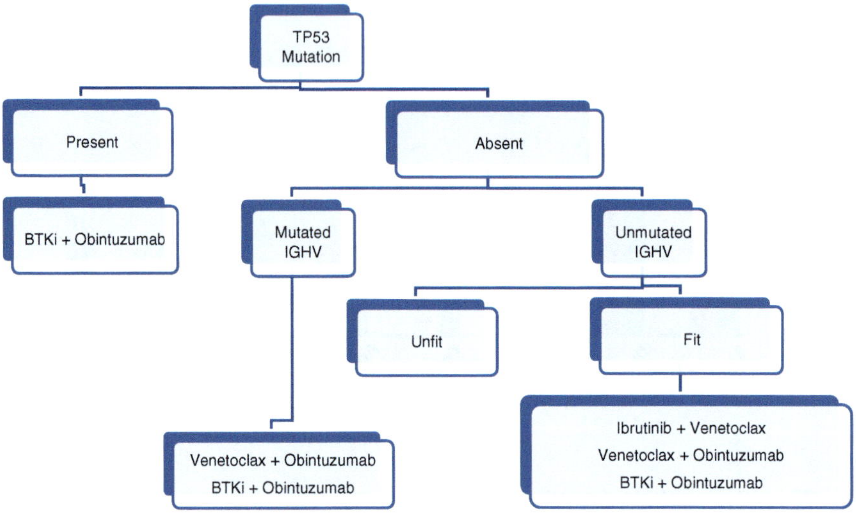

Fig. 27.7 Treatment algorithm—newly diagnosed CLL

27.9 Clinical Case (Continued)

For the CLL case concerned, BTKi and BCL2 inhibitor–based therapy are appropriate options as PFS and OS are better over CIT. BTKi monotherapy needs continuous treatment, whereas combination with BCL 2 inhibitor can be given for a fixed duration. His tumor load is very high, with mild impairment of renal function, which favors BTKi therapy but at the cost of continuous treatment. On the other hand, factors favoring fixed-duration BCL2 inhibitor-based regimens are his cardiac comorbidity and hypertension. These options with pros and cons were discussed with the patient, and he opted for a fixed-duration therapy. Since the patient is hypertensive with underlying coronary artery disease and on an antiplatelet drug, a combination of venetoclax and zanubrutinib is considered for him.

27.10 Conclusions

The introduction of targeted agents has revolutionized the treatment of CLL, regardless of risk factors or age. Indeed, BTKi and venetoclax, with or without the anti-CD20 monoclonal antibody obinutuzumab, were convincingly shown to represent relatively safe and effective agents. Though PFS was much better with these agents, a survival advantage over CIT has not been documented. Thus, today, personalized treatment of CLL patients is possible, and the choice of a fixed-duration approach based on venetoclax-containing regimens or a continuous treatment approach with BTKi should be discussed with every patient. Therapeutic decisions should be guided by coexisting medical conditions, logistics, efficacy of the agents, and treatment goals.

References

1. An international prognostic index for patients with chronic lymphocytic leukaemia (CLL-IPI): a meta-analysis of individual patient data. The Lancet Oncol. 17:779–90.
2. 457| Hematology 2024 | ASH Education Program.
3. Hallek M, Cheson BD, Catovsky D, et al. iwCLL guidelines for diagnosis, indication for treatment, response assessment, and supportive management of CLL. Blood. 2018;131(25):2745–60.
4. Vetrie D, Vorˇechovsky I, Sideras P, et al. The gene involved in X-linked agammaglobulinaemia is a member of the src family of protein-tyrosine kinases. Nature. 1993;361:226–33.
5. Lewis KL, Cheah CY. Non-covalent BTK inhibitors—the new BTKids on the block for B-cell malignancies. J Pers Med. 2021;11:764.
6. Brandhuber B, Gomez E, Smith S, et al. LOXO- 305, a next generation reversible BTK inhibitor,for overcoming acquired resistance to irreversible BTK inhibitors. Clin Lymphoma Myeloma Leuk. 2018;18:S216.
7. Roberts AW, Davids MS, Pagel JM, Kahl BS, Puvvada SD, Gerecitano JF, Kipps TJ, Anderson MA, Brown JR, Gressick L, et al. Targeting BCL2 with venetoclax in relapsed chronic lymphocytic leukemia. N Engl J Med. 2016;374:311–22.
8. Sutanto F, Konstantinidou M, Domling A. Covalent inhibitors: a rational approach to drug discovery. RSC Med Chem. 2020;11:876–84.
9. Byrd JC, Brown JR, O'Brien S, et al. Ibrutinib versus ofatumumab in previously treated chronic lymphoid leukemia. N Engl J Med. 2014;371:213–23.
10. Byrd JC, Hillmen P, O'Brien S, et al. Longterm follow-up of the RESONATE phase 3 trial of ibrutinib vs ofatumumab. Blood. 2019;133:2031–42.
11. Burger JA, Tedeschi A, Barr PM, et al. Ibrutinib as initial therapy for patients with chronic lymphocytic leukemia. N Engl J Med. 2015;373:2425–37.
12. Burger JA, Barr PM, Robak T, et al. Long-term efficacy and safety of first-line ibrutinib treatment for patients with CLL/SLL: 5 years of follow-up from the phase 3 RESONATE-2 study. Leukemia. 2020;34:787–98.
13. Woyach JA, Ruppert AS, Heerema NA, et al. Ibrutinib regimens versus chemoimmunotherapy in older patients with untreated CLL. N Engl J Med. 2018;379:2517–28.
14. Byrd JC, Furman RR, Coutre SE, et al. Ibrutinib treatment for first-line and relapsed/refractory chronic lymphocytic leukemia: final analysis of the pivotal phase Ib/II PCYC-1102 study. Clin Cancer Res. 2020;26:3918–27.
15. Shanafelt TD, Wang XV, Kay NE, et al. Ibrutinib-rituximab or chemoimmunotherapy for chronic lymphocytic leukemia. N Engl J Med. 2019;381:432–43.
16. Byrd JC, Harrington B, O'Brien S, et al. Acalabrutinib (ACP-196) in relapsed chronic lymphocytic leukemia. N Engl J Med. 2016;374(4):323–32. https://doi.org/10.1056/NEJMoa1509981.
17. Barf T, Covey T, Izumi R, et al. Acalabrutinib (ACP-196): a covalent bruton tyrosine kinase inhibitor with a differentiated selectivity and in vivo potency profile. J Pharmacol Exp Ther. 2017;363(2):240LP252. https://doi.org/10.1124/jpet.117.242909.
18. Ghia P, Pluta A, Wach M, et al. Acalabrutinib vs rituximab plus Idelalisib (IdR) or Bendamustine (BR) by investigator choice in relapsed/refractory (RR) chronic lymphocytic leukemia: phase 3 ASCEND study. Hematol Oncol. 2019;37(S2):86–7. https://doi.org/10.1002/hon.54_2629.
19. Sharman JP, Banerji V, Fogliatto LM, et al. ELEVATE TN: phase 3 study of acalabrutinib combined with obinutuzumab (O) or alone vs O plus chlorambucil (Clb) in patients (Pts) with treatment-naive chronic lymphocytic leukemia (CLL). Blood. 2019;134(Supplement_1):31. https://doi.org/10.1182/blood-2019-128404.
20. Sharman JP, Egyed M, Jurczak W, et al. Acalabrutinib ± obinutuzumab versusn obinutuzumab + chlorambucil in treatmentnaive chronic lymphocytic leukemia: elevate-TN four-year follow up. J Clin Oncol. 2021;39:7509.
21. Byrd JC, Hillmen P, Ghia P, Kater AP, Chanan-Khan A, Furman RR, O'Brien S, Yenerel MN, Illés A, Kay N, et al. Acalabrutinib versus Ibrutinib in previously treated chronic lymphocytic leukemia: results of the first randomized phase III trial. J Clin Oncol. 2021;39:3441–52.

22. Rogers KA, Thompson PA, Allan JN, Coleman M, Sharman JP, et al. Phase II study of acalabrutinib in ibrutinib intolerant patients with relapsed/refractory chronic lymphocytic leukemia. Haematologica. 2021;106(9):2364–73.
23. Brown JR, Eichhorst B, Hillmen P, Jurczak W, Kaźmierczak M, Lamanna N, O'Brien SM, Tam CS. Zanubrutinib or Ibrutinib in relapsed or refractory chronic lymphocytic leukemia. N Engl J Med. 2023;388:319–32.
24. Shadman M, Munir T, Robak T, Brown JR, Kahl BS, Ghia P, Giannopoulos K, Šimkovič M, Österborg A, Laurenti L, Walker PA. Zanubrutinib versus bendamustine and rituximab in patients with treatment-naïve chronic lymphocytic leukemia/small lymphocytic lymphoma: median 5-year follow-up of SEQUOIA. J Clin Oncol. 43(7):781.
25. Woyach JA, Furman RR, Liu T-M, et al. Resistance mechanisms for the Bruton's tyrosine kinase inhibitor ibrutinib. N Engl J Med. 2014;370:2286–94.
26. Mato AR, Shah NN, Jurczak W, et al. Pirtobrutinib in relapsed or refractory B-cell malignancies (BRUIN): a phase 1/2 study. Lancet. 2021;397:892–901.
27. Chanan-Khan A, Cramer P, Demirkan F, et al. Ibrutinib combined with bendamustine and rituximab compared with placebo, bendamustine, and rituximab for previously treated chronic lymphocytic leukaemia or small lymphocytic lymphoma (HELIOS): a randomised, double-blind, phase 3 study. Lancet Oncol. 2016;17:200–11.
28. Fraser GAM, Chanan-Khan A, Demirkan F, et al. Final 5-year findings from the phase 3 HELIOS study of ibrutinib plus bendamustine and rituximab in patients with relapsed/refractory chronic lymphocytic leukemia/small lymphocytic lymphoma. Leuk Lymphoma. 2020;61:3188–97.
29. Jain N, Thompson P, Burger J, et al. Ibrutinib, fludarabine, cyclophosphamide, and obinutuzumab (iFCG) regimen for chronic lymphocytic leukemia (CLL) with mutated IGHV and without TP53 aberrations. Leukemia. 2021;35:3421–9.
30. WG, Allan JN, Siddiqi T, et al. Ibrutinib plus venetoclax for first-line treatment of chronic lymphocytic leukemia: primary analysis results from the minimal residual disease cohort of the randomized phase II CAPTIVATE study. J Clin Oncol. 2021;39:3853–65.
31. Tedeschi A, Ferrant E, Flinn IW, *et al.* Zanubrutinib in combination with venetoclax for patients with treatment-naive (TN) chronic lymphocytic leukemia (CLL) or small lymphocytic lymphoma (SLL) with del(17p): early results from Arm D of the SEQUOIA (BGB-3111-304) trial. Blood 2021;138:67.
32. Rogers KA, Huang Y, Ruppert AS, et al. Phase II study of combination obinutuzumab, ibrutinib,and venetoclax in treatment-naive and relapsed or refractory chronic lymphocytic leukemia. J Clin Oncol. 2020;38:3626–37.
33. Davids MS, Lampson BL, Tyekucheva S, et al. Acalabrutinib, venetoclax, and Obinutuzumab as frontline treatment for chronic lymphocytic leukaemia: a single-arm, open-label, phase 2study. Lancet Oncol. 2021; 22: 1391–1402.
34. Soumerai JD, Mato AR, Dogan A, et al. Zanubrutinib, obinutuzumab, and venetoclax with minimal residual disease-driven discontinuation in previously untreated patients with chronic lymphocytic leukaemia or small lymphocytic lymphoma: a multicentre, singlearm, phase 2 trial. Lancet Haematol. 2021;8:e879–90.
35. O'Brien SM, Brown JR, Byrd JC, et al. Monitoring and managing BTK inhibitor treatment-related adverse events in clinical practice. Front Oncol. 2021;11:720704.
36. Ghez D, Calleja A, Protin C, et al. Early-onset invasive aspergillosis and other fungal infections in patients treated with ibrutinib. Blood. 2018;131:1955–9.
37. Sun C, Gao J, Couzens L, et al. Seasonal influenza vaccination in patients with chronic lymphocytic leukemia treated with ibrutinib. JAMA Oncol. 2016;2:1656–7.
38. Pleyer C, Ali MA, Cohen JI, et al. Effect of Bruton tyrosine kinase inhibitor on efficacy of adjuvanted recombinant hepatitis B and zoster vaccines. Blood. 2021;137:185–9.
39. Shadman M, Ujjani C. Vaccinations in CLL: implications for COVID-19. Blood. 2021;137:144–6.

40. Mock J, Kunk PR, Palkimas S, et al. Risk of major bleeding with ibrutinib. Clin Lymphoma Myeloma Leuk. 2018;18:755–61.
41. Kamel S, Horton L, Ysebaert L, et al. Ibrutinib inhibits collagen-mediated but not ADPmediated platelet aggregation. Leukemia. 2015;29:783–7.
42. Brown JR, Moslehi J, O'Brien S, et al. Characterization of atrial fibrillation adverse events reported in ibrutinib randomized controlled registration trials. Haematologica. 2017;102:1796–805.
43. Lampson BL, Yu L, Glynn RJ, et al. Ventricular arrhythmias and sudden death in patients taking ibrutinib. Blood. 2017;129:2581–4.
44. Byrd JC, Hillmen P, Ghia P, et al. Acalabrutinib versus ibrutinib in previously treated chronic lymphocytic leukemia: results of the first randomized phase III trial. J Clin Oncol. 2021;39:3441–52.
45. Hillmen P, Eichhorst B, Brown JR, et al. First interim analysis of ALPINE study: results of a phase 3 randomized study of zanubrutinib vs ibrutinib in patients with relapsed/refractory chronic lymphocytic leukemia/small lymphocytic lymphoma. In: 2021 European Hematology Association Virtual Congress, 11 June 2021, pp. 9–17.
46. Liu N, Rowley BR, Bull CO, et al. BAY 80-6946 is a highly selective intravenous PI3K inhibitor with potent p110α and p110δ activities in tumor cell lines and xenograft models. Mol Cancer Ther. 2013;12:2319–30.
47. Mato AR, Nabhan C, Thompson MC, et al. Toxicities and outcomes of 616 ibrutinib-treated patients in the United States: a real-world analysis. Haematologica. 2018;103:874–9.
48. Tam CS, Robak T, Ghia P, et al. Zanubrutinib monotherapy for patients with treatment naïve chronic lymphocytic leukemia and 17p deletion. Haematologica. 2020;106:2354–63.
49. Imbruvica (ibrutinib) [package insert]. Sunnyvale: Pharmacyclics, Inc., 2020.
50. Calquence (acalabrutinib) [package insert]. Wilmington: AstraZeneca Pharmaceuticals LP; 2019.
51. Brukinsa (zanubrutinib) [package insert]. San Mateo: BeiGene USA, Inc., 2021.

Chapter 28
Management of Aggressive Non-Hodgkins Lymphoma: Case-Based Approach

Vaishnavi Gupta, Mukesh Kumar Singh, Mofizur Rahman Khan, R. N. Tagore, and Avinash Kumar Singh

Abstract Aggressive non-Hodgkin's lymphoma (NHL) represents a diverse group of rapidly proliferating hematologic malignancies, with diffuse large B-cell lymphoma (DLBCL) being the most common subtype, followed by Burkitt lymphoma and peripheral T-cell lymphomas (PTCLs). These cancers, although treatable with chemotherapy and immunotherapy, remain a significant cause of morbidity and mortality, especially in patients who present with advanced disease or experience relapse. Advances in molecular biology have provided insights into the pathogenesis of these cancers, paving the way for more personalized treatment strategies.

This chapter explores the clinical management of aggressive B-cell and T-cell NHLs, focusing on treatment strategies for both newly diagnosed and relapsed/refractory patients. In addition, it examines the role of molecular profiling in risk stratification, emphasizes the importance of emerging therapies such as CAR T-cell therapy, bispecific antibodies, and antibody-drug conjugates (ADCs), and discusses global guidelines for the treatment of NHL, with particular attention to the adaptation of these guidelines in resource-limited settings. Illustrative case studies are used to underscore the clinical decision-making process, guiding the practitioner in tailoring treatment to the individual patient's needs. The chapter concludes with a discussion on future research directions and the ongoing challenges in the management of aggressive NHL.

Keywords Aggressive non-Hodgkin's lymphoma · DLBCL · PTCL · CAR T-cell therapy · Molecular profiling · Global guidelines

---

V. Gupta · M. K. Singh · A. K. Singh (✉)
Department of Hematology, PARAS HMRI Hospital, Patna, Bihar, India

M. R. Khan · R. N. Tagore
Department of Medical Oncology, PARAS HMRI Hospital, Patna, Bihar, India

H. P. Pati et al. (eds.), *Clinical Hematology and Hemato-Oncology*,
https://doi.org/10.1007/978-981-92-1167-8_28

Learning Objectives
- Understand classification and risk stratification.
- Apply treatment for newly diagnosed and R/R NHL.
- Integrate novel/emerging therapies.
- Evaluate global and Indian guidelines.

28.1 Introduction

Aggressive non-Hodgkin's lymphomas (NHLs) are a heterogeneous group of lymphoid malignancies characterized by rapid progression, high proliferative index, and significant morbidity and mortality if left untreated. The most common subtype is diffuse large B-cell lymphoma (DLBCL), accounting for approximately 30–40% of all NHL cases worldwide [1]. The management of aggressive NHLs has evolved significantly over the past few decades, primarily due to advances in diagnostic techniques, molecular profiling, and the development of targeted therapies.

The standard initial therapy for most patients with aggressive NHL is immunochemotherapy, with the R-CHOP regimen (rituximab, cyclophosphamide, doxorubicin, vincristine, and prednisone) considered the gold standard for DLBCL [2]. This regimen achieves long-term remission in a substantial proportion of patients. However, up to 40% of patients either relapse or are refractory to first-line treatment, necessitating salvage therapies and potentially autologous stem cell transplantation (ASCT) [3].

Molecular subtyping of DLBCL into germinal center B-cell-like (GCB) and activated B-cell-like (ABC) phenotypes has prognostic implications and is increasingly guiding therapeutic decisions [4]. More recently, next-generation sequencing has revealed the complex genetic landscape of aggressive lymphomas, uncovering mutations and pathways that may serve as therapeutic targets.

The advent of novel agents such as CAR T-cell therapy, bispecific antibodies, and small molecule inhibitors (e.g., BTK, BCL2, and PI3K inhibitors) has expanded treatment options, particularly for relapsed or refractory disease [5, 6]. These therapies offer promise but also bring challenges, including toxicity management, cost, and accessibility.

T-cell lymphomas are a heterogeneous and relatively uncommon subset of non-Hodgkin lymphomas (NHL), accounting for approximately 10–15% of all NHL cases worldwide [7, 8]. These malignancies arise from mature (peripheral) T-cells and are broadly categorized as peripheral T-cell lymphomas (PTCL), which include multiple distinct clinicopathologic entities such as PTCL-not otherwise specified (PTCL-NOS), angioimmunoblastic T-cell lymphoma (AITL), anaplastic large cell lymphoma (ALCL), and extranodal NK/T-cell lymphoma, nasal type [1]. Unlike their B-cell counterparts, T-cell lymphomas often have an aggressive clinical course, limited response to conventional chemotherapy, and a poorer overall prognosis.

The pathogenesis of T-cell lymphomas is complex and involves dysregulation of immune signaling pathways, epigenetic alterations, and viral associations, particularly Epstein-Barr virus (EBV) in certain subtypes [9]. Diagnosis is challenging due to overlapping morphological and immunophenotypic features, necessitating expert hematopathological evaluation and comprehensive immunophenotyping. Standard first-line therapy, often anthracycline-based (e.g., CHOP), has limited efficacy in many subtypes, highlighting the need for novel therapeutic approaches [10–12]. Recent advances in molecular profiling and the development of targeted therapies are gradually improving outcomes, although treatment remains an area of unmet clinical need.

28.1.1 Classification of Aggressive Non-Hodgkin Lymphomas [8]

Aggressive NHL can be categorized into aggressive B NHL and aggressive T NHL, which includes subtypes as follows:

- Aggressive B NHL has the following subtypes.
  1. Diffuse large B-cell lymphoma (DLBCL), NOS—most common; GCB and ABC subtypes.
  2. High-grade B-cell lymphoma with MYC and BCL2 and/or BCL6 rearrangements- Previously termed "double/triple-hit"; requires intensified therapy.
  3. High-grade B-cell lymphoma, NOS.
  4. Burkitt lymphoma.
  5. Primary mediastinal large B- cell lymphoma (PMBCL).
  6. Large B-cell lymphoma with IRF4 rearrangement.
  7. Mantle cell lymphoma (blastoid/pleomorphic variant).
- Aggressive T cell NHL has the following subtypes.
  1. Peripheral T-cell lymphoma, NOS, is the most common, heterogenous and poor-prognosis.
  2. Angioimmunoblastic T-cell lymphoma (AITL)-derived from T-follicular helper (TFH) cells; systemic symptoms.
  3. Anaplastic large cell lymphoma (ALCL), ALK-positive-CD30+, better prognosis.
  4. ALCL, ALK-negative-CD30 + more aggressive than ALK positive.
  5. Adult T-cell leukemia/lymphoma (ATLL)-HTLV1 associated with more aggressive.
  6. Extranodal NK/T-cell lymphoma, nasal type-EBV driven; highly aggressive.

28.2 Emerging Therapies

Recent advances in the molecular understanding of aggressive NHL have ushered in a new era of targeted and immune-based therapies. These emerging strategies aim to address unmet needs in both B-cell and T-cell lymphomas, particularly in the relapsed/refractory setting. All therapies are outlined in Fig 28.1.

High-grade B-cell lymphomas with aggressive features, especially those lacking MYC/BCL2/BCL6 rearrangements but exhibiting high proliferation, may benefit from intensified regimens like DA-EPOCH-R. Double-hit and double-expressor subtypes are differentiated based on cytogenetic and immunohistochemical findings, guiding therapy intensity. While interim PET scans are valuable for response assessment, routine PET-adapted treatment changes are not yet standard. Genomic classifiers are emerging as future tools for tailored therapy [29, 30].

In B-cell NHL, chimeric antigen receptor (CAR) T-cell therapies targeting CD19, such as axicabtagene ciloleucel and tisagenlecleucel, have demonstrated durable responses in patients with refractory DLBCL. Despite challenges such as cytokine release syndrome (CRS) and neurotoxicity, these therapies offer hope for long-term remission in previously incurable cases. Bispecific antibodies, including glofitamab and epcoritamab, simultaneously engage CD3+ T-cells and CD20+ malignant B-cells, showing high response rates with manageable toxicity profiles. Antibody-drug conjugates (ADCs) such as polatuzumab vedotin (targeting CD79b) and loncastuximab tesirine (targeting CD19) are being integrated into salvage regimens or combined with rituximab-based therapies to improve outcomes [31, 32].

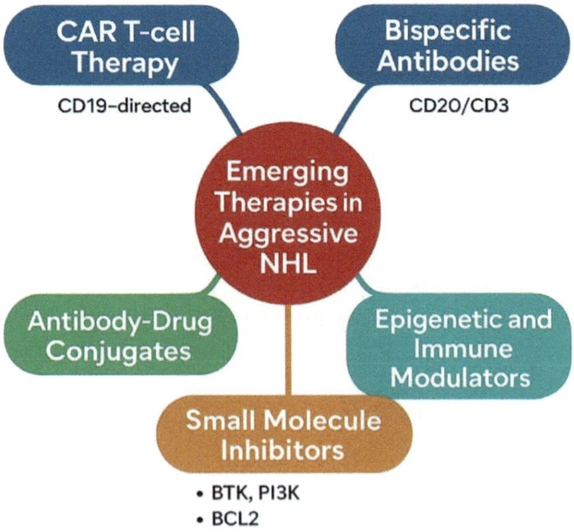

Fig. 28.1 Emerging therapeutic options for aggressive NHL

For T-cell NHL, particularly PTCL, treatment remains challenging due to intrinsic chemoresistance and the lack of targetable antigens. However, progress has been made with agents like brentuximab vedotin in CD30-positive subtypes such as ALCL and some PTCL-NOS cases. Histone deacetylase (HDAC) inhibitors (e.g., romidepsin, belinostat) and antifolates (e.g., pralatrexate) are approved for relapsed PTCL, offering modest response rates with tolerable side effects [19–22, 28]. Combinatorial strategies and rational sequencing of these agents are under investigation.

Furthermore, immunomodulatory drugs (IMiDs) like lenalidomide, when combined with tafasitamab (an anti-CD19 monoclonal antibody), have shown promise in relapsed DLBCL. Novel cellular therapies targeting antigens beyond CD19, including CD22 and CD70, are in early-phase trials. Epigenetic modulators, checkpoint inhibitors, and small molecule inhibitors targeting PI3K, JAK/STAT, and NF-κB pathways are also being explored [30].

In India, access to these therapies may be limited by cost and availability. Nonetheless, select centers are participating in global clinical trials, and generic or biosimilar versions of some agents are becoming more accessible.

Overall, emerging therapies are reshaping the treatment landscape of aggressive NHL. While B-cell lymphomas have seen more robust advancements to date, the field of T-cell lymphomas is evolving rapidly, and continued translational research and trial enrollment are essential to bring these options to the bedside.

28.3 Global and Regional Guidelines

NCCN, ESMO, BSH, and Indian guidelines offer harmonized frameworks. Indian consensus recommends R-CHOP as standard for DLBCL and CHOP/CHOEP for PTCL, with preference for cost-effective diagnostics and therapies in resource-limited settings [33]. Different treatment recommendations are given in Table 28.1.

Table 28.1 Recommended treatment of aggressive B- and T-cell non-Hodgkin lymphomas

Subtype	Setting	Recommended treatment	Guideline/ reference
DLBCL (GCB/ABC)	Newly diagnosed	R-CHOP x6 cycles	NCCN 2024 [34]
DLBCL (double/triple-hit)	Newly diagnosed	DA-EPOCH-R	NCCN 2024 [34], Dunleavy et al. [35]
DLBCL	Relapsed/ refractory (transplant eligible)	Salvage chemo (R-ICE/R-DHAP) → ASCT	Gisselbrecht et al. [36]
DLBCL	Relapsed/ refractory (post-ASCT or Ineligible)	CAR T-cell therapy (axi-cel, liso-cel)	NCCN 2024 [34], Locke et al. [37]
DLBCL	Relapsed/ refractory (non-transplant)	Polatuzumab + bendamustine + rituximab	Sehn et al. [24]
MCL	Newly diagnosed, fit younger	Cytarabine-containing induction (e.g., R-CHOP/R-DHAP) → ASCT ± rituximab maintenance	NCCN 2024 [34]
MCL	Relapsed/ refractory	BTK inhibitors (ibrutinib, acalabrutinib, zanubrutinib); CAR T-cell therapy (brexu-cel)	NCCN 2024 [34]
PTCL-NOS	Newly diagnosed	CHOP or CHOEP ± ASCT consolidation	NCCN 2024 [34], Reimer et al. [38]
CD30+ PTCL (e.g., ALCL)	Newly diagnosed	Brentuximab vedotin + CHP	Horwitz et al. [39]
PTCL	Relapsed/ refractOry	Romidepsin, pralatrexate, belinostat, BV (CD30+)	Coiffier et al. [40], NCCN 2024 [34]
PTCL (chemosensitive, eligible)	Relapsed/ refractory	Allogeneic stem cell transplant	Shustov et al. [41]

28.4 Illustrative Clinical Case 1: Newly Diagnosed Diffuse Large B-Cell Lymphoma

A 62-year-old man presents with a rapidly enlarging right cervical mass and B symptoms (fever, night sweats, weight loss). Imaging reveals bulky disease involving cervical, mediastinal, and abdominal lymph nodes. Excisional biopsy confirms diffuse large B-cell lymphoma (DLBCL), germinal center B-cell (GCB) subtype. PET-CT shows stage III disease. ECOG performance status is 1.

Diagnostic and Prognostic Assessment
DLBCL is the most common aggressive NHL subtype. Diagnosis requires histopathologic confirmation with immunohistochemistry and/or molecular classification into GCB and activated B-cell (ABC) subtypes, which have prognostic relevance [8]. PET-CT is the standard imaging modality for staging [13]. The International Prognostic Index (IPI) remains a key tool for risk stratification [14].

Treatment Approach
Standard first-line therapy for most patients is R-CHOP (rituximab, cyclophosphamide, doxorubicin, vincristine, and prednisone) for 6 cycles [15]. For bulky disease, consolidative radiotherapy may be considered based on interim PET response.

Management
- R-CHOP × 6 cycles.
- Interim PET-CT after 2–4 cycles.
- Post-treatment PET to assess response.

In this case, the patient achieved a complete metabolic response after 6 cycles of R-CHOP, with sustained remission at 2-year follow-up.

28.4.1 Commentary

Diffuse large B-cell lymphoma (DLBCL) represents the most common subtype of aggressive non-Hodgkin's lymphoma, accounting for approximately 30–40% of adult cases globally. This case illustrates a prototypical presentation—rapidly progressive nodal enlargement with B symptoms in a middle-aged man—highlighting the urgency and complexity of diagnosis and treatment initiation.Immunophenotyping and molecular characterization have significantly improved the classification of DLBCL into biologically distinct subtypes. The germinal center B-cell (GCB) and activated B-cell (ABC) subtypes, as identified by gene expression profiling or immunohistochemical algorithms (e.g., Hans classifier), carry prognostic implications, with the GCB subtype generally associated with better outcomes following R-CHOP [16]. However, molecular studies have further refined risk assessment through the identification of high- grade B-cell lymphomas with rearrangements in MYC, BCL2, and/or BCL6 (so-called "double- hit" or "triple-hit" lymphomas), which confer poor prognosis and require more intensive therapy, such as dose-adjusted EPOCH-R [16].

Staging with PET-CT and IPI scoring remains foundational for risk stratification and treatment planning. In this case, the patient's stage III disease and good performance status (ECOG 1) place him in an intermediate-risk category per the IPI. R-CHOP remains the standard-of-care first-line regimen, offering cure rates of 60–70% in patients with favorable to intermediate-risk profiles [17]. The use of interim PET-CT allows for early identification of non-responders, although the role of modifying therapy based on interim PET findings remains investigational outside clinical trials.

This case underscores the importance of integrating clinical, pathological, and molecular data to guide therapy. With the incorporation of rituximab and advances in supportive care, long-term disease-free survival is achievable for most patients with DLBCL. Future approaches may involve individualized frontline therapy based on molecular risk profiling and minimal residual disease monitoring to optimize outcomes.

28.5 Clinical Case 2: Primary Mediastinal B-Cell Lymphoma in a Young Adult

A 28-year-old woman presents with cough and chest pain. CT reveals a large anterior mediastinal mass with compression of vascular structures. Biopsy confirms primary mediastinal large B-cell lymphoma (PMBCL).

Treatment and Outcome
PMBCL, a distinct subtype of DLBCL, often affects young women and exhibits favorable outcomes with dose-adjusted EPOCH-R (DA-EPOCH-R), eliminating the need for radiotherapy in many patients [18].

Management:
- DA-EPOCH-R × 6 cycles.
- PET-CT after therapy; no radiotherapy required with complete response.

The patient achieved a complete response without radiotherapy and remains disease-free at 3 years.

28.6 Clinical Case 3: Newly Diagnosed Peripheral T-Cell Lymphoma (NOS)

Clinical scenario: A 52-year-old man presents with generalized lymphadenopathy and pruritus. Biopsy reveals peripheral T-cell lymphoma, not otherwise specified (PTCL-NOS). PET-CT shows stage IV disease. Bone marrow is involved.

Treatment Approach
PTCLs account for 10–15% of aggressive NHLs and generally have a poor prognosis. CHOP remains the standard first-line therapy, though outcomes are inferior to B-cell counterparts [19]. Consideration of stem cell transplant in first remission is standard for fit patients [20].

Management:

- CHOP × 6 cycles.
- Achieved partial response.
- Underwent autologous stem cell transplantation (ASCT) in first remission.

28.6.1 Commentary

Peripheral T-cell lymphomas (PTCLs) are a rare and heterogeneous group of aggressive NHLs, accounting for approximately 10–15% of cases in adults. PTCL-NOS is the most prevalent subtype within this group and is characterized by an aggressive clinical course, poor response to standard chemotherapy, and a high relapse rate. Unlike B-cell lymphomas, the addition of targeted monoclonal antibodies like rituximab is not applicable, limiting therapeutic options.

This case highlights the challenges in managing PTCL-NOS, particularly the modest efficacy of CHOP, which remains the most commonly used regimen despite limited evidence of durable benefit. The patient achieved a partial response after 6 cycles, and due to the high risk of early relapse, underwent autologous stem cell transplant (ASCT) in first remission—a strategy supported by retrospective and prospective studies demonstrating improved progression-free survival [19–22].

Current research efforts are directed at refining risk stratification using molecular profiling and identifying actionable mutations (e.g., TET2, RHOA) to guide future therapies.

Enrollment in clinical trials is strongly encouraged, given the unmet need in this population. Novel agents such as brentuximab vedotin (for CD30+ disease) and epigenetic therapies are showing promise in relapsed settings and may shift toward frontline use in the coming years.

28.7 Clinical Case 4: Relapsed/Refractory DLBCL Post-R-CHOP

A 70-year-old man relapses 10 months after initial complete remission with R-CHOP. Biopsy confirms DLBCL, ABC subtype. He is ineligible for high-dose therapy due to comorbidities.

Management Strategy

For fit patients, salvage chemoimmunotherapy followed by autologous stem cell transplant remains the standard [22, 23]. For transplant-ineligible patients, options include:

- Polatuzumab vedotin + bendamustine + rituximab (Pola-BR) [24]
- Tafasitamab + lenalidomide (for non-double/triple-hit DLBCL) [25]

- CD19-directed CAR T-cell therapy in eligible patients [26] Management
- Treated with Pola-BR
- Achieved partial response and maintained stable disease at 8 months

28.8 Clinical Case 5: Relapsed Peripheral T-Cell Lymphoma

A 45-year-old woman with relapsed PTCL-NOS after CHOP. She is transplant-ineligible.

Management Approach
There is no standard salvage regimen for R/R PTCL. Options include:

- Pralatrexate
- Romidepsin
- Brentuximab vedotin (for CD30+ PTCL) [27]
- Clinical trials (e.g., duvelisib, belinostat} [28]

  Management:

- Treated with romidepsin
- Achieved stable disease but progressed after 5 months
- Enrolled in a clinical trial of duvelisib

28.8.1 Commentary

This case highlights the formidable challenges associated with managing refractory PTCL in elderly patients. PTCL encompasses a diverse and biologically heterogeneous group of disorders, many of which are intrinsically resistant to conventional chemotherapy. In this context, the patient's poor response to CHOP and subsequent progression underscores the urgent need for more effective therapeutic strategies in this population. Novel agents such as romidepsin, pralatrexate, and belinostat offer modest single-agent activity and are particularly valuable for patients ineligible for intensive regimens or stem cell transplantation [27, 28]. The patient's comorbidities and advanced age limit curative options, reinforcing the importance of balancing efficacy with tolerability. Clinical trials remain crucial to advancing the treatment landscape in this setting. Additionally, there is growing interest in targeted therapies, immunomodulators, and antibody-drug conjugates, such as brentuximab vedotin, especially in CD30-positive subtypes [27]. This case also raises important considerations around goals of care, quality of life, and early integration of palliative care. As the population ages, similar cases will become increasingly common, demanding more personalized, tolerable, and effective approaches to refractory T-cell lymphomas

28.9 Conclusion

Aggressive non-Hodgkin's lymphomas encompass a diverse group of diseases with variable outcomes. Timely diagnosis, risk stratification, and appropriate use of chemoimmunotherapy remain the foundation of treatment. For relapsed/refractory disease, novel therapies including CAR T-cell therapy, bispecific antibodies, and targeted agents offer new hope. Individualized treatment based on disease biology and patient factors is crucial, and clinical trial enrollment should be considered whenever feasible.

References

1. Swerdlow SH, Campo E, Harris NL, et al. WHO classification of tumours of haematopoietic and lymphoid tissues. Revised 4th ed. Lyon: IARC; 2016.
2. Coiffier B, Lepage E, Briere J, et al. CHOP chemotherapy plus rituximab compared with CHOP alone in elderly patients with diffuse large-B-cell lymphoma. N Engl J Med. 2002;346(4):235–42.
3. Philip T, Guglielmi C, Hagenbeek A, et al. High-dose therapy and autologous bone marrow transplantation after failure of conventional chemotherapy in adults with intermediate- grade or high-grade non-Hodgkin's lymphoma. N Engl J Med. 1995;333(23):1540–5.
4. Alizadeh AA, Eisen MB, Davis RE, et al. Distinct types of diffuse large B-cell lymphoma identified by gene expression profiling. Nature. 2000;403(6769):503–11.
5. Locke FL, Neelapu SS, Bartlett NL, et al. Phase 1 results of ZUMA-1: a multicenter study of KTE-C19 anti-CD19 CAR T-cell therapy in refractory aggressive lymphoma. Mol Ther. 2017;25(1):285–95.
6. Schuster SJ, Bishop MR, Tam CS, et al. Tisagenlecleucel in adult relapsed or refractory diffuse large B-cell lymphoma. N Engl J Med. 2019;380(1):45–56.
7. Vose J, Armitage J, Weisenburger D. International peripheral T-cell and natural killer/T- cell lymphoma study: pathology findings and clinical outcomes. Blood. 2008;111(12):5078–87.
8. Swerdlow SH, Campo E, Harris NL, et al. WHO classification of tumours of haematopoietic and lymphoid tissues. 4th ed. Lyon: IARC; 2017.
9. Vose J, Armitage J, Weisenburger D. International peripheral T-cell and natural killer/T- cell lymphoma study: pathology findings and clinical outcomes. J Clin Oncol. 2008;26(25):4124–30.
10. Horwitz S, O'Connor OA, Pro B, et al. Brentuximab vedotin with chemotherapy for CD30-positive peripheral T-cell lymphoma (ECHELON-2): a global, double-blind, randomised, phase 3 trial. N Engl J Med. 2019;380(18):1726–37.
11. Savage KJ. Prognosis and treatment of peripheral T-cell lymphomas in the modern era. Hematology Am Soc Hematol Educ Program. 2014;2014(1):313–9.
12. Horwitz SM, Ansell SM, Ai WZ, et al. NCCN guidelines insights: T-cell lymphomas, version 2.2018. J Natl Compr Cancer Netw. 2018;16(2):123–31.
13. Cheson BD, Fisher RI, Barrington SF, et al. Recommendations for initial evaluation, staging, and response assessment of Hodgkin and non-Hodgkin lymphoma. J Clin Oncol. 2014;32(27):3059–68.
14. Ziepert M, Hasenclever D, Kuhnt E, et al. Standard International Prognostic Index remains a valid predictor in DLBCL. J Clin Oncol. 2010;28(14):2373–80.
15. Coiffier B, Thieblemont C, Van Den Neste E, et al. Long-term outcome of R-CHOP in elderly DLBCL. J Clin Oncol. 2010;28(27):4527–33.

16. Sarkozy C, Sehn LH. Molecular pathogenesis and risk stratification in DLBCL. Hematology Am Soc Hematol Educ Program. 2018;2018(1):494–507.
17. Fox CP, Chaganti S, McIlroy G, et al. The management of newly diagnosed large B-cell lymphoma: a British Society for Haematology Guideline. Br J Haematol. 2024;204(4):1178–92.
18. Dunleavy K, Pittaluga S, Maeda LS, et al. Dose-adjusted EPOCH-R in primary mediastinal B-cell lymphoma. N Engl J Med. 2013;368(15):1408–16.
19. Savage KJ, Harris NL, Vose JM, et al. Peripheral T-cell lymphoma, NOS. Blood. 2004;103(7):2464–71.
20. d'Amore F, Relander T, Lauritzsen GF, et al. Upfront autologous stem-cell transplantation in peripheral T-cell lymphoma: NLG-T-01. J Clin Oncol. 2012;30(25):3093–9.
21. Reimer P, Rüdiger T, Geissinger E, et al. Autologous stem-cell transplantation as first-line therapy in peripheral T-cell lymphomas. J Clin Oncol. 2009;27(1):106–13.
22. Philip T, Guglielmi C, Hagenbeek A, et al. High-dose therapy with autologous stem-cell transplantation in aggressive lymphoma. N Engl J Med. 1995;333(23):1540–5.
23. Hutchings M, Morschhauser F, Iacoboni G, et al. Glofitamab in relapsed or refractory DLBCL: phase I/II study. N Engl J Med. 2021;385(8):727–40.
24. Sehn LH, Herrera AF, Flowers CR, et al. Polatuzumab vedotin plus bendamustine and rituximab in relapsed/refractory DLBCL. J Clin Oncol. 2020;38(2):155–65.
25. Salles G, Duell J, González Barca E, et al. Tafasitamab plus lenalidomide in relapsed/refractory DLBCL. Lancet Oncol. 2020;21(7):978–88.
26. Neelapu SS, Locke FL, Bartlett NL, et al. Axicabtagene ciloleucel CAR T-cell therapy in refractory large B-cell lymphoma. N Engl J Med. 2017;377(26):2531–44.
27. Horwitz SM, Ansell S, Ai WZ, et al. Brentuximab vedotin with chemotherapy in CD30- positive peripheral T-cell lymphomas. J Clin Oncol 2014;32(32):3281–3287.
28. O'Connor OA, Horwitz S, Masszi T, et al. Belinostat in relapsed or refractory peripheral T- cell lymphoma. J Clin Oncol. 2015;33(23):2492–9.
29. Olszewski AJ, Kurt H, Evens AM. Aggressive large B-cell lymphoma: defining and treating high-grade B-cell lymphoma, NOS. Blood. 2024;143(10)
30. British Society for Haematology. Diagnosis and management of diffuse large B-cell lymphoma—2024 update. Br J Haematol. 2024;
31. Budde LE, Sehn LH, Matasar MJ, et al. Mosunetuzumab in relapsed/refractory B-cell non-Hodgkin lymphoma. J Clin Oncol. 2022;40(5):481–91.
32. Zinzani PL, Santoro A, Gritti G, et al. Nivolumab combined with brentuximab vedotin for relapsed/refractory primary mediastinal large B-cell lymphoma: CheckMate 436. J Clin Oncol. 2019;37(33):3081–9.
33. Indian Academy of Pediatrics. IAP guidelines for the management of lymphoma. Indian J Hematol Blood Transfus. 2020;36(Suppl 1):S1–20.
34. National Comprehensive Cancer Network. NCCN Clinical Practice Guidelines in Oncology: B-cell Lymphomas. Version 1.2024. Plymouth Meeting, PA: NCCN; 2024. https://www.nccn.org
35. Dunleavy K, Roschewski M, Abramson JS, et al. Differential efficacy of dose-adjusted EPOCH-R in DLBCL subtypes. Blood. 2014;123(22):3565–70.
36. Gisselbrecht C, Glass B, Mounier N, et al. Salvage regimens with autologous transplantation for relapsed large B-cell lymphoma. N Engl J Med. 2010;362(12):1035–44.
37. Locke FL, Ghobadi A, Jacobson CA, et al. Long-term safety and activity of axicabtagene ciloleucel in refractory large B-cell lymphoma. Lancet Oncol. 2019;20(1):31–42.
38. Reimer P, Krug U, Tinhofer I, et al. Autologous stem-cell transplantation and risk- adapted therapy in PTCL. Blood. 2009;113(23):5864–71.
39. Horwitz S, Ansell S, Fanale M, et al. Brentuximab vedotin in CD30-positive PTCL: results of a phase 2 trial. Lancet. 2019;393(10168):229–40.
40. Coiffier B, Pro B, Prince HM, et al. Results from a pivotal, open-label, phase II study of romidepsin in relapsed or refractory PTCL. J Clin Oncol. 2012;30(6):631–6.
41. Shustov AR, Somlo G, Harris B, et al. Autologous transplantation for T-cell lymphoma: a report from the CIBMTR. Biol Blood Marrow Transplant. 2010;16(3):426–34.

Chapter 29
MGUS and Its Clinical Variants

Nitin Gupta

Abstract Monoclonal gammopathy of undetermined significance (MGUS) represents a premalignant plasma cell disorder characterized by the presence of a small clone of plasma cells producing monoclonal immunoglobulin in the absence of overt organ damage. Most individuals with MGUS remain asymptomatic and never develop clinically significant disease. Nevertheless, a subset of patients may progress to multiple myeloma or related lymphoproliferative disorders over time. In recent years, it has become evident that monoclonal proteins may themselves cause tissue injury even when diagnostic criteria for hematologic malignancy are not fulfilled. These disorders are collectively described as monoclonal gammopathies of clinical significance (MGCS). Renal involvement is the most frequently recognized manifestation and is termed monoclonal gammopathy of renal significance (MGRS). Other organs that may be affected include the peripheral nervous system, skin, eyes, and components of the hemostatic system.

This chapter provides an overview of MGUS and reviews the spectrum of organ-specific disorders associated with pathogenic monoclonal proteins.

Keywords MGUS · MGCS · MGRS · POEMS syndrome · CIDP

N. Gupta (✉)
Clinical Hematology and Bone Marrow/Stem Cell Transplant, Sir Ganga Ram Hospital/
Ganga Ram Institute of Post Medical Education and Research, New Delhi, India
e-mail: nitin.gupta@sgrh.com

H. P. Pati et al. (eds.), *Clinical Hematology and Hemato-Oncology*,
https://doi.org/10.1007/978-981-92-1167-8_29

Learning Objectives
After reading this chapter, the reader should be able to:

- Describe the biological and clinical features of MGUS.
- Understand the concept of monoclonal gammopathies of clinical significance.
- Recognize organ-specific complications related to monoclonal proteins.
- Outline principles of evaluation and management of these conditions.

29.1 MGUS Introduction

Monoclonal gammopathy of undetermined significance (MGUS) is defined by the detection of a serum monoclonal immunoglobulin at a concentration below 3 g/dL together with fewer than 10% clonal plasma cells in the bone marrow and no evidence of end-organ damage attributable to plasma cell dyscrasia. End-organ involvement includes hypercalcemia, renal insufficiency, anemia, and lytic bone lesions.

Three major categories of MGUS are recognized:

1. *Non-IgM MGUS,* typically associated with IgG or IgA monoclonal proteins
2. IgM MGUS
3. Light-chain MGUS

Non-IgM MGUS is generally considered a precursor state for multiple myeloma, whereas IgM MGUS may evolve into lymphoplasmacytic lymphoma or Waldenström macroglobulinemia. Light-chain MGUS represents an early stage that may precede light-chain multiple myeloma or AL amyloidosis [1].

29.2 Epidemiology

MGUS is relatively common in the aging population. Population-based studies indicate that approximately *3–4% of individuals older than 50 years* harbor a detectable monoclonal protein. The prevalence increases steadily with age and may exceed *7% in individuals older than 80 years.* Men are affected slightly more frequently than women [2].

A number of environmental and genetic factors have been implicated in the development of MGUS. Increased prevalence has been reported among first-degree relatives of patients with multiple myeloma, suggesting a possible genetic susceptibility. Other associated factors include obesity, chronic immune stimulation, and certain occupational exposures such as pesticides or industrial chemicals [3].

29.3 Risk of Progression

Although MGUS itself is usually asymptomatic, it carries a measurable risk of transformation into malignant plasma cell or lymphoid disorders. The average rate of progression is approximately *1% per year*. Risk stratification models have been developed to identify patients with a greater likelihood of disease evolution. One commonly used model incorporates three clinical variables:

- Non-IgG monoclonal protein type.
- Serum monoclonal protein concentration ≥ 1.5 g/dL.
- Abnormal serum free light-chain ratio.

Individuals possessing all three risk factors have a risk of progression at 20 years of 58%, whereas the risk is 37%, 21%, and 5% when two, one, and none of the risk factors are present, respectively [4].

29.4 Monoclonal Gammopathies of Clinical Significance

The traditional view of MGUS as an entirely benign condition has changed in recent years. It is now recognized that monoclonal immunoglobulins may cause tissue damage through a variety of mechanisms despite the absence of overt hematologic malignancy. Such conditions are collectively termed *monoclonal gammopathies of clinical significance (MGCS)* [5]. Organ injury in these disorders may occur through mechanisms including deposition of immunoglobulin fragments, autoimmune activity of the paraprotein, or activation of inflammatory pathways.

MGCS can involve several organ systems including:

- Kidneys
- Peripheral nerves
- Skin
- Eyes
- Hematologic and coagulation systems
- Multisystem syndromes

Once monoclonal gammopathy is detected in a patient with an unexplained syndrome, attention is given to demonstrate a causal association between the paraprotein and the end- organ dysfunction. Given the high frequency of MGUS in the aging population, a large subset of patients in whom MGCS is considered will, in fact, have MGUS after the diagnostic evaluation is complete. Management typically focuses on targeting the underlying plasma cell or B-cell clone responsible for producing the pathogenic immunoglobulin.

29.5 Monoclonal Gammopathy of Renal Significance (MGRS)

Clinical case 1: A 44-year-old male patient with1 month history of headache, weakness, and swelling of feet presents to a general physician and is found to have hypertension, mild anemia (10.90gm/dL), mildly elevated creatinine (1.46 mg/dL), and proteinuria 2+. Further evaluation by a nephrologist revealed a 24-hour urine protein of 1258 mg/day. Renal biopsy showed diffuse dominant staining for kappa light chains along the glomerulus and focally along the tubular basement membrane and blood vessels with concurrent negativity for lambda light chains, IgA, IgG, IgM, C3 and Clq. The Congo red stain was negative. He was then referred to a clinical hematologist for further treatment of light chain deposition disease.

MGRS refers to renal disorders caused by monoclonal immunoglobulins produced by a small clonal B-cell or plasma cell population that does not meet criteria for multiple myeloma or lymphoma. Despite the small clone size, the monoclonal protein may exert direct nephrotoxic effects, leading to significant kidney damage. A broad spectrum of renal pathologies has been recognized in association with monoclonal gammopathy of renal significance (MGRS) (Fig. 29.1). In these conditions, the pattern of kidney injury is determined primarily by the biochemical and structural properties of the monoclonal immunoglobulin rather than by the type of hematologic clone responsible for its production. The classification proposed by the International Kidney and Monoclonal Gammopathy (IKMG) Research Group relies largely on immunofluorescence findings and the ultrastructural characteristics of deposits identified on electron microscopy [6]. MGRS-associated renal lesions are initially categorized according to whether monoclonal immunoglobulin deposits are present. Disorders with deposits are further divided into those with *organized* and *non-organized* structures. Organized deposits are then subclassified based on their ultrastructural morphology into *fibrillar*, *microtubular*, and *crystalline or inclusion-type deposits* (Fig. 29.2).

1. Organized Monoclonal Deposits

Organized monoclonal deposits can be grouped into three ultrastructural patterns: *fibrillar*, *microtubular*, and *crystalline/inclusion forms*.

Fibrillar deposits are characteristically seen in *light-chain or heavy-chain amyloidosis* and in *monoclonal fibrillary glomerulonephritis (FGN)*. In contrast, microtubular deposits exhibit hollow cores and relatively larger diameters; these are typically observed in *immunotactoid glomerulonephritis* and *cryoglobulinemic glomerulonephritis*. The crystalline or inclusion category includes entities such as *light chain proximal tubulopathy (LCPT)*, *crystal-storing histiocytosis*, and *crystalglobulin-associated glomerulonephritis*.

2. Non-organized Monoclonal Deposits

Non-organized monoclonal deposits are characteristic of *monoclonal immunoglobulin deposition disease (MIDD)* and *proliferative glomerulonephritis with*

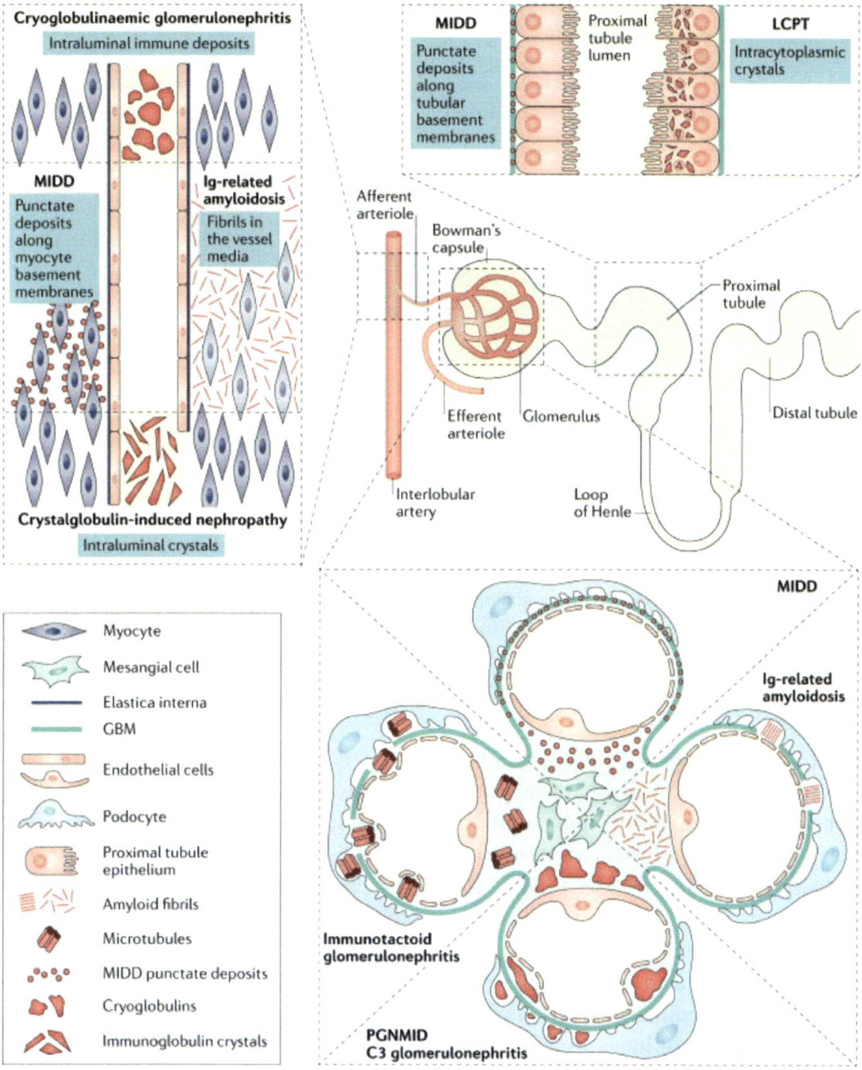

Fig. 29.1 Localization of MGRS-associated renal lesions. Monoclonal gammopathy of renal significance (MGRS)-associated lesions can involve one or more renal compartments. In immunotactoid glomerulonephritis, C3 glomerulopathy, and proliferative glomerulonephritis with monoclonal immunoglobulin deposits (PGNMID), MGRS-associated lesions involve only the glomeruli, whereas in light-chain proximal tubulopathy (LCPT), MGRS-associated lesions involve only the proximal tubules. MGRS-associated lesions in cryoglobulinemic glomerulonephritis mainly involve the glomeruli but can occasionally affect blood vessels in the form of intravascular cryoglobulin thrombi or endovasculitis. Immunoglobulin-related amyloidosis and monoclonal immunoglobulin deposition disease (MIDD) usually affect all renal compartments, including glomeruli, vessels, and the tubulointerstitium. GBM, glomerular basement membrane [6]

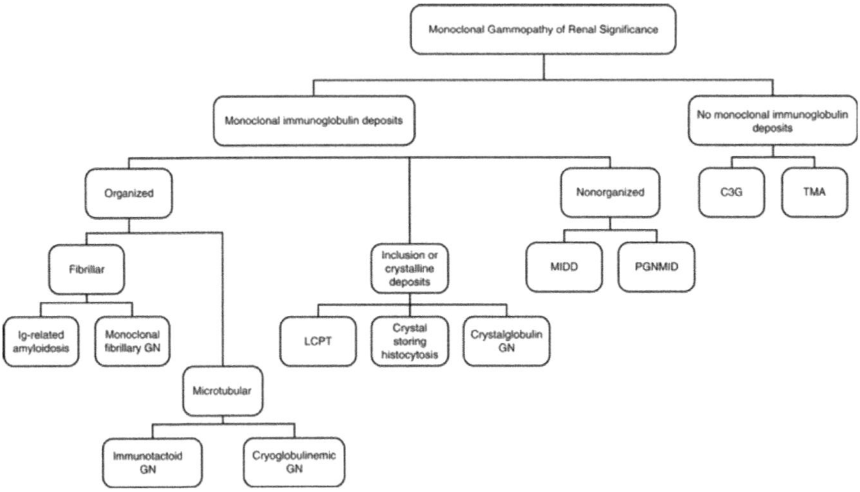

Fig. 29.2 Classification of monoclonal gammopathy of renal significance. C3G, C3 glomerulopathy with monoclonal gammopathy; Ig, immunoglobulin; GN, glomerulonephritis; LCPT, light chain proximal tubulopathy; MIDD, monoclonal immunoglobulin deposit disease; PGNMID, proliferative glomerulonephritis with monoclonal immunoglobulin deposits; TMA, thrombomicroangiopathy with monoclonal gammopathy [6]

monoclonal immunoglobulin deposits (PGNMID). MIDD encompasses a group of disorders characterized by linear deposition of monoclonal immunoglobulin components along renal basement membranes. Depending on the deposited component, these disorders are classified as *light chain deposition disease (LCDD)*, *heavy chain deposition disease (HCDD)*, or *light- and heavy-chain deposition disease (LHCDD)*. In many cases of MIDD, the deposited immunoglobulin lacks the first constant domain and is commonly a truncated IgG1 molecule. In contrast, PGNMID is most frequently associated with the IgG3 subclass. The deposits are typically restricted to glomeruli, predominantly involving the mesangial and subendothelial regions, and generally consist of intact immunoglobulin molecules.

3. MGRS Without Immunoglobulin Deposits

Certain renal disorders associated with monoclonal gammopathy do not demonstrate immunoglobulin deposition but are still considered within the spectrum of MGRS. Examples include *C3 glomerulopathy (C3G) associated with monoclonal gammopathy and thrombotic microangiopathy (TMA)*.

In C3G associated with monoclonal gammopathy, glomerular deposits consist predominantly of complement component C3 fragments rather than immunoglobulins. The condition is categorized as MGRS because a circulating monoclonal gammopathy is detected in approximately 60–80% of patients older than 50 years with C3G.

Thrombotic microangiopathy has been proposed as a provisional MGRS entity. It may present with microangiopathic hemolytic anemia and can occur in patients with MGUS, multiple myeloma, or Waldenström macroglobulinemia.

29.6 Diagnostic Evaluation of MGRS

MGRS should be suspected when individuals with a known monoclonal gammopathy or B-cell lymphoproliferative disorder develop otherwise unexplained renal dysfunction or significant proteinuria. Among patients with monoclonal gammopathy who undergo kidney biopsy, nearly *40%* are found to have lesions attributable to MGRS. Accurate diagnosis requires a *combined nephrological and hematological assessment*, with *renal biopsy serving as a key diagnostic step*. The presence of MGUS or monoclonal B-cell lymphocytosis in association with kidney impairment alone is insufficient to establish the diagnosis.

Distinguishing MGRS from other renal pathologies is essential because management is directed toward the underlying clonal disorder in order to preserve renal function. If bone marrow evaluation fails to identify a pathogenic clone, imaging studies may be performed to detect extramedullary plasmacytoma or lymphadenopathy amenable to biopsy. Notably, in certain conditions, such as *PGNMID*, a circulating monoclonal protein is detected in only *20–30% of patients*, making clone identification challenging.

29.7 Treatment of MGRS

The IKMG recommends initiating therapy for MGRS even when overt hematologic malignancy is absent. Due to the rarity and heterogeneity of these disorders, robust prospective trials are lacking, and current treatment strategies are largely derived from case reports, small series, and retrospective analyses. The primary objective of therapy is preservation of renal function and prevention of further organ damage. At present, there are no therapies specifically designed to remove monoclonal immunoglobulin deposits from the kidney or other affected tissues. Conventional immunosuppressive therapies are generally ineffective. Instead, treatment targets the pathologic clone responsible for producing the nephrotoxic monoclonal protein, which may be of plasma cell, lymphoplasmacytic, or B-cell origin. Clinical outcomes strongly correlate with the depth of hematologic response; deeper responses are associated with improved renal survival [7].

Management of *MIDD*, particularly LCDD, often parallels that of *AL amyloidosis*, with favorable outcomes reported using bortezomib-based regimens and autologous stem cell transplantation (ASCT). *Immunotactoid glomerulopathy* frequently arises from an underlying *CLL clone* in up to half of cases, making *rituximab-based therapy* a reasonable approach. In *PGNMID*, identification of a clonal population is frequently difficult despite the presence of monotypic immunoglobulin deposition in the kidney. In one series, 10 out of 16 patients lacked a detectable bone marrow clone and were treated empirically: eight received rituximab-based regimens, while two were treated with either alkylator-based therapy or bortezomib. Among these empirically treated patients, three achieved complete renal responses and five partial responses [8]. Similarly, in a cohort of 50 patients with *C3 glomerulopathy associated with monoclonal gammopathy*, treatment approaches included chemotherapy in 29 patients, immunosuppressive therapy in 8, and supportive care in the remaining patients. Patients receiving clone-directed chemotherapy who achieved hematologic responses demonstrated superior renal response rates and longer renal survival [9].

Renal transplantation may be considered in selected patients with MGRS. However, the risk of disease recurrence in the transplanted kidney must be carefully evaluated. A case series of 28 patients who underwent kidney transplantation between 1987 and 2016—including those with LCDD ($n = 10$), C3 glomerulopathy with monoclonal gammopathy ($n = 5$), and LCPT ($n = 4$)—demonstrated a high rate of recurrence in the allograft when adequate hematologic remission had not been achieved prior to transplantation. Recurrence rates were 57.8% in LCDD, 100% in C3G, and 75% in LCPT [10].

In our patient, further evaluation revealed a small monoclonal spike of 0.20 g/dL corresponding to IgG-kappa, along with a markedly abnormal serum free light-chain ratio (kappa 979 mg/L, lambda 20.30 mg/L; ratio 48.22). Bone marrow examination demonstrated 17% plasma cells, and PET-CT imaging did not reveal lytic skeletal lesions. Electron microscopy of the renal biopsy showed approximately 40% effacement of podocyte foot processes and marked expansion of the mesangial matrix. Sparse subendothelial and mesangial electron-dense deposits were identified, without a definitive substructure on high-magnification examination. Additionally, there was prominent subendothelial widening with accumulation of granular material. Based on these findings, a diagnosis of kappa light chain deposition disease (LCDD) was established. The patient received four cycles of bortezomib, lenalidomide, and dexamethasone (VRd), achieving a complete hematologic response accompanied by resolution of proteinuria. He subsequently underwent autologous stem cell transplantation using high-dose melphalan (200 mg/m^2) as conditioning, followed by lenalidomide maintenance therapy for two years. At 3.5 years post-transplant, the patient remains in complete remission.

29.8 Monoclonal Gammopathy of Neurological Significance (MCNS)

A 51-year-old man presented to a neurologist with gradually progressive weakness of the lower limbs accompanied by paresthesia and gait disturbance. Laboratory evaluation showed a hemoglobin level of 16.5 g/dL, a total leukocyte count of 7.5 × 10 [9]/L (neutrophils 70%, lymphocytes 25%, monocytes 5%), and thrombocytosis with a platelet count of 480 × 10 [9]/L. Metabolic investigations, including iron studies, vitamin B12, folate levels, and screening for heavy metals, were within normal limits. Nerve conduction studies demonstrated distal symmetrical sensorimotor polyneuropathy involving large nerve fibers, with mixed axonal and demyelinating features, predominantly affecting the lower extremities compared with the upper limbs. Autoimmune testing, including anti–myelin-associated glycoprotein (MAG) antibodies, was negative. However, serum protein electrophoresis identified an Ig lambda monoclonal protein measuring 0.87 g/dL. Serum free light-chain analysis showed kappa 29.6 mg/L, lambda 44.5 mg/L, with a kappa/lambda ratio of 0.67. The patient was subsequently referred to a hematooncologist. Bone marrow examination revealed 5–6% CD138-positive plasma cells with lambda light-chain restriction. Whole-body PET-CT demonstrated FDG-avid lytic lesions with peripheral sclerosis involving the left iliac bone and an additional lesion in the posterior aspect of the right fifth rib. Based on the constellation of findings, a diagnosis of POEMS syndrome was established.

Monoclonal gammopathy of neurological significance (MGNS) represents a challenging clinical entity from both diagnostic and therapeutic perspectives. The heterogeneity of clinical manifestations and the frequent absence of tissue biopsy confirmation—unlike other monoclonal gammopathies of clinical significance (MGCS)—often complicate the diagnostic process. Furthermore, treatment strategies are not standardized and few prospective studies have evaluated therapeutic interventions. Neurological deficits may also become irreversible if diagnosis and treatment are delayed. When evaluating a patient with suspected MGNS, the first step is to exclude common secondary causes of polyneuropathy, including *diabetes mellitus, vitamin B12 deficiency, chronic alcohol consumption, and hepatitis C infection*. The prevalence of a detectable monoclonal protein in patients with peripheral neuropathy is estimated to be 3–10%. Several mechanisms have been proposed to explain neuropathy in these patients, including demyelination mediated by monoclonal immunoglobulins, antibody binding to myelin-associated glycoprotein, and antiganglioside antibody activity [11]. All patients presenting with peripheral neuropathy in association with a monoclonal gammopathy should undergo a comprehensive evaluation. This typically includes bone marrow examination, serum and urine monoclonal protein studies, and nerve conduction studies with or without electromyography. Importantly, alternative non-plasma-cell-related causes of neuropathy must always be ruled out, especially in individuals with IgG or IgA MGUS, where the monoclonal protein may be an incidental finding. In contrast, neuropathy occurring in the setting of IgM MGUS is more frequently directly related to the monoclonal protein.

In cases of demyelinating neuropathy, testing for specific autoantibodies such as anti-MAG antibodies and anti-disialosyl ganglioside antibodies is recommended. Patients with axonal or mixed neuropathy should be evaluated for AL amyloidosis and cryoglobulinemic vasculitis. If these conditions are excluded, the neuropathy is generally considered unrelated to the monoclonal gammopathy.

Major MGCS entities that may present with neuropathy include *AL amyloidosis, POEMS syndrome, cryoglobulinemia, CANOMAD syndrome, distal acquired demyelinating symmetric neuropathy associated with monoclonal protein (DADS-M), and sporadic late-onset nemaline myopathy*. The first three conditions typically involve multiple organ systems, whereas the latter disorders predominantly affect the peripheral nervous system.

29.9 Chronic Inflammatory Demyelinating Polyneuropathy Associated with MGUS

Chronic inflammatory demyelinating polyneuropathy (CIDP) is an immune-mediated disorder characterized by progressive or relapsing weakness and sensory dysfunction due to peripheral nerve inflammation. One recognized subtype occurs in association with MGUS, most commonly involving IgM monoclonal proteins directed against myelin-associated glycoprotein. These antibodies cause demyelination of distal large-fiber sensorimotor nerves. Nerve biopsy in such cases often demonstrates separation of myelin lamellae along with deposition of IgM and complement (C3d) on myelin sheaths. Standard treatment approaches include plasmapheresis, intravenous immunoglobulin (IVIG), and corticosteroids, sometimes combined with cyclophosphamide. Interestingly, CIDP associated with MGUS appears to respond more favorably to plasma exchange than other CIDP variants, with response rates approaching 70% [12].

A related entity is *distal acquired demyelinating symmetric neuropathy with monoclonal protein (DADS-M)*, which predominantly affects older men. This condition mainly involves large sensory fibers, leading to *sensory ataxia*, diminished sensory responses, reduced motor conduction velocity, and prolonged distal latencies. Muscles of the face, trunk, and proximal limbs are usually spared. A high frequency of the *MYD88 L265P mutation* has been reported in these patients.

More than half of individuals with *IgM MGUS–associated neuropathy* demonstrate autoantibody activity, most commonly directed against MAG, although antibodies against *GM1 ganglioside* may also be present. Antibody titers do not correlate well with clinical severity and are therefore not reliable markers for treatment response. Patients with mild distal sensory symptoms without gait impairment can often be managed conservatively with physiotherapy and balance training. However, those with gait instability, falls, or progressive weakness require early treatment to prevent permanent axonal injury. Therapies such as rituximab, IVIG, or corticosteroids often provide limited benefit. More effective strategies include rituximab-based immunochemotherapy combined with cyclophosphamide and prednisolone or targeted agents such as ibrutinib. In a prospective study, the combination of acalabrutinib and rituximab produced hematologic responses in 86% of patients and neurological improvement in 57% patients [13]. In the absence of standardized treatment protocols, management generally follows therapeutic principles used for Waldenström macroglobulinemia. Some patients lacking anti-MAG antibodies exhibit antibodies directed against *gangliosides*. Those with *anti-GM1 antibodies* typically develop *multifocal motor neuropathy*, in which *rituximab monotherapy* is often recommended as first-line treatment, while *ibrutinib* may be considered in refractory disease [15].

29.10 POEMS Syndrome

POEMS syndrome is a rare paraneoplastic condition driven by excessive cytokine production, particularly vascular endothelial growth factor (VEGF). The acronym represents the major clinical components: *polyneuropathy, organomegaly, endocrinopathy, monoclonal gammopathy, and skin changes*. The disorder most commonly affects individuals in their fifth decade of life, with a slight male predominance. The defining clinical manifestation is a *symmetrical ascending sensorimotor neuropathy*. The monoclonal immunoglobulin is almost invariably of the lambda light-chain subtype. Elevated VEGF levels lead to increased vascular permeability and angiogenesis, contributing to manifestations such as peripheral edema, papilledema, and cutaneous hemangiomas. Skeletal involvement typically consists of *focal osteosclerotic lesions*, and radiotherapy directed at these lesions can result in significant disease control. Diagnosis requires *both mandatory major criteria* (polyneuropathy and a monoclonal plasma-cell disorder), along with *at least one additional major criterion* (sclerotic bone lesions, elevated VEGF levels, or Castleman disease) and *one minor criterion*, such as organomegaly, endocrinopathy, skin changes, papilledema, thrombocytosis, or extravascular volume overload. Treatment aimed at eliminating the plasma-cell clone reduces VEGF production and is usually accompanied by clinical improvement. Prognosis is favorable with appropriate therapy, with median survival exceeding 12 years, although neurological recovery may be slow. Radiotherapy can be curative in patients with isolated plasmacytoma. Systemic therapy has traditionally included autologous stem cell transplantation, but lenalidomide-dexamethasone, proteasome inhibitors, and anti-CD38 monoclonal antibodies such as daratumumab are increasingly used with good outcomes [29].

29.11 CANOMAD Syndrome

CANOMAD (chronic ataxic neuropathy, ophthalmoplegia, IgM paraprotein, cold agglutinins, and disialosyl antibodies) represents another rare neurological disorder associated with MGUS. The pathogenesis involves *IgM autoantibodies directed against disialosyl gangliosides*, which affect sensory, ocular, and bulbar nerves. Patients commonly present with gait instability, paresthesia, ophthalmoplegia, and progressive muscle weakness. The disease course is typically chronic with intermittent relapses. Evidence from case reports and small series suggests that IVIG and rituximab-based therapies are the most effective treatment options. In a French multicenter retrospective study of 45 patients, clinical responses were observed in 53%

with IVIG and 52% with rituximab, whereas conventional immunosuppressive agents were generally less effective [14].

29.12 Sporadic Late-Onset Nemaline Myopathy

Sporadic late-onset nemaline myopathy (SLOMN) is characterized by progressive proximal muscle weakness, myalgia, and muscle wasting involving the limbs, neck, and facial muscles. Clinical features may include *head drop, dysphagia, dysarthria, and respiratory insufficiency*, and the disease may lead to severe cardiopulmonary complications. Histologically, *nemaline rods* are observed within muscle fibers. The disorder typically affects middle-aged adults, and more than half of affected individuals have an associated *MGUS* [16]. Although the exact pathophysiological mechanism remains unclear, treatment directed at the plasma-cell clone has shown benefit. *Autologous hematopoietic stem cell transplantation* is considered first-line therapy for eligible patients and has produced favorable hematologic and neuromuscular responses in a significant proportion of cases. For patients who are not candidates for transplantation, *plasma-cell–directed regimens* such as *lenalidomide-dexamethasone, cyclophosphamide-based therapy, or bortezomib-containing regimens* may be effective. [17]

Patients with IgM MGUS–associated neuropathy who lack identifiable autoantibodies often present with slowly progressive distal sensory neuropathy, sometimes accompanied by tremor or ataxia. Electrophysiological studies generally reveal a demyelinating pattern. For individuals with mild symptoms, conservative management may be appropriate. However, patients with significant disability or progressive disease may benefit from IVIG as an initial therapeutic approach, while plasmapheresis, rituximab (alone or with alkylating agents), or ibrutinib may be considered in refractory cases [15].

Our patient received four cycles of bortezomib, lenalidomide, and dexamethasone, achieving complete hematologic remission. Neurological symptoms improved rapidly, and the patient regained the ability to walk independently without support. Although autologous stem cell transplantation was recommended, the patient declined this option and was subsequently maintained on bortezomib and dexamethasone for one year. Over time, he experienced near-complete neurological recovery and continues to remain clinically stable.

29.13 MGUS-Associated Cutaneous Manifestations

The skin represents one of the organ systems frequently affected by monoclonal gammopathies. Cutaneous manifestations may arise through several mechanisms, including deposition of monoclonal immunoglobulins within tissues, cytokine-mediated inflammation, or direct pathogenic activity of paraproteins. These mechanisms can lead to a wide spectrum of dermatologic disorders.

1. Scleromyxedema

Scleromyxedema is an uncommon form of *cutaneous mucinosis* that occurs in association with monoclonal gammopathy. The disorder typically affects middle-aged adults and presents with widespread papular eruptions accompanied by skin thickening and induration. These changes result from mucin accumulation within the dermis together with fibrosis. Although primarily a dermatologic condition, scleromyxedema can involve multiple organ systems, including the cardiovascular, gastrointestinal, pulmonary, renal, musculoskeletal, and nervous systems, which accounts for its substantial morbidity and mortality. The underlying pathogenesis involves fibroblast proliferation and increased mucin production, likely driven by cytokine dysregulation and the presence of monoclonal immunoglobulins, most commonly IgG with lambda light chains.

Current evidence from observational studies suggests that intravenous immunoglobulin (IVIG) in combination with systemic corticosteroids represents the preferred first-line therapy. High-dose IVIG (2 g/kg administered over five consecutive days every 4–6 weeks) can induce remission in patients with non-severe disease lacking cardiac or central nervous system involvement. Responses may persist for months or even years; therefore, maintenance infusions every 6–12 weeks are often required [12]. For patients with severe disease or those who fail IVIG therapy, plasma-cell–directed treatments are recommended. Lenalidomide is generally favored over thalidomide due to a more favorable toxicity profile. In refractory cases, bortezomib-based regimens or autologous stem cell transplantation have been reported to produce clinical improvement [18, 19].

2. Necrobiotic Xanthogranuloma

Necrobiotic xanthogranuloma (NXG) is a rare form of non-Langerhans cell histiocytosis predominantly affecting older adults. It manifests as yellowish, violaceous, or reddish papules and nodules that gradually enlarge to form infiltrated plaques. The periorbital region is the most commonly involved site. In addition to cutaneous lesions, extracutaneous involvement may occur, affecting the eyes, respiratory tract, cardiovascular system, or other organs. Approximately 80% of patients with NXG have an associated monoclonal gammopathy. Management remains challenging due to the absence of standardized treatment guidelines. Corticosteroids combined with IVIG are frequently used as initial therapy. Alternative options include alkylating agents such as chlorambucil, as well as bortezomib or immunomodulatory drugs like lenalidomide or thalidomide. For refractory disease, plasmapheresis or autologous hematopoietic stem cell transplantation may be considered [20].

3. Acquired Cutis Laxa

Acquired cutis laxa is an uncommon connective tissue disorder characterized by loose, inelastic skin resulting from degradation of elastic fibers in the dermis.

Patients often appear to have *prematurely aged skin with prominent wrinkling*. The condition has been reported in association with systemic inflammatory diseases, drug exposure, hematologic malignancies, and monoclonal gammopathies, most frequently involving IgG with lambda or kappa light chains. Management focuses primarily on treating the underlying hematologic disorder, as no specific medical therapy exists for the cutaneous changes. Cosmetic interventions such as reconstructive surgery or laser-based skin tightening procedures may be considered for symptomatic relief.

4. Neutrophilic Dermatoses

Neutrophilic dermatoses comprise a heterogeneous group of inflammatory skin disorders characterized by *dense neutrophilic infiltration of the dermis or epidermis*. Clinically, they may present with *pustules, ulcers, nodules, or painful plaques*. Although these conditions may occur in the context of systemic inflammatory diseases and can involve extracutaneous organs, they are not caused by infection or vasculitis. Several variants of neutrophilic dermatosis have been linked to IgA monoclonal gammopathy, including pyoderma gangrenosum, erythema elevatum diutinum, subcorneal pustular dermatosis, Sweet syndrome, and neutrophilic urticarial dermatosis. Treatment strategies depend on the specific subtype but typically involve systemic corticosteroids, often combined with other immunosuppressive agents [12].

29.14 MGUS-Associated Ocular Manifestations

Ocular complications related to monoclonal gammopathy are uncommon but well-documented. Both *corneal and retinal structures* may be affected even in the absence of overt plasma cell or lymphoproliferative malignancy.

1. Paraproteinemic Keratopathy

Paraproteinemic keratopathy—also referred to as *keratopathy associated with monoclonal gammopathy or immunotactoid keratopathy*—results from bilateral corneal deposition of monoclonal immunoglobulins, most frequently IgG-kappa. These deposits produce characteristic corneal opacities, which may appear either as crystalline structures (crystalline keratopathy) or as non-crystalline patterns such as peripheral bands, granular deposits, or lattice-like changes. In patients with progressive ocular involvement or progression of the underlying monoclonal gammopathy, systemic therapy targeting the plasma cell clone, including chemotherapy or autologous hematopoietic cell transplantation, may halt disease progression and improve symptoms. Surgical interventions such as *keratoplasty or corneal transplantation* can temporarily restore vision; however, recurrence within the graft is common [22].

2. Maculopathy Associated with Monoclonal Gammopathy

Maculopathy represents a much rarer ocular complication of monoclonal gammopathy. Patients may develop serous retinal detachment affecting one or both eyes, potentially resulting in progressive visual impairment. The exact pathophysiological mechanism remains uncertain. Proposed explanations include direct deposition of monoclonal immunoglobulins within retinal structures or autoantibody activity directed against macular tissues. In many reported cases, treatment of the underlying monoclonal gammopathy has resulted in resolution or improvement of retinal pathology [23].

29.15 Multisystem Syndromes Associated with MGCS

While some monoclonal gammopathies of clinical significance affect a single organ system, others present as complex multisystem disorders with distinctive pathophysiological mechanisms. Here, we describe six representative multi-organ MGCS syndromes.

1. Clarkson Disease (Systemic Capillary Leak Syndrome)

Systemic capillary leak syndrome, also known as *Clarkson disease*, was first described in 1960. It is characterized by *recurrent episodes of severe hypotension and generalized edema* caused by widespread leakage of plasma from the intravascular compartment into surrounding tissues. These episodes lead to hemoconcentration and hypoalbuminemia, frequently resulting in hypovolemic shock. The underlying mechanism remains poorly understood, although IgG MGUS is detected in a large proportion of patients. Management of acute attacks focuses on careful fluid replacement and hemodynamic stabilization. Long-term prevention strategies have evolved, and intravenous immunoglobulin therapy has shown promising results. In a study involving 69 patients, IVIG significantly reduced both mortality and recurrence rates compared with treatment using terbutaline over a median follow-up of five years [21].

2. Acquired C1 Inhibitor Deficiency

Acquired C1 inhibitor deficiency, also known as *acquired angioedema*, is a rare disorder characterized by *recurrent episodes of swelling involving the skin, gastrointestinal tract, and upper airway*. Although clinically similar to hereditary angioedema, this condition typically occurs in individuals older than 40 years. The pathogenesis involves autoantibodies directed against the C1 esterase inhibitor, resulting in dysregulation of the complement pathway. Monoclonal gammopathy is detected in approximately 30–40% of cases. Acute episodes may be treated with C1 inhibitor replacement therapy, fresh frozen plasma, icatibant, or ecallantide. Preventive strategies include antifibrinolytic agents such as tranexamic acid, corticosteroids, androgens such as danazol, or regular administration of C1 inhibitor concentrate. There are also reports describing the successful use of rituximab in refractory cases [24].

3. Crystal-Storing Histiocytosis

Crystal-storing histiocytosis (CSH) is a rare disorder in which abnormal immunoglobulins accumulate as crystalline inclusions within lysosomes of histiocytes.

This process can result in localized or systemic organ damage, affecting the kidneys, eyes, lungs, bone marrow, gastrointestinal tract, or spleen. Treatment is directed at the underlying plasma cell or lymphoid malignancy, and regimens such as bortezomib-based therapy, daratumumab-containing combinations, or R-CHOP chemotherapy have been associated with clinical improvement [26].

4. Schnitzler Syndrome

Schnitzler syndrome is a rare autoinflammatory condition characterized by *chronic urticarial rash, monoclonal gammopathy (usually IgM-kappa), osteosclerotic bone lesions, lymphadenopathy, and hepatosplenomegaly*. The disorder most often develops during the fifth decade of life and occurs slightly more frequently in men. The urticarial rash is typically intermittent and migratory, changing distribution over time. Because there is no definitive test confirming the causal relationship between the monoclonal protein and the inflammatory manifestations, diagnosis relies on clinical criteria known as the Strasbourg criteria, after excluding other possible conditions. The disease is believed to result from inflammasome activation and excessive production of interleukin-1 (IL-1). Whether the monoclonal protein directly triggers the inflammatory cascade or represents a secondary phenomenon remains uncertain. IL-1 blockade with anakinra is considered the treatment of choice and often results in rapid and sustained symptom relief [27].

5. TEMPI Syndrome

TEMPI syndrome is an uncommon plasma-cell-associated disorder characterized by five principal clinical features: *telangiectasia, markedly elevated erythropoietin levels with erythrocytosis, monoclonal gammopathy, perinephric fluid accumulation, and intrapulmonary shunting* [30]. Cutaneous telangiectasias are frequently visible on the face, trunk, and upper limbs. Patients typically exhibit striking elevations of serum erythropoietin and progressive erythrocytosis. Although the precise pathophysiology remains uncertain, it has been proposed that the monoclonal protein contributes to tissue hypoxia and abnormal vascular responses. Importantly, therapies directed toward the underlying plasma-cell clone have been shown to improve or reverse several clinical manifestations of the syndrome, suggesting a causal relationship between the paraprotein and disease features.

6. Cryoglobulinemia

Cryoglobulinemia refers to the presence of immunoglobulins that precipitate at low temperatures and dissolve upon warming. These proteins can form immune complexes that deposit in blood vessels and trigger inflammatory vasculitis. Three main categories of cryoglobulinemia are recognized:

- *Type I,* consisting of monoclonal immunoglobulin, is often associated with plasma cell or lymphoid malignancies.
- *Type II,* involving monoclonal immunoglobulin with rheumatoid factor activity interacting with polyclonal IgG.
- *Type III,* composed of polyclonal immune complexes, typically arising in inflammatory or infectious conditions.

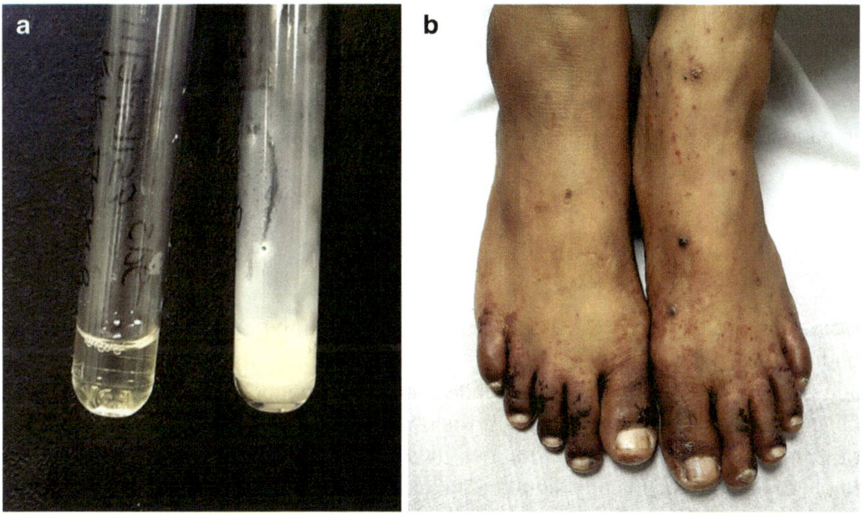

Fig. 29.3 A serum showing precipitation of cryoglobulins at 4° C temperature in the right tube. B. Necrotic vasculitic skin ulceration due to cryoglobulinemic vasculitis and bluish discoloration of toes

Clinical manifestations may include purpura, livedo reticularis, painful skin ulceration, peripheral neuropathy, and arthritis (Fig. 29.3) [33]. Renal involvement may occur in some patients. Management of types I and II cryoglobulinemia requires identification and treatment of the underlying clonal disorder responsible for producing the pathogenic immunoglobulin [31].

29.16 Hematologic Manifestations of MGCS

Certain monoclonal gammopathies predominantly affect the hematologic or coagulation systems. These include:

- Acquired von Willebrand syndrome
- Cold agglutinin disease
- Monoclonal gammopathy of thrombotic significance

29.17 Acquired von Willebrand Syndrome

Acquired von Willebrand syndrome (aVWS) can develop in association with several conditions, including cardiovascular disorders, Wilms tumor, autoimmune diseases, hypothyroidism, and hematologic malignancies. In some patients, the disorder is linked to MGUS or other lymphoproliferative diseases. Clinical manifestations resemble those of inherited von Willebrand disease and include mucocutaneous bleeding, easy bruising, and excessive bleeding during surgical procedures. Treatment strategies are similar to those used for congenital von Willebrand disease. Intravenous immunoglobulin therapy has demonstrated favorable responses in patients in whom the disorder is associated with monoclonal gammopathy [25].

29.18 Cold Agglutinin Disease

Cold agglutinin disease (CAD) is an autoimmune hemolytic anemia caused by antibodies that bind to red blood cells at low temperatures. Most cases occur in older adults and are associated with an underlying IgM monoclonal gammopathy produced by a small B-cell clone. Diagnosis is established through laboratory evidence of hemolytic anemia together with identification of cold-reactive antibodies exhibiting high titers and clinically significant thermal amplitude. Therapeutic approaches aim to suppress the pathogenic B-cell clone. Rituximab is frequently used as initial therapy, while combination regimens such as bendamustine–rituximab or targeted agents may be required for refractory disease [32].

29.19 Monoclonal Gammopathy of Thrombotic Significance

Monoclonal gammopathy of thrombotic significance (MGTS) is a recently recognized entity characterized by recurrent thrombosis associated with monoclonal immunoglobulins that activate platelets. In this disorder, the monoclonal protein acts as an antibody directed against *platelet factor 4*, triggering platelet activation and promoting clot formation even in the absence of heparin exposure. The clinical picture may resemble heparin-induced thrombocytopenia. Management includes anticoagulation along with therapies aimed at suppressing the clonal B-cell or plasma-cell population responsible for producing the pathogenic immunoglobulin [28].

29.20 Conclusion

Patients found to have monoclonal gammopathy should undergo careful clinical evaluation to determine whether the monoclonal protein is contributing to organ dysfunction. Although MGUS is often asymptomatic, a growing number of disorders are now recognized in which the monoclonal immunoglobulin itself plays a pathogenic role. The concept of *monoclonal gammopathies of clinical significance* highlights the importance of identifying these conditions early. Treatment strategies are individualized and generally focus on suppressing the responsible plasma-cell or B-cell clone. In certain cases, adjunctive therapies targeting immune pathways may also be beneficial. Continued research into the mechanisms underlying these disorders and prospective clinical trials will be essential for improving diagnostic strategies and optimizing management for affected patients.

References

1. Rajkumar SV, Dimopoulos MA, Palumbo A, Blade J, Merlini G, Mateos MV, et al. International Myeloma Working Group updated criteria for the diagnosis of multiple myeloma. Lancet Oncol. 2014;15(12):e538–48. https://doi.org/10.1016/S1470-2045(14)70442-5. Epub 2014 Oct 26. PMID: 25439696
2. Kyle RA, Therneau TM, Rajkumar SV, Larson DR, Plevak MF, Offord JR, Dispenzieri A, Katzmann JA, Melton LJ 3rd. Prevalence of monoclonal gammopathy of undetermined significance. N Engl J Med. 2006;354(13):1362–9. https://doi.org/10.1056/NEJMoa054494.
3. Greenberg AJ, Rajkumar SV, Vachon CM. Familial monoclonal gammopathy of undetermined significance and multiple myeloma: epidemiology, risk factors, and biological characteristics. Blood. 2012;119(23):5359–66. https://doi.org/10.1182/blood-2011-11-387324.
4. Kyle RA, Durie BG, Rajkumar SV, Landgren O, Blade J, Merlini G, et al. International Myeloma Working Group. Monoclonal gammopathy of undetermined significance (MGUS) and smoldering (asymptomatic) multiple myeloma: IMWG consensus perspectives risk factors for progression and guidelines for monitoring and management. Leukemia. 2010;24(6):1121–7. https://doi.org/10.1038/leu.2010.60.
5. Dispenzieri A. Monoclonal gammopathies of clinical significance. Hematology Am Soc Hematol Educ Program. 2020;2020(1):380–8.
6. Leung N, Bridoux F, Batuman V, et al. The evaluation of monoclonal gammopathy of renal significance: a consensus report of the International Kidney and Monoclonal Gammopathy Research Group. Nat Rev Nephrol. 2019;15(1):45–7.
7. Bridoux F, Nasr SH, Arnulf B, Leung N, Sirac C, Jaccard A. Renal manifestations of MGUS. Hematology Am Soc Hematol Educ Program. 2024;2024(1):489–98. https://doi.org/10.1182/hematology.2024000573. PMID: 39644070
8. Gumber R, Cohen JB, Palmer MB, et al. A clone-directed approach may improve diagnosis and treatment of proliferative glomerulonephritis with monoclonal immunoglobulin deposits. Kidney Int. 2018;94(1):199–205.
9. Chauvet S, Fremeaux-Bacchi V, Petitprez F, et al. Treatment of B-cell disorder improves renal outcome of patients with monoclonal gammopathy associated C3 glomerulopathy. Blood. 2017;129(11):1437–47.
10. Heybeli C, Alexander MP, Bentall AJ, et al. Kidney transplantation in patients with monoclonal gammopathy of renal significance (MGRS) associated lesions: a case series. Am J Kidney Dis. 2022;79(2):202–16.
11. Chaudhry HM, Mauermann ML, Rajkumar SV. Monoclonal Gammopathy-associated peripheral neuropathy: diagnosis and management. Mayo Clin Proc. 2017;92(5):838–50.
12. Oganesyan A, Gregory A, Malard F, Ghahramanyan N, Mohty M, Kazandjian D, Mekinian A, Hakobyan Y. Monoclonal gammopathies of clinical significance (MGCS): in pursuit of optimal treatment. Front Immunol. 2022;13:1045002. https://doi.org/10.3389/fimmu.2022.1045002.

13. Sarosiek SR, Branagan AR, Doughty C, Flynn CA, Little M, Stockman K, White TP, Meid K, Treon SP, Castillo JJ. Prospective study of Acalabrutinib with rituximab in patients with symptomatic anti-MAG mediated IgM peripheral neuropathy. Blood. 2023;142(Supplement 1):213. https://doi.org/10.1182/blood-2023-185113.
14. Le Cann M, Bouhour F, Viala K, Simon L, Tard C, Rossi C, et al. CANOMAD: a neurological monoclonal gammopathy of clinical significance that benefits from b-cell–targeted therapies. Blood. 2020;136(21):2428–36. https://doi.org/10.1182/blood.2020007092.
15. Cibeira MT, Rodríguez-Lobato LG, Alejaldre A, Fernández de Larrea C. Neurological manifestations of MGUS. Hematology Am Soc Hematol Educ Program. 2024;2024(1):499–504. https://doi.org/10.1182/hematology.2024000665.
16. Schnitzler LJ, Schreckenbach T, Nadaj-Pakleza A, Stenzel W, Rushing EJ, Van Damme P, et al. Sporadic late-onset nemaline myopathy: clinico-pathological characteristics and review of 76 cases. Orphanet J Rare Dis. 2017;12(1):1–2. https://doi.org/10.1186/s13023-017-0640-.
17. Kansagra AJ, et al. Outcomes of Autologous Hematopoietic Stem Cell Transplant in Sporadic Late Onset Nemaline Myopathy with Associated Monoclonal Gammopathy of Unknown Significance. Biol Blood Marrow Transpl. 24(3):S124–5.
18. Yeung CK, Loong F, Kwong YL. Scleromyxedema due to a plasma cell neoplasm: rapid remission with bortezomib, thalidomide and dexamethasone. Br J Haematol. 2012;157(4):411. https://doi.org/10.1111/j.1365-2141.2012.09088.
19. Donato ML, Feasel AM, Weber DM, Prieto VG, Giralt SA, Champlin RE, et al. Scleromyxedema: role of high-dose melphalan with autologous stem cell transplantation. Blood. 2006;107(2):463–6. https://doi.org/10.1182/blood-2004-12-4870.
20. Steinhelfer L, Kühnel T, Jägle H, Mayer S, Karrer S, Haubner F, Schreml S. Systemic therapy of necrobiotic xanthogranuloma: a systematic review. Orphanet J Rare Dis. 2022;17(1):132. https://doi.org/10.1186/s13023-022-02291-z.
21. de Chambrun MP, Gousseff M, Mauhin W, Lega JC, Lambert M, Rivière S, et al. Intravenous immunoglobulins improve survival in monoclonal gammopathy-associated systemic capillary-leak syndrome. Am J Med. 2017;130(10):1219–e19. https://doi.org/10.1016/j.amjmed.2017.05.023.
22. Wasielica-Poslednik J, Gericke A, Desuki A, Schlötzer-Schrehardt U, Pfeiffer N, Lisch W. Recurrence of paraproteinemic keratopathy after penetrating keratoplasty and its assessment with confocal microscopy. Am J Ophthalmol Case Rep. 2018;11:87–91. https://doi.org/10.1016/j.ajoc.2018.06.014.
23. Mansour AM, Arevalo JF, Badal J, Moorthy RS, Shah GK, Zegarra H, Pulido JS, Charbaji A, Amselem L, Lavaque AJ, Casella A, Ahmad B, Paschall JG, Caimi A, Staurenghi G. Paraproteinemic maculopathy. Ophthalmology. 2014;121(10):1925–32. https://doi.org/10.1016/j.ophtha.2014.04.007.
24. Branellec A, Bouillet L, Javaud N, Mekinian A, Boccon-Gibod I, Blanchard-Delaunay C, et al. Acquired C1-inhibitor deficiency: 7 patients treated with rituximab. J Clin Immunol. 2012;32(5):936–41. https://doi.org/10.1007/s10875-012-9691-2.
25. Abou-Ismail MY, Rodgers GM, Bray PF, Lim MY. Acquired von willebrand syndrome in monoclonal gammopathy–a scoping review on hemostatic management. Res Pract Thromb haemostasis. 2021;5(2):356–65. https://doi.org/10.1002/rth2.12481.
26. Hu X, Liu J, Bai C, Wang J, Song X. Bortezomib combined with thalidomide and dexamethasone is effective for patient with crystal-storing histiocytosis associated with monoclonal gammopathy of undermined significance. Eur J Haematol. 2012;89(2):183–4. https://doi.org/10.1111/j.1600-0609.2012.01800.x.
27. Iberri D, Liedtke M. MGCS: where do we stand today? Hematology Am Soc Hematol Educ Program. 2024;2024(1):482–8. https://doi.org/10.1182/hematology.2024000572.
28. Gkalea V, Fotiou D, Dimopoulos MA, Kastritis E. Monoclonal Gammopathy of thrombotic significance. Cancers (Basel). 2023;15(2):480. https://doi.org/10.3390/cancers15020480. PMID: 36672429

29. Dispenzieri A. POEMS syndrome: update on diagnosis, risk-stratification, and management. Am J Hematol. 2023;98(12):1934–50. https://doi.org/10.1002/ajh.27081. Epub 2023 Sep 21
30. Sykes DB, O'Connell C, Schroyens W. The TEMPI syndrome. Blood. 2020;135(15):1199–203. https://doi.org/10.1182/blood.2019004216.
31. Killeen RB, Awais M, Mikes BA. Cryoglobulinemia. In: StatPearls [Internet]. Treasure Island (FL): StatPearls Publishing; 2025. PMID: 32491538.
32. Berentsen S. How I treat cold agglutinin disease. Blood. 2021;137(10):1295–303. https://doi.org/10.1182/blood.2019003809.
33. Gupta N, Rao S, Agarwal P. Multiple myeloma presenting as cryoglobulinaemic vasculitis. Br J Haematol. 2019;185(5):818. https://doi.org/10.1111/bjh.15868.

Chapter 30
Multiple Myeloma: Risk Stratification and Management

Gurleen Oberoi and Rajiv Kumar

Abstract Multiple myeloma is the second most common hematological malignancy. Rapid strides in prognostication and therapy have dramatically improved survival. The revised IMWG diagnostic criteria has already expanded the definition of MM. Molecular cytogenetic classification and the subsequent genetic risk stratification have helped to better define the disease and take appropriate therapeutic decisions in the various risk groups. WB PET CT scan has provided a quick and complete assessment of bone and extramedullary disease and is being increasingly used in place of whole body MRI. Minimal Residual Disease assessment is helping refine the intensity and duration of therapies, thereby reducing adverse drug effects. Phenomenal breakthroughs in the field of immunotherapy, in the form of CAR T cell therapy and BiTE antibodies, are providing new avenues of therapy to relapse-refractory disease patients post multiple lines of therapy. This article summarizes the current status of diagnostic workup, risk stratification, and therapeutic approaches in multiple myeloma.

Keywords Myeloma · ASCT · IMWG · BiTEs · CART · Risk stratification · ISS

Learning Objectives
- Approach to newly diagnosed and relapse/refractory multiple myeloma.
- Diagnostic work up.
- Risk stratification.
- Management and the role of ASCT and of newer drugs.

G. Oberoi
Consultant Hematopathology, Medanta Hospital, Gurgaon, India

R. Kumar (✉)
Consultant Clinical Hematology, Army Hospital (Research and Referral), New Delhi, India

H. P. Pati et al. (eds.), *Clinical Hematology and Hemato-Oncology*,
https://doi.org/10.1007/978-981-92-1167-8_30

30.1 Introduction

Multiple myeloma (MM) is a malignancy caused by the proliferation of neoplastic clonal plasma cells, usually producing monoclonal antibodies, and can lead to osteolytic lesions, fractures, renal impairment, and anemias. For many years, MM was considered to be an incurable disease; however, recent breakthroughs in diagnostic techniques, therapy, and a deeper understanding of the molecular biology of the disease have transformed it into one that is manageable, with much improved quality of life, outcomes, and potentially curable in some cases. The key to this evolution can be attributed to early diagnosis, improved risk stratification, and availability of new treatment modalities, allowing clinicians to tailor personalized therapies that maximize efficacy while minimizing side effects.

This chapter will focus on the diagnosis, risk stratification, and management of multiple myeloma, including the latest updates that have contributed to a better understanding of disease prognosis and the personalization of treatment plans.

30.2 Diagnosis of Multiple Myeloma

Early and accurate diagnosis is crucial and the first step for effective management of multiple myeloma. The diagnostic approach combines clinical evaluation, serological tests, imaging, and histopathological examination. Recent advancements in diagnostic techniques have provided more sensitive and specific tools for identifying MM, enabling earlier detection and better disease characterization.

1. Clinical Presentation

Multiple myeloma presentation is often nonspecific, with symptoms ranging from back pain, bone pains, and fatigue to renal insufficiency and infections. Common and classic presentations include:

1. *Bone pain:* This is often the most common presenting symptom, particularly in the central or axial skeleton (spine, ribs, pelvis, and vertebrae), due to osteolytic lesions, which are detected in a routine skeletal survey. These osteolytic lesions are the cause of bone pains and pathological fractures with trivial trauma in these patients.
2. *Anemia:* MM often leads to anemia because of the disruption of normal hematopoiesis in the bone marrow and sometimes a relative deficiency of erythropoietin. Rarely there is macrocytic anemia due to vitamin B12 deficiency.
3. *Hypercalcemia:* Elevated calcium levels are due to bone resorption and demineralization, leading to the release of calcium into the bloodstream. It is also suggested that if serum calcium level is elevated but there are no symptoms of hypercalcemia, then ionized calcium should be measured, as this increase can occur due to binding of calcium with M protein.

4. *Renal disease or failure:* Renal failure can be a presenting feature of myeloma. This occurs as a result of the deposition of light chains (a component of the monoclonal protein) in the kidneys, leading to renal impairment. This leads to raised serum creatinine levels.

The above-mentioned common presentations are thus included in diagnostic criteria as myeloma-defining events. As we know, the acronym "CRAB" is used to remember it, which goes as: calcium elevation, renal insufficiency, anemia, and bone disease. Infections (partly due to decreased normal immunoglobulin [Ig] production), bleeding, neurological manifestations due to spinal cord compression or peripheral neuropathy, and hyperviscosity can be other presenting features [1].

2. Laboratory Tests

When a patient is suspected of MM on the basis of the clinical presentation discussed above, further physical examination and initial screenings are planned. Physical examination includes a detailed neurologic examination. Complete blood count, serum calcium, serum creatinine, and detection and quantification of M protein are performed.

The following are the common initial laboratory tests in patients suspected of MM:

1. *Complete Blood Count (CBC) and peripheral smear examination:* A CBC often reveals anemia, neutropenia, and thrombocytopenia, all of which can result from bone marrow infiltration by malignant plasma cells. Peripheral smear examination shows Rouleaux formation and can show leucoerythroblastic blood picture and circulating plasma cells.
2. *Serum Beta-2 Microglobulin (β2M):* Elevated levels of β2M are associated with increased tumor burden and poor prognosis in MM. This biomarker is used as part of the International Staging System (ISS) for MM.
3. *Creatinine and Calcium Levels:* Hypercalcemia and elevated creatinine levels may indicate bone destruction and renal impairment, both of which are common complications of MM, and they are included in diagnostic criteria (as mentioned in Fig. 30.1).
4. Detection of Monoclonal protein: Majority of MM patients (~97%) show the presence of monoclonal (M) protein, which can be detected by protein electrophoresis of the serum (SPEP) and/or urine (UPEP) from a 24-hour collection, serum free light chain (FLC) analysis (Table 30.1). It can be combined with immunofixation of the serum and urine, which confirms the presence of M band and determines its type. Mass spectrometry (MS) is presently being considered as a technique to detect and quantify the M-protein with high sensitivity and specificity.

Of the 20% cases with no M band on SPEP, the majority of these patients can have light chain myeloma. The FLC assay and sometimes UPEP with immunofixation help in detecting these cases 2–3% of all the myeloma cases are non-secretory as there is impaired secretion, thus showing absence of M band by serum/urine immunofixation; however, production is there as demonstrated by

Diagnostic criteria for plasma cell myeloma (PCM) : Adapted from the International Myeloma Working Group (IMWG) updated criteria for the diagnosis of multiple myeloma

Both criterias must be met:

- **Clonal bone marrow plasma cells ≥10%** or biopsy-proven bony or extramedullary plasmacytoma
- Any **one or more** of the following **myeloma defining events:**
  - ❑ Evidence of end-organ damage that can be attributed to the underlying plasma cell proliferative disorder, specifically:
    - **Hypercalcemia**: serum calcium >0.25 mmol/L (>1 mg/dL) higher than the upper limit of normal or >2.75 mmol/L (>11 mg/dL).
    - **Renal insufficiency**: creatinine clearance <40 mL per minute or serum creatinine >177 µmol/L (>2 mg/dL)
    - **Anemia**: hemoglobin value of >2 g/dL below the lower limit of normal, or a hemoglobin value <10 g/dL.
    - **Bone lesions: one or more osteolytic lesions** on skeletal radiography, computed tomography (CT), or positron emission tomography-CT (PET-CT).
  - ❑ ≥ 1 of the following biomarkers of malignancy:
    1. **Clonal bone marrow plasma cell percentage ≥ 60%.**
    2. **Involved: uninvolved serum free light chain (FLC) ratio ≥ 100** (involved free light chain level must be ≥100 mg/L).
    3. **>1 focal lesions on magnetic resonance imaging** (MRI) studies (at least 5 mm in size)

Fig. 30.1 Diagnostic criteria for diagnosing multiple myeloma (revised IMWG) [1]

Table 30.1 Monoclonal protein detection in MM

S. NO.	Methodology	Sensitivity
1.	SPEP	80%
2.	SPEP + IFE	90%
3.	SPEP + IFE + Sflc	97%

immunohistochemistry showing presence of cytoplasmic M protein/immunoglobin. Acquired mutations in the immunoglobulin light chain variable genes and light chain constant region are known to be the pathogenesis of these cases. In around two-thirds of these cases has elevated serum free light chains and an abnormal ratio making them minimal/oligosecretary myeloma. Also, 15% of these are non-producer myeloma with no cytoplasmic immunoglobulin synthesis [1].

30.3 Bone Marrow Evaluation

Bone marrow evaluation, including aspiration and biopsy, immunophenotyping, conventional cytogenetics, and especially fluorescence in situ hybridization (FISH) are planned for the patient. Presence of chromosomal abnormalities like t(11;14), t(4;14), t(14;16), t(6;14), t(14;20), trisomies, and del(17p) detected by FISH, provides insights into prognosis and risk stratification.

A bone marrow biopsy is the gold standard for confirming the presence of malignant plasma cells. A sample of bone marrow is aspirated and examined for the percentage of plasma cells, with a threshold of ≥10% clonal plasma cells being indicative of MM. Due to the patchy nature of the disease, bone marrow biopsy becomes crucial for establishing a diagnosis of multiple myeloma when a lower percentage of plasma cells are detected on bone marrow aspirate. Also, when the plasma cell percentage is variable between biopsy and aspirate a higher percentage is taken into consideration. Immunohistochemistry (IHC), immunofluorescence and flow cytometry can be used to establish clonality by demonstrating kappa and lambda light chain restriction [1, 2].

30.4 Imaging Techniques

Modern imaging techniques help to identify bone lesions, measure disease burden, and evaluate extramedullary involvement, thus becoming crucial for the diagnostics and follow-up of MM. Cross-sectional imaging, like whole-body low-dose computed tomography (CT) without contrast, whole-body combined 18F-FDG PET/CT, and whole-body MRI, are more sensitive than plain radiographs for detecting bone involvement in patients suspected of MM

(a) *X-rays:* Traditionally used to detect osteolytic lesions in bones, though they may not detect small lesions or soft tissue involvement.
(b) *MRI and Whole-Body MRI:* It offers a more sensitive method for detecting bone marrow infiltration and skeletal lesions, including those in the spine and pelvis. Whole-body MRI is particularly effective in detecting early-stage disease and in monitoring treatment response.
(c) *PET-CT Scans:* Positron emission tomography (PET) combined with computed tomography (CT) is an excellent tool for detecting active disease and extramedullary plasmacytomas. PET-CT scans can provide a more comprehensive picture of disease activity, especially in relapsed cases.

Utilizing the above modalities along with the diagnostic criteria mentioned in Fig. 30.1, the diagnosis of MM is established.

30.5 Genetic and Molecular Profiling

Multiple myeloma is a collection of several cytogenetically distinct entities. Approximately 40% of multiple myeloma has trisomies (hyperdiploid multiple myeloma), the rest of the patients have translocations involving the immunoglobulin heavy chain (IgH) locus on chromosome 14q32, and a very small proportion of

Table 30.2 Primary molecular cytogenetic classification of MM

Subtype	Gene(s)/chromosomes affected	Approximate percentage of myeloma patients
Hyperdiploid multiple myeloma[a]	Recurrent trisomies involving odd-numbered chromosomes with the exception of chromosomes 1, 13, and 21	45
IgH translocated multiple myeloma		40
t(11;14) (q13;q32)	*CCND1* (cyclin D1)	20
t(6;14) (p21;q32)	*CCND3* (cyclin D3)	5
t(4;14) (p16;q32)	*NSD2*	10
t(14;16) (q32;q23)	*C-MAF*	4
t(14;20) (q32;q11)	*MAFB*	<1
Other IgH translocations, other cytogenetic abnormalities, or normal		5

patients have both trisomies and IgH translocations. Trisomies and IgH translocations are primary abnormalities as they occur in the initial course (MGUS). The secondary cytogenetic abnormalities like gain(1q), del(1p), del(17p), del(13), and secondary translocations involving MYC are acquired later in the disease course of multiple myeloma; however, both primary and secondary cytogenetic abnormalities can influence disease outcome, course, response to therapy, and prognostication (Table 30.2). Thus, genetic testing is increasingly gaining importance in the diagnosis and prognosis of MM [2, 4].

These include:

- *Fluorescence* In Situ *Hybridization (FISH):* FISH is used to identify chromosomal abnormalities such as translocations (e.g., t(4;14), t(14;16)) and deletions (e.g., del(17p)) that are associated with high-risk disease.
- *Next-Generation Sequencing (NGS):* NGS enables the comprehensive analysis of genetic mutations, copy number alterations, and epigenetic changes in MM cells. Key mutations, including those in TP53, NRAS, and KRAS, are associated with poor prognosis and are useful for risk stratification.

30.6 Risk Stratification in Multiple Myeloma

In MM, risk stratification and staging play a crucial role in guiding treatment decisions and identifying patients who may benefit from more aggressive or personalized treatment regimens. Overall survival and prognostication are mostly dependent on host/patient characteristics, disease staging, biological characteristics of disease (especially, cytogenetic abnormalities), and response to therapy. Additionally, elevated serum lactate dehydrogenase and circulating plasma cells detected by peripheral smear examination (plasma cell leukemia) are known to be associated with aggressive disease.

Durie-Salmon staging system, International Myeloma Working Group (IMWG)-2014 staging system, the International Staging System (ISS) were the earlier systems used for stratifying the patients. The now-revised International Staging System (R-ISS) is the most favored risk stratification. It has been a game-changer as it integrates genetic abnormalities and other molecular markers that better reflect the biological behavior of the disease compared to the previous systems [1].

1. International Staging System (ISS)

The ISS, introduced in 2005, has been one of the most widely used systems for risk stratification in MM. It is based on two parameters:

- *Serum Beta-2 Microglobulin (β2M):* High levels of β2M are associated with a poor prognosis.
- *Serum Albumin Levels:* Low albumin levels correlate with worse survival, as they reflect the overall health of the patient and the presence of inflammatory processes.

The ISS stages MM into three categories:

- Stage I: Low-risk (β2M $<$ 3.5 mg/L, albumin $\geq$3.5 g/dL).
- Stage II: Intermediate-risk (neither stage I nor stage III criteria).
- Stage III: High-risk (β2M $\geq$ 5.5 mg/L).

2. Revised International Staging System (R-ISS)

The Revised International Staging System (RISS) integrates aspects of tumor burden from the International Staging System (ISS) and disease biology, including the presence of high-risk cytogenetic abnormalities or elevated lactate dehydrogenase (LDH) levels. This comprehensive approach forms a unified prognostic index, providing a more accurate reflection of the patient's overall risk and likely disease progression.

The R-ISS incorporates the following additional prognostic factors (Table 30.3), such as:

Table 30.3 Stages of R-ISS for myeloma

Stages	Criteria
I	Serum albumin $\geq$3.5 gm/dl Serum beta-2-microglobulin <3.5 mg/L No high-risk cytogenetics, standard-risk cytogenetics Normal serum lactate dehydrogenase level
II	Intermediate features: Not fitting Stage I or III
III	Both of the following: Serum beta-2-microglobulin >5.5 mg/L High risk cytogenetics [t(4;14), t(14;16), or del(17p)] or elevated serum lactate dehydrogenase level

- *Cytogenetic Abnormalities:* The presence of high-risk genetic mutations, such as del(17p), t(4;14), and t(14;16), is now part of the staging system. These mutations are associated with a poor prognosis.
- *Lactate Dehydrogenase (LDH):* Elevated LDH levels indicate high tumor burden and correlate with worse outcomes.

3. Genetic Risk Stratification

Fluorescence in situ hybridization (FISH) is the preferred technique for detecting specific chromosomal abnormalities in multiple myeloma (MM), as it allows for molecular-level detection. The most commonly used method is interphase FISH on bone marrow plasma cells, with two primary techniques: interphase FISH on purified plasma cells and light chain-restricted plasma cell cytoplasmic immunoglobulin-enhanced FISH.

Trisomies of odd-numbered chromosomes, resulting in hyperdiploidy, are widely recognized as indicating a favorable prognosis. High-risk genetic abnormalities are associated with shorter median survival when treated with standard therapies.

Key genetic markers of high-risk MM include:

- *Del(17p):* Deletion of the short arm of chromosome 17, which includes the tumor suppressor gene TP53, is one of the most significant high-risk factors in MM.
- *t(4;14):* Translocation between chromosomes 4 and 14 leads to the overexpression of the FGFR3 gene, which is associated with poor prognosis.
- *t(14;16):* This translocation results in the dysregulated expression of the MAF gene and is also associated with poor survival.
- *Mutations in TP53, NRAS, and KRAS:* These mutations contribute to disease progression and resistance to treatment.

Deletion 13 and hypodiploidy are considered to have an adverse prognosis when detected by conventional cytogenetics; they are not independent predictors when identified using FISH.

These genetic findings are included in Updated mSMART 3.0 (Mayo stratification for Myeloma and Risk Adapted Therapy 3.0) (Table 30.4).

Chromosome 1 abnormalities, such as 1q gain (three copies), 1q amplification (four or more copies), 1p deletion, and 1q21 aberrations, are linked to poor prognosis and disease progression. The second revision of the International Staging System (R2-ISS) has incorporated 1q gain/amplification as a key prognostic factor [2, 4].

By analyzing the coordinates of the translocation breakpoints in the NSD2 gene, subsets of multiple myeloma (MM) with t(4;14) can be identified using next-generation sequencing (NGS). Research has shown that these subsets, which differ by the location of the breakpoints, exhibit varying median overall survival (OS) rates. These subsets are categorized as early disruption, late disruption, or no disruption. NGS has also identified recurrent mutations in key genes such as KRAS, NRAS, BRAF, and TP53, which contribute to disease progression and treatment resistance. Furthermore, NGS has made it possible to detect clonal evolution and

Table 30.4 Updated mSMART 3.0 (Mayo stratification for Myeloma and Risk Adapted Therapy 3.0) (2024)

Risk groups	Percentage of newly diagnosed patients with the abnormality
Standard risk	60%
Trisomies t(11;14) (most common) t(6;14)	
High risk	40%
High risk genetic abnormalities t(4;14) t(14:16) t(14;20) del(17p) Gain(1q) del(1p) Double-hit myeloma: Any 2 High risk factors Triple-hit myeloma: Any 3 or more high risk factors RISS stage 3 High plasma cell S-phased GEP: High risk signature	

Note: Presence of concurrent trisomies may ameliorate the high risk effect

minimal residual disease, providing a more accurate approach to monitoring the disease.

By combining clinical, genetic, and molecular data, clinicians can categorize MM patients into different risk groups, enabling the development of tailored treatment strategies.

Future directions in risk stratification and prognostication:

The following are being increasingly used and considered to be included in mainstream prognostication and risk stratification systems:

1. *Immunophenotypic Markers:* Markers like CD28, CD56, CD38, CD138, and SLAMF7 are under investigation for their prognostic and therapeutic implications in multiple myeloma (MM). Targeting SLAMF7 is found to be promising in improving survival outcomes for patients with certain immune profiles. Recent studies have also suggested that CD56-negative MM cells are associated with a more aggressive disease course, higher relapse risk, and a diminished response to therapy. These findings have led to a deeper focus on understanding the clinical significance of these markers and how they might help predict patient responses to emerging therapies, including immune-based treatments and monoclonal antibodies. Ongoing research aims to validate their role in refining risk stratification and guiding therapeutic decisions.
2. *Minimal Residual Disease (MRD):* The novel and efficient therapies, including monoclonal antibodies and CAR T cells, have now made prolonged survival possible in the majority of MM patients. With the advent of highly sensitive and

specific methods, including Next-generation flow cytometry and Next-generation sequencing, the detection of minimal residual disease (MRD) during or after treatment has become robust. In multiple myeloma, the detection of minimal residual disease (MRD) has become a key prognostic indicator in recent years. It is now known that achieving MRD-negative status after treatment is closely associated with longer progression-free survival (PFS) and overall survival (OS), offering a more precise measure of treatment success compared to traditional metrics like complete response [3].

As a result, MRD monitoring is being increasingly integrated into clinical practice, allowing for a more personalized approach to patient care. MRD assessment is particularly useful for identifying high-risk groups that may remain MRD-positive even after aggressive therapy. For instance, patients with high-risk cytogenetic abnormalities such as del(17p) or t(4;14) may not achieve MRD negativity despite initial responses, highlighting the need for more intensive or novel treatment options. Recent research also suggests that patients who achieve sustained MRD-negative status after induction therapy can be safely offered a potential strategy to reduce treatment burden and side effects. As MRD testing becomes more commonplace, ensuring the standardization of testing methods is essential [3].

3. *MicroRNAs:* MicroRNAs, such as miR-15a, are being increasingly recognized for their involvement in the progression of MM and their contribution to poor prognosis (Gabay et al. 2024). These small RNA molecules can influence tumor biology by regulating gene expression, and their dysregulation in MM patients has been linked to disease progression and treatment resistance. As part of a broader effort to enhance personalized treatment, combining microRNAs with other biomarkers is providing a more comprehensive risk profile. These biomarkers, along with circulating tumor DNA (ctDNA), are being explored for their potential to monitor minimal residual disease (MRD), and they may eventually become integral to guiding clinical decisions, such as whether to intensify or de-escalate treatment regimens based on MRD status [2].
4. *Circulating Tumor DNA (ctDNA):* ctDNA analysis offers a non-invasive method for monitoring tumor burden, tracking emerging resistance mutations, detecting MRD, and identifying early signs of disease relapse. Recent advancements have improved the sensitivity of ctDNA testing, making it a promising tool for monitoring treatment efficacy and identifying patients at risk of relapse earlier than traditional methods. Studies have shown that ctDNA dynamics correlate with clinical outcomes, suggesting that ctDNA could be a critical tool in decision-making regarding treatment adjustments. This technology is rapidly evolving and may soon be incorporated into routine clinical practice for more personalized management of MM, especially as part of ongoing efforts to improve MRD detection and monitor response to novel therapies [4].

30.7 Management of Multiple Myeloma

The approach to treatment of multiple myeloma is guided by prognostic risk stratification and the stage at which it presents to the physician. In view of multiple approved therapies being available today it is important to use evidence-based guidelines to sequence the therapies correctly to get the optimum results in the long term. The various group of drugs currently available is given in Table 30.5.

The most important factors guiding the choice of therapy include newly diagnosed versus relapsed disease, age, frailty, and R-ISS risk stratification. The treatment paradigm is evolving rapidly, and combination therapies are the standard of care.

Table 30.5 Commonly used drugs in MM and combination regimens

S no	Drug	Dose and route of administration	Common combination protocol regimens
1	Bortezomib	1.3 mg/m^2, IV & SC	VRd, VTd, VPd, Vd
2	Carfilzomib	20 mg/m^2 first dose followed by 27 mg/m^2 IV twice weekly OR 56–70 mg/m^2 weekly	KRd, KPd, DKd, Kd
3	Ixazomib	4 mg PO on days 1,8, and 15 of each 28-day cycle	IRd, IPd
4	Thalidomide	200 mg HS	VTd, MPT
5	Lenalidomide	25 mg OD on days 1–21 of each cycle, 10 mg OD in maintenance	VRd, KRd, DRd, Rd
6	Pomalidomide	4 mg OD on days 1–21 of each cycle, 2 mg OD in maintenance	VPd, KPd, DPd
7	Daratumumab IV	16 mg/kg IV weekly in split doses or one dose followed by fortnightly after the first 8 doses	DVRd, DVd, DKRd, DPd,
8	Melphalan oral	7 mg/m^2 OR 0.18 mg/kg for days 1–4 of 28-day cycle	MPT, MPR, Mel-Dex

30.8 Treatment of Newly Diagnosed Multiple Myeloma

The treatment of a patient with newly diagnosed myeloma involves a very early decision-making at the time of diagnosis regarding the eligibility/fitness of the patient to undergo an Autologous Stem Cell Transplant (ASCT). Age is an important factor in this decision-making and most of the centers take an age cut-off of 65 years, above which ASCT is not offered. However, in addition to age, various frailty scores are used to determine the fitness of patients to undergo ASCT. In the United States, more patients are deemed fit for ASCT as compared to Europe.

30.9 Fit for ASCT

Patients deemed fit to undergo ASCT are further risk-stratified based on the R-ISS risk scores. Patients in the standard risk group are preferably treated with a four-drug regimen consisting of Dara-VRd or Isa-VRd for 3–4 cycles and then taken up for ASCT. Response rates, MRD negative rates, and progression-free survival (PFS) are superior with Dara-VRd when compared to bortezomib, lenalidomide, and dexamethasone (VRd). Bortezomib is commonly administered as a weekly dose of 1.3 mg/m^2 subcutaneously, and dexamethasone is given as a single 40 mg weekly dose or each 40 mg dose is split into 20 mg each on consecutive days. Lenalidomide is administered as a 25 mg once daily dose given on 21 days on and 7 days off, a four-weekly protocol. Early ASCT before any relapse and delayed ASCT post relapse have been shown to be of equal benefit, and hence there is an option of cryopreservation of mobilized hematopoietic stem cells and continuation of therapy as above for another 5–8 cycles. This is followed by single drug maintenance therapy with lenalidomide for a period of 2 years or till relapse. Patients not tolerating lenalidomide can alternatively be given maintenance therapy with bortezomib [1].

Patients in the high-risk group are also treated with Dara-VRD or Isa-VRD for 3–4 cycles and taken up for early ASCT. This is followed by 02-drug maintenance with bortezomib and lenalidomide till relapse. During maintenance, bortezomib is used as 1.3 mg/m^2 SC once fortnightly and lenalidomide is given at a dose of 10 mg OD. Dose is often titrated on the lower side in case of intolerance, like cytopenias or neuropathy.

In patients with renal dysfunction at diagnosis, the use of lenalidomide is contraindicated, alternative protocols are used. The most common combination drug protocol used is Dara-VCD or Dara-VTD.

ASCT is carried out with high-dose melphalan (HDM-140-200 mg/m^2) and stem cell rescue. Stem cell mobilization is done with a 5-day GCSF-based protocol. The use of lenalidomide for 4–6 cycles often limits the stem cell mobilization, and hence, plerixafor, a CXCR4 antagonist, is commonly added to the GCSF mobilization protocol. Daratumumab also reduces stem cell mobilization, as hematopoietic stem cells also express CD38.

In addition to the four-drug induction protocol, till recently, a 3-drug protocol consisting of VRd was the standard of care and continues to be a reasonable combination in countries where daratumumab is not available or not affordable. In addition, DRd, VCd, and VTd protocols can be used in countries where lenalidomide is not available or contraindicated due to renal failure. In patients presenting with severe neuropathy, the use of bortezomib is contraindicated due to the adverse effect profile of bortezomib, and in such cases, carfilzomib can be used as a KRd combination. However, KRd has not been found to be superior to VRd (ENDURANCE Trial) in newly diagnosed multiple myeloma. The other active regimens in patients with aggressive disease in the form of plasma cell leukemia and multiple extramedullary plasmacytomas include the PAD (bortezomib, doxorubicin, dexamethasone) regimen and the VDT-PACE (bortezomib, dexamethasone, thalidomide, cisplatin, doxorubicin, cyclophosphamide, and etoposide) regimen [5].

30.10 Unfit for ASCT

In patients who are considered unfit for ASCT at the time of initial diagnosis, the further choice of the therapeutic protocol is based on frailty. Various frailty scores have been used to risk-stratify the patients. Karnofsky Performance Status (KPS), Charlson Comorbidity Index (CCI), and ECOG Performance Scale are commonly used general frailty scores in use. In addition, myeloma-specific frailty scores like IMWG score, Simplified IMWG score, and UK Myeloma score can also be used. Patients who are considered not frail are treated with a four-drug regimen, Dara-VRd or Isa-VRd, for 8–12 cycles, irrespective of standard or high risk. However, patients in the high-risk group are further treated with a 2-drug maintenance regimen of bortezomib and lenalidomide. Patients in the standard risk group are treated with a lenalidomide-based maintenance regimen. In the frail subgroup of ASCT-ineligible patients, a 3-drug regimen is preferred. 8–12 cycles of VRd protocol followed by one or two drug maintenance is used in the standard and high-risk groups, respectively. In the standard risk frail group, there is an option to use the DRd protocol till relapse. Dose modifications in elderly frail patients should be considered in the form of a dexamethasone dose of 20 mg and a lower dose of lenalidomide. Patients having problems with frequent hospital visits for parenteral drug administration, can be considered for oral ixazomib and dexamethasone. The VCd regimen remains a viable alternative for patients with renal dysfunction or in countries where lenalidomide is unavailable. The details of commonly used protocols/regimen in MM are given in Table 30.4 [1, 12].

30.11 Stem Cell Transplantation

Autologous stem cell transplantation (ASCT) typically consists of administration of high-dose melphalan (HDM) in doses of 140–200 mg/m^2 followed by stem cell rescue. ASCT improves the median OS by 12 months. Higher doses of stem cell infusion may be associated with better PFS. However, randomized trials have shown no benefit in the OS between an early or a delayed ASCT (IFM trial, DETERMINATION trial). An early ASCT is generally done after 4 cycles of initial therapy, whereas a delayed ASCT is done at the time of relapse as salvage therapy. Tandem ASCT, which consists of double or two consecutive transplants, has conflicting data with respect to any survival benefit, and the results are at best inconclusive and hence are no longer considered by most of the centers today. Despite the availability of newer drugs, ASCT continues to be a standard of care in transplant-eligible patients with MM. Post-transplant consolidation therapy consisting of two or more drugs for 1–2 cycles is considered in patients who do not achieve a CR post ASCT. However, the BMT CTN-0702 trial did not show any benefit with such a therapy, and direct initiation of maintenance therapy post ASCT is preferable in most of the cases.

Allogenic Stem Cell transplantation, mostly non-myeloablative, is still an experimental procedure in MM patients, as the results show a transplant-related mortality of 10–20% and high rates of GVHD. However, in young patients with high-risk relapsed disease, it may still be considered in patients who are willing to accept the TRM risks.

30.12 Maintenance Therapy

Maintenance therapy is the standard of care for patients receiving ASCT or no ASCT. Lenalidomide has been shown to improve both PFS and OS and is initiated post 8–12 cycles of triplet therapy in patients unfit for ASCT and post ASCT in fit patients. The maintenance therapy is commonly given till relapse. However, time-limited lenalidomide maintenance for 2 years is also used as an alternative. Further studies are ongoing to determine the exact benefits of long-term lenalidomide maintenance, as there is a 2–three-fold risk of second cancers. In patients not tolerating lenalidomide or with severe renal dysfunction, bortezomib maintenance given every alternate week is the standard of care. In patients with del 17(p), bortezomib maintenance may improve OS. In patients with high-risk MM, two-drug maintenance with bortezomib and lenalidomide is the preferred regimen given till relapse. The role of daratumumab in patients who received it as part of upfront therapy is unclear, and its combination with lenalidomide maintenance is not routinely recommended at present [9].

30.13 Supportive Therapy

Bisphosphonates, which suppress the osteoclastic activity and improve bone health, are indicated in all patients with MM. Zoledronic acid and pamidronate are the most commonly used. Zoledronic acid is administered in a 4 mg IV monthly schedule; however, a 3–4 monthly schedule may provide equal benefit with reduced side effects. In patients with significant renal dysfunction, Denosumab, a monoclonal antibody RANKL inhibitor, is the preferred agent to inhibit osteoclastic activity.

Prevention of infections is a cornerstone in the management of MM. Prophylactic Levofloxacin in the first 3–4 months of therapy may reduce the incidence of infections. Prophylaxis against herpes with daily oral acyclovir and pneumocystic jeroveci with cotrimoxazole is routinely used. IVIg prophylaxis in patients with hypogammaglobulinemia and recurrent infections may be considered [11].

30.14 Treatment of Relapsed Multiple Myeloma

MM is an incurable hematological malignancy, and relapse is the norm. Initiation of therapy at first and subsequent relapse are determined by the timing of relapse, response to prior therapy, aggressiveness of the relapse, and performance status. Choice of therapy is largely determined by the likely resistance to lenalidomide and daratumumab and the use of prior ASCT. As most of the patients are likely to have been treated upfront with a triplet therapy (like VRd, VCd, VTd) OR a daratumumab-containing regimen followed by lenalidomide or other maintenance therapy, it is important to determine the likelihood of Bortezomib/lenalidomide/daratumumab resistance. The relapse regimen should consist of a triplet regimen with at least two new drugs to which the disease is likely to be sensitive [8].

The drugs available for use at first relapse consist of carfilzomib, daratumumab, and Pomalidomide. The daratumumab regimens used are DVd, DPd, DRd, and DKd. Carfilzomib is a novel keto-epoxide tetrapeptide proteasome inhibitor that is effective even in bortezomib-refractory patients. In comparison to Bortezomib, the neurotoxicity is less but it can have severe cardiac side effects in some patients (5%).

Pomalidomide is an analogue of lenalidomide, which has activity in patients refractory to lenalidomide.

The other drugs available in MM include elotuzumab, isatuximab, selinexor, and ixazomib. These drugs are not currently available in India and many other countries. Elotuzumab is a monoclonal antibody targeting the signaling lymphocytic activation molecule F7 (SLAMF7). It is active in combination with pomalidomide as an EPd regimen. Ixazomib is an oral proteasome inhibitor with once-weekly oral administration active in newly diagnosed as well as relapsed and refractory settings. It is approved for use as an IRd combination regimen. Selinexor blocks exportin 1(XPO1), leading to inhibition of NFkB. In combination regimen as SVd, it has shown improved PFS in comparison to Vd. Isatuximab is a monoclonal antibody targeting the CD38 antigen. In the combination regimen, as Isa-PD, it has shown better PFS in comparison to PD. Also, Isa-Kd has shown comparable efficacy to DKd in trials [10].

30.15 Chimeric Antigen Receptor-T (CAR-T) Cell Therapy

Chimeric antigen receptor therapy is a new immunotherapy option for patients with MM. The antigen foremost to be targeted in MM is B cell maturation antigen (BCMA). BCMA, a tumor necrosis factor receptor superfamily member 17 (TNFRSF17), is preferentially expressed on plasma cells but not on CD34+ hematopoietic stem cells, making it a promising antigenic target. Currently, 02 CART products targeted against BCMA have been approved by the US FDA and include Idecabtagene vicleucel (Ide-cel) and ciltacabtagene autoleucel (cilta-cel). Ide-cel has an ORR of 73% with a CR rate of 33% in relapse-refractory multiple myeloma (RRMM) patients. Cilta-cel has shown an ORR of 97% and a sCR rate of 67% in RRMM. Ide-cel was studied in the KarMMa trial, while the pivotal trial that studied Cilta-cel was CARTITUDE-1. Cytokine release syndrome is the most common adverse effect of both products. In addition, ICANS/neurotoxicity is also seen. The high cost of these therapies is a major impediment to their availability for patients with RRMM [7].

The other potential targets for CART in MM, which are currently being studied, include SLAMF7, CD38, NKGD2, GPRC5D, and Kappa (k) light chain.

30.16 Bispecific Antibodies

Bispecific antibodies are dual antigen targeting constructs that engage the T cells to plasma cells through various target antigens like B-cell membrane antigen (BCMA), G-protein-coupled receptor family C group 5 member D (GPRC5D), and Fc receptor-homolog 5 (FcRH5). BiTEs (Bispecific T cell engagers) are engineered constructs of two single-chain variable fragments (ScFv) that act as a dual-targeting molecule. This immunological synapse causes T-cell activation and degranulation, which causes MM cell wall perforation, leading to apoptosis through perforin and granzyme B. These agents have proven to induce deep and durable responses in heavily pre-treated myeloma patients with a predictable safety profile and the ease of off-the-shelf availability [6].

Two BCMA-targeting bispecific antibodies, teclistamab and elranatamab, have been approved for use in patients with relapsed myeloma in patients who have received at least four prior regimens. Teclistamab was approved based on the MajesTEC-1 trial. Erlanatamab was approved following the MagnetisMM-3 trial.

Talquetamab is a bispecific antibody that targets GPRC5D and can hence be valuable even in patients who have been previously treated with BCMA-directed therapy. It has been approved for use following the MonumenTAL-1 study.

Cytokine release syndrome, neurotoxicity, infections, and cytopenias are the most important adverse effects of bispecific antibodies [1, 5].

30.17 Other Drugs

Venetoclax, a Bcl-2 inhibitor, has single-agent activity specifically in patients with t(11;14) subtype of multiple myeloma. However, it is not yet approved for use in MM as a higher mortality was seen with this drug despite deeper responses and better PFS.

Belantamab Mafodotin is a humanized anti-BCMA antibody that is conjugated to monomethyl auristatin-F, a microtubule-disrupting agent. In a phase II trial, it showed a response in 33% patients who had failed at least 3 previous lines of therapy. However, the drug was withdrawn from the market due to a very high incidence of Keratopathy (25%) in the treated patient population [5, 8].

30.18 Conclusion

The diagnostic workup and management of multiple myeloma have seen rapid advances over the last decade, which have significantly improved the survival of patients and their quality of life. ASCT continues to have a place in the management of the disease despite the introduction of newer drugs. The risk-stratified management algorithm in parallel with frailty scores has helped intensify therapy in a significant subset, leading to better outcomes. Myeloma remains an incurable disease, and with multiple new lines of drugs being available and many in the pipeline, it is a challenge to sequence the drugs in a given patient to achieve optimum outcomes in the various risk subgroups. BiTEs and CART cell therapy are already changing the landscape of previously untreatable relapse-refractory disease patients who had received multiple lines of therapy.

References

1. Rajkumar SV. Multiple myeloma: 2024 update on diagnosis, risk-stratification, and management. Am J Hematol. 2024;99(9):1802–24. https://doi.org/10.1002/ajh.27422. Epub 2024 Jun 28. PMID: 38943315; PMCID: PMC11404783
2. Veryaskina YA, Titov SE, Skvortsova NV, Kovynev IB, Antonenko OV, Demakov SA, Demenkov PS, Pospelova TI, Ivanov MK, Zhimulev IF. Multiple myeloma: genetic

and epigenetic biomarkers with clinical potential. Int J Mol Sci. 2024;25:13404. https://doi.org/10.3390/ijms252413404.
3. Szalat R, Anderson K, Munshi N. Role of minimal residual disease assessment in multiple myeloma. Haematologica. 2024;109(7):2049–59. https://doi.org/10.3324/haematol.2023.284662. PMID: 38328864; PMCID: PMC11215375
4. Mejia Saldarriaga M, Darwiche W, Jayabalan D, Monge J, Rosenbaum C, Pearse RN, Niesvizky R, Bustoros M. Advances in the molecular characterization of multiple myeloma and mechanism of therapeutic resistance. Front Oncol. 2022;12:1020011. https://doi.org/10.3389/fonc.2022.1020011. PMID: 36387095; PMCID: PMC9646612
5. Rajkumar SV, Kumar S. Multiple myeloma current treatment algorithms. Blood Cancer J. 2020;10:94.
6. Devasia AJ, Chari A, Lancman G. Bispecific antibodies in the treatment of multiple myeloma. Blood Cancer J. 2024;14:158. https://doi.org/10.1038/s41408-024-01139-y.
7. Sheykhhasan M, Ahmadieh-Yazdi A, Vicidomini R, et al. CAR T therapies in multiple myeloma: unleashing the future. Cancer Gene Ther. 2024;31:667–86. https://doi.org/10.1038/s41417-024-00750-2.
8. Dimopoulos MA, Moreau P, Terpos E, et al. Multiple myeloma: EHA-ESMO Clinical Practice Guidelines for diagnosis, treatment and follow-up. Ann Oncol. 2021;32(3):309–22. https://doi.org/10.1016/j.annonc.2020.11.014.
9. Kumar SK, Callander NS, Adekola K, et al. Multiple Myeloma, Version 2.2024. JNCCN. 2023;21(12):1281–301.
10. Costa LJ, Banerjee R, Mian H, et al. international myeloma working group immunotherapy committee recommendation on sequencing immunotherapy for treatment of multiple myeloma. Leukemia. https://doi.org/10.1038/s41375-024-02482-6.
11. Geraldes C, Roque A, Sarmento-Ribeiro AB, et al. Practical management of disease-related manifestations and drug toxicities in patients with multiple myeloma. Front. Oncol. 14:1282300. https://doi.org/10.3389/fonc.2024.1282300.
12. Möller M-D, Gengenbach L, Graziani G, et al. Geriatric assessments and frailty scores in multiple myeloma patients: a needed tool for individualized treatment. Curr Opin Oncol. 2021;33:648–57.

Part V
Myeloid Malignancies

Chapter 31
Who-HEM5 and ICC(2022) Classifications for Myeloid Neoplasms

Sanjeev Kumar Gupta and Gadha Krishna Leons

Abstract The latest 5th edition of the World Health Organization classification of hematolymphoid neoplasms (WHO-HEM5) (2022) and the International Consensus Classification (ICC) (2022) of myeloid neoplasms provide the basic framework and guidance for sub-classification of various myeloid proliferations and neoplasms. The updated biological information defined by the underlying genetic abnormalities has been given due consideration in the current classifications of myeloid neoplasms. Although the broad underlying principles of the WHO-HEM5 and ICC classifications of myeloid neoplasms are similar, however, there are minor differences. So, in addition to enumerating the WHO-HEM5 and ICC sub-classes of myeloid neoplasms, the key differences of these classifications have been highlighted in this chapter. The differences leading to the diagnostic challenges have also been highlighted with the help of a few clinical scenarios, particularly for acute myeloid leukemia (AML) and myelodysplastic neoplasms (MDS).

Keywords WHO-HEM5 classification · ICC classification. Myeloid neoplasm · Acute myeloid leukemia (AML) · Myelodysplastic neoplasm (MDS) · Myelodysplastic syndrome (MDS) · Myeloproliferative neoplasm (MPN)

S. K. Gupta (✉) · G. K. Leons
Laboratory Oncology, Dr BRA IRCH, All India Institute of Medical Sciences (AIIMS), New Delhi, India

H. P. Pati et al. (eds.), *Clinical Hematology and Hemato-Oncology*,
https://doi.org/10.1007/978-981-92-1167-8_31

Learning Objectives:
- To know the 5th edition of World Health Organization classification of myeloid neoplasms (WHO-HEM5)
- To know the latest International Consensus Classification (ICC) of myeloid neoplasms
- To understand the key differences in the WHO-HEM5 and ICC classification of myeloid neoplasms.
- To understand the diagnostic challenges due to the variations in the WHO-HEM5 and ICC classification of myeloid neoplasms through clinical scenarios.

31.1 Introduction

Myeloid neoplasms are a diverse group of clonal hematopoietic disorders distinguished by the proliferation and accumulation of abnormal myeloid cells in the bone marrow, blood, and other tissues. These disorders encompass a wide spectrum of diseases, including acute myeloid leukemia (AML), myelodysplastic neoplasm (MDS) (myelodysplastic syndrome according to ICC), myeloproliferative neoplasm (MPN), and overlap syndrome such as MDS/MPN, among others. Accurate classification of myeloid neoplasms is essential for diagnosis, treatment planning, and prognosis. In addition, it facilitates research by enabling consistent disease definitions and comparison across studies. Two major classification systems are being used for this purpose: the World Health Organization Classification (5th edition, WHO-HEM5) (2022) [1] and the International Consensus Classification (ICC) (2022) [2] of myeloid neoplasms.

The dominant biological attributes defined by the underlying cytogenetic and molecular aberrations have been updated in the current classifications of myeloid neoplasms. This was guided by a relatively better understanding of the biology of myeloid neoplasms and also necessitated by the advances in the field of high-throughput sequencing techniques and adoption of many targeted therapies based on the genetic aberrations in the current era of individualized therapy. Although the broad underlying principles of the WHO-HEM5 and ICC classifications of myeloid neoplasms are similar, however, they sometimes diverge in terms of diagnostic criteria, sub-classification, blast criteria, and specific genomic alteration integration. So, in addition to enumerating the WHO-HEM5 and ICC sub-classes of myeloid neoplasms, the key differences of these classifications have been highlighted in this chapter. The differences leading to the diagnostic challenges have also been highlighted with the help of clinical scenarios, particularly for AML and MDS. Figure 31.1 provides a schematic diagram of representative myeloid neoplasms, their inter-relationship and a brief overview of their key clinicopathological features.

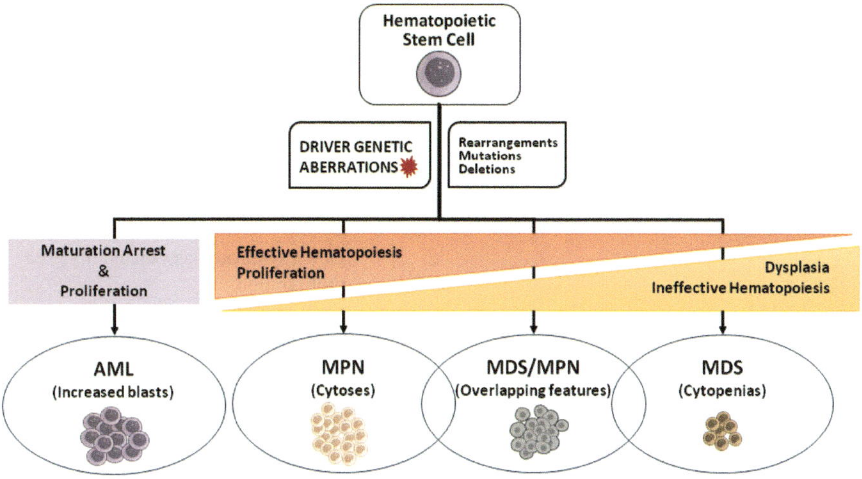

Fig. 31.1 Schematic diagram showing key features of representative myeloid neoplasms and their inter-relationship

Table 31.1 Categories of myeloid neoplasms as per WHO-HEM5

Myeloid precursor lesions (clonal hematopoiesis)
Myeloproliferative neoplasms (MPN)
Mastocytosis
Myelodysplastic neoplasms (MDS)
Myelodysplastic/myeloproliferative neoplasms (MDS/MPN)
Acute myeloid leukemia (AML)
Secondary myeloid neoplasms (MN post cytotoxic therapy; MN associated with germline predisposition; MN associated with down syndrome)
Myeloid/lymphoid neoplasms (M/L neoplasms with eosinophilia and tyrosine kinase gene fusions; acute leukemias of mixed lineage)

31.1.1 World Health Organization (WHO-HEM5) Classification of Myeloid Neoplasms

The WHO-HEM5 classification system is a globally recognized framework for the diagnosis and classification of hematologic malignancies, including myeloid neoplasms. The WHO-HEM5 system emphasizes a multidisciplinary approach, combining morphology, immunophenotyping, cytogenetics, molecular genetics, and clinical data to classify myeloid neoplasms. The most recent edition, WHO-HEM5, updated in 2022, incorporates advances in molecular genetics and morphology to further refine diagnostic criteria, improve disease categorization, predict disease behavior, and guide therapy, e.g., the specific genetic alterations, such as mutations in FLT3, NPM1, CEBPA, etc., define distinct subtypes of AML. Table 31.1 lists the categories of myeloid neoplasms as per WHO-HEM5

Table 31.2 Categories of myeloid neoplasms as per ICC

Myeloproliferative neoplasms (MPN)
Mastocytosis
Myelodysplastic/myeloproliferative Neoplasms (MDS/MPN)
Myelodysplastic syndromes (MDS) and premalignant clonal cytopenias
Acute myeloid leukemia (AML)
Pediatric and/ or germline disorders
Down syndrome-associated myeloid proliferation
Myeloid or lymphoid neoplasms with tyrosine kinase gene fusions and eosinophilia
Acute leukemia of ambiguous lineage
Blastic plasmacytoid dendritic cell neoplasm

31.1.2 International Consensus Classification (ICC) of Myeloid Neoplasms

The ICC is a complementary classification system developed by an international panel of experts. The ICC recommends integrating the morphological, clinical, and genomic data for classification and aims to provide a more precise and clinically relevant framework for diagnosing myeloid neoplasms. Similar to WHO-HEM5, there is a categorization of disease categories to better reflect their biology and clinical behavior. Table 31.2 lists the categories of myeloid neoplasms as per ICC.

31.1.3 Comparison of WHO-HEM5 and ICC Classifications

While both the WHO-HEM5 and ICC classifications aim to provide a comprehensive framework for classification of myeloid neoplasms with integration of morphological, clinical and genomic findings, there are minor differences between the two system, pertaining to the diagnostic criteria, nomenclature and disease sub--categories. The similarities and differences in the individual classes of myeloid neoplasms, as per the WHO-HEM5 and ICC classifications, have been examined in the following sections [3, 4].

31.2 Myeloid Precursor Lesions (Clonal Hematopoiesis)

Clonal hematopoiesis may occur as a common age-dependent occurrence in healthy people without a diagnosed hematological disorder. The latest classifications have incorporated the categories of clonal hematopoiesis including premalignant conditions like clonal hematopoiesis of indeterminate potential (CHIP) and clonal cytopenia of undetermined significance (CCUS). The definitions of various conditions relevant to clonal hematopoiesis are provided below.

- *Clonal hematopoiesis (CH)*: Clonal hematopoiesis is a clonal growth of hematopoietic cells from affected progenitor cells, irrespective of the underlying cause.
- *Age-related clonal hematopoiesis (ARCH)*: Clonal hematopoiesis associated with ageing in absence of any diagnosed hematological disorder or cytopenia. It may be detected in peripheral blood (PB) or bone marrow (BM) and does not refer to specific gene alterations or quantitative criteria reflecting clonal abundance.
- *Clonal hematopoiesis of indeterminate potential (CHIP)*: Clonal hematopoiesis with detection of leukemia-related gene variants at ≥2% allelic burden without clinical hematological disease manifestations or persistent cytopenias.
- *Clonal cytopenia of undetermined significance (CCUS)*: Identification of clonal hematopoiesis alongside sustained, unexplained cytopenia(s) that fail to fulfill diagnostic thresholds for established myeloid malignancies.
- *Idiopathic cytopenia of unknown significance (ICUS)*: Persistent and unexplained cytopenia without detectable hematological malignancy-associated driver mutations.
- *VEXAS syndrome*: is a hematopoiesis-derived inflammatory disorder stemming from acquired mutations in the X-linked UBA1 gene, characterized by progressive multi-system autoinflammation affecting cutaneous, pulmonary, vascular, musculoskeletal, and cartilaginous tissues, frequently accompanied by hematological abnormalities including cytopenias.

31.3 Myeloproliferative Neoplasms (MPNs)

Myeloproliferative neoplasms (MPNs) are characterized by excessive production of mature white blood cells, erythrocytes, and/or platelets. The main disease subtypes remain unchanged from the prior edition of WHO classification and includes chronic myeloid leukemia (CML), polycythemia vera (PV), essential thrombocythemia (ET), and primary myelofibrosis (PMF) (Table 31.3).

Table 31.3 Myeloproliferative neoplasms (MPN) in WHO-HEM5 and ICC

MPN (WHO-HEM5)	MPN (ICC)
Chronic myeloid leukemia	Chronic myeloid leukemia
Polycythemia vera	Polycythemia vera
Essential thrombocythemia	Essential thrombocythemia
Primary myelofibrosis	Primary myelofibrosis
Chronic neutrophilic leukemia	Chronic neutrophilic leukemia
Chronic eosinophilic leukemia	Chronic eosinophilic leukemia, NOS
Juvenile myelomonocytic leukemia	–
MPN, NOS	MPN, unclassifiable

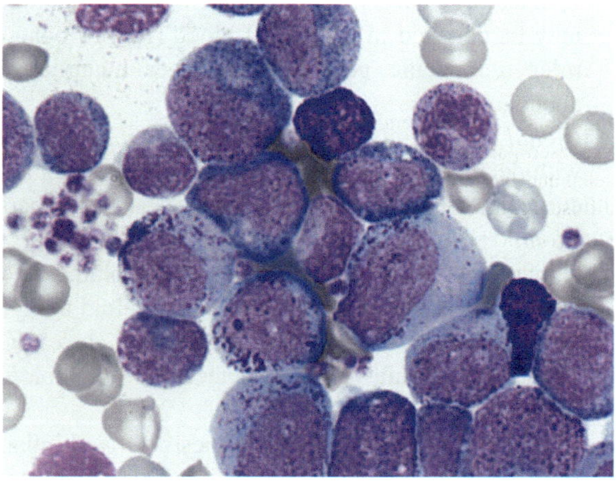

Fig. 31.2 Peripheral blood smear microphotograph in chronic myeloid leukemia, chronic phase showing neutrophilic granulocytosis in all stages of maturation and basophils

31.3.1 Chronic Myeloid Leukemia (CML)

CML is an MPN characterized by BCR::ABL1 fusion and neutrophilic granulocytosis in all stages of maturation (Fig. 31.2). The ICC retains the three, pre-TKI era, disease phases of CML, i.e., chronic, accelerated and blast phases, but the WHO-HEM5 has omitted the "accelerated phase" and consolidated the disease into two phases- chronic and blast, highlighting the chronic phase risk features (Table 31.4).

.

31.3.2 Polycythemia Vera (PV)

PV is an MPN marked by erythrocytosis, often with leukocytosis and/or thrombocytosis, and typically in association with JAK2 mutations. The latest WHO classification has eliminated red blood cell (RBC) mass as a major criterion for diagnosis

Table 31.4 Chronic myeloid leukemia (CML) accelerated phase and blast phase diagnostic criteria

	CML (WHO-HEM5)	CML (ICC)
Accelerated phase	Omitted	Blasts 10% to 19% 20% or more basophils in blood Additional clonal cytogenetic abnormality in Ph + cells (second Ph chromosome, trisomy 8, isochromosome 17q, trisomy 19, 3q abnormalities, complex karyotype)
Blast phase	20% or more myeloid blasts, or Extramedullary blast proliferation, or Lymphoblasts, even when <10%	20% or more blasts Myeloid sarcoma To consider lymphoblastic crisis if >5% lymphoblasts (>5%) present

Table 31.5 Polycythemia vera (PV) diagnostic criteria

PV (WHO-HEM5)	PV (ICC)
Major criteria	*Major criteria*
1. Increased hemoglobin (Hb) (> 16.5 g/dL in males, > 16.0 g/dL in females) or raised hematocrit (> 49% in males (>52% in absence of JAK2 mutation), > 48% in females) 2. Hypercellular bone marrow biopsy with tri-lineage proliferation of erythroid cells, granulocytes, and mature megakaryocytes 3. JAK2 V617F or exon 12 mutation	1. Increased Hb or hematocrit (HCT) or red blood cell (RBC) mass (>16.5 g/dL in males and > 16.0 g/dL in females; HCT: >49% in males and > 48% in females; RBC mass: >25% increment) 2. JAK2 V617F or exon 12 mutation 3. Hypercellular bone marrow biopsy with tri-lineage proliferation of erythroid cells, granulocytes, and mature megakaryocytes without atypia
Minor criterion	*Minor criterion*
Reduced erythropoietin (EPO)	Reduced erythropoietin (EPO)
All three major or first two major and minor criteria[a] *needed for PV diagnosis*	*All three major or first two major and minor criteria*[a] *needed for PV diagnosis*

[a]BM biopsy is not required if there is persistent erythrocytosis (Hb >18.5 g/dL in males or > 16.5 g/dL in females and HCT >55.5% in males or > 49.5% in females) and the presence of a JAK2 V617F or exon 12 mutation with the presence of a minor criterion

because RBC mass is an uncommon investigation in current clinical practice. ICC recommends more sensitive JAK2 V617F tests with <1% sensitivity and testing for non-canonical or uncommon JAK2 mutations in exons 12 to 15 in cases negative for JAK2 V617F. The rest of the diagnostic criteria for PV are almost similar as per WHO-HEM5 and ICC (Table 31.5).

Table 31.6 Essential thrombocythemia (ET) diagnostic criteria

ET (WHO-HEM5)	ET (ICC)
Major criteria	*Major criteria*
Platelet count >/= 450 × 10^9/L Bone marrow with proliferation of large, mature megakaryocytes and hyperlobulation of nuclei without significant increase in neutrophils or erythroid cells; in the absence of or minor (grade 1) increase in marrow reticulin Diagnostic criteria not met for other MPNs Mutations in JAK2, CALR, or MPL	Platelet count >/= 450 × 10^9/L Bone marrow with proliferation of large, mature megakaryocytes and hyperlobulation of nuclei without significant increase in neutrophils or erythroid cells; no relevant BM fibrosis. Diagnostic criteria not met for other MPNs Mutations in JAK2, CALR, or MPL
Minor criteria	*Minor criteria*
Clonal marker present OR Reactive thrombocytosis excluded	Clonal marker present OR Reactive thrombocytosis excluded
ET diagnosis requires all major or the first three major plus the minor criteria	*ET diagnosis requires all major or the first three major plus the minor criteria*

31.3.3 Essential Thrombocythemia (ET)

ET is an MPN marked by a persistent unexplained increase in platelet count with normocellular marrow showing increased large, mature megakaryocytes. ICC recommends sensitive assays for JAK2 V617F (<1% sensitivity) and CALR and MPL (1–3% sensitivity), and to consider testing for non-canonical JAK2 and MPL mutations in negative cases. The diagnostic criteria for ET are almost similar as per WHO-HEM5 and ICC (Table 31.6).

31.3.4 Primary Myelofibrosis (PMF)

PMF is an MPN marked by the proliferation of megakaryocytes and granulocytes along with marrow fibrosis, bone sclerosis, and extramedullary hematopoiesis. There are prefibrotic and fibrotic stages of PMF. There is atypia in the megakaryocytes with small to giant forms showing maturation defects like cloud-like nuclei, hypolobulation, and hyperchromasia of nuclei, and abnormal dense clustering of megakaryocytes. For the driver mutation analysis, ICC recommends sensitive assays for JAK2 V617F (<1% sensitivity) and CALR and MPL (1–3% sensitivity) and testing for non-canonical JAK2 and MPL mutations in negative cases. The diagnostic criteria are almost similar for prefibrotic PMF (Table 31.7) and fibrotic PMF (Table 31.8) as per WHO-HEM5 and ICC. Both WHO-HEM5 and ICC recommend the detection of mutations associated with myeloid neoplasms (e.g., ASXL1, EZH2, TET2, IDH1, SRSF2, IDH2, SF3B1 mutations) to determine the clonality of the disease in the absence of the three major clonal mutations.

Table 31.7 Diagnostic criteria for primary myelofibrosis (PMF), prefibrotic

PMF, prefibrotic (WHO-HEM5)	PMF, early/prefibrotic stage (pre-PMF) (ICC)
Major criteria	*Major criteria*
Hypercellular marrow with megakaryocytic proliferation and atypia, minimal fibrosis (up to grade 1), proliferation of granulocytes, and often a reduction in erythropoiesis Diagnostic criteria not met for other MPNs Mutation in JAK2, CALR, MPL, or another clonal marker or exclusion of reactive marrow fibrosis	Hypercellular marrow with megakaryocytic proliferation and atypia, minimal fibrosis (up to grade 1), proliferation of granulocytes, and often a reduction in erythropoiesis Diagnostic criteria not met for other MPNs Mutation in JAK2, CALR, MPL, or another clonal marker or exclusion of reactive marrow fibrosis
Minor criteria	*Minor criteria*
Anemia not due to any other cause Leukocytosis (at least 11 × 10^9/L) Palpable splenomegaly or detected by imaging Increased LDH	Anemia not due to any other cause Leukocytosis (at least 11 × 10^9/L) Palpable splenomegaly or detected by imaging Increased LDH
Prefibrotic PMF diagnosis requires all three major criteria and at least one minor criterion in two consecutive observations.	*Prefibrotic PMF diagnosis requires all three major criteria and at least one minor criterion in two consecutive observations.*

Table 31.8 Diagnostic criteria for primary myelofibrosis (PMF), fibrotic stage

PMF, fibrotic stage (WHO-HEM5)	PMF, overt fibrotic stage (ICC)
Major criteria	*Major criteria*
Megakaryocytic atypia with proliferation and reticulin and/or collagen fibrosis grade 2 or 3 Diagnostic criteria not met for other MPNs Mutation in JAK2, CALR, MPL, or another clonal marker or exclusion of reactive marrow fibrosis	Megakaryocytic atypia with proliferation and reticulin and/or collagen fibrosis grade 2 or 3 Diagnostic criteria not met for other MPNs Mutation in JAK2, CALR, MPL, or another clonal marker or exclusion of reactive marrow fibrosis
Minor criteria	*Minor criteria*
Anemia not due to any other cause Leukocytosis (at least 11 × 10^9/L) Palpable splenomegaly or detected by imaging Increased LDH Leukoerythroblastosis	Anemia not due to any other cause Leukocytosis (at least 11 × 10^9/L) Palpable splenomegaly or detected by imaging Increased LDH Leukoerythroblastosis
Overt PMF diagnosis requires all three major criteria and at least one minor criterion in two consecutive observations	*Overt PMF diagnosis requires all three major criteria and at least one minor criterion in two consecutive observations*

31.3.5 Chronic Neutrophilic Leukemia (CNL)

CNL is an MPN marked by persistent neutrophilia with CSF3R mutations in majority of cases, in absence of dysplasia or BCR::ABL1 fusion. The minimum leukocyte count requirements are 25 × 10^9/L per WHO-HEM5 and 13 × 10^9/L per ICC criteria of CNL (Table 31.9).

Table 31.9 Diagnostic criteria for chronic neutrophilic leukemia (CNL)

CNL (WHO-HEM5)	CNL (ICC)
Leukocytosis (at least 25 × 10^9/L) 80% or more segmented neutrophils plus bands; <10% Neutrophil precursors; < 10% monocytes not meeting criteria for CMML; absence of dysgranulopoiesis	Leukocytosis (at least 13 × 10^9/L; at least 25 × 10^9/L in cases lacking CSF3R mutation) 80% or more segmented neutrophils plus bands; <10% Neutrophil precursors; < 10% monocytes; absence of dysgranulopoiesis
Hypercellular marrow with increase in neutrophils with normal maturation; blasts <5%	Hypercellular marrow with an increase in neutrophils with normal maturation
Reactive neutrophilia excluded and diagnostic criteria of other MPN not met; Absence of PDGFRA, PDGFRB, FGFR1 rearrangement, and no PCM1::JAK2 fusion	Diagnostic criteria of other MPN not met
CSF3R T618l or other CSF3R mutation, OR, Persistent neutrophilia (for at least 3 months), splenomegaly, and exclusion of reactive neutrophilia; to demonstrate clonality of myeloid cells if a plasma cell neoplasm is present	CSF3R T618I or other CSF3R mutation or persistent neutrophilia (for at least 3 months), splenomegaly, and exclusion of reactive neutrophilia; to demonstrate clonality of myeloid cells if a plasma cell neoplasm is present

Table 31.10 Diagnostic criteria for chronic eosinophilic leukemia (CEL)

CEL (WHO-HEM5)	CEL, not otherwise specified (ICC)
Hypereosinophilia, with more than 1.5 × 10^9/L eosinophils on at least two occasions over 4 weeks; evidence of clonality; abnormal BM morphology; diagnostic criteria for other myeloid or lymphoid neoplasms not met	1. Hypereosinophilia, with at least 1.5 × 10^9/L eosinophils and are at least 10% of WBCs 2. Blasts <20% & not meeting other diagnostic criteria for AML 3. No BCR::ABL1, PDGFRA, FGFR1, PDGFRB, JAK2 rearrangements 4. Criteria for other MPN; CMML, or systemic mastocytosis not met 5. Hypercellular marrow with dysplasia in megakaryocytes; often increased fibrosis with eosinophils or increased blasts (at least 5% in marrow and/or at least 2% in blood) 6. Clonal abnormality &/or somatic mutation(s) or, persistent eosinophilia with exclusion of reactive eosinophilia
	The diagnosis of CEL requires all 6 criteria.

31.3.6 Chronic Eosinophilic Leukemia (CEL)

CEL is an MPN marked by clonal proliferation of eosinophilic precursors causing persistent eosinophilia (Table 31.10).

31.3.7 Juvenile Myelomonocytic Leukemia (JMML)

JMML is an MPN of early childhood driven by RAS pathway activation, leading to increased granulocytes and monocytes, frequently with organ infiltration. WHO-HEM5 has included JMML as MPN, whereas ICC classifies it under the group of pediatric and/or germline mutation-associated disorders, with similar diagnostic criteria (Table 31.11).

31.3.8 Myeloproliferative Neoplasm (MPN) Not Otherwise Specified (NOS)

MPN, NOS (unclassifiable) in WHO-HEM5 and MPN-U in ICC includes cases having definite features of an MPN but fail to meet the diagnostic criteria for any of the specific types of MPN.

Table 31.11 Diagnostic criteria for juvenile myelomonocytic leukemia (JMML)

JMML (WHO-HEM5)	JMML (ICC)
Clinical, hematological, and laboratory criteria (all five criteria are required): Monocytosis (at least 1 × 10^9/L) Blasts and promonocytes <20% Organ infiltration, frequently splenomegaly Absence of BCR:: ABL1 Absence of KMT2A rearrangement *Genetic criteria (one criterion required):* RAS pathway mutation: Clonal PTPN11, KRAS, or NRAS mutation, or Clonal NF1 mutation, or Clonal CBL mutation Non-canonical clonal RAS pathway pathogenic alterations causing activation of ALK, PDGFRB, ROS1 genes *Other criteria:* At least two of the following criteria should be met in addition to the clinical, hematological, and laboratory criteria if the listed genetic criteria are not met or not evaluated HbF raised for age Myeloid and erythroid precursors in blood Platelets reduced with hypercellular marrow with or without dysplasia GM-CSF hypersensitivity	*Clinical and hematologic features* (the first 2 features are present in most cases; the last 2 are required) Monocytosis (at least 1 × 10^9/L) Splenomegaly Blasts <20% Absence of BCR::ABL1 *Genetic studies (1 finding required)* PTPN11 or KRAS or NRAS or RRAS mutation Germline mutation of NF1 or clinical NF1 Germline CBL mutation

Table 31.12 Subtypes of mastocytosis

Mastocytosis (WHO-HEM5)	Mastocytosis (ICC)
Cutaneous mastocytosis	*Cutaneous mastocytosis*
Urticaria pigmentosa/maculopapular cutaneous mastocytosis	Urticaria pigmentosa/maculopapular cutaneous mastocytosis
Diffuse cutaneous mastocytosis	Diffuse cutaneous mastocytosis
Cutaneous mastocytoma	Mastocytoma of skin
Systemic mastocytosis	*Systemic mastocytosis*
Bone marrow mastocytosis	Indolent systemic mastocytosis (includes BM mastocytosis)
Indolent systemic mastocytosis	Smoldering systemic mastocytosis
Smoldering systemic mastocytosis	Aggressive systemic mastocytosis
Aggressive systemic mastocytosis	Mast cell leukemia
Systemic mastocytosis with associated hematologic neoplasm (SM-AHN)	Systemic mastocytosis with associated myeloid neoplasm (SM-AMN)
Mast cell leukemia	*Mast cell sarcoma*
Mast cell sarcoma	
Extracutaneous mastocytoma	

31.4 Mastocytosis

Mastocytosis is a heterogeneous group of disorders characterized by the abnormal mast cells proliferation in various organs or tissues. KIT D816 mutation is found in more than 80% of systemic mastocytosis. This disease category includes cutaneous mastocytosis, systemic mastocytosis (SM), and mast cell sarcoma by WHO-HEM5 and ICC (Table 31.12). The "SM with an associated hematologic neoplasm" (SM-AHN) category in WHO-HEM5 is restricted to myeloid neoplasms and renamed as "SM with associated myeloid neoplasm" (SM-AMN) in ICC classification.

31.5 Myelodysplastic Neoplasms (MDS)

Myelodysplastic neoplasms (MDS) are clonal hematopoietic stem cell neoplasms, characterized by cytopenias and morphological dysplasia, and clinically marked by ineffective hematopoiesis and an increased AML risk. The WHO-HEM5 classification adopts the name myelodysplastic neoplasm in place of myelodysplastic syndrome (MDS) to emphasize the neoplastic nature of the disease; however, it retains the abbreviation MDS rather than MDN, due to the phonetic similarity and thus a likelihood of confusion of MDN with MPN. WHO-HEM5 subdivides the cases into genetically defined and morphologically defined groups and retains ≥15% ring sideroblasts as a substitute for SF3B1 mutation in MDS with low blasts. WHO-HEM5 omits the classes based solely on the morphological dysplasia involving one (single lineage dysplasia, SLD) or more (multilineage dysplasia, MLD) hematopoietic lineages; however, ICC retains these classes. In addition, ICC introduces the category of MDS/AML for 10–19% blasts in PB or BM (Table 31.13 and Fig. 31.3).

Table 31.13 Myelodysplastic neoplasms (MDS) subtypes

Myelodysplastic neoplasms (MDS) (WHO-HEM5)	Premalignant clonal cytopenias and myelodysplastic syndromes (MDS) (ICC)
MDS with defining genetic abnormalities MDS with low blasts and isolated 5q deletion[a] (MDS-5q) (blasts <5% in marrow and < 2% in blood) MDS with low blasts and SF3B1 mutation (MDS-SF3B1) (blasts <5% in marrow and < 2% in blood) MDS with biallelic TP53 inactivation (MDS-biTP53) (<20% blasts) *MDS, morphologically defined* MDS with low blasts (MDS-LB) (<5% BM and < 2% PB blasts) MDS, hypoplastic (</=25% age adjusted BM cellularity) (MDS-h) MDS with increased blasts (MDS-IB) MDS-IB1 (5–9% blasts in marrow or 2–4% in blood) MDS-IB2 (10–19% blasts in marrow or 5–19% in blood or Auer rods) MDS with fibrosis (MDS-f) (5–19% blasts in marrow; 2–19% in blood)	Clonal cytopenia of undetermined significance MDS with mutated SF3B1 (VAF at least 10%) MDS with del(5q) [alone, or with 1 additional abnormality except monosomy 7 or 7q deletion] MDS with mutated TP53 (VAF more than 10%) MDS, not otherwise specified (MDS, NOS) Without dysplasia With single lineage dysplasia With multilineage dysplasia MDS with excess blasts (5–9% BM, 2–9% PB blasts) MDS/acute myeloid leukemia (MDS/AML) (10–19% BM or PB blasts) MDS/AML with mutated TP53 MDS/AML with myelodysplasia-related gene mutations MDS/AML with myelodysplasia-related cytogenetic abnormalities MDS/AML, not otherwise specified
MDS of childhood Childhood MDS with low blasts (<5% blasts in marrow; <2% in blood) Hypocellular Not otherwise specified Childhood MDS with increased blasts (5–19% blasts in marrow; 2–19% in blood)	Refractory cytopenia of childhood (persistent cytopenias; dysplasia and blasts <5% blasts in marrow; <2% in blood)

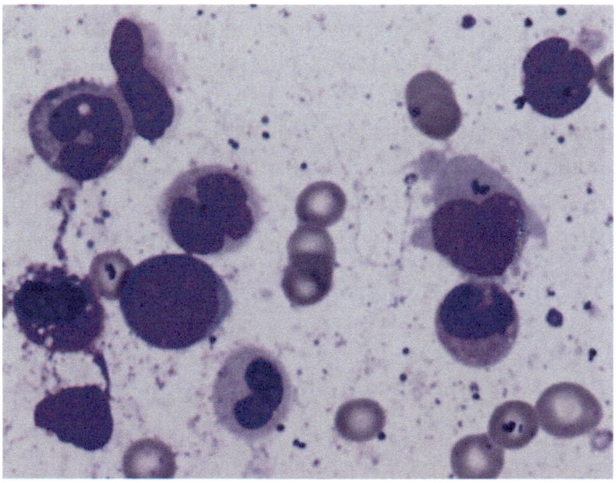

Fig. 31.3 Peripheral blood smear microphotograph in a case with myelodysplastic neoplasm (MDS), showing dysplastic granulocytes and increased blasts

Case Scenario

A 65-year-old male presented with fatigue and pallor for 3 years. His laboratory work-up revealed low hemoglobin (9.1 g/dL), low-normal platelets (120×10^9/L), and low white blood cells (3.5×10^9/L). PB smear showed dimorphic RBCs, and BM aspirate revealed mild dyserythropoiesis, ring sideroblasts (10% of erythroid precursors), and 4% blasts. The biochemical analysis, including B12 and folate levels, was normal.

Diagnosis considered before molecular analysis report: MDS with low blasts (MDS-LB) as per WHO-HEM5 and MDS, NOS with single lineage dysplasia (SLD) as per ICC

Molecular testing: Positive for SF3B1 mutation.

Final diagnosis according to WHO-HEM5: MDS with low blasts and SF3B1 mutation. (MDS-SF3B1)

Diagnosis according to ICC Classification: MDS with mutated SF3B1

Comment: While both systems recognize SF3B1 mutation as a defining genetic abnormality of MDS, associated with favorable prognosis and may warrant the use of luspatercept, however, they differ in that detection of 15% or more ring sideroblasts may substitute for SF3B1 mutation as per WHO-HEM5, however there is no such provision in the ICC classification.

31.6 Myelodysplastic/Myeloproliferative Neoplasms (MDS/MPN)

MDS/MPN is a category of myeloid neoplasms marked by overlapping criteria, pathological and molecular features of myelodysplastic neoplasms (MDS) and myeloproliferative neoplasms (MPN), with cytopenias as well as cytoses combinations. Atypical chronic myeloid leukemia in the ICC classification has been renamed as myelodysplastic/myeloproliferative neoplasm with neutrophilia in the WHO-HEM5 classification. ICC has also introduced a category of "Clonal monocytosis of undetermined significance" for the cases with persistent monocytosis and myeloid mutation(s), however, not meeting the criteria for CMML. Clonal cytopenia and monocytosis of undetermined significance have cytopenia in addition. In the ICC, MDS/MPN with isochromosome 17q has been added as a provisional subtype under MDS/MPN-NOS (Table 31.14).

31.6.1 Chronic Myelomonocytic Leukemia (CMML)

CMML is an MDS/MPN, marked by persistent monocytosis and mutations involving epigenetic regulation, signal transduction, and spliceosome genes (Table 31.15).

Table 31.14 Subtypes of myelodysplastic/myeloproliferative neoplasms (MDS/MPN)

MDS/MPN (WHO-HEM5)	MDS/MPN (ICC)
CMML	CMML
	Clonal cytopenia with monocytosis of undetermined significance
	Clonal monocytosis of undetermined significance
MDS/MPN with neutrophilia *(previously known as atypical chronic myeloid leukemia)*	Atypical chronic myeloid leukemia
MDS/MPN with SF3B1 mutation and thrombocytosis	MDS/MPN with thrombocytosis and SF3B1 mutation
	MDS/MPN with ring sideroblasts and thrombocytosis, not otherwise specified
MDS/MPN, NOS	MDS/MPN, NOS *New provisional entity: MDS/MPN with isolated isochromosome 17q*

Table 31.15 Diagnostic criteria of chronic myelomonocytic leukemia (CMML)

CMML (WHO-HEM5)	CMML (ICC)
Prerequisite criteria 1. Persistent monocytosis, with at least 0.5 × 10^9/L monocytes, which are at least 10% of WBCs. 2. Less than 20% blasts 3. Diagnostic criteria of CML or other MPNs not met. 4. Diagnostic criteria of myeloid/lymphoid neoplasms with tyrosine kinase fusions not met. *Supporting criteria* 1. Myelodysplasia 2. Acquired clonal genetic abnormality. 3. Abnormal monocyte subsets partitioning. *Requirements for diagnosis* All cases should have pre-requisite criteria. One or more supporting criteria must be met if monocytosis is 1 × 10^9/L or more. Supporting criteria 1 and 2 must be met if monocytosis is between 0.5 and 1 × 10^9/L. *Subtyping criteria* Myelodysplastic CMML (MD-CMML): WBC less than 13 × 10^9/L Myeloproliferative CMML (MP-CMML): WBC 13 × 10^9/L or more *Subgrouping criteria* (based on % of blasts and promonocytes) CMML-1: <5% in PB and < 10% in BM CMML-2: 5–19% in PB and 10–19% in BM	Monocytosis, with at least 0.5 × 10^9/L monocytes, which are at least 10% of WBCs Cytopenia Less than 20% blasts (including promonocytes) Clonal genetic marker and/or myeloid mutation with VAF =/>10% In the absence of clonality marker, monocytosis (at least 1.0 × 10^9/L and >10%), and increased blasts (including promonocytes) (>/=5% in BM and/or >/=2% in PB), or dysplasia, or abnormal immunophenotype suggestive of CMML needed for diagnosis. Hypercellular marrow with myeloid proliferation often with increased monocytes Absence of BCR::ABL1 or other disease--defining genetic abnormalities

31.6.2 Myelodysplastic/Myeloproliferative Neoplasm with Neutrophilia (MDS/MPN-N)

MDS/MPN-N, formerly known as atypical chronic myeloid leukemia (still the same in ICC), is a myeloid neoplasm with overlap of myelodysplastic and myeloproliferative features with persistent neutrophilia and left shift of neutrophils (Table 31.16).

31.7 Acute Myeloid Leukemia (AML)

The WHO-HEM5 and ICC systems updated their classifications of AML, with the addition of many AML-defining recurrent genetic categories. ICC has lowered the diagnostic blast threshold for AML with recurrent genetic abnormalities, e.g., RUNX1::RUNX1T1, to 10% blasts; however, according to the WHO-HEM5 classification, such cases are diagnosed irrespective of blast count. However, AML with BCR::ABL1 diagnosis needs 20% blasts as per both WHO-HEM5 and ICC. Another key feature of the ICC classification is the blurring of blast% boundaries between AML and MDS to recognize the biological continuity between these two entities and the introduction of a new category of MDS/AML for cases with 10–19% blasts (Table 31.17, Figs. 31.4 and 31.5).

Case Scenario

A 45-year-old female presented with fatigue, bruising, and recurrent infections for 4 months. Her laboratory work-up revealed low hemoglobin (8.5 g/dL), low platelets (50×10^9/L), and increased white blood cells (15×10^9/L). Peripheral blood smear showed 6% blasts and the BM aspirate revealed a hypercellular marrow with

Table 31.16 Diagnostic criteria of myelodysplastic/myeloproliferative neoplasm with neutrophilia (MDS/MPN-N)

Myelodysplastic/myeloproliferative neoplasm with neutrophilia (MDS/MPN-N) (WHO-HEM5)	Atypical chronic myeloid leukemia (aCML) (ICC)
Myeloid neoplasm with both myelodysplastic and myeloproliferative features with persistent neutrophilia and left shift of neutrophils	Leukocytosis (at least 13 × 10^9/L, with increased neutrophils and at least 10% neutrophilic precursors Cytopenia <20% blasts Dysgranulopoiesis Less than 10% monocytes Less than 10% eosinophils Hypercellular marrow with proliferation and dysplasia of granulocytes Absence of BCR::ABL1 or other disease--defining genetic abnormalities

Table 31.17 Classification of acute myeloid leukemia (AML)

Acute myeloid leukemia (AML) (WHO-HEM5)	AML (ICC)
AML with defining genetic abnormalities Acute promyelocytic leukemia with PML::RARA fusion AML with RUNX1::RUNX1T1 AML with CBFB::MYH11 AML with DEK::NUP214 AML with RBM15::MRTFA AML with BCR::ABL1 AML with KMT2A rearrangement AML with NUP98 rearrangement AML with MECOM rearrangement AML with CEBPA mutation AML with NPM1 mutation AML, myelodysplasia-related AML with other defined genetic alterations *Acute myeloid leukemia, defined by differentiation* AML with minimal differentiation AML without maturation AML with maturation Acute basophilic leukemia Acute myelomonocytic leukemia Acute monocytic leukemia Acute erythroid leukemia Acute megakaryoblastic leukemia Myeloid sarcoma	Acute promyelocytic leukemia (APL) with PML::RARA APL with other RARA rearrangements AML with RUNX1::RUNX1T1 AML with CBFB::MYH11 AML with MLLT3::KMT2A AML with other KMT2A rearrangements AML with DEK::NUP214 AML with GATA2; MECOM(EVI1) AML with other MECOM rearrangements AML with other rare recurring translocations AML with BCR::ABL1 AML with in-frame bZIP CEBPA mutations AML with mutated NPM1 AML and MDS/AML with mutated TP53 10–19% (MDS/AML) and >/= 20% (AML) AML and MDS/AML with myelodysplasia-related gene mutations 10–19% blasts (MDS/AML) and >/= 20% blasts (AML) (Characterized by mutations in ASXL1, RUNX1, BCOR, EZH2, SF3B1, SRSF2, U2AF1, STAG2, etc.) AML with myelodysplasia-related cytogenetic abnormalities 10–19% blasts (MDS/AML) and >/= 20% blasts (AML) (characterized by detecting a complex karyotype, del(5q), −7/del(7q), +8, del(12p), i(17q), del(20q), etc.) AML not otherwise specified (NOS) 10–19% blasts (MDS/AML) and >/= 20% blasts (AML) Myeloid sarcoma

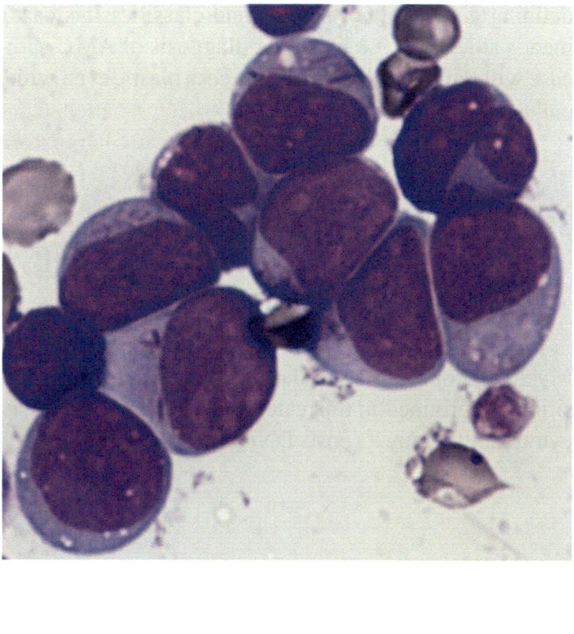

Fig. 31.4 Peripheral blood smear microphotograph in acute myeloid leukemia, showing myeloblasts with moderate cytoplasm, open chromatin with nucleoli, and some with Auer rods

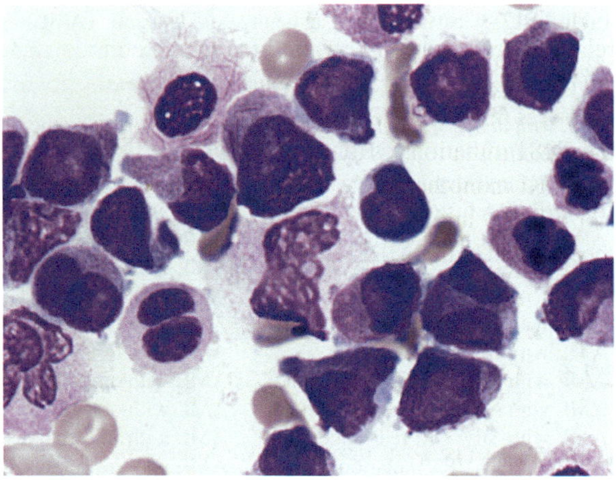

Fig. 31.5 Bone marrow smear microphotograph in acute promyelocytic leukemia, showing abnormal granular promyelocytes, some with bilobed nuclei, and Faggot cells with multiple Auer rods

dysmyelopoiesis and 8% blasts. On flow cytometry, these blasts were confirmed to be of myeloid lineage.

Diagnosis considered before molecular analysis report: MDS with increased blasts1 (MDS-IB1) as per WHO-HEM5 and MDS, with excess blasts as per ICC

Molecular testing: Positive for NPM1 mutation; negative for FLT3-ITD.

Final diagnosis according to WHO-HEM5: AML with NPM1 mutation. (subtype of AML with defining genetic abnormalities)

Diagnosis according to ICC Classification: MDS, with excess blasts

(At least ≥10% blasts required for diagnosis of AML with mutated NPM1 as per ICC)

Comment: While both systems recognize NPM1 mutation as a defining genetic abnormality and its association with favorable prognosis, however, they differ in that WHO-HEM5 does not have any minimum blast requirement for AML with defining genetic abnormalities and classifies this case as AML while ICC recommends at least ≥10% blasts for diagnosis of AML with mutated NPM1 and so, this case will remain as MDS, with excess blasts, even with NPM1 mutation being present, according to ICC.

31.8 Secondary Myeloid Neoplasms (Myeloid Neoplasms and Proliferations Associated with Antecedent or Predisposing Conditions)

Myeloid neoplasms secondary to cytotoxic therapy exposure or germline predisposition are grouped in this category per WHO-HEM5 as "Myeloid Neoplasms, post cytotoxic therapy" (post DNA-damaging therapy for an unrelated condition),

"Hematologic Neoplasms with Germline Predisposition" (arising in individuals with genetic conditions associated with increased risk of myeloid malignancies), and "Myeloid proliferation associated with Down Syndrome" (like transient abnormal myelopoiesis (TAM) and myeloid leukemia associated with Down syndrome (ML-DS)). The main subtypes of myeloid neoplasms with germline predisposition are listed in Table 31.18.

Table 31.18 Subtypes of myeloid neoplasms associated with germline predisposition

Myeloid neoplasms with germline predisposition (WHO-HEM5)	Hematologic neoplasms with germline predisposition (ICC)
Myeloid neoplasms with germline predisposition without a preexisting platelet disorder or organ dysfunction	*Hematologic neoplasms with germline predisposition without a constitutional disorder affecting multiple organ systems*
CEBPA variant	CEBPA mutation
DDX41 variant	DDX41 mutation
TP53 variant (li-Fraumeni syndrome)	TP53 mutation
Myeloid neoplasms with germline predisposition and pre-existing platelet disorder	*Hematologic neoplasms with germline predisposition*
RUNX1 variant	*Associated with a constitutional platelet disorder*
ANKRD26 variant	ANKRD26 mutation
ETV6 variant	RUNX1 mutation
Myeloid neoplasms with germline predisposition and potential organ dysfunction	ETV6 mutation
GATA2 variant	*Hematologic neoplasms with germline predisposition*
BM failure syndromes	*Associated with a constitutional disorder affecting multiple organ systems*
Severe congenital neutropenia	GATA2 mutation
Schwachman-diamond syndrome	SAMD9L mutation
Fanconi anemia	SAMD9 mutation
Telomere biology disorders	Myeloid neoplasms associated with BM failure syndromes
RASopathies (NF1, CBL syndrome, Noonan syndrome)	Fanconi anemia
Down syndrome	Diamond-Blackfan anemia
SAMD9 variant (MIRAGE syndrome)	Schwachman-diamond syndrome
SAMD9L variant (SAMD9L-related ataxia pancytopenia syndrome)	Severe congenital neutropenia
BLM variant (bloom syndrome)	Telomere biology disorders including dyskeratosis congenita
	JMML associated with neurofibromatosis
	JMML associated with Noonan-syndrome--like disorder (CBL-syndrome)
	Down syndrome
	ALL with germline predisposition
	PAX5 mutation
	IKZF1 mutation

31.9 Myeloid/Lymphoid Neoplasms

31.9.1 Myeloid/Lymphoid Neoplasms with Eosinophilia and Tyrosine Kinase Gene Fusions

This disease category includes myeloid and lymphoid neoplasms driven by rearrangements involving genes encoding tyrosine kinases leading to fusion products in which the kinase domain is constitutively activated, resulting in cell signaling dysregulation that promotes proliferation and survival. Myeloid/lymphoid neoplasms with eosinophilia and tyrosine kinase gene fusions subtypes are similar as per WHO-HEM5 and ICC (Table 31.19).

31.9.2 Acute Leukemias of Ambiguous Lineage

Acute leukemias of ambiguous lineage leukemias that do not show differentiation along a single lineage and may have a combination of myeloid and lymphoid components. These are classified based on the defining genetic abnormalities or immunophenotypically in the absence of a defining genetic lesion (Table 31.20).

Table 31.19 Myeloid/lymphoid neoplasms with eosinophilia and tyrosine kinase gene fusions (WHO-HEM5 and ICC)

Genetic abnormalities defining myeloid/lymphoid neoplasms with eosinophilia and tyrosine kinase gene fusions (WHO-HEM5 and ICC)
Myeloid/lymphoid (M/L) neoplasm with PDGFRA rearrangement
M/L neoplasm with PDGFRB rearrangement
M/L neoplasm with FGFR1 rearrangement
M/L neoplasm with JAK2 rearrangement
M/L neoplasm with FLT3 rearrangement
M/L neoplasm with ETV6::ABL1
Other defined tyrosine kinase fusions
ETV6::FGFR2; ETV6::LYN; ETV6::NTRK3; RANBP2::ALK; BCR::RET; FGFR1OP::RET

Table 31.20 Acute leukemias of ambiguous lineage

Acute leukemias of ambiguous lineage (WHO-HEM5)	Acute leukemias of ambiguous lineage (ICC)
Acute leukemia of ambiguous lineage (ALAL) with defining genetic abnormalities Mixed-phenotype acute leukemia (MPAL) with BCR::ABL1 MPAL with KMT2A rearrangement ALAL with other defined genetic alterations ZNF384 rearrangement BCL11B rearrangement *ALAL, immunophenotypically defined* MPAL, B/myeloid MPAL, T/myeloid MPAL, rare types ALAL, not otherwise specified Acute undifferentiated leukemia	Acute undifferentiated leukemia Mixed phenotype acute leukemia (MPAL) with BCR::ABL1 MPAL, with KMT2A rearrangement MPAL, B/myeloid, NOS MPAL, T/myeloid, NOS

31.10 Blastic Plasmacytoid Dendritic Cell Neoplasm (BPDCN)

Blastic plasmacytoid dendritic cell neoplasm (BPDCN) is a myeloid neoplasm in the ICC classification; however, it has been categorized under dendritic cell and histiocytic neoplasms in WHO-HEM5, which is a separate category from myeloid neoplasms.

31.11 Summary

The table given below summarizes the key differences between the WHO-HEM5 and ICC classification of myeloid neoplasms (Table 31.21).

To summarize, the WHO-HEM5 and ICC classifications of myeloid neoplasms represent evolving frameworks that reflect advances in molecular genetics, morphology, and clinical medicine. While the WHO-HEM5 classification remains the most widely accepted system globally in academic as well as clinical settings, the ICC offers a complementary approach that offers a more clinically relevant framework and stringent molecular testing advisory for actionable genetic information for certain disease entities. Both systems emphasize the importance of genetic and molecular data in defining disease entities, guiding treatment, and predicting outcomes. As our understanding of myeloid neoplasms continues to evolve, these classification systems will likely undergo further refinement to improve diagnostic accuracy and patient care.

Table 31.21 Summary of the key differences between WHO-HEM5 and ICC classification of myeloid neoplasms

Category	WHO-HEM5	ICC
Chronic myeloid leukemia	Accelerated phase not recognized	Accelerated phase is recognized
Polycythemia Vera	Red cell mass eliminated as a major criterion	Red cell mass still included as a major criterion Sensitive assays for JAK2 V617F and to consider non-canonical or atypical JAK2 mutations in negative cases
Essential thrombocythemia and primary myelofibrosis	No specific recommendation	Sensitive assays for JAK2 V617F and CALR and MPL and to consider non-canonical JAK2 and MPL mutations in negative cases
Chronic neutrophilic leukemia	The minimum blood WBC count required for diagnosis is 25 × 10^9/L	The minimum blood WBC count required for diagnosis is 13 × 10^9/L
Juvenile myelomonocytic leukemia	Classified as myeloproliferative neoplasm	Classified under pediatric and/or germline mutation-associated disorders
Myelodysplastic neoplasms	Removed SLD and MLD categories, defined on the basis of morphological dysplasia. 15% or more ring sideroblasts act as a substitute for the SF3B1 mutation Introduced hypoplastic MDS (MDS-h), identified by age-adjusted hypocellularity in childhood	Morphological categories retained based on single or multilineage dysplasia
MDS/MPN	Atypical chronic myeloid leukemia (aCML) category has been renamed as MDS/MPN with neutrophilia	Atypical chronic myeloid leukemia (aCML) name retained. Introduced "Clonal monocytosis of undetermined significance," "Clonal cytopenia and monocytosis of undetermined significance" and a provisional category "MDS/MPN with i(17q)"
Acute myeloid leukemia	Eliminates the 20% blast requirement for AML diagnosis for most AML cases with defining genetic abnormalities. The 20% blast cut-off has been retained for AML with *BCR::ABL1* & *CEBPA* mutation. WHO-HEM5 requires "increased" blasts for a diagnosis of AML with defining genetic abnormalities, but does not apply a precise numeric threshold	Requires at least 10% blasts for AML with recurrent genetic abnormalities. However, AML with *BCR::ABL1* still requires 20% blasts. The ICC identifies an intermediate disease state of MDS/AML with a BM or PB blast enumeration of 10–19% in the absence of AML-defining genetic alterations

(continued)

Table 31.21 (continued)

Category	WHO-HEM5	ICC
AML with myelodysplasia-related changes (AML-MR)	The term AML with myelodysplasia-related changes (AML-MRC) with AML has been replaced by myelodysplasia-related (AML-MR). Defined by myelodysplasia--related gene mutations and myelodysplasia-related cytogenetic abnormalities. Morphological dysplasia alone is omitted as a criterion for AML-MR.	Separates AML-MRC into two categories: AML with myelodysplasia-related gene mutations and cytogenetic abnormalities. *RUNX1* included as a myelodysplasia-related mutation. Morphological dysplasia alone is omitted as a criterion for AML-MR, similar to WHO-HEM5
NPM1-mutated AML	NPM1-mutated AML is diagnosed as AML irrespective of the blast count	Requires >/=10% blasts in the PB or BM for AML diagnosis with *NPM1* mutation
CEBPA-mutated AML	Requires 20% blasts and includes biallelic (*biCEBPA*) and single mutations in the basic leucine zipper (bZIP) region of CEBPA (*smbZIP-CEBPA*)	Requires >/=10% blasts and only includes in-frame bZIP *CEBPA* mutations
Secondary myeloid neoplasms	Myeloid neoplasms arising secondary to cytotoxic therapy or germline predisposition	Considered diagnostic qualifiers rather than classifiers, e.g., therapy-related (prior chemotherapy, radiotherapy, etc.); or Progressing from MDS; or MDS/MPN; or germline predisposition
TP53-mutated AML	Does not specify mutated *TP53* as a distinct entity	AML with mutated *TP53* is a distinct entity
Acute erythroid leukemia (AEL)	The diagnosis of AEL supersedes AML-MR	Most pure erythroid leukemia (PEL) cases will now be classified as AML with mutated *TP53*
BPDCN	Categorized under dendritic cell and histiocytic neoplasms separately from myeloid neoplasms	Categorized under myeloid neoplasms

References

1. Khoury JD, Solary E, Abla O, Akkari Y, Alaggio R, Apperley JF, et al. The 5th edition of the World Health Organization classification of haematolymphoid tumours: myeloid and histiocytic/dendritic neoplasms. Leukemia. 2022;36(7):1703–19.
2. Arber DA, Orazi A, Hasserjian RP, Borowitz MJ, Calvo KR, Kvasnicka HM, et al. International consensus classification of myeloid neoplasms and acute leukemias: integrating morphologic, clinical, and genomic data. Blood. 2022;140(11):1200–28.
3. Chandra DJ, Lachowiez CA, Loghavi S. Practical considerations in clinical application of WHO 5th and ICC classification schemes for acute myeloid leukemia. Blood Rev. 2024;64:101156.
4. Xiao W, Nardi V, Stein E, Hasserjian RP. A practical approach on the classifications of myeloid neoplasms and acute leukemia: WHO and ICC. J Hematol Oncol. 2024;17(1):56.

Chapter 32
Risk Stratification and Updates in Management of MDS

Tuphan Kanti Dolai and Kaustav Ghosh

Abstract Myelodysplastic syndromes (MDS) are a heterogeneous group of clonal hematopoietic stem cell disorders characterized by ineffective hematopoiesis, resulting in cytopenia's and an increased risk of progression to acute myeloid leukemia. The diagnosis and classification of MDS have evolved significantly, with the 2022 WHO classification delineating subtypes based on molecular, genetic, and morphological criteria. Risk stratification using the Revised International Prognostic Scoring System and the more recent Molecular International Prognostic Scoring System has enabled more accurate prognosis and personalized treatment strategies. Supportive care—including transfusions, infection prophylaxis, iron chelation, and vaccination remains foundational, particularly in lower-risk MDS. Disease-modifying therapies for lower-risk MDS include erythropoiesis-stimulating agents, lenalidomide, luspatercept, and hypomethylating agents. High-risk MDS patients benefit from more aggressive approaches, including allogeneic hematopoietic stem cell transplantation, which remains the only curative option. Bridging therapy, conditioning regimens, and post-transplant monitoring play vital roles in optimizing transplant outcomes. In less fit or frail patients, hypomethylating agents such as azacitidine and decitabine provide disease control with acceptable tolerability. Emerging targeted therapies—directed at molecular abnormalities offer promising avenues for personalized treatment, especially in relapsed or refractory settings. This review comprehensively discusses the evolving classification, prognostication, and management of MDS, integrating conventional and novel therapeutic modalities, and highlighting current evidence and clinical practice recommendations, with a special focus on the Indian healthcare context.

Keywords Myelodysplastic syndromes · Risk stratification · Hypomethylating agents · Allogeneic hematopoietic stem cell transplantation · Targeted therapies

T. K. Dolai (✉) · K. Ghosh
Department of Hematology, Nil Ratan Sircar Medical College and Hospital (NRSMCH), Kolkata, West Bengal, India

H. P. Pati et al. (eds.), *Clinical Hematology and Hemato-Oncology*,
https://doi.org/10.1007/978-981-92-1167-8_32

Learning Objectives

- Understand the classification of myelodysplastic syndromes (MDS) based on WHO and its implications for clinical management.
- Describe the key prognostic scoring systems, including the Revised International Prognostic Scoring System (IPSS-R), and Molecular International Prognostic Scoring System (IPSS-M), and how they stratify risk in MDS.
- Identify clinical, cytogenetic, and molecular factors that influence prognosis and guide therapeutic decision-making in MDS.
- Differentiate between lower-risk and higher-risk MDS, including their treatment goals.
- Evaluate current therapeutic strategies for both lower-risk and higher-risk MDS, including hypomethylating agents, supportive care, and disease-modifying therapies.
- Understand the indications for hematopoietic stem cell transplantation and the considerations influencing transplant eligibility.
- Assess the latest evidence on novel therapies for relapsed/refractory and high-risk MDS, including targeted agents.
- Integrate recent updates and evolving guidelines into individualized patient care plans for optimal management of MDS.

32.1 Illustrative Clinical Case

32.1.1 Patient Profile

A 56-year-old male presented with pallor associated with persistent fatigue and generalized weakness for the past six months. No history of fever, rash, bleeding, joint pain, yellowish discoloration of eyes or urine, and blood transfusion

32.1.2 Initial Evaluation

Complete blood count revealed macrocytic anemia (Hb: 7.8 g/dL, MCV: 105 fL), mild leukopenia (WBC: 3.8 × 10^9/L, ANC 2.8 × 10^9/L), and normal platelet counts. A peripheral smear showed dysplastic changes in red cells and occasional hypogranular neutrophils. Iron profile, vitamin B12 and folate levels were normal. Bone marrow biopsy revealed a hypercellular marrow with dysplasia in erythroid and myeloid lineages and <5% blasts. Cytogenetics showed a normal karyotype, and molecular testing was negative for high-risk mutations. Based on these findings, he was diagnosed with lower-risk myelodysplastic syndrome (MDS) under the 2022 WHO classification, and scored as intermediate risk and low risk according to the IPSS-R and IPSS-M, respectively.

32.1.3 Initial Management

He was started on erythropoiesis-stimulating agent therapy. Over the next six months, his hemoglobin stabilized around 9.5–10 g/dL, and he reported improved energy levels and quality of life.

32.1.4 Disease Progression

At the 18-month follow-up, he presented with worsening fatigue and a new onset of petechiae. Blood counts showed pancytopenia (Hb: 7.2 g/dL, WBC: 2.4×10^9/L (ANC 0.9×10^9/L), platelets: 34×10^9/L). Repeat bone marrow biopsy revealed 12% blasts, dysmegakaryopoiesis, and a new cytogenetic abnormality—monosomy 7. He was reclassified as having higher-risk MDS (IPSS-R high; IPSS-M very high).

32.1.5 Escalation of Treatment

Given the progression, he was started on azacitidine at 75 mg/m^2 subcutaneously for 7 days in a 28-day cycle. After 6 cycles, he achieved hematologic improvement with blast reduction to <5% and transfusion independence. He was deemed to be in clinical remission.

32.1.6 Transplant Decision and Procedure

Given his relatively young age, good performance status, and availability of a matched sibling unrelated donor. He underwent reduced-intensity conditioning followed by allogeneic hematopoietic stem cell transplantation. His post-transplant course was uneventful, with neutrophil engraftment by day +18 and no acute graft-versus-host disease.

32.1.7 *Follow-Up*

At his 9-month post-transplant follow-up, he remains in molecular remission, with normal blood counts and undetectable measurable residual disease. He continues regular monitoring, and immunosuppressive therapy tapering is underway.

32.2 Introduction

Myelodysplastic syndromes (MDS) are disorders of the hematopoietic stem cells characterized by dysplasia, leading to reduced blood cell counts (cytopenias) and a significant risk of progression to acute myeloid leukemia (AML). Diagnosis typically involves bone marrow aspiration and biopsy, along with cytogenetic and molecular studies. Prognostic evaluation is performed using the revised international prognostic scoring system (IPSS-R), which categorizes MDS into lower-risk (IPSS-R score ≤ 3.5) and higher-risk (IPSS-R score ≥ 4.0) groups [1]. Morphological classification of MDS has traditionally been guided by the French-American-British (FAB) and World Health Organization (WHO) systems. Under current WHO criteria, cases with 20–30% bone marrow blasts are now categorized as AML, and chronic myelomonocytic leukemia is recognized as a separate condition. In the fifth edition of the WHO classification, MDS is divided into two primary categories: those associated with specific genetic alterations (such as MDS with isolated 5q deletion, MDS with SF3B1 mutations, and MDS with TP53 mutations) and those classified based on morphology, including MDS with low blast count, hypoplastic MDS, MDS with increased blasts, and MDS with associated fibrosis [2]. WHO 2022 Classification of MDS is summarized in Table 32.1 [2].

Table 32.1 WHO 2022 classification of MDS[1]

	Blasts	Cytogenetics	Mutation
MDS with defining genetic abnormalities			
MDS with low blasts and isolated 5q deletion (MDS-5q)	<2% Peripheral blood and <5% bone marrow	5q deletion alone, or with 1 other abnormality other than monosomy 7 or 7q deletion	
MDS with low blasts and SF3B1 mutation (MDS-SF3B1) [a]	<2% Peripheral blood and <5% bone marrow	Absence of 5q deletion, monosomy 7, or complex karyotype	SF3-B1
MDS with biallelic TP53 inactivation (MDS-biTP53)	<20% Peripheral blood and bone marrow	Usually complex	Two or more TP53 mutations, or 1 mutation with evidence of TP53 copy number loss or neutral loss of heterozygosity

(continued)

Table 32.1 (contiuned)

	Blasts	Cytogenetics	Mutation
MDS with low blasts (MDS-LB)	<2% Peripheral blood and <5 % bone marrow		
MDS, hypoplastic (MDS-h)[b]	<2% Peripheral blood and <5% bone marrow		
MDS with increased blasts (MDS-IB):			
A) MDS-IB1	2–4% Peripheral blood or 5–9% bone marrow		
B) MDS-IB2	5–9% Peripheral blood or 10–19% bone marrow or auer rods		
C) MDS with fibrosis (MDS-f)	2–19% Peripheral blood; 5–19% bone marrow		
	Blasts		
Childhood MDS with low blasts	<2% Peripheral blood; <5% bone marrow		
Hypocellular			
Not otherwise specified			
Childhood MDS with increased blasts	2–19% peripheral blood; 5–19% bone marrow		

MDS morphologically defined
[a]Detection of ≥15% ring sideroblasts may substitute for SF3B1 mutation
[b]By definition, ≤25% bone marrow cellularity, age adjusted

Key Differences in WHO 2022 MDS Classification Compared to WHO 2016 classification

- Updated terminology and diagnostic criteria for specific MDS subtypes, including new categories for MDS associated with bone marrow hypoplasia or fibrosis
- The WHO guidelines maintain the distinction between MDS and most types of AML based on a threshold of 20% blasts
- The classification "MDS, unclassifiable" has been removed
- Treatment-related myeloid neoplasms are now categorized under "Myeloid neoplasms post-cytotoxic therapy."
- MDS with germline pathogenic variants remains classified under MDS
- Childhood MDS is now recognized as a distinct category in the classification

32.3 Risk Stratification

Following the introduction of the International Prognostic Scoring System (IPSS) in 1997, various revisions and new prognostic models were proposed to better reflect differences in clinical outcomes among MDS patients. These updates aimed to enhance the accuracy of prognosis by incorporating additional clinical variables and enabling dynamic use throughout the disease course [3]. Figure 32.1 shows the evolution of prognostic models in MDS.

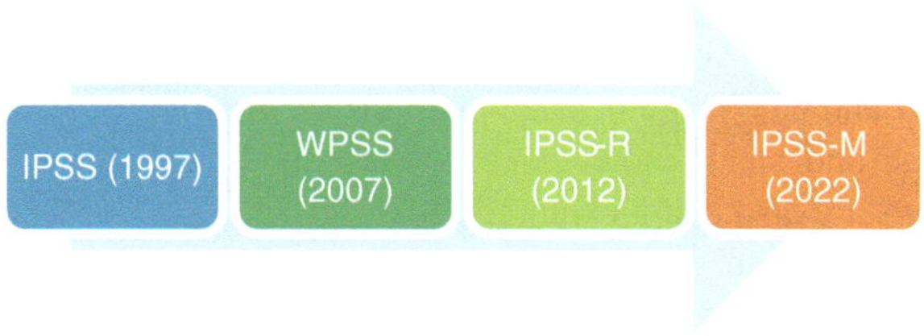

Fig. 32.1 Evolution of prognostic models in MDS (Abbreviations: IPSS, International Prognostic Scoring System; WPSS, WHO-based Prognostic Scoring System; IPSS-R, Revised International Prognostic Scoring System; IPSS-M, Molecular International Prognostic Scoring System)

32.3.1 Currently Widely Used Risk Stratification is Based on IPSS-R [4]

Calculation—A value from 0 to 4 is determined for each of five variables:

- *Bone marrow blasts*—(0 points) ≤2 percent; (1 point) >2 to <5 percent; (2 points) 5 to 10 percent; (3 points) >10 percent
- *Karyotype*
  - *Very good karyotype*—(0 points) includes -Y or del(11q)
  - *Good karyotype*—(1 point) includes normal karyotype, del(5q), del(12p), del(20q), or a double abnormality including del(5q)
  - *Intermediate karyotype*—(2 points) includes del(7q), +8, +19, i(17q), and any other single or double independent clones
  - *Poor karyotype*—(3 points) includes −7, inv.(3)/t(3q)/del(3q), double abnormalities including −7/del(7q), or three abnormalities

    Very poor karyotype—(4 points) includes complex karyotype (>3 abnormalities)
- *Hemoglobin (g/dL)*—(0 points) ≥10; (1 point) 8 to <10; (1.5 points) <8
- *Platelets (cells/microL)*—(0 points) ≥100,000; (0.5 points) 50,000 to 100,000; (1 point) <50,000
- *Absolute neutrophil count (ANC; cells/microL)*—(0 points) ≥800; (0.5 points) <800

There are five IPSS-R prognostic categories: very low, low, intermediate-1 (MDS Lower risk); intermediate-2, and high risk (MDS Higher risk)

- *Very low risk (≤1.5 points)*—Overall survival (OS) 8.8 years; AML-t25 (time for 25% patients to progress to AML) >14.5 years
- *Low risk (>1.5 to 3 points)*—OS 5.3 years; AML-t25 > 10.8 years

- *Intermediate risk (>3 to 4.5 points)*—OS 3.0 years; AML-t25 3.2 years
- *High risk (>4.5 to 6 points)*—OS 1.6 years; AML-t25 1.4 years
- *Very high risk (>6 points)*—OS 0.8 year; AML-t25 0.7 year

The IPSS-R has been a global standard for patient risk stratification since 2012 for clinical trial design, correlative analyses, and treatment recommendations, relying on hematologic and cytogenetic features; however, it does not consider the potential role of gene mutations. Marrow samples from 2701 patients with MDS were profiled for mutations in 156 genes. Feature selection was applied to determine the set of independent molecular IPSS (IPSS-M) prognostic variables (depth of cytopenia, marrow blast percentage, IPSS-R version of cytogenetic risk groups, and new genomic variables) [5]. The 31 genes considered in the IPSS-M are categorized into two groups:

1. *Primary Mutations (16 genes)*: These mutations have a significant impact on prognosis and include: ASXL1, CBL, DNMT3A, ETV6, EZH2, FLT3 (including ITD and TKD), IDH1, IDH2, MLL-PTD (MLL partial tandem duplication), NPM1, NRAS, RUNX1, SF3B1, SRSF2, TP53 (multi-hit), U2AF1.
2. *Secondary Mutations (15 genes)*: These mutations contribute to prognosis but are less impactful individually: BCOR, BCORL1, CEBPA, ETNK1, EZH2, GATA2, GNB1, IDH1, MLL-PTD, NF1, PHF6, PPM1D, PTPN11, PRPF8, SETBP1, STAG2, TP53 (single-hit), U2AF1, WT1.

   *IPSS-M stratifies patients into *six risk categories*: Very Low, Low, and Moderate-Low categories are Lower risk MDS; Moderate-High, High, and Very High are higher risk MDS*

Clinical Significance

A. *Enhanced Prognostic Accuracy*

- Delivers more precise predictions for OS and leukemia-free survival (LFS)
- Clarifies risk variation within IPSS-R subgroups

B. *Tailored Treatment Strategies*

- Aids in the early detection of high-risk individuals who might benefit from allogeneic stem cell transplantation
- Informs optimal timing and selection of hypomethylating agents or targeted treatments

C. *Advancement in Research and Clinical Trials*

- Enables more refined patient stratification for clinical studies
- Supports the development of personalized medicine strategies for managing MDS

32.4 Treatment of MDS

32.4.1 Supportive Care

It encompasses safe and appropriate blood transfusion practices, infection prevention and early intervention, and management of iron overload. Supportive care practices differ across healthcare centers and are often guided by the patient's clinical condition and its severity.

A. *Transfusions:*

- Red blood cell (RBC) transfusions. Blood transfusions are mainly administered to ease symptoms caused by anemia and to reduce the risk of complications, particularly in individuals with heart, lung, or neurological conditions.
  The decision to transfuse depends on factors such as the patient's age, symptoms, and existing health issues. While there is no universally accepted standard, many healthcare facilities choose to transfuse asymptomatic patients when their hemoglobin levels are at or below 8 g/dL [6].
- Platelet transfusions are used to manage or prevent bleeding in patients who have either a low platelet count or dysfunctional platelets. Preventive transfusions are commonly given when platelet levels drop below 10,000/microL. However, a higher transfusion threshold (around 20,000/microL) is preferred in patients experiencing active bleeding, fever, serious infections, lung issues, clotting disorders, or neurological symptoms. If bleeding persists despite platelet transfusions or in cases of severe, unresponsive low platelet counts, antifibrinolytic medications such as tranexamic acid or aminocaproic acid may be considered [7].

B. *Iron chelation:* Iron chelation therapy has not been shown to provide clear clinical benefits in patients with myelodysplastic syndromes (MDS), and there is no agreed-upon standard regimen. In patients with serum ferritin levels over 1000 ng/mL and a history of receiving 15 to 75 units of packed red blood cells, the use of iron chelators has been associated with a 36.4% decrease in event-free survival [8].

C. *Infections:* Patients with an absolute neutrophil count (ANC) below 500/microL who develop a fever or show signs of infection require urgent evaluation. Empiric antibiotic treatment should begin immediately after blood cultures are drawn, even before other tests are completed. Filgrastim (a granulocyte-colony stimulating factor, or G-CSF) may be added to antibiotic therapy for cases of neutropenic fever. There is no evidence that giving G-CSF prophylactically, in the absence of infection, improves survival or other clinical outcomes in MDS patients. However, it may be considered for those with frequent or difficult-to-treat infections. Routine use of antimicrobial prophylaxis is not supported in neutropenic MDS patients. However, clinical judgment should guide its use in individuals receiving therapies such as azacitidine, decitabine, or lenalidomide—particularly if they cause neutropenia—or before invasive procedures like surgery or dental work [9].

D. *Vaccination:* Vaccination is recommended for patients with myelodysplastic MDS to help prevent specific infections. While individuals with MDS can safely receive inactivated or recombinant vaccines, live vaccines are typically avoided due to the risk they pose to those who are immunocompromised [9].

32.4.2 Lower Risk MDS (LR-MDS)

A. *Asymptomatic patients: Regularly monitor and assess complete blood count every one to three months until disease progression or symptoms [10].*

B. *Symptomatic patients*:

   I. *Isolated anemia (hemoglobin < 10gm/dl, transfusion dependent (>2 Unit/8 weeks)*

   - *Erythropoiesis-stimulating agents (ESAs)*, such as recombinant erythropoietin and darbepoetin alfa, are the main treatments for anemia in patients with LR-MDS who have serum EPO levels of 500 U/L or less. The aim of ESA therapy is to keep hemoglobin levels between 10 and 12 g/dL, achieve an increase in hemoglobin of at least 1.5 g/dL, or decrease the need for red blood cell transfusions by at least 4 units over an 8-week period. Response rates to ESAs range from 20% to 40% over 18 to 24 months. If there is no response, alternative treatments such as lenalidomide or luspatercept (for MDS with ring sideroblasts) may be considered [11].
   - *Luspatercept (LUSPA)*: In MDS, increased SMAD2/3 signaling in early blood-forming cells interferes with red blood cell development. Luspatercept (ACE-536) is a novel recombinant fusion protein composed of a modified activin receptor type IIB linked to the Fc portion of human immunoglobulin. It works by selectively binding specific ligands from the transforming growth factor β (TGF-β) family, thereby reducing SMAD2/3 signaling and enhancing the maturation of late-stage red blood cell precursors. The FDA approved luspatercept in April 2020 for use in patients with MDS who have ring sideroblasts and an SF3B1 mutation and who require regular blood transfusions, based on the MEDALIST trial [12].
   - *Lenalidomide (LEN)*: It triggers p53-dependent cell cycle arrest and apoptosis in cells carrying heterozygous CSNK1A1 mutations. In patients with del(5q) myelodysplastic syndromes (MDS), overexpression of CSNK1A1 decreases sensitivity to lenalidomide in bone marrow cells, a pattern not seen in MDS patients with a normal karyotype or in healthy individuals. Lenalidomide is the standard therapy for lower-risk, transfusion-dependent MDS with del(5q), leading to transfusion independence in about 67% of patients, with responses typically lasting 2 to 3 years. However, those with both del(5q) and TP53 mutations tend to have lower response rates and shorter response durations [13].

II. *Isolated thrombocytopenia (platelet count < 20,000/cu mm, or < 50,000/cu mm with bleeding)*: In LR-MDS, bleeding risk is increased due to both dysfunctional megakaryocytes and common medications used in older adults, such as aspirin and NSAIDs. Active bleeding should be managed with platelet transfusions and antifibrinolytics. However, transfusions offer only temporary benefit, often trigger immune reactions, and may lead to spleen enlargement.
Thrombopoietin receptor agonists—romiplostim and eltrombopag—are the preferred treatments for thrombocytopenia in LR-MDS. Romiplostim (750 μg weekly via subcutaneous injection) has been shown to improve platelet counts and reduce bleeding. Eltrombopag (150–300 mg orally daily) has similar effects. These therapies should not be used if the blast percentage exceeds 5% [14, 15].

III. *Isolated neutropenia (ANC < 500/cu mm)*: Other causes, such as large granular lymphocytic leukemia, paroxysmal nocturnal hemoglobinuria, cyclic neutropenia, and autoimmune disorders, must be ruled out. G-CSF and GM-CSF are generally not recommended, unless there is febrile neutropenia. Vaccinations, including influenza and pneumococcal, should be up to date. If infections recur, consider antiviral or antibiotic prophylaxis [9].

IV. *Multi-lineage cytopenias*: LR-MDS patients who do not respond to initial first-line therapies may be considered for immunosuppressive therapy (IST) targeting T-cells or for treatment with hypomethylating agents (HMAs) such as azacitidine or decitabine.

- *IST*: For those presenting with pancytopenia and features resembling bone marrow failure—like acquired aplastic anemia with a hypocellular marrow (hypoplastic MDS)—IST using horse anti-thymocyte globulin (hATG) combined with oral cyclosporine (CSA) can be an option. Patients most likely to benefit from IST are typically younger, have hypocellular bone marrow, fewer than 5% blasts, normal cytogenetics, are HLA-DR positive, and have had only a short duration of transfusion dependence. The overall response rate to IST in LR-MDS is around 29%, but this increases to about 50% in those with hypoplastic MDS. While IST use is limited in hypoplastic MDS, hATG with CSA remains a valid option for younger LR-MDS patients unresponsive to erythropoiesis-stimulating agent (ESA) therapy [16].
- *HMA*: In patients of LR-MDS refractory to first-line therapies, HMA therapy can be used. Dose-reduced regimens (i.e., 3–5 days of azacitidine [AZA] 75 mg/m^2 per day or 3 days of 50 mg/m2 per day decitabine [DAC]) are generally used. AZA and DAC show similar effectiveness and side effect profiles. The choice between them typically depends on the method and schedule of administration, as well as patient and physician preferences. Some prefer decitabine for its shorter intravenous administration schedule, especially when an IV access device is available, while others favor azacitidine for its subcutaneous delivery and minimal time in infu-

sion centers. Treatment usually consists of at least six cycles, but therapy may be continued indefinitely until it loses effectiveness or causes significant side effects. For patients achieving complete remission after six cycles, ongoing therapy can be continued or paused and resumed upon relapse. In patients with ≥5% blasts, treatment should be maintained as long as tolerated. If adverse effects arise, dose adjustments or brief interruptions are preferred over discontinuation, such as shortening the treatment days or extending the interval between cycles [17].

A phase 2 trial comparing low-dose, three-day-per-cycle regimens in 113 patients with LR- MDS or MDS/MPN showed no significant difference in one-year overall survival (87% with decitabine vs. 83% with azacitidine), event-free survival, or red blood cell transfusion independence. Both drugs were well-tolerated [18].

In the first and only Indian study, the outcome of low-dose AZA (three-day-per-cycle) in patients with LR-MDS was evaluated. An overall response and one-year overall survival were achieved in 55% and 95% of the patients, respectively, in 20 LR-MDS after six cycles of AZA. Transfusion independence and improvement in ECOG performance status were achieved in 55% and 62.5% of the patients, respectively, at the end of one year [19].

Oral dac/ced is an oral agent that combines decitabine with the cytidine deaminase inhibitor cedazuridine, and is under development [20].

- *Hematopoietic stem cell transplant (HSCT)*: Allogeneic stem cell transplantation (alloSCT) is generally not recommended at the initial presentation for patients with LR-MDS. Candidates who have already undergone multiple lines of therapy—such as growth factors, lenalidomide, or hypomethylating agents—should be assessed for potential transplantation. These individuals may also be suitable for enrollment in clinical trials. In younger patients with hypoplastic MDS, upfront consideration for alloSCT is warranted given their disease characteristics and potential for durable benefit.

V. *Relapsed/ refractory (R/R) cases*

- ESA failure: HMA
- Thrombocytopenia: HMA
- Hypoplastic anemia R/R to IST: HMA
- Targeted therapy (Del 5q, IDH1, IDH2, TP53, SF3B1)
- HMA failure: No approved drug, consider clinical trials, alloSCT or emerging therapies discussed below

VI. *Emerging therapies* 21]

- Roxadustat (oral hypoxia inducible factor (HIF) inhibitor) for non-del 5q LR
  MDS with low transfusion burden and EPO ≤ 400 U/L

- Imetelstat (intravenous telomerase inhibitor) for non-del 5q LR MDS with high transfusion burden and failure to respond to ESA
  H3B-8800 (oral spliceosomal inhibitor) for LR MDS associated with spliceosome mutation
- APR-246/ Eprenetapopt (intravenous TP53 modifier) for treatment naïve MDS patients with TP53 mutation
- Ivosidenib and Olutasidenib (oral IDH1 inhibitor) with relapsed or refractory MDS with IDH1mutation
- Enasidenib (oral IDH2 inhibitor) with relapsed or refractory (R/R) MDS with IDH2 mutation
- KER-050 (TGF beta inhibitor), in LR-MDS patients R/R to ESA
- Canakinumab (IL-1β inhibitor), in cases R/R to ESA, HMA
- Emavusertib (IRAK4 inhibitor), in treatment naïve and R/R (ESA) LR-MDS
- BMS-986253 (IL8 inhibitor) for LR-MDS R/R (ESA, LEN, LUSPA)
- SX-682 (CXCR1 and 2 inhibitor) for LR-MDS R/R (ESA, LEN)
- Tomaralimab (TLR2 inhibitor) for LR-MDS R/R (ESA, LEN)

Figure 32.2 summarizes the treatment algorithm for LR-MDS

32.4.3 Higher Risk MDS (HR-MDS)

For medically fit patients, intensive chemotherapy followed by alloSCT is the preferred approach. Non-transplant approaches, including less intensive chemotherapy and supportive care, are preferred in less fit [Eastern Cooperative Oncology Group Performance Status (ECOG PS): 3, Modified Charlson Comorbidity Index (CCI): ≥3] and frail patients (ECOG PS: 3 or 4, Modified CCI: ≥4) [22].

I. *Medically fit patients*

- *Hematopoietic stem cell transplant (HSCT)*: AlloSCT is considered the only potentially curative option for patients with higher-risk MDS, with 30% to 50% of patients achieving prolonged disease-free survival DFS following the procedure. Bridging therapy is typically used when graft acquisition takes 2–3 months or longer, with some experts recommending cytoreductive treatment in cases of high disease burden (e.g., ≥10% blasts), particularly for patients not receiving myeloablative conditioning [23].

  A. *Indications* 24]

  - All medically fit higher-risk MDS
  - LR-MDS with progressive cytopenias, increasing transfusion burden, failure of HMA/IST, high-risk cytogenetics, and molecular features
  - Therapy-related MDS
  - Hypoplastic MDS with progressive cytopenias, increasing transfusion burden, failure of IST, high-risk cytogenetics, and molecular features

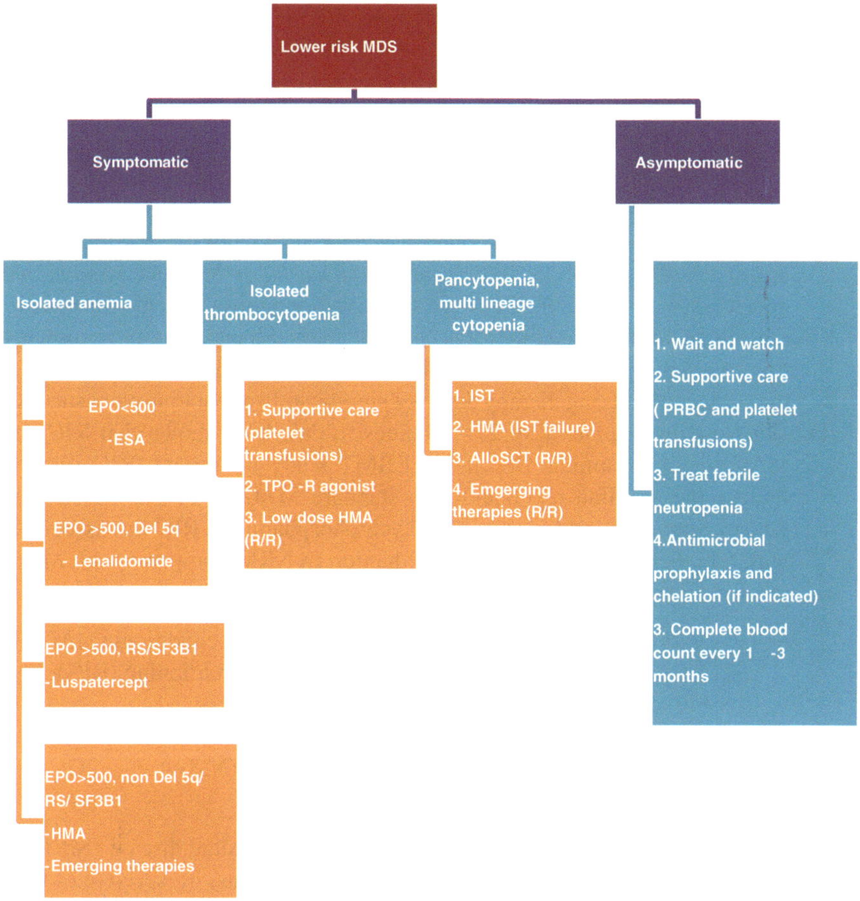

Fig. 32.2 Treatment algorithm for LR-MDS (Abbreviations: MDS myelodysplastic syndromes; ESA erythropoietin stimulating agents; RS ring sideroblasts; HMA hypomethylating agents; TPO-R thrombopoietin receptor; IST immunosuppressive therapy; AlloSCT allogenic stem cell transplantation; R/R relapsed/refractory; PRBC packed red blood cell)

- Progression to acute myeloid leukemia
  MDS following inherited bone marrow failure syndrome

B. *Choice of donor* [24]—Matched sibling donors (MSD) and matched unrelated donors (MUD), and HLA-matched sibling donors remain standard choices for stem cell transplantation in MDS. However, the use of haploidentical donors has grown due to wider availability. In contrast, unrelated cord blood transplants are less favored because of limited cell doses and delayed hematologic and immune recovery. Encouraging outcomes with haploidentical transplants are seen, though they still fall short of those seen with fully matched donors, mainly due to higher non-relapse mortality. Donor age also impacts outcomes, with younger donors offering better results—especially relevant in older MDS patients

C. *Bridging therapy* [25]—HMA-based therapy, with or without venetoclax, and intensive chemotherapy [infusional cytarabine plus an anthracycline (e.g., so-called "7 + 3" therapy, or CPX-351 (liposomal daunorubicin-cytarabine)] are commonly used as bridging treatments before alloHCT in MDS patients. A study involving 265 such patients found no significant difference in post-transplant outcomes based on the type of pre-transplant therapy received. Specifically, three-year overall survival (OS), relapse rates, and non-relapse mortality (NRM) were similar among those treated with azacitidine alone (48 patients), intensive chemotherapy (98 patients), or a combination of azacitidine and intensive chemotherapy (17 patients), suggesting that the choice of bridging therapy does not significantly affect transplant success.

D. *Conditioning regimen* [26, 27]—Studies to date have shown that RIC and MAC result in similar OS. In an EBMT study comparing RIC (mainly fludarabine-busulfan regimens) with standard MAC (total body irradiation with cyclophosphamide or busulfan-cyclophosphamide), RIC was associated with a higher risk of relapse but a reduction in NRM compared with MAC, resulting in similar PFS and OS

- *Less than 55 years, very fit*- Consider myeloablative conditioning (MAC), e.g., 8 Gy TBI, fludarabine, or reduced intensity conditioning (RIC), e.g., TreoFlu or FluMel.
- *Less than 70 years, fit*- RIC, e.g., TreoFlu or FluMel
  More than/equal to 70 years—Non myeloablative (NMA), e.g., 2Gy TBI, fludarabine

E. *Post transplant* [27]—Assessment of measurable residual disease (MRD) is advised following allogeneic HCT in all MDS patients, irrespective of their risk category. However, current evidence is inadequate to support routine use of prophylactic or maintenance therapy post-transplant. For patients with detectable MRD or relapse after transplant, therapeutic options include hypomethylating agents (HMAs) and donor lymphocyte infusions (DLI).
Factors associated with poor outcomes post-transplant are:

- Mutations of TP53, JAK2, or RAS pathway genes
- Detectable MRD pre-transplant followed by RIC
- Age > 75 years

Outcome of HSCT in MDS in different studies conducted in India

- *Baranwal et al.* [28]—Prognostic utility of therapy-related AML/MDS, pre- and post-allo-SCT was studied. The 3-year OS for high-risk patients, defined by pathogenic variants in TP53/BCOR/IDH1/GATA2/BCORL1, was 0%, while standard-risk patients had 64.6% OS ($P = 0.001$). A complex karyotype consistently negatively impacted survival. In t-MDS, monosomy 5 and monosomy 17 before alloSCT were associated with higher relapse incidence (RI). Post-alloSCT OS did not differ between t-MDS and t-AML, but t-MDS had significantly higher 3-year RI. These findings suggest that while alloSCT can be curative in some therapy-related myeloid neoplasm patients, outcomes remain poor, especially in high-risk cases. Relapse risk is notably higher for t-MDS patients with persistent disease before alloSCT.

Karumathil et al. [29]—154 patients with MDS—including 22 children and both HR (86) and LR (68) cases—underwent HSCT at a median age of 36 years. MAC was used in 97 patients, and reduced-intensity regimens in 53. Most transplants (92%) utilized peripheral blood stem cells. HLA-MSD accounted for 113 cases, while 41 involved alternate donors. Engraftment was achieved in 81.9% at a median of 15 days; 12.9% died before engraftment, and 5.2% experienced primary graft failure. Complications included sinusoidal obstruction syndrome (17.5%) and grade 2–4 acute GVHD in 46.3%, with grade 3–4 GVHD in 34.9%. Chronic GVHD occurred in 69.4%. Infection rates included bacterial (24.6%), viral (20.1%, mainly CMV), and fungal (17.5%). After a median follow-up of 33 months, 65 patients were alive. Five-year overall and event-free survival rates were 41.7% and 40.8%, respectively, with significantly better outcomes in children (71%) and MRD transplants (45%) compared to alternate donors (29%). Outcomes improved over decades, reaching 51% for MRDs in 2011–2021. Poorer survival was linked to older age, blood group mismatches, and haploidentical donors.

II. *Less fit patients*

- *HMA*: Azacitidine and decitabine, both HMAs, are commonly used to manage HR-MDS in patients who are not candidates for alloSCT. These agents can lead to hematologic improvement, symptom control, and better quality of life with relatively low toxicity. However, only azacitidine has been shown to improve overall survival (OS) in this group. There are no head-to-head randomized trials comparing the two drugs. Preferences between them often depend on administration routes: azacitidine is given subcutaneously, which allows outpatient treatment but may cause pain or bruising in patients with low platelet counts, while decitabine is administered intravenously, often preferred for patients with central venous access [17].

  A. *AZA*: It is typically administered at a dose of 75 mg/m^2 per day subcutaneously on days 1 through 7 of a 28-day cycle. Alternative dosing schedules are also used, such as the "5-2-2" regimen, which involves five consecutive days of treatment, two days off, and then two additional days of dosing within the same 28-day period. Treatment with azacitidine should be continued for a minimum of four to six cycles. In the AZA-001 trial, most patients responded by the sixth cycle, though up to 50% required as many as 12 cycles to achieve their optimal response [30].

B. *DAC*: It is given at a dose of 20 mg/m /day intravenously for five days every four weeks. Treatment should continue for at least four to six cycles. Following a phase I trial of decitabine at MD Anderson Cancer Center (MDACC), a Bayesian randomized phase II trial was conducted to compare three different dosing regimens. This study found that a 5-day schedule of intravenous decitabine at 20 mg/m^2 per day was more effective than either a 10-day regimen or a subcutaneous administration [31]. Additionally, the oral formulation of decitabine combined with cedazuridine received approval based on findings from the Ascertain trial (NCT03306264), for the same clinical indications as intravenous decitabine [32].
C. *AML-like chemotherapy*: In HR-MDS, AML-like treatment protocols (anthracycline and cytarabine) tend to yield lower CR rates (approximately 40–60%), shorter remission durations (around 10–12 months), and are associated with more prolonged marrow aplasia compared to their use in AML. Their feasibility is further limited by the older median age of MDS patients. The key predictors of response are cytogenetic profile and TP53 mutation status—patients with adverse karyotypes (such as monosomy 7, del(7q), or complex karyotypes) or TP53 mutations typically have low CR rates and brief remissions. AML-like therapy is currently reserved for younger patients with favorable cytogenetics who are potential candidates for alloSCT [17].
D. *IDH1/2 inhibitor*: Mutant IDH1 inhibitors (such as ivosidenib and olutasidenib) and the IDH2 inhibitor enasidenib are approved for use in AML, although their effectiveness in treating MDS remains unclear. Currently, ivosidenib has received FDA approval specifically for patients with relapsed or refractory MDS harboring a susceptible IDH1 mutation [17].
E. *Low-dose cytarabine*: Low-dose cytarabine has not shown a clearly established benefit in treating higher-risk MDS and is not approved for this indication by the FDA or EMA. In one study, administering cytarabine at 10 mg/m^2 subcutaneously twice daily for 21 days resulted in a 32% response rate, a median response duration of six months, and reduced transfusion needs compared to best supportive care. However, it was associated with a higher incidence of infections and showed no improvement in overall survival or time to disease progression [33]. Additionally, the AZA-001 trial demonstrated that outcomes with low-dose cytarabine were inferior to those achieved with azacitidine [30].

III. *Frail patients*: For patients who are medically frail, the main goal of care is to ease symptoms and enhance their quality of life. Supportive care should be provided to all individuals in this category. Some may opt for less intensive treatments aimed at relieving symptoms and improving overall well-being.
IV. *Relapsed/ refractory (R/R) cases* [17]

- *Relapse after alloSCT*: Options include DLI or a second allogeneic transplant
- *No prior use of HMA*: Patients who relapse following allogeneic transplant or intensive chemotherapy but haven't been treated with an HMA may be considered for azacitidine or decitabine
- *Relapse after HMA therapy*: Venetoclax, a BCL2 inhibitor, can be added to an HMA. In cases of MDS with IDH1 or IDH2 mutations, a targeted therapy can be combined with an HMA. For patients who acquire a FLT3 mutation, gilteritinib may be a treatment option
- *Changing HMAs or adding other drugs*: There is no strong evidence that switching between HMAs or adding other agents like lenalidomide or vorinostat improves outcomes in patients with high-risk MDS

V. *Emerging therapies* [34, 35]

- Azacitidine with *Pevonedistat* (NEDD8-activating enzyme inhibitor)
- Azacitidine with *Venetoclax* (BCL-2 inhibitor)
- Azacitidine with *Sabatolimab* (Anti-TIM-3 monoclonal antibody)
- Azacitidine with *Magrolimab* (Anti-CD47 monoclonal antibody)
- Azacitidine with *Lenalidomide*
- Azacitidine with *Durvalumab* (Immune checkpoint inhibitor)
- Azacitidine with *Vorinostat* (HDAC inhibitor)
- APR-246/ *Eprenetapopt (Intravenous TP53 modifier)*
- *Ivosidenib and Olutasidenib* (Oral IDH1 inhibitor) with relapsed or refractory (R/R) MDS with IDH1mutation
- *Enasidenib* (Oral IDH2 inhibitor) with R/R MDS with IDH2 mutation
- *Gilteritinib* (Oral FLT3 inhibitor) for MDS with FLT3 mutation
- *Rigosertib* (Multikinase inhibitor / RAS-mimetic)
- CPX-351, liposomal cytarabine combined with daunorubicin

Fig. 32.3 summarizes the treatment algorithm for HR-MDS

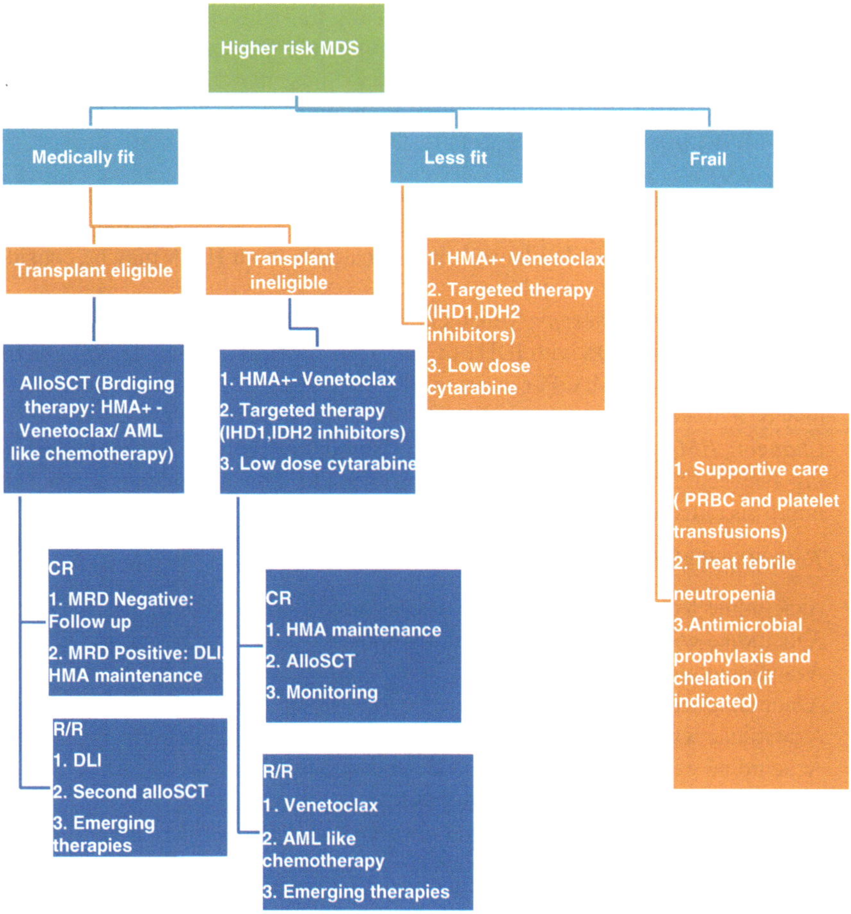

Fig. 32.3 Treatment algorithm for HR-MDS (Abbreviations: MDS myelodysplastic syndromes; HMA hypomethylating agents; AlloSCT allogenic stem cell transplantation; PRBC packed red blood cell; CR complete response; R/R relapse/refractory)

32.5 Response Criteria [36]

1. *Complete remission (CR)-*
   BM: <5% myeloblasts; dysplasia may persist, PB: Hb ≥10 g/dL, platelets ≥100 × 10^9/L; neutrophils ≥1.0 × 10^9/L; blasts 0%
2. *CR equivalent-* Patients with <5% BM blasts at baseline
   BM: <5% myeloblasts; dysplasia may persist, PB: Hb ≥10 g/dL, platelets ≥100 × 10^9/L; neutrophils ≥1.0 × 10^9/L; blasts 0%, Full cytogenetic clearance of baseline abnormalities

3. *Partial remission (PR)*- All CR criteria if previously abnormal, but marrow blasts decreased by ≥50% from pre-treatment value and to a level between 5% and 10%.

   Persistent dysplasia allowed. No progression in other parameters.
4. *CRl (CR with limited count recovery)*- BM: <5% myeloblasts; dysplasia may persist, PB: blasts 0%

   CRuni (CR unilineage): PB, not meeting CR but only 1 of the following: Hb ≥10 g/dL; platelets ≥100 × 10^9/L; neutrophils ≥1.0 × 10^9/L

   CRbi (CR bilineage): PB, not meeting CR but only 2 of the following: Hb ≥10 g/dL; platelets ≥100 × 10^9/L; neutrophils ≥1.0 × 10^9/L
5. *CRh (CR with partial hematologic recovery)*- BM: <5% myeloblasts; dysplasia may persist, PB: Not meeting criteria for CR or CRL, no Hb threshold required, platelets ≥50 × 10^9/L; neutrophils ≥0.5 × 10^9/L; blasts 0%
6. *Hematological improvement (HI)*- Defined separately for each lineage:

   Erythroid (HI-E): Increase in hemoglobin by ≥1.5 g/dL, or Reduction in RBC transfusions by ≥4 units over 8 weeks (compared to pretreatment).

   Platelet (HI-P): Absolute increase of ≥30 × 10^9/L for baseline <100 × 10^9/L, or become transfusion-independent.

   Neutrophil (HI-N): At least 100% increase and an absolute increase >0.5 × 10^9/L for baseline <1.0 × 10^9/L.
7. *Overall response rate (ORR)* = CR (or CR equivalent) + PR + CRL + CRh + HI

32.6 Conclusion

MDS comprises a diverse group of hematologic disorders, each with a variable prognosis and treatment approach. The 2022 WHO classification has significantly improved diagnostic accuracy by incorporating genetic and molecular markers—such as 5q deletion and mutations in TP53 or SF3B1—enhancing the alignment with precision medicine. This advancement facilitates personalized treatment and is supported by prognostic models like IPSS-M, which integrates mutational data for more accurate survival predictions.

The management of MDS is now tailored according to the patient's risk level. For LR-MDS, the primary goals are symptom management and slowing disease progression, with treatments including erythropoiesis-stimulating agents, lenalidomide for del(5q), and luspatercept for ring sideroblasts. Additionally, HMAs and immunosuppressive therapies are utilized for cases with refractory or multilineage cytopenias.

HR-MDS demands prompt treatment due to the increased likelihood of leukemic transformation. Allogeneic stem cell transplantation remains the only curative option, but it is limited to eligible patients. Successful outcomes depend on strategies like bridging therapies, conditioning regimens, and post-transplant monitoring, including MRD evaluation. For patients who are not candidates for transplantation,

HMAs are the standard treatment, and the increasing use of oral formulations enhances patient accessibility. Despite progress, relapse continues to be a challenge. Targeted therapies for mutations like TP53 and IDH1/2, along with experimental drugs such as imetelstat and spliceosome modulators, show potential. In India, research has demonstrated positive outcomes with low-dose azacitidine, reduced-intensity transplants, and haploidentical donors, though challenges remain regarding diagnostics and infrastructure.

In conclusion, advancements in diagnostics, prognostic tools, and treatments point to improved MDS management, highlighting the importance of greater access to care and continued research, especially in resource-limited areas.

References

1. Malcovati L, Hellström-Lindberg E, Bowen D, Adès L, Cermak J, Del Cañizo C, et al. Diagnosis and treatment of primary myelodysplastic syndromes in adults: recommendations from the European Leukemia Net. Blood. 2013;122(17):2943–64.
2. Khoury JD, Solary E, Abla O, Akkari Y, Alaggio R, Apperley JF, et al. The 5th edition of the World Health Organization classification of haematolymphoid tumours: myeloid and histiocytic/dendritic neoplasms. Leukemia. 2022;36(7):1703–19.
3. Greenberg P, Cox C, LeBeau MM, Fenaux P, Morel P, Sanz G, et al. International scoring system for evaluating prognosis in myelodysplastic syndromes. Blood. 1997;89(6):2079–88.
4. Greenberg PL, Tuechler H, Schanz J, Sanz G, Garcia-Manero G, Solé F, et al. Revised international prognostic scoring system for myelodysplastic syndromes. Blood. 2012;120(12):2454–65.
5. Bernard E, Tuechler H, Greenberg PL, Hasserjian RP, Arango Ossa JE, Nannya Y, et al. Molecular international prognostic scoring system for myelodysplastic syndromes. NEJM evidence. 2022;1(7):EVIDoa2200008.
6. Tanasijevic AM, Revette A, Klepin HD, Zeidan A, Townsley D, DiNardo CD, et al. Consensus minimum hemoglobin level above which patients with myelodysplastic syndromes can safely forgo transfusions. Leuk Lymphoma. 2020;61(12):2900–4.
7. Antun AG, Gleason S, Arellano M, Langston AA, McLemore ML, Gaddh M, et al. Epsilon aminocaproic acid prevents bleeding in severely thrombocytopenic patients with hematological malignancies. Cancer. 2013;119(21):3784–7.
8. Angelucci E, Li J, Greenberg P, Wu D, Hou M, Montaňo Figueroa EH, et al. Iron chelation in transfusion-dependent patients with low-to intermediate-1–risk myelodysplastic syndromes: a randomized trial. Ann Intern Med. 2020;172(8):513–22.
9. Toma A, Fenaux P, Dreyfus F, Cordonnier C. Infections in myelodysplastic syndromes. Haematologica. 2012;97(10):1459.
10. Carraway HE, Saygin C. Therapy for lower-risk MDS. Hematology 2014, the American Society of Hematology Education Program Book. 2020;2020(1):426–33.
11. Hellström-Lindberg E, Gulbrandsen N, Lindberg G, Ahlgren T, Dahl IM, Dybedal I, et al. A validated decision model for treating the anaemia of myelodysplastic syndromes with erythropoietin+ granulocyte colony-stimulating factor: significant effects on quality of life. Br J Haematol. 2003;120(6):1037–46.
12. Fenaux P, Platzbecker U, Mufti GJ, Garcia-Manero G, Buckstein R, Santini V, et al. The Medalist trial: results of a phase 3, randomized, double-blind, placebo-controlled study of luspatercept to treat anemia in patients with very low-, low-, or intermediate-risk myelodysplastic syndromes (MDS) with ring sideroblasts (RS) who require red blood cell (RBC) transfusions. Blood. 2018;132:1.

13. List AF, Bennett JM, Sekeres MA, Skikne B, Fu T, Shammo JM, et al. Extended survival and reduced risk of AML progression in erythroid-responsive lenalidomide treated patients with lower-risk del (5q) MDS. Leukemia. 2014;28(5):1033–40.
14. Kantarjian HM, Fenaux P, Sekeres MA, Szer J, Platzbecker U, Kuendgen A, et al. Long-term follow-up for up to 5 years on the risk of leukaemic progression in thrombocytopenic patients with lower-risk myelodysplastic syndromes treated with romiplostim or placebo in a randomised double-blind trial. Lancet Haematol. 2018;5(3):e117–26.
15. Oliva EN, Alati C, Santini V, Poloni A, Molteni A, Niscola P, et al. Eltrombopag versus placebo for low-risk myelodysplastic syndromes with thrombocytopenia (EQoL-MDS): phase 1 results of a single-blind, randomised, controlled, phase 2 superiority trial. Lancet Haematol. 2017;4(3):e127–36.
16. Stahl M, DeVeaux M, De Witte T, Neukirchen J, Sekeres MA, Brunner AM, et al. The use of immunosuppressive therapy in MDS: clinical outcomes and their predictors in a large international patient cohort. Blood Adv. 2018;2(14):1765–72.
17. Garcia-Manero G. Myelodysplastic syndromes: 2023 update on diagnosis, risk-stratification, and management. Am J Hematol. 2023;98(8):1307–25.
18. Jabbour E, Short NJ, Montalban-Bravo G, Huang X, Bueso-Ramos C, Qiao W, et al. Randomized phase 2 study of low-dose decitabine vs low-dose azacitidine in lowerrisk MDS and MDS/MPN. Blood. 2017;130(13):1514.
19. Ghosh K Sr, Dolai TK, Mandal PK, Jena R. Outcome of low dose Azacitidine in patients of lower risk myelodysplastic syndromes. Blood. 2024 Nov;5(144):6697.
20. Garcia-Manero G, Griffiths EA, Steensma DP, Roboz GJ, Wells R, McCloskey J, et al. Oral cedazuridine/decitabine for MDS and CMML: a phase 2 pharmacokinetic/pharmacodynamic randomized crossover study. Blood. 2020;136(6):674–83.
21. Sébert M. Next-generation therapy for lower-risk MDS. Hematology. 2023;2023(1):59–64.
22. Lin RJ, Artz AS. Allogeneic hematopoietic cell transplantation for older patients. Hematology. 2021;2021(1):254–63.
23. Chang C, Storer BE, Scott BL, Bryant EM, Shulman HM, Flowers ME, et al. Hematopoietic cell transplantation in patients with myelodysplastic syndrome or acute myeloid leukemia arising from myelodysplastic syndrome: similar outcomes in patients with de novo disease and disease following prior therapy or antecedent hematologic disorders. Blood. 2007;110(4):1379–87.
24. Sureda A, Corbacioglu S, Greco R, Kröger N, Carreras E. The EBMT handbook: hematopoietic cell transplantation and cellular therapies. 2024.
25. Damaj G, Duhamel A, Robin M, Beguin Y, Michallet M, Mohty M, et al. Impact of azacitidine before allogeneic stem-cell transplantation for myelodysplastic syndromes: a study by the Societe Francaise de Greffe de Moelle et de Therapie-Cellulaire and the Groupe-Francophone des Myelodysplasies. J Clin Oncol. 2012;30(36):4533–40.
26. Bischof L, Ussmann J, Platzbecker U, Jentzsch M, Franke GN. Allogeneic stem cell transplantation for MDS—clinical issues, choosing preparative regimens and outcome. Leuk Lymphoma. 2025:1–4.
27. Gurnari C, Robin M, Adès L, Aljurf M, Almeida AM, Duarte FB, et al. Clinical-genomic profiling of MDS to inform allo-HSCT: recommendations from an international panel on behalf of the EBMT. Blood J. 2025:blood-2024025131.
28. Baranwal A, Chhetri R, Yeung D, Clark M, Shah S, Litzow MR, et al. Factors predicting survival following alloSCT in patients with therapy-related AML and MDS: a multicenter study. Bone Marrow Transplant. 2023;58(7):769–76.
29. Karumathil S, Kulkarni U, Selvarajan S, Lionel S, Devasia AJ, Aboobacker FN, et al. Outcomes in patients undergoing hematopoietic stem cell transplantation for myelodysplastic syndromes. Blood Cell Ther. 2025;8(1):147.
30. Silverman LR, Fenaux P, Mufti GJ, Santini V, Hellström-Lindberg E, Gattermann N, et al. Continued azacitidine therapy beyond time of first response improves quality of response in patients with higher-risk myelodysplastic syndromes. Cancer. 2011;117(12):2697–702.

31. Kantarjian H, Oki Y, Garcia-Manero G, Huang X, O'Brien S, Cortes J, et al. Results of a randomized study of 3 schedules of low-dose decitabine in higher-risk myelodysplastic syndrome and chronic myelomonocytic leukemia. Blood. 2007;109(1):52–7.
32. Savona MR, Odenike O, Amrein PC, Steensma DP, DeZern AE, Michaelis LC, et al. An oral fixed-dose combination of decitabine and cedazuridine in myelodysplastic syndromes: a multicentre, open-label, dose-escalation, phase 1 study. Lancet Haematol. 6(4):e194–203.
33. Miller KB, Kim K, Morrison FS, Winter JN, Bennett JM, Neiman RS, et al. The evaluation of low-dose cytarabine in the treatment of myelodysplastic syndromes: a phase-III intergroup study. Ann Hematol. 1993;66(164):1993–70.
34. Koenig KL, Borate U. New investigational combinations for higher-risk MDS. Hematology. 2022;2022(1):368–74.
35. Sallman DA, Xie Z. Frontline treatment options for higher-risk MDS: can we move past azacitidine? Hematology. 2023;2023(1):65–72.
36. Zeidan AM, Platzbecker U, Bewersdorf JP, Stahl M, Adès L, Borate U, et al. Consensus proposal for revised International Working Group 2023 response criteria for higher-risk myelodysplastic syndromes. Blood. 2023;141(17):2047–61.

Chapter 33
Management of Chronic Myeloid Leukemia in Adults and Children

Swapnil Tripathi and Narendra Agrawal

Abstract Chronic myeloid leukemia (CML) is a clonal myeloproliferative neoplasm characterized by presence of the BCR::ABL1 fusion gene. The introduction of tyrosine kinase inhibitors (TKIs) has revolutionized CML management, leading to a dramatic improvement in overall survival and transforming CML into a chronic, manageable condition for most patients. Recent advances have focused on achieving deeper molecular responses and enabling treatment-free remission (TFR), which is now a key therapeutic goal. Novel agents and combination strategies continue to be explored to overcome resistance and improve long-term outcomes. However, the management of CML during pregnancy and in pediatric populations presents unique challenges, with limited prospective data and a lack of standardized guidelines. This chapter reviews the evolving landscape of CML therapy across adult and pediatric populations, highlighting recent developments, clinical decision-making strategies, and areas in need of further research.

Keywords Chronic myeloid leukemia · Tyrosine kinase inhibitor · Treatment-free remission · Novel agents

Learning Objectives

- Understand the role of first, second, and third generation TKIs in achieving DMR and TFR in adult and pediatric CML, especially in Indian settings.
- Assess timing and indications for allo-HSCT in TKI-resistant CML, including challenges in pediatric and low-resource contexts.
- Recognize resistance mechanisms like BCR::ABL1 mutations and apply mutation-guided TKI selection in practice.
- Identify management strategies for pediatric and pregnant CML patients where guidelines are limited and evolving.

S. Tripathi · N. Agrawal (✉)
Department of Hemato-oncology and BMTU, RGCIRC, New Delhi, India

H. P. Pati et al. (eds.), *Clinical Hematology and Hemato-Oncology*,
https://doi.org/10.1007/978-981-92-1167-8_33

33.1 Introduction

Chronic myeloid leukemia (CML) is a clonal myeloproliferative neoplasm originating at the level of the hematopoietic stem cell, pathognomonically characterized by the presence of the BCR::ABL1 fusion gene, a consequence of the reciprocal translocation t(9;22)(q34;q11), commonly known as the Philadelphia chromosome. This molecular aberration results in the constitutive activation of the ABL1 tyrosine kinase, driving unregulated proliferation and impaired apoptosis of myeloid progenitor cells. CML has held a pivotal place in hematologic oncology, not only as one of the earliest described leukemias but also as a paradigm for molecularly targeted therapy.

Historically, CML was first clinically characterized in the 1840s through the pioneering work of David Craigie and John Hughes Bennett in Scotland, and independently by Rudolf Virchow in Germany. However, the disease's cytogenetic hallmark—the Philadelphia chromosome—was not discovered until 1960, when Peter Nowell and David Hungerford identified it as the first consistent chromosomal abnormality linked to cancer. This discovery laid the foundation for modern cancer cytogenetics and was later expanded with the elucidation of the BCR::ABL1 fusion transcript in the 1980s [1].

Epidemiologically, CML accounts for approximately 15–20% of adult leukemias [2]. The median age at diagnosis ranges from 55 to 65 years, with a higher prevalence in males (male-to-female ratio of approximately 1.3–1.7:1) [2]. Its global incidence is estimated at 1–2 cases per 100,000 population annually, with slightly lower rates reported in some Asian regions, including India, where studies suggest an incidence of 0.8–2.2 per 100,000 [3]. While ionizing radiation remains the only well-established environmental risk factor, most cases arise sporadically, without identifiable causative exposures. With the advent of tyrosine kinase inhibitors (TKIs), particularly imatinib, the therapeutic landscape of CML has transformed dramatically, converting what was once a uniformly fatal disease into a chronic, manageable condition for the vast majority of patients.

33.2 Clinical Features

Chronic myeloid leukemia (CML) most often presents in the chronic phase, during which up to 50% of patients are asymptomatic and diagnosed incidentally through routine blood counts. Among symptomatic individuals, clinical manifestations are generally nonspecific and reflect hypermetabolism or splenic involvement. Fatigue (34%), weight loss (20%), excessive sweating (15%), and early satiety or abdominal fullness (15%) are common presenting complaints [4]. These symptoms correlate with expanding disease burden and cytokine-mediated effects. Splenomegaly is a hallmark, reported in 48–76% of patients in case series, and may cause left upper quadrant pain, early satiety, or referred pain in the left shoulder due to diaphragmatic irritation. In some cases, sternal tenderness from active marrow expansion is present, and less commonly, acute gouty arthritis may result from hyperuricemia due to high cellular turnover. Thrombocytosis is frequently observed, but paradoxically, 21% of patients may experience bleeding symptoms attributable to qualitative platelet dysfunction. Bone pain is seen in approximately 7% of cases.

As CML progresses to the accelerated phase (AP) or blast phase (BP), clinical features shift significantly. AP is marked by increasing blasts (10–19%), worsening cytopenias or thrombocytosis refractory to therapy, progressive splenomegaly, and increasing basophilia. BP resembles acute leukemia, with >20% blasts in blood or marrow, and patients may present with constitutional symptoms, anemia, infections, and bleeding. Extramedullary involvement—including lymphadenopathy, skin, soft tissue masses, and central nervous system disease—is typically restricted to BP and indicates poor prognosis.

33.3 Diagnosis

Chronic phase chronic myeloid leukemia (CML-CP) is typified by marked leukocytosis, often exceeding 100,000/μL, with a full spectrum of granulocytic precursors visible in the peripheral blood. The "myelocyte bulge," wherein myelocytes surpass metamyelocytes in number, and a blast count under 2% are distinguishing features [5]. Basophilia is nearly universal, eosinophilia is present in the majority, and mild anemia and thrombocytosis are common; thrombocytopenia is atypical and should prompt reconsideration of the diagnosis.

Bone marrow examination reveals hypercellularity with prominent granulocytic proliferation and suppressed erythropoiesis, resulting in a myeloid:erythroid ratio that may exceed 20:1. Megakaryocytes are increased but characteristically small and hypolobated. Dysplasia is absent in the chronic phase but signals disease acceleration if present. While diagnosis can be confirmed with peripheral BCR::ABL1 testing, marrow evaluation remains critical for accurate disease staging and detection of fibrosis or advanced transformation. Bone marrow aspirate is also sent for cytogenetics to look for the defining translocation and also to look for additional chromosomal abnormalities. Also, bone marrow examination gives information on the grade of reticulin fibrosis, which has been associated with decreased major molecular response rate in the first year of tyrosine kinase inhibitor therapy.

Cytogenetically, the defining lesion is the t(9;22)(q34;q11.2) translocation generating the BCR::ABL1 fusion gene, most commonly producing a p210 transcript (e13a2/e14a2), with rarer variants such as p190 or p230 identified by RT-PCR [6]. Over 90% of cases show the Philadelphia chromosome by conventional karyotyping; cryptic rearrangements necessitate FISH or RT-PCR. Additional chromosomal abnormalities (ACAs), present in 10–15% at baseline, often indicate clonal evolution and may include trisomy 8, i(17q), extra Ph chromosomes, or 22q deletions. These ACAs confer a significantly elevated risk of progression and adverse outcomes independent of clinical risk scores [7]. Notably, integrating ACA status with tools like the ELTS score enhances prognostic precision. The identification of ACAs at diagnosis has assumed renewed relevance in the TKI era, necessitating routine cytogenetic analysis for all newly diagnosed patients.

33.4 Diagnostic Criteria

The diagnosis of CML is established by demonstrating:

- t(9;22)(q34;q11.2) via karyotyping or FISH, *and/or*
- *BCR::ABL1* fusion by RT-PCR from peripheral blood or bone marrow granulocytes

Peripheral blood is sufficient for diagnosis in typical CP cases, but bone marrow biopsy is required to define disease phase and assess for adverse features such as fibrosis or excess blasts. The presence of myeloid sarcoma or lymphoid aggregates may indicate blast phase.

33.5 Disease Phase Classification

Classification systems differ in their definitions of disease phases

- *International Consensus Classification (ICC)* [8]:
  - *Chronic Phase (CP):* No advanced-phase features.
  - *Accelerated Phase (AP):* One or more of the following: 10–19% blasts in blood/marrow, basophils ≥20%, or major additional chromosomal abnormalities (e.g., +8, i(17q), 3q26).
  - *Blast Phase (BP):* ≥20% blasts, myeloid sarcoma, or >5% lymphoblasts (confirmed by immunophenotyping).
- *WHO fifth Edition (WHO5)* [9]:
  - *Chronic Phase (CP):* Absence of blast phase features.
  - *Blast Phase (BP):* ≥20% blasts in blood/marrow, extramedullary blast proliferation (e.g., myeloid sarcoma), or increased lymphoblasts (no defined threshold).

Accurate phase classification guides therapy intensity and prognostication, particularly in the context of tyrosine kinase inhibitor (TKI) selection or consideration of hematopoietic stem cell transplantation.

33.6 Management of CML—CP

The treatment of CML has significantly improved over time. In the early days of the disease, the treatment was confined to cytoreductive agents such as busulfan and hydroxyurea, which targeted proliferative excess without affecting the underlying leukemogenic clone [10]. Busulfan, an alkylating agent, induced myelosuppression but led to unpredictable cytopenias and cumulative marrow damage. Hydroxyurea, by inhibiting ribonucleotide reductase, provided better hematologic control with fewer long-term toxicities and became the frontline therapy. However, both agents failed to induce cytogenetic remissions or alter the disease's natural trajectory toward blast crisis.

The introduction of interferon-alpha (IFN-α) in the 1980s marked a pivotal advance, as it demonstrated the capacity to induce partial and complete cytogenetic responses in a subset of patients (~15–25%) [11]. IFN-α exerted its anti-leukemic effects through both immunomodulatory and direct anti-proliferative actions, including modulation of MHC expression, suppression of BCR-ABL mRNA, and promotion of apoptosis. Additionally, IFNα, unlike TKI, preferentially targets CML stem cells. Combination therapy with low-dose cytarabine (Ara-C) showed synergistic effects in small studies. The Baccarani criteria were established during this period to stratify response to therapy. However, toxicity and variable tolerability limited its broader application. Median survival with IFN-α increased modestly compared to hydroxyurea (from ~3–5 years to ~6–7 years), but long-term cure remained elusive.

The molecular revolution in CML therapy began with the elucidation of the BCR-ABL fusion gene, a constitutively active tyrosine kinase resulting from the Philadelphia chromosome translocation t(9;22)(q34;q11). This discovery paved the way for targeted therapy. The first such agent, imatinib mesylate (Gleevec), a selective ATP-competitive inhibitor of the ABL tyrosine kinase domain, demonstrated unprecedented efficacy. The IRIS trial confirmed its superiority over IFN-α plus cytarabine, with 5-year overall survival of >85% and major cytogenetic response (MCyR) in >90% of patients [12]. Imatinib-induced deep molecular responses (MR3 or greater) became achievable and durable in the majority of chronic-phase patients. Trials of TKsI in newly diagnosed CML are tabulated below (Table 33.1).

Resistance to imatinib, due to point mutations in the ABL kinase domain (e.g., Y253H, E255K/V, T315I) or BCR-ABL gene amplification, led to the development of second-generation TKIs such as dasatinib (a dual ABL/SRC inhibitor) and nilotinib (a more potent ABL inhibitor with higher affinity). These agents achieved more rapid and deeper molecular responses and became first-line options, particularly in high-risk patients (Sokal, Hasford, or ELTS score). Subsequently, bosutinib and ponatinib were introduced, with ponatinib uniquely retaining activity against the T315I gatekeeper mutation. Each successive generation of TKI expanded the therapeutic landscape and allowed tailored therapy based on resistance mutation profiling via Sanger or next-generation sequencing (NGS).

Table 33.1 Landmark trial of tyrosine kinase inhibitor for newly diagnosed CML-CP

Trial name	TKI studied	Comparator	Phase	Response
IRIS (2003) [12]	Imatinib	IFN-α + Cytarabine	III	MCyR: 87%, MMR: 40% at 12 months;
DASISION (2010) [13]	Dasatinib	Imatinib	III	MMR: 46% vs. 28% at 12 months; CCyR at 12 months—77% vs. 66%, $P = 0.007$
ENESTnd (2010) [14]	Nilotinib (300 & 400 mg BID)	Imatinib	III	MMR: 44% (300 mg) vs. 22% at 12 months; lower progression to AP/BC
BFORE (2017) [15]	Bosutinib (400 mg QD)	Imatinib	III	MMR: 47% vs. 37% at 12 months; improved early molecular response rates
ASC4FIRST (2023) [16]	Asciminib (80 mg QD)	Investigator's choice (Imatinib, Nilotinib, Dasatinib, Bosutinib)	III	MMR at 48 weeks: 68.3% vs. 49.2%; superior efficacy with favorable safety profile

The current post-2020 era is witnessing the advent of next-generation ABL inhibitors (e.g., asciminib), which target the myristoyl pocket of ABL (STAMP inhibitor), representing a novel allosteric approach. Asciminib has demonstrated efficacy in patients with prior TKI failure, including T315I-positive cases. In parallel, there is renewed interest in combining TKIs with immunotherapies, BCL2 inhibitors (e.g., venetoclax), or autologous cell-based approaches to potentially eradicate leukemic stem cells and achieve a functional cure.

33.7 How to Choose First Line

The selection of a frontline tyrosine kinase inhibitor (TKI) in chronic myeloid leukemia (CML) is guided by multiple factors, including therapeutic goals, patient age, comorbid conditions, financial considerations, and the individual's CML risk stratification. The overarching objectives of treatment are to normalize life expectancy and, in selected cases, achieve a sustained deep molecular response (DMR)—defined as MR4 or MR4.5 maintained for several years—potentially allowing for treatment-free remission (TFR). While long-term survival benefits have been shown to be comparable between imatinib and second-generation TKIs in numerous randomized trials, this equivalence assumes optimal treatment adherence, early identification and management of resistance, and appropriate switching strategies. However, if the therapeutic aim is to expedite DMR and enable TFR, second-generation TKIs may offer an advantage due to their faster and deeper molecular responses. Therefore, in younger patients or those prioritizing TFR, second-generation agents may be preferred as initial therapy.

33.7.1 TKI Resistance

With the widespread use of commercially available tyrosine kinase inhibitors (TKIs) and the rising prevalence of chronic myeloid leukemia (CML), treatment resistance has become an increasingly important clinical challenge. Approximately 15%–25% of patients experience TKI intolerance after 10 years of therapy, which is the leading cause for switching TKIs [17]; however, intolerance can often be managed with dose modifications. True resistance occurs in about 10% of patients over the same period and is characterized by BCR::ABL1 transcript levels remaining above 1% at 12 months, loss of hematologic or cytogenetic responses, or disease progression.

Resistance is frequently driven by mutations in the BCR::ABL1 kinase domain (KD) that impair TKI binding and efficacy. Second-generation TKIs can overcome many imatinib-resistant mutations; however, certain mutations, notably the T315I "gatekeeper" mutation, confer resistance to all TKIs except ponatinib, asciminib, and olverembatinib. Therefore, mutation testing is critical to guide therapy selection, especially in patients with suboptimal response or disease progression.

Before diagnosing resistance, clinicians must evaluate patient adherence and potential drug interactions, as poor adherence—especially adherence below 90%—is strongly linked to reduced molecular responses and inferior clinical outcomes. Younger patients and those experiencing side effects or requiring dose escalations are particularly at risk for adherence challenges.

33.7.1.1 TKD Mutation Testing Methods [18]

- *Sanger Sequencing*: Traditional method with sensitivity around 10–20%, used widely to detect known and novel mutations.
- *Next-Generation Sequencing (NGS)*: Offers higher sensitivity (down to 1%) and the ability to detect low-level mutations and compound mutations.
- *When to Test*: Recommended at the time of treatment failure, suboptimal response, or progression to advanced phases.

33.7.1.2 Clinical Implications of Mutation Testing

- Identification of specific mutations helps tailor TKI therapy (e.g., ponatinib for T315I).
- Detecting compound or multiple mutations may predict a poorer prognosis and guide aggressive treatment or consideration of allogeneic stem cell transplantation.
- Monitoring emerging mutations allows for early intervention before overt clinical resistance develops.

33.8 Managing TKI Adverse Effects

Tyrosine kinase inhibitors (TKIs) have revolutionized the treatment of chronic myeloid leukemia (CML), but long-term therapy is often associated with a spectrum of adverse effects (AEs) that can impact adherence, quality of life, and clinical outcomes [19]. Effective management of these toxicities is crucial to maintaining therapy and achieving optimal responses. (Table 33.2).

Every TKI has the potential of causing cytopenia resulting in treatment interruption. Management of ANC drops to less than 1000/cumm and platelet count <50,000/cumm involves drug interruption, and once these parameters are improved, restarting the drug [20]. In case of recurrent cytopenia, dose reduction is advised. Some of the TKI-specific adverse effects are tabulated below.

Table 33.2 Adverse effects of TKIs and its management

Drug	Common adverse effects	Pathogenesis	Management
Imatinib	Leg cramps, fluid retention/edema, myelosuppression, rash, hepatotoxicity	Leg cramps: electrolyte imbalance, muscle toxicity; edema: capillary permeability; myelosuppression: bone marrow suppression; rash: hypersensitivity; hepatotoxicity: direct toxicity	Leg cramps: hydration, electrolytes (Mg, K), calcium channel blockers, stretching; Edema: diuretics, salt restriction; Myelosuppression: dose adjustment, G-CSF; Rash: topical steroids, antihistamines; Hepatotoxicity: monitor LFTs, dose adjustment
Dasatinib	Myelosuppression, pleural effusion, rash, hepatotoxicity, QT prolongation	Myelosuppression: bone marrow suppression; pleural effusion: vascular permeability; rash: hypersensitivity; hepatotoxicity: hepatocyte toxicity; QT prolongation: cardiac ion channel blockade	Myelosuppression: dose adjustment, G-CSF; pleural effusion: diuretics, steroids, drainage; rash: topical steroids; hepatotoxicity: LFT monitoring; QT prolongation: ECG monitoring, electrolyte correction
Nilotinib	Rash, myelosuppression, hepatotoxicity, pancreatitis, QT prolongation, cardiovascular events	Rash: hypersensitivity; myelosuppression: bone marrow toxicity; hepatotoxicity: hepatocyte damage; pancreatitis: pancreatic inflammation; QT prolongation: ion channel blockade; cardiovascular: endothelial/cardiac toxicity	Rash: topical steroids; myelosuppression: dose adjustment; hepatotoxicity: LFT monitoring; pancreatitis: discontinue drug; QT prolongation: ECG monitoring; cardiovascular: risk factor control, possible drug switch

(continued)

Table 33.2 (continued)

Drug	Common adverse effects	Pathogenesis	Management
Bosutinib	Diarrhea, myelosuppression, hepatotoxicity, rash	Gastrointestinal toxicity; bone marrow suppression; liver toxicity; hypersensitivity	Diarrhea: anti-diarrheal agents, hydration; myelosuppression: dose adjustment; hepatotoxicity: monitor LFTs; rash: topical treatments
Ponatinib	Myelosuppression, cardiovascular events, hepatotoxicity, rash	Bone marrow suppression; vascular toxicity causing thrombosis; hepatocyte toxicity; hypersensitivity	Cardiovascular: aggressive risk management, dose adjustment; myelosuppression: dose reduction; hepatotoxicity: monitor; Rash: topical therapy
Asciminib	Fatigue, headache, elevated lipase	Targets myristoyl pocket with fewer off-target effects; metabolic enzyme elevation	Supportive care, monitoring, dose adjustment if needed

33.9 Monitoring

Monitoring in chronic myeloid leukemia (CML) is essential for assessing treatment response, guiding therapeutic decisions, and identifying candidates for treatment-free remission (TFR). It involves sequential evaluation of hematologic, cytogenetic, and molecular responses. While hematologic and cytogenetic monitoring were foundational in the pre-TKI era, molecular monitoring using quantitative PCR for BCR::ABL1 transcripts (on the International Scale) is now the gold standard. Key milestones include achieving BCR::ABL1 $\leq$10% at 3 months (early molecular response) and $\leq$ 0.1% (major molecular response) by 12 months [21]. Sustained deep molecular responses (MR4 or MR4.5) are crucial for considering TFR. Regular and standardized monitoring enables early detection of suboptimal response or resistance, allowing timely therapeutic modifications. Table 33.3 highlights the basic monitoring parameters.

Table 33.3 Monitoring parameters for CML-CP

Type of monitoring	Parameter assessed	Response definition	Timepoints	Clinical significance
Hematologic	CBC, spleen size	Complete hematologic response (CHR): normalization of WBC, platelets, no blasts, no splenomegaly	Within 3 months of therapy	Indicator of initial disease control
Cytogenetic	% of Ph + metaphases in bone marrow (karyotyping/ FISH)	Complete cytogenetic response (CCyR): 0% Ph + metaphases Partial (PCyR): 1–35% Minor: 36–95%	Every 6–12 months (or earlier if PCR unavailable)	Surrogate for progression-free survival (PFS); largely supplanted by molecular monitoring
Molecular	BCR::ABL1 transcript levels (IS—International Scale)	Major molecular response (MMR): BCR::ABL1 $\leq$ 0.1% MR4: $\leq$ 0.01% MR4.5: $\leq$ 0.0032% Complete molecular response (CMR): undetectable BCR::ABL1	At 3, 6, 12 months, then every 3 months	Key marker for long-term disease control and eligibility for TFR
Early Molecular Response (EMR)	BCR::ABL1 at 3 and 6 months	Optimal: $\leq$10% at 3 months. Warning: >10%	3 and 6 months	Strong predictor of long-term outcomes; failure is associated with poor prognosis
Deep Molecular Response (DMR)	Sustained MR4 or deeper	$\geq$2 years of stable MR4 or MR4.5	After $\geq$2 years on TKI	Required for TKI discontinuation (TFR attempt)
Treatment-Free Remission (TFR)	Sustained molecular remission off TKI	BCR::ABL1 remains undetectable or below the MMR threshold without treatment	Post-TKI discontinuation (monitor monthly x6, then less frequent)	Emerging goal of therapy: ~40–60% can maintain TFR with careful selection

33.10 Role of HSCT in CML CP

Since the advent of BCR::ABL1 tyrosine kinase inhibitors (TKIs), the number of patients undergoing allo-HSCT for CML-CP in India has declined substantially. However, the overall burden of CML continues to rise, and approximately 1–2% of patients develop resistance to multiple TKIs annually, necessitating allo-HSCT [22]. In India, allo-HSCT retains a vital role, especially in patients with advanced phases of CML (AP/BP) or TKI resistance.

Cost considerations are paramount in India, where healthcare resources vary widely. While allo-HSCT can cost between $14,000 and $20,000 in India—significantly less than in Western countries—this remains a substantial financial burden for many patients [23]. Meanwhile, generic imatinib and other TKIs are available at much lower costs (around $40-50 per year), which has improved accessibility and long-term outcomes for many Indian patients. Nonetheless, for patients resistant to second- or third-generation TKIs, allo-HSCT is a potentially curative and cost-effective option in the Indian context, especially when TKI therapy costs escalate beyond affordability.

Pediatric CML in India accounts for a small but important subset of cases. Pediatric patients often present with advanced disease due to delayed diagnosis or limited access to specialized care. In this population, allo-HSCT remains a critical treatment modality, particularly when TKI intolerance or resistance occurs. Indian pediatric transplant centers report overall survival rates post-allo-HSCT in the range of 65–80%, which is comparable to international data. The long-term follow-up of children transplanted in India shows encouraging disease-free survival, although challenges such as donor availability, infections, and post-transplant care infrastructure remain. Given the potential toxicities of lifelong TKI therapy in growing children and adolescents, allo-HSCT is often considered earlier in suitable pediatric patients, balancing curative potential and quality of life [24].

Overall, in India, treatment decisions must weigh the cost and availability of TKIs versus allo-HSCT, patient age, disease phase, and socioeconomic factors. For many patients, particularly younger ones or those with TKI-resistant disease, allo-HSCT remains an essential curative approach.

33.11 Treatment Free Remission

Treatment-free remission (TFR) in chronic myeloid leukemia (CML) is an emerging and meaningful therapeutic goal that allows selected patients to discontinue tyrosine kinase inhibitors (TKIs) after achieving and maintaining a deep molecular response (DMR) [25]. Landmark clinical trials (Table 33.4) such as STIM, EURO-SKI, and ENESTfreedom have shown that 40–60% of eligible patients can sustain remission without ongoing therapy. The Latin American expert consensus reinforces these findings and provides region-specific guidance, emphasizing that TFR should only be attempted in patients in the first chronic phase of CML who have typical BCR-ABL1 transcripts (b3a2 or b2a2), no history of TKI resistance (though prior intolerance is acceptable), and consistent access to standardized, sensitive qPCR monitoring using the International Scale. Patients should have received TKI therapy for at least 5 years and must demonstrate stable MR^4.5 (BCR-ABL1 $\leq 0.0032\%$) sustained over at least 2 years, confirmed by four separate qPCR results over a 12-month period [25]. Although a high Sokal score is not an absolute contraindication, patients with such risk profiles should be counseled about the potentially higher risk of relapse.

Table 33.4 Trials of treatment-free remission

Trial name	TKI used	Eligibility (DMR duration)	Patients (n)	TFR success rate	Follow-up duration
STIM [26]	Imatinib	≥2 years MR4.5	100	~39% at 2 years	Median 77 months
EURO-SKI [27]	Imatinib	≥1 year MR4.5	755	~50% at 2 years	Median 24 months
ENESTfreedom [28]	Nilotinib	≥1 year MR4.5	215	~51.6% at 2 years	192 weeks
DASFREE [29]	Dasatinib	≥1 year MR4.5	84	~48% at 2 years	2 years
TRAD [30]	Imatinib	≥2 years MR4.5	54	~63% at 1 year	Median 20 months

Table 33.5 Disease criteria for trial of treatment-free remission

Criteria	Details
Chronic phase CML	No history of accelerated/blast phase
TKI therapy duration	≥5 years (ideally), with at least 3 years of sustained DMR
Molecular response	Deep molecular response (DMR), defined as MR^4 (BCR-ABL1 ≤ 0.01%) or MR^4.5, for ≥2 years
Molecular monitoring access	Reliable and frequent qRT-PCR testing available (<0.0032% sensitivity)
Adherence history	Good adherence and understanding of follow-up requirements

Successful TFR management requires meticulous molecular monitoring and psychosocial readiness (Table 33.5). Prior to TKI discontinuation, patients should undergo a comprehensive psychosocial assessment to ensure they understand the implications and are equipped to cope with potential relapse. Post-cessation, molecular relapse—defined as the loss of major molecular response (MMR, BCR-ABL1 > 0.1%)—typically occurs within the first 6 months, necessitating monthly qPCR during this period, followed by qPCR every 2–3 months for up to 1 year, and every 3 months thereafter indefinitely. Reinitiation of TKI therapy upon relapse usually results in rapid re-achievement of MMR or DMR, validating the safety of this approach when conducted under strict surveillance. TFR offers clear advantages, including reduced long-term toxicity, improved quality of life, and economic benefits. Ongoing research aims to enhance TFR success through better predictive markers—such as natural killer (NK) cell profiles or BCR-ABL1 transcript variants—and therapeutic strategies like immune modulation or induction of deeper molecular responses. Nonetheless, patients should be made aware that TFR does not equate to a cure and requires lifelong monitoring and clinical vigilance.

33.12 Management in Special Scenarios

33.12.1 *Pregnancy*

Antepartum Management

During pregnancy, especially in the first trimester, the use of tyrosine kinase inhibitors (TKIs) is generally avoided due to their potential teratogenic effects, with the risk being highest during organogenesis. A summary of various studies reporting the outcomes of pregnancy in patients who received TKIs during pregnancy has been tabulated in Table 33.6. In patients with chronic-phase CML and low leukemic burden, treatment can often be deferred or substituted with safer alternatives. Interferon-alpha (IFN-α) is the preferred agent during pregnancy, as it does not cross the placenta and is considered safe throughout gestation [31]. In situations with high white blood cell counts, hydroxyurea may be used briefly prior to conception or during the first trimester, balancing maternal benefit and fetal risk. Leukapheresis offers a non-pharmacologic option for urgent cytoreduction. After the first trimester, particularly if maternal disease control becomes inadequate, reintroduction of a TKI may be cautiously considered under close monitoring and after detailed counseling. Aspirin and low-molecular-weight heparin may be indicated in patients with marked thrombocytosis or leukocytosis to reduce thrombotic complications.

Table 33.6 Summary of tyrosine kinase inhibitor (TKI) exposure during pregnancy and associated outcomes

Study/Registry	TKIs studied/N	Exposure timing	Key adverse outcomes/anomalies	Clinical insights
Pye et al. (UK) [32]	Imatinib (*N* = 180)	Preconception/first trimester	~12% congenital anomalies: exencephaly, encephalocele, renal agenesis, skeletal malformations	Recommends stopping imatinib preconception; limited safety in early gestation
Conchon et al. (Brazil) [33]	Imatinib, Dasatinib (*N* = 12)	Variable	One case of fetal hydrops (dasatinib); 8 live births without anomalies	Advises TKI discontinuation prior to conception; dasatinib is at particularly high risk
Abruzzese et al. (Italy) [34]	Imatinib, Nilotinib (*N* = 40)	Mostly first trimester	~10% anomalies: hypospadias, cardiac defects, low-set ears	Supports IFN or leukapheresis as safer alternatives during pregnancy
EUTOS Registry [35]	Various TKIs (*N* > 300)	Any trimester	Anomalies mainly with first trimester exposure; no new safety signals post-organogenesis	Advocates planned conception; interferon is the safest option across all trimesters

Postpartum Management
Following delivery, patients with prior deep molecular response who experienced TKI cessation during pregnancy are closely monitored with frequent molecular testing. TKIs are typically reinitiated if there is any evidence of molecular relapse or loss of response. Breastfeeding is discouraged while on TKI therapy due to the risk of drug excretion into breast milk and potential neonatal exposure, although some reports suggest that short-term exposure may have minimal effects [31]. Women with CML considering future pregnancies are encouraged to achieve a stable deep molecular remission and plan conception in coordination with their care team, ensuring appropriate timing of TKI discontinuation and close follow-up.

Not much data is available on the use of ponatinib and asciminib during pregnancy.

33.13 Children

Chronic myeloid leukemia (CML) in children is rare, comprising approximately 2% of leukemias in children under 15 and 9% in adolescents aged 15–19 years [38]. The annual incidence is about 1 case per million in children and 2.2 per million in adolescents. Although pediatric CML has been hypothesized to differ biologically from adult disease, no definitive distinctions have been established.

Diagnosis in children mirrors that of adults: complete blood count, peripheral smear, and BCR-ABL1 testing via RT-PCR. However, prognostic scoring systems used in adults—such as Sokal, Hasford, and EUTOS—are not validated for pediatric use and are therefore not recommended for risk stratification in children, as per the Children's Oncology Group (COG).

33.13.1 Tyrosine Kinase Inhibitors (TKIs) in Pediatric CML

Imatinib was the first TKI approved for pediatric CP-CML. Dasatinib and nilotinib are now FDA-approved for use in children, with evidence favoring faster and deeper responses, though no survival benefit has yet been demonstrated [36]. Ponatinib remains investigational in children and is primarily considered for T315I-mutated cases, though safe pediatric dosing is undefined. Asciminib, a STAMP inhibitor, is under study in the ASC4KIDS trial, showing promising pharmacokinetic and safety results [37]. Table 33.7 shows the doses and approval years of TKIs in the pediatric population.

The choice of TKI therapy in children is largely extrapolated from adult data, but pediatric-specific concerns—particularly long-term toxicity—demand careful consideration. Active growth and hormonal development in children make them susceptible to unique adverse effects such as impaired linear growth and pubertal delay. Table 33.8 shows the specific adverse effects to be monitored in the pediatric population.

Table 33.7 TKIs doses and approval status in pediatric population [39]

TKI	Dosage	FDA approval year
Imatinib	340 mg/m^2 once daily	2003
Dasatinib	60 mg/m^2 once daily	2017
Nilotinib	230 mg/m^2 twice daily	2018
Bosutinib	300 mg/m^2 twice daily	Not approved
Ponatinib	25 mg/m^2 once daily	Not approved
Asciminib	1.3 mg/kg twice daily with food	Investigational

Table 33.8 System-specific adverse effects and monitoring

System	Potential adverse effects	Recommended monitoring and interventions
Linear growth	Growth deceleration Short stature	Serial measurement of height and weight at each clinical visit Calculate growth velocity and compare to age-appropriate norms Estimate predicted adult height using mid-parental height Endocrinology referral for growth hormone (GH) stimulation testing if indicated
Bone Health	Impaired bone remodeling Low bone mineral density Increased fracture risk	Consider DEXA scanning in cases of unexplained fractures or clinical/radiographic signs of osteopenia Assess serum calcium, phosphate, and 25-hydroxyvitamin D Refer to endocrinology for metabolic bone disease evaluation
Thyroid Function	Subclinical or overt hypothyroidism Less commonly, hyperthyroidism	Measure TSH and free T4 at baseline, every 4–6 weeks after therapy initiation, then every 6–12 months or as clinically indicated Refer to endocrinology for persistent dysfunction Initiate thyroid hormone replacement as needed
Pubertal Development	Delayed onset or progression of puberty Hypogonadism	Periodic Tanner staging to assess pubertal progression Evaluate gonadotropins (LH, FSH) and sex steroids (testosterone or estradiol) if delayed puberty or suspected gonadal dysfunction Refer to pediatric endocrinology as needed
Fertility	Impaired gonadal function Reduced fertility potential	Discuss fertility preservation prior to or during treatment, especially in pubertal males Offer sperm cryopreservation when appropriate
Pregnancy Considerations	Teratogenic risk in exposed pregnancies	Conduct pregnancy testing before initiation in females of reproductive age Provide contraceptive counseling In future adulthood, consider planned TKI discontinuation to allow for safer conception and pregnancy

The management of pediatric CML continues to evolve with newer agents like asciminib under evaluation. Pediatric-specific data and long-term safety monitoring are critical for optimizing outcomes while minimizing late toxicities.

33.14 Investigational Combination Therapies in Chronic Myeloid Leukemia (CML)

Although tyrosine kinase inhibitors (TKIs) have revolutionized CML management, they often fail to eradicate quiescent leukemic stem cells, which can lead to relapse after therapy discontinuation. To overcome this, novel combination therapies targeting both BCR::ABL1 and other survival pathways are under investigation.

33.14.1 Dasatinib Plus Venetoclax [40]

Venetoclax, a BCL-2 inhibitor, was combined with dasatinib in clinical trials to enhance apoptosis in resistant CML stem cells. Among 65 patients treated with dasatinib 50 mg daily plus venetoclax added after 3 months, molecular response rates (MMR 86%, MR4 53%, MR4.5 45% at 12 months) were similar to dasatinib monotherapy, with excellent 4-year event-free and overall survival. However, improvements in durable deep molecular responses (DMR) and treatment-free remission (TFR) remain uncertain.

33.14.2 Decitabine Combinations [41]

Decitabine, a hypomethylating agent, has shown activity in advanced-phase CML as monotherapy and combined with TKIs. A phase I/II trial combining decitabine and dasatinib in accelerated or blast phase CML demonstrated major hematologic response rates of 48% and a median overall survival of 13.8 months. Oral decitabine/cedazuridine (ASTX727) plus low-dose dasatinib (50 mg/day) is currently being studied in newly diagnosed chronic phase CML.

33.14.3 Other Combination Approaches

Several trials are exploring agents to deepen molecular responses and target leukemic stem cells, including pegylated interferon-alpha (IFN-α), JAK2 inhibitors, immune checkpoint inhibitors, and dendritic cell vaccines. The TIGER trial demonstrated that nilotinib combined with pegylated IFN-α improved molecular remission rates and 2-year TFR compared to nilotinib alone, but at the cost of increased adverse events [42]. Addition of the JAK1/2 inhibitor ruxolitinib to TKIs showed promising increases in deep molecular responses in patients with residual disease.

33.15 Management of CML: Advanced Phase

Advanced-phase chronic myeloid leukemia (CML), which includes the accelerated phase (AP) and blast phase (BP), is associated with significantly poorer outcomes compared to chronic phase (CP). Initial treatment in CML-AP and CML-BP typically involves tyrosine kinase inhibitors (TKIs), with newer generation TKIs such as dasatinib or ponatinib preferred over imatinib due to better efficacy in advanced disease. The goal is to reduce disease burden and prepare patients for early allogeneic hematopoietic stem cell transplantation (allo-HSCT), the only curative option in these phases.

Combination therapy using TKIs plus chemotherapy achieves response rates of approximately 40% in myeloid (non-lymphoid) blast phase and 70–80% in lymphoid blast phase CML. Despite this, the median survival remains limited to 6–12 months for myeloid BP and 12–24 months for lymphoid BP. Allo-HSCT after achieving remission improves long-term survival; reported survival rates post-transplant are around 15–40% in accelerated phase and 10–20% in blast phase patients.

In patients with CML-AP evolving from CP, the median survival is less than 3 years, while de novo CML-AP patients have significantly better outcomes, with an estimated 8-year survival of 60–80%. However, survival in the accelerated phase remains inferior to chronic phase, even for high-risk chronic phase patients, where 10-year overall survival (OS) rates were reported as 56% for de novo AP vs. 69% for high-risk CP.

The presence of additional cytogenetic abnormalities (ACAs), particularly the 3q26/MECOM translocation, indicates a very poor prognosis and demands urgent consideration of allo-HSCT [43, 44]. Genetic mutations outside the BCR::ABL1 kinase domain, notably ASXL1 mutations, are found in up to 40% of AP and 13% of CP patients and correlate with poor response and increased risk of progression. Patients harboring ASXL1 mutations tend to have lower rates of molecular response and more frequent TKI interruptions due to myelosuppression.

The current optimal strategy for CML-BP involves combining intensive chemotherapy (e.g., FLAG-IDA) with ponatinib, followed by allo-HSCT once complete remission is achieved, then followed by TKI maintainence post transplant [44]. De novo accelerated phase patients who achieve an optimal response (complete cytogenetic response with BCR::ABL1 < 1% by 6 months) on second-generation TKIs may continue on indefinite TKI therapy. Others, including those with evolved AP or BP, are candidates for allo-HSCT.

Overall, advanced-phase CML management hinges on potent TKIs, chemotherapy as appropriate, and timely allo-HSCT, with molecular and cytogenetic factors guiding prognosis and therapeutic decisions. Long-term survival remains limited, underscoring the need for continued research into novel approaches.

33.16 Illustrative Clinical Case

A 10-year-old girl presented with progressive abdominal distention and generalized weakness. Clinical examination revealed splenomegaly extending 6 cm below the left costal margin. Peripheral blood counts showed marked leukocytosis with a left shift and basophilia. Molecular testing confirmed the presence of the BCR::ABL1 fusion transcript (p210 isoform), establishing the diagnosis of chronic-phase CML. At the time of diagnosis, imatinib was the only approved tyrosine kinase inhibitor (TKI) for pediatric patients, and therapy was initiated accordingly. However, due to failure to achieve molecular remission, she was transitioned to dasatinib. Subsequent mutation analysis (IMRA) identified the presence of a T315I mutation, prompting a switch to ponatinib, the only TKI effective against this resistant clone. Despite this, her BCR::ABL1 transcript levels remained >10%, indicating suboptimal molecular response. She is currently 27 years old and being treated with a combination of asciminib and ponatinib, yet her BCR::ABL1 level remains persistently elevated at 7%, reflecting a highly refractory disease course. This case underscores the therapeutic challenges and limited treatment options in pediatric CML with T315I mutation, and highlights the emerging role of combination TKI strategies in such difficult-to-treat scenarios.

33.17 Conclusion

The management of chronic myeloid leukemia (CML) has undergone a paradigm shift with the introduction of tyrosine kinase inhibitors (TKIs), transforming what was once a fatal disease into a chronic, controllable condition. Newer-generation TKIs have improved molecular response rates and outcomes but also bring unique adverse effect profiles, posing fresh clinical challenges beyond those seen with imatinib. Special populations—particularly pregnant and lactating women—continue to pose therapeutic dilemmas, as no TKI is approved in this setting, and interferon-alpha remains the only safe option. While international trials have explored combination TKI strategies, monotherapy remains the standard, as combination approaches have not demonstrated a clear benefit.

In the Indian context, accessibility, affordability, and long-term compliance continue to influence treatment decisions significantly. The widespread implementation of treatment-free remission (TFR) remains limited due to logistical challenges, the cost of serial molecular monitoring, and a lack of awareness or structured national protocols. There is a need for robust Indian data on TFR, mutation-guided therapy, and adverse event monitoring in diverse real-world settings. Tailored strategies that balance efficacy, safety, and socio-economic feasibility will be crucial in improving long-term outcomes for CML patients in India.

References

1. Goldman JM. Chronic myeloid leukemia: a historical perspective. Semin Hematol. 2010;47(4):302–11. https://doi.org/10.1053/j.seminhematol.2010.07.001.
2. Siegel RL, Miller KD, Jemal A. Cancer statistics, 2015. CA Cancer J Clin. 2015;65(1):5–29. https://doi.org/10.3322/caac.21254.
3. Ganesan P, Kumar L. Chronic myeloid leukemia in India. J Glob Oncol. 2016;3(1):64–71. Published 2016 Jul 20. https://doi.org/10.1200/JGO.2015.002667.
4. Savage DG, Szydlo RM, Goldman JM. Clinical features at diagnosis in 430 patients with chronic myeloid leukaemia seen at a referral centre over a 16-year period. Br J Haematol. 1997;96(1):111–6. https://doi.org/10.1046/j.1365-2141.1997.d01-1982.x.
5. Spiers AS, Bain BJ, Turner JE. The peripheral blood in chronic granulocytic leukaemia. Study of 50 untreated Philadelphia-positive cases. Scand J Haematol. 1977;18(1):25–38.
6. Baccarani M, Castagnetti F, Gugliotta G, et al. The proportion of different BCR-ABL1 transcript types in chronic myeloid leukemia. An international overview. Leukemia. 2019;33(5):1173–83. https://doi.org/10.1038/s41375-018-0341-4.
7. Hehlmann R, Lauseker M, Voskanyan A, et al. Impact of emerging ACA on survival in chronic myeloid leukemia (CML). Leukemia. 2022;36:2544–7. https://doi.org/10.1038/s41375-022-01681-3.
8. Gianelli U, Thiele J, Orazi A, et al. International consensus classification of myeloid and lymphoid neoplasms: myeloproliferative neoplasms. Virchows Arch. 2023;482(1):53–68. https://doi.org/10.1007/s00428-022-03480-8.
9. Khoury JD, Solary E, Abla O, et al. The 5th edition of the World Health Organization classification of haematolymphoid tumours: myeloid and histiocytic/dendritic neoplasms. Leukemia. 2022;36(7):1703–19. https://doi.org/10.1038/s41375-022-01613-1.
10. Hehlmann R, Heimpel H, Hasford J, et al. Randomized comparison of busulfan and hydroxyurea in chronic myelogenous leukemia: prolongation of survival by hydroxyurea. The German CML Study Group. Blood. 1993;82(2):398–407.
11. Talpaz M, Hehlmann R, Quintás-Cardama A, Mercer J, Cortes J. Re-emergence of interferon-α in the treatment of chronic myeloid leukemia. Leukemia. 2013;27(4):803–12. https://doi.org/10.1038/leu.2012.313.
12. O'Brien SG, Deininger MW. Imatinib in patients with newly diagnosed chronic-phase chronic myeloid leukemia. Semin Hematol. 2003;40(2 Suppl 2):26–30. https://doi.org/10.1053/shem.2003.50058.
13. Kantarjian HM, Shah NP, Cortes JE, et al. Dasatinib or imatinib in newly diagnosed chronic-phase chronic myeloid leukemia: 2-year follow-up from a randomized phase 3 trial (DASISION). Blood. 2012;119(5):1123–9. https://doi.org/10.1182/blood-2011-08-376087.
14. Giles FJ, Rosti G, Beris P, et al. Nilotinib is superior to imatinib as first-line therapy of chronic myeloid leukemia: the ENESTnd study. Expert Rev Hematol. 2010;3(6):665–73. https://doi.org/10.1586/ehm.10.61.
15. Cortes JE, Gambacorti-Passerini C, Deininger MW, et al. Bosutinib versus Imatinib for newly diagnosed chronic myeloid leukemia: results from the randomized BFORE trial. J Clin Oncol. 2018;36(3):231–7. https://doi.org/10.1200/JCO.2017.74.7162.

16. Cortes JE, Hochhaus A, Takahashi N, et al. Asciminib monotherapy for newly diagnosed chronic myeloid leukemia in chronic phase: the ASC4FIRST phase III trial. Future Oncol. 2022;18(38):4161–70. https://doi.org/10.2217/fon-2022-0923.
17. Haddad FG, Kantarjian H. Navigating the management of chronic phase CML in the era of generic BCR::ABL1 tyrosine kinase inhibitors. J Natl Compr Cancer Netw. 2024;22(1):e237116.
18. Soverini S. Resistance mutations in CML and how we approach them. Hematology Am Soc Hematol Educ Program. 2023;2023(1):469–75. https://doi.org/10.1182/hematology.2023000447.
19. Bauer S, Comer H, Ramsey B, Thomas K. Management of adverse events associated with tyrosine kinase inhibitor use in adult patients with chronic myeloid leukemia in chronic phase: an advanced practice perspective. J Adv Pract Oncol. 2021;12(5):521–33. https://doi.org/10.6004/jadpro.2021.12.5.7.
20. Steegmann JL, Baccarani M, Breccia M, et al. European LeukemiaNet recommendations for the management and avoidance of adverse events of treatment in chronic myeloid leukaemia. Leukemia. 2016;30(8):1648–71. https://doi.org/10.1038/leu.2016.104.
21. Shanmuganathan N, Hughes TP. Molecular monitoring in CML: how deep? How often? How should it influence therapy? Hematology Am Soc Hematol Educ Program. 2018;2018(1):168–76. https://doi.org/10.1182/asheducation-2018.1.168.
22. Elmakaty I, Saglio G, Al-Khabori M, et al. The contemporary role of hematopoietic stem cell transplantation in the management of chronic myeloid leukemia: is it the same in all settings? Cancers (Basel). 2024;16(4):754. Published 2024 Feb 12. https://doi.org/10.3390/cancers16040754.
23. Sharma SK, Choudhary D, Gupta N, et al. Cost of hematopoietic stem cell transplantation in India. Mediterr J Hematol Infect Dis. 2014;6(1):e2014046. Published 2014 Jul 1. https://doi.org/10.4084/MJHID.2014.046.
24. Andolina JR, Neudorf SM, Corey SJ. How I treat childhood CML. Blood. 2012;119(8):1821–30. https://doi.org/10.1182/blood-2011-10-380774.
25. Pavlovsky C, Abello Polo V, Pagnano K, et al. Treatment-free remission in patients with chronic myeloid leukemia: recommendations of the LALNET expert panel. Blood Adv. 2021;5(23):4855–63. https://doi.org/10.1182/bloodadvances.2020003235.
26. Mahon FX, Réa D, Guilhot J, et al. Discontinuation of imatinib in patients with chronic myeloid leukaemia who have maintained complete molecular remission for at least 2 years: the prospective, multicentre Stop Imatinib (STIM) trial. Lancet Oncol. 2010;11(11):1029–35. https://doi.org/10.1016/S1470-2045(10)70233-3.
27. Mahon FX, Pfirrmann M, Dulucq S, et al. European stop tyrosine kinase inhibitor trial (EURO-SKI) in chronic myeloid leukemia: final analysis and novel prognostic factors for treatment-free remission. J Clin Oncol. 2024;42(16):1875–80. https://doi.org/10.1200/JCO.23.01647.
28. Hochhaus A, Masszi T, Giles FJ, et al. Treatment-free remission following frontline nilotinib in patients with chronic myeloid leukemia in chronic phase: results from the ENESTfreedom study. Leukemia. 2017;31(7):1525–31. https://doi.org/10.1038/leu.2017.63.
29. Shah NP, García-Gutiérrez V, Jiménez-Velasco A, et al. Dasatinib discontinuation in patients with chronic-phase chronic myeloid leukemia and stable deep molecular response: the DASFREE study. Leuk Lymphoma. 2020;61(3):650–9. https://doi.org/10.1080/10428194.2019.1675879.
30. Perusini MA, Novitzky-Basso I, Atenafu EG, et al. Final report of TKI discontinuation trial with dasatinib for the second attempt of treatment-free remission after failing the first attempt with imatinib: Treatment-free Remission Accomplished by Dasatinib (TRAD) study. Br J Haematol. 2023;203(5):781–91. https://doi.org/10.1111/bjh.19058.
31. Robertson HF, Apperley JF. Treatment of CML in pregnancy. Hematology Am Soc Hematol Educ Program. 2022;2022(1):123–8. https://doi.org/10.1182/hematology.2022000330.
32. Pye SM, Cortes J, Ault P, et al. The effects of imatinib on pregnancy outcome. Blood. 2008;111(12):5505–8. https://doi.org/10.1182/blood-2007-10-114900.

33. Conchon M, Sanabani SS, Serpa M, et al. Successful pregnancy and delivery in a patient with chronic myeloid leukemia while on Dasatinib therapy. Adv Hematol. 2010;2010:136252. https://doi.org/10.1155/2010/136252.
34. Abruzzese E, Aureli S, Bondanini F, et al. Chronic myeloid leukemia and pregnancy: when dreams meet reality. State of the art, management and outcome of 41 cases, Nilotinib placental transfer. J Clin Med. 2022;11(7):1801. Published 2022 Mar 24. https://doi.org/10.3390/jcm11071801.
35. Chelysheva E, Apperley J, Turkina A, et al. Chronic myeloid leukemia diagnosed in pregnancy: management and outcome of 87 patients reported to the European LeukemiaNet international registry [published correction appears in Leukemia. 2024;38(11):2514. 10.1038/s41375-024-02412-6.]. Leukemia 2024;38(4):788–795. https://doi.org/10.1038/s41375-024-02183-0.
36. Ata F, Benkhadra M, Ghasoub R, et al. Tyrosine kinase inhibitors in pediatric chronic myeloid leukemia: a focused review of clinical trials. Front Oncologia. 2023;13:1285346. Published 2023 Dec 20. https://doi.org/10.3389/fonc.2023.1285346.
37. Hijiya N, Mauro MJ. Asciminib in the treatment of Philadelphia chromosome-positive chronic myeloid leukemia: focus on patient selection and outcomes. Cancer Manag Res. 2023;15:873–91. Published 2023 Aug 23. https://doi.org/10.2147/CMAR.S353374.
38. Ries LAG, Smith M, Gurney JG, et al. Cancer incidence and survival among children and adolescents: United States SEER program 1975–1995. In: National Cancer Institute, vol. 99. Bethesda, MD: SEER Program; 1999. p. 46–9.
39. Carofiglio F, Lopalco A, Lopedota A, et al. Bcr-Abl tyrosine kinase inhibitors in the treatment of pediatric CML. Int J Mol Sci. 2020;21(12):4469. Published 2020 Jun 23. https://doi.org/10.3390/ijms21124469.
40. Jabbour E, Haddad FG, Sasaki K, et al. Combination of dasatinib and venetoclax in newly diagnosed chronic phase chronic myeloid leukemia. Cancer. 2024;130(15):2652–9. https://doi.org/10.1002/cncr.35317.
41. Abaza Y, Kantarjian H, Alwash Y, et al. Phase I/II study of dasatinib in combination with decitabine in patients with accelerated or blast phase chronic myeloid leukemia. Am J Hematol. 2020;95(11):1288–95. https://doi.org/10.1002/ajh.25939.
42. Hochhaus A, Burchert A, Saußele S, et al. S157: Nilotinib vs. Nilotinib + peg-interferon αlpha induction and Nilotinib or peg-interferon αlpha maintenance therapy for newly diagnosed chronic myeloid leukemia patients. The Tiger trial. Hemasphere. 2023;7(Suppl):e4695659. Published 2023 Aug 8. https://doi.org/10.1097/01.HS9.0000967540.46956.59.
43. Haddad FG, Sasaki K, Issa GC, Jabbour E, Kantarjian H. The presence of additional cytogenetic abnormalities (ACAs) or Philadelphia chromosome variants do not adversely affect the achievement of treatment-free remission in chronic myeloid leukemia. Am J Hematol. 2024;99(6):1175–6. https://doi.org/10.1002/ajh.27307.
44. Copland M. Treatment of blast phase chronic myeloid leukaemia: a rare and challenging entity. Br J Haematol. 2022;199(5):665–78. https://doi.org/10.1111/bjh.18370.

Chapter 34
NonBCR: ABL MPN: Diagnosis, Risk Stratification, and Management

Bhushan Asthana, Pawan Kumar Singh, Shilpi Saxena, and Isha Gambhir

Abstract BCR::ABL1-negative myeloproliferative neoplasms (MPNs) are a heterogeneous group of clonal hematopoietic disorders characterized by excessive myeloid proliferation. The classical *BCR::ABL1*-negative MPN subtypes include polycythemia vera (PV), essential thrombocythemia (ET), and primary myelofibrosis (PMF). The others are chronic neutrophilic leukemia (CNL), chronic eosinophilic leukemia (CEL), and juvenile myelomonocytic leukemia (JMML). Recent advancements in molecular genetics and diagnostic techniques have refined the classification, risk stratification, and management of these disorders.

The 2022 World Health Organization (WHO) and International Consensus Classification (ICC) updates emphasize the integration of clinical, morphological, and molecular criteria in MPN diagnosis. Molecular testing plays a pivotal role with JAK2, CALR, and MPL mutations serving as key diagnostic markers on one hand, while emerging non-driver mutations (e.g., ASXL1, SRSF2, U2AF1Q157) influencing prognosis on the other.

Risk stratification has evolved with the development of novel prognostic models, such as the Mutation-Enhanced International Prognostic Scoring System (MIPSS70+ v2.0) and the Genetically Inspired Prognostic Scoring System (GIPSS) for PMF, which integrate genetic and clinical factors to refine outcome predictions. For ET and PV, thrombotic risk assessment remains crucial for therapeutic decision-making, with treatment strategies planned based on molecular and clinical risk factors.

The primary goal of treatment in MPN is to prevent the thrombotic complications and symptom control and not to modify the outcome of the disease, except in some cases where allogenic BMT is resorted to cure the disease and prevent leukemic transformation.

B. Asthana (✉)
Army Medical Corps, Military Hospital Shillong, Shillong, Meghalaya, India

P. K. Singh · I. Gambhir
Hematology & BMT, Yatharth Group of Hospitals, Noida, Uttar Pradesh, India

S. Saxena
Command Hospital, Panchkula, Haryana, India

H. P. Pati et al. (eds.), *Clinical Hematology and Hemato-Oncology*,
https://doi.org/10.1007/978-981-92-1167-8_34

This chapter presents a case-based discussion of recent updates in diagnostic criteria, molecular profiling, risk stratification models, and treatment algorithms for BCR::ABL1-negative MPNs, highlighting their clinical implications and future directions. The integration of next-generation sequencing, emerging biomarkers, and targeted therapies holds promise for improved disease classification, prognostication, and personalized treatment approaches.

Keywords BCR::ABL1-negative myeloproliferative neoplasms · Polycythemia vera · Essential thrombocythemia · Primary myelofibrosis · Risk stratification

Learning Objectives
At the end of reading the chapter, the reader should be able to:

1. Understand the classification of BCR::ABL1-negative MPNs.
2. Diagnostic criteria for BCR::ABL1-negative MPNs, highlighting the role of molecular and genetic testing in these disorders.
   - Discuss clinical, hematological, morphological, and molecular features.
   - The importance of driver mutations (JAK2, CALR, MPL) and other genetic markers,
   - Recognize the emerging role of high-throughput sequencing and next--generation molecular diagnostics in classifying these disorders.
3. Understand risk stratification models in MPNs.
   - Describe thrombotic risk stratification in PV and ET.
   - International prognostic scoring systems (IPSS, DIPSS, MIPSS70+, GIPSS) for PMF.
   - Highlight the significance of genetic risk factors (e.g., ASXL1, SRSF2, U2AF1 mutations) in governing prognosis.
4. Application of current knowledge to clinical scenarios to improve outcomes.
   - Adopt a systematic approach to diagnosing MPNs, while appreciating the need to follow up those cases.
   - Interpret risk stratification models as a guide for prognosis and treatment-related decisions.
   - Identify suitable treatment modalities for these patients to benefit from interventions such as cytoreductive therapy, JAK inhibitors, or stem cell transplantation.

34.1 Introduction

BCR::ABL1-negative myeloproliferative neoplasms (MPNs), a diverse group of hematological neoplasms, encompass a spectrum of hematologic disorders resulting from clonal proliferation of myeloid cells. The classical *BCR::ABL1*-negative MPN subtypes include polycythemia vera (PV), essential thrombocythemia (ET), and primary myelofibrosis (PMF), while others are chronic neutrophilic leukemia (CNL), chronic eosinophilic leukemia (CEL), myeloproliferative neoplasm, unclassifiable (MPN-U), and juvenile myelomonocytic leukemia (JMML). Recent advancements offering refined diagnostic criteria and risk stratification methods have enhanced our understanding and management approaches towards these disorders. With the incorporation of genetic and molecular findings in these neoplasms, further refinement of risk stratification and prognosis is possible. In ET and PV, risk stratification primarily focuses on thrombotic risk; whereas in PMF, it centers around the likelihood of disease progression and overall survival. In this chapter, the case-based approach and risk stratification of various BCR::ABL1-negative MPNs are discussed.

34.2 Diagnosis

The 2016 revision of the World Health Organization (WHO) classification introduced updated diagnostic criteria for MPNs [1] which emphasized the integration of clinical features, bone marrow morphology, and molecular studies. For instance, the presence of Janus Kinase 2 (JAK2), Calreticulin (CALR), or Myeloproliferative Leukemia (MPL) mutations is defined as the driver mutation for MPN and plays a pivotal role in confirming diagnoses. JAK2 (V617F) mutations are found in more than 96% of PV patients, while CALR exon 9 insertions or deletions are present in about 20%–25% of ET patients [2, 3]. Triple-negative ET is found in less than 15% of all ET cases, and triple-negative PMF (TN-PMF) is less than 20% of all PMF cases [4, 5].

In WHO 2022 classification, the following refinements were made in the previous classification:

(a) Inclusion of JMML under the MPN category [6].
(b) Determination of red cell mass deleted from diagnostic criterion of PV.
(c) Changes incorporated in the diagnostic criteria of CEL:
    (i) The time interval for defining sustained hypereosinophilia reduced from 6 months (24 weeks) to 4 weeks.
    (ii) Inclusion of both clonality and abnormal bone marrow morphology (e.g., megakaryocytic or erythroid dysplasia) as an essential diagnostic criteria.
    (iii) Elimination of increased blasts {($\geq$2% in peripheral blood (PB) or 5–19% in bone marrow (BM)} as an alternative to clonality.

The ICC 2022 criteria closely align with the WHO 2022 classification, with a few modifications [7].

A comparative update in the diagnostic criteria for BCR-ABL1-negative MPNs, as mentioned in WHO 2022 and ICC 2022, is presented in Table 34.1.

JMML has been included in the category of MPN under the WHO 2022 classification, with the following defining criteria:

Table 34.1 Diagnostic criteria for BCR-ABL1–negative MPNs according to WHO 2022 and ICC 2022 classifications

Category	WHO 2022 [6] diagnostic criteria	ICC 2022 [7] diagnostic criteria
PV	Major criteria 1. Hemoglobin concentration >16.5 g/dL (men), >16 g/dL (women), or elevated hematocrit (HCT)# >49% in men & >48% in women. 2. BM biopsy showing age-adjusted hypercellularity with trilineage growth (panmyelosis), including prominent erythroid, granulocytic, and megakaryocytic lineages with pleomorphic mature megakaryocytes*. 3. Presence of JAK2V617F or JAK2 exon 12 mutation Minor criteria: 1. Subnormal serum erythropoietin (EPO) level Diagnosis: Requires the presence of all three major criteria or the first two major criteria plus the minor criterion #HCT for diagnosis in the presence of JAK2 mutation. *BM biopsy may not be required in patients with sustained absolute erythrocytosis: (hemoglobin >18.5 g/dL in men or >16.5 g/dL in women or HCT values of >55.5% in men or >49.5% in women) If JAK2 V617F or JAK2 exon 12 mutation and the minor criteria are present.	Major criteria 1. Hemoglobin >16.5 g/dL in men or >16.0 g/dL in women or HCT >49% in men or >48% in women or red blood cell mass >25% above mean normal predicted value 2. BM biopsy showing age-adjusted hypercellularity with trilineage proliferation (panmyelosis), including prominent erythroid, granulocytic, and an increase in pleomorphic, mature megakaryocytes without atypia* 3. Presence of JAK2 V617F or JAK2 exon 12 mutation** Minor criteria 1. Subnormal serum erythropoietin level Diagnosis: Requires the presence of all three major criteria or the first two major criteria plus the minor criterion. *BM biopsy may not be required in patients with sustained absolute erythrocytosis: (hemoglobin >18.5 g/dL in men or >16.5 g/dL in women and HCT values of >55.5% in men or >49.5% in women) and the presence of a JAK2 V617F or JAK2 exon 12 mutation. However, initial MF (present in as many as 20% of patients) can only be detected by BM, and this finding may predict a more rapid progression to overt myelofibrosis (post-PV myelofibrosis). **It is recommended to use highly sensitive assays for JAK2 V617F with a sensitivity level <1% and CALR and MPL with sensitivity levels 1–3%. In negative cases, consider searching for non-canonical JAK2 mutations

Post-PV MF	Required criteria 1. Previously established diagnosis of PV 2. BM fibrosis of grade 2 or 3 Additional criteria: 1. Anemia (i.e., below the reference range given age, sex, and altitude considerations) Or Sustained loss of requirement of either phlebotomy (in the absence of cytoreductive therapy) or cytoreductive treatment for erythrocytosis 2. Leukoerythroblastosis 3. Spleen enlargement greater than 5 cm from baseline or development of newly palpable splenomegaly 4. Development of any two (or all three) of the following constitutional symptoms: > 10% weight loss in 6 months, Night sweats, Unexplained fever (>37.5 °C) Diagnosis: All required criteria plus at least two additional criteria are necessary to determine the post-PV MF	Required criteria 1. Previous established diagnosis of PV 2. BM fibrosis of grade 2 or 3 Additional criteria 1. Anemia (i.e., hemoglobin below the reference range adjusted for age, sex, and altitude or sustained absence of phlebotomy requirement, in the absence of cytoreductive treatment for erythrocytosis) 2. Leukoerythroblastosis 3. Increase in palpable splenomegaly of >5 cm from baseline or the development of a newly palpable splenomegaly 4. Development of any two (or all three) of the following constitutional symptoms: >10% weight loss in 6 months Night sweats Unexplained fever (>37.5 °C) Diagnosis: requires meeting all the required criteria and at least two additional criteria

(continued)

Table 34.1 (continued)

Category	WHO 2022 [6] diagnostic criteria	ICC 2022 [7] diagnostic criteria
ET	Major criteria 1. Platelet count >450 × 10^9/L 2. BM biopsy showing proliferation mainly of the megakaryocytic lineage, with increased numbers of enlarged, mature megakaryocytes with hyperlobulated staghorn-like nuclei, infrequently dense clusters; no significant increase or left shift in neutrophil granulopoiesis or erythropoiesis; no relevant BM fibrosis 3. Diagnostic criteria for BCR-ABL1-positive CML, PV, PMF, or other myeloid neoplasms are not met 4. JAK2, CALR, or MPL Mutation present Minor criteria: Presence of a clonal marker or absence of evidence of reactive thrombocytosis Diagnosis requires either all major criteria or the first 3 major criteria plus the minor criteria	Major criteria 1. Platelet count ≥450 × 10^9/L 2. BM biopsy showing proliferation mainly of the megakaryocytic lineage, with increased numbers of enlarged, mature megakaryocytes with hyperlobulated staghorn-like nuclei, infrequently dense clusters; no significant increase or left shift in neutrophil granulopoiesis or erythropoiesis; no relevant BM fibrosis 3. Diagnostic criteria for *BCR::ABL1*-positive CML, PV, PMF, or other myeloid neoplasms are not met 4. *JAK2*, *CALR*, or *MPL* mutation Minor criteria Presence of a clonal marker or absence of evidence of reactive thrombocytosis Diagnosis requires either all major criteria or the first 3 major criteria plus the minor criteria
Post ET MF	Required criteria: 1. Prior documentation of WHO-defined ET 2. BM fibrosis grade ≥ 2 Additional criteria: 1. Anemia and a ≥ 2 g/dL decrease in hemoglobin from baseline 2. Leukoerythroblastic blood smear 3. Increasing palpable splenomegaly of >5 cm from baseline or new palpable splenomegaly 4. Increased serum lactate dehydrogenase (LDH) 5. Development of constitutional symptoms: (a) >10% weight loss in 6 months, (b) Night sweats, (c) Unexplained fever (>37.5 °C) Diagnosis: requires either both of the required criteria or at least two additional criteria	Required criteria: 1. Previously established diagnosis of ET 2. BM fibrosis of grade 2 or 3 Additional criteria: 1. Anemia (i.e., below the reference range for given age, sex, and altitude) and a > 2 g/dL decrease from the baseline hemoglobin concentration 2. Leukoerythroblastosis 3. Increase in palpable splenomegaly of >5 cm from baseline or the development of a newly palpable splenomegaly 4. Elevated LDH level 5. Development of any 2 (or all 3) of the following constitutional symptoms:>10%weight loss in 6 months, night sweats, unexplained fever (>37.5 °C) Diagnosis: All required criteria plus at least two additional criteria

Pre PMF	Major criteria 1. BM biopsy showing megakaryocytic proliferation and atypia, without reticulin fibrosis >grade I, accompanied by increased age-adjusted BM cellularity, granulocytic proliferation, and often decreased erythropoiesis 2. JAK2, CALR, or MPL mutations or the presence of another clonal marker or the absence of minor reactive BM reticulin fibrosis 3. Not meeting WHO criteria for BCR::ABL1-positive CML, PV, ET, myelodysplastic syndromes, or other myeloid neoplasms Minor criteria 1. Anemia not attributed to a comorbid condition 2. Leukocytosis $\geq 11 \times 10^9$/L 3. Splenomegaly: detected clinically and/or by imaging 4. LDH above the reference range Diagnosis requires all three major criteria and at least one minor criterion to be confirmed in two consecutive determinations	Major criteria (same as WHO 2022) 1. BM biopsy showing megakaryocytic proliferation and atypia, BM fibrosis grade < 2, increased age-adjusted BM cellularity, granulocytic proliferation, and (often) decreased erythropoiesis 2. *JAK2*, *CALR*, or *MPL* mutation† or presence of another clonal marker‡ or absence of reactive BM reticulin fibrosis 3. Diagnostic criteria for *BCR::ABL1*-positive CML, PV, ET, Myelodysplastic syndromes, or other myeloid neoplasms are not met Minor criteria 1. Anemia not attributed to a comorbid condition 2. Leukocytosis $\geq 11 \times 10^9$/L 3. Palpable splenomegaly 4. LDH above the reference range Diagnosis requires three major criteria and at least one minor criterion confirmed in two consecutive determinations
PMF (overt fibrotic stage)	Major criteria 1. BM biopsy showing megakaryocytic proliferation and atypia, accompanied by reticulin and/or collagen fibrosis grades 2 or 3 2. JAK2, CALR, or MPL mutation or presence of another clonal marker or absence of reactive BM reticulin fibrosis 3. Diagnostic criteria for *BCR::ABL1* positive CML, PV, ET, myelodysplastic syndromes, or other defined myeloid neoplasms are not met. Minor criteria Serial numbers 1–4 in minor diagnostic criteria are the same as PMF (prefibrotic) 5. Leukoerythroblastosis Diagnosis: same criteria as Prefibrotic PMF	Major criteria 1. Megakaryocytic proliferation and atypia, accompanied by reticulin and/or collagen fibrosis grades 2 or 3 2. JAK2, CALR, or MPL mutation or presence of another clonal marker or absence of reactive myelofibrosis. 3. Diagnostic criteria for ET, PV, BCR-ABL1-positive CML, myelodysplastic syndrome, or other myeloid neoplasms are not met Minor criteria: 1. Anemia not attributed to a comorbid condition 2. Leukocytosis $\geq 11 \times 10^9$/L 3. Palpable splenomegaly 4. LDH level above the reference range 5. Leukoerythroblastosis Diagnosis: same criteria as Prefibrotic PMF

(continued)

Table 34.1 (continued)

Category	WHO 2022 [6] diagnostic criteria	ICC 2022 [7] diagnostic criteria
CNL	1. PB WBC count >/=25 × 10^6/L. Segmented neutrophils plus banded neutrophils constitute >80% of WBCs; no dysgranulopoiesis. Neutrophil precursors (promyelocytes, myelocytes, and metamyelocytes) constitute <10% of the white blood cells. Monocyte <10% of all leukocytes. 2. Hypercellular BM (increased neutrophil granulocytes; myeloblast<5%) 3. Not meeting criteria for CML, PV, ET, or PMF and exclusion of reactive neutrophilia. 4. No rearrangement of *PDGFRA*, *PDGFRB*, or *FGFR1*, and no *PCM1-JAK2* fusion 5. *CSF3R* T618I or another activating *CSF3R* mutation Or Persistent neutrophilia (>/=3 months), splenomegaly, and no identifiable cause of reactive neutrophilia, including absence of a plasma cell neoplasm or, if a plasma cell neoplasm is present, demonstration of clonality of myeloid cells by cytogenetic or molecular studies.	1. PB WBC count ≥13 × 10^9/L * for cases with CSF3R mutation. Segmented neutrophils plus banded neutrophils constitute >80% of WBCs. No significant dysgranulopoiesis. Neutrophil precursors (promyelocytes, myelocytes, and metamyelocytes) constitute <10% of the white blood cells. Monocyte count <10% of all leukocytes. Circulating blasts are only rarely observed (10–19% blasts in PB or BM represent CNL in accelerated phase; >20% blasts: blast phase) 2. Hypercellular BM with increased neutrophil granulocytes showing normal maturation. 3. CSF3RT618I or another activating CSF3R mutation or persistent neutrophilia (≥3 months), splenomegaly, and no identifiable cause of reactive neutrophilia, including absence of a plasma cell neoplasm or, if a plasma cell neoplasm is present, demonstration of clonality of myeloid cells by cytogenetic or molecular studies. 4. Not meeting diagnostic criteria for BCR::ABL1-positive CML, PV, ET, PMF, or of a myeloid/lymphoid neoplasm with eosinophilia and tyrosine kinase gene fusions. *PB WBC at least 25 × 10^9/L in cases lacking CSF3R T618I or another activating CSF3R mutation

CEL, NOS	CEL: Essential: 1. Hypereosinophilia (eosinophil count ≥1.5×10^9/L) on at least two occasions over an interval of at least 4 weeks 2. Evidence of clonality 3. Abnormal BM morphology 4. Not meeting criteria for other myeloid or lymphoid neoplasms	CEL, NOS: The diagnosis requires all 6 criteria 1.Eosinophilia (absolute eosinophil count >1.5×10^9/L and eosinophils >10% of white blood cells) 2. The blasts in the PB and BM are less than 20%, and inv.(16)(p13.1q22), t(16;16)(p13;q22), and other diagnostic features of AML are absent 3. No tyrosine kinase gene fusion including BCR::ABL1, other ABL1, PDGFRA, PDGFRB, FGFR1, JAK2, or FLT3 fusions 4. Not meeting criteria for other well-defined MPN; CMML, or SM 5. BM shows increased cellularity with dysplastic megakaryocytes with or without dysplastic features in other lineages and often significant fibrosis, associated with an eosinophilic infiltrate or increased blasts >/= 5% in the BM and/or >2% in the PB 6. Demonstration of a clonal cytogenetic abnormality and/or somatic mutation(s)* * In the absence of a clonal cytogenetic abnormality and/or somatic mutation(s) or increased blasts, BM findings supportive of the diagnosis will suffice in the presence of persistent eosinophilia, provided other causes of eosinophilia have been excluded

(continued)

Table 34.1 (continued)

Category	WHO 2022 [6] diagnostic criteria	ICC 2022 [7] diagnostic criteria
MPN-U	A. Requires all of the following: 1. Presence of any one of the following features: 1. Clinical and hematological features of MPN (e.g., splenomegaly, leucocytosis, thrombocytosis) in the absence of significant monocytosis and significant eosinophilia 2. BM hypercellularity with megakaryocytic hyperplasia and varying degrees of granulocytic and erythroid hyperplasia, without dysplastic features 3. Clinical and morphological features can be discrepant 2. Not meeting criteria for any other MPN, MDS, MDS/MPN, or myeloid/lymphoid neoplasm with eosinophilia and tyrosine kinase gene fusions 3. Presence of driver mutations JAK2, CALR, or MPL or another clonal marker B. Requires absence of both of the following: 1. Insufficient clinical data or inadequate bone marrow specimen for accurate evaluation and classification 2. Recent history of cytotoxic or growth factor therapy	Requires all three criteria 1. Clinical and hematological features of an MPN are present (Exclude reactive causes of BM fibrosis) 2. JAK2, CALR, or MPL mutation * or presence of another clonal marker ** 3. Diagnostic criteria for any other MPN, MDS, MDS/MPN #, or BCR::ABL1-positive CML are not met * It is recommended to use highly sensitive assays for JAK2 V617F (sensitivity level, 1%) and CALR and MPL (sensitivity level 1% to 3%); in negative cases, consider searching for noncanonical JAK2 and MPL mutations **Assessed by cytogenetics or sensitive NGS techniques; detection of mutations associated with myeloid neoplasms (e.g., ASXL1, EZH2, IDH1, IDH2, SF3B1, SRSF2, and TET2 mutations) supports the clonal nature of the disease #In cases presenting with myelodysplastic features, the effects of any previous treatment, severe comorbidity, and changes during the natural progression of the disease process must be carefully excluded

A. Clinical, Hematologic, and Laboratory Criteria (all five criteria are required):

1. PB monocyte count is ≥1 × 10^9/L.
2. Blasts and promonocytes constitute <20% of PB and BM.
3. Clinical evidence of organ infiltration, most commonly splenomegaly.
4. Absence of BCR::ABL1.
5. Absence of a *KMT2A* rearrangement.

B. Genetic Criteria (One Criterion is Sufficient for Diagnosis).

1. A variant in a component or a regulator of the canonical RAS pathway:

(a) A clonal somatic variant in *PTPN11*, *KRAS*, or *NRAS*.
(b) A clonal somatic or germline variant in *NF1* and a loss of heterozygosity or compound heterozygosity in *NF1*.
(c) A clonal somatic or germline variant in *CBL* and a loss of heterozygosity in *CBL*b.

2. A noncanonical clonal RAS pathway pathogenic variant or fusions that activate genes located upstream of the RAS pathway, such as *ALK*, *PDGFRB*, and *ROS1*.

C. Other Criteria (2 or More Are Required for Diagnosis).

1. Circulating myeloid (promyelocytes, myelocytes, metamyelocytes) and erythroid precursors.
2. Increased HbF for age.
3. Thrombocytopenia with hypercellular bone marrow, often with megakaryocytic hypoplasia; dysplastic features may or may not be evident.
4. Myeloid progenitors are hypersensitive to GM-CSF (detected by clonogenic assays or by measuring STAT5 phosphorylation in the absence or with low doses of exogenous GM-CSF).

JMML, however, does not feature in ICC 2022 criteria under the MPN category and is separately categorized under "pediatric and/or germline mutation-associated disorders".

34.3 Polycythaemia Vera (PV)

Clinical Case 1 A 61-year-old male who presented with elevated hemoglobin of 19.1 g/dL and hematocrit of 57.5%, with a mean corpuscular volume (MCV) of 85.1 fL and red cell distribution width (RDW) of 14.1%. The total leukocyte count (TLC) was 13.2 × 10^3/μL, with an absolute neutrophil count (ANC) of 8.1 × 10^3/μL. The platelet count was markedly elevated at 620 × 10^3/μL with a mean platelet width (MPV) of 8.7 fL. Serum erythropoietin was subnormal (2.6 mU/mL). Molecular analysis of PB revealed a JAK2V617F variant allele frequency (VAF) of 34%. Cytogenetic analysis revealed a normal karyotype.

The BM aspirate and biopsy were performed; the representative images of the BM biopsy are shown in Fig. 34.1.

The patient was managed with phlebotomy, hydroxyurea, and aspirin. However, he defaulted in his treatment and after a year, reported with thrombotic CVA. On evaluation, he had anemia and thrombocytopenia, and his peripheral blood smear showed a leucoerythroblastic picture with grade 2 fibrosis on BM biopsy. The patient was offered palliative care and finally succumbed to his illness.

PV is primarily diagnosed by the presence of clonal erythrocytosis. It can present with symptoms of pruritus, systemic symptoms like headache and dizziness, and raised hemoglobin, leukocytosis, thrombocytosis, and splenomegaly. It carries an elevated risk of thrombotic events and can rarely progress to post-polycythemic myelofibrosis (post-PV MF) or acute myeloid leukemia (AML) [8, 9]. Since nearly all patients with polycythemia vera (PV) carry a JAK2 mutation, testing for this mutation is the initial step in establishing a diagnosis.

If PV is suspected clinically, serum erythropoietin (EPO) is subnormal, and *JAK2* mutations are absent, a BM examination is recommended to identify histological features associated with MPN. Although rarely found in PV, additional testing for MPN-associated driver mutations (*CALR* and *MPL*) should be performed (1). *LNK* mutations can be detected in approximately 5.3% patients with *JAK2-negative* erythrocytosis (2). The diagnostic algorithm for PV is given in Fig. 34.2:

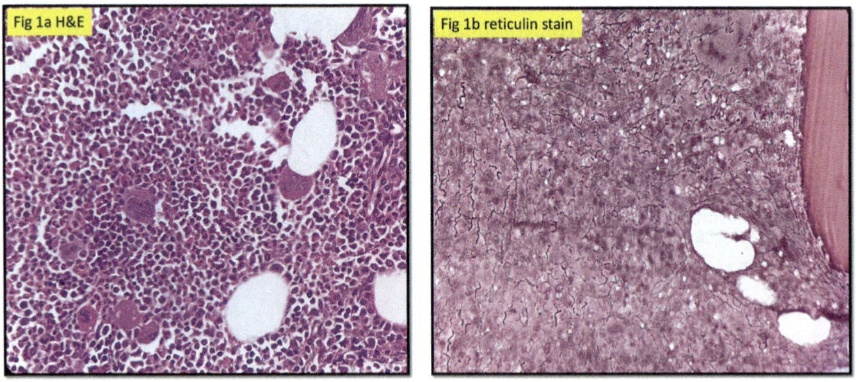

Fig. 34.1 (**a**) Hypercellular bone marrow with increased megakaryocytes (loose clusters of large and small megakaryocytes), erythroid and myeloid precursors (panmyelosis) (400×, H&E). (**b**) Bone marrow with grade 1 fibrosis (400× Reticulin stain)

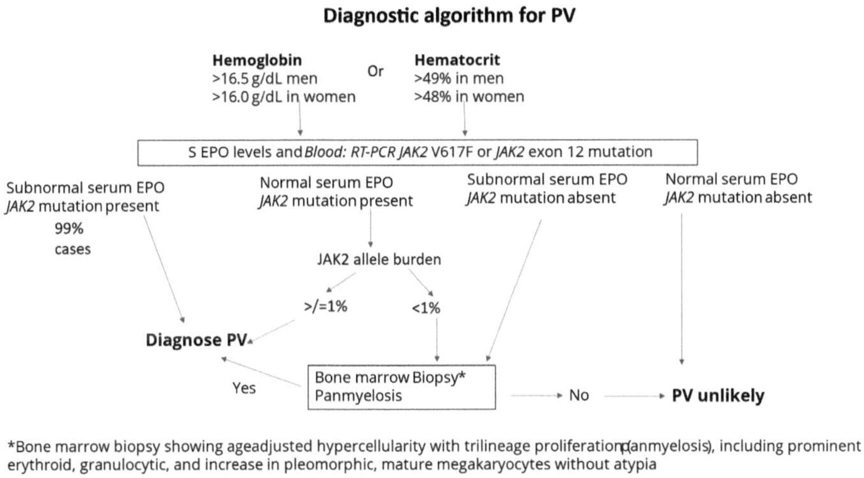

Fig. **34.2** Diagnostic algorithm for PV

34.4 Risk Stratification in PV

In PV (as also in ET), the risk stratification can be utilized to predict risk of thrombosis, leukemic or MF transformation, and survival.

The thrombotic risk assessment is used to categorize patients into various risk groups to serve as a guide for therapeutic decision-making.

(a) Low risk (age <60 years and no history of thrombosis).
(b) High risk (age >60 years or history of thrombosis).

The collective risk for leukemic transformation in PV is 2.3% and 5.5% at 10 years and 15 years, respectively. The risk factors for leukemic transformation are older age, TLC $\geq 15 \times 10^9$/L, abnormal karyotype, and treatment exposure to pipobroman/ chlorambucil. The risk factors for progression to MF include JAK2V617F allele burden of >50%, presence of BM fibrosis at the time of diagnosis, persistent leukocytosis, and palpable splenomegaly [2, 10].

Age is the most important predictor of survival in PV. Further, age-independent risk factors for overall survival are leukocytosis [11], venous thrombosis, and abnormal karyotype. Thus, cytogenetic studies are recommended to be done at baseline in PV [8, 9].

Mutation-enhanced international prognostic score for PV (MIPSS-PV)

(a) Age >67 years (2 points).
(b) SRSF2 mutation (2 points); (incidence: 3%).
(c) TLC >11,000/uL (1 point); (incidence is 50%).
(d) Abnormal karyotype (1 point) (20%).

Risk category (MIPSS-PV)	Points	Median survival (years)
Low	0–1	24
Intermediate	2–3	13
High	>3	3.2

Treatment of PV will be discussed along with ET.

34.5 Essential Thrombocythemia (ET)

Case 2 A 37-year-old asymptomatic lady, during routine lab investigations, was incidentally found to have thrombocytosis, with a platelet count of 1067 × 10^3/µL. The platelet distribution width (PDW) was 50.1%, and the MPV was 8.4 fL. Her hemoglobin was 13.1 g/dL with a HCT of 39.4%, MCV of 84.5 fL, and RDW of 13.2%. The TLC was 8.2 × 10^3/µL, with an ANC of 5.74 × 10^3/µL. Peripheral blood smear showed thrombocytosis with normocytic normochromic red blood cells. Ultrasonography (USG) of the abdomen revealed splenomegaly (16.4 cm). BM aspirate was normocellular, with increased megakaryocytes exhibiting large hyper-lobated nuclei; the myeloid-to-erythroid (M:E) ratio was 4:1 with 2% blasts, and no evidence of dysmyelopoiesis. BM biopsy showed a normocellular marrow with increased megakaryocytes arranged in loose clusters and bearing hyperlobated nuclei (Fig. 34.3). Molecular analysis for BCR-ABL1, JAK2, CALR, and MPL mutations was negative

The reactive thrombocytosis was excluded by detailed history and extensive laboratory workup for infection, inflammatory diseases, medications, and malignancy. The patient was diagnosed as triple-negative ET. She is on regular follow-up with no thrombotic event.

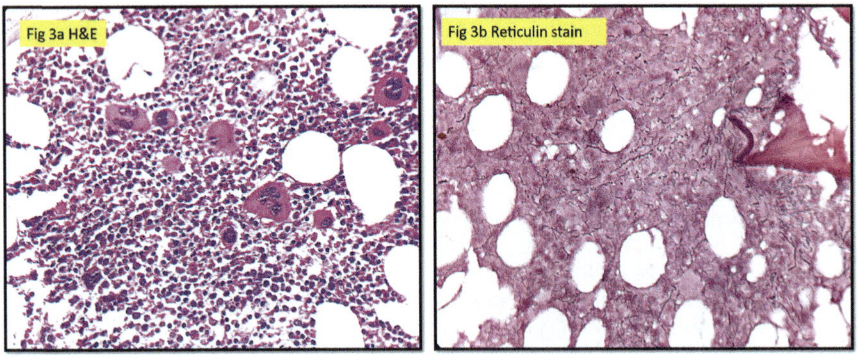

Fig. 34.3 (**a**) Normocellular BM biopsy with loose clusters of megakaryocytes showing stag horn nuclei of megakaryocytes (400×, H&E). (**b**) Bone marrow with grade 0 fibrosis (400×, Reticulin stain)

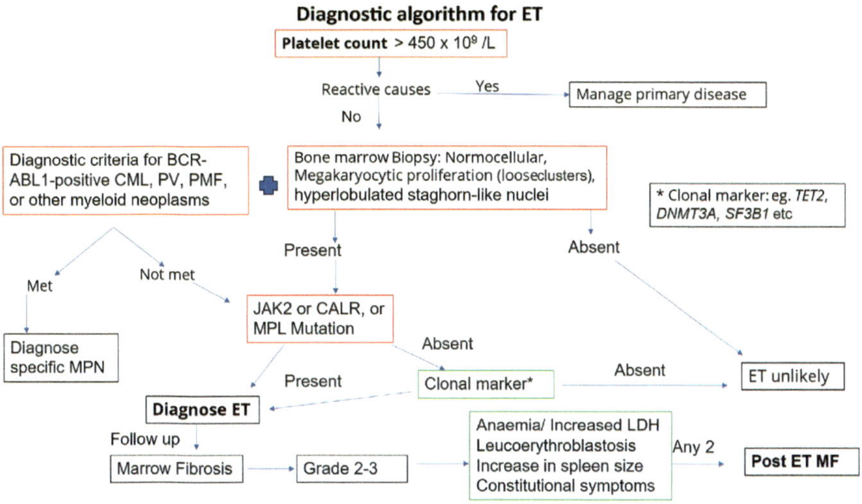

Fig. 34.4 Diagnostic algorithm for ET

ET is characterized by autonomous megakaryocytic proliferation in the BM due to genetic mutations in hematopoietic stem cells, resulting in a sustainable increase in platelets in the PB. The recurrent mutations in ET include *JAK2*, *CALR,* and *MPL* in 50–60%, 30%, and 3% of ET cases, respectively. The triple-negative genotype is found in around 10% of ET patients and is associated with a better prognosis [12]. About 50% of ET patients harbor other mutations, the most frequent being ten-eleven-ten {(*TET2)* (9–11%)}, additional sex combs like {(*ASXL1)* (7–20%)}, DNA methyltransferase {(*DNMT3A)* (7%)}, and Splicing factor 3B subunit 1 {(*SF3B1)* (5%)}. Abnormal karyotype is seen in <10% of patients and includes +9/20q−/13q- (12). The diagnostic algorithm for ET is given in Fig. 34.4.

34.5.1 Risk Stratification of ET

Survival of ET patients: The two models for survival in ET patients (triple A model and Mutation-enhanced international prognostic system) are shown in Table 34.2.

In ET, independent risk factors for MF-free survival include age >60 years, male gender, palpable splenomegaly, *CALR-1* or *MPL* mutation, and *JAK2*V617F VAF >35%. *CALR* VAF of >60% in ET patients shows a higher risk of progression to MF [15].

Table 34.2 The two models for survival in ET patients

	Risk category	Points	Median survival (years)
A. Triple A model [13] Parameters Age Age >70 years (4 pts) Age 50–70 years (2 pts) Absolute neutrophil count: ≥8 × 10^9/L (1 point) Absolute lymphocyte count: <1.7 × 10^9/L (1 point)	Low	0–1	47
	Intermediate 1	2–3	21
	Intermediate 2	4	14
	High	5–6	8
B. Mutation-enhanced international prognostic system for ET [14] Parameters Age >60 years (4 points) Male gender (1 point) WBC ≥11 × 10^9/L (1 point) Adverse mutations (2 points) (*SF3B1/SRSF2/U2AF1/TP53*)	Low	0–1	34.4
	Intermediate 1	2–3	14.1
	Intermediate 2	4	
	High	5–6	7.9

34.5.2 Prognosis in ET Patients

Mutation	Association
MPL and *CALR-1*	Increased risk of progression to MF
Spliceosome	Inferior overall (OS) and MF-free survival
TP53	Leukemic transformation
*JAK2*V617F	Thrombosis

Risk factors for thrombosis and bleeding in ET

1. Thrombotic risk assessment in ET patients: (same as PV).

   Low-risk (age <60 years and no history of thrombosis).
   High-risk (age >60 years or history of thrombosis).

2. Revised-International Prognostic Score of Thrombosis for ET (IPSET-thrombosis) [16]—identified independent prothrombotic role for cardiovascular (CV) risk factors (hypertension, diabetes mellitus, and active smoking) and *JAK2*V617F mutation as "additional modifiers," in addition to age and history of thrombosis identified earlier.

   The revised risk stratification scheme includes four categories:

(a) "Very low risk'=" (no thrombosis history, age ⩽60 years and *JAK2*-unmutated);
(b) "Low risk" (no thrombosis history, age ⩽60 years and *JAK2*-mutated);
(c) "Intermediate risk" (no thrombosis history, age >60 years and *JAK2*-unmutated);
(d) "High risk (thrombosis history or age >60 years with *JAK2* mutation)."

Table 34.3 Effect of cardiovascular risk factors and JAK2 mutation on vascular event rates in low- and high-risk ET

Risk category (IPSET-thrombosis)	Additional risk factors	Risk of thrombosis patients/year (%)
Low	None	0.44
	Cardiovascular risk factor	1.05
	JAK2V617F mutation	1.59
	Both	2.57
High	None	1.44
	Cardiovascular risk factor	1.64
	JAK2V617F mutation	2.36
	Both	4.17

The impact of cardiovascular risk factors and JAK2 mutation on vascular event rates among low- and high-risk patients in ET patients is presented in Table 34.3.

34.5.3 Management of PV and ET

The treatment algorithm, similar in PV and ET, based on risk stratification as discussed above, primarily aims at prevention of thrombotic complications and is as shown in Fig. 34.5. All patients are given antiplatelet agents [17] and the addition of cytoreductive therapy [18] is based on risk profile and aims at maintaining HCT <45% in PV [19]. Aspirin, in twice-daily dosing, helps in reducing microvascular symptoms like erythromelalgia and headaches [20]. Twice daily dosing is also recommended in low-risk cases with uncontrolled microvascular symptoms, with once daily dosing or where the risk of thrombosis is more but not enough to warrant cytoreductive therapy. First-line cytoreductive therapy is hydroxyurea with interferon-α and busulfan or ruxolitinib (JAK inhibitor) as second-line options [21–23]. None of these agents has been implicated with an increased risk of leukemic transformation [8]. For second-line therapy, Interferon- α is preferred in younger patients, while Busulfan is preferred in older patients.

PMF is a clonal MPN characterized by the proliferation of abnormal megakaryocytes and granulocytes in the BM associated with significant fibrosis. Compared to other MPNs, this entity has a shorter overall survival and a higher incidence of leukemic transformation.

Clinical Case 3 A 68-year-old male presented with complaints of easy fatigability and early satiety for 3 months. No history of autoimmune diseases or any medication. Clinical examination revealed pallor and splenomegaly, which was confirmed on abdominal USG, measuring 17.5 cm. Laboratory investigations showed pancytopenia. The hemoglobin level was 8.1 g/dL and HCT of 24.4%, normocytic indices (MCV 87 fL), and elevated RDW of 17.8%. The TLC was reduced at $3.82 \times 10^3/\mu L$, with an ANC of $1.10 \times 10^3/\mu L$. Platelet count was also decreased at $48 \times 10^3/\mu L$,

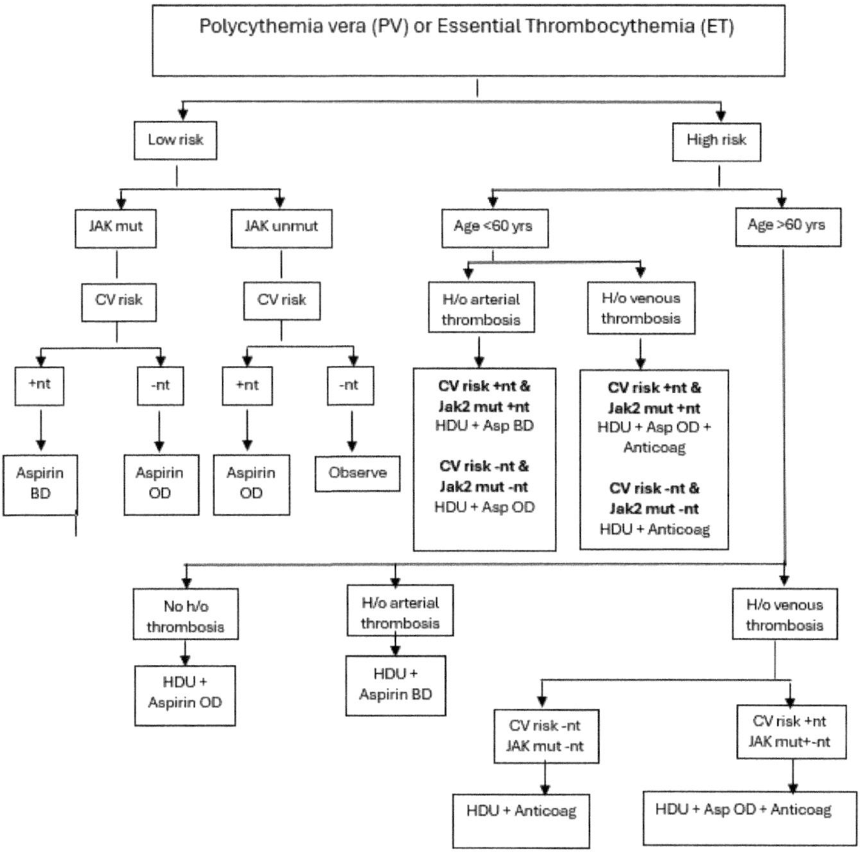

Fig. 34.5 Treatment algorithm for polycythemia vera and essential thrombocythemia

with an MPV of 8.6 fL. BM aspirate was dilute. BM biopsy revealed atypical megakaryocytes and grade 2 reticulin fibrosis (Fig. 34.6), consistent with PMF.

34.5.4 Risk Stratification in PMF

Prognostic models developed for risk stratification in overt primary myelofibrosis (PMF) incorporate genetic and clinical factors to guide treatment decisions, which are aimed at a more personalized approach to patient management, ranging from active surveillance in low-risk cases to allogeneic hematopoietic stem cell transplantation for high-risk patients.

The risk categories are as shown in Tables 34.4 and 34.5.

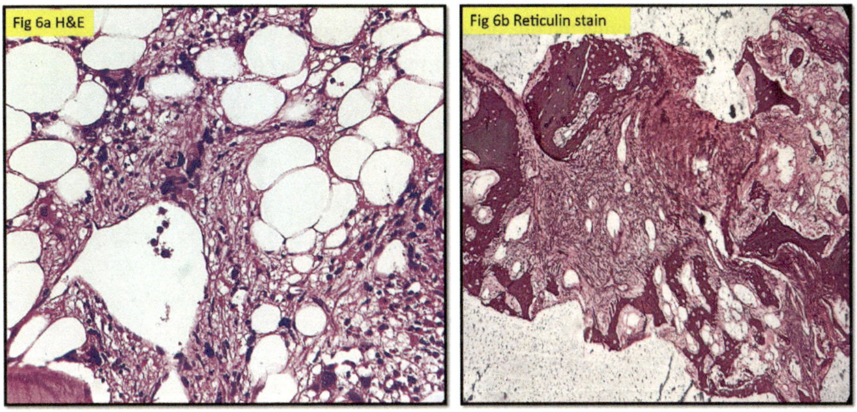

Fig. 34.6 (**a**) Bone marrow biopsy with increased megakaryocytes, a tight cluster of atypical megakaryocytes, and intrasinusoidal hematopoiesis (400×, H&E). (**b**) Bone marrow with grade 2 fibrosis (100×, Reticulin stain)

Table 34.4 Risk stratification in primary myelofibrosis according to the three prognostic scores (IPSS, DIPSS, and DIPSS-plus)

Variable	IPSS (2009)		DIPSS (2010)		DIPSS-plus (2011)	
Age >65 years	✓		✓		✓	
Constitutional symptoms	✓		✓		✓	
Hb <10 gm/dl	✓		✓		✓	
WBC >25,000/dl	✓		✓		✓	
Circulating blasts >1%	✓		✓		✓	
Platelet count <1,00,000/dl					✓	
RBC transfusion need					✓	
Unfavorable karyotype					✓	
Score calculation	1 point for each variable		2 points for Hb and 1 point each for others		1 point for each variable	
Risk group	Points	Median survival (yrs)	Points	Median survival (yrs)	Points	Median survival (yrs)
Low	0	11.3	0	NR	0	15.4
Intermediate-1	1	7.9	1–2	14.2	1	6.5
Intermediate-2	2	4.0	3–4	4	2–3	2.9
High	≥3	2.3	5–6	1.5	≥4	1.3

Unfavorable karyotype includes + 8, 7q−, translocations not involving chromosome 1, two abnormalities not including a VHR abnormality, 5q−, complex karyotype without a VHR abnormality, monosomal karyotype without a VHR abnormality

IPSS International Prognostic Scoring System, *DIPSS* Dynamic International Prognostic Scoring System, *NR* not reached

Table 34.5 Comparative overview of PMF risk stratification systems—MIPSS70, MIPSS70+ v2.0, and GIPSS—highlighting the role of genetic and molecular testing

Variable	MIPSS70		MIPSS70 + version2.0		GIPSS	
Clinical variable						
Hb <10 gm/dl	✓					
WBC >25,000/dl	✓					
Platelet count <1,00,000/dl	✓					
Circulating blasts >2%	✓		✓			
Constitutional symptoms	✓		✓			
Marrow fibrosis ≥2	✓					
Severe anemia[a]			✓			
Moderate anemia[b]			✓			
Genetic variables						
One HMR mutation	✓		✓			
≥2 HMR mutations	✓		✓			
Type 1/ 1-like CALR mutation absent	✓		✓		✓	
VHR karyotype			✓		✓	
Unfavorable karyotype			✓		✓	
ASXL1 mutation					✓	
SRSF2 mutation					✓	
U2AF1Q157 mutation					✓	
Score calculation	2 points: High WBC, Low platelet count ≥ 2 HMR mutations 1 point: For each variable		4 points: VHR karyotype, 3 points: Unfavorable karyotype and 2 HMR mutations, 2 points: 1 HMR mutation, Type 1/Type 1-like CALR absent, Constitutional symptoms 1 point each: other two variables		2 points for VHR karyotype 1 point for each other variable	
Risk group	Points	Median survival (yrs)	Points	Median survival (yrs)	Points	Median survival (yrs)
Very low			0	NR		
Low	0–1	NR	1–2	16.4	0	26.4

(continued)

Table 34.5 (continued)

Variable		MIPSS70		MIPSS70 + version2.0		GIPSS	
Intermediate	1	2–4	6.3	3–4	7.7	1	8
Intermediate	2					2	4.2
High		≥5	3.1	5–8	4.1	≥3	2
Very high				≥9	1.8		

MIPSS70- for patients <70 yrs age (transplant eligible);
MIPSS70+ version 2.0- Mutation and karyotype enhanced International Prognostic Scoring System.
GIPSS- Genetically Inspired International Prognostic Scoring System.
HMR- High Risk Mutations include ASXL1, SRSF2, EZH2, IDH1 & IDH2; U2AF1Q157 is also included in MIPSS70+ and GIPSS; CALR- Calreticulin.
VHR- Very high risk; these include -7/7q-, i(17q), inv(3), -5/5q-, 12p-, +8, 11q23 rearrangements, single/multiple autosomal trisomies other than +8 or +9 (e.g., +21, +19)
[a]Severe anemia: hemoglobin <9 gm/dl in men and <8 gm/dl in women
[b]Moderate anemia: hemoglobin 9–10.9 gm/dl in men and 8–9.9 gm/dl in women

Unfavorable karyotype is also associated with a higher risk of leukemic transformation, with a reported 5-year risk of 46% versus 7% in patients with "favorable" karyotype.

34.5.5 Management of PMF

For PMF, the treatment decision is relatively simple with allogenic BMT being offered in Intermediate-2 and high-risk cases or with high-risk genetic features, as shown in Fig. 34.7. The rest of the cases are being managed symptomatically. Five-year survival was 37% in matched sibling donor transplant and 30% from unrelated donor transplant [24]. Previous use of ruxolitinib has shown better outcomes after transplant, and the role of ruxolitinib as maintenance therapy post BMT is being studied.

34.5.6 Symptomatic Treatment in PMF

Splenomegaly and constitutional symptoms: The most common agent used to treat these symptoms is hydroxyurea, and it is very effective in alleviating these symptoms. But the responses are usually short-lived and long-term usage is not possible due to myelosuppression [25, 26]. Ruxolitinib is the JAK inhibitor that is approved in intermediate- and high-risk patients for splenomegaly and constitutional symptom improvement based on two randomized controlled trials (Comfort-I & II) [27–29]. In resistant and intolerant cases, Fedratinib, Pacritinib, and Momelotinib are found promising.

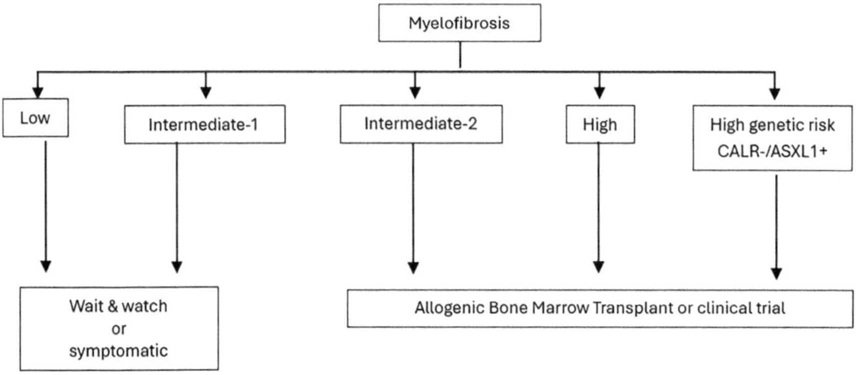

Fig. 34.7 Treatment algorithm for primary myelofibrosis

Anemia: For treatment of anemia, erythropoietin stimulating agents have shown response rates of 45–60% and are mostly seen in patients with serum EPO levels less than 100 U/L [30, 31]. Danazol is also effective in improving anemia in patients with PMF [32]. Another good option is thalidomide [33] or lenalidomide [34] with low-dose prednisolone, which helps in improving the cytopenia. These are very good alternatives in patients who present with thrombocytopenia, where ruxolitinib cannot be given.

34.5.7 Allogenic BMT in PMF

Allogenic BMT is the only curative option in PMF but is offered only in DIPSS-Plus Intermediate-2 and high-risk cases, because in these, the benefit-to-risk ratio is better [35]. MSD allogenic BMT has the best outcome, but in high-risk cases, alternative donor transplant like MUD or Haplo can also be offered. Pre-transplant use of ruxolitinib helps in improving splenomegaly and performance status of the patient, in-fact it is recommended to continue to give till peri-transplant phase too [36].

34.6 Chronic Neutrophilic Leukemia (CNL)

It is a rare MPN defined by persistent mature neutrophilic leukocytosis, BM granulocytic proliferation and hepatosplenomegaly. Specific genetic mutations, particularly in the colony-stimulating factor 3 receptor (*CSF3R*), classically T618I gene, are detected in >60% of cases [6].

Case 4 A 65-year-old male presented with easy fatigability. The clinical examination revealed pallor and splenomegaly. USG revealed splenomegaly measuring 17.5 cm. His CBC showed mild anemia with a hemoglobin of 11.5 g/dL and HCT of 34.6%, characterized as normocytic normochromic. He had marked leukocytosis with a TLC of 26.1 × 10^3/uL, neutrophilia (ANC of 23.8 × 10^3/uL), and 2% myelocytes and 3% metamyelocytes were noted. His platelet count was normal at 196 × 10^3/uL. A BM aspirate revealed hypercellularity with a markedly increased myeloid-to-erythroid ratio of 23:1 and 2% blasts, but no dysmyelopoiesis was observed. Genetic testing for BCR-ABL1, JAK2, CALR, or MPL mutations was negative; however, a *CSF3RT618I mutation was positive.*

The Mayo Clinic CNL risk model for survival of CNL patients is mentioned in Table 34.6 [37].

CSF3RT618I-mutation is frequently associated with older age at diagnosis, lower Hb level and platelet count, higher WBC count, and abnormal karyotype as compared to "other" *CSF3R*-mutations [38]. The leukemic transformation rate of CNL is ~10–25%, and overall survival is 15–31 months. It is emphasized that despite the rarity of CNL, an unusually high incidence of plasma cell neoplasms has been reported to be associated with CNL. Hematopoietic stem cell transplant is the only potentially curative modality and should be considered in eligible patients. Recent genetic profiling has disclosed CBL, CEBPA, EZH2, NRAS, TET2, and U2AF1 to represent high-risk mutations in CNL. Mutations in NRAS/KRAS and ETNK1 genes have also been identified, supporting novel agents targeting involved pathways.

The median overall survival in CSF3R T618I-positive CNL is reported to be 24 months [39]. The risk of transformation to leukemia is 10–21% in various studies [40, 41]. There was no standard of care for CNL, and mostly it was managed symptomatically, till ruxolitinib [42] showed promising results. Other agents used in this series included interferon-alpha (IFN-a), hypomethylating agents, thalidomide, cladribine, and imatinib, and these can be decided based on the algorithm in Fig. 34.8.

Table 34.6 Risk stratification CNL

Parameters	Low risk	High risk
1. Platelets: <160 × 10^9/L (2 points) 2. Leucocytes >60 × 10^9/L (1 point) 3. ASXL1 mutation (1 point)	0–1 point	2–4 points

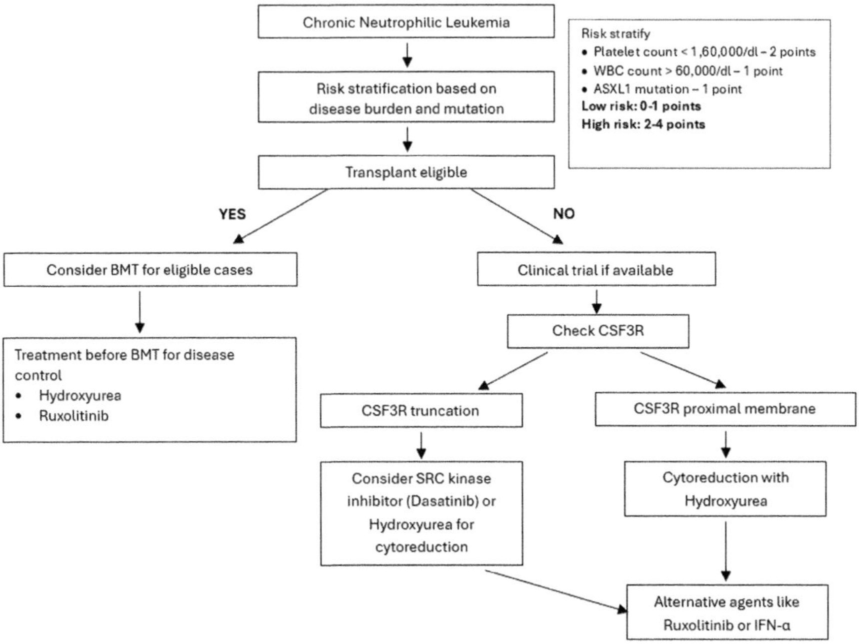

Fig. 34.8 The algorithm for the management of chronic neutrophilic leukemia

34.7 Chronic Eosinophilic Leukemia (CEL)

Case 5 A 75-year-old male presented with easy fatigability, weight loss, and cough, along with a history of hypertension and Type II diabetes mellitus. Clinical examination revealed pallor and splenomegaly. USG revealed splenomegaly (18 cm). Hematological investigations showed anemia (hemoglobin 10.1 g/dL, hematocrit 30.6%) with a MCV of 98.2 fL. His TLC was elevated at 19.8 × 10^3/uL, notably with marked eosinophilia (absolute eosinophil count of 7.52 × 10^3/uL). Peripheral blood smear revealed eosinophils with hypolobated nuclei and sparse granules (Fig. 34.9). The BM aspirate was hypercellular with a myeloid-to-erythroid ratio of 23:1. The aspirate revealed 7% blasts, and increased eosinophils and their precursors (30%). Both *dysmyelopoiesis* and *dysmegakaryopoiesis* were observed. Genetic testing for BCR-ABL1, JAK2, CALR, MPL, PDGFRA, PDGFRB, FGFR1, or PCM1-JAK2 rearrangements was all negative. However, an *ASXL1 mutation was positive* with a VAF of 16%.

The patient denied any history of allergic disorders, drug reactions, or autoimmunity. The workup for infectious diseases (including filariasis), lymphoproliferative disorders, and solid tumors was negative. The patient was diagnosed as CEL and managed with corticosteroids and hydroxyurea.

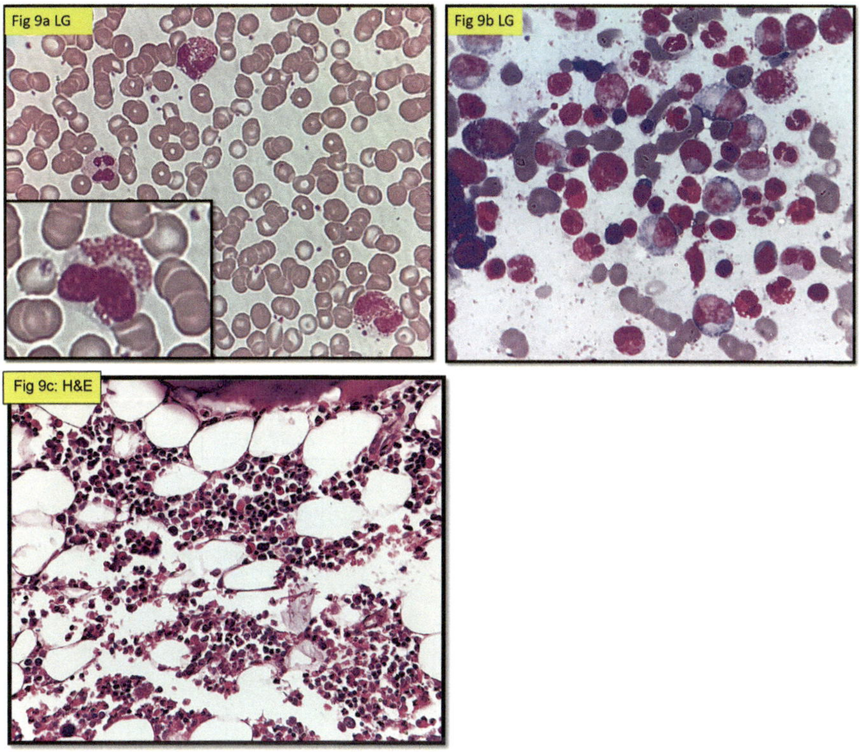

Fig. 34.9 (**a**) Peripheral blood film shows eosinophilia, (400×, LG stain) (inset: eosinophil with sparse granules and abnormal lobulation); (**b**) bone marrow smear—with eosinophilia; (**c**) bone marrow trephine biopsy: hypercellular for age with preponderance of cells of neutrophil and eosinophil lineages (400×, H&E). Reticulin was not increased

Management: Usually, it is very difficult to diagnose CEL when a patient is being evaluated for hypereosinophilic syndrome, but with newer diagnostic tools, especially NGS, it has become a bit easier. So, the better algorithm is based on the management of HES [43] rather than CEL, as mentioned in Fig. 34.10. Detailed evaluation should be done to rule out secondary causes, and if found, they must be treated. In secondary causes, once the primary problem is treated, the eosinophilia resolves too.

34.7.1 Risk Stratification

The prognosis of CEL patients is poor, with a median survival of around 2 years [6]. The cause of death is infection, disease-related organ failure, and bleeding. STAT5B p.N642H mutation alone or in combination with SF3B1 has longer OS as compared to STAT5B p.N642H combined with other mutations [44].

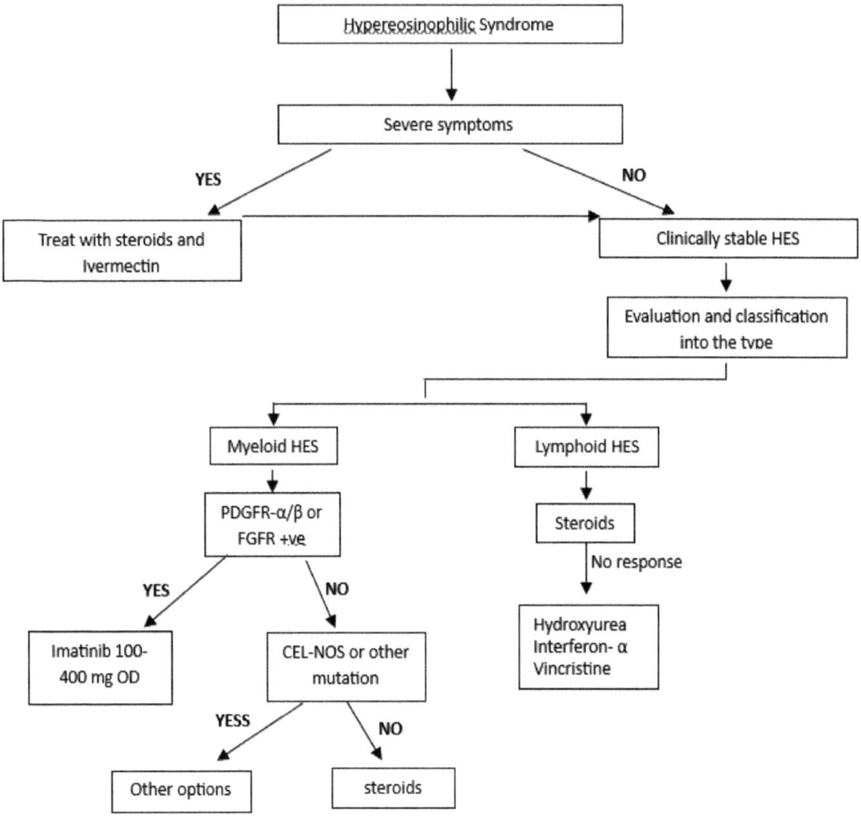

Fig. 34.10 Management algorithm of hypereosinophilic syndrome

34.8 Juvenile Myelomonocytic Leukemia

Case 6 An 8-month-old male infant, weighing 5 kg, presented with *fever* and *failure to thrive*. Clinical examination revealed *splenomegaly,* and ultrasound confirmed *hepatosplenomegaly*. His hemogram showed *anemia* with a hemoglobin of 8.7 g/dL, MCV of 70.1 fL, and RDW of 19.2%. He had marked *leukocytosis* with a TLC of 53.74 × 10^3/uL with an ANC of 32.07 × 10^3/uL and 7% myelocytes and metamyelocytes, and an absolute monocyte count of 3.9 × 10^3/uL. His *platelet count was low* at 35 × 10^3/uL. Peripheral blood smear showed a leucoerythroblastic picture with monocytosis and 2% blasts (Fig. 34.11a). Hemoglobin electrophoresis revealed raised HbF. The BM aspirate revealed 9% blasts (Fig. 34.11b). Flow cytometry identified myeloid blasts (CD117, CD33, CD13, and CD7 positive; negative for MPO, CD19, CD10, CD79A and Cytoplasmic CD3). Genetic testing for BCR-ABL1, JAK2, CALR, or MPL mutations was negative. However, his *karyotype revealed Monosomy 7,* and the *PTPN11 mutation was positive*.

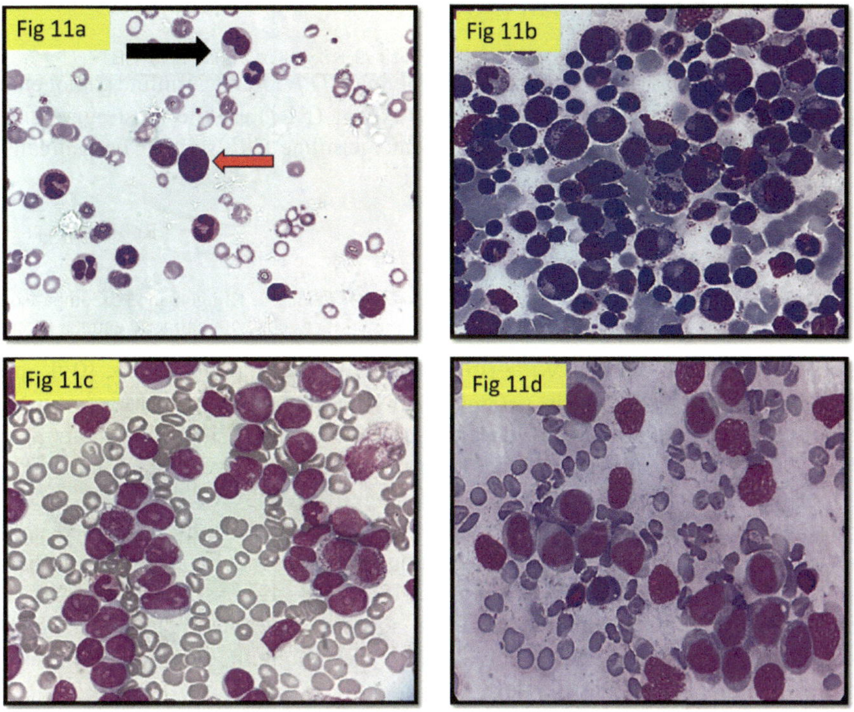

Fig. 34.11 (**a**) PBS at the initial presentation with monocyte (black arrow) and blast 2% (red arrow). (**b**) BM aspirate at the presentation showing proliferation of myeloid cells, increased monocytes, and 9% blasts. The patient progressed to AML after 10 months, as shown in PBS (**c**) and BMA (**d**)

The infant was managed initially with supportive care, hydroxyurea, and later with azacytidine, awaiting an allogeneic BM transplant. Within 1 year, he developed acute myeloid leukemia (Fig. 34.11c and d) and succumbed to the disease in less than 2 years of diagnosis.

JMML is the most common MPN observed in young children, presenting at a median age of approximately 1.8 years, with a male-to-female ratio of approximately 2.5:1 [45].

Compared to the earlier diagnostic criteria of JMML mentioned in the WHO 2016, the updates in the WHO 2022 diagnostic criteria include:

(a) Elimination of monosomy 7 as a cytogenetic criterion,
(b) KMT2A (MLL1) gene rearrangements need to be excluded and,
(c) Emphasis on the significance of diagnostic molecular studies, particularly those aimed at demonstrating RAS pathway activation [6].

34.8.1 Risk Stratification in JMML

The cases harboring somatic mutations involving *PTPN11* and germline pathogenic variants associated with neurofibromatosis type 1 (NF1) are the most aggressive types. Some cases associated with pathogenic germline *CBL* variants occasionally undergo spontaneous remission.

34.8.2 Non-transplanted JMML Children

The liver size (≥2 cm below the rib) and initial platelet count $<40 \times 10^9$/L are factors that affect survival in patients with RAS mutations [46]. Meyran et al. reported a predictive model to prognosticate outcomes in JMML patients post HSCT. Four adverse prognostic factors are: age at diagnosis ≥2 years, monocyte count at diagnosis $>7.2 \times 10^9$/L, time from diagnosis to HSCT ≥6 months, and the presence of ≥1 additional genetic alteration [47]. Additionally, increased age-adjusted hemoglobin F levels are also a poor prognostic feature. These are associated with lesser EFS and OS, even after HSCT [48, 49]. Associated secondary mutations and/or a hypermethylated DNA signature have an unfavorable prognosis with EFS rates of approximately 25%, so they should be offered HSCT early and/or a clinical trial, if available.

On the contrary, rare patients with a single mutated gene (NRAS or KRAS) or with germline CBL syndrome with a hypomethylated signature can be put on wait & watch or may be treated with a hypomethylating agent. They usually present during infancy and have higher platelet counts and normal fetal hemoglobin levels, and thus can be categorized in the intermediate category [50].

Usually, spontaneous resolution occurs in patients with germline CBL or PTPN11 mutations, so they should be put on a wait-and-watch. However, if they are symptomatic because of splenomegaly, leukocytosis, anemia, or thrombocytopenia, they can be given oral 6-mercaptopurine (50 mg/m^2/d) with or without cis-retinoic acid (100 mg/m^2/d). These agents will only alleviate the symptoms and don't improve the outcome [51, 52].

High-risk patients having multiple mutations, age >1 year, or elevated fetal hemoglobin are treated by 1–2 cycles of moderate intensity therapy with fludarabine (30 mg/m^2/d for 5 days) and cytarabine (2 g/m^2/d for 5 days) and then consolidated with allogenic BMT. The algorithm for management of JMML is shown in Fig. 34.12.

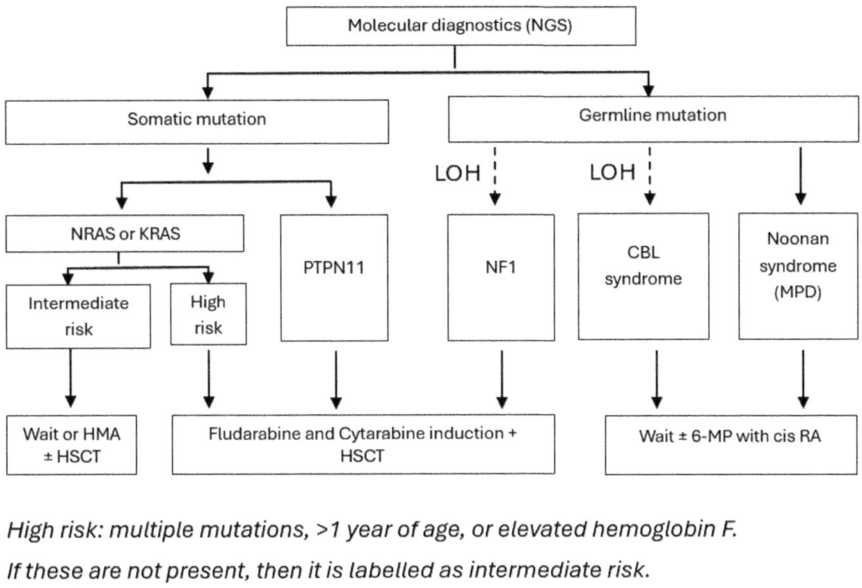

Fig. 34.12 Algorithm for management of Juvenile Myelomonocytic Leukemia (JMML)

34.8.3 Myeloproliferative Neoplasm, Unclassifiable (MPN—U)

This entity is a diagnosis of exclusion and is defined as an MPN that fails to meet the diagnostic criteria for any of the other defined 'classical' or 'non-classical' MPNs after a complete diagnostic workup. Most cases constitute very early-stage diseases, in which differentiation between various above-mentioned MPNs may be difficult. Most of the cases have MPN driver mutations (the most common is *JAK2*, followed by *CALR*), the rest of the cases have mutations in non-driver genes (*TET2*, *ASXL1*, SRSF2, *RUNX1*, and *DNMT3A*).

The prognosis of MPN-U depends on the following parameters:

1. Patient age: Advanced age-poor prognosis.
2. Co-morbid conditions.
3. Morphology (indicators of poor prognosis are).
   (a) Increase in myeloblasts.
   (b) Extensive fibrosis.
   (c) Extramedullary hematopoiesis.
4. Mutation landscape, e.g., ASXL1 mutations: poor prognosis.
5. Cytogenetic abnormalities.

Presently, allogeneic hematopoietic stem cell transplantation alone offers a long-term survival option.

34.9 Conclusion

The integration of molecular genetics into the diagnostic and prognostic frameworks of BCR::ABL1-negative MPNs represents a significant advancement in hematology. These developments enable more precise diagnoses and tailored treatment strategies, ultimately improving patient outcomes.

References

1. Arber DA, Orazi A, Hasserjian R, Thiele J, Borowitz MJ, Le Beau MM, et al. The 2016 revision to the World Health Organization classification of myeloid neoplasms and acute leukemia. Blood. 2016;127(20):2391–405.
2. Passamonti F, Rumi E, Pietra D, Elena C, Boveri E, Arcaini L, et al. A prospective study of 338 patients with polycythemia vera: the impact of JAK2 (V617F) allele burden and leukocytosis on fibrotic or leukemic disease transformation and vascular complications. Leukemia. 2010;24(9):1574–9.
3. Klampfl T, Gisslinger H, Harutyunyan AS, et al. Somatic mutations of calreticulin in myeloproliferative neoplasms. N Engl J Med. 2013;369(25):2379–90. https://doi.org/10.1056/NEJMoa13113474.
4. Alimam S, Villiers W, Dillon R, et al. Patients with triple- negative, JAK2V617F and CALR-mutated essential thrombocythemia share a unique gene expression signature. Blood Adv. 2021;5(4):1059–68. https://doi.org/10.1182/bloodadvances.2020003172.
5. Al-Ghamdi YA, Lake J, Bagg A, et al. Triple-negative primary myelofibrosis: a bone marrow pathology group study. Mod Pathol. 2023;36(3):100016. https://doi.org/10.1016/j.modpat.2022.100016. Epub 2023 Jan 10
6. Khoury JD, Solary E, Abla O, et al. The 5th edition of the World Health Organization classification of haematolymphoid tumours: myeloid and histiocytic/dendritic neoplasms. Leukemia. 2022;36(7):1703–19.
7. Arber DA, Orazi A, Hasserjian RP, et al. International Consensus Classification of myeloid neoplasms and acute leukemias: integrating morphologic, clinical, and genomic data. *Blood.* 2022;140(11):1200–28. https://doi.org/10.1182/blood.2022015850.
8. Tefferi A, Rumi E, Finazzi G, et al. Survival and prognosis among 1545 patients with contemporary polycythemia vera: an international study. Leukemia. 2013;27(9):1874–81.
9. Passamonti F, Thiele J, Girodon F, et al. A prognostic model to predict survival in 867 World Health Organization-defined essential thrombocythemia at diagnosis: a study by the International Working Group on Myelofibrosis Research and Treatment. Blood. 2012;120(6):1197–201.
10. Barraco D, Cerquozzi S, Hanson CA, Ketterling RP, Pardanani A, Gangat N, et al. Prognostic impact of bone marrow fibrosis in polycythemia vera: validation of the IWG-MRT study and additional observations. Blood Cancer J. 2017;7(3):e538.
11. Bonicelli G, Abdulkarim K, Mounier M, et al. Leucocytosis and thrombosis at diagnosis are associated with poor survival in polycythaemia vera: a population-based study of 327 patients. Br J Haematol. 2013;160(2):251–4.
12. Tefferi A, Vannucchi AM, Barbui T. Essential thrombocythemia: 2024 update on diagnosis, risk stratification, and management. Am J Hematol. 2024;99(4):697–718. https://doi.org/10.1002/ajh.27216.
13. Tefferi A, Loscocco GG, Farrukh F, et al. A globally applicable "triple A" risk model for essential thrombocythemia based on Age, Absolute neutrophil count, and Absolute lymphocyte count. Am J Hematol. 2023;98(12):1829–37. https://doi.org/10.1002/ajh.27079.

14. Tefferi A, Guglielmelli P, Lasho TL, et al. Mutation-enhanced international prognostic systems for essential thrombocythaemia and polycythaemia vera. Br J Haematol [Internet]. 2020 [cited 2025 Feb 23];189(2). Available from: https://pubmed.ncbi.nlm.nih.gov/31945802/
15. Guglielmelli P, Szuber N, Gangat N, et al. CALR variant allele frequency in essential thrombocythemia: molecular associations and impact on disease phenotype and outcome. Blood. 2023;142(Suppl 1):6328. https://doi.org/10.1182/blood-2023-174076.
16. Barbui T, Vannucchi AM, Buxhofer-Ausch V, et al. Practice-relevant revision of IPSET-thrombosis based on 1019 patients with WHO-defined essential thrombocythemia. Blood Cancer J. 2015;5(11):e369. https://doi.org/10.1038/bcj.2015.94.
17. Landolfi R, Marchioli R, Kutti J, et al; European Collaboration on Low-Dose Aspirin in Polycythemia Vera Investigators. Efficacy and safety of low-dose aspirin in polycythemia vera. N Engl J Med. 2004; b350(2):114–124.
18. Cortelazzo S, Finazzi G, Ruggeri M, et al. Hydroxyurea for patients with essential thrombocythemia and a high risk of thrombosis. N Engl J Med. 1995;332(17):1132–6.
19. Marchioli R, Finazzi G, Specchia G, et al; CYTO-PV Collaborative Group. Cardiovascular events and intensity of treatment in polycythemia vera. N Engl J Med. 2013;368(1):22–33.
20. Alvarez-Larrán A, Cervantes F, Pereira A, et al. Observation versus antiplatelet therapy as primary prophylaxis for thrombosis in low-risk essential thrombocythemia. Blood. 2010;116(8):1205–10.
21. Shvidel L, Sigler E, Haran M, et al. Busulphan is safe and efficient treatment in elderly patients with essential thrombocythemia. Leukemia. 2007;21(9):2071–2.
22. Kiladjian JJ, Chomienne C, Fenaux P. Interferon-α therapy in bcr-abl-negative myeloproliferative neoplasms. Leukemia. 2008;22(11):1990–8.
23. Quintás-Cardama A, Kantarjian H, Manshouri T, et al. Pegylated interferon alfa-2a yields high rates of hematologic and molecular response in patients with advanced essential thrombocythemia and polycythemia vera. J Clin Oncol. 2009;27(32):5418–24.
24. Ballen KK, Shrestha S, Sobocinski KA, et al. Outcome of transplantation for myelofibrosis. Biol Blood Marrow Transplant. 2010;16(3):358–67.
25. Martinez-Trillos A, Gaya A, Maffioli M, et al. Efficacy and tolerability of hydroxyurea in the treatment of the hyperproliferative manifestations of myelofibrosis: results in 40 patients. Ann Hematol. 2010;89:1233–7.
26. Mesa RA. The evolving treatment paradigm in myelofibrosis. Leuk Lymphoma. 2013;54:242–51.
27. Verstovsek S, Mesa RA, Gotlib J, et al. A double-blind, placebo-controlled trial of ruxolitinib for myelofibrosis. N Engl J Med. 2012;366:799–807.
28. Harrison C, Kiladjian JJ, Al-Ali HK, et al. JAK inhibition with ruxolitinib versus best available therapy for myelofibrosis. N Engl J Med. 2012;366:787–98.
29. Cervantes F, Vannucchi AM, Kiladjian JJ, et al. Three-year efficacy, safety, and survival findings from COMFORT-II, a phase 3 study comparing ruxolitinib with best available therapy for myelofibrosis. Blood. 2013;122:4047–53.
30. Huang J, Tefferi A. Erythropoiesis stimulating agents have limited therapeutic activity in transfusion-dependent patients with primary myelofibrosis regardless of serum erythropoietin level. Eur J Haematol. 2009;83:154–5.
31. Cervantes F, Alvarez-Larran A, Hernandez-Boluda JC, et al. Erythropoietin treatment of the anaemia of myelofibrosis with myeloid metaplasia: results in 20 patients and review of the literature. Br J Haematol. 2004;127:399–403.
32. Cervantes F, Isola IM, Alvarez-Larran A, et al. Danazol therapy for the anemia of myelofibrosis: assessment of efficacy with current criteria of response and long-term results. Ann Hematol. 2015;94:1791–6.
33. Mesa RA, Steensma DP, Pardanani A, et al. A phase 2 trial of combination low-dose thalidomide and prednisone for the treatment of myelofibrosis with myeloid metaplasia. Blood. 2003;101:2534–41.

34. Mesa RA, Yao X, Cripe LD, et al. Lenalidomide and prednisone for myelofibrosis: Eastern Cooperative Oncology Group (ECOG) phase 2 trial E4903. Blood. 2010;116:4436–8.
35. McLornan DP, Mead AJ, Jackson G, Harrison CN. Allogeneic stem cell transplantation for myelofibrosis in 2012. Br J Haematol. 2012;157:413–25.
36. Salit RB, Scott BL, Stevens EA, Baker KK, Gooley TA, Deeg HJ. Pre-hematopoietic cell transplant Ruxolitinib in patients with primary and secondary myelofibrosis. Bone Marrow Transplant. 2020;55:70–6.
37. Szuber N, Orazi A, Tefferi A. Chronic neutrophilic leukemia and atypical chronic myeloid leukemia: 2024 update on diagnosis, genetics, risk stratification, and management. Am J Hematol. 2024;99(7):1360–87. https://doi.org/10.1002/ajh.27321.
38. Szuber N, Elliott M, Tefferi A. Chronic neutrophilic leukemia: 2022 update on diagnosis, genomic landscape, prognosis, and management. Am J Hematol. 2022;97(4):491–505. https://doi.org/10.1002/ajh.26481.
39. Cui YJ, Jiang Q, Liu JQ, et al. The clinical characteristics, gene mutations and prognosis of chronic neutrophilic leukemia. Zhonghua Xue Ye Xue Za Zhi. 2017;38(1):28–32.
40. Elliott MA. Chronic neutrophilic leukemia and chronic myelomonocytic leukemia: WHO defined. Best Pract Res Clin Haematol. 2006;19(3):571–93.
41. Szuber N, Finke CM, Lasho TL, et al. CSF3R-mutated chronic neutrophilic leukemia: long-term outcome in 19 consecutive patients and risk model for survival. Blood Cancer J. 2018;8(2):21.
42. Dao KT, Gotlib J, Deininger MMN, et al. Efficacy of Ruxolitinib in patients with chronic neutrophilic leukemia and atypical chronic myeloid leukemia. J Clin Oncol. 2020;38(10):1006–18.
43. Klion AD. How I treat Hypereosinophilic syndrome. Blood. 2015;27(126):1069–77.
44. Helbig G, Soja A, Bartkowska-Chrobok A, Kyrcz-Krzemień S. Chronic eosinophilic leukemia-not otherwise specified has a poor prognosis with unresponsiveness to conventional treatment and high risk of acute transformation. Am J Hematol. 2012;87(6):643–5. https://doi.org/10.1002/ajh.23193.
45. Passmore SJ, Chessells JM, Kempski H, et al. Paediatric myelodysplastic syndromes and juvenile myelomonocytic leukaemia in the UK: a population-based study of incidence and survival. Br J Haematol. 2003;121(5):758–67. https://doi.org/10.1046/j.1365-2141.2003.04361.x.
46. ChenY,WangX,LiuC,ZhuX,YangW.GeneticcharacteristicsandclinicalprognosisofJMMLwith RAS mutations. *Blood.* 2024;144(Suppl 1):4569. https://doi.org/10.1182/blood-2024-204751.
47. Meyran D, Arfeuille C, Chevret S, et al. A predictive classifier of poor prognosis in transplanted patients with juvenile myelomonocytic leukemia: a study on behalf of the Société Francophone de Greffe de Moelle et de Thérapie Cellulaire. Haematologica. 2024;109(9):2908–19. https://doi.org/10.3324/haematol.2023.284103.
48. Passmore SJ, Hann IM, Stiller CA, et al. Pediatric myelodysplasia: a study of 68 children and a new prognostic scoring system. Blood. 1995;85(7):1742–50.
49. Dvorak CC, Loh ML. Juvenile myelomonocytic leukemia: molecular pathogenesis informs current approaches to therapy and hematopoietic cell transplantation. Front Pediatr. 2014;2:25.
50. Stieglitz E, Mazor T, Olshen AB, et al. Genome-wide DNA methylation is predictive of outcome in juvenile myelomonocytic leukemia. Nat Commun. 2017;8(1):2127.
51. Dvorak CC, Satwani P, Stieglitz E, et al. Disease burden and conditioning regimens in ASCT1221, a randomized phase II trial in children with juvenile myelomonocytic leukemia: a Children's Oncology Group study. Pediatr Blood Cancer. 2018;65(7):e27034.
52. Hecht A, Meyer J, Chehab FF, et al. Molecular assessment of pretransplant chemotherapy in the treatment of juvenile myelomonocytic leukemia. Pediatr Blood Cancer. 2019;66(11):e27948.

Chapter 35
Recent Advances in Management of Acute Myeloid Leukaemia

Tejasvini Vaid and Nitin Sood

Abstract Recent advances in AML have introduced targeted therapies and immunotherapies that significantly enhance disease management. Among targeted agents, Revumenib, a menin inhibitor, shows efficacy in KMT2A-rearranged and NPM1-mutated AML. Ivosidenib and olutasidenib target mutated IDH1, restoring differentiation pathways, while venetoclax, a BCL-2 inhibitor, improves survival when combined with hypomethylating agents. FLT3 inhibitors such as gilteritinib and quizartinib have reshaped treatment for FLT3-mutated AML. Tamibarotene, a synthetic retinoid, is effective in acute promyelocytic leukaemia.

Immunotherapies have emerged as complementary approaches. Peptide and dendritic cell vaccines targeting leukaemia-associated antigens like WT1 and PRAME show promise in inducing antigen-specific T-cell responses and preventing relapse. Immune checkpoint inhibitors (e.g., nivolumab, sabatolimab) are being evaluated in combination with standard therapies. Anti-CD47 antibody magrolimab enhances macrophage-mediated phagocytosis, and antibody-drug conjugates like pivekimab sunirine demonstrate potent activity in high-risk patients. Radioimmunoconjugates and CAR T-cell therapies represent innovative strategies under investigation, despite challenges with toxicity and antigen specificity.

These advancements signal a shift towards precision medicine in AML, with ongoing clinical trials aiming to optimize therapy combinations, improve patient selection, and extend survival in this aggressive disease.

Keywords Acute myeloid leukaemia · Targeted therapy · Immunotherapy · Precision medicine · Novel therapies

T. Vaid · N. Sood (✉)
Department of Medical and Hemato-Oncology, Medanta-The Medicity, Gurugram, Haryana, India

H. P. Pati et al. (eds.), *Clinical Hematology and Hemato-Oncology*, https://doi.org/10.1007/978-981-92-1167-8_35

Learning Objectives

1. Understand the molecular targets and mechanisms of newly approved AML therapies.
2. Evaluate the clinical efficacy and side effects of targeted agents, including menin, IDH, FLT3, and BCL-2 inhibitors.
3. Describe the role and limitations of investigational immunotherapies such as vaccines, checkpoint inhibitors, and CAR T-cell therapies in AML.
4. Analyse ongoing challenges in AML treatment, including resistance, toxicity, and patient selection.

35.1 Introduction

Acute myeloid leukaemia (AML) is a heterogeneous hematologic malignancy with historically limited treatment options and poor prognosis. Recently, there have been a lot of advances in the management of AML. These largely include targeted therapies and immunotherapies that significantly affect disease management. In this chapter, we predominantly address their role in AML management.

35.2 Illustrative a Clinical Case

A 48-year-old female with no co-morbidities presented with generalized weakness and fever. There was no obvious focus of infection. The patient did not report and bleeding manifestations or any masses or swellings. Physical examination was unremarkable. Routine tests revealed Hb 7gm/dl, TLC 26,000/mcl, platelets 60,000/mcl with 20% blasts in the peripheral smear. Bone marrow aspiration, biopsy, flowcytometry were done, and a diagnosis of AML was confirmed. FLT3-ITD was mutated on the AML comprehensive panel. She was started on tumour lysis prophylaxis (TLS) along with antifungal and varicella prophylaxis. Baseline HRCT thorax and 2D ECHO were normal. She underwent induction therapy with 7 + 3 regimen (cytarabine 100 mg/m^2 continuous infusion for 7 days plus daunorubicin 60 mg/m^2 for 3 days) combined with midostaurin 50 mg twice daily from day 8 to 21. She achieved a complete remission and proceeded to consolidation with high-dose cytarabine (HiDAC, 3 g/m^2 every 12 h on days 1, 3, and 5) plus midostaurin from day 8 to 21. During her second consolidation cycle, the patient experienced a relapse with 25% blasts in peripheral smear and persistence of the FLT3-ITD mutation. Given the high-risk molecular profile, she was started on Gilteritinib 120 mg daily as salvage therapy. The patient demonstrated a rapid hematologic response with blast clearance on day 28, achieving a second remission. This remission facilitated proceeding to alloHSCT with a matched sibling donor with a myeloablative conditioning regimen (FluBu4). Due to the lack of availability of Quizartinib, Gilteritinib, though not approved, was considered for post-transplant maintenance to reduce relapse risk, pending engraftment and tolerance, in line with emerging data supporting FLT3 inhibitor maintenance in this high-risk population.

35.3 Targeted Therapies in AML

35.3.1 *Menin Inhibitor*

Revumenib

(a) *Mechanism of action:* Revumenib is a selective menin inhibitor targeting KMT2A-rearranged (MLLr) and NPM1-mutated acute leukaemia's. These leukemias are driven by abnormal transcriptional pathways that are maintained due to the interaction of the menin-KMT2A fusion protein. Menin acts as the scaffold that tethers KMT2A to the chromatin and recruits key cofactors, including DOT1L, resulting in sustained expression of MEIS1, HOXA9, and other transcriptional targets. This results in a differentiation block and leukemic transformation of the cell involved. Revumenib binds to menin and prevents its interaction with KMT2A fusion proteins. This block downregulates the HOX and MEIS1 gene expression, which are critical for maintaining leukemic stem cell survival and self-renewal [1].

(b) *Indication:* It is currently approved by the FDA for relapse or refractory (R/R) acute leukaemia with KMT2A rearrangement in adults and children 1 year of age or older.

(c) *Dosage:* The standard dose of revumenib in adults who weigh >40 kg is 270 mg twice a day in the absence of a strong CYP inhibitor and 160 mg twice a day in the presence of a strong CYP inhibitor. The dose varies as per body surface area in individuals <40 kg. The treatment should be continued till there is evidence of disease progression or unacceptable toxicity occurs. In patients who do not experience disease progression or unacceptable toxicity, treatment should be continued for a minimum of 6 months to allow for clinical response.

(d) *Side effects:* Differentiation syndrome, QTc prolongation, neutropenia, anaemia, haemorrhage, hepatic dysfunction.

(e) *Clinical trial data:* The AUGMENT-101 trial is a multi-centre Phase 1/2 study that evaluated Revumenib in patients with R/R acute leukaemia's with KMT2A rearrangements (KMT2Ar) or NPM1 mutations. The combined complete remission (CR) and complete remission with partial hematologic recovery (CRh) rate was approximately 30% [1, 2].

35.3.2 *IDH1 Inhibitors*

In normal cells, wild-type (isocitrate dehydrogenase-1) IDH1 catalyses the conversion of isocitrate to alpha-ketoglutarate (α-KG). However, a gain-of-function mutation of IDH1 results in conversion of α-KG to D-2-hydroxyglutarate (2-HG). Elevated 2-HG levels impair cellular differentiation through epigenetic modifications. It leads to inhibition of α-KG–dependent dioxygenases such as TET2 and histone demethylases, thus promoting leukemogenesis. IDH1 inhibitors selectively inhibit the mutated IDH1 enzyme, leading to the blockage of 2-HG production. This reduction in 2-HG levels results in normalization of differentiation pathways leading to disease remission [3].

A. *Ivosidenib:*

   (a) *Mechanism of action:* Ivosidenib is a first-in-class reversible and selective IDH1 inhibitor.
   (b) *Indication:* It is approved for the treatment of newly diagnosed patients with AML who are 75 years of age or older or patients who have co-morbidities that preclude the use of intensive chemotherapy. It is also approved for use in R/R AML.
   (c) *Dosage:* 500 mg orally once a day with or without food. The medication should be taken until unacceptable toxicity or disease progression. Avoid consuming a high-fat meal. Avoid concomitant use with strong CYP inhibitors.
   (d) *Side effects:* Differentiation syndrome, QTc prolongation, hepatotoxicity, Guillain–Barré syndrome.
   (e) *Clinical trial data:* The Phase III AGILE trial conducted in patients with newly diagnosed AML compared ivosidenib in combination with azacitidine to azacytidine plus placebo. It revealed a median OS of 24 months in the ivosidenib plus azacitidine arm compared to 7.9 months in the azacitidine and placebo arm (HR: 0.44; p value <0.001) [4].

B. *Olutasidenib.*

   (a) *Mechanism of action:* It is a selective, reversible allosteric IDH1 inhibitor.
   (b) *Indication:* Olutasidenib is currently approved by the FDA for *the* treatment of adult patients with R/R AML who have a susceptible IDH1 mutation.
   (c) *Dosage:* The dose of olutasidenib is 150 mg orally twice daily, taken on an empty stomach at least 1 h before or 2 h after food. The drug should be continued until there is evidence of disease progression or unacceptable toxicity occurs. For patients without disease progression or unacceptable toxicity, treatment should be continued for a minimum of 6 months to allow time for clinical response.
   (d) *Side effects:* Differentiation syndrome, QTc prolongation, neutropenia, anaemia, haemorrhage, hepatic dysfunction.
   (e) *Clinical trial data:* The 2102-HEM-101 trial was a pivotal Phase 1/2 clinical trial designed to evaluate the safety and efficacy of olutasidenib in patients with R/R AML with an IDH1 mutation. In the Phase 2 portion of the trial, olutasidenib was administered at a dose of 150 mg twice a day, as per the dose established in Phase 1 of the trial. A composite complete remission (CR + CRh) rate of approximately 18%, with a median duration of response of 25.9 months, was noted. The median time taken to develop a response was 1.9 months. The safety profile was similar to that of other IDH1 inhibitors, with common adverse events including fatigue, nausea, elevated liver enzymes, and differentiation syndrome. Trials investigating olutasidenib in combination with azacitidine are underway [5].

35.3.3 IDH2 Inhibitor

Enasidenib

(a) *Mechanism of action:* Enasidenib is a selective isocitrate dehydrogenase inhibitor 2 (IDH2) inhibitor. Mutations in IDH2 lead to neomorphic enzyme activity that converts α-KG to 2-HG, and elevated levels of 2-HG impair cell differentiation by altering histone methylation. Enasidenib inhibits the mutated IDH2, thus releasing the differentiation block.
(b) *Indication:* It is FDA approved (but not EMA approved) for the treatment of R/R AML in adults.
(c) *Dosage:* 100 mg orally once a day with or without food. Treatment should be continued till disease progression or unacceptable toxicity.
(d) *Side effects:* differentiation syndrome, hepatotoxicity, leukocytosis and TLS, nausea, vomiting.
(e) *Clinical trial data:* The pivotal data for enasidenib came from the open-label Phase I/II AG221-C-001 trial conducted in patients with R/R AML with IDH2 mutation. The trial revealed a CR of 19% and an overall response rate (ORR) of 40%. However, the subsequent Phase III IDHENTIFY trial, where enasidenib was compared to a conventional regimen in patients with R/R AML, failed to demonstrate any survival advantage. The median OS was 6.5 months in the enasidenib arm and 7.3 months in the control arm [6].

35.3.4 Tamibarotene

(a) *Mechanism of action:* Tamibarotene is a synthetic retinoid that selectively binds and activates the retinoic acid receptor alpha (RARα). By binding RARα with high affinity, tamibarotene promotes the transcription of genes involved in cell differentiation and apoptosis. This results in normal differentiation of the leukemic promyelocytes into mature neutrophils.
(b) *Approval:* Tamibarotene is approved in Japan for the treatment of acute promyelocytic leukaemia (APL).
(c) *Dosage:* The dosage of tamibarotene is 3 mg/m^2 twice daily. Treatment is usually continued until CR is achieved or for a defined treatment duration (often up to 8 weeks), depending on response and side effects.
(d) *Side effects:* differentiation syndrome, pseudotumor cerebri, hepatic dysfunction, anaemia, thrombocytopenia, neutropenia, rash, dry skin.
(e) *Clinical trial data:* A Phase 2 trial conducted in Japan by Shigeno et al. evaluated the efficacy and safety of tamibarotene in patients with R/R APL who had previously been treated with all-trans retinoic acid (ATRA) and chemotherapy. An overall response (OS) rate of 58%, with about 33% of patients achieving complete remission and a median remission duration of 14.6 months, was noted. Tamibarotene was generally well tolerated, with manageable side effects, including differentiation syndrome [7]. A Phase 3 randomized trial by Asou

et al. compared tamibarotene with ATRA as maintenance therapy in patients with newly diagnosed APL who had achieved remission. The trial demonstrated that tamibarotene significantly reduced relapse rates compared to ATRA, particularly in patients with high-risk disease, and improved relapse-free survival [8].

35.3.5 BCL-2 Inhibitor

Venetoclax

(a) *Mechanism of action:* Venetoclax is a selective inhibitor of BCL-2, an anti-apoptotic protein that is often overexpressed in AML. By binding with high affinity to BCL-2, venetoclax displaces pro-apoptotic proteins like BIM and BAX, which are normally bound by BCL-2 to prevent apoptosis. The release of these proteins leads to an increase in mitochondrial outer membrane permeability, resulting in the release of cytochrome c and subsequent activation of the caspase cascade, culminating in programmed cell death. Venetoclax effectively induces apoptosis in AML blasts that rely on BCL-2 for survival, restoring the normal apoptotic process in these cells [9].
(b) *Indication:* It is approved in combination with azacitidine, decitabine, or low-dose cytarabine (LDAC), for the treatment of newly diagnosed AML in adults who are 75 years or older, or in individuals who have comorbidities that preclude the use of intensive induction chemotherapy.
(c) *Dosage:* The dosing regimen for AML begins with a 3-day ramp-up phase to reduce the risk of TLS: 100 mg on day 1, 200 mg on day 2, and 400 mg on day 3. From day 4 onward, the dose is 400 mg once a day in combination with azacitidine or decitabine, and 600 mg once a day in combination with low-dose cytarabine. These regimens are part of a 28-day treatment cycle and are continued until disease progression or unacceptable toxicity occurs. Dosage needs modification when taken with strong CYP inhibitors. Dose reduction for haematological adverse effects is not uncommon.
(d) *Side effects:* TLS, anaemia, neutropenia, thrombocytopenia, diarrhoea, nausea, vomiting.
(e) *Clinical trial data:* The VIALE-A and VIALE-C trials are Phase III trials that compared venetoclax in combination with hypomethylating agents (HMAs) or LDAC to HMAs with placebo or LDAC with placebo, respectively, for patients with AML who were ineligible for intensive chemotherapy.

In the VIALE-A trial, the median OS was 14.7 months for the venetoclax-azacitidine arm versus 9.6 months for the placebo-azacitidine arm, with a hazard ratio (HR) of 0.66 (95% confidence interval [CI], 0.52–0.85; $P < 0.001$) [10].

In the VIALE-C trial, the primary analysis did not reveal a statistically significant increase in OS; however, a 6-month follow-up revealed a median OS of

8.4 months for the venetoclax-LDAC arm versus 4.1 months for the placebo-LDAC arm, with an HR of 0.70 (95% CI, 0.50–0.99; $P = 0.040$) [11].

Recent advancements in AML treatment have explored triple-drug regimens incorporating venetoclax to enhance therapeutic efficacy, particularly in patients with specific genetic mutations.

A phase I/II study (NCT04140487) evaluated the combination of venetoclax, azacytidine, and gilteritinib in newly diagnosed and R/R FLT3-mutated AML patients who were unfit for intensive chemotherapy. The CR rate and 18-month OS in patients with newly diagnosed AML was 90% and 72%, respectively; however, dose reduction due to myelosuppression was common [12]. A phase Ib study combining venetoclax and azacitidine with ivosidenib (an IDH1 inhibitor) in newly diagnosed IDH1-mutated AML patients showed a composite CR rate of 53% and a median OS of 24 months, outperforming single-agent azacitidine [13].

35.3.6 FLT3 Inhibitors

FLT3 mutations, particularly internal tandem duplications (ITD) and tyrosine kinase domain (TKD) point mutations, are among the most common genetic alterations in AML, occurring in approximately 30% of cases. These mutations are associated with a poor prognosis due to high relapse rates and reduced OS [14]. The advent of targeted therapies, especially FLT3 inhibitors, has significantly transformed the treatment landscape for FLT3-mutated AML.

FLT2-ITD and FLT3-TKD mutations lead to constitutive activation of the FLT3 receptor leading to uncontrolled proliferation, survival, and resistance to apoptosis due to activation of downstream pathways such as STAT5, RAS/MAPK, and PI3K/AKT. FLT3 inhibitors bind to the ATP binding site of the receptor, thus preventing the phosphorylation and activation of these downstream pathways, which leads to disruption of cell growth and induced apoptosis [15].

First-Generation FLT3 Inhibitors

A. *Midostaurin*

(a) *Mechanism of action:* It is a multi-targeted kinase inhibitor that inhibits both FLT3-ITD and FLT3-TKD.
(b) *Indication:* Newly diagnosed AML with FLT3 mutation in combination with cytarabine and daunorubicin (7 + 3) induction and cytarabine consolidation.
(c) *Dosage:* 50 mg orally twice a day from day 8 to day 21 of every cycle of induction and consolidation. It is metabolized by CYP3A4, and strong CYP3A4 inhibitors can lead to increased drug levels. Medication should be taken with food to enhance absorption.
(d) *Side effects:* nausea, vomiting, QTc prolongation, hepatotoxicity are common side effects.

(e) *Clinical trial data:* The Phase III RATIFY trial demonstrated that adding midostaurin to chemotherapy improved OS compared to chemotherapy alone. The median OS was 74.7 months and 25.6 months in the midostaurin arm and placebo arm, respectively [16].

Second-Generation FLT3 Inhibitors

B. *Gilteritinib.*

(a) *Mechanism of action:* It is a type 1 FLT3 inhibitor that inhibits both FLT3-ITD as well as FLT3-TKD.
(b) *Indication:* Approved for R/R FLT3-mutated AML.
(c) *Dosage:* 120 mg orally once a day with or without food. The drug should be continued until disease progression or until unacceptable side effects. A minimum time duration of 6 months is needed to allow for clinical response. Avoid usage with a strong CYP3A inhibitor. If unavoidable, then monitor closely for gilteritinib-associated side effects.
(d) *Side effects:* QTc prolongation, posterior reversible encephalopathy syndrome (PRES), differentiation syndrome, pancreatitis, hepatotoxicity, cytopenias.
(e) *Clinical trial data:* In the Phase III ADMIRAL trial, gilteritinib demonstrated a median OS of 9.3 months as compared to 5.6 months for those receiving salvage chemotherapy (HR 0.64; 95% CI: 0.48–0.83; p: 0.0004). Combined CR and CR with partial haematological (CRh) recovery was 21% [17].

C. *Quizartinib*

(a) *Mechanism of action:* It is a selective FLT3-ITD inhibitor.
(b) *Indication:* It is FDA approved for adults with newly diagnosed AML with FLT3-ITD mutation in combination with standard cytarabine and daunorubicin (7 + 3) induction and cytarabine consolidation and maintenance monotherapy after consolidation chemotherapy.
(c) *Dosage:* 35.4 mg orally once a day from day 8 to 21 during induction and day 6 to 19 during consolidation. A dose of 26.5 mg once a day for days 1–14 followed by an escalation to 53 mg once a day, provided QTcF is less than or equal to 450 ms. If the QTcF is >450 ms, a dose of 26.5 mg once a day should be continued. It is taken daily with no interruptions up to 36 cycles.
(d) *Side effects:* QTc prolongation, neutropenia, diarrhoea, mucositis, etc.
(e) *Clinical trial data:* In the Phase III QuANTUM-First trial, the median OS was 31.9 months in the quizartinib arm as compared to 15.1 months in the placebo arm (HR 0.78; 95% CI 0.62–0.98; p value: 0.032). The addition of quizartinib to chemotherapy resulted in a significant improvement in median OS in comparison to chemotherapy alone. However, its use requires careful monitoring due to potential QT prolongation [18].

35.4 Immunotherapy in AML

35.4.1 Peptide-Based Vaccines in AML

Peptide-based vaccines are a form of immunotherapy designed to elicit an antigen-specific cytotoxic T lymphocyte (CTL) response against leukaemia-associated antigens (LAAs). These vaccines are composed of synthetically produced peptides derived from LAAs, which are administered in combination with adjuvants to stimulate an adaptive immune response [19].

Wilms' Tumour 1 (WT1) is a transcription factor that is highly overexpressed in AML and associated with disease progression and is one of the most thoroughly investigated LAAs. A Phase I/II trial, NCT01266083, assessed the WT1 peptide vaccine galinpepimut-S (GPS) in patients with AML in CR1. In this trial, 22 patients received 6 GPS injections twice a week with the option of boosters at 6 months. WT1-specific $CD8^{+}$ T-cell response was noted in 64% patients and the median relapse free survival was 16.9 months [20]. The subsequent Phase III study, known as the REGAL trial (NCT04229979), compares GPS to the investigator's choice of maintenance treatment in AML patients in CR2 or higher and is underway [21].

Other LAAs under investigation include PRAME (preferentially Expressed Antigen In Myeloma), a cancer antigen with restricted expression on normal antigen, and RHAMM (Receptor for Hyaluronic Acid Mediated Motility) R3 peptide, which stimulated HLA-A2 restricted CTLs that have AML-specific cytotoxicity [22].

35.4.2 Dendritic Cell (DC) Vaccines in AML

DC vaccines are an emerging immunotherapeutic strategy in AML that leverage potential antigen-presenting properties of DCs to stimulate leukaemia-specific CTLs. Despite high remission rates with chemotherapy, AML patients are prone to relapse. Due to its typically low mutational burden and immune evasion characteristics, effective post-remission strategies that increase immune surveillance are urgently needed. DC vaccines are designed to boost anti-leukemic immunity by loading autologous or allogeneic DCs with LAAs such as WT1, PRAME, RHAMM, or whole tumour lysates. These antigen-loaded DCs are then reintroduced into other patients to prime T cells against residual leukaemia cells [23].

A well-studied approach uses autologous monocyte-derived DCs pulsed with WT1 peptides or AML blast lysates. In a pivotal Phase I/II trial (NCT00834002), Anguille et al. demonstrated that AML patients in CR1 who received WT1-loaded DCs developed sustained WT1-specific T-cell responses, achieving a 43% leukaemia-free survival rate at 2 years- significantly higher than historical controls [24].

Another key trial used autologous DCs electroporated with WT1 mRNA in AML patients in remission after one or more courses of polychemotherapy and at a high risk of relapse. This phase I/II trial (NCT00965224) reported that 13 of 30 patients showed vaccine-induced WT1-specific T-cell responses. The 5-year OS was 53.8% and 25% in responders vs non-responders. Patients who received the vaccine in CR1 had a 5-year relapse-free survival of 50% among those who responded, as compared to 7.7% among those who did not exhibit any response. The vaccine was well-tolerated with few side effects [25].

Additionally, a trial using leukaemia-derived apoptotic bodies to load DCs (NCT01373515) demonstrated the feasibility and immunogenicity of a multivalent, patient-specific DC vaccine. It elicited both $CD4^+$ and $CD8^+$ responses and showed promising disease-free survival in early-phase testing [26].

To address the challenge of immune escape, recent studies have focused on a multi-antigen vaccine strategy. The ongoing phase I trial NCT01734304 is evaluating a DC vaccine consisting of WT-1 and PRAME peptides in AML patients in remission. Interim data revealed durable T -cell responses and encouraging one-year relapse-free survival outcomes [27].

While DC vaccines have shown excellent safety and immune activation profiles, their efficacy is currently being tested in large cohorts in combination with immune checkpoint inhibitors or HMAs to enhance response durability [28].

35.4.3 Checkpoint Inhibitors

Checkpoint inhibitors (CPIs) are monoclonal antibodies that target immune regulatory pathways such as PD-1/PD-L1, CTLA-4, and TIM3, aiming to restore anti-tumour immunity of exhausted T cells. While CPIs have revolutionized treatment in solid tumours and lymphoid malignancies, their application in AML has been more challenging due to the immunosuppressive bone marrow microenvironment and the relatively low mutational burden of AML.

AML cells exploit immune checkpoint pathways to evade immune surveillance. Upregulation of PD-L1 on blasts and PD-1 on T cells has been observed, particularly during or after treatment, contributing to T-cell exhaustion and disease persistence. The rationale for the use of CPI in AML is thus based on reversing this immune dysfunction and enhancing T-cell-mediated leukaemia clearance [29].

Early-phase trials have investigated anti-PD-1 agents such as nivolumab, pembrolizumab, and anti-CTLA-4 agents like ipilimumab in R/R AML and in post-transplant relapse. In a Phase II study (NCT02397720), nivolumab combined with azacitidine in R/R AML showed an overall response rate (ORR) of 33%, with a subset of patients achieving durable remissions. Immune-related adverse events were observed, however [30].

Ipilimumab monotherapy was studied in a Phase I trial (NCT00027870) in patients with post-allogeneic stem cell transplant relapse. Results showed clinical responses in AML patients, including complete remissions, and expansion of leukaemia-reactive T-cell clones, suggesting a graft-versus-leukaemia (GvL) effect without severe graft-versus-host disease (GVHD) [31].

More recently, dual checkpoint blockade (e.g., nivolumab + ipilimumab) and combinations with hypomethylating agents or vaccines are under active investigation (e.g., NCT04284787) [32]. Use of decitabine with venetoclax in the management of AML leads to upregulation of PD1 in T cells. Trial evaluating the combination of venetoclax, decitabine, and nivolumab for the treatment of AML is underway. Despite initial promise, PD-1 and CTLA-4 inhibitors in AML require careful patient selection due to side effects, risks of GVHD post-transplant, and variable response rates [33].

T-cell immunoglobulin and mucin-domain containing-3 (TIM-3) is an effective immunotherapeutic target in AML because it is highly expressed not only on exhausted T cells but also on leukaemia stem cells (LSCs), which are thought to drive relapse and resistance. Moreover, TIM-3 is not frequently expressed on normal hematopoietic stem cells, making it a selective marker for targeting the malignant stem cell population. TIM-3 signalling also promotes immune evasion by suppressing T-cell responses, contributing to an immunosuppressive microenvironment. Therefore, blocking TIM-3 may both reinvigorate anti-leukemic immunity and directly impair the survival of LSCs, offering a dual therapeutic benefit [34].

Sabatolimab is a monoclonal antibody targeting TIM-3. Clinical trials have primarily explored its use in combination with other therapies like venetoclax and azacitidine. In an early-phase clinical trial (NCT02608268), sabatolimab, when combined with venetoclax and azacitidine, showed a promising ORR of 57% in R/R AML, with a manageable safety profile. These results suggest that targeting TIM-3, alongside epigenetic and BCL-2 inhibition, may enhance treatment outcomes in AML [35]. Sabatolimab is also being studied in combination with PD-1 inhibitors and other immunomodulatory agents in ongoing clinical trials.

35.4.4 Anti-CD47 Monoclonal Antibodies

Magrolimab is a humanized monoclonal antibody against CD47. CD47 is a transmembrane protein overexpressed on AML cells that delivers a "don't eat me" signal to macrophages via interaction with signal regulatory protein alpha (SIRPα). By blocking this interaction, magrolimab promotes phagocytosis of AML cells [36]. When combined with hypomethylating agents like azacitidine, which upregulate pro-phagocytic signals, the anti-leukemic effect is further potentiated.

In a Phase 1b study (NCT03248479), magrolimab was used in combination with azacitidine and demonstrated promising activity in treatment-naïve AML patients ineligible for intensive chemotherapy. In this trial, 82.8% patients had TP53 mutations. The overall CR rate was 32.2%. The median OS was 9.8 months and 18.9 months in TP53-mutated and TP53 wild-type patients, respectively. The combination was generally well tolerated; common adverse events included gastrointestinal symptoms and anaemia [37, 38].

These encouraging results led to the initiation of several Phase 3 trials. ENHANCE-2 (NCT04778397) evaluated magrolimab plus azacitidine versus standard therapy in TP53-mutant AML [39]. ENHANCE-3 (NCT05079230) evaluated magrolimab in combination with azacitidine and venetoclax in newly diagnosed AML patients who were unfit for intensive therapy. However, interim analyses revealed that magrolimab-containing protocols were associated with increased mortality due to infections and respiratory failure [40, 41].

35.4.5 Antibody-Drug Conjugate-Pivekimab Sunirine

Pivekimab sunirine (IMGN632) is an investigational antibody-drug conjugate (ADC) against CD123, a transmembrane protein overexpressed on leukemic blasts and LSCs in AML, while sparing normal hematopoietic stem cells. It consists of a high-affinity anti-CD123 antibody linked to an indolinobenzodiazepine pseudodimer (IGN), which induces DNA alkylation and single-strand breaks without cross-linking. When the ACD binds the CD123 on the cell surface, it is internalized. Once inside the cell, the linker is cleaved by intracellular proteases and the IGN exerts its cytotoxic effect on the DNA [42].

In a Phase 1/2 study involving patients with R/R AML, pivekimab sunirine monotherapy demonstrated an ORR of 21%, including a complete remission (CR) rate of 17%. The treatment was generally well-tolerated, with manageable adverse events such as febrile neutropenia, infusion reactions, and anaemia [43]. Building upon these findings, a Phase 1b/2 study evaluated pivekimab sunirine in combination with venetoclax and azacitidine in patients with newly diagnosed AML who are unfit for intensive chemotherapy. This triplet regimen yielded a CR rate of 54% and a minimal residual disease (MRD) negativity rate of 76%. Notably, patients with TP53 mutations exhibited a CR rate of 88% and an MRD negativity rate of 80% [44]. Ongoing trials are evaluating the efficacy and safety of pivekimab sunirine in various combinations and dosing schedules, including its integration with the FLAG-Ida chemotherapy regimen in newly diagnosed adverse-risk AML patients [45].

35.4.6 Radioimmunoconjugates in AML

Radioimmunoconjugates are a class of targeted therapeutics that combine monoclonal antibodies with a radionuclide to deliver localized radiation to malignant cells. In AML, these agents aim to selectively irradiate leukemic blasts and LSCs while sparing healthy tissues. The antibodies are typically directed against surface antigens overexpressed in AML, such as CD33, CD45, and CD123, which are expressed on leukemic cells but have limited expression on normal hematopoietic progenitors.

One of the earliest and most studied radioimmunoconjugates is I-131-apamistamab, which targets CD45 and delivers iodine-131 to hematopoietic cells. It is being developed for patients with R/R AML as a myeloablative conditioning regimen prior to allogeneic stem cell transplantation (allo-HSCT). In the Phase III SIERRA trial (NCT02665065), patients with R/R AML >55 years of age who achieved CR were randomized in a 1:1 ratio to receive either conventional care followed by allo-HSCT or I-131-apamistamab followed by allo-HSCT. The durable CR rate was significantly higher with ^{131}I-apamistamab (17.1% [95% CI, 9.4 to 27.5]) than conventional care (0% [95% CI, 0 to 4.7]; $P < 0.0001$) with favourable OS HR and EFS HR. [46]

Similarly, lintuzumab-Ac225, an anti-CD33 antibody-based radioimmunoconjugate linked to actinium-225, an alpha-emitting radionuclide. Alpha particles offer high linear energy transfer and potent cytotoxicity within a short path length, minimizing off-target effects. Early-phase trials have shown promising anti-leukemic activity, although myelosuppression remains a dose-limiting toxicity [47–49].

35.4.7 CART Cell Therapy in AML

CAR T-cell therapy has revolutionized the treatment of B-cell malignancies. In AML, the strategy involves engineering T-cells to target antigens overexpressed on leukemic blasts and LSCs. Common targets being investigated include CD33, CD123, CLL-1, and CD70. However, since these antigens are also expressed on normal hematopoietic stem cells, such therapies carry the risk of off-tumour side effects, on-target side effects, and prolonged myelosuppression [50].

Early-phase clinical trials have demonstrated the potential of CAR T-cell therapy in AML:

- CD123-Directed CAR T-Cells: In a Phase I trial (NCT02623582), patients with R/R AML were treated with an autologous anti-CD123 CAR T-cell product. While some patients exhibited anti-leukemic responses, the trial was terminated due to adverse events, including cytokine release syndrome (CRS) and on-target, off-tumour toxicity [51].
- Allogeneic CAR T-Cells: UCART123, an "off the shelf" allogeneic anti-CD123 CAR T-cell product created by genetically modifying non-HLA-matched healthy donor T cells, was evaluated in a Phase I trial (NCT03190278). The study faced challenges, including patient mortality due to CRS, leading to protocol modifications and dose adjustments [52].

Several obstacles hinder the widespread application of CAR T-cell therapy in AML:

- Antigen Specificity: In the absence of an AML-specific antigen, production of CAR-T cells that target leukemic cells without affecting normal HSPCs has not been possible. This has led to prolonged cytopenias and increased infection risk.

- Antigen Heterogeneity and Loss: AML exhibits significant antigenic heterogeneity, and leukemic cells may downregulate target antigens, leading to immune escape and disease relapse [53].
- Immunosuppressive Microenvironment: The AML microenvironment is characterized by immunosuppressive factors, including regulatory T-cells and myeloid-derived suppressor cells, which can inhibit CAR T-cell function and persistence [54].
- Manufacturing Challenges: Producing CAR T-cells from heavily pretreated AML patients can be difficult due to T-cell dysfunction and low yields, complicating the manufacturing process [55].

35.5 Summary

Recent advances in AML management have led to significant improvements in patient outcomes through the approval of targeted therapies that address specific genetic mutations. Agents like Revumenib (menin inhibitor), Ivosidenib and Olutasidenib (IDH1 inhibitors), Enasidenib (IDH2 inhibitor), Venetoclax (BCL-2 inhibitor), and FLT3 inhibitors such as Midostaurin, Gilteritinib, and Quizartinib have improved remission rates and overall survival, particularly when used in combination with hypomethylating agents or chemotherapy. These therapies have transformed treatment paradigms for patients who were previously limited to conventional chemotherapy. Meanwhile, investigational strategies are focusing on novel immune and molecular pathways. These include vaccines targeting leukaemia-associated antigens, checkpoint inhibitors (e.g., sabatolimab, nivolumab) to reverse T-cell exhaustion, and agents like Magrolimab and Pivekimab Sunirine that target CD47 and CD123, respectively, enhancing immune-mediated clearance of leukaemia cells. Additionally, radioimmunoconjugates and CAR T-cell therapies are being developed to deliver highly targeted cytotoxicity. Together, these evolving strategies are expanding therapeutic options and offering hope for better long-term disease control in AML.

References

1. Issa GC, Aldoss I, JF DP, et al. Safety and clinical activity of the menin inhibitor revumenib (SNDX-5613) in KMT2A-rearranged or NPM1-mutated acute leukemias (AUGMENT-101). N Engl J Med. 2023;388(22):1987–98.
2. DiNardo CD, Stein EM, de Botton S, et al. Menin inhibitor revumenib in KMT2A-rearranged or NPM1-mutated leukemia: updated phase I results. J Clin Oncol. 2024;42(15):1671–82.
3. Dang L, Yen K, Attar EC. IDH mutations in cancer and progress toward development of targeted therapeutics. Ann Oncol. 2016;27(4):599–608.
4. Montesinos P, DiNardo CD, Daver N, et al. Ivosidenib plus azacitidine for IDH1-mutated acute myeloid leukaemia (AGILE). N Engl J Med. 2022;386(16):1519–31.

5. de Botton S, Stein EM, CD DN, et al. Olutasidenib for relapsed or refractory IDH1-mutated AML: results of the 2102-HEM-101 phase II study. Leukemia. 2023;37(8):1683–93.
6. Stein EM, CD DN, Pollyea DA, et al. Enasidenib in mutated IDH2 relapsed/refractory AML: long-term follow-up of the AG221-C-001 trial. Blood. 2019;134(9):662–73.
7. Shigeno K, Naito K, Sahara N, et al. Multicentre phase II study of tamibarotene in all-trans-retinoic-acid-resistant relapsed APL. Br J Haematol. 2004;127(5):691–700.
8. Asou N, Kishimoto Y, Takemoto Y, et al. Randomised phase III study of tamibarotene vs ATRA for maintenance in newly diagnosed APL. Blood. 2014;123(9):1290–8.
9. Pan R, Ruvolo V, Mu H, et al. Leukemia cell dependence on BCL-2 is determined by cellular differentiation state. Cancer Discov. 2014;4(3):362–75.
10. CD DN, Jonas BA, Pullarkat V, et al. Azacitidine and venetoclax in previously untreated AML (VIALE-A). N Engl J Med. 2020;383(7):617–29.
11. Wei AH, Montesinos P, Ivanov V, et al. Venetoclax plus low-dose cytarabine for older/unfit AML (VIALE-C). Blood Adv. 2022;6(12):3442–54.
12. DiNardo CD, Aldoss I, Kantarjian HM, et al. Triple therapy with venetoclax-azacitidine-gilteritinib for FLT3-mutated AML: phase I/II (NCT04140487). Leukemia. 2024;38(3):642–50.
13. Pratz KW, Pollyea DA, DiNardo CD, et al. Venetoclax-azacitidine-ivosidenib in newly diagnosed IDH1-mutated AML: phase Ib results. J Clin Oncol. 2023;41(17):3051–62.
14. Kottaridis PD, Gale RE, Frew ME, et al. The presence of a FLT3 internal tandem duplication in patients with acute myeloid leukemia (AML) adds important prognostic information and predicts relapse. Blood. 2001;98(6):1752–9.
15. Levis M, Small D. FLT3: ITDoes matter in leukemia. Leukemia. 2003;17(9):1738–52.
16. Stone RM, Mandrekar SJ, Sanford BL, et al. Midostaurin plus chemotherapy for FLT3-mutated AML (CALGB 10603/RATIFY). N Engl J Med. 2017;377(5):454–64.
17. Perl AE, Martinelli G, Cortes JE, et al. Gilteritinib or salvage chemotherapy for relapsed/refractory FLT3-mutated AML (ADMIRAL). N Engl J Med. 2019;381(18):1728–40.
18. Erba HP, Montesinos P, Kim HJ, et al. Quizartinib plus chemotherapy in newly diagnosed FLT3-ITD-positive AML (QuANTUM-first). Lancet. 2023;401(10388):1571–83.
19. Oka Y, Tsuboi A, Kawakami M, et al. Cancer immunotherapy targeting WT1 peptide. Leukemia. 2008;22(5):797–805.
20. Keilholz U, Letsch A, Busse A, et al. WT1 peptide vaccination in AML patients: a phase I/II clinical trial. Blood. 2013;122(21):1589.
21. ClinicalTrials.gov. A Phase III Study of Galinpepimut-S (GPS) in AML (REGAL) - NCT04229979.
22. Rezvani K, Yong ASM, Mielke S, et al. Leukemia-associated antigens and their use in immunotherapy of myeloid leukemias. Blood Rev. 2011;25(5):185–93.
23. Anguille S, Lion E, Smits EL, et al. Clinical use of dendritic cells for cancer therapy. Lancet Oncol. 2014;15(10):e257–67.
24. Anguille S, Van de Velde A, Smits EL, et al. WT1 peptide-loaded dendritic cell vaccination in AML patients in remission: a phase I/II trial. Blood. 2017;129(10):1357–65.
25. Molldrem JJ, Lee PP, Wang C, et al. WT1 mRNA-electroporated dendritic cell vaccine in AML: immune responses and survival data. Blood. 2011;117(26):7111–20.
26. Borg C, Terme M, Taieb J, et al. Dendritic cell vaccination with leukemic apoptotic bodies elicits CD4+ and CD8+ T cell responses in AML. J Clin Invest. 2016;126(1):329–38.
27. Schroers R, Weinschenk T, et al. Multi-antigen dendritic cell vaccine targeting WT1 and PRAME in AML: interim results of a phase I trial. J Immunother Cancer. 2020;8(2):e000925.
28. Daver N, Garcia-Manero G, Basu S, et al. Efficacy, safety, and biomarkers of response to immune checkpoint inhibitors in AML: current status and future directions. Leukemia. 2020;34(2):278–92.
29. Zhang H, Su S, Li K, et al. Immune checkpoint blockade in acute myeloid leukemia: opportunities and challenges. Front Immunol. 2020;11:570097.
30. Daver N, Garcia-Manero G, Basu S, et al. Efficacy, safety, and biomarkers of response to azacitidine and nivolumab in relapsed/refractory acute myeloid leukemia: a phase II study. Cancer Discov. 2019;9(5):370–83.

31. Bashey A, Medina B, Corringham S, et al. CTLA-4 blockade with ipilimumab to treat relapse of malignancy after allogeneic hematopoietic stem cell transplantation. Blood. 2016;127(2):258–65.
32. ClinicalTrials.gov. Study of Nivolumab Plus Ipilimumab in AML - NCT04284787.
33. Garcia-Manero G, Daver NG, Takahashi K, et al. Safety and efficacy of azacitidine, venetoclax, and nivolumab in patients with AML. Blood Adv. 2021;5(9):2459–69.
34. Zhu C, Anderson AC, Schubart A, et al. The Tim-3 ligand galectin-9 negatively regulates T helper type 1 immunity. Nat Immunol. 2005;6(12):1245–52.
35. Garcia-Manero G, et al. Phase 1b study of sabatolimab in combination with hypomethylating agents and venetoclax in AML and MDS. Blood. 2021;138(Suppl 1):639.
36. Chao MP, Weissman IL, Majeti R. The CD47–SIRPα pathway in cancer immune evasion and potential therapeutic implications. Curr Opin Immunol. 2012;24(2):225–32.
37. Sallman DA, Asch AS, Al Malki MM, et al. The first-in-class anti-CD47 antibody magrolimab in combination with azacitidine for the treatment of patients with AML: results of a phase 1b study. J Clin Oncol. 2021;39(15_suppl):7008.
38. Sallman DA, Asch AS, Al Malki MM, et al. Magrolimab + azacitidine in AML with TP53 mutations: clinical efficacy and biomarker insights. Blood Adv. 2022;6(13):3692–700.
39. ClinicalTrials.gov. Study of Magrolimab + Azacitidine vs Physician's Choice in TP53-Mutant AML—NCT04778397.
40. ClinicalTrials.gov. Study of Magrolimab + Azacitidine + Venetoclax in Untreated AML—NCT05079230.
41. Fierce Biotech. Gilead scraps two phase 3 trials of magrolimab in AML after safety signals; 2024.
42. Kovtun Y, Jones GE, Adams S, et al. A CD123-targeting antibody-drug conjugate, IMGN632, designed to eradicate AML while sparing normal bone marrow progenitors. Blood Adv. 2018;2(8):848–58.
43. Daver NG, Montesinos P, Stein EM, et al. Pivekimab sunirine (IMGN632), a novel CD123-targeting antibody–drug conjugate, in relapsed or refractory acute myeloid leukaemia: a phase 1/2 study. Lancet Oncol. 2024;25(3):388–99. https://doi.org/10.1016/S1470-2045(23)00674-5.
44. Daver N, Maiti A, DiNardo CD, et al. Pivekimab sunirine (PVEK, IMGN632), a CD123-targeting antibody-drug conjugate, in combination with azacitidine and venetoclax in patients with CD123+ newly diagnosed AML unfit for intensive chemotherapy. Blood. 2023;142(Suppl 1):2906.
45. ClinicalTrials.gov. Study of pivekimab sunirine (IMGN632) in combination with FLAG-Ida in patients with acute myeloid leukemia or other high grade myeloid neoplasms [Internet]. Bethesda (MD): National Library of Medicine (US); 2023. Report No.: NCT06034470
46. Pagel JM, Appelbaum FR, O'Donnell PV, et al. Randomized phase III SIERRA trial of 131I-Apamistamab before allogeneic hematopoietic cell transplantation for relapsed or refractory acute myeloid leukemia. J Clin Oncol. 2024;42(12):1234–45.
47. Jurcic JG, Rosenblat TL, McDevitt MR, et al. Phase I trial of alpha-particle immunotherapy with 225Ac-lintuzumab (anti-CD33) for relapsed or refractory acute myeloid leukemia. J Nucl Med. 2016;57(6):872–9.
48. Scheinberg DA, MR MD. Actinium-225-labeled anti-CD33 monoclonal antibody (lintuzumab) for treatment of acute myeloid leukemia. Blood. 2013;122(21) Abstract 405
49. O'Hear CE, Pandit-Taskar N, Larson SM, et al. Targeted alpha-particle therapy with 225Ac-lintuzumab and low-dose cytarabine in older patients with untreated acute myeloid leukemia. J Nucl Med. 2019;60(9):1221–7.
50. Mardiana S, Gill S. CAR T cells for acute myeloid leukemia: state of the art and future directions. Front Oncol. 2020;10:697.
51. Wermke M, Kraus S, Ehninger A, et al. Proof-of-concept for UniCAR-T-CD123 switchable CAR T therapy in R/R AML. Blood. 2021;137(22):3145–8.

52. Pe Sallman DA, DeAngelo DJ, Pemmaraju N, et al. AMELI-01: a phase I trial of UCART123v1.2, an anti-CD123 allogeneic CAR-T cell product, in adult patients with relapsed or refractory (R/R) CD123+ acute myeloid leukemia (AML). Blood. 2022;140(Suppl 1):2371–3.
53. Yang M, Tang X, Zhang Z, Gu L. Antigen escape mechanisms and their implications for CAR T-cell therapy in acute myeloid leukemia. Blood. 2024;145(7):657–69.
54. Zhou J, Zhao Y, Su Y, Li Y, Lv H, Meng X, et al. Immune suppressive microenvironment in acute myeloid leukemia: challenges and therapeutic opportunities. Front Immunol. 2020;11:605085.
55. Wang W, Wu Z, Liu Y, Han W. Manufacturing challenges and strategies for CAR T cells in acute myeloid leukemia. J Hematol Oncol. 2021;14(1):46.

Chapter 36
Management of Elderly AML

Ashish Dixit and Jhansi Jayachandran

Abstract Acute myeloid leukemia (AML) has established treatment plans in young and fit patients. They are usually treated with intensive chemotherapy (IC) followed by post-remission consolidation with either intermediate-high dose cytarabine or hematopoietic stem cell transplantation (HSCT) based on genetic risk stratification. However, being a disease that predominantly affects the elderly, there is a lack of standard therapy in this subset. They are rarely candidates to take IC owing to comorbidity and frailty. Besides, adverse cytogenetic mutations seem to occur in elder AML patients more than in younger ones, making complications that follow IC not worth it, given the risks of resistant disease (RD) and relapses. Therapy with a hypomethylating agent (HMA) and targeted therapy forms the most suitable plan for elders. The latest World Health Organization (WHO) 2022 AML classification has adequately emphasized genetic and molecular profiling, which has paved the way for the identification of many more potential targets and therapies. This article provides an overview of the evolution of treatment in elderly AML from the past, currently available options, and various targeted therapies already available and in the pipeline.

Keywords Acute myeloid leukemia · Azacitidine · Decitabine · Hypomethylating agents · targeted therapies

Abbreviation

ADC	Antibody-drug conjugate
AML	Acute myeloid leukemia
ASCT	Allogeneic stem cell transplantation

A. Dixit (✉)
Manipal Hospital, Bangalore & Adjunct Prof, Manipal University, KMC, Manipal, Karnataka, India

J. Jayachandran
Manipal Hospital Whitefield, Bengaluru, Karnataka, India

H. P. Pati et al. (eds.), *Clinical Hematology and Hemato-Oncology*,
https://doi.org/10.1007/978-981-92-1167-8_36

ASH	American Society of Hematology
BCL-2	B cell leukemia/lymphoma
BiTEs	Bispecific T cell engagers
BSC	Best supportive care
CAR-T	Chimeric Antigen Receptor T
CCR	Conventional care regimens
CDA	Cytidine deaminase
CR	Complete remission
DS	Differentiations syndrome
ELN	European Leukemia Net
EMA	European Medical Association
FDA	Food and Drug Administration
FLT3	FMS-Like Tyrosine Kinase 3
G-CSF	Granulocyte- colony stimulating factor
HMA	Hypomethylating agent
HSCT	Hematopoietic stem cell transplantation
IC	Intensive chemotherapy
ICC	International consensus classification
ID	Induction deaths
IDH	Isocitrate Dehydrogenase
LDAC	Low dose cytarabine
LSC	Leukemia stem cell
MAC	Myeloablative chemotherapy
MDS	Myelodysplastic syndrome
MRD	Minimal residual disease
NKCEs	Natural Killer Cell Engagers
NPM1	Nucleophosmin
OS	Overall survival
PFS	Progression-free survival
R/R	Relapsed/Refractory
RD	Resistant disease
RIC	Reduced intensity chemotherapy
t-AML	therapy-related AML
TLS	Tumor lysis syndrome
TRM	Treatment-related mortality
WHO	World health organization

Learning Objectives

- Adequate knowledge of assessing eligibility for intensive chemotherapy in the elderly.
- Counseling elderly AML patients with details on risks and benefits in various treatment plans.
- Assessing eligibility for allogeneic stem cell transplantation.
- Encourage clinical trials incorporating targeted therapies.

36.1 Introduction

AML is a heterogeneous, aggressive hematological neoplasm of myeloblasts. Young and fit patients are treated with IC, consisting of a combination of cytarabine and anthracycline with or without allogeneic stem cell transplantation (ASCT). Treatment of AML in the elderly is challenging as they are not fit for conventional IC in view of frailty and medical comorbidity. Moreover, identification of poor risk features like adverse cytogenetics, TP53 mutation, complex karyotype, and antecedent myelodysplastic syndrome (MDS) is often seen in the elderly [1]. Such disease biology responds poorly to IC, hence giving a skewed risk-benefit ratio and a treatment-related mortality (TRM) of 10–25%. Hence, treatment of AML in the elderly is an area of active research, more so given that the median age of AML is 68 years.

Tremendous advancements have been made in the mutational profile of AML, decoding its molecular biology and paving the way for major modifications in the disease classification and risk stratification from the WHO and the international consensus classification (ICC) in 2022. This arena of targeted therapy is more relevant in the elderly who don't have a suitable alternative to IC [2].

36.2 Evolution of Treatment Strategies

In the past, elderly patients with AML were treated with various treatment regimens. IC with standard induction regimen 7 + 3 (Daunorubicin 60 mg/m^2 for 3 days; Cytarabine 100–200 mg/ m^2 for 7 days) was used in various studies, and the outcome was dismal. Although complete remission (CR) rates ranged from 35% to 65%, induction deaths (ID) occurred in 10–20% patients, and RD was identified in 25–45% cases, even in patients without unfavorable cytogenetics, as shown in the Table 36.1 below.

Given these unsatisfactory results, less intensive approaches were tried, like best supportive care (BSC), including Hydroxurea. The MRC study evaluated the efficacy of low-dose cytarabine (LDAC) versus BSC. LDAC in this study consisted of

Table 36.1 Trials with intensive chemotherapy used as induction in elderly AML

Study group	Number of patients	Median age	CR rate	ID rate	RD rate
EORTC-HOVON	489	68 years	42%	18%	40%
MRC	1311	66 years	55%	19%	26%
CALGB (1990–1993)	388	69 years	53%	25%	22%
EORTC-GIMEMA	722	68 years	55%	14%	31%
HOVON-MRC	419	67 years	51%	15%	34%
CALGB (1998–2002)	669	71 years	46%	NA	NA
ALFA	416	72 years	57%	10%	33%

CR complete remission, *ID* induction death, *RD* resistant disease, *NA* not available cytarabine 20 mg/m^2 twice daily for 10 consecutive days every 4 weeks for at least 4 cycles. Although the study demonstrated higher CR and overall survival (OS), at the end of 1 year, only 25% patients were alive, making LDAC a poor standard choice for treatment of AML in the elderly as well as a poor comparator for trials. Overall, BSC-only or LDAC were associated with median OS of only 5 and 12 months, respectively, prompting the need for further research for better treatment of AML in the elderly [3].

36.3 Current Treatment Strategies

36.3.1 Hypomethylating Agents (HMA)

When it was discovered that methylation was involved in the silencing of tumor suppressor genes and eventually played a role in AML pathogenesis, research on inhibitors of DNA methyltransferase gained popularity. HMA, like Azacitidine and Decitabine, later began being investigated as the standard of care for AML in the elderly.

Fenaux et al. published a subset analysis of the phase 3 AZA-001 trial evaluating the efficacy of Azacitidine as compared with conventional care regimens (CCR), including BSC only, LDAC, or intensive therapy, in AML with low blast count (20–30% blasts). Azacitidine was administered subcutaneously in a dosage of 75 mg/m^2/day for 7 days of every 28-day cycle. The study showed that Azacitidine has significantly prolonged OS compared with CCR [Median OS, 24.5 months versus 16.0 months; $P = 0.005$]. The OS difference was significant between Azacitidine and BSC, but there was no significant difference in OS between Azacitidine and LDAC or intensive chemotherapy in the study [4]. A similar study was published in AML with high blast count (>30% blasts) by Dombert et al. Although the OS difference was not significant, it was higher in the Azacitidine arm compared to the CCR arm (10.4 vs 6.5 months; $p = 0.1009$) [5]. Azacitidine has been approved by the Food and Drug Administration (FDA) for MDS since 2004 and for AML with 20–30% blasts based on the extended analysis of the AZA-001 trial since 2009.

In a DACO-016 study by Kantarjian et al., Decitabine was compared with the treatment of choice, which was either supportive care or LDAC with cytarabine 20 mg/ m^2 for 10 consecutive days every 4 weeks. Decitabine was given in a dosage of 20 mg/ m^2/day for 5 days every 4 weeks. Although results showed that the difference in median OS was not significant (7.7 months vs 5 months, $p = 0.108$), the difference in CR was significant (17.8% vs 7.8%, $p = 0.001$) [6]. Becker et al., in a subgroup analysis of the 06011 study, compared Decitabine with BSC in the AML subgroup and showed that Decitabine use yielded longer progression-free survival (PFS) [7]. Decitabine is approved for MDS, including patients with 20–30% blasts, by the FDA and is approved for AML by the European Medicines Agency (EMA). Decitabine is not formally approved by the FDA for AML but remains to be used off-label [8].

Direct trials comparing the efficacy of both HMAs don't exist, although conclusions were made based on trials comparing Azacitidine vs CCR and Decitabine vs CCR. Decitabine showed higher efficacy with respect to CR rates compared to Azacitidine, but the latter resulted in less cytopenia than the former [9].

To avoid the burden of travel and time spent in the hospital, intravenous (IV) therapy was changed to oral HMAs. CC-486, an oral formulation of Azacitidine and oral Decitabine, was investigated. Unfortunately, cytidine deaminase (CDA) from liver and gut degrades oral Decitabine, an inhibitor of CDA, Cedazuridine, an inhibitor of CDA, was introduced as an oral fixed dose combination (FDC) (35 mg Decitabine with 100 mg Cedazuridine). Exposure to the patient was equivalent to IV Decitabine 20 mg/m^{2}for 5 days [10].

36.3.2 B Cell Leukemia/Lymphoma (Bcl-2) Inhibitors

Overexpression of BCL-2 in AML confers chemotherapy resistance, making the selective inhibitor of BCL-2, Venetoclax, a great choice for AML therapy. Earlier research on BCL-2 inhibitors predominantly used Navitoclax, a BH3-mimetic, which was a non-selective inhibitor of BCL-2 along with BCLXL and BCL-W. The latter caused severe thrombocytopenia, limiting its utility, as megakaryocytes are BCL-XL dependent. Venetoclax lacked any such side effects as it does not have affinity for BCL-XL and was selective for BCL-2 [11].

Venetoclax as a single agent, used in doses of 400–800 mg, produced leukemia-free survival of 2.3 months and median OS of 4.7 months [12]. Although it was well tolerated, it seemed to have limited efficacy. In combination with HMA like Azacitidine, which is an inhibitor of MCL-1, Venetoclax showed significant efficacy in preclinical models. Phase 1b trial comparing combinations of Venetoclax, with Azacitidine and with Decitabine showed that CR was achieved in 27% of Venetoclax + Azacitidine arm and 35% of Venetoclax + Decitabine arm [13]. After few phase 2 trials showing similar CR rates, VIALE-A was a remarkable phase 3 trial. The trial included elderly >75 years or younger AML patients unfit for IC, and excluded favorable cytogenetics and compared the combination of Azacitidine with Venetoclax with Azacitidine with placebo. Response rate and OS were superior in the Azacitidine + Venetoclax arm compared to Azacitidine + placebo (CR: 66% vs 28%; OS: 14.7 months vs 9.6 months). This led to FDA approval of Venetoclax in combination with HMA in November 2014 [14]. Studies assessing the efficacy of Venetoclax with Decitabine in a phase 2 trial also showed promising results with CR/complete response with incomplete hematological recovery (CRi) rates of 84% [15]. A combination of Venetoclax with Cytarabine was studied in patients with de novo AML and with patients progressing on HMA therapy. Median OS was 4.1 months and 13.1 months, with and without prior HMA, respectively [16]. The same was proved in phase 3 VIALE-C trial, where 48% in the venetoclax plus low-dose cytarabine arm attained CR/CRi rate compared to 13% in cytarabine alone arm. Although initially not evident, an extended survey also proved a survival benefit in the venetoclax plus low-dose cytarabine arm [17]. Venetoclax for maintenance therapy is also an area of active research, but potential risks of myelosuppression and infections remain. Its potential use post-allogeneic stem cell transplantation for AML is still under trials. Overall, current therapy for elderly AML involving a combination of Venetoclax and HMA is given in doses of 100 mg Venetoclax ramped up to 400 mg, along with 7 days of Azacitidine at a dose of 75 mg/m^{2}or 5 days Decitabine at a dose of 20 mg/m^{2}until disease progression or unacceptable toxicity.

Although approval of Venetoclax has revolutionized the treatment of AML in the elderly, it comes with a serious side effect profile. 30–50% patients developed febrile neutropenia, 45% patients developed grade 3–4 cytopenia. It is prudent to administer initial therapy as an inpatient due to the risk of tumor lysis syndrome (TLS). Current treatment strategies recommend bone marrow assessment during cycle 1 to assess blast clearance and discontinuation of Venetoclax or targeted therapy to allow for marrow recovery. If there is a response, growth factors like Granulocyte-colony stimulating factor (G-CSF) can be used to boost blood counts and enable fitness for subsequent cycles. Subsequent response assessment marrows are planned after cycle 4 and thereon every 3 cycles [18].

36.3.3 FMS-Like Tyrosine Kinase 3 (FLT3) Inhibitors

FLT3 mutations are usually associated with aggressive AML biology and confer poor prognosis [19]. Data for frontline use of FLT3 inhibitors like Midostaurin and Quizartinib in young patients with AML is vast. RATIFY trial compared IC with and without Midostaurin (50 mg orally twice daily) in young patients with AML and showed that the Midostaurin arm significantly improved OS (74.7 months vs 25.6 months, $p = 0.009$) [20]. QUANTUM-First trial evaluated efficacy of Quizartinib in AML patients and showed that in comparison with IC alone, combination with Quizartinib significantly improved OS (31.9 months vs 15.1 months, $p = 0.032$). These trials led to the approval of Midostaurin and Quizartinib in young AML as frontline therapy by the FDA [21].

For elderly AML, data on FLT3 inhibitors are not sufficient. RATIFY trial excluded patients with AML >60 years. QUANTUM- First trial did include patients aged 60–75 years, and they constituted about 40% of the study population. However, the OS benefit of Quizartinib did not apply to this subset (17.5 months vs 14.2 months). Following the success of Gilteritinib in the relapsed/refractory AML setting in the ADMIRAL trial, the LACEWING study incorporated Gilteritinib in combination with Azacitidine as opposed to Azacitidine alone for AML patients >65 years of age and inferred that the Gilteritinib arm resulted in significantly higher composite CR than the Azacitidine alone arm, although OS did not differ significantly between the arms [22].

FLT3-mutated AMLs are also resistant to venetoclax-based therapies because FLT3 mutations reduce BCL-2 and upregulate BCL-xl and MCL-1 [23]. Several trials incorporating a combination of FLT3 inhibitors in combination with Venetoclax were undertaken. A combination of Azacitidine, Venetoclax, and Gilteritinib (80 mg daily) was evaluated for older AML patients in a prospective trial. Although only 30 patients were included in the trial, 100% had composite CR, and the 2-year OS rate was 71% [24]. FLT3 inhibitors like Sorafenib and Midostaurin were studied in a maintenance setting post-transplantation in trials like SORAMIN and RADIUS, respectively. Both drugs showed longer relapse-free survival (RFS). But these are still phase 2 trials [25, 26]. Further research on the use of FLT3 inhibitors in elderly AML will be needed to definitively prove their benefit.

36.3.4 Isocitrate Dehydrogenase (IDH) Inhibitors

IDH mutations are commonly observed in AML, IDH1 and IDH2 mutations being noted in about 8% and 12%, respectively. IDH1 and IDH2 mutations are usually associated with older age at presentation, making them all the more important targets for therapy that this population needs [27]. While initial trials with Enasidenib, an IDH2 inhibitor, were focused on relapse/refractory AML, trials in newly diagnosed AML cases began subsequently. The original AG221–001 study involving 39 elderly patients with newly diagnosed IDH2-mutated AML reported a CR rate of 18% and a median OS of 11.3 months with Enasidenib [28]. Following this, AG 221–005 phase 2 trial compared Azacitidine + Enasidenib versus Azacitidine alone in 101 elderly AML. 53% and 12% had attained CR in the Azacitidine + Enasidenib arm, as compared to the Azacitidine alone arm, respectively. 71% in the combination attained an overall response rate (ORR), with only 42% attaining ORR in the Azacytidine arm. The difference between the two groups with respect to OS was not significant [29]. As a result of these trials, approval of Enasidenib by the FDA was restricted to relapsed/refractory (R/R) AML, and the dose of Enasidenib was determined to be 100 mg daily.

Studies incorporating the IDH1 inhibitor, Ivosidenib, started with 33 patients, and the CR rate was 30% with a median OS of 12.6 months [30]. A combination of Ivosidenib and Azacitidine was studied in a phase 1b trial, demonstrating a CR rate of 61% and a 12-month OS of 82% [31]. A large phase 3 AGILE study comparing a combination of Azacytidine with Ivosidenib with Azacytidine alone showed an impressive and significant difference in event-free survival (EFS) ($p = 0.002$) with 37% estimated probability that at 1 year, a patient would remain event-free in the Ivosidenib + Azacitidine group compared to 12% in the Azacitidine alone group. OS difference was also significant (24 months vs 7.9 months, $p = 0.001$), favoring the combination [32]. Ivosidenib was approved both as monotherapy and in combination with Azacitidine by the FDA for newly diagnosed AML patients above 75 years old who are not fit for IC in May 2019 and May 2022, respectively. Olutasidenib is an IDH1 inhibitor approved only for R/R AML based on CR rates and ORR of 32% and 48%, respectively, in a single-arm study, and use in newly diagnosed AML is not established [33].

The recommended dose of Ivosidenib was established at 500 mg daily. Adverse events associated with IDH inhibitors include indirect hyperbilirubinemia in Enasidenib and QTC prolongation in Ivosidenib. Both drugs were associated with differentiation syndrome (DS).

36.3.5 Other Approved Targeted Therapy-Glasdegib, Gemtuzumab Ozagamicin (Go), and Cpx-351

Glasdegib is an inhibitor of the Sonic Hedgehog pathway, which is active in AML [34]. In combination with LDAC, glasdegib resulted in significantly longer CR and OS as compared to LDAC alone (8.8 months vs 4.9 months, 17% vs 1%, respectively) [35].

GO is an anti-CD33 immuno-conjugate, composed of a humanized immunoglobulin attached to calicheamicin with anti-mitotic activity. After evidencing its efficacy in low and intermediate- risk AML, trials on elderly AML were conducted [36]. Phase 3 ALFA 0701 trial compared standard therapy with and without GO and concluded that EFS was better in the GO arm (40.8% vs 17.1%; $p = 0.0003$). OS was also favoring the GO arm (53.2% vs 41.9%, $p = 0.0368$). Toxicity in the GO arm mainly comprised hematological ones with cytopenia and were more common than in the standard treatment arm. Hence, for favorable risk AML with CD 33 positivity, GO is a prudent addition to standard IC [37].

CPX-351 injection combines two efficient chemotherapy agents—cytarabine and Daunorubicin in a molar ratio of 5:1 within a liposomal formulation. It was approved by the FDA for therapy-related AML (t-AML) and AML with myelodysplasia-related changes. In the elderly, in such AML, CPX-351 use resulted in significantly prolonged OS (median OS 9.56 months vs 5.95 months), hence making it an ideal choice for t-AML and AML with myelodysplasia-related changes, even in the elderly [38, 39].

36.4 Hematopoietic Stem Cell Transplantation (HSCT) and Post-remission Therapy

While so many trials and treatment strategies emerged due to dissatisfaction with the option of IC, the question of allogeneic HSCT seems to be apparently off the table. For the few elderly AML patients who are eligible for IC, is the option of allogeneic HSCT acceptable as consolidation therapy? High burden of comorbidities and intense complications post-IC make HSCT a less attractive option for the elderly, given that TRM might be higher. Various comorbidity-based prognostic models include age as a variable [40]. In a trial analyzing 1321 patients who were diagnosed to have AML >60 years and had undergone HSCT in CR1, 3-year OS for cohorts of age 60–64, 65–69, and >70 years were 49.4%, 42.3%, and 44.7%, respectively (p = 0.026). Conditioning regimen was chosen prudently with both reduced intensity chemotherapy (RIC) and myeloablative chemotherapy (MAC) used only for the 60–69 years age group, and 3-year OS was reported as 46% for RIC and 49% for MAC in this group. MAC was rarely used for patients over 70 years old [41]. While HSCT is an excellent curative option for all patients, including those above 60 years of age, careful selection of patients, keeping in mind comorbidities, prior myelosuppression, organ functions, and, most importantly, understanding of the risks and consequences, is important.

For those elders who attain remission after IC and are not fit for HSCT, post-remission treatment with consolidation therapy was advised, as published in the American Society of Hematology (ASH) 2020 guidelines [42]. Various consolidation therapies were used earlier for elderly AML, including intensive therapy with the same IC regimen used during induction or ambulatory therapy like a 6-monthly course with Daunorubicin or Idarubicin in doses of 45 mg/m^2 and 9 g/m^2, respectively, in combination with 60 mg/m^2/12th hourly cytarabine as subcutaneous infusion at home for 5 days. Median ages of the arms were 72 years and 71 years, respectively. Ambulatory therapy proved superior to intensive therapy with respect to OS, disease-free survival (DFS), hence advocating less intensive consolidation therapy [43].

Later, cytarabine alone was tried as consolidation therapy in various trials [44] [45]. Azevedo et al. published a trial underlying the importance of cytarabine consolidation therapy in AML, wherein 22% of 311 patients were in the >60 years age group. In this study, very high dose cytarabine (total dose of >27 g/m^2) had significantly higher survival in all the patients, and there was no statistical difference in EFS between the subgroups divided based on whether age was more than or less than 60 years [46].

Elderly AML patients who receive Azacitidine and Decitabine as upfront therapy will need to continue them indefinitely or until progression, despite achieving adequate control after 2–4 cycles. They are also used as consolidation or maintenance therapy after CR in elderly AML [47].

36.5 Relapsed/Refractory (R/R) AML

Usually, relapse of AML in the elderly is considered to carry a very poor prognosis with mostly palliative treatment. Investigational approaches and participation in clinical trials should be encouraged after a complete understanding of the risks, benefits, and feasibility of options [48, 49].

36.6 Newer Therapy and Ongoing Research

There is enormous ongoing research on developing newer targeted therapies for AML, as there are still a lot of gaps to be filled in the therapeutic management of AML in the elderly (Fig. 36.1). Targeted therapies approved so far have led to a significant improvement in remission and survival rates, but there is still a long way to go. As the biology of AML becomes clearer, several newer targets to hit are being identified.

Menin is a protein, the expression of which results from a historically deemed poor prognosis KMT2A fusion. It also results from Nucleophosmin (NPM1) and NUP98 fusion genes, which are considered as good risk and relatively adverse risk mutations, respectively, as per European Leukemia Net (ELN) 2022 AML classification. It results from the altered expression of Hox genes, which is important for leukemogenesis. Menin inhibitors like Revumenib and Ziftomenib are being investigated in clinical trials on R/R AML currently. Revumenib was studied in the phase 1 AUGMENT-101 trial that included KMT2A rearranged and NPM1 mutated R/R AML, and CR rates of 33% and 21% are reported in the respective mutations. KOMET-001 trial evaluated and showed the efficacy of Ziftomenib in R/R AML with KMT2A rearrangement and NPM1 mutation, with 16.7% and 30% CR in the respective subgroups. Trial on recent menin inhibitor JNJ-75276617 also showed similar results. The SAVE regimen, which includes all oral combinations of Revumenib, Decitabine/Cedazuridine, and Venetoclax, underwent a phase 1 trial in R/R AML, and results were impressive with 100% ORR and 50% CR rates. The

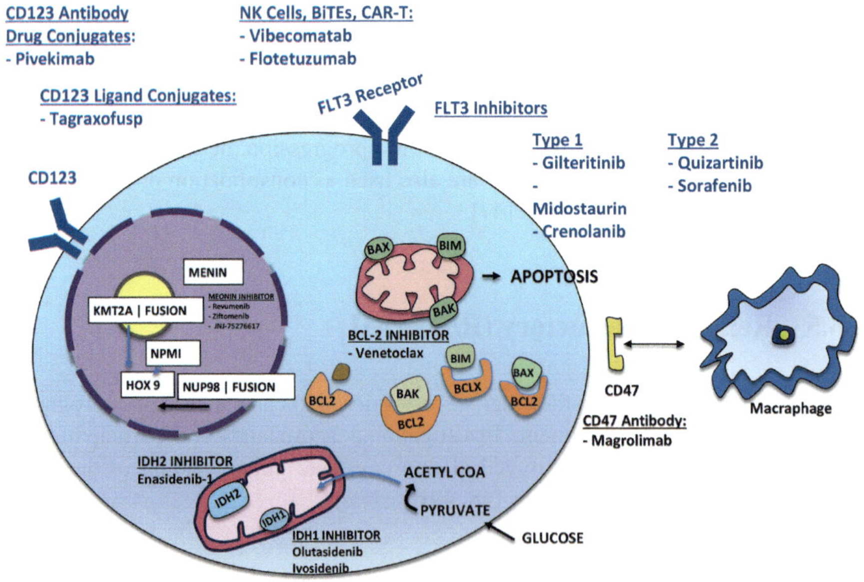

Fig. 36.1 Potential targeted therapy in elderly AML

success story of menin inhibitors is only hampered by the early relapses reported if patients are not taken up for timely HSCT [50].

AML myeloblasts also express CD123, which is considered a leukemia stem cell (LSC) marker. CD 123 is an integral part of the human interleukin-3 (IL-3) receptor and forms its alpha chain. These are expressed much more on LSC than in normal stem cells, making it a selective target for AML. Talacotuzumab was the first targeted therapy against CD123. While this was a naked antibody, subsequently, an antibody-drug conjugate (ADC) called Pivekimab was developed and studied in R/R AML. Piveimab yielded a disappointing 20% ORR rate. Hence, it was then tried in combination with the Azacitidine/Venetoclax combination, and that yielded 51% ORR.

Various advanced modalities where immune cells are engaged in accelerated blast destruction have gained popularity recently, like Bispecific T cell engagers (BiTEs) and Natural Killer Cell Engagers (NKCEs). BiTEs targeting CD123 were all set to rise to fame, but Vibecomatab and Flotetuzumab were already discontinued. NKCEs targeting CD 123 have been developed, studied, and, in fact, report on efficacy in R/R AML, which was even published in ASCO 2023, but again, the CR rate was only 13%. Chimeric Antigen Receptor T cells (CAR-T cells) against CD123 underwent a phase 1 trial with 16 patients and need further study. Tagraxofusp is a drug containing an IL-3 ligand conjugated with diphtheria toxin (DT). Due to unattractive results as a single agent, combinations with HMA/Venetoclax are being tried [51].

Anti-CD 47 Magrolimab blocks the "don't-eat me" signal that AML and other cells with CD 47 give to macrophages, thereby facilitating phagocytosis of cells. Currently, Magrolimab is being tried in combination with Azacitidine in phase 1b/2 trials. 87 patients were enrolled, and 28 (32.2%) achieved CR, which included 23 (31.9%) patients with TP53 mutation. Phase 3 trials evaluating the efficacy of this combination, like ENHANCE 2 and ENHANCE 3, are underway [52].

36.7 Case Scenario

A 68 years old man was admitted with 3 days history of fever. There was no comorbidity other than diabetes mellitus (DM), which was in control. On examination, he was physically fit. There was no lymphadenopathy or splenomegaly. Baseline blood investigations showed pancytopenia with a white blood cell (WBC) count of 15,800 and 89% blasts in the differential. Bone marrow revealed 92% blasts, which were positive for Myeloperoxidase (MPO). The immunophenotype of the cells was evaluated in flow cytometry, and the final diagnosis of AML with CD33 negativity was confirmed. Cytogenetic study revealed normal 46 XY cytogenetics, and further molecular analysis revealed biallelic mutations of both CEBPA, making it a favourable risk AML.

Treatment plan with IC (7 days cytarabine 100 mg/m^2 daily for 7 days and daunorubicin 45 mg/ m^2) on each of days 1, 2, and 3 was undertaken. He had significant neutropenia and sepsis, which eventually resolved with supportive care including G-CSF and transfusions. After complete count recovery, a repeat bone marrow was done, which showed morphological CR and minimal residual disease (MRD) negativity. After 7 weeks, consolidation therapy with intermediate-dose cytarabine (1000 mg/m^2 every 12 h on days 1, 3, and 5) was given. The same was continued for 3 more cycles. Other than febrile neutropenia between cycles, no further complications occurred. He is being followed up, and there has been no relapse in 3 years now.

Discussion: Given that the patient was above 60 years of age, the options of IC for induction therapy were carefully chosen. As this patient had no comorbidity other than DM and was physically fit, he was still a candidate for IC, despite his age. The option of GO and FLT3 inhibitors could not be considered with IC, as CD33 was negative on flow cytometry, and FLT3 mutation was not reported in the molecular study. If he were not fit, his option would have been HMA with Venetoclax. As IDH mutations were not reported, IDH inhibitors could not be considered. Since it was a favorable risk AML, post-remission consolidation with cytarabine was given. However, given the age and sepsis during induction, high-dose cytarabine was not opted. If he relapses on follow-up, detailed counseling for various options must be given. His options would be HMA with Venetoclax. Fitness for Fludarabine, cytarabine, G-CSF, and Idarubicin (FLAG-IDA) would generally come with a higher threshold for patients above 60 years, especially after having observed significant complications during induction. Such intense therapies are usually avoided in the elderly. By the time of relapse, a fresh assessment of comorbidities must be done with respect to fitness for HSCT, which must be a combined decision after weighing in the patient's needs, risks, and understanding.

36.8 Diagnostic Algorithm (Fig. 36.2)

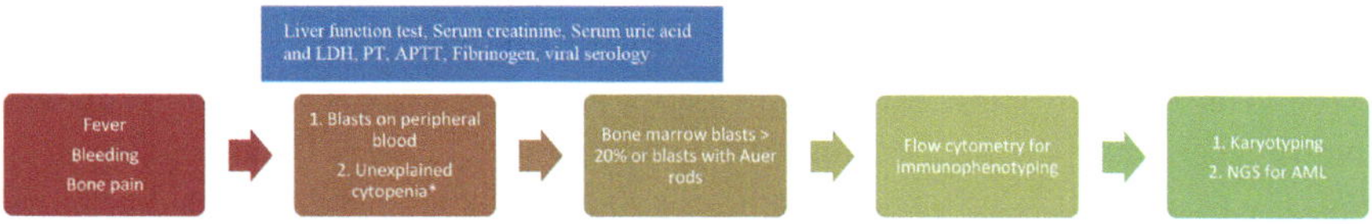

Fig. 36.2 Diagnostic workup in elderly AML. * For the possibility of aleukemic AML. LDH lactate dehydrogenase, PT prothrombin time, APTT activated partial thromboplastin time, NGS next generation sequencing

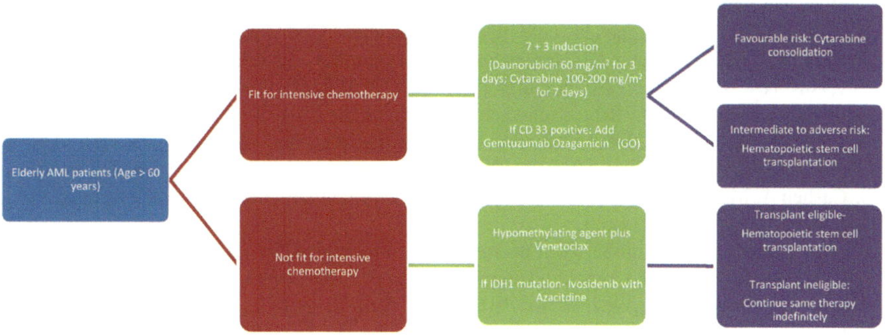

Fig. 36.3 Treatment algorithm in elderly AML

36.9 Treatment Algorithm (Fig. 36.3)

36.10 Short Summary

Treatment of AML in the elderly is challenging in view of comorbidities, which in turn makes the option of IC questionable. However, elderly fit patients should still be offered IC and may even be considered for HSCT if eligible. For those who are not fit for IC, ever-growing research has yielded various treatment options, including combinations of HMA and Venetoclax, several targeted therapies like IDH inhibitors, FLT3 inhibitors, Gladegib, and so on. Although with these therapies, there are alternative and satisfactory regimens for the elderly, none of them can be deemed perfect for the elderly. Further research and trials will pave the way for even better and customized therapies in the elderly [53].

References

1. Bazinet A, Kadia TM. Changing paradigms in the treatment of acute myeloid leukemia in older patients. Clin Adv Hematol Oncol. 2022;20(1):37–46.
2. Lai C, Bhansali RS, Kuo EJ, Mannis G, Lin RJ. Older adults with newly diagnosed AML: hot topics for the practicing clinician. Am Soc Clin Oncol Educ Book. 2023;(43):e390018.
3. Dombret H, Raffoux E, Gardin C. Acute myeloid leukemia in the elderly. Semin Oncol. 2008;35(4):430–8.
4. Fenaux P, Mufti GJ, Hellström-Lindberg E, Santini V, Gattermann N, Germing U, et al. Azacitidine prolongs overall survival compared with conventional care regimens in elderly patients with low bone marrow blast count acute myeloid leukemia. J Clin Oncol. 2010;28(4):562–9.
5. Dombret H, Seymour JF, Butrym A, Wierzbowska A, Selleslag D, Jang JH, et al. International phase 3 study of azacitidine vs conventional care regimens in older patients with newly diagnosed AML with >30% blasts. Blood. 2015;126(3):291–9.
6. Kantarjian HM, Thomas XG, Dmoszynska A, Wierzbowska A, Mazur G, Mayer J, et al. Multicenter, randomized, open-label, phase III trial of decitabine versus patient choice, with

physician advice, of either supportive care or low-dose cytarabine for the treatment of older patients with newly diagnosed acute myeloid leukemia. J Clin Oncol. 2012;30(21):2670–7.
7. Becker H, Suciu S, Rüter BH, Platzbecker U, Giagounidis A, Selleslag D, et al. Decitabine versus best supportive care in older patients with refractory anemia with excess blasts in transformation (RAEBt)—results of a subgroup analysis of the randomized phase III study 06011 of the EORTC Leukemia Cooperative Group and German MDS Study Group (GMDSSG). Ann Hematol. 2015;94(12):2003–13.
8. Cashen A, Malik P. Decitabine in the treatment of acute myeloid leukemia in elderly patients. Cancer Manag Res. 2014;6:53.
9. Ma J, Ge Z. Comparison between decitabine and azacitidine for patients with acute myeloid leukemia and higher-risk myelodysplastic syndrome: a systematic review and network meta-analysis. Front Pharmacol. 2021;12:701690.
10. Garcia-Manero G, McCloskey JK, Griffiths EA, Yee K, Zeidan AM, Al-Kali A, Deeg HJ, Patel P, Sabloff M, Keating MM, Dao KH, Zhu N, Gabrail NY, Fazal S, Maly J, Odenike O, Kantarjian H, DeZern AE, O'Connell CL, Roboz GJ, Busque L, Wells RA, Amin H, Randhawa JK, Leber B, Hao Y, Keer HN, Azab M, Savona MR. Oral decitabine/cedazuridine in patients with lower risk myelodysplastic syndrome: a longer-term follow-up of from the ascertain study. Blood. 2021;138:66.
11. Gangat N, Tefferi A. Venetoclax-based chemotherapy in acute and chronic myeloid neoplasms: literature survey and practice points. Blood Cancer J. 2020;10(11):122.
12. Guerra VA, DiNardo C, Konopleva M. Venetoclax-based therapies for acute myeloid leukemia. Best Pract Res Clin Haematol. 2019;32(2):145–53.
13. DiNardo CD, Pratz K, Pullarkat V, Jonas BA, Arellano M, Becker PS, et al. Venetoclax combined with decitabine or azacitidine in treatment-naive, elderly patients with acute myeloid leukemia. Blood. 2019;133(1):7–17.
14. CD DN, Jonas BA, Pullarkat V, Thirman MJ, Garcia JS, Wei AH, et al. Azacitidine and venetoclax in previously untreated acute myeloid leukemia. N Engl J Med. 2020;383(7):617–29.
15. DiNardo CD, Maiti A, Rausch CR, Pemmaraju N, Naqvi K, Daver NG, et al. 10-day decitabine with venetoclax for newly diagnosed intensive chemotherapy ineligible, and relapsed or refractory acute myeloid leukaemia: a single-centre, phase 2 trial. Lancet Haematol. 2020;7(10):e724–36.
16. Wei AH, Strickland SA, Hou JZ, Fiedler W, Lin TL, Walter RB, et al. Venetoclax combined with low-dose cytarabine for previously untreated patients with acute myeloid leukemia: results from a phase Ib/II study. J Clin Oncol. 2019;37(15):1277–84.
17. Wei AH, Montesinos P, Ivanov V, DiNardo CD, Novak J, Laribi K, et al. Venetoclax plus LDAC for newly diagnosed AML ineligible for intensive chemotherapy: a phase 3 randomized placebo-controlled trial. Blood. 2020;135(24):2137–45.
18. Maiti A, Konopleva MY. How we incorporate venetoclax in treatment regimens for acute myeloid leukemia. Cancer J. 2022;28(1):2–13.
19. Perl AE, Larson RA, Podoltsev NA, Strickland S, Wang ES, Atallah E, et al. Outcomes in patients with FLT3-mutated relapsed/ refractory acute myelogenous leukemia who underwent transplantation in the phase 3 ADMIRAL trial of gilteritinib versus salvage chemotherapy. Transplant Cell Ther. 2023;29(4):265.e1–265.e10.
20. Stone RM, Mandrekar SJ, Sanford BL, Laumann K, Geyer S, Bloomfield CD, et al. Midostaurin plus chemotherapy for acute myeloid leukemia with a *FLT3* mutation. N Engl J Med. 2017;377(5):454–64.
21. Perl A, Erba HP, Montesinos P, Vrhovac R, Patkowska E, Kim H, et al. Quantum-first trial: FMS-like tyrosine kinase 3-internal tandem duplication (*FLT3* -ITD)-specific measurable residual disease (MRD) clearance assessed through induction (IND) and consolidation (CONS) is associated with improved overall survival (OS) in newly diagnosed (nd) *FLT3* -ITD+ AML patients (pts). Blood. 2023;142(Suppl 1):832.
22. Wang ES, Montesinos P, Minden MD, Lee JH, Heuser M, Naoe T, et al. Phase 3 trial of gilteritinib plus azacitidine vs azacitidine for newly diagnosed *FLT3* mut+ AML ineligible for intensive chemotherapy. Blood. 2022;140(17):1845–57.

23. Short NJ, Nguyen D, Ravandi F. Treatment of older adults with FLT3-mutated AML: emerging paradigms and the role of frontline FLT3 inhibitors. Blood Cancer J. 2023;13(1):142.
24. Short NJ, et al. Azacitidine, venetoclax, and gilteritinib in newly diagnosed and relapsed or refractory FLT3-mutated AML. JCO. 2024;42:1499–508.
25. Burchert A, Bug G, Fritz LV, Finke J, Stelljes M, Röllig C, et al. Sorafenib maintenance after allogeneic hematopoietic stem cell transplantation for acute myeloid leukemia with *FLT3* –internal tandem duplication mutation (SORMAIN). J Clin Oncol. 2020;38(26):2993–3002.
26. Maziarz RT, Levis M, Patnaik MM, Scott BL, Mohan SR, Deol A, et al. Midostaurin after allogeneic stem cell transplant in patients with FLT3-internal tandem duplication-positive acute myeloid leukemia. Bone Marrow Transplant. 2021;56(5):1180–9.
27. Issa GC, DiNardo CD. Acute myeloid leukemia with IDH1 and IDH2 mutations: 2021 treatment algorithm. Blood Cancer J. 2021;11(6):107.
28. Pollyea DA, Tallman MS, De Botton S, Kantarjian HM, Collins R, Stein AS, et al. Enasidenib, an inhibitor of mutant IDH2 proteins, induces durable remissions in older patients with newly diagnosed acute myeloid leukemia. Leukemia. 2019;33(11):2575–84.
29. Cai SF, Huang Y, Lance JR, Mao HC, Dunbar AJ, SN MN, et al. A study to assess the efficacy of enasidenib and risk-adapted addition of azacitidine in newly diagnosed *IDH2* -mutant AML. Blood Adv. 2024;8(2):429–40.
30. Roboz GJ, CD DN, Stein EM, De Botton S, Mims AS, Prince GT, et al. Ivosidenib induces deep durable remissions in patients with newly diagnosed IDH1-mutant acute myeloid leukemia. Blood. 2020;135(7):463–71.
31. DiNardo CD, Stein AS, Stein EM, Fathi AT, Frankfurt O, Schuh AC, et al. Mutant Isocitrate dehydrogenase 1 inhibitor Ivosidenib in combination with Azacitidine for newly diagnosed acute myeloid leukemia. J Clin Oncol. 2021;39(1):57–65.
32. Montesinos P, Recher C, Vives S, Zarzycka E, Wang J, Bertani G, et al. Ivosidenib and azacitidine in *IDH1* -mutated acute myeloid leukemia. N Engl J Med. 2022;386(16):1519–31.
33. Venugopal S, Watts J. Olutasidenib: from bench to bedside. Blood Adv. 2023;7(16):4358–65.
34. Niscola P, Gianfelici V, Catalano G, Giovannini M, Mazzone C, Noguera NI, et al. Acute myeloid leukemia in older patients: from new biological insights to targeted therapies. Curr Oncol. 2024;31(11):6632–58.
35. Cortes JE, Heidel FH, Hellmann A, Fiedler W, Smith BD, Robak T, et al. Randomized comparison of low dose cytarabine with or without glasdegib in patients with newly diagnosed acute myeloid leukemia or high-risk myelodysplastic syndrome. Leukemia. 2019;33(2):379–89.
36. Ciotti G, Marconi G, Sperotto A, Giannini MB, Gottardi M, Martinelli G. Biological therapy in elderly patients with acute myeloid leukemia. Expert Opin Biol Ther. 2023;23(2):175–94.
37. Castaigne S, Pautas C, Terré C, Raffoux E, Bordessoule D, Bastie JN, et al. Effect of gemtuzumab ozogamicin on survival of adult patients with de-novo acute myeloid leukaemia (ALFA-0701): a randomised, open-label, phase 3 study. The Lancet. 2012;379(9825):1508–16.
38. Arellano M, Carlisle JW. How I treat older patients with acute myeloid leukemia. Cancer. 2018;124(12):2472–83.
39. Abdallah M, Xie Z, Ready A, Manogna D, Mendler JH, Loh KP. Management of Acute Myeloid Leukemia (AML) in older patients. Curr Oncol Rep. 2020;22(10):103.
40. Shouval R, Fein JA. The sum of the parts: what we can and cannot learn from comorbidity scores in allogeneic transplantation. Hematology. 2023;2023(1):715–22.
41. Maakaron JE, Zhang MJ, Chen K, Abhyankar S, Bhatt VR, Chhabra S, et al. Age is no barrier for adults undergoing HCT for AML in CR1: contemporary CIBMTR analysis. Bone Marrow Transplant. 2022;57(6):911–7.
42. Sekeres MA, Guyatt G, Abel G, Alibhai S, Altman JK, Buckstein R, et al. American Society of Hematology 2020 guidelines for treating newly diagnosed acute myeloid leukemia in older adults. Blood Adv. 2020;4(15):3528–49.
43. Gardin C, Turlure P, Fagot T, Thomas X, Terre C, Contentin N, et al. Postremission treatment of elderly patients with acute myeloid leukemia in first complete remission after inten-

sive induction chemotherapy: results of the multicenter randomized Acute Leukemia French Association (ALFA) 9803 trial. Blood. 2007;109(12):5129–35.
44. Magina KN, Pregartner G, Zebisch A, Wölfler A, Neumeister P, Greinix HT, et al. Cytarabine dose in the consolidation treatment of AML: a systematic review and meta-analysis. Blood. 2017;130(7):946–8.
45. Wang L, Zhao N, Zhou L, Tong J, Xue L, Zhang L, et al. Standard-intensity induction and intermediate/high-dose cytarabine consolidation can improve survival for elderly patients with newly diagnosed acute myeloid leukemia: a retrospective cohort study. Clin Interv Aging. 2022;17:55–64.
46. Azevedo MC, Velloso EDRP, Buccheri V, Chamone DAF, Dorlhiac-Llacer PE. Possible benefit of consolidation therapy with high-dose cytarabine on overall survival of adults with non-promyelocytic acute myeloid leukemia. Braz J Med Biol Res. 2015;48(2):178–85.
47. Wang ES. Treating acute myeloid leukemia in older adults. Hematology. 2014;2014(1):14–20.
48. De Leeuw DC, Ossenkoppele GJ, Janssen JJWM. Older patients with acute myeloid leukemia deserve individualized treatment. Curr Oncol Rep. 2022;24(11):1387–400.
49. Dennis M, Copland M, Kaur H, Kell J, Nikolousis E, Mehta P, et al. Management of older patients with frailty and acute myeloid leukaemia: a British Society for Haematology good practice paper. Br J Haematol. 2022;199(2):205–21.
50. Wysota M, Konopleva M, Mitchell S. Novel therapeutic targets in acute myeloid leukemia (AML). Curr Oncol Rep. 2024;26(4):409–20.
51. Lane AA, Garcia JS, Raulston EG, Garzon JL, Galinsky I, Baxter EW, et al. Phase 1b trial of tagraxofusp in combination with azacitidine with or without venetoclax in acute myeloid leukemia. Blood Adv. 2024;8(3):591–602.
52. Daver NG, Vyas P, Kambhampati S, Al Malki MM, Larson RA, Asch AS, et al. Tolerability and efficacy of the anticluster of differentiation 47 antibody magrolimab combined with azacitidine in patients with previously untreated AML: phase Ib results. J Clin Oncol. 2023;41(31):4893–904.
53. Shimony S, Stahl M, Stone RM. Acute myeloid leukemia: 2025 update on diagnosis, risk-stratification, and management. Am J Hematol. 2025;100(5):860–91.

Chapter 37
Venetoclax: A Magic Drug for Hematological Malignancies

Jina Bhattacharyya, Damodar Das, and Sewali Deka Talukdar

Abstract Venetoclax is a highly selective B-cell lymphoma-2 (BCL-2) inhibitor. It helps in overcoming the apoptotic potential of the cancer cells. BCL-2 is overexpressed in many hematological malignancies, and thus, with the introduction of venetoclax, there is a revolutionary change in the therapeutic approach to hematological malignancies like AML, CLL, multiple myeloma, and others. Based on data from MUANO and CLL 14 studies in CLL patients, VIALLE in AML patients, and Bellini in patients with multiple myeloma, venetoclax has been included in the standard treatment protocol of these malignancies in many centers worldwide. Even though the drug does not result in a cure of the disease and is associated with side effects, including tumor lysis syndrome, because of its increasing use in a wide spectrum of hematological disorders, venetoclax has been considered, as the magic drug. Emerging resistance has been a concern; different combination regimens are being tried in different trials to get maximum benefit from this wonder drug.

Keywords BH3 mimetics · BCL 2 inhibitor · Venetoclax · AML · CLL · Multiple myeloma · Lymphoma · MDS · ALL · Tumor lysis · Resistance

---

J. Bhattacharyya (✉)
Department of Clinical Hematology, Gauhati Medical College Hospital, Guwahati, Assam, India

D. Das
Department of Medicine, Assam Medical College Hospital, Dibrugarh, Assam, India

S. D. Talukdar
Department of Clinical Hematology, Gauhati Medical College Hospital, Guwahati, Assam, India

H. P. Pati et al. (eds.), *Clinical Hematology and Hemato-Oncology*, https://doi.org/10.1007/978-981-92-1167-8_37

Learning Objectives

- Apoptotic and anti-apoptotic pathways and their role in the pathogenesis of cancer.
- B cell lymphoma 2 (BCL 2) family and its role in apoptosis.
- Development of BCL 2 inhibitor, its pharmacokinetic properties, mechanism of action, and different uses in hematological malignancies, both in adult and pediatric populations.
- Different phases of clinical trials leading to approval of and off-label use of venetoclax in different hematological malignancies.
- Standard first-line treatment regimens for different hematological malignancies.
- Toxicities of venetoclax and drug interactions. Need for giving antibiotic and antifungal prophylaxis with venetoclax.
- Tumor lysis syndrome and ramp up dosing schedule of venetoclax in AML and CLL.
- Development of resistance to venetoclax.

37.1 Introduction

B cell lymphoma 2 (BCL-2) family, which includes BCL-2, BCL extra-large (XL), and myeloid cell leukemia-1 (MCL-1), are anti-apoptotic proteins; these are overexpressed in many hematological cancers, and this is the primary mechanism of escaping cell death by these cancer cells. Venetoclax is a drug that selectively inhibits BCL-2, and thus it restores the apoptotic signaling leading to the death of cancer cells.

The role of BCL 2 in cancer cell survival was initially identified in the research works carried out by scientists in the Walter and Eliza Hall Institutes (WEHI) of Medical Research, and later on, BH3 mimetics were developed by them in collaboration with other centers. Initial BH3 mimetics had broad-spectrum activity resulting in thrombocytopenia; subsequent research works led to the development of ABT-99, a highly potent and selective BCL 2 inhibitor, named as venetoclax [1].

The advent of venetoclax has revolutionized the treatment of many hematological malignancies. It is approved as a chemo-free treatment in the first line and relapsed and refractory settings of chronic lymphocytic leukemia and in combination with hypomethylating agents or low-dose cytarabine in the treatment of AML in older adults who are not fit for standard intensive chemotherapy. The use of venetoclax in many other hematological conditions is undergoing different phases of clinical trial and is also used off-label in other conditions. Table 37.1 shows the approved and off-label use of venetoclax in different hematological malignancies.

We would discuss venetoclax and its uses in different hematological malignancies, starting with an illustrative case.

Table 37.1 Indications of venetoclax in hematological malignancies

Indication	Approved/ off-label	Details
Chronic lymphocytic leukemia (CLL)	Approved	Approved as monotherapy and in combination with obinutuzumab or rituximab for CLL/SLL, including in patients with 17p deletion.
Small lymphocytic lymphoma (SLL)	Approved	Treated similarly to CLL; included in the same approval indications.
Acute myeloid leukemia (AML)	Approved	Approved in combination with azacitidine, decitabine, or low-dose cytarabine for newly diagnosed AML in patients ≥75 years or with comorbidities precluding intensive chemotherapy.
Multiple myeloma (MM)	⊘ Off-label	Investigational, particularly in t(11;14) subtype due to BCL-2 overexpression. Clinical trials show promising activity. Not FDA approved yet.
Non-Hodgkin lymphoma (NHL)	⊘ Off-label	Studied in DLBCL, FL, MCL, and others. Limited efficacy as monotherapy; combination regimens under investigation. Not FDA approved.
Mantle cell lymphoma (MCL)	⊘ Off-label	Some activity observed, especially in R/R disease. Often studied in combination with BTK inhibitors. Not approved.
T-cell lymphomas	⊘ Off-label	Experimental use; limited data. Some preclinical rationale, but minimal clinical trial support.
Myelodysplastic syndromes (MDS)	⊘ Off-label	Being explored in combination with HMAs in higher-risk MDS. Early-phase studies ongoing.
Hairy cell leukemia (HCL)	⊘ Off-label	Preclinical data suggests potential role; not widely studied in clinical trials. Not approved.

37.2 Illustrative Clinical Case

A 61-year-old female presented with fever, cough, and weakness of 2 weeks' duration on July 29, 2023. She was febrile, pale, and dyspneic on admission with no lymphadenopathy or organomegaly. Her complete blood count (CBC) had shown leukocytosis (TLC 26,500/cumm) with 20% blast on the peripheral blood, morphologically myeloblast, which was later confirmed by immunophenotyping (IPT) as acute myeloid leukemia (AML). Her hemoglobin was 9 g/dl, and platelet count was 160,000/cumm. Bone marrow aspiration (BMA) had 50% blasts (Fig. 37.1); she had t(8;21), Trisomy 8, and deletion of X on karyotype (Fig. 37.2), and next generation sequencing (NGS) had shown RUNX1::RUNX1T1 and ETV6 {p(Y17C) coding c.50A > G in 51.73%}. In view of her age and presence of infection and patient's choice, azacytidine and venetoclax (AZA-Ven) were started in the regimen of Aza infusion for 7 days and venetoclax orally 100 mg daily for 21 days, repeated every 28 days; dose could not be ramped up to 400 mg due to neutropenia and recurrent infection, and therefore she was continued with 100 mg venetoclax daily.

Except for leucopenia and related infections, she tolerated her treatment well and did not require any blood component support. At the end of the fourth cycle, her

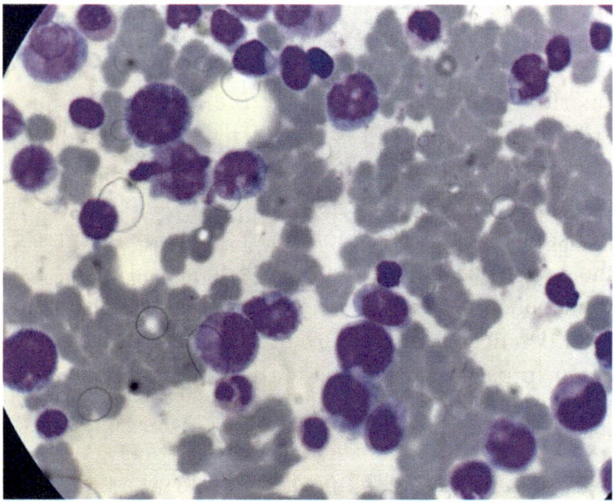

Fig. 37.1 100× bone marrow aspirate showing blasts

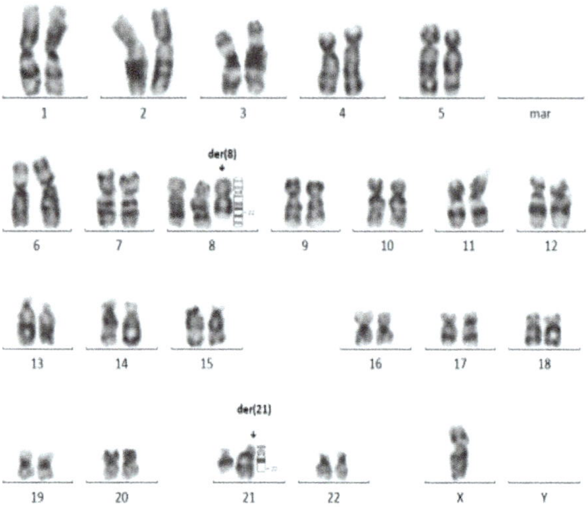

Fig. 37.2 Patient's karyotype at diagnosis

CBC was within normal limits; bone marrow assessment was done, which was in complete remission (CR) (Fig. 37.3); minimal residual disease (MRD) by IPT was O.93% (Fig. 37.4). Her karyotype was normal (Fig. 37.5). She was continued on Aza Ven; a repeat bone marrow at the end of 1 year showed persistent CR with normal karyotype and MRD negativity by IPT (Fig. 37.6). However, RUNX1::RUNX1T1 in NGS persisted. The patient has completed 2 years of AZA-Ven and continues to be in bone marrow and cytogenetic remission till her last follow-up on May 2, 2025.

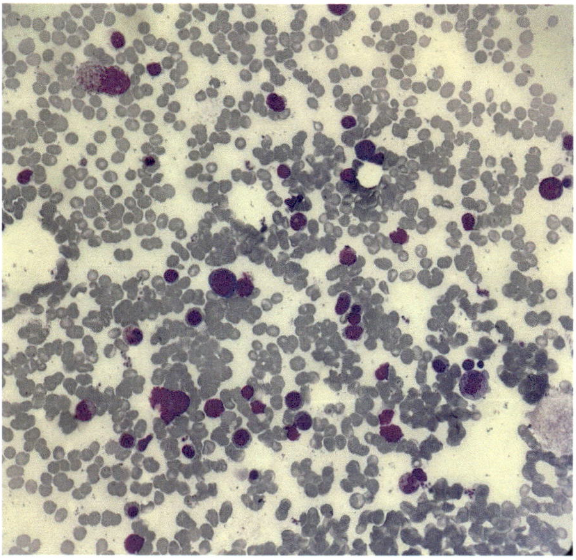

Fig. 37.3 40× morphological remission

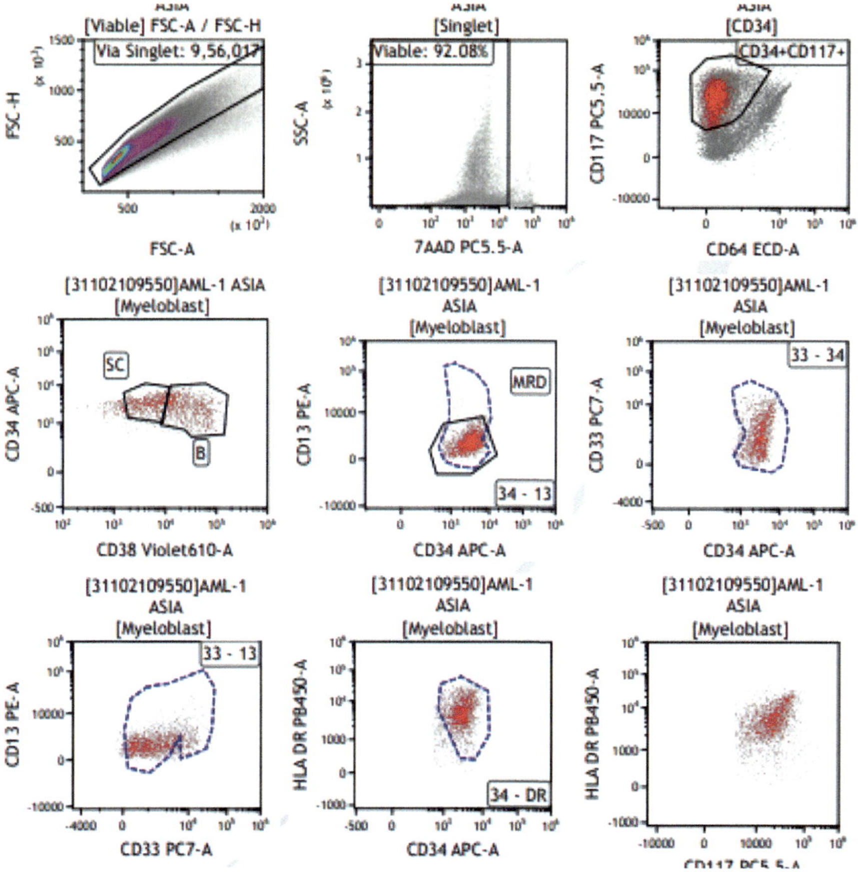

Fig. 37.4 MRD positivity by flow cytometry (0.93%) after four cycles of AZA Ven

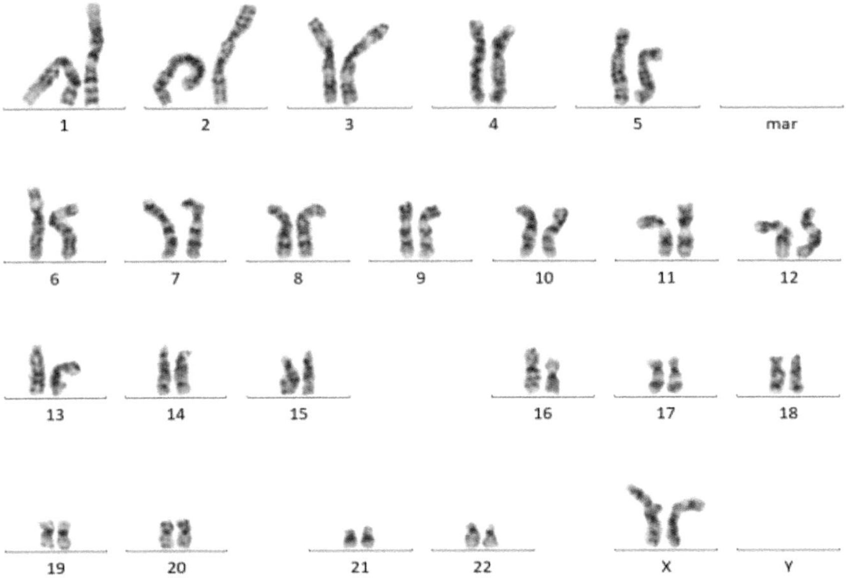

Fig. 37.5 Patient's karyotype after four cycles of Aza-Ven

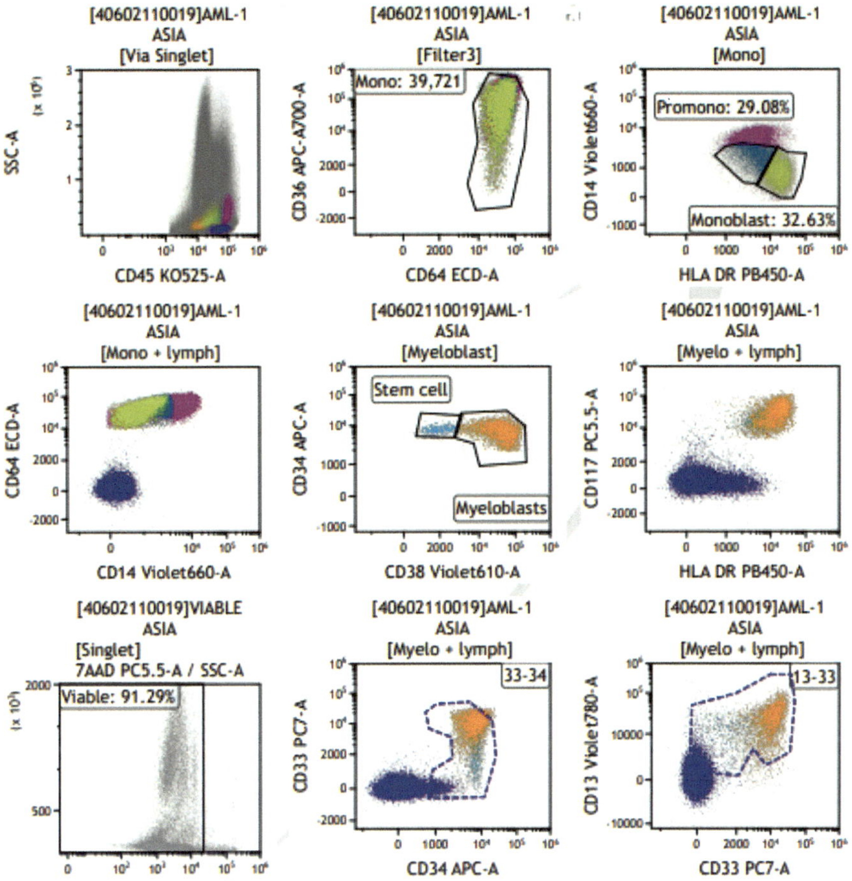

Fig. 37.6 MRD negativity in Nov 2024 by flow cytometry (<0.1%)

37.3 Venetoclax in CLL/SLL

CLL cells express high levels of BCL2 in the marrow and cytogenetic remission, resulting in resistance to apoptosis. Venetoclax, being a BCL-2 inhibitor, leads to apoptosis of these cells. It has changed the chemo-free treatment landscape of CLL from a continuous treatment approach to a fixed-dose treatment approach.

On May 15, 2019, the Food and Drug Administration approved venetoclax (VENCLEXTA, AbbVie Inc. and Genentech Inc.) for adult patients with chronic lymphocytic leukemia (CLL) or small lymphocytic lymphoma (SLL).

Approval was based on CLL14 (NCT02242942), a randomized (1:1), multicenter, open-label, actively controlled trial of venetoclax in combination with obinutuzumab (VEN + G) versus obinutuzumab in combination with chlorambucil (GClb) in 432 patients with previously untreated CLL with coexisting medical conditions [2]. The trial demonstrated a statistically significant improvement in PFS for patients who received VEN + G compared with those who received GClb (HR 0.33; 95% CI: 0.22, 0.51; $p < 0.0001$). Median PFS was not reached in either arm after a median follow-up duration of 28 months. The overall response rate was 85% in the VEN + G arm compared to 71% in the GClb arm, $p = 0.0007$. The trial also demonstrated statistically significant improvements in rates of minimal residual disease negativity (less than one CLL cell per 10^4 leukocytes) in bone marrow and peripheral blood.

The first clinical trial to establish the role of venetoclax in CLL was the phase I/II M12–175 trial in relapsed and refractory CLL patient and had established its role in CLL; the trial showed an objective overall response(ORR) of 77% with a median time to see ORR of 6 weeks and a median progression-free survival of 25 months. It had also first recommended the ramp-up dose of venetoclax [3]. This was followed by the M13–982 trial in relapsed and refractory CLL and also 17p deleted/TP53 mutated untreated CLL; the trial showed an overall response rate (ORR) of 77% with PFS and OS at 24 months being 54% and 73%, respectively. Thirty percent (30%) of patients received minimal residual disease (MRD) negativity [4]. The MURANO trial, which was a landmark trial, had compared chemoimmunotherapy (Rituximab and Bendamustine) with rituximab and venetoclax after a phase II trial [5] of venetoclax and rituximab combination had shown significant response benefit; the patient population in the MURANO trial was relapsed and refractory CLL, including 17p deleted/TP53 mutated CLL patients. The PFS at 2 years was significantly prolonged in the venetoclax arm as compared to the BR arm (84.9% vs 36.3%), and also the MRD negativity at 9 months (62.4% vs 13.3%) [6]. A four-year update of the MURANO trial has shown persistence of PFS benefit even after discontinuation of therapy with an overall survival benefit(OS) at 4 years of 85.3% with the venetoclax arm vs 66.8% with the BR arm [7].

In preclinical studies, obintuzumab and venetoclax combination had shown better response than the venetoclax rituximab combination [8]. This led to the Phase 3 CLL14 trial to compare venetoclax obintuzumab (VO) and chlorambucil obintuzumab (CO); twelve cycles were given to elderly and medically unfit patients with CLL. The outcome of this trial led to the approval of this drug, as mentioned above. The six-year follow-up of this trial has shown long-term survival benefits, achievement of undetectable measurable residual disease (uMRD), and an improved quality of life (QoL) [9].

CLL 13 trial with VO was carried out in younger fit patients as first-line treatment and had shown a one-year fixed-duration VO regimen as superior to chemo immunotherapy [10].

The combination of Ibrutinib and venetoclax (VI) was shown to be synergistic in preclinical studies with minimal overlapping toxicities [11]. MD Anderson Cancer Centre had undertaken a phase II study using this combination for a total of 24 cycles; at the end of 12 cycles, CR/Cri was 88% with 61% being MRD negative with an estimated PFS and OS being 98% and 99%, respectively [12]. Subsequently, the GLOW trial compared VI with CO; patients with 17p deletion/TP53 mutations were not enrolled. At the end of 27.7 months, the VI arm had significantly higher

PFS (84.4% vs 44.1%) and higher MRD negativity (55.7% vs 21%) as compared to the CO arm. The VI regimen has been approved as the first line treatment of CLL by the European Medicines Agency(EMA) based on Phase 3 GLOW trial data [13]. Phase 2 CAPTIVATE study was carried out in younger patients with similar benefits, validating the GLOW trial data [14].

Besides being time-limited, fixed-duration therapies secondarily lead to improved quality of life, less treatment-related toxicities, and less risk of occurrence of resistance.

Based on these studies, fixed-duration therapy of venetoclax and obintuzumab has been advocated to be the regimen of choice as first-line treatment of CLL, irrespective of TP53 mutation/17p deletion or IVGH mutation status, and a combination of venetoclax and Rituximab for the second line treatment [15].

ESMO, in its recently updated guideline, has also advocated for fixed-duration therapies for CLL. Other ongoing studies, including the CLL 17 trial, are looking at further refinement of CLL treatment. Studies are comparing BTK inhibitor monotherapy, combination regimens, and fixed duration regimens with the aim to define optimal treatment approaches to specific subgroups of CLL and tailor treatment, based on molecular and clinical characteristics in previously untreated CLL patients [16].

Triple therapy with obituzumab, a BTKi inhibitor, and venetoclax in untreated high-risk CLL patients harboring TP53 or 17p deletion, has been undergoing different phases of clinical trial and has shown promising results [17]. The phase 2 CLL2-GIVe trial has shown 36-month progression-free survival of 79.9%, and the 36-month overall survival of 92.6% [18].

37.4 Venetoclax in Acute Myeloid Leukemia

Till recently, treatment for AML was only 3 + 7 intensive chemotherapy and was the only treatment available for more than 50 years. Elderly patients who were unfit and also younger patients with co-morbidities, making them unfit for intensive chemotherapy, were offered only supportive treatment. With the approval of venetoclax-based therapy for these patient populations, the treatment of patients with AML who are not fit for intensive chemotherapy has been revolutionized.

BCL-2 is overexpressed in leukemic CD34+ progenitor cells. Preclinical studies have shown that AML cell lines express BCL2 and are dependent on it for their survival; these studies have exhibited sensitivity to Ven treatment and also have shown synergistic effects of Ven with azacytidine [19]. The first clinical trial with BCL 2 inhibitor, venetoclax, was carried out in relapsed and refractory AML patients and had shown an overall response rate of 19%, including 6% CR and 36% overall survival at 6 months; an important observation of this trial was that patients with IDH mutations had shown better results [20]. This followed a combination of venetoclax with hypomethylating agents in a phase 1b trial; patients above 65 years of age, unfit for standard treatment, were enrolled [21]. At 15 months follow up CR rate was 67% with 29% MRD negativity. When compared to a historical cohort, where a hypomethylating agent was used alone, the combination was found to have a significantly better outcome (CR 67% vs 30%). Subgroup analysis of this study also showed better outcomes in patients having Nucleophosmin 1 (NPM1) and IHD I mutations. These results led to the accelerated approval of venetoclax in ND AML patients unfit for intensive chemotherapy in November 2018; full approval was given in 2020 following the phase III VIALLE-A study results [22].

The landmark VIALLE-A phase III trial ($n = 431$) was carried out to compare the combination of azacytidine and venetoclax ($n = 286$) vs azacytidine alone ($n = 145$). In this study, 67% achieved CR/Cri (CR 37%) with significantly higher OS (median:14.7 mo vs 9.6 mo). Thus, VIALLE–A had confirmed the superior benefit observed in earlier studies. VIALLE C compared low-dose cytarabine with a combination of low-dose cytarabine and venetoclax and had shown better OS in the combination group on extended follow-up [23, 24]. These trial results led to the FDA approval of these combinations in older patients with newly diagnosed AML who are unfit for standard chemotherapy or younger patients with co-morbid conditions. Long-term follow-up of the VIALLE A (43.2mo) has confirmed the superior benefit of the ven combinations therapy; in the subgroup analysis, it has been shown that survival benefit was better in those with IDH 1 and IDH 2 mutated AML and those with MRD negativity.

With revolutionary change in treatment of unfit ND AML patients, studies were started with the addition of Ven to intensive chemotherapy in high-risk AML patients or patients who have relapsed or are refractory (r/r AML). These studies have resulted in a CR rate of 91%, MRD negativity of 97%, with an estimated EFS of 72% and estimated OS of 97% [25].

The CAVEAT trial investigated the addition of venetoclax to an attenuated 5 + 2 regimen of cytarabine and idarubicin in older fit ND AML, resulting in a CRc rate of 72% and a median OS of 11.2 months. This venetoclax plus a modified intensive chemotherapy regimen offers an effective, well-tolerated, time-limited approach in this patient population. Complete response rates were highest for patients who had *IDH1/2* or *NPM1* mutations, at 75% and 81%, respectively, and lowest for patients with *TP53* mutations at 27%. The two-year OS rate was highest in patients with *IDH1/2*, *SRSF2*, or *NPM1* mutation at 76%, 72%, and 69%, respectively, and lowest in patients with *TP53* mutation at 13% [26].

MD Anderson group has published the long-term results of use of venetoclax along with intensive chemotherapy (FLAG IDA) in both newly diagnosed (ND) and relapsed and refractory (R/R) AML patients (138 patients;77 vs 61). In the ND cohort, the overall response rate (ORR) was 97%, with a composite complete remission (CRc) rate of 95%, and undetectable measurable residual disease (MRD) status by flow cytometry was 90%. The 3-year OS and EFS rates were 66% and 64%, respectively. In the RR cohort, the ORR was 67%; CRc rate 41%, and the flow negative MRD rate was 74%; the response was particularly favorable in patients with wild-type TP53 status, with an ORR of 79%, CRc rate of 74%, and 3-year OS rate of 51%. It was concluded that FLAG-IDA + VEN is effective for remission induction in both ND and RR AML [27].

37.5 Venetoclax in Pediatric Myeloid Neoplasm

With the revolutionization of treatment of AML in older adults, unfit for intensive chemotherapy, venetoclax use has been undergoing clinical trial in younger patients, including pediatric patients in relapsed and refractory AML, therapy-related MDS (tMDS/AML) and advanced MDS (MDS-EB) patients, mostly as a bridge to hematopoietic stem cell transplantation (HSCT).

Pediatric AML is a biologically heterogeneous disease, and it is important to characterize the disease at baseline biologically so that risk stratification and treatment can be planned; with better characterization, outcomes have improved with OS reaching up to 70%. However, the disease relapses in 30–40% of cases, and standard treatment is not available for relapsed cases; available intensive chemotherapy in this group results in only 20–30% OS.

VENAML is a phase I dose escalating trial in r/r AML where venetoclax was used with intensive chemotherapy; the dose of venetoclax was identified as 360 mg/m^2 (maximum 600 mg), and 70% achieved CR and 80% achieved CR/PR [28]. The use of HMA and venetoclax can be a good option as a bridge to allogenic hematopoietic stem cell transplantation in this pediatric patient population. Studies [29, 30] have shown that 25% to up to 100% patients were bridged to HSCT after 1–2 cycles of HMA and venetoclax, of which 50–70% patients are alive and disease-free at last follow-up. A combination of venetoclax and Daratumumab also were added to a preparative myeloablative conditioning regimen in children with refractory AML, with an OS and EFS at 2 years being 65% and 44% respectively [31]. Due to lack of phase 3 trials no clear recommendations about schedule, no of cycles, time of response assessment, venetoclax interruption etc. are yet to be defined; majority of the trials use venetoclax at 21 day or 28 day cycles and it has been observed in phase 1 trial that >50% blast reduction after the first cycle is associated with achieving CR with MRD negativity after the second cycle [28].

In newly diagnosed pediatric AML patients, the addition of venetoclax to standard induction regimen has also shown better outcomes across all risk groups. In the first reported study from China in ND pediatric AML, the CR rates are as high as 94.7% in the low/middle-risk group and 80.8% in the high-risk group, while MRD-negative rates were 52.6% and 38.5%, respectively; the overall CR rate following a single course of venetoclax-based induction therapy was 86.7%, surpassing the CR rate attained after two courses of traditional chemotherapy induction. Even MRD negativity was higher in spite of a higher number of high-risk patients in this study, as compared to traditional induction therapy [32].

This study has established the potential of venetoclax in improving response rates in newly diagnosed pediatric AML patients.

The role of venetoclax combination in de novo MDS, therapy-related MDS, and MDR-AML is also increasing as a bridge to HSCT, as this regimen is associated with less infection-related toxicity. In patients associated with congenital bone marrow failure syndromes like Fanconi's anemia and Schwachman- Diamond Syndrome, this regimen may be particularly useful. In primary advanced childhood

AML and MDR-AML, it has been shown that if the patients do not proceed to HSCT, they invariably relapse; in therapy-related AML who were bridged to HSCT, all are alive and disease-free. None of the studies have reported toxicity-related deaths, major toxicities being tumor lysis, neutropenia, and infection. Issues like no of cycles, the best combinations, best clinical endpoint to proceed to HSCT are still undefined; a phase 3 clinical trial would be needed to define these.

Use of venetoclax in pediatric AML patients with specific mutations is also undergoing initial phases of trial. Rearrangements of KMT2A gene are frequent in children and infants with AML, conferring an adverse prognosis; in KMT2A pediatric AML, >/+ 10% blast is sufficient to make a diagnosis of AML [33]. A potent menin inhibitor, Revumenib, has been shown to give remission in KMT2A-mutated pediatric AML patients; use of venetoclax plus azacytidine with menin inhibitors has shown high efficacy in the preliminary results of an ongoing trial in KMT2A rearranged, NPM mutated AML patients and has confirmed the synergistic effect of venetoclax and menin inhibitors in preclinical studies [34, 35]. In FLT 3-positive AML patients, a triplet approach with FLT 3 inhibitor, venetoclax, and chemotherapy or HMA is suggested based on preclinical studies showing a synergistic effect of FLT 3 inhibitor and venetoclax [36].

To optimize the use of venetoclax in Pediatric patients with AML and MDS, even though the studies have shown promising results, prospective data is a must to get approval from the regulatory bodies; like in adults, development of resistance is a concern, and possible strategies to overcome these are being studied. Optimal duration and number of cycles of ven-based combination also need to be studied. Venetoclax use has been reported in the treatment of other myeloid neoplasm like juvenile myelomonocytic leukemia [37].

37.6 Venetoclax in Relapsed/Refractory Mantle Cell Lymphoma

Amongst the relapsed and refractory non Hodgkin lymphoma (NHL) patients with, mantle cell lymphoma has been shown (phase I study) to have the best response to venetoclax based treatment [38].

A phase II trial (AIM trial) was conducted with ibrutinib and venetoclax in patients with relapsed/refractory mantle cell lymphoma and those with untreated mantle cell lymphoma who were unfit for standard cytotoxic therapy. Patients received ibrutinib at 560 mg once daily for the first 4 weeks, followed by a ramp-up schedule of venetoclax. The steady-state dose was 400 mg once daily; the dose of venetoclax was increased to 800 mg in the patients who did not achieve a CR. The median follow-up was 15.9 months. The CR rate was 42% (without PET assessment) at week 16, which was significantly superior to the results obtained with ibrutinib in the historical cohort (9%; $P < 0.001$); the response was 62% when PET assessment was done. MRD negativity was seen in 67% patients. The median PFS and OS were not reached, PFS and OS at 12 months were 75% (95% CI, 60–94%) and 79% (95% CI, 64–97%), respectively, and at 18 months were 57% (95% CI, 40–82%) and 74% (95% CI, 57–95%), respectively [39].

This and other studies have confirmed the benefit of a combination of venetoclax and BTKi in patients with mantle cell lymphoma who have failed first-line treatment.

37.6.1 Venetoclax in DLBCL

Overexpression of BCL2 and BCL2 rearrangements confer poor prognosis in patients with diffuse large B-cell lymphoma (DLBCL); trials are therefore being taken up to target this. The single-arm phase IB CAVALLI trial used venetoclax with R-CHOP and was compared with a historic cohort of the GOYA study [40]. PFS was significantly higher in the venetoclax trial (80% vs 67%) at a median follow-up of 32 months.

In another single-center phase IB-2 study, the regimen of venetoclax, ibrutinib, prednisone, obinutuzumab, and lenalidomide (ViPOR) was used in relapsed or refractory DLBCL; ViPOR was given every 21 days for 6 cycles. With a median follow-up of 40 months, 2-year PFS and OS were 34% (95% confidence interval [CI], 21–47) and 36% (95% CI, 23–49), respectively. The side effects were reversible, and the study concluded that treatment with ViPOR was associated with durable remissions in patients with specific molecular DLBCL subtypes [41].

37.6.2 Venetoclax in Multiple Myeloma

It has been shown in preclinical studies that myeloma cell lines have increased sensitivity to venetoclax, especially in the presence of t(11;14), the latter has overexpression of BCL-2. A phase I trial of venetoclax single agent in relapsed and refractory multiple myeloma had shown ORR of 21%; in the subset with t(11;14), the ORR was 40% [42]. Venetoclax when combined with bortezomib and dexamethasone in subsequent phase I trial, had shown ORR of 67% confirming a synergistic effects between them [43]. BELLINI trial, which was a phase 3 double-blind randomized trial, was conducted in relapsed and refractory MM patients using either venetoclax or placebo in combination with bortezomib and dexamethasone; 114 patients, either with t(11;14) or BCL-2 overexpression (PCR-based) were enrolled. PFS was not reached in the venetoclax arm with an ORR of 85% and MRD negativity of 19%, whereas in the placebo group, PFS was 9.9 months with 70% ORR and 0% MRD negativity [44]. This has led to the recommendation of venetoclax in combination with bortezomib and dexamethasone in R/RMM patients.

This was validated in a retrospective study done at Mayo Clinic [45]. This retrospective study evaluated the efficacy and safety of Ven-based therapies in 232 MM patients without concurrent AL amyloidosis treated between Jan 2015 and Dec 2023. Triple-class refractoriness was defined as resistance to at least one proteasome inhibitor (PI), one immunomodulatory drug (IMID), and one anti-CD38 monoclonal antibody. Penta-drug refractory disease was defined as resistance to at least two IMIDs, two PIs, and one anti-CD38 monoclonal antibody. Patients had received a median of three prior lines of therapy before starting the venetoclax regimen. Of the total participants, 65% (n = 152) were triple-class refractory (TCR), and 27.2% (n = 63) were penta-drug refractory.

The ORR for the entire cohort was 57%. In patients with t(11;14), the ORR was 64% compared to 27% in those without t(11;14) ($p < 0.001$). Within the t(11;14) cohort, patients with 1q gain/amplification or del(17p) had an ORR of 57%, whereas those without these abnormalities had an ORR of 71% ($p = 0.04$). In the non-t(11;14) cohort, patients with 1q gain/amplification or del(17p) had an ORR of 15%, whereas those without these abnormalities had an ORR of 43%.

In patients with t(11;14) and high-risk cytogenetic abnormalities (e.g., del(17p) and 1q gain/amplification), PFS with venetoclax-based regimens was inferior compared to t(11;14) patients without these abnormalities.

With this evidence of significant better outcomes in patients of relapsed and refractory MM in the subgroup harboring t (11;14), there is increasing importance of venetoclax combination regimens in this setting.

37.7 Venetoclax in Acute Lymphoblastic Leukemia (ALL)

Relapsed and refractory ALL in adults or newly diagnosed ALL in older adults have a poor outcome to treatment due to resistant disease and toxicity to conventional chemotherapy.

Lymphoblasts have been shown to be sensitive to venetoclax, and because of this property, it was hypothesized that if venetoclax is used with chemotherapy, it can enhance the efficacy of chemotherapy by allowing dose reduction and thereby lowering toxicity and enhancing tolerability. In a phase 1b multicentric trial conducted at the Dana-Farber Cancer Institute (Boston, MA) and the University of Texas MD Anderson Cancer Center (Houston, TX) venetoclax was given with modified dose of chemotherapy; it had enrolled 19 patients with ALL either newly diagnosed (aged ≥60 years, n = 11 [B-cell, n = 8; T-cell, n = 3]) or relapsed/refractory (R/R; aged ≥18 years, n = 8 [B-cell, n = 3; T-cell, n = 5]). Venetoclax was given for 21 days with each cycle of mini–hyper-CVD (mini-HCVD; cyclophosphamide, vincristine, dexamethasone alternating with methotrexate and cytarabine). The trial, even though limited by its small sample, has concluded that venetoclax and low-dose chemotherapy is a promising combination for newly diagnosed older adults and also relapsed and refractory adult ALL patients [46]. Table 37.2 shows dosing schedules of venetoclax and mini HCVD.

Table 37.2 Venetoclax with mini hyper CVAD in ALL

Patients	Regimen	Dose	Toxicity	Result
B- & T-cell newly diagnosed ALL >60 years	*Venetoclax* 21d/cycle + *Mini Hyper* CVAD + *Rituximab* (if CD20+) + *Intrathecal MTX*	Ven 600 mg/day	Infection was most common No TLS	De Novo: CR 90% MRD negative 100%
R/R adult ALL				R/R: CR 38%, MRD negative 67%

37.8 Other Off-label Use of Venetoclax

Venetoclax has shown good response when used in relapsed and refractory hairy cell leukemia (HCL) patients. In vitro studies have shown proapoptotic activity of venetoclax in hairy cells from patients with hairy cell leukemia. Based on these observations, six hairy cell leukemia patients who had failed both chemotherapy and targeted treatment with BRAF inhibitor vemurafenib in combination with rituximab, were given venetoclax for 12 cycles every 28 days with or without rituximab; all patients except one had achieved CR with MRD negativity in one. Duration of progression-free survival was 23–53-plus months in all 5 patients. Thus, this study concluded that venetoclax is safe and efficacious as salvage therapy in relapsed and refractory conditions of HCL [47].

Initial phases of trials are ongoing in relapsed and refractory marginal zone lymphomas also [48].

Myelodysplastic syndrome (MDS) is a heterogeneous disease, and the only curative treatment option is hematopoietic stem cell transplantation (HSCT); however, the majority of patients are not eligible for HSCT. For higher risk MDS (HR-MDS), a hypomethylating agent is the first line of treatment; however, overall survival remains poor. After the approval of Aza Ven in the treatment of AML, trials are ongoing in patients with HR-MDS who are treatment-naive. In a phase 1 b trial, the best response of CR or marrow CR was observed in 29.9% and 50.5% (mOR, 80.4%), respectively. Median OS was 26.0 months, with 1- and 2-year survival estimates of 71.2% and 51.3%, respectively [49].

A phase 3 trial (VERONA) is ongoing to confirm these responses in HR-MDS patients. (clinicalTrials.gov: NCT04401748).

37.9 Dosing Schedule of Venetoclax

In VIALE –A study protocol, ven is scheduled at 28 days; however, the majority of patients had significant toxicities. Willekens et al., in a retrospective study, report a comparative outcome with 7 days of venetoclax with azacytidine (7 + 7 regimen) vs standard dose ven + HMA and reported similar CR/Cri (72% in both) and OS (11.2

vs 10 months) with lowering of platelet requirements (62% vs 77%) and early mortality at 8 weeks (6% vs 16%) in ND AML patients [50].

Mayo Clinic also has reported similar observations in ND –AML patients ($n = 270$) in schedules of 14 days ($n = 40$), 21 days ($n = 41$), and 28 days ($n = 189$). CR/Cri was similar in all the schedules (68 vs 66 vs 62% respectively in ven 14d vs 21 d vs 28d schedule respectively. However, in the patients with adverse karyotype (ELN), showed higher CR/Cri rates in ven 21 (60%) vs Ven 28 (44%) vs Ven 14(22%) [51]. Ongoing Phase 2 randomized trial comparing toxicity and efficacy of ven, 28 vs ven 14 days would confirm the efficacy and safely of 14 d vs 28d ven schedule in patients with ND AML Another phase 2 study with decitabine sc (0.2 mg/kg/day) weekly with ven 400 mg weekly has shown 90% treatment continuation without interruption with 52% CR/Cri and 47% MRD negativity [52].

These studies have observed that a shorter course of Ven in NDAML is less myelotoxic and might be as efficacious as the standard dosing schedule (28d). General recommendation in patients with a high risk of infectious complications is a 14-day dosing schedule; and since sensitivity to ven is strongly associated with the genetic profile of the patient, an individualized dosing strategy is recommended. Ongoing studies will further confirm the dosing schedule for ND AML.

37.10 Pharmacokinetics, Side Effects, Dosage, and Administration of Venetoclax

Venetoclax is available in tablet form in different strengths starting from 20 mg, 50 mg, and 100 mg. It is well absorbed orally, and bioavailability is significantly better with high-fat meals. Therefore, it is recommended to take venetoclax with food to ensure consistent absorption.

Following oral administration, the maximum concentration is reached 5–8 h after the dose. It is highly bound to plasma proteins and is metabolized in the liver by cytochrome P450 3A (CYP3A) enzymes and mostly eliminated in the feces. Bioavailability in Asean patients is higher than in non-Asians; however, there is no difference in the toxicity profile.

Patients are at risk of tumor lysis syndrome (TLS), and therefore, it is administered in a ramp-up fashion in AML and CLL. Table 37.3 shows the ramp-up schedule in AML and CLL.

The common side effects of the drug are infection and neutropenia affecting about 15–20% of the patients with AML and CLL, with grade ¾ cytopenia occurring in>5% of the patients. The most common serious adverse events are pneumonia, sepsis, and febrile neutropenia occurring in >2% of patients.

Patients are risk-stratified for TLS; Table 37.4 shows risk stratification in CLL patients. If patients are at high risk, they are hospitalized for at least 24 h for monitoring. Following the first ramp-up dose, parameters for TLS are assessed after 6–8 h; the next day's dose is not started till parameters are available. In case of

Table 37.3 Ramp-up schedule of venetoclax in CLL and AML

CLL	Venetoclax
Week 1	20 mg
Week 2	50 mg
Week 3	100 mg
Week 4	200 mg
Week 5	400 mg
AML	
Day 1	100 mg
Day 2	200 mg
Day 3	400 mg
Day 4	400 mgwith AZA/600 mg with Ara C

Table 37.4 Risk stratification for TLS in CLL

Risk group	Factors
Low risk	LN <5 cm & ALC <25 × 10^9/L
Intermediate risk	LN 5–10 cm & ALC >25 × 10^9/L
High risk	>10 cm LN or LN >5 cm & ALC >25 × 10^9/L

LN Lymph Node, *ALC* Absolute Lymphocyte Count

laboratory TLS, the next day's dose is withheld till the parameters become normal. For AML patients, the total leucocyte count should be less than 25,000/cumm and there should not be any laboratory TLS before starting venetoclax.

With a larger indication of venetoclax use, resistance to venetoclax has become a concern. Studies are ongoing to understand the mechanism of venetoclax resistance [53].

37.11 Summary

Venetoclax is a BCL-2 inhibitor that acts against antiapoptotic pathways, leading to apoptosis of cancer cells. Preclinical studies have identified the anti-apoptotic potential of this molecule in cancer cells of different hematological malignancies. This observation led to the initiation of different phases of clinical trials, one of the first being in CLL cells. Landmark randomized trials followed, after the exciting response in the early phases to see efficacy and safety of venetoclax in CLL, AML, and others; these led to the approval of the drug by the regulatory bodies in CLL and AML, both in newly diagnosed and relapsed and refractory settings. More evidence in other malignancies like multiple myeloma, Mantle cell lymphoma, DLBCL, ALL, HCL, MZL, and MDS led to off-label use of this magic molecule in combination and alone. The risk of tumor lysis is high, and hence TLS prophylaxis is a must; therefore, a ramp-up dose is given in both CLL and AML patients. The most significant toxicity is neutropenia. Which can be severe and can lead to neutropenic sepsis, pneumonia, and other infectious complications. As a prophylaxis to TLS, a ramp-up dosing schedule is followed, and antibacterial and antifungal agents are recommended as infection prophylaxis. The long-term results are emerging from different randomized trials establishing the superiority of venetoclax combinations over the standard treatment of many hematological diseases. In pediatric myeloid malignancies, this regimen has been identified as an ideal bridging to HSCT. The concern is emerging resistance; trials are underway to understand the emergence of resistance and to overcome it.

References

1. Souers AJ, Leverson JD, Boghaert ER, Ackler SL, Catron ND, Chen J, et al. ABT-199, a potent and selective BCL-2 inhibitor, achieves antitumor activity while sparing platelets. Nat Med. 2013;19:202–8.
2. Al-Sawaf O, Zhang C, Tandon M, Sinha A, Fink AM, Robrecht S, Samoylova O, Liberati AM, Pinilla-Ibarz J, Opat S, Sivcheva L, Le Dû K, Fogliatto LM, Niemann CU, Weinkove R, Robinson S, Kipps TJ, Tausch E, Schary W, Ritgen M, Wendtner CM, Kreuzer KA, Eichhorst B, Stilgenbauer S, Hallek M, Fischer K. Venetoclax plus obinutuzumab versus chlorambucil plus obinutuzumab for previously untreated chronic lymphocytic leukaemia (CLL14): follow-up results from a multicentre, open-label, randomised, phase 3 trial. Lancet Oncol. 2020;21(9):1188–200. https://doi.org/10.1016/S1470-2045(20)30443-5.
3. Roberts AW, Davids MS, Pagel JM, Kahl BS, Puvvada SD, Gerecitano JF, et al. Targeting BCL2 with venetoclax in relapsed chronic lymphocytic leukemia. N Engl J Med. 2016;374:311–22.
4. Stilgenbauer S, Eichhorst B, Schetelig J, Coutre S, Seymour JF, Munir T, et al. Venetoclax in relapsed or refractory chronic lymphocytic leukaemia with 17p deletion: a multicentre, open-label, phase 2 study. Lancet Oncol. 2016;17:768–78.
5. Seymour JF, Ma S, Brander DM, Choi MY, Barrientos J, Davids MS, et al. Venetoclax plus rituximab in relapsed or refractory chronic lymphocytic leukaemia: a phase 1b study. Lancet Oncol. 2017;18:230–40.
6. Seymour JF, Kipps TJ, Eichhorst B, Hillmen P, D'Rozario J, Assouline S, et al. Venetoclax–Rituximab in relapsed or refractory chronic lymphocytic leukemia. N Engl J Med. 2018;378:1107–20.
7. Kater AP, Seymour JF, Hillmen P, Eichhorst B, Langerak AW, Owen C, et al. Fixed duration of venetoclax-rituximab in relapsed/refractory chronic lymphocytic leukemia eradicates minimal residual disease and prolongs survival: post-treatment follow-up of the MURANO Phase III study. J Clin Oncol. 2019;37:269–77.
8. Flinn IW, Gribben JG, Dyer MJS, Wierda W, Maris MB, Furman RR, et al. Phase 1b study of venetoclax-obinutuzumab in previously untreated and relapsed/refractory chronic lymphocytic leukemia. Blood. 2019;133:2765.
9. Al-Sawaf O, Robrecht S, Zhang C, et al. Venetoclax-obinutuzumab for previously untreated chronic lymphocytic leukemia: 6-year results of the randomized phase 3 CLL14 study. Blood. 2024;144(18):1924–35. https://doi.org/10.1182/blood.2024024631.
10. ürstenau M, Kater A, Robrecht S, et al. First-line venetoclax combinations versus chemoimmunotherapy in fit patients with chronic lymphocytic leukaemia (GAIA/CLL13): 4-year follow-up from a multicentre, open-label, randomised, phase 3 trial. Lancet Oncol. 2024;25(6):744–59. https://doi.org/10.1016/S1470-2045(24)00196-7.
11. Cervantes-Gomez F, Lamothe B, Woyach JA, Wierda WG, Keating MJ, Balakrishnan K, et al. Pharmacological and protein profiling suggests venetoclax (ABT-199) as optimal partner with ibrutinib in chronic lymphocytic leukemia. Clin Cancer Res. 2015;21:3705–15.

12. Jain N, Keating M, Thompson P, Ferrajoli A, Burger J, Borthakur G, et al. Ibrutinib and venetoclax for first-line treatment of CLL. N Engl J Med. 2019;380:2095–103.
13. Niemann C, Munir T, Moreno C, et al. Fixed-duration ibrutinib–venetoclax versus chlorambucil–obinutuzumab in previously untreated chronic lymphocytic leukaemia (GLOW): 4-year follow-up from a multicentre, open-label, randomised, phase 3 trial. Lancet Oncol. 2023;24(12):1423–33. https://doi.org/10.1016/S1470-2045(23)00452-7.
14. Wierda W, Allan J, Siddiqi T, et al. Ibrutinib plus venetoclax for first-line treatment of chronic lymphocytic leukemia: primary analysis results from the minimal residual disease cohort of the randomized phase II CAPTIVATE study. J Clin Oncol. 2021;39(34):3853–65.
15. Rajendra A, Sengar M. Venetoclax: a narrative drug review. Cancer Res Stat Treat. 2022;5(3):519–32. https://doi.org/10.4103/crst.crst_179_22.
16. Molica M, Perrone S. Venetoclax and beyond: New Horizons in CLL and AML therapy. Expert Review of Anticancer Therapy. 2025;25(1):1–4.
17. Rogers KA, Woyach JA. The evolving frontline management of CLL: are triplets better than doublets? How will we find ou? Hematol Am Soc Hematol Educ Program. 2024;2024(1):467–73.
18. Huber H, Tausch E, et al. Final analysis of the CLL2-GIVe trial: obinutuzumab, ibrutinib, and venetoclax for untreated CLL with del(17p)/*TP53*mut. Blood. 2023;142(11):961–72.
19. Vo TT, Ryan J, Carrasco R, Neuberg D, Rossi DJ, Stone RM, et al. Relative mitochondrial priming of myeloblasts and normal HSCs determines chemotherapeutic success in AML. Cell. 2012;151:344–55.
20. Konopleva M, Pollyea DA, Potluri J, Chyla B, Hogdal L, Busman T, et al. Efficacy and biological correlates of response in a phase II study of venetoclax monotherapy in patients with acute myelogenous leukemia. Cancer Discov. 2016;6:1106–17.
21. DiNardo CD, Pratz K, Pullarkat V, Jonas BA, Arellano M, Becker PS, et al. Venetoclax combined with decitabine or azacitidine in treatment-naive, elderly patients with acute myeloid leukemia. Blood. 2019;133:7 17.
22. DiNardo CD, Jonas BA, Pullarkat V, Thirman MJ, Garcia JS, Wei AH, et al. Azacitidine and venetoclax in previously untreated acute myeloid leukemia. N Engl J Med. 2020;383:617 29.
23. Wei AH, Montesinos P, Ivanov V, DiNardo CD, Novak J, Laribi K, et al. Venetoclax plus LDAC for newly diagnosed AML ineligible for intensive chemotherapy:A phase 3 randomized placebo-controlled trial. Blood. 2020;135(2137):45.
24. Wei AH, Montesinos P, Ivanov V, Dinardo CD, Novak J, Laribi K, et al. A phase III study of venetoclax plus low-dose cytarabine in previously untreated older patients with acute myeloid leukemia (VIALE-C): a six-month update. J Clin Oncol. 2020;38(15_suppl):7511
25. Wang H, Mao L, Yang M, Qian P, Lu H, Tong H, et al. Venetoclax plus 3+7 daunorubicin and cytarabine chemotherapy as first-line treatment for adults with acute myeloid leukaemia: a multicentre, single-arm, phase 2 trial. Lancet Haematol. 2022;9:e415 24.
26. Chua CC, Loo S, et al. Final analysis of the phase 1b chemotherapy and Venetoclax in elderly acute myeloid leukemia trial (CAVEAT). Blood Adv. 2025;9(8):1827–35.
27. Long term results of venetoclax combined with FLAG-IDA induction and consolidation for newly diagnosed and relapsed or refractory acute myeloid leukemia. Leukemia. 2025 April;39(4):854–63. https://doi.org/10.1038/s41375-025-02531-8.
28. Karol SE, Alexander TB, Budhraja A, et al. Venetoclax in combination with cytarabine with or without idarubicin in children with relapsed or refractory acute myeloid leukaemia: a phase 1, dose-escalation study. Lancet Oncol. 2020;21(4):551–60.
29. Pfeiffer T, Li Y, Karol SE, et al. Venetoclax-based combination therapy as a bridge to allogeneic hematopoietic stem cell transplant in children with relapsed/refractory AML. Transplant Cell Ther. 2022;28(3):S120–1.
30. Masetti R, Baccelli F, Leardini D, et al. Venetoclax-based therapies in pediatric advanced MDS and relapsed/refractory AML: a multicenter retrospective analysis. Blood Adv. 2023;7(16):4366–70.
31. Klimentova M, Shelikhova L, Ilushina M, et al. Targeted therapy with venetoclax and daratumumab as part of HSCT preparative regimen in children with chemorefractory acute myeloid leukemia. Transplant Cell Ther. 2023;29(2):127.e1–9.

32. Wen X, Lu Y, Li Y, et al. Remission rate, toxicity and pharmacokinetics of venetoclax-based induction regimens in untreated pediatric acute myeloid leukemia. npj Precis Onc. 2024;8:248.
33. Arber DA, Orazi A, Hasserjian R, et al. The 2016 revision to the World Health Organization classification of myeloid neoplasms and acute leukemia. Blood. 2016;127(20):2391–405.
34. Issa GC, Cuglievan B, CD DN, et al. Early results of the phase I/II study investigating the all-oral combination of the menin inhibitor revumenib (SNDX-5613) with decitabine/cedazuridine (ASTX727) and venetoclax in acute myeloid leukemia (SAVE). Blood. 2023;142(suppl 1):58.
35. Fiskus W, Boettcher S, Daver N, et al. Effective menin inhibitor-based combinations against AML with MLL rearrangement or NPM1 mutation (NPM1c). Blood Cancer J. 2022;12(1):5–11.
36. Ma J, Zhao S, Qiao X, et al. Inhibition of Bcl-2 synergistically enhances the antileukemic activity of midostaurin and gilteritinib in preclinical models of FLT3-mutated acute myeloid leukemia. Clin Cancer Res. 2019;25(22):6815–26.
37. Wu Y, Zehnle PMA, Rajak J, et al. BH3 mimetics and azacitidine show synergistic effects on juvenile myelomonocytic leukemia. Leukemia. 2024;38(1):136148.
38. Davids MS, Roberts AW, Seymour JF, Pagel JM, Kahl BS, Wierda WG, et al. Phase I first-in-human study of venetoclax in patients with relapsed or refractory non-hodgkin lymphoma. J Clin Oncol. 2017;35:826–33.
39. Tam CS, Anderson MA, Pott C, Agarwal R, Handunnetti S, Hicks RJ, et al. Ibrutinib plus venetoclax for the treatment of mantle-cell lymphoma. N Engl J Med. 2018;378:1211 23.
40. Zelenetz AD, Salles G, Mason KD, Casulo C, Le Gouill S, Sehn LH, et al. Venetoclax plus R- or G-CHOP in non-Hodgkin lymphoma: results from the CAVALLI phase 1b trial. Blood. 2019;133:1964 76.
41. Melani C, Lakhotia R, Pittaluga S, et al. Combination targeted therapy in relapsed diffuse large B-cell lymphoma. N Engl J Med. 2024;390:2143–55.
42. Kumar S, Kaufman JL, Gasparetto C, Mikhael J, Vij R, Pegourie B, et al. Efficacy of venetoclax as targeted therapy for relapsed/refractory t (11;14) multiple myeloma. Blood. 2017;130:2401 9.
43. Moreau P, Chanan-Khan A, Roberts AW, Agarwal AB, Facon T, Kumar S, et al. Promising efficacy and acceptable safety of venetoclax plus bortezomib and dexamethasone in relapsed/refractory MM. Blood. 2017;130(2392):400.
44. Kumar SK, Harrison SJ, Cavo M, de la Rubia J, Popat R, Gasparetto C, et al. Venetoclax or placebo in combination with bortezomib and dexamethasone in patients with relapsed or refractory multiple myeloma (BELLINI): a randomised, double-blind, multicentre, phase 3 trial. Lancet Oncol. 2020;21:1630–42.
45. Bolarinwa A, Nagaraj M, Zanwar S, et al. Venetoclax-based treatment combinations in relapsed/refractory multiple myeloma: practice patterns and impact of secondary cytogenetic abnormalities on outcomes. Blood Cancer J. 2025;15:57.
46. Luskin MR, Shimony S, Keating J, et al. Venetoclax plus low-intensity chemotherapy for adults with acute lymphoblastic leukemia. Blood Adv. 2025;9(3):617–26.
47. Vereertbrugghen A, Colado A, Gargiulo E, et al. *In vitro* sensitivity to venetoclax and microenvironment protection in hairy cell leukemia. Front Oncol. 2021;11:598319.
48. Tiacci E, De Carolis L, Santi A, Falini B. Venetoclax in relapsed or refractory hairy-cell leukemia. N Engl J Med. 2023;388(10):952–4.
49. Garcia JS, Platzbecker U, Odenike O, et al. Efficacy and safety of venetoclax plus azacitidine for patients with treatment-naive high-risk myelodysplastic syndromes. Blood. 2025;145(11):1126–35.
50. Willekens C, Bazinet A, Chraibi S, et al. Reduced venetoclax exposure to 7 days vs standard exposure with hypomethylating agents in newly diagnosed AML patients. Blood Cancer J. 2025;15(1):68.
51. Karrar O, Abdelmagid M, Rana M, Iftikhar M, et al. Venetoclax duration (14 vs. 21 vs. 28 days) in combination with hypomethylating agent in newly diagnosed acute myeloid leukemia: comparative analysis of response, toxicity, and survival. Am J Hematol. 2024;99(2):E63–6.

52. Goldfinger M, Mantzaris I, Shastri A, et al. A weekly low-dose regimen of decitabine and venetoclax is efficacious and less myelotoxic in a racially diverse cohort. Blood. 2024;144(22):2360–3.
53. Nair R, Vu AH, Freer AK, et al. Heme promotes venetoclax resistance in multiple myeloma through MEK-ERK signaling and purine biosynthesis. Blood. 2025;145(7):732–47.

Chapter 38
CAR-T Cell Therapy in Haematologic Malignancies

Rahul Bhargava, Shrinidhi Nathany, Nikhil M. Kumar, and Anusha Swaminathan

Abstract Chimeric Antigen Receptor T-cell (CAR-T) therapy has emerged as a revolutionary modality in cancer immunotherapy, particularly transforming the prognosis of relapsed/refractory haematologic malignancies. This chapter offers a comprehensive overview of CAR-T cell therapy, tracing its evolution, mechanistic underpinnings, and current clinical applications. It begins by detailing the structural domains of a CAR construct and categorizing its development into five generations, alongside newer variants like universal CARs, TanCARs, and inhibitory CARs aimed at enhancing precision and safety. The historical timeline outlines major milestones in adoptive cell therapy, culminating in current FDA-approved CAR-T products for B-cell malignancies and multiple myeloma. Key challenges such as tumour escape via antigen loss, immune exhaustion, and bone marrow microenvironment resistance are discussed, highlighting the need for strategic combinatorial approaches. Manufacturing techniques—both ex vivo and in vivo—are described, along with regulatory considerations. Clinical indications and FDA-approved products are tabulated with their trial data. The chapter further addresses unique CAR-T-related complications, including cytokine release syndrome (CRS), immune effector cell-associated neurotoxicity syndrome (ICANS), infections, hypogammaglobulinemia, cytopenias, and secondary hemophagocytic lymphohistiocytosis (sHLH), along with evidence-based management protocols. Monitoring strategies for CAR-T persistence, immune reconstitution, and minimal residual disease (MRD) are outlined, emphasizing their prognostic and therapeutic implications. Finally, the chapter explores long-term follow-up frameworks modelled on allogeneic transplant clinics, detailing common late effects and the importance of multidisciplinary care. As CAR-T therapy expands to solid tumours and autoimmune diseases, this chapter underscores the pivotal role of innovation in design, post-infusion strategies, and real-world data integration to ensure sustained efficacy and safety.

Keywords CAR T cells · B ALL · Multiple myeloma · Lymphoma

R. Bhargava (✉) · S. Nathany · N. M. Kumar · A. Swaminathan
Hematology and BMT, Fortis Memorial Research Institute, Gurugram, Haryana, India

H. P. Pati et al. (eds.), *Clinical Hematology and Hemato-Oncology*,
https://doi.org/10.1007/978-981-92-1167-8_38

Learning Objectives

- Understand the molecular structure and mechanistic function of CAR-T constructs.
- Describe the evolution and classification of CAR-T generations and variants.
- Identify FDA-approved CAR-T products and their indications.
- Recognize the mechanisms of tumour escape and resistance.
- Manage acute and chronic CAR-T-related toxicities.
- Understand immune monitoring, MRD assessment, and long-term follow-up protocols.
- Evaluate future directions, including solid tumours, novel constructs, and maintenance strategies.

38.1 Introduction

Succeeding the paradigm brought about by immunotherapy in cancer, the newest kid on the block is the CAR T cell therapy, which is revolutionizing the prognostic spectrum of myriad malignancies [1]. This cellular therapy has been USFDA-approved for the treatment of relapses/refractory cases of various haematological malignancies, and is making its way to the frontline soon. Many products suchlike are also under development for solid organ malignancies as well [2]. This chapter provides a comprehensive overview and detailed aspects of this therapy from the principle of development, to clinical aspects, as well as regulatory requirements that govern the manufacturing and administration of the product [3].

38.2 Understanding the Building Blocks of CART Therapy: Domains of a CART

CART cell therapy is a form of cellular therapy, which is one of the pillars of adoptive T cell therapy (ACT). ACT currently entails three main forms: a) tumour-infiltrating lymphocytes, b) CART, c) T cell receptor therapy [4].

The concept of CAR is prototypical of T cells, but not exclusive. They are called chimeric as they are composed of different antibody parts, and are capable of conveying the specificity of engineered cells against target antigens, while concurrently enhancing their activation [5]. They are expressed on the surface of immune effector cells and are reprogrammed either ex vivo or in situ.

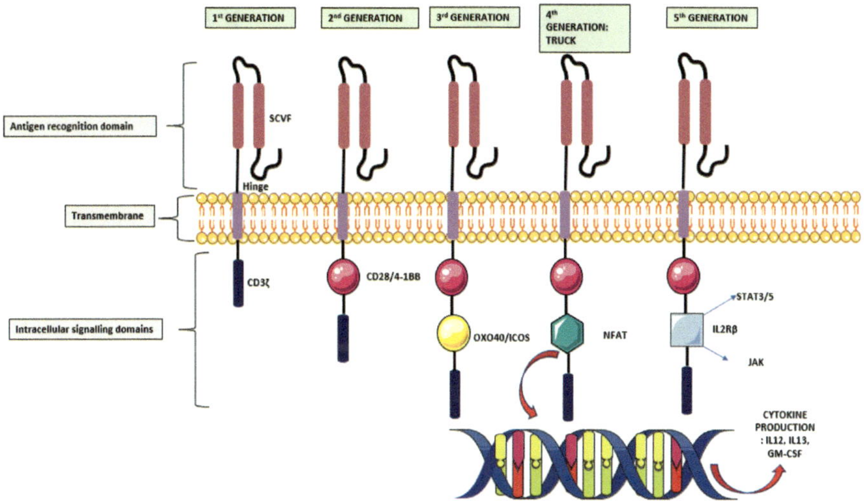

Fig. 38.1 Various generations of CART

A simplified schema of what a typical CART consists of is depicted in Fig. 38.1. To better understand the CART product has four domains:

1. *Extracellular domain*: This is responsible for recognition of the antigen and is composed of a single chain variable fragment (SCVF) of immunoglobulin.
2. *Hinge/spacer region.*
3. *Transmembrane domain*: This binds the extracellular and intracellular domains and determines the final flexibility and conformation of the CAR to specifically bind the targeted epitope/antigen for which it has been reprogrammed [6].
4. *Intracellular domain*: This is involved in facilitating the signal transduction upon antigen binding.

38.3 Generations of CART

Based on the intracellular domain composition, various generations of CART have been described. The intracellular domain comprises the T cell activation domain of CD3ζ (CD3 Zeta), and the signalling domains of the costimulatory molecules CD28, 4-1BB (CD137), and OX-40 (CD134) [7]. There are 5 generations of CART and some variants which have been described and are depicted in Fig. 38.2. The currently approved ones are the second generation for clinical use. The exact indications and clinical uses are discussed later in this chapter.

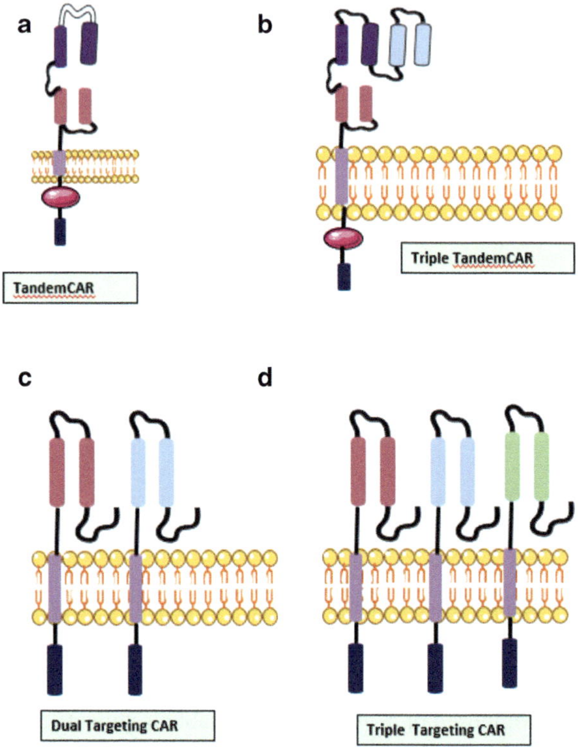

Fig. 38.2 Additional variations of CART

38.4 Additional Variations in CAR

In the process of continued development to enhance the specificity, potency, accuracy, antigen recognition, and patient safety, many variants of CAR have also been developed, which are listed as follows:

(a) *Universal CAR & Universal CART cells*: This variant uses a third-party intermediary between the transmembrane and extracellular domains, which is expected to increase the antigen recognition range. Examples include BBIR CAR, Universal CAR, and SUPRA CAR. The cells are derived from healthy donors and are manipulated in a way to avoid immune rejection on infusion. A detailed discussion on this is beyond the scope of the chapter. Readers are encouraged to access the references cited.

(b) *The Tandem CAR (TanCAR)*: This variant has two SCVF for two different tumour antigens connected to one transgenic receptor. Any generation can be adapted to make this variant.

(c) *The Triple SCVF:* This is like the TanCAR but with three SCVF.

(d) *Dual CAR:* This variant can recognize two different tumour antigens simultaneously but is engineered on two separate CARs, each with its own intracellular domain, on the same T cell [8].

(e) *Switchable, Inhibitory, AND-gate CAR:* This has the regulatory control in case there are severe side effects or unwanted toxicities. The switch can be activated in order to turn off the CAR. Gate Car uses a modular receptor, Syn NOTCH, and only when both the SCVF bind to tumour antigens simultaneously, the CAR is activated. In the Inhibitory CAR, there is a traditional CAR and an iCAR. The iCAR recognizes the non-tumour cells and enables them to evade the killing by T cells, thus protecting the non-tumour cells from the damage.

38.5 History and Major Milestones in CART Development

The concept of modulating the immune system for cancer therapy dates back to the 1960s, and the use of adoptive T cell therapy commenced with the use of TILs in the late 1980s. Since then, continuous development in this space has been ongoing with remarkable results and outcomes, especially in the CART therapy for haematolymphoid malignancies [9]. Fig. 38.3 is a chronological schematic depiction of these milestones in the space of adoptive T cell therapy.

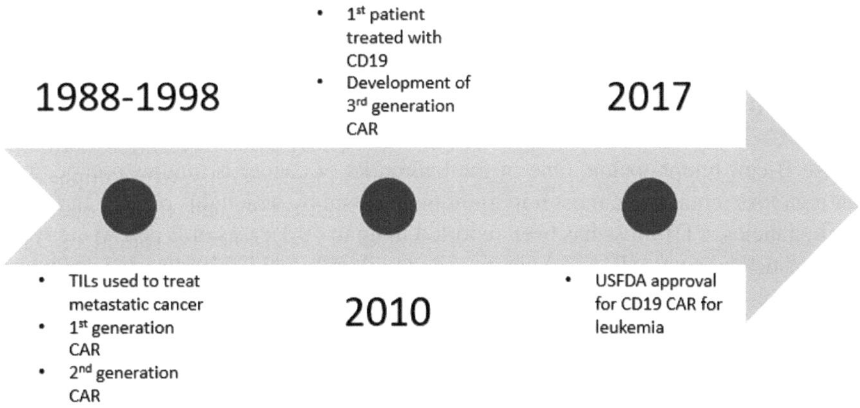

Fig. 38.3 Timeline of milestones achieved in CART development

38.6 Genetic Engineering and Manufacturing Processes [3]

CART can be manufactured ex vivo and in vivo, with the main problem being the high manufacturing cost, stringent quality control procedures, and regulatory guidelines. The regulatory guidelines pertaining to India are briefly summarized in a later section of this chapter [10].

(a) Ex vivo: The patient's T cells are isolated and reprogrammed ex vivo, expanded, and then infused into the patient's bloodstream and tumour cell destruction [11].
(b) In vivo: This strategy entails the engineering of the CART directly inside the patient's body. In this, the required genetic material is infused into the patient's T cells in vivo, which reprograms into CART, in vivo. This approach simplifies the manufacturing process and reduces the risk of graft versus host disease [6, 12].

38.7 Good Tumour Antigen and Tumour Escape

The majority of the CART products available do not recognize tumour-specific antigens, but are directed towards pan B antigens like CD19, CD20, CD22, or BCMA, which is a maturation antigen [13]. These usually serve as ideal antigens since the depletion of B cells is usually well tolerated, in contrast to endogenous T cell receptors, which are HLA-restricted [14]. Therefore, to be designated as a good tumour antigen, the antigen should not be present on non-malignant cells, should have a consistent expression in all cells, and should be expressed in the extracellular space and therefore readily accessible for CAR reprogramming [15].

All CAR products approved to date are lineage-specific antigen CARs, which cause B cell lymphopenia. One of the hallmarks of cancer is tumour escape, and antigen loss remains the most important mechanism by which this occurs. In B cell malignancies, CD19 loss has been reported in up to 40% cases of B cell Acute lymphoblastic leukaemia (B-ALL) when treated with different CD19-directed products. These are attributed to point mutations in CD19 and alternatively spliced CD19 mRNA, which lead to non-anchorage of a functional CD19 protein to the cell membrane and hence antigen loss. Similarly, the same is reported in33% cases [16]. In myeloma, for those treated with BCMA products, anecdotal reports have revealed biallelic molecular mechanisms in the BCMA gene. However, in the KarMMa trial, only 4% cases relapsed without an increase in soluble BCMA, which is considered a biomarker for resistance to CART [17].

The other mechanism is immune dysregulation and exhaustion, which may lead to tumour escape during CART. It has been reported that in patients of DLBCL, expression of interferon signalling, high blood levels of IL-6, and monocytic myeloid-derived suppressor cells, were associated with lack of demonstrable response [18–20]. Upregulation of interferon and downregulation of JAK2 can cause CART resistance, as upregulation of interferon causes expression of PDL1 on lymphoma cells, which leads to CART resistance. This theory holds a direct implication for the design of the CART. This necessitates approaches that combine CART with immune checkpoint blockade either through genetic engineering or co-infusion.

The third mechanism is microenvironment-mediated resistance. The concept here is that the bone marrow microenvironment is known to upregulate antiapoptotic mechanisms, and the tumour lysis by T and NK cells is also driven by activation of the extrinsic and intrinsic apoptotic pathways. It has been demonstrated that the interaction of myeloma cells with bone marrow mesenchymal stem cells protects the myeloma cells from cytotoxicity, which is caused by T cells as well as through daratumumab-directed reprogrammed NK cells [21].

38.8 Clinical Indications for CART

CAR-T cell therapy has emerged as a transformative treatment for relapsed/refractory (R/R) haematologic malignancies, particularly B-cell malignancies and multiple myeloma. The approval of CAR-T therapies was based on high response rates and durable remissions in landmark clinical trials. Table 38.1 depicts the available CARs, with USFDA-approved indications, and the associated clinical trial [22, 23].

Table 38.1 The various products available, along with their approved clinical indications and approval status

CART product	Target	Clinical Trial (NCT#)	Indication	Approval year
Tisagenlecleucel (Kymriah)	CD19	ELIANA (NCT02435849), JULIET (NCT02445248)	B-ALL: Paediatric and young adult, R/R DLBCL	2017
Axicabtagene ciloleucel (Yescarta)	CD19	ZUMA-1 (NCT02348216)	R/R large B cell lymphoma	2017
Brexucabtagene autoleucel (Tecartus)	CD19	ZUMA-2 (NCT02601313)	R/R mantle cell lymphoma	2020
Lisocabtagene maraleucel (Breyanzi)	CD19	TRANSCEND (NCT02631044)	R/R large B cell lymphoma	2021
Idecabtagene vicleucel (Abecma)	BCMA	KarMMa (NCT03361748)	R/R multiple myeloma	2021
Ciltacabtagene autoleucel (Carvykti)	BCMA	CARTITUDE-1 (NCT03548207)	R/R multiple myeloma	2022

38.9 Complications of CART and Their Management

This section discusses the complications that are unique to CART and their management as recommended. However, a detailed discussion on pathophysiology as well as other complications related to specific clinical scenarios is beyond the scope of this chapter.

(a) *Cytokine Release Syndrome (CRS)* [24]: CRS results from massive cytokine release (IL-6, IL-1, IFN-γ, TNF-α) due to T-cell activation, leading to systemic inflammation and capillary leak syndrome. The frequency and severity of CRS after CAR-T cell therapy vary between products (any grade: 37–93%, G3/4: 1–23%). CRS occurred in 77% of patients in the ELIANA trial (B-ALL) and 94% in ZUMA-1 (DLBCL). This usually manifests as fever preceding or with concurrent symptoms like headache, malaise, arthralgia, tachypnoea, tachycardia, hypotension, arrhythmia, hypoxia, eventually culminating in shock, cardiorespiratory failure, and organ dysfunction [25]. The CRS is graded and managed based on ASTCT criteria [26]. The same is depicted in Table 38.2.
(b) *Immune Effector Cell-Associated Neurotoxicity Syndrome (ICANS)* [27, 28]: ICANS results from endothelial activation, blood-brain barrier (BBB) disruption, and cytokine-driven neuroinflammation, manifesting as encephalopathy, aphasia, seizures, and cerebral oedema. ICANS was reported in 64% of patients in ZUMA-1 (DLBCL) and 10% in CARTITUDE-1 (MM) [29].
(c) *Hypogammaglobulinemia:* The pathophysiology here is that CD19-directed CAR-T therapy leads to B-cell aplasia, resulting in hypogammaglobulinemia and increased susceptibility to infections [30]. It has been reported in >80% of patients post-CD19 CAR-T therapy (Maude et al., 2018). Monitoring IgG levels and IV IG therapy with treatment of infections is recommended.
(d) *Myelotoxicity and Prolonged Cytopenias:* CAR-T therapy leads to bone marrow suppression due to conditioning chemotherapy (fludarabine/cyclophosphamide) and inflammatory milieu. Prolonged cytopenias (>30 days) were reported in 40–50% of patients in the ZUMA-1 and JULIET trials [31].

Table 38.2 Grading system of cytokine release syndrome and their management

Grade	Clinical features	Management
1	Fever (not attributable to any other cause), no hypotension/hypoxia	In the absence of response in 3 days to supportive care/antipyretics, consider tocilizumab
2	Hypotension(responsive to fluids), hypoxia (responsive to low flow O2 < 6litres/minute)	Tocilizumab (IL-6 inhibitor) ± steroids
3	Vasopressor requiring hypotension, hypoxia requiring high flow O_2	Tocilizumab (IL-6 inhibitor) ± steroids (dexamethasone), ICU monitoring
4	Life-threatening organ dysfunction, ventilator/ECMO support	Tocilizumab, high-dose steroids (dexamethasone, consider switch to methylprednisolone), ICU admission

(e) *Infectious Complications:* Patients undergoing CAR-T therapy are at high risk for infections, particularly during the first 3 months post-infusion, due to B-cell aplasia, neutropenia, and steroid use. The majority of the infections occur in the first 28 days, with bacterial being the most common, followed by viral and fungal. Late complications around 90 days may result due to respiratory viruses [32]. Around 1–5% cases also develop invasive fungal infections: yeasts and moulds showing almost equal incidence [33]. The use of antiviral, antifungal, and anti-pneumocystis (PCP) prophylaxis to reduce the risk of infections post-CAR-T cell therapy is recommended; however, there is no consensus on the optimal choice and duration of prophylaxis. Patients undergoing CAR-T cell therapy typically receive antiviral prophylaxis with acyclovir or valacyclovir, along with antifungal prophylaxis targeting either yeast or mould infections, and co-trimoxazole for *Pneumocystis jirovecii* pneumonia (PCP) prevention. Individuals identified as high-risk for mould infections—such as those with pre-existing neutropenia before CAR-T infusion, a history of mould infections within the past 6 months, prior allogeneic stem cell transplantation, or a diagnosis of acute leukaemia—should receive mould-active prophylaxis. Additionally, patients who experience grade 3 or higher cytokine release syndrome (CRS) or immune effector cell-associated neurotoxicity syndrome (ICANS) post-infusion, as well as those requiring prolonged corticosteroid or immunosuppressive therapy, should also be provided with mould-active antifungal prophylaxis [34]. In cases where these high-risk factors are absent, prophylaxis targeting yeast infections may be sufficient, with close surveillance for mould infections recommended.

Antifungal prophylaxis is typically continued until neutrophil recovery and discontinuation of immunosuppressive therapy. PCP prophylaxis is generally maintained for 6 months or until the CD4 T-cell count exceeds 200 cells/μL [35]. For patients with persistent severe hypogammaglobulinemia and a history of recurrent infections, monthly intravenous immunoglobulin (IVIG) administration may be considered. Management of confirmed or suspected infections following CAR-T cell therapy should align with institutional protocols and closely resemble infection management strategies used after stem cell transplantation.

The effectiveness of vaccinations following CD19- or BCMA-targeted CAR-T cell therapy remains uncertain. However, patients should be evaluated for vaccination at 6 months post-infusion, with decisions guided by post-vaccine antibody titres. Implementing comprehensive infection prevention and management strategies is essential to improving patient outcomes after CAR-T cell therapy. Table 38.3 depicts the various grades of ICANS and their management strategies.

(f) *Secondary HLH/macrophage activation syndrome*: This is a life-threatening hyperinflammatory syndrome, and differentiation of the same from CRS may be clinically difficult. These symptoms often present as fever, cytopenia affecting multiple cell lineages, and multiorgan failure. In patients with persistent fever without a confirmed infectious cause, or worsening fever despite appro-

Table 38.3 Grades of immune effector cell-associated neurotoxicity syndrome (ICANS) and their management strategies

Grade	Clinical features	Management
1	Mild confusion, tremors, headache	Seizure prophylaxis with levetiracetam (750 mg twice daily) should be initiated. Medications that contribute to central nervous system depression should be avoided. A neurology specialist should be consulted for further evaluation and management. Supportive care should be provided as required. Fundoscopic examination should be performed to assess for papilledema. Brain MRI with contrast is recommended, with brain CT as an alternative if MRI is not feasible. If appropriate, a diagnostic lumbar puncture should be considered to measure opening pressure and analyse cerebrospinal fluid (CSF) for culture and sensitivity, cytology, biochemistry, and viral studies. In patients with focal peripheral neurological deficits, spinal MRI should be performed. An electroencephalogram (EEG) may be indicated to assess for seizure activity. Tocilizumab at a dose of 8 mg/kg should only be administered in the presence of concurrent cytokine release syndrome (CRS). Neurocognitive assessments should be conducted twice daily using the immune effector cell-associated encephalopathy (ICE) score, and neurotoxicity should be graded according to the immune effector cell-associated neurotoxicity syndrome (ICANS) criteria
2	Moderate encephalopathy, impaired handwriting	Investigations and supportive care should be conducted as recommended for grade 1 cases. The use of high-dose dexamethasone with a rapid taper should be considered. Transfer to the intensive care unit (ICU) may be warranted based on the patient's condition
3	Severe encephalopathy, seizures	Investigations and supportive care should be provided in accordance with management recommendations for grade 1 cases. Dexamethasone should be administered at a dose of 10–20 mg intravenously every 6 h, or an equivalent dose of methylprednisolone, until symptoms improve to grade 1, followed by a gradual taper. Seizures should be managed with lorazepam (0.5 mg IV) or an alternative benzodiazepine as needed, followed by loading with levetiracetam or another appropriate anticonvulsant. If fundoscopy reveals stage 1 or 2 papilledema with a cerebrospinal fluid (CSF) opening pressure exceeding 20 mmHg, urgent consultation with a neurologist should be sought. For patients with persistent grade 3 or higher immune effector cell-associated neurotoxicity syndrome (ICANS), repeat neuroimaging with CT or MRI should be considered every 2–3 days to monitor disease progression

(continued)

Table 38.3 (continued)

Grade	Clinical features	Management
4	Unresponsive, cerebral oedema	Investigations and supportive care should be conducted in accordance with management guidelines for grade 1 cases. The patient should be transferred to the intensive care unit (ICU), with consideration given to mechanical ventilation for airway protection if necessary. Seizure management should follow the protocols established for grade 3 cases. In the event of convulsive status epilepticus, urgent consultation with a neurologist should be sought. Methylprednisolone should be administered at a dose of 1000 mg per day for 3 days, followed by a gradual tapering regimen of 250 mg every 12 h for 2 days, then 125 mg every 12 h for 2 days, and finally 60 mg every 12 h for 2 days. For the management of elevated intracranial pressure, treatment options should include the administration of acetazolamide at an initial dose of 1000 mg IV, followed by 250–1000 mg IV every 12 h, along with supportive measures such as elevating the head of the bed, hyperventilation, and hyperosmolar therapy with mannitol

Table 38.4 H score and its criteria for secondary hemophagocytic lymphohistiocytosis

Parameter	Criteria for scoring
Temperature	0 (<38), 33 (38.4–39.4), 49 (>39.4)
Organomegaly	0 (no), 23 (hepatomegaly or splenomegaly),38 (hepatomegaly &splenomegaly)
No. of cytopenias	0 (1), 24 (2), 34 (3)
Ferritin (ng/ml)	0 (<2000), 35 (2000–6000), 50 (>6000)
Triglycerides (mmoles/l)	0 (<1.5), 44 (1.5–4), 64 (>4)
Fibrinogen (gm/l)	0 (>2.5), 30 (≤2.5)
SGOT	0 (<30), 19 (>30)
Bone marrow aspirate	0 (no), 35 (yes)

priate antimicrobial treatment, secondary hemophagocytic lymphohistiocytosis (sHLH) or macrophage activation syndrome (MAS) should be considered as a potential diagnosis. Serum ferritin serves as a useful and easily accessible biomarker for identifying sHLH/MAS and can also be utilized to assess response to treatment. Neelapu et al. proposed diagnostic criteria for sHLH/MAS in patients with CRS post-CAR-T cell therapy, demonstrating a peak serum ferritin measurement of >10,000 μg/L and two of the following findings: a grade >3 increase in serum transaminase or bilirubin; grade >3 oliguria or increase in serum creatinine; grade >3 pulmonary oedema or histological evidence of haemophagocytosis in the bone marrow or organs. Table 38.4 depicts the H scores that have been published and adapted to CART.

The primary treatment consists of intravenous methylprednisolone (IVMP) at a dose of 1 g per day for 3–5 days, combined with intravenous immunoglobulin (IVIG) at 1 g/kg for 2 days, with the option to repeat the IVIG dose on day 14 if necessary [36, 37]. If secondary hemophagocytic lymphohistiocytosis (sHLH) or macrophage activation syndrome (MAS) is confirmed or if the patient shows signs of clinical deterioration, anakinra is introduced at an initial dose of 1–2 mg/kg daily, which can be increased up to 8 mg/kg per day based on response. Cyclosporine A (CSA) may be considered in cases of early or steroid-resistant disease. For refractory cases, etoposide is an option; however, its use may be complicated by the presence of pre-existing cytopenias, which are common in patients with sHLH/MAS following CAR-T cell therapy. Additionally, potential underlying triggers, such as Epstein-Barr virus (EBV), bacterial infections, or malignancies—particularly lymphoma—should be identified and appropriately treated [38].

38.10 Immune Monitoring

38.10.1 Tracking CAR-T Cell Persistence and Expansion

The expansion and persistence of CAR-T cells play a crucial role in determining long-term outcomes. Flow cytometry and polymerase chain reaction (PCR)-based methods are used to monitor the presence of CAR-T cells in peripheral blood and bone marrow. Studies have shown that peak CAR-T cell expansion typically occurs within 10–14 days post-infusion, with persistence varying from a few months to over a year [39]. Longer persistence has been correlated with better response rates, particularly in B-cell malignancies, where ongoing B-cell aplasia serves as an indicator of functional CAR-T cell activity.

38.10.2 Monitoring for Minimal Residual Disease and Relapse Risk

Minimal residual disease (MRD) assessment post-CAR-T therapy has emerged as a valuable tool for early relapse detection. Next-generation sequencing (NGS) and flow cytometry-based MRD monitoring have demonstrated that MRD-negative status at 1–3 months post-infusion is associated with improved progression-free survival. Patients who remain MRD-positive at 6 months post-CAR-T therapy exhibit a high risk of relapse and may benefit from preemptive maintenance strategies such as bispecific antibodies, lenalidomide, or checkpoint inhibitors.

38.10.3 Assessing Immune Reconstitution and Infection Risk

CAR-T cell therapy is associated with profound and prolonged immune suppression, leading to increased susceptibility to infections. B-cell aplasia following CD19-directed CAR-T therapy results in hypogammaglobulinemia, necessitating regular monitoring of immunoglobulin levels and intravenous immunoglobulin (IVIG) replacement in cases of recurrent infections. Furthermore, patients receiving CAR-T therapy often experience prolonged cytopenias due to conditioning chemotherapy, with neutropenia persisting for weeks to months post-infusion. Granulocyte colony-stimulating factor (G-CSF) is frequently used in cases of persistent neutropenia, while antimicrobial prophylaxis against bacterial, fungal, and viral infections is recommended for high-risk patients [40].

38.11 Follow-Up and Long-Term Monitoring

38.11.1 Follow-Up and Specialized Programs

In Europe, CAR-T cell therapy is typically provided through a hub-and-spoke model, where patients are referred from local hospitals to specialized cellular therapy centres for treatment. Long-term follow-up can be integrated into existing accredited allogeneic hematopoietic stem cell transplantation (allo-HCT) late effects clinics, which already have structured protocols for systematically evaluating patients over time for delayed toxicities [41]. These clinics follow a checklist-based approach to ensure patients receive comprehensive and consistent monitoring. As the number of long-term CAR-T cell therapy survivors increases, establishing dedicated CAR-T late effects clinics may become necessary. Additionally, service-level agreements (SLAs) between CAR-T centres and referral institutions should define shared care responsibilities and outreach services [42].

38.11.2 Long-Term Complications Following CAR-T Therapy

CAR-T cell therapy recipients may experience a range of late-onset adverse effects, requiring close monitoring and early intervention. These include cytopenias, hypogammaglobulinemia, infections, secondary malignancies, and neurological or psychiatric complications [43]. Table 38.5 depicts the late effects, their incidence and, and management strategies after CART therapy.

Multidisciplinary team (MDT) input is essential in CAR-T late effects clinics to manage these complications. Such teams should include CAR-T specialists, clinical nurse specialists, psychologists, data managers, and clinical trial staff [44]. Given that patients receiving CAR-T therapy have undergone extensive prior treatments,

Table 38.5 Common late effects after CAR T cell therapy and their management

Late effect	Incidence	Management
Prolonged cytopenias (especially neutropenia)	~50% at 2 months, ~20% beyond 2 months	Transfusions, growth factor support, and infection prophylaxis
Hypogammaglobulinemia	~50%, may persist for years	IV immunoglobulin (IVIG) therapy
Infections (mainly bacterial, affecting the upper respiratory tract)	>50%	IVIG, antibiotics, viral screening, vaccinations
Secondary malignancies (solid tumours > haematologic malignancies)	Low incidence	Surveillance and early detection
Neurological complications (neuropathy, cerebrovascular events)	~10%	Supportive care, multidisciplinary management
Psychiatric issues (depression, anxiety)	~10%	Psychological support, psychiatric consultation
Immune-related disorders (alveolitis, pneumonitis, dermatitis, myositis, arthralgia)	<10%	Corticosteroids, immunosuppressive therapy

both physical and psychological long-term effects should be addressed, including CAR-T cell persistence, risk of secondary malignancies, autoimmune conditions, endocrine and reproductive health, bone health, and patient-reported outcomes such as quality of life [45]. Studies conducted thus far suggest that quality-of-life metrics following CAR-T therapy are comparable to those of the general population [46].

38.11.3 Follow-Up Schedule

The frequency of follow-up depends on the patient's underlying disease status [47]. During the first year post-infusion, monthly follow-ups are necessary to monitor remission status and any short-term complications. Long-term follow-up typically occurs every 6months for the next 2 years, then annually until year 15, and possibly indefinitely for high-risk patients [48]. Individuals who undergo additional hematopoietic stem cell transplantation (HSCT), cytotoxic therapy, or further immune effector cell therapy should follow established post-HSCT monitoring guidelines (Majhail et al., 2012).

Case Study TP53 and BCL2 Mutated Transformed Follicular Lymphoma Responding to CAR-T with Longitudinal ctDNA Monitoring.

A 55-year-old female with a history of Grade 1–2 follicular lymphoma diagnosed in May 2017 presented with constitutional symptoms and bulky lymphadenopathy in February 2023, raising suspicion of histologic transformation. She had initially received 6 cycles of R-CVP, followed by rituximab maintenance until 2020, with a sustained partial response. In February 2023, PET-CT revealed extensive FDG-avid lymphadenopathy and a standardized uptake value (SUV) > 15 in the retroperitoneal mass. Excisional biopsy confirmed transformation to DLBCL (GCB type, MYC negative). Immunohistochemistry showed Ki-67 > 90%. She received R-ICE x 3 cycles, followed by BEAM conditioning and autologous stem cell transplantation in June 2023. She experienced biochemical relapse in November 2023, confirmed on PET-CT and biopsy. A custom 75-gene NGS panel revealed:

- TP53 p.R248Q (VAF 75%)—confirmed somatic by skin fibroblast culture.
- BCL2 p.G101V (VAF 51%)—known to confer resistance to venetoclax. No EZH2, MYD88, or CARD11 mutations were seen.

The patient was ineligible for allogeneic SCT due to age, donor unavailability, and cardiac comorbidities. She was enrolled in a CAR-T cell therapy program using tisa-cel (tisagenlecleucel), a second-generation CD19-directed CAR-T. Before lymphodepletion, a peripheral blood plasma sample was collected. ctDNA concentration was 4.5 ng/μL, and ultra-deep error-corrected sequencing confirmed TP53 R248Q at 2.1% VAF and BCL2 G101V at 1.5% VAF. The patient underwent FLU/CY conditioning and received CAR-T infusion in January 2024 at 5.8×10^6 cells/kg. She tolerated the infusion well with only grade 1 CRS, managed with supportive care alone. ctDNA-based MRD monitoring showed:

- Day +28 (Post-CAR-T):ctDNA concentration dropped to 1.2 ng/μL: TP53 VAF: 0.5%, BCL2 VAF: 0.3%; PET-CT showed partial metabolic response (Deauville 4).
- Day +56: ctDNA concentration: 0.6 ng/μL, TP53: 0.2%, BCL2: 0.1%; PET: further shrinkage of nodes, with borderline residual activity.
- Day +90:ctDNA: 0.2 ng/μL, no detectable mutations;PET-CT: Complete Metabolic Response (Deauville 2).

The patient remains in molecular remission at the last follow-up in April 2025. This is the first time she achieved undetectable ctDNA despite multiple prior lines of therapy, and serial ctDNA assessment is being continued every 6 weeks to preempt relapse.

Teaching Points & Future Implications: TP53 hotspot mutation R248Q is associated with poor prognosis and therapy resistance in transformed lymphomas. Longitudinal ctDNA profiling offered a minimally invasive, dynamic biomarker for CAR-T response assessment and may serve as an early predictor of relapse. Dual mutation in TP53 and BCL2 did not preclude durable molecular and metabolic remission, highlighting CAR-T as a transformative strategy in poor-risk lymphoma subsets.

38.12 Summary

CAR-T cell therapy has transformed the treatment landscape for relapsed and refractory haematologic malignancies, offering unprecedented response rates and durable remissions in patients with otherwise limited therapeutic options. Since the approval of CD19- and BCMA-directed CAR-T therapies, significant progress has been made in improving efficacy, refining patient selection criteria, and managing associated toxicities. However, challenges remain, including cytokine release syndrome (CRS), immune effector cell-associated neurotoxicity syndrome (ICANS), prolonged cytopenias, infections, and relapse due to antigen escape or CAR-T cell exhaustion. Rigorous immune monitoring and structured follow-up often ensure optimal outcomes.

Ongoing research aims to optimize CAR-T cell persistence, expand therapeutic indications to acute myeloid leukaemia (AML), solid tumours, and autoimmune diseases, and develop novel constructs such as dual-targeting, armoured, and allogeneic CAR-T cells to enhance safety and efficacy. Additionally, post-infusion maintenance strategies utilizing bispecific antibodies, small-molecule inhibitors, and checkpoint blockade may improve long-term outcomes and reduce relapse rates.

As CAR-T therapy becomes more widely adopted, standardized long-term follow-up programs will be essential to monitor late toxicities, ensure immune reconstitution, and mitigate long-term risks such as secondary malignancies and autoimmune complications. The integration of multidisciplinary care teams, accreditation frameworks (FACT-JACIE), and real-world data collection (EBMT Registry, PASS programs) will further refine patient management and regulatory oversight.

Despite these challenges, CAR-T therapy represents a paradigm shift in oncology and personalized medicine. The continued evolution of this field—driven by advancements in genetic engineering, immune modulation, and combination strategies—will likely broaden its clinical applications, ultimately improving survival and quality of life for patients with haematologic and potentially solid malignancies.. Evolving innovations and integrated care pathways will further expand its therapeutic scope.

References

1. World Health Organization. Available online: https://www.who.int/health-topics/cancer#tab=tab_1. Accessed on 4 July 2023.
2. Zhang X, Zhu L, Zhang H, Chen S, Xiao Y. CAR-T cell therapy in hematological malignancies: current opportunities and challenges. Front Immunol. 2022;13:927153.
3. Poirot L, Philip B, Schiffer-Mannioui C, Le Clerre D, Chion-Sotinel I, Derniame S, Potrel P, Bas C, Lemaire L, Galetto R, Lebuhotel C. Multiplex genome-edited T-cell manufacturing platform for "off-the-shelf" adoptive T-cell immunotherapies. Cancer Res. 2015;75(18):3853–64.
4. Park JH, Rivière I, Gonen M, Wang X, Sénéchal B, Curran KJ, Sadelain M. Long-term follow-up of CD19 CAR therapy in acute lymphoblastic leukemia. N Engl J Med. 2018;5:449–59. https://doi.org/10.1056/NEJMoa1709919.

5. Rosenberg SA, Restifo NP, Yang JC, Morgan RA, Dudley ME. Adoptive cell transfer: a clinical path to effective cancer immunotherapy. Nat Rev Cancer. 2008;8(4):299–308.
6. Kowolik CM, Topp MS, Gonzalez S, Pfeiffer T, Olivares S, Gonzalez N, Smith DD, Forman SJ, Jensen MC, Cooper LJ. CD28 costimulation provided through a CD19-specific chimeric antigen receptor enhances in vivo persistence and antitumor efficacy of adoptively transferred T cells. Cancer Res. 2006;66(22):10995–1004.
7. Strohl WR, Naso M. Bispecific T-cell redirection versus chimeric antigen receptor (CAR)-T cells as approaches to kill cancer cells. Antibodies. 2019;8(3):41.
8. Stopeck AT, Gessner A, Miller TP, Hersh EM, Johnson CS, Cui H, Frutiger Y, Grogan TM. Loss of B7. 2 (CD86) and intracellular adhesion molecule 1 (CD54) expression is associated with decreased tumor-infiltrating T lymphocytes in diffuse B-cell large-cell lymphoma. Clin Cancer Res. 2000;6(10):3904–9.
9. Wang Y, Qi K, Cheng H, Cao J, Shi M, Qiao J, Yan Z, Jing G, Pan B, Sang W, Li D. Coagulation disorders after chimeric antigen receptor T cell therapy: analysis of 100 patients with relapsed and refractory hematologic malignancies. Biol Blood Marrow Transplant. 2020;26(5):865–75.
10. Ghassemi S, Prachi P, Scholler J, Nunez-Cruz S, Barrett DM, Bedoya F, Fraietta JA, Lacey SF, Levine BL, Grupp SA, June CH. Minimally ex vivo manipulated gene-modified T cells display enhanced tumor control. Blood. 2016;128(22):4549.
11. Lum LG, Thakur A, Al-Kadhimi Z, Colvin GA, Cummings FJ, Legare RD, Dizon DS, Kouttab N, Maizel A, Colaiace W, Liu Q. Targeted T-cell therapy in stage IV breast cancer: a phase I clinical trial. Clin Cancer Res. 2015;21(10):2305–14.
12. Lamers CH, Willemsen R, van Elzakker P, van Steenbergen-Langeveld S, Broertjes M, Oosterwijk-Wakka J, Oosterwijk E, Sleijfer S, Debets R, Gratama JW. Immune responses to transgene and retroviral vector in patients treated with ex vivo–engineered T cells. Blood J Am Soc Hematol. 2011;117(1):72–82.
13. Ruella M, Barrett DM, Kenderian SS, Shestova O, Hofmann TJ, Perazzelli J, Klichinsky M, Aikawa V, Nazimuddin F, Kozlowski M, Scholler J. Dual CD19 and CD123 targeting prevents antigen-loss relapses after CD19-directed immunotherapies. J Clin Invest. 2016;126(10):3814–26.
14. Droste P, Frenzel A, Steinwand M, Pelat T, Thullier P, Hust M, Lashuel H, Dübel S. Structural differences of amyloid-β fibrils revealed by antibodies from phage display. BMC Biotechnol. 2015;15:1–3.
15. Kochenderfer JN, Wilson WH, Janik JE, Dudley ME, Stetler-Stevenson M, Feldman SA, Maric I, Raffeld M, Nathan DA, Lanier BJ, Morgan RA. Eradication of B-lineage cells and regression of lymphoma in a patient treated with autologous T cells genetically engineered to recognize CD19. Blood J Am Soc Hematol. 2010;116(20):4099–102.
16. Scholler N, Garvik B, Quarles T, Jiang S, Urban N. Method for generation of in vivo biotinylated recombinant antibodies by yeast mating. J Immunol Methods. 2006;317(1–2, 132):–43.
17. Yan Z, Cao J, Cheng H, Qiao J, Zhang H, Wang Y, Shi M, Lan J, Fei X, Jin L, Jing G. A combination of humanised anti-CD19 and anti-BCMA CAR T cells in patients with relapsed or refractory multiple myeloma: a single-arm, phase 2 trial. Lancet Haematol. 2019;6(10):e521–9.
18. Xin T, Cheng L, Zhou C, Zhao Y, Hu Z, Wu X. In-vivo induced CAR-T cell for the potential breakthrough to overcome the barriers of current CAR-T cell therapy. Front Oncol. 2022;12:809754.
19. Irving M, Lanitis E, Migliorini D, Ivics Z, Guedan S. Choosing the right tool for genetic engineering: clinical lessons from chimeric antigen receptor-T cells. Hum Gene Ther. 2021;32(19–20):1044–58.
20. Zhang J, Hu Y, Yang J, Li W, Zhang M, Wang Q, Zhang L, Wei G, Tian Y, Zhao K, Chen A. Non-viral, specifically targeted CAR-T cells achieve high safety and efficacy in B-NHL. Nature. 2022;609(7926):369–74.

21. Boissel L, Betancur M, Lu W, Wels WS, Marino T, Van Etten RA, Klingemann H. Comparison of mRNA and lentiviral based transfection of natural killer cells with chimeric antigen receptors recognizing lymphoid antigens. Leuk Lymphoma. 2012;53(5):958–65.
22. Gross G, Waks T, Eshhar Z. Expression of immunoglobulin-T-cell receptor chimeric molecules as functional receptors with antibody-type specificity. Proc Natl Acad Sci. 1989;86(24):10024–8.
23. Yuan J, Maserejian N, Liu Y, Devine S, Gillis C, Massaro J, Au R. Severity distribution of Alzheimer's disease dementia and mild cognitive impairment in the Framingham Heart Study. J Alzheimer's Dis. 2021;79(2):807–17.
24. Schuster SJ, Svoboda J, Chong EA, Nasta SD, Mato AR, Anak Ö, Brogdon JL, Pruteanu-Malinici I, Bhoj V, Landsburg D, Wasik M. Chimeric antigen receptor T cells in refractory B-cell lymphomas. N Engl J Med. 2017;377(26):2545–54.
25. Faridar A, Thome AD, Zhao W, Thonhoff JR, Beers DR, Pascual B, Masdeu JC, Appel SH. Restoring regulatory T-cell dysfunction in Alzheimer's disease through ex vivo expansion. Brain communications. 2020;2(2):fcaa112.
26. Hoyos V, Savoldo B, Quintarelli C, Mahendravada A, Zhang M, Vera J, Heslop HE, Rooney CM, Brenner MK, Dotti G. Engineering CD19-specific T lymphocytes with interleukin-15 and a suicide gene to enhance their anti-lymphoma/leukemia effects and safety. Leukemia. 2010;24(6):1160–70. Brentjens RJ, Latouche JB, Santos E, Marti F, Gong MC, Lyddane C, King PD, Larson S, Weiss M, Rivière I, Sadelain M. Eradication of systemic B-cell tumors by genetically targeted human T lymphocytes co-stimulated by CD80 and interleukin-15. Nat Med. 2003;9(3):279–86
27. Hassan R, Kreitman RJ, Pastan I, Willingham MC. Localization of mesothelin in epithelial ovarian cancer. Appl Immunohistochem Mol Morphol. 2005;13(3):243–7.
28. June CH, Sadelain M. Chimeric antigen receptor therapy. N Engl J Med. 2018;379(1):64–73.
29. Coiffier B, Lepage E, Brière J, Herbrecht R, Tilly H, Bouabdallah R, Morel P, Van Den Neste E, Salles G, Gaulard P, Reyes F. CHOP chemotherapy plus rituximab compared with CHOP alone in elderly patients with diffuse large-B-cell lymphoma. N Engl J Med. 2002;346(4):235–42.
30. Lee DW, Gardner R, Porter DL, Louis CU, Ahmed N, Jensen M, Grupp SA, Mackall CL. Current concepts in the diagnosis and management of cytokine release syndrome. Blood J Am Soc Hematol. 2014;124(2):188–95.
31. Lanitis E, Poussin M, Hagemann IS, Coukos G, Sandaltzopoulos R, Scholler N, Powell DJ. Redirected antitumor activity of primary human lymphocytes transduced with a fully human anti-mesothelin chimeric receptor. Mol Ther. 2012;20(3):633–43.
32. Milone MC, Fish JD, Carpenito C, Carroll RG, Binder GK, Teachey D, Samanta M, Lakhal M, Gloss B, Danet-Desnoyers G, Campana D. Chimeric receptors containing CD137 signal transduction domains mediate enhanced survival of T cells and increased antileukemic efficacy in vivo. Mol Ther. 2009;17(8):1453–64.
33. Davenport AJ, Jenkins MR, Cross RS, Yong CS, Prince HM, Ritchie DS, Trapani JA, Kershaw MH, Darcy PK, Neeson PJ. CAR-T cells inflict sequential killing of multiple tumor target cells. Cancer Immunol Res. 2015;3(5):483–94.
34. Brandes M, Willimann K, Moser B. Professional antigen-presentation function by human γδ T cells. Science. 2005;309(5732):264–8.
35. Gronski MA, Boulter JM, Moskophidis D, Nguyen LT, Holmberg K, Elford AR, Deenick EK, Kim HO, Penninger JM, Odermatt B, Gallimore A. TCR affinity and negative regulation limit autoimmunity. Nat Med. 2004;10(11):1234–9.
36. Beecham EJ, Ma Q, Ripley R, Junghans RP. Coupling CD28 co-stimulation to immunoglobulin T-cell receptor molecules: the dynamics of T-cell proliferation and death. J Immunother. 2000;23(6):631–42.
37. Casalegno Garduño R, Däbritz J. New insights on CD8+ T cells in inflammatory bowel disease and therapeutic approaches. Front Immunol. 2021;12:738762.
38. Aghajanian H, Rurik JG, Epstein JA. CAR-based therapies: opportunities for immunomedicine beyond cancer. Nat Metab. 2022;4(2):163–9.

39. Levine BL, Bernstein WB, Connors M, Craighead N, Lindsten T, Thompson CB, June CH. Effects of CD28 costimulation on long-term proliferation of CD4+ T cells in the absence of exogenous feeder cells. J Immunol. 1997;159(12):5921–30.
40. Uckun FM, Jaszcz W, Ambrus JL, Fauci AS, Gajl-Peczalska K, Song CW, Wick MR, Myers DE, Waddick K, Ledbetter JA. Detailed studies on expression and function of CD19 surface determinant by using B43 monoclonal antibody and the clinical potential of anti-CD19 immunotoxins. Blood. 1988;71(1):13–29.
41. Sun L, Su Y, Jiao A, Wang X, Zhang B. T cells in health and disease. Signal Transduct Target Ther. 2023;8(1):235.
42. Mantovani S, Palermo B, Garbelli S, Campanelli R, Robustelli della Cuna G, Gennari R, Benvenuto F, Lantelme E, Giachino C. Dominant TCR-α requirements for a self antigen recognition in humans. J Immunol. 2002;169(11):6253–60.
43. Avanzi MP, Yeku O, Li X, Wijewarnasuriya DP, van Leeuwen DG, Cheung K, Park H, Purdon TJ, Daniyan AF, Spitzer MH, Brentjens RJ. Engineered tumor-targeted T cells mediate enhanced anti-tumor efficacy both directly and through activation of the endogenous immune system. Cell Rep. 2018;23(7):2130–41.
44. Baek H, Ye M, Kang GH, Lee C, Lee G, Choi DB, Jung J, Kim H, Lee S, Kim JS, Lee HJ. Neuroprotective effects of CD4+ CD25+ Foxp3+ regulatory T cells in a 3xTg-AD Alzheimer's disease model. Oncotarget. 2016;7(43):69347.
45. Sorg C, Myers N, Redel P, Bublak P, Riedl V, Manoliu A, Perneczky R, Grimmer T, Kurz A, Förstl H, Drzezga A. Asymmetric loss of parietal activity causes spatial bias in prodromal and mild Alzheimer's disease. Biol Psychiatry. 2012;71(9):798–804.
46. Saetzler V, Riet T, Schienke A, Henschel P, Freitag K, Haake A, Heppner FL, Buitrago-Molina LE, Noyan F, Jaeckel E, Hardtke-Wolenski M. Development of beta-amyloid-specific CAR-tregs for the treatment of alzheimer's disease. Cells. 2023;12(16):2115.
47. Van Oekelen O, Aleman A, Upadhyaya B, Schnakenberg S, Madduri D, Gavane S, Teruya-Feldstein J, Crary JF, Fowkes ME, Stacy CB, Kim-Schulze S. Neurocognitive and hypokinetic movement disorder with features of parkinsonism after BCMA-targeting CAR-T cell therapy. Nat Med. 2021;27(12):2099–103.
48. Carpenter RO, Evbuomwan MO, Pittaluga S, Rose JJ, Raffeld M, Yang S, Gress RE, Hakim FT, Kochenderfer JN. B-cell maturation antigen is a promising target for adoptive T-cell therapy of multiple myeloma. Clin Cancer Res. 2013;19(8):2048–60.

Part VI
Hematopoietic Stem Cell Transplant

Chapter 39
Present Status of Stem Cell Transplant in Acute Leukemia in Children and Adults

Sanjeev Kumar Sharma and Anamika Bakliwal

Abstract The stem cell transplant (SCT) has long been considered a standard of care for patients who have high-risk or relapsed/refractory leukemia. The role of allogeneic (allo) SCT has recently been blurred with the development of newer and targeted agents and with the availability of CAR-T cell therapy. However, allo SCT still holds a crucial role in the treatment of leukemia. This chapter highlights the current status of allo SCT in pediatric and adult leukemia patients. The prognosis of acute lymphoblastic leukemia (ALL) is different in children compared to adults, whereas acute myeloid leukemia (AML) has a nearly similar prognosis, though prognosis worsens with aging in all leukemias as adult/elderly patients have high-risk cytogenetics and tolerate chemotherapy poorly. Though there has been advancement in the newer modalities for the treatment of leukemias, there has been simultaneous improvement in the transplant outcomes because of innovative strategies for the management of GVHD and infections. Patients with relapsed or refractory leukemia have poor survival if they do not undergo SCT. Though matched sibling donor (MSD) allo SCT is the preferred SCT, those patients who lack MSD can be offered matched unrelated donor (MUD) or haploidentical SCT. Recently, the availability of CAR-T cell therapy has challenged the requirement for allo SCT in B-cell ALL. For T-cell ALL and AML patients, CAR-T cell therapy is still in the early phase of development, and allo SCT is the only curative hope. The real benefits of allo SCT are based on two principles, the first is the replacement of mutagenic host stem cells with donor's healthy stem cells (genetically mediated effect) and the second is the provision of graft-versus-leukemia (GVL) effect by donor's T cells (adoptive-T cell immune-mediated effect).

S. K. Sharma (✉) · A. Bakliwal
Department of Hemato-oncology and Bone Marrow Transplant, BLK-MAX Superspeciality Hospital, New Delhi, India

H. P. Pati et al. (eds.), *Clinical Hematology and Hemato-Oncology*,
https://doi.org/10.1007/978-981-92-1167-8_39

Keywords Stem cell transplant · Acute lymphoblastic leukemia · Acute myeloid leukemia · Chemotherapy · Inotuzumab · CAR-T cell therapy · Relapsed or refractory acute leukemia

Learning Objectives
- Children with acute lymphoblastic leukemia (ALL) who are in first complete remission (CR) do not require transplant
- Role of allogeneic stem cell transplant (allo SCT) in adults with ALL is still debatable, with high-risk patients usually considered for allo SCT, whereas low-risk patients can be managed with chemo/immunotherapy alone. Relapsed and refractory ALL patients can be treated with either chimeric antigen receptor (CAR)-T cell therapy or allo SCT. Availability of novel agents has revolutionized the management of such patients.
- Adults with T-cell ALL should be given priority for allo SCT over continued chemotherapy
- Standard risk AML patients are treated with chemotherapy, whereas intermediate and high-risk AML patients are considered for allo SCT
- Patients with relapsed/refractory AML are candidates for allo SCT
- Patients not fit for myeloablative SCT should be considered for reduced intensity allo SCT
- Patients who lack a matched sibling donor should be considered for haploidentical or matched unrelated donor allo SCT

39.1 Acute Lymphoblastic Leukemia

Leukemias are heterogenous diseases. ALL originates from lymphoid progenitors and has been further divided based on certain genetic and molecular signatures [1]. The treatment and prognosis of each subcategory of ALL differ in different age groups. ALL with molecular markers and cytogenetic features associated with poor prognosis include hypodiploidy with less than 44 chromosomes, Ph-positive ALL, KMT2A gene rearrangement, Ph-like ALL, intrachromosomal amplification of chromosome 21, CRLF2 gene rearrangement, and early T-cell precursor (ETP) ALL [2].

Among children, ALL is the most common hematological malignancy and treatment guidelines are well described. They have the best long-term survival and cure rates. However, contrary to pediatric ALL, adults with ALL have a poor response to the available treatment options and most patients relapse. With current multi-agent induction chemotherapy, more than 80–85% of children with ALL can be cured, whereas adults have survival rates of 30–40% only, despite augmenting the protocols [3]. There are multiple reasons for these differences between adult and pediatric responses to available chemotherapeutic agents, including age, high-risk genetic features, poor drug metabolism, and multiple co-morbidities in adult patients. The majority of children with ALL have B-cell precursor ALL, are surface antigen CD10 (CALLA) positive, and are hyperdiploid. All these features are associated with a very good response to chemotherapy. Hyperdiploidy, which is a good prognostic feature, is seen in about 30% of pediatric ALL but is present in less than 5% of adult ALL patients. A genetic abnormality that is seen more commonly in adults and is associated with a poorer prognosis is the Philadelphia chromosome (Ph positive ALL). Its frequency increases with age and is seen in 25–30% adult ALL patients, whereas it is infrequent in childhood ALL (3–5%). Although 60–80% of adults with ALL achieve CR, more than 60–70% of them relapse, and these patients have a very dismal prognosis [4]. The options for these patients are novel agents, CAR-T cell therapy, or allo SCT, or a combination of these. Only about 25–30% of patients get HLA-matched sibling donors (MSD). So, the rest of the patients who do not have an MSD are candidates for alternate donor SCT, like matched unrelated donor (MUD), mismatched unrelated donor (MMUD), or haploidentical donor.

In the treatment of ALL, one of the most important variables that is taken into consideration while deciding about upgrading the treatment is measurable residual disease (MRD). It is used as a tool for assessment of remission status after initial therapy and during various phases of treatment to check for the relapse risk or impending relapse. The MRD can be assessed by flow cytometry, immunoglobulin/T-cell receptor (Ig/TCR) sequences measurement by polymerase chain reaction (PCR), or by molecular markers (e.g., BCR-ABL, MLL-AF4).

39.2 Consolidation/Intensification Phase

The consolidation/intensification phase is the treatment given after achieving initial remission. It is an important part of the whole treatment as patients not given consolidation usually relapse because of persistence of minimal residual disease, which is not morphologically evident. The type of consolidation is based on the risk-stratification of the leukemia, such that patients having low-risk leukemia are given less intensive consolidation, in order to avoid unnecessary toxicity, whereas high-risk patients are given more intensive consolidation that may include allo SCT. SCT can be deferred in standard-risk patients who are minimal residual disease (MRD) negative. Patients with positive MRD are categorized as a high-risk group, and such patients are considered for allo SCT as consolidation therapy.

The role of allo SCT in adults with ALL is still a matter of debate, with some groups favoring SCT for all adults (patients over 35 years age) while others advocating SCT only for those with matched sibling donors or having high-risk features [5]. This controversy has further escalated with the availability of novel targeted agents and CAR-T cell therapy. Allo SCT is the preferred treatment for ALL patients in second CR achieved by either novel agents or, in some cases, post CAR-T cell therapy. MRD monitoring can also guide physicians in determining which patients might require a transplant and at what stage.

39.3 Transplant of Adolescents and Young Adults (Aya)

Allo SCT is not recommended for standard-risk adolescents and young adult (AYA) ALL patients who have been treated with intensive pediatric-based protocols and who have achieved MRD-negative response [6]. For AYA patients, the recommendation is treatment with intensive chemotherapy alone. Allo SCT is reserved for patients in the second CR. However, patients with persistent MRD after induction are candidates for upfront consolidation with allo SCT [7]. In such cases, novel agents can be used for achieving MRD-negative remission. According to the National Comprehensive Cancer Network (NCCN), all adult ALL patients (>39 years) who have received less intense regimens should be considered for allo SCT in first CR [8].

39.4 Role of Novel Treatment Strategies

The broad expression of CD19 and CD22 on B-cell ALL blasts makes them an attractive therapeutic target. The recent development of targeted therapies, including antibody–drug conjugates, bi-specific antibodies, and CAR-T cell therapy, has revolutionized B-ALL management [9]. CAR-T cell therapy is a new form of adoptive T-cell immunotherapy, which requires the infusion of genetically engineered autologous T cells that are made to persist in vivo for a longer duration, providing durable disease control. Blinatumomab or inotuzumab have revolutionized the treatment of B-ALL patients in significantly reducing leukemic burden before allo SCT.

In the ALL patients with MRD positivity or if the patient relapses after a prior allo-SCT, the options include chemotherapy, blinatumomab, inotuzumab, CAR-T cell therapy, or a second allo-SCT. Blinatumomab is a novel bi-specific T-cell engager (BiTE) having an anti–CD19–directed CD3 BiTE antibody [9]. Compared to conventional chemotherapy, blinatumomab has a relatively better safety profile, and this is particularly important for older ALL patients, where toxicity is a major limitation for administering conventional multi-agent chemotherapy. Inotuzumab ozogamicin is an antibody-drug conjugate, which consists of an antibody directed towards glycoprotein CD22 on the cell surface, attached with a cytotoxin calicheamicin. Inotuzumab is usually combined with chemotherapy and/or blinatumomab, with the goal of increasing the depth of response (MRD negativity) and thus the survival outcomes. Blinatumomab consolidation can also be considered as a bridge to SCT. Further treatment options include tisagenlecleucel (CD19 CAR-T) either as final therapy or as a bridge to allo SCT.

39.5 Conditioning Regimens for Allo SCT

The type of conditioning regimen also plays an important role in deciding about allo SCT for ALL, with a total body irradiation (TBI) based regimen being most preferred. This is because of its ability to eradicate radio-sensitive leukemic blasts within the central nervous system and other medullary and extra-medullary sites. Cyclophosphamide-TBI is the most widely used myeloablative conditioning (MAC) regimen for allo SCT; however, due to radiation-related toxicities, like late secondary malignancies, cataracts, and growth impairment, particularly in children and young adults, TBI-free conditioning regimens (most commonly busulfan-cyclophosphamide) have also been utilized [10]. For elder population, less intensive reduced intensity conditioning (RIC) regimens like fludarabine/melphalan, fludarabine/busulfan maybe good choice who are not eligible for MAC allo SCT or have co-morbidities.

39.6 Ph Positive ALL

For Ph-positive ALL patients, incorporation of tyrosine kinase inhibitors (TKIs) with chemotherapy regimens has improved both the rate and the depth of remissions [5]. This has allowed the patients to proceed to allo SCT, whereas those who are not fit for SCT or are frail and elderly can be continued on TKIs. Ph positivity is considered as a high-risk disease, and most adult patients are considered for allo SCT. Patients who have been treated with ponatinib and hyper CVAD and have achieved remission can be treated with this regimen only. TKIs have also been combined with blinatumumab with very good results in elderly patients and can provide a chemotherapy-free regimen for treating Ph-positive ALL in the elderly.

39.7 T -Cell ALL

Studies in adults with T-cell ALL, unlike those in B-cell ALL, have shown that allo SCT should be considered upfront in all such patients as they have a high chance of relapse if continued on chemotherapy alone [11]. This is probably because T-cell ALL is a high-risk disease, and there is a lack of availability of novel targeted therapies. Most of these patients present with high WBC count and extramedullary disease. T-cell ALL patients lacking MSD can be considered for MUD-SCT or a haplo SCT. Nelarabine has shown good efficacy in relapsed/refractory T-cell ALL.

39.8 Early T Precursor ALL

The early T precursor ALL (ETP-ALL) is considered to have an inferior overall survival among all T-ALL subtypes. This is probably because the majority of ETP-ALL patients contain mutations which are not commonly seen in non-ETP-ALL like EZH2, RAS, FLT3 ITD, and RUNX1 [12]. These patients have poor survival with standard chemotherapy, and, therefore, they need different approaches. Allo SCT in first remission is recommended for ETP-ALL in view of poor response to available treatment options.

39.9 Relapsed B-ALL

The most common challenge in the management of hematological malignancies is the treatment of relapsed or refractory disease, as the prognosis worsens with relapses. The same holds true for ALL.

The reason for the relapse, other than being a high-risk disease, is the inability to treat adult patients as aggressively as children. The treatment of relapse also depends upon multiple factors, including the age of the patient, duration of remission, genetic risk factors, co-morbidities, and prior therapies.

Children with relapsed ALL are typically treated with re-induction therapy in an attempt to induce a second CR. Further treatment options after achieving CR are based on MRD status and risk factors. Most of the early relapses are treated with allo SCT, though CAR-T cell therapy is also an option. Adults and elderly patients are treated with novel agents, including inotuzumab, blinatumumab, or CAR-T cell therapy. Allo SCT is an option for fit adult ALL patients in second CR.

39.10 Mixed Phenotype Acute Leukemia

Mixed phenotype acute leukemia (MPAL) is also considered as a high-risk leukemia. Mostly, it behaves like lymphoblastic leukemia with better treatment response to ALL-like regimens. Patients who are treated with ALL-based chemotherapy appear to relapse less than patients treated with AML-like chemotherapy [13]. Adult patients with MPAL are candidates for allo SCT in first CR. However, in children, the response to ALL-like intensive therapy is good, and allo SCT should not be considered upfront, and is reserved for relapsed or refractory cases [14]. Allo SCT in MPAL shows graft-versus-leukemia effect and thus can lead to a potential cure.

39.11 Indications for Stem Cell Transplant in Pediatric ALL

Upfront allo SCT is not indicated in pediatric ALL, unless the child has MRD positivity after certain time-points (Table 39.1), unlike in adults, where SCT is one of the important treatment options. This is because pediatric ALL patients have a very good prognosis with aggressive chemotherapy. The indications for SCT have evolved over time. The conventional risk factors, like cytogenetics, which were earlier considered as high-risk features, have now been replaced by MRD [8, 10]. For example, for Ph-positive pediatric B-cell ALL, the addition of TKI to the intensive chemotherapy has dramatically improved the outcomes such that allo SCT in first CR has taken a backstage. Site of relapse also has some clinical implications: if the child has only bone marrow relapse, then it is considered to have a poor prognosis; isolated central nervous system or other extramedullary relapse has a better prognosis, whereas combined marrow and extramedullary relapse is considered to have an intermediate prognosis.

39.12 Indications for Allo SCT in Adult ALL

The need for allo SCT can be decreased in adult ALL patients (<35 years of age) if they have been treated with pediatric-inspired intensive chemotherapy regimens. Those patients who present with high-risk cytogenetics, have MRD positivity, or are over 35 years of age, and all relapsed or refractory patients should be considered for consolidation with allo SCT. Even in standard-risk adult ALL patients, studies have shown that SCT significantly improves leukemia-free survival (Table 39.2) [5, 8]. For Ph-positive adult ALL, allo SCT is preferred in CR1. Since there are limited treatment options in T-ALL, consolidation with SCT in first CR should be considered upfront.

Table 39.1 The indications for allo SCT in pediatric ALL include

(a) Children with MRD $\geq$0.01% at the end of consolidation
(b) T-ALL with MRD levels high ($\geq$0.1%) at the end of consolidation
(c) In the relapsed ALL setting, depending on the time and site of relapse. Late B-ALL relapses can be treated with chemo/immunotherapy, sparing them of allo SCT, while all patients with early relapsed B-cell ALL and all relapsed T-cell ALL should be considered for allo SCT
(d) Children with 2 or more relapses
(e) Some centers have offered allo SCT following remission after CAR-T-cell therapy. It has been used as a consolidation or salvage treatment

Table 39.2 Indications of allo SCT in adult ALL

(a) MRD-positive ALL
(b) High-risk adult ALL (including Ph-positive ALL)
(c) Adult ALL in second remission
(d) Relapsed/refractory ALL

39.13 Role of allo SCT in the Era of CAR-T Cell Therapy

The innovation of chimeric antigen receptor-T (CAR-T) cell therapy has revolutionized the treatment of relapsed or refractory B-ALL, offering an alternative for patients who previously had limited options. CAR-T therapy mainly involves the gene modification of autologous T cells outside the body to express engineered receptors, which are targeted toward tumor-associated antigens, like e.g., CD19 and CD22. The antigens chosen are those that are widely expressed on B cells and can be easily targeted. Upon reinfusion, these CAR-T cells actively fight and eliminate blasts through various cytotoxic mechanisms. CAR-T cell therapy has also been used as a bridge to allo SCT with the potential to induce remissions. Though the remission rates and durability of response have increased, relapse after CAR-T therapy still occurs in 20–50% of responding patients. Relapse, however, can occur as blasts develop various mechanisms such as antigen escape, lineage switching, antigen splicing, or insufficient persistence of CAR-T cells. It has been suggested that young B ALL patients who can achieve CR after CD19-CAR T cell therapy should be taken up for allo-SCT, in particular when there is fear of loss of functionality of the CD19-CARTs (i.e., loss of B-cell aplasia) is detected within two months of treatment [15]. Sequential use of allo-SCT after CAR-T cell therapy has also been used to achieve durable remissions in B-ALL patients, achieving MRD-negative CR [16]. However, not all patients receiving CAR-T cell therapy need allo SCT and there is still ongoing debate on who should be considered for consolidation with allo SCT.

39.14 Acute Myeloid Leukemia

39.14.1 Induction Therapy

Acute myeloid leukemia (AML) is the malignancy of myeloid progenitors and is commonly seen in the elderly population, but can also present in the pediatric age group. The most preferred induction treatment for AML includes 3 days of daunorubicin and 7 days of cytarabine (continuous infusion), termed "3 + 7" chemotherapy, and with this regimen, about 60–70% patients can achieve CR [17]. Another regimen, which has been used more commonly recently, is azacytidine (hypomethylating agent) plus venetoclax (bcl 2 inhibitor), particularly in elderly patients not fit for intensive induction. Moreover, targeted strategies can also be added to either the 3 + 7 or azacytidine plus venetoclax regimen (e.g., midostaurin for FLT3-mutated AML).

39.14.2 Consolidation Therapy

The induction remission in AML is followed by consolidation with either chemotherapy or allo SCT. Without further post remission or consolidation, leukemia usually recurs within 3–6 months. Therefore, consolidation therapy is absolutely necessary for the treatment of AML. Consolidation for low-risk disease includes intermediate-dose or high-dose cytarabine. Allo SCT is the preferred consolidation for intermediate and high-risk AML patients [18].

Patients with AML in first CR should proceed to SCT and usually do not need pre-transplant consolidation. Bridging consolidation chemotherapy can be considered while searching for a donor. Studies suggest that the MAC regimen should be preferred over the RIC regimen in fit young patients with MRD positivity before allo SCT [19].

Low-risk AML patients should receive an allo SCT in second CR. Patients with AML in second CR without MSD can be considered for either MUD or identical transplant. The preferred MAC regimens are busulfan/cyclophosphamide (Bu/Cy) and cyclophosphamide/TBI, and they have similar response rates [20], though BuCy is commonly used.

39.15 Primary Refractory AML

Primary refractory AML has been defined as failure to achieve CR after at least two cycles of induction. Patients who undergo allo SCT with persistent disease have poorer overall survival than those who are in CR. However, even with active disease, approximately 20–25% AML patients can achieve long-term survival after an allo SCT [21]. Similarly, about 30–40% of children with refractory AML can be cured with aggressive salvage therapies followed by allo SCT [22].

39.15.1 Indications for Allo SCT in AML

Allo SCT has been shown to significantly improve survival in patients with intermediate and high-risk AML (Table 39.3). The European LeukemiaNet (ELN) has suggested that if there is disease-free survival improvement of atleast 10% by allo SCT, then it should be recommended, and this has been shown in intermediate and high-risk AML patients [23]. Refractory/relapsed AML is another category of AML patients, which has a very poor prognosis, and allo SCT is the only hope of survival in such

Table 39.3 Indications of allo SCT in AML

(a) Intermediate and high-risk AML
(b) Persistent MRD-positive low-risk AML
(c) Relapsed/refractory AML
(d) Chronic myeloid leukemia in blast crises

patients. In AML patients, the studies have suggested that outcomes of haploidentical SCTs are comparable to those of MUD and mismatched unrelated (MMUD) transplants [24]. Similar to ALL, treatments based on MRD are being prioritized in AML patients and those with MRD-positive disease can be considered for allo SCT [23].

39.15.2 Indications for SCT in Low-Risk AML

SCT is not advocated in the first CR in the favorable risk AML. These AML include patients with core-binding factors have translocations t(8;21), inv. [16], t(16;16) and NPM1 mutation with wild-type FLT3-ITD. Though ASBMT guidelines [25] do not recommend allo SCT for favorable risk AML, the EBMT group [26] allows the use of SCT in favorable risk AML patients if MRD is positive after initial treatment. Infantile AML and in children with FAB M0, M6, or M7 AML are considered high-risk disease and can be indications for SCT in first CR [27]. MRD has become an important tool to guide therapeutic decisions in AML patients, similar to ALL patients, and can allow allo SCT in favorable risk AML patients with persistent MRD positivity. MRD monitoring can also be done by measuring quantitative polymerase chain reaction (qPCR) CBF fusion gene transcripts (RUNX1-RUNX1T1 and CBFB-MYH11), and by the next-generation sequencing (NGS) technique. The issue with CBF fusion gene transcripts is that low levels of these fusion gene transcripts may persist even after the end of treatment and this may not affect survival, however, failing to achieve a marked reduction (of >3-log reduction) in CBF fusion transcript by qPCR after 2 cycles of induction chemotherapy is a poor indicator and is associated with a high risk of relapse and these patients can be given the option of allo SCT [28].

39.15.3 Treatment of High-Risk AML

High-risk AML includes patients with unfavorable cytogenetics defined as complex karyotype (with more than three abnormalities, excluding trisomies) or t(6;11)(q27;q23), t(11;19)(q23;p13.1), inv. [3](q21q26), t(6;9)(p23;q34), monosomy 7, or those with the FLT3-ITD or MLL gene mutation. These patients are candidates for allo SCT with MSD, MUD, or haploidentical donors in first remission. Auto SCT should be avoided in high-risk AML patients. All patients in second CR and those having relapsed-refractory AML are candidates for allo SCT [23, 24].

39.15.4 Treatment of AML Relapsed After First SCT

One of the important causes of treatment failure after SCT is the relapse of the disease. After initial SCT, the disease is monitored by MRD and chimerism at regular intervals, and these can guide the management as predictors of impending relapse. The relapses are more frequent in the initial 3 years of SCT [23, 24]. About 30–40% of AML patients after allo SCT relapse, and such patients have high mortality with a 2-year survival of less than 10–20% [29]. Risk factors in relapsed AML after allo SCT that indicate poor prognosis are: a) relapse happening within 6 months of transplant, b) relapse associated with ongoing active GVHD, c) unfavorable risk cytogenetics, and d) age more than 40 years. Treatment of patients with impending relapse includes donor lymphocyte infusion (DLI), azacytidine therapy, FLT3 inhibitors, or other novel agents. DLI, by virtue of generating an immunological response, can induce remission through graft-versus-leukemia (GVL) effect [30]. Prophylactic DLI can be given in patients assumed to be at high risk of relapse, high-risk cytogenetics, or where no GVHD has developed after SCT. DLI can also be administered pre-emptively when MRD is showing a rising trend, or chimerism shows a decreasing trend without frank relapse. If the relapse has developed early after the first SCT, then doing a second allo SCT carries a high risk of treatment-related mortality. RIC regimens can be used for conditioning in such patients compared to MAC regimens. CAR-T cell therapy is not yet available for AML at present, but it may be an option in the future.

39.16 Indications of SCT in Chronic Myeloid Leukemia with Blast Crises

The introduction of tyrosine kinase inhibitors (TKI) has revolutionized the treatment of CML, whereby in the pre-TKI era, SCT was the norm, but now, with more than 90% long-term survival with TKIs, SCT has only few indications in CML. Poor tolerance to TKIs or disease progression of CML-CP (e.g., in T315I mutation) are indicators for SCT in CML-CP. In patients with CML blast crises (CML-BC), allo SCT should be done after achieving the second chronic phase (CP) with chemo/immunotherapy (based on whether it is myeloid or lymphoid blast crises) without the need for deep cytogenetic or molecular responses. In contrast to adult CML-BC patients, the majority of children and adolescents with CML-BC present with a lymphoid phenotype. Prior to SCT, the patient with CML-BC should be treated with induction therapy along with TKI to achieve morphological remission [31]. Allo SCT should be performed immediately after hematologic remission (second CP) has been achieved [31]. As for all allo SCTs, if MSD is not available, then MUD or haploidentical SCT should be considered for patients with CML-BC.

39.17 Clinical Cases

Case 1 A 7-year-old male child presented with generalized lymphadenopathy and bony pains. He was evaluated and found to have pancytopenia. Bone marrow examination and flow cytometry confirmed B-cell ALL. He was treated with the BFM 2009-based protocol and achieved MRD-negative complete remission (CR) after induction therapy. Six months after starting maintenance chemotherapy, he developed gum bleeding and bony pains, and a repeat bone marrow examination revealed relapse of the disease. He was treated with BFM-REZ-based protocol and achieved morphological remission, but was MRD positive. He was treated with inotuzumab and achieved MRD negativity after one cycle, and was taken up for haploidentical SCT with his father as the donor. He is in remission 2 years post SCT.

Case 2 A 42-year-old male was diagnosed as a case of Ph-negative B-cell ALL and was treated with a hyper CVAD-based protocol. He was refractory to induction therapy and inotuzumab was added to the regimen. He was given inotuzumab–mini Hyper CVD and achieved MRD negative disease, but after 2 months, his MRD became positive. He underwent CAR-T cell therapy with fludarabine—cyclophosphamide as the bridging therapy. He became MRD negative, but after 3 months of CAR-T therapy, he had B-cell recovery. He was still MRD negative, but considering impending relapse, he was taken up for haploidentical SCT with his brother as the donor. He developed stage II acute GVHD and later chronic GVHD and is disease-free (MRD negative) 11 months post SCT.

Case 3 A 58-years-old male was diagnosed as a case of high-risk AML. He underwent induction chemotherapy with the 3 + 7 protocol and achieved complete remission. He had a full match with his brother and underwent MSD allo SCT. Thirteen months post SCT, he relapsed and was given salvage chemotherapy with FLAG-venetoclax and achieved CR. He underwent a second transplant with his son as a haploidentical donor. He developed limited chronic GVHD and is in remission 2 years post SCT.

39.18 Summary

Hematopoietic stem cell transplant holds a major role in the management of acute leukemias. In B-cell ALL, despite the availability of novel agents and CAR-T cell therapy, allo SCT plays a major role both as consolidation after relapse or in refractory cases. These novel therapies are still considered a bridge to transplant, though CAR-T cell therapy can replace allo SCT as the definitive cure for B-cell ALL. In T-cell ALL and AML patients, allo SCT has not been replaced by any novel agent, and eligible patients are treated with allo SCT, which can also be offered to those who cannot tolerate MAC regimens or those who do not have fully matched sibling donors. RIC regimens and haploidentical SCT have broadened the applicability of SCT in such patients. Except for pediatric ALL, most of the other acute leukemias in children and adults may require allo SCT at some stage of the disease course.

References

1. Sharma SK. What a clinical hematologist should know about T cells? Int Blood Res Rev. 2020:20–32.
2. Hunger SP, Mullighan CG. Acute lymphoblastic leukemia in children. N Engl J Med. 2015;373(16):1541–52.
3. Gökbuget N, Hoelzer D. Treatment of adult acute lymphoblastic leukemia. Semin Hematol. 2009;46(1):64–75.
4. Gökbuget N, Stanze D, Beck J, Diedrich H, et al. Outcome of relapsed adult lymphoblastic leukemia depends on response to salvage chemotherapy, prognostic factors, and performance of stem cell transplantation. Blood. 2012;120(10):2032–41.
5. Sharma SK. Stem cell transplant for acute lymphoblastic leukemia. In: Basics of hematopoietic stem cell transplant. Singapore: Springer Nature Singapore; 2023. p. 479–500.
6. Tosi M, Spinelli O, Leoncin M, Cavagna R, et al. MRD-based therapeutic decisions in genetically defined subsets of adolescents and young adult Philadelphia-negative ALL. Cancer. 2021;13(9):2108.
7. DeFilipp Z, Advani AS, Bachanova V, Cassaday RD, et al. Hematopoietic cell transplantation in the treatment of adult acute lymphoblastic leukemia: updated 2019 evidence-based review from the American Society for Transplantation and Cellular Therapy. Biol Blood Marrow Transplant. 2019;25(11):2113–23.
8. Leonard JT, Hayes-Lattin B. Reduced intensity conditioning allogeneic hematopoietic stem cell transplantation for acute lymphoblastic leukemia; current evidence, and improving outcomes going forward. Curr Hematol Malig Rep. 2018;13(4):329–40.
9. Brivio E, Bautista F, Zwaan CM. Naked antibodies and antibody-drug conjugates: targeted therapy for childhood acute lymphoblastic leukemia. Haematologica. 2024;109(6):1700–12.
10. Shi-Xia X, Xian-Hua T, Hai-Qin X, Bo F, Xiang-Feng T. Total body irradiation plus cyclophosphamide versus busulphan with cyclophosphamide as conditioning regimen for patients with leukemia undergoing allogeneic stem cell transplantation: a meta-analysis. Leuk Lymphoma. 2010;51(1):50–60.
11. Marks DI, Paietta EM, Moorman AV, Richards SM, et al. T-cell acute lymphoblastic leukemia in adults: clinical features, immunophenotype, cytogenetics, and outcome from the large randomized prospective trial (UKALL XII/ECOG 2993). Blood. 2009;114(25):5136–45.
12. Castaneda Puglianini O, Papadantonakis N. Early precursor T-cell acute lymphoblastic leukemia: current paradigms and evolving concepts. Ther Adv Hematol. 2020;11:2040620720929475.
13. Batra S, Ross AJ. Pediatric mixed-phenotype acute leukemia: what's new? Cancer. 2021;13(18):4658.
14. Munker R, Labopin M, Esteve J, Schmid C, Mohty M, Nagler A. Mixed phenotype acute leukemia: outcomes with allogeneic stem cell transplantation. A retrospective study from the Acute Leukemia Working Party of the EBMT. Haematologica. 2017;102(12):2134–40.
15. Ramos CA. Should CD19 CAR-T cells for ALL be followed by allogeneic stem cell transplant? Transplant Cell Ther. 2022;28(1):1–2.
16. Yang T, Dong Y, Shi J, et al. Sequential allogeneic HSCT after CAR-T therapy for relapsed/refractory acute lymphoblastic leukemia patients: a long-term follow-up result. J Adv Res. 2025;78:461.

17. Rowe JM. Optimal induction and post-remission therapy for AML in first remission. Am Soc Hematol Educ Progr. 2009:396–405.
18. Sharma SK, Choudhary D, Doval D, et al. Hematopoietic stem cell transplant for hematological malignancies: experience from a tertiary care center in Northern India and review of Indian data. South Asian J Cancer. 2021;11:062.
19. Hourigan CS, Dillon LW, Gui G, Logan BR, et al. Impact of conditioning intensity of allogeneic transplantation for acute myeloid leukemia with genomic evidence of residual disease. J Clin Oncol. 2020;38(12):1273–83.
20. Jethava YS, Sica S, Savani B, Socola F, et al. Conditioning regimens for allogeneic hematopoietic stem cell transplants in acute myeloid leukemia. Bone Marrow Transplant. 2017;52(11):1504–11.
21. Craddock C, Labopin M, Pillai S, Finke J, et al. Factors predicting outcome after unrelated donor stem cell transplantation in primary refractory acute myeloid leukaemia. Leukemia. 2011;25(5):808–13.
22. Karlsson L, Cheuk D, De Moerloose B, Hasle H, et al. Characteristics and outcome of primary resistant disease in paediatric acute myeloid leukaemia. Br J Haematol. 2023;201:757.
23. Döhner H, Wei AH, Appelbaum FR, Craddock C, et al. Diagnosis and Management of AML in Adults: 2022 ELN Recommendations from an International Expert Panel. Blood. 2022;7.
24. Brissot E, Labopin M, Ehninger G, Stelljes M, et al. Haploidentical versus unrelated allogeneic stem cell transplantation for relapsed/refractory acute myeloid leukemia: a report on 1578 patients from the Acute Leukemia Working Party of the EBMT. Haematologica. 2019;104(3):524–32.
25. Kanate AS, Majhail NS, Savani BN, Bredeson C, et al. Indications for hematopoietic cell transplantation and immune effector cell therapy: guidelines from the American Society for Transplantation and Cellular Therapy. Biol Blood Marrow Transplant. 2020;26(7):1247–56.
26. Duarte RF, Labopin M, Bader P, Basak GW, et al. Indications for haematopoietic stem cell transplantation for haematological diseases, solid tumours and immune disorders: current practice in Europe, 2019. Bone Marrow Transplant. 2019;54(10):1525–52.
27. Creutzig U, Zimmermann M, Bourquin JP, Dworzak MN, et al. Favorable outcome in infants with AML after intensive first- and second-line treatment: an AML-BFM study group report. Leukemia. 2012;26(4):654–61.
28. Borthakur G, Kantarjian H. Core binding factor acute myelogenous leukemia—2021 treatment algorithm. Blood Cancer J. 2021;11(6):114.
29. Tsirigotis P, Byrne M, Schmid C, Baron F, et al. Relapse of AML after hematopoietic stem cell transplantation: methods of monitoring and preventive strategies. A review from the ALWP of the EBMT. Bone Marrow Transplant. 2016;51(11):1431–8.
30. Kolb HJ, Schattenberg A, Goldman JM, Hertenstein B, et al. Graft-versus-leukemia effect of donor lymphocyte transfusions in marrow grafted patients. Blood. 1995;86(5):2041–50.
31. Sembill S, Ampatzidou M, Chaudhury S, Dworzak M, et al. Management of children and adolescents with chronic myeloid leukemia in blast phase: international pediatric CML expert panel recommendations. Leukemia. 2023;37:27.

Chapter 40
Management of Acute and Chronic GVHD: Current Status and Recent Advances

Sumeet Mirgh and Shaikh Mohd Rizwan

Abstract Graft-versus-host disease (GVHD) is an immune complication post-allogeneic stem-cell transplant, which is associated with mortality and morbidity. Conventional GVHD prophylaxis includes a calcineurin inhibitor with methotrexate for matched related, with the addition of ATG for unrelated transplants. Post-transplant cyclophosphamide has expanded its utility for prophylaxis from haploidentical to matched transplants. With respect to the diagnosis of acute GVHD, the staging and grading system reported by the Mount Sinai Acute GVHD International Consortium has superseded previous systems. Various biomarkers (ST2, REG3α, amphiregulin) have emerged which can prognosticate acute GVHD at multiple time-points—prior to its development, at the time of diagnosis of acute GVHD, and 1 week after systemic treatment of acute GVHD. Moreover, the last decade has seen a multitude of new drugs (ruxolitinib, ibrutinib, belumosudil, axatilimab) that have changed the treatment landscape of both acute and chronic GVHD. The field of GVHD has never been as exciting as present. It suffers the problem of plenty—for prophylaxis, prognostication, and treatment. Herein, we review the recent advances in the field of acute and chronic GVHD.

Keywords Graft-versus-host disease (GVHD) · Post-transplant cyclophosphamide (PTCy) · Prophylaxis · Biomarkers · Steroid-refractory

S. Mirgh (✉)
Adult Hematolymphoid and BMT, Advanced Centre for Treatment, Research and Education in Cancer (ACTREC) Tata Memorial Centre, Mumbai, Maharashtra, India

Homi Bhabha National Institute, Mumbai, Maharashtra, India

S. M. Rizwan
Department of Clinical Hematology, Seth GS Medical College and KEM Hospital, Mumbai, Maharashtra, India

H. P. Pati et al. (eds.), *Clinical Hematology and Hemato-Oncology*,
https://doi.org/10.1007/978-981-92-1167-8_40

Learning Objectives
1. Understand the endpoints used in trials in acute GVHD
2. GVHD prophylaxis——the current standard and the emergence of novel regimens like post-transplant cyclophosphamide and abatacept
3. Diagnosis and staging of acute GVHD—MAGIC staging
4. Early prognostication—use of biomarkers for risk stratification and prognostication
5. Treatment of acute GVHD—the emergence of ruxolitinib
6. To understand staging and newer approvals for chronic GVHD

40.1 Introduction

Allogeneic hematopoietic stem-cell transplantation (Allo-HSCT) remains one of the most individualized and curative forms of cellular and immune therapy. However, one of its drawbacks remains the development of graft-versus-host disease (GVHD), which contributes to morbidity and non-relapse mortality (NRM). GVHD is a complex immune complication post-HSCT which involves activation of host antigen-presenting cells (APCs), stimulation of donor T-cells, followed by a complex cascade of inflammatory cytokines and cellular effectors which cause tissue damage. The typical target organs are skin, gut and liver (organs with maximum antigenic load). Hence, it typically presents with a maculopapular rash, diarrhoea, and jaundice [1].

The number of allo-HSCTs continue to increase across the world. From 2006 to 2016, it almost doubled from 20,333 to 38,425. The segregation of GVHD into acute (aGVHD) vs chronic (cGVHD), has been conventionally as per time-line—before/after 100 days post-HSCT, respectively. As per the National Institute of Health (NIH) consensus, this distinction is based on clinical features and history, rather than time-line. Those with acute manifestations only can be classic or late-onset (first episode within or after 100 days post-HSCT, respectively), recurrent (patient with prior aGVHD develops a new episode), or persistent (manifestations persisting >100 days post-HSCT). When both acute and chronic GVHD are present, it is called "overlap" syndrome. Those that fulfil the NIH definition are labelled as cGVHD, irrespective of time-frame [2].

After allo-HSCT, approximately half the patients develop grade 2–4 aGVHD, of which half develop severe aGVHD, i.e., grade 3–4, in spite of GVHD prophylaxis. Amongst patients with ≥grade-3 GVHD, only half will respond to systemic steroids. Patients who are steroid refractory (sr-aGVHD) have dismal outcomes with a median survival of less than 1 year and NRM rates as high as 40% [1]. Hence, it is important to know the latest advances with respect to GVHD management.

40.2 End-Points in Acute GVHD

Survival end-points of trials in aGVHD (similar to non-transplant trials) have focused on overall survival (OS), progression-free survival (PFS), and event-free survival (EFS). For EFS, the definition of "event" is variable. It typically includes progression, death due to any cause, and may include grade 3–4 adverse events (AEs), institution of new therapy, or development of another malignancy. Survival or cure after allo-HSCT is modulated by mortality due to relapse and other causes. Other causes include severe GVHD, infections, regimen-toxicity (e.g. cardiotoxicity due to high-dose cyclophosphamide), or miscellaneous causes which are clubbed together and called NRM. Hence, OS is modulated by NRM and relapse-mortality. However, a patient may survive and still have morbidity due to cGVHD, especially if it requires systemic immunosuppression. Efforts to reduce GVHD [viz. anti-thymocyte globulin (ATG) or T-cell depletion] may overcome GVHD, at the cost of an increase in relapse. Similarly, practices to overcome relapse, like intensive chemo/radiotherapy, may consequently increase the likelihood of NRM. Hence, composite end-points which include NRM, relapse-mortality, and morbidity of GVHD are increasingly used. One such end-point is GVHD-free and relapse-free survival (GRFS). *GRFS is defined as time to grade 3–4 aGVHD, cGVHD needing systemic immunosuppression, relapse, or death, whichever occurs first* (Fig. 40.1). Thus, it is more holistic and represents survival without morbidity [3]. While GRFS is useful, all its components carry equal weightage, which may not be true. For example—relapse in an acute leukaemia has a higher risk of mortality than grade-3 aGVHD, which has a 50% chance of response to systemic therapy. Moreover, GRFS

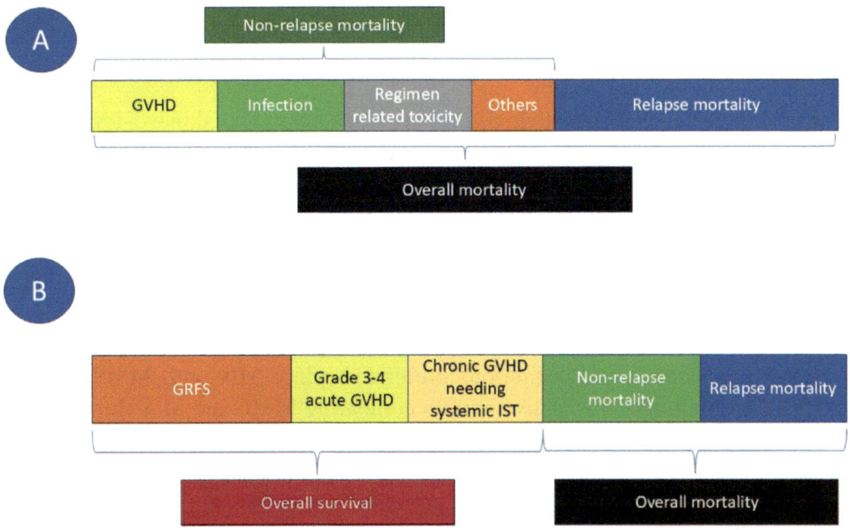

Fig. 40.1 Panel (**a**)—Causes of overall mortality post allo-HSCT, Panel (**b**)—Concept of GRFS (GVHD-free and relapse-free survival) and OS (overall survival)

stops at the first event, and subsequent events are not accounted. For example—in a patient who develops GVHD followed by death, only the GVHD will be counted in GRFS. Thus, all the components of a composite end-point should be analysed [4].

40.3 Case Scenarios

40.3.1 How Can We Effectively Prevent GVHD

Case 40.1
A 50-year-old male underwent allo-HSCT in first complete remission (CR1) for high-risk AML. His donor was his haploidentical sister (5/10) aged 51-years. He was conditioned with Fludarabine + Melphalan followed by GCSF-mobilized PBSCs, and PTCy (post-transplant cyclophosphamide) + Tacrolimus + Mycophenolate mofetil (MMF) as GVHD prophylaxis. He developed grade-3 oral mucositis on day + 7. On day + 46, he developed a maculopapular skin rash over both arms and the upper trunk. He received topical steroids and had significant clinical improvement.

Risk factors for aGVHD in the above patient were—female donor (also multiparous) for male recipient, stem-cell source [peripheral blood (PB) graft > bone marrow (BM)], haploidentical donor (over-matched related/unrelated donor), and older donor age. Other risk factors include the type of GVHD prophylaxis (lower with ATG, alemtuzumab, PTCy) and conditioning intensity [Myeloablative conditioning (MAC) > reduced-intensity conditioning (RIC)] [2].

40.3.1.1 What's Known

The principle of GVHD prophylaxis is to prevent activation of donor T-lymphocytes in the peri/post-transplant phase. Typically, calcineurin inhibitor (CNI) [Cyclosporine (CsA) or Tacrolimus (Tac)] + anti-metabolite [methotrexate (Mtx)] combination forms the backbone of GVHD prophylaxis for matched related (MRD) and unrelated donor (MUD) transplants (Table 40.1). In a randomized phase-3 trial (RCT), Tac/Mtx showed a lower incidence of grade 2–4 aGVHD versus CsA/Mtx, albeit without any difference in survival. In view of the absence of a survival benefit, the choice between CsA and Tac is as per institutional preference [1]. In view of toxicities like mucositis, some institutions prefer to replace Mtx with MMF. A meta-analysis of multiple retrospective studies comparing MMF and Mtx showed lower mucositis and earlier engraftment with MMF; however, without any difference in grade 2–4 aGVHD or OS. In the absence of RCT, Mtx is still preferred along with CNI, except in cord blood transplant, wherein earlier engraftment would be required [2].

Table 40.1 Summary of current practice of GVHD prophylaxis regimens, as per donor type

Donor type	Standard GVHD prophylaxis
Matched related donor (MRD)	CNI + Mtx (Tac/Mtx = CsA/Mtx)
Matched unrelated donor (MUD)	CNI + Mtx + ATG
Haploidentical HSCT	PTCy/CsA/MMF

Abbreviations: *ATG* anti-thymocyte globulin, *CNI* calcineurin inhibitor, *CsA* cyclosporine, *MMF* mycophenolate mofetil, *Mtx* methotrexate, *PTCy* post-transplant cyclophosphamide, *Tac* tacrolimus

On the other hand, for MUD transplants, ATG is added (Table 40.1). Rabbit ATG, which is typically used for GVHD prophylaxis, comes in two formulations—thymoglobulin (rATG or ATG-T) and ATLG (Anti-T lymphocyte globulin or Grafalon; formerly called ATG-Fresenius). While the first one is polyclonal globulin made by immunising with human thymocytes, the source for the second one is the human Jurkat T-cell line. Both have not been compared in a randomized manner to date. However, a network meta-analysis [5] and a recent study [6] which compared Thymoglobulin and ATLG, showed that ATLG was better for GVHD prevention.

With respect to haploidentical transplants, PTCy has become the standard of care (Table 40.1). Pioneered by Johns-Hopkins group, PTCy has made allo-HSCT possible across all HLA donors. Their rationale was that high doses of cyclophosphamide target "alloreactive T-cells" thereby preventing GVHD. It also "spares" the stem cells and T-regulatory cells, thereby preserving engraftment and preventing GVHD, respectively. Its ability to spare stem-cells and T-regulatory cells stems from the high content of aldehyde dehydrogenase in stem-cells, which gives it the ability to metabolize cyclophosphamide faster to an inactive metabolite. In view of greater HLA mismatch in haploidentical HSCT, three immunosuppressants are used for GVHD prophylaxis, i.e., PTCy+CsA + MMF, unlike MRD transplants [7].

40.3.1.2 What's New

PTCy outside haploidentical transplant (Table 40.2)

In a practice-changing RCT (BMT-CTN-1703), PTCy/Tac/MMF was compared with the standard Tac/Mtx in 8/8 MRD and 8/8 or 7/8 MUD transplants. There was significantly better GRFS in the PTCy arm, driven by a reduction of severe acute/chronic GVHD, without any difference in relapse rates and OS. However, it should be remembered that despite having two-thirds MUD donors as a graft source, ATG was not used as GVHD prophylaxis. Although there was delayed platelet engraftment with a higher incidence of grade-2 infections, PTCy fared significantly better. Additional advantages include that cyclophosphamide is the cheapest oncology drug, and needs to be administered for a short duration of 48 hours, unlike CNIs [8].

Unlike RIC, there is no RCT of PTCy with MAC for matched donors. A phase-2 study explored the role of PTCy/Tac/MMF after MAC with TBI alone or Flu-Bu4 (Fludarabine+4 days of iv busulfan) in 7–8/8 matched donor transplants (55%

Table 40.2 Novel regimens for GVHD prophylaxis

Study	Conditioning	Graft source	GVHD prophylaxis	GVHD-related end-points	Survival end-points
PTCy					
Bolaños-Meade J, et al. NEJM 2023 (randomized phase 3) [8]	RIC (Flu-Bu2; Flu-Mel; Flu-Cy ± 2Gy TBI)	MRD; MUD (8/8 or 7/8)	PTCy/Tac/MMF vs Tac/Mtx	[a]1 yr. GRFS—52.7% vs 34.9% [a]1 yr. grade 3–4 aGVHD - 6.3% vs 14.7% [a]1 yr. cGVHD 21.9% vs 35.1%	1 yr. OS 76.8% vs 72% 1 yr. relapse rates—21% vs 20%
Jurdi NE, et al. TCT 2023 (single arm) [9]	MAC (13.2 Gy TBI; Flu-Bu4)	MRD; MUD (8/8 or 7/8)	PTCy/Tac/MMF	1 yr. cGVHD needing systemic IST 5.5% 6 month aGVHD 2–4 17.5% 6 month aGVHD 3–4 5.5%	2 yr. OS 73.7% 2 yr. GRFS 52.2% 2 yr. RR 39.1% 2 yr. NRM 10.2%
Abatacept					
Watkins J, et al. JCO 2021 (Randomized phase 2) [11]	MAC (Flu-Bu, Bu-Cy, Cy/TBI, Flu/Mel)	MUD (8/8 or 7/8)	CNI/Mtx + Abatacept vs CNI/Mtx	Day+100 grade 3–4 aGVHD (8/8) 7% vs 14%; [a](7/8) 2.3% vs 30% [a]Day+180 severe GVHD free survival (8/8) 93% vs 82%; (7/8) 97% vs 58%	2 yr. OS (8/8) 74% vs 64%; [a](7/8) 74% vs 45%
Sitagliptin					

(continued)

Table 40.2 (continued)

Study	Conditioning	Graft source	GVHD prophylaxis	GVHD-related end-points	Survival end-points
Farag SS et al. NEJM 2021 [13]	MAC (Cy/TBI or Cy-Thiotepa)	10/10 MUD or 6/6 MRD	Sitagliptin + Tacrolimus + Sirolimus	Day+100 Grade 2–4 aGVHD 5%; day+100 Grade 3–4 aGVHD 3%; 1 year GRFS 46%	1 yr. NRM 0% 1 yr. relapse rate 26% 1 yr. cGVHD 37%
Vedolizumab					
Chen YB, et al. Nature Medicine 2024 [15]	MAC and RIC; ATG used in 42% patients	7–8/8 UD HSCT	Vedolizumab + CNI/Mtx or CNI/MMF	[a]Day+180 Lower gut aGVHD-free-survival 85.5% vs 70.9% No difference in acute GVHD of the upper gut, liver or skin	Day+180 PFS 83.1% vs 77.6% Day+180 OS 89.7% vs 84.4% Day+180 NRM 93.9% vs 88%
PTCy + Abatacept					
Samer Al-Homsi A, et al. Blood Advances 2023 [17]	MAC (54%), RIC (11%), NMA (35%)	Haploidentical HSCT	PTCy/ Tac + Abatacept	C.I. of grade 2–4 aGVHD 17% C.I. of grade 3–4 aGVHD 4% 1 yr. moderate-severe cGVHD 15%	1 yr. PFS 84% 1 yr. OS 86% 1 yr. GRFS 66%

Abbreviations: *aGVHD* acute graft-versus-host disease, *ATG* anti-thymocyte globulin, *Bu* busulfan, *cGVHD* chronic graft-versus-host disease, *C.I.* cumulative incidence, *CNI* calcineurin inhibitor, *CsA* cyclosporine, *Cy* cyclophosphamide, *Flu* fludarabine, *GRFS* GVHD-free and relapse-free survival, *IST* immunosuppressive therapy, *MAC* myeloablative conditioning, *Mel* melphalan, *MMF* mycophenolate mofetil, *MRD* matched related donor, *Mtx* methotrexate, *MUD* matched unrelated donor, *NMA* non myeloablative conditioning, *NRM* non-relapse mortality, *OS* overall survival, *PFS* progression free survival, *PTCy* post-transplant cyclophosphamide, *RIC* reduced intensity conditioning, *RR* relapse risk, *TBI* total body irradiation, *Tac* tacrolimus, *UD HSCT* unrelated donor hematopoietic stem cell transplant

[a]Statistically significant

MRD). The primary end-point of this study - 1-year incidence of cGVHD needing systemic immunosuppression was only 5.5%. However, there were important drawbacks. Three-fourths of patients developed mucositis needing TPN, higher incidence of bacteraemia and *C. difficile* infection, 14% required intubation and 6% developed arrhythmias. Importantly, the median day of neutrophil and platelet engraftment was 16 days and 26 days, respectively, which is later as compared to conventional CNI/Mtx-based GVHD prophylaxis. Secondly, the relapse rate was as high as 40%, with predominance of these cases in paediatric patients. Thus, PTCy should be used with caution, in the context of MAC, especially in paediatric patients conditioned with TBI [9].

Abatacept (Table 40.2)
T-cells, in addition to their T-cell receptor, require co-stimulatory receptors which sustain its action. The CD28 co-stimulatory receptor on T-cells binds to CD80/CD86 on APCs, which mediate its action. Abatacept blocks co-stimulation by blocking the CD28-CD80/CD86 interaction. Abatacept is a unique fusion-protein formed by combining the antigen-binding portion of CTLA4 (Cytotoxic T-lymphocyte-associated protein 4) with the Fc portion of the IgG molecule. While the former gives it specificity for its target, the latter prolongs its half-life. Hence, it is also called as CTLA4-Ig molecule [10].

In 7–8/8 UD-HSCT, an RCT of CNI + Mtx with or without abatacept was published in 2021. Abatacept (Day-1,+5,+14,+28 at 10 mg/kg) showed a significantly lower rate of grade 3–4 aGVHD by day+100, which also translated into a significant severe GVHD-free survival by day+180. The magnitude of benefit for the reduction of severe GVHD was much higher in 7/8 than in 8/8 UD transplants, which translated to an OS benefit, too. Importantly, the control arm of 7/8 UD-HSCT was a matched cohort from CIBMTR, which did not include ATG. However, a post-hoc analysis that included ATG in the control group also showed similar results [11]. Importantly, similar results were replicated in a real-world analysis, outside of a trial setting, which affirms the value of abatacept [12].

Sitagliptin (Table 40.2)
Apart from CD28 described above, other co-stimulatory molecules like CD26, aka DPP-4 (dipeptidyl peptidase 4), are also present on the T-cell surface. CD26/DPP4 interacts with its ligand caveolin on APCs, which in turn upregulates CD86 on APCs [13]. A recent study from India showed that lower expression of CD26 on different immune-cell subsets in donor PBSCs was associated with less GVHD and better survival. They concluded that CD26 inhibitors should be used in trials to test this observation [14]. A selective DPP-4 inhibitor, already approved for type-2 diabetes mellitus (T2DM), called Sitagliptin, was tested in a single-arm, phase 2 study. In spite of a small sample size (n = 36), the results of grade 2–4 aGVHD rates of 5% at day+100, and 0% 1-year NRM were excellent. Even in the absence of ATG (two-thirds UD-HSCTs), the incidence of grade 2–4 GVHD was only 5%. Interestingly, in spite of using 12 times higher dose of Sitagliptin, i.e., 600 mg BD (Dose in T2DM is 100 mg OD), there were no reports of hypoglycaemia. Taking these many tablets after a TBI-based MAC conditioning, which has a 50% risk of severe

mucositis, is challenging. Nonetheless, in spite of the excellent outcomes, results of this study have not been practice-changing, and would need an RCT in the future [13].

Vedolizumab (Table 40.2)
α4β7 is an integrin that is expressed on the surface of lymphocytes (naïve and activated), which facilitates homing to the gut. Vedolizumab is a humanized monoclonal antibody against α4β7, which blocks its docking with MAdCAM-1 on the endothelial cells of gut lymphoid tissue and disrupts the homing of lymphocytes to the gut. It was compared in a randomized fashion with placebo to the backbone of CNI/Mtx or CNI/MMF. Vedolizumab was given 300 mg IV on day-1, day+13, and then every 28 days till day+153 (maximum 7 doses). Importantly, vedolizumab decreases the incidence of all grades and severe lower-gut GVHD, without any effect on other organ GVHD, relapse, NRM or survival. However, there were numerically higher Clostridioides infections in the vedolizumab group, albeit without any increased incidence of colitis. It should be remembered that although 40% patients in this group received ATG, their dosing and schedule were not specified. Moreover, gut-GVHD was diagnosed clinically, without any central review committee or endoscopic correlation. However, the fact that it was a double-blind trial probably overcomes that limitation [15].

Prevention of GVHD Without Any Pharmacological Prophylaxis
A long-standing dream of a transplant physician has been to develop regimens for GVHD prevention without any medications. Instead of in vivo T-cell depletion, ex vivo manipulation of a graft is possible, wherein T-cells are depleted from the graft, referred to as "T-cell depletion" or "CD34 enrichment" or "CD34-selected" grafts. This strategy (CD34-selected grafts) was compared in an RCT to two other strategies - PTCy-based prophylaxis with a BM graft and conventional Tac/Mtx with a BM graft. Importantly, while CD34-selected grafts had significantly lower moderate-severe cGVHD, OS was lower in that arm—driven by higher NRM due to infection and organ failure. Thus, it is important that while analysing outcomes in transplant trials, one must also look at the NRM and overall mortality (Fig. 40.1) due to other causes, before making a change in clinical practice. A serendipitous finding of this study was the second arm (PTCy-arm). CNI-free single-agent PTCy-based prophylaxis after a MAC followed by MRD-transplant provided comparable OS with better GRFS than the standard arm [16].

40.3.1.3 Combination Regimens

PTCy + Abatacept (Table 40.2)
With the hypothesis that abatacept will prevent aGVHD, and PTCy will prevent cGVHD, investigators combined PTCy (50 mg/kg/day day+3,+4) + abatacept (10 mg/kg-3/4 doses) along with short-course tacrolimus (day+5 till day+90; taper beginning from day+60). This was called the CAST (PTCy, Abatacept, Short course Tacrolimus) regimen by the authors. This study enrolled 46 patients with a median

age of 60 years. Intriguingly, the cumulative incidence (C.I.) of grade 2–4 aGVHD was 17%, and grade 3–4 aGVHD was 4.4%. The findings of grade 2–4 aGVHD and 1-year moderate-severe cGVHD rate of less than 20% were astonishing. However, this was a single-arm study, without formal comparison to the established standard in haplo-HSCT, i.e., PTCy/Tac/MMF [17]. Hence, to bridge this gap—a propensity-matched comparison was done which compared the CAST regimen (PTCy/Abatacept/Short-course-tacrolimus) with a contemporaneous CIBMTR cohort of PTCy/Tac/MMF. Importantly, the rates of aGVHD grades 2–4 at day+120 and 1-year GRFS were 16.7% and 66.7% in the CAST cohort versus 28.6% and 47.6% in the control group, respectively. Moreover, CAST was associated with a significantly reduced incidence of relapse (9.5% versus 26.2%, P = 0.045) with improved disease-free survival (85.7% versus 61.9%, P = 0.01) [18]. With such encouraging results, authors sought to reduce the PTCy dose [25 mg/kg/day (day+3,+4)] (re-CAST study). However, in the re-CAST study, C.I. of ≥grade-2 aGvHD and moderate-severe cGvHD was 29.4% and 67.4%, respectively. Hence, authors cautioned against reducing the dose of PTCy [19].

JAK Inhibitors
In a phase 2 study of itacitinib+Tac/sirolimus, rates of ≥grade-3 aGVHD was 5%, with 1-year GRFS of 51%. Ruxolitinib has been administered in the peri-transplant period, with a variable duration of 3–12 months post-transplant. Importantly, these trials have shown ≥grade-3 aGVHD rates of <15%, with longer duration ruxolitinib showing benefit for reducing moderate-severe cGVHD [20]. An RCT in haploidentical-HSCT patients, reported in ASH 2024, replicated similar results. While the incidence of both acute and chronic GVHD was significantly reduced in the ruxolitinib arm, PTCy was not a part of the control arm. Hence, the absolute benefit of ruxolitinib in this study is questionable [21].

40.3.1.4 Precision-Engineered Cellular Therapy

Orca-T and Orca-Q
Conventional allo-HSCT involves infusing a graft that has more than 50 cell types. With the help of high-throughput cell-sorting technology, a company called "Orca-Bio" modified the PBSC graft, which was composed of a 1:1 mix of T-regulatory cells and conventional T-cells (Orca-T). After mobilizing the donor with G-CSF, recipients received a product comprised of HSCs+ T-regulatory cells (dose of three million/kg). On day +2, an additional product of conventional T-cells (dose of three million/kg) was infused, followed by tacrolimus from day +3 [1]. This means that there is a 2-log reduction in the dose of conventional T-cells, as compared to standard allo-HSCT. Moreover, infusing T-regs 48 hours prior gives them a lead-time bias, time to expand, and thereby suppresses the alloreactive T-cells. Based on encouraging results from the phase-2 study, a phase-3 study was conducted, which compared Orca-T versus conventional PBSC graft (followed by Tac/Mtx) after MAC in matched donors. One-year GRFS rates of 63.1% and 30.9% significantly

favoured the experimental arm [22]. Similar to Orca-T, Orca-Q was manufactured with a mild difference in the T-cell subsets, which were added back. It also had a population of invariant NK-T cells for GVHD control. Preliminary results in the haplo-HSCT setting after MAC showed an excellent 1-year GRFS of 83%. Importantly, the above study used single-agent Tac, without PTCy. PTCy after MAC is challenging, as it increases the morbidity due to acute toxicities. Hence, Orca-Q holds promise as a novel PTCy-free regimen for MAC haplo-HSCT [23].

40.3.2 Diagnosis of Acute GVHD

Case 40.2

A 30-year-old male underwent allo-HSCT for Ph + B-ALL in CR1. He received TBI-based MAC, PBSCs from a matched sibling (25-year male), followed by CsA/ Mtx GVHD prophylaxis. On day + 40, he developed a maculopapular itchy rash involving 55% BSA. 24 hours later, he developed two episodes of semi-solid stools, which could not be quantified. Stool infectious workup was negative. He was started on oral prednisolone 2 mg/kg/day. His baseline ST2 (suppressor of tumorigenesis 2) and REG3α (regenerating islet-derived protein 3a) were high, although his gut-GVHD was stage-0 (<500 ml and < 3 episodes), but skin was stage-2 (overall grade-2). On day 7 steroids, his stools were normal, his itching had resolved, but he still had erythema, which was present > 50% BSA. In labelling a response, itching is not considered and his gut-GVHD was grade-0 to begin with. Since there is no decrease in stage or grade of GVHD, this would qualify as absence of response by day 7 with respect to skin. His ST2, REG3α had normalized by day7. He was continued on the same steroid dose, and by day 14—his erythema decreased. Steroid taper was started after day 14 and completely stopped by day 40. He did not have any recurrence of GVHD and continues to do well at one-year follow-up. One week after systemic treatment, as compared to clinical response, biomarker response has a better specificity and can more correctly identify patients at lower risk of NRM.

What's Known

The initial Glucksberg criteria for aGVHD staging/grading were framed in 1974, which were subsequently modified in 1997. However, staging/grading of aGVHD still varies across studies, as some use the modified Glucksberg system, while some use the CIBMTR system. Hence, in order to homogenize data collection, an international research consortium was formed called MAGIC (Mount Sinai Acute GVHD International Consortium), which refined the guidelines for staging [24].

What's New

Each organ involved is staged from 0–4 (with 4 being the worst); and a composite of staging of all organs is used to label an overall clinical "grade" [24]. Staging of individual organs is largely clinical, unless for liver manifestations wherein absolute values of bilirubin (stage 1—2-3 mg/dl; stage 2—3.1 - 6 mg/dl; stage 3—6.1—15 mg/ dl; stage 4 - >15 mg/dl) are considered. With respect to clinical staging of skin—the amount of body surface area with erythema (<25% - stage 1; 25–50% - stage 2; >50% - stage 3) is considered. Unlike Glucksberg, MAGIC staging counts only areas of "erythema" in skin GVHD. For stage-4 skin GVHD, the presence of bullae should be present in >5% of BSA, in addition to generalized erythroderma to label as "stage-4" skin GVHD. Transaminitis, previously considered in Glucksberg, is no longer included in MAGIC staging. Additionally, performance status is removed, as there are multiple factors that lead to morbidity and consequently impact the performance status. Moreover, for upper-gut involvement, biopsy is not required. The upper gut is considered to be clinically involved if symptoms of nausea last >72 hours, and anorexia is associated with weight loss. For lower-gut involvement, diarrhoea volume is not required in stage-4, as severe abdominal pain +/− ileus or gastrointestinal bleeding are sufficient to stage it as severe. However, for earlier stages (1–3), it is important to quantify the diarrhoeal volume. Adults with diarrhoeal volumes are quantified as—500—999 ml—stage 1; 1000–1500 ml—stage 2; and more than 1500 ml as stage 3. At times, patients may not have watery stools which make it difficult for volume quantification, and hence the number of episodes of stools (3–5—stage 1; 5–7—stage 2; >7—stage 3) is added for staging severity. It is also important to note that histopathological grading of any organ need not correlate with clinical severity, in view of patchy involvement of disease in mucosa or skin. Hence, staging should be done as per clinical severity [24, 25]. For overall grading; ≤stage 2 skin without any other organ is "grade 1", stage 3 skin with(out) stage 1 of other organs is "grade 2", stage 2–3 liver / lower-gut with stage 0–3 skin is "grade 3"; while any organ (skin/liver/lower gut) stage 4 is called "grade 4".

In aGVHD, overall response rate (ORR) at day 28 correlates with long-term survival. However, this is a clinical response, and waiting for one month can be detrimental. Hence, in real-world practice, one-week clinical response is often utilized to decide on treatment changes; although it has a poor correlation with long-term outcomes [26]. It would be prudent to see if any baseline parameters at the onset of GVHD predict the likelihood of poor long-term outcome. MacMillan et al. reported in 2015 a clinical grading (*Minnesota risk-stratification*) which predicted NRM, based on aGVHD severity and number of organs involved. Sixteen percent of the entire cohort had a Minnesota high-risk. These patients had significantly lower day 28 ORR, higher TRM, and higher all-cause mortality. Table 40.3 simplifies the findings of MacMillan et al. [27]. Additionally, having biomarkers that diagnose the likelihood of severe GVHD or predict NRM before clinical parameters worsen, are an unmet need [26].

The MAGIC is a group of 25 transplant centres conducting GVHD research with the prime objective of discovering and validating GVHD biomarkers. In the last two decades, they have reported on the prognostic role of two biomarkers—*ST2* and *REG3α*. Amongst all organs, the gastrointestinal tract (GIT) is the primary site of severe GVHD, and within the GIT, the "crypts" are the epicentre of damage. In gut-GVHD, epithelial, endothelial, and stromal damage release IL-33, an alarmin which binds to soluble ST2, overwhelms it, and then binds to ST2 on T-cells. Binding ST2 on T-cells activates it and thereby causes more release of IFN-γ and other cytokines.

Table 40.3 Criteria for Minnesota high-risk score[a] [27]

Minnesota high-risk
Single organ involvement
Any organ stage 4
Lower GIT stage ≥3
Any stage of isolated liver involvement
Two organ involvement
Liver + lower GI involvement (any stage)
Lower GIT stage ≥2 + any skin involvement
Any combination of three organ involvement

Abbreviations: *GIT* gastrointestinal tract
[a]All others are labelled as Minnesota standard risk

On the other hand, Paneth cells, located at the base of crypts, secrete many antimicrobial peptides, one of which is REG3α. Paneth cells, due to their antimicrobial properties, are called "guardians of the crypts". In gut-GVHD, inflammatory crypt damage kills the Paneth cells, which release REG3α in the bloodstream. MAGIC has validated the combination of these two biomarkers in peripheral blood at single time-points of—day7 post-HSCT (even before the onset of any clinical GVHD), at the time of onset of GVHD, and 7 days after treatment of aGVHD (Fig. 40.2). In all these scenarios, authors showed high and low-risk groups predictive of *6-month NRM*. This combination of biomarkers (calculated by a logarithmic score), which could efficiently predict 6-month NRM, was called as *MAGIC algorithm probability (MAP)* score. Importantly, when measured at the time of GVHD diagnosis, the MAP score could separate patients into three different groups (called as *Ann-Arbor scores*) which stratified patients into different risks of NRM. Since these biomarkers predict long-term clinical outcomes (over clinical response at 7 days), they are considered as "liquid biopsy" of the GIT. When measured at 1-week post-treatment, even those without diarrhoea (clinical standard-risk) but high MAP scores (17% patients) i.e., biomarker high-risk, had worse outcomes (42% vs 8%; $p < 0.001$). On the other hand, in patients with persistent diarrhoea >500 ml/day (clinical high-risk) but low MAP scores (34%), NRM was lower (20% vs 70%; $p < 0.001$). This implied the discordance with clinical response, as the extent and dynamics of crypt damage would be better predicted by biomarker response [28, 29]. Similar to ST2 and REG3α, amphiregulin—a tissue repair ligand secreted by innate lymphoid cells, and gut-associated lymphoid tissue—has also been studied in GVHD. Etra et al. reported that the ST2 + REG3α combination and amphiregulin alone were able to delineate outcomes in patients with Minnesota standard-risk and high-risk aGVHD patients, respectively. This implies that biomarkers can identify a group of patients with high NRM amongst Minnesota-standard-risk and those with low NRM amongst Minnesota-high-risk patients. In clinical practice, this would imply treatment intensification and avoidance of treatment change in patients who are otherwise standard-risk and high-risk patients, respectively [30].

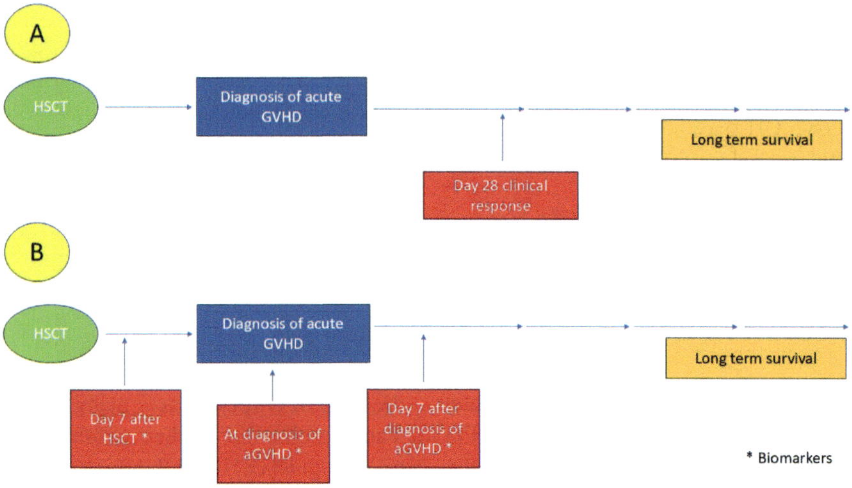

Fig. 40.2 Prediction of long-term outcomes as per: Panel (**a**)—Day 28 response (conventional knowledge), Panel (**b**)—Biomarker-based response assessments

40.4 Treatment of Acute GVHD

Case 40.3

A 35-year-old male with early thymic precursor-acute lymphoblastic leukaemia (ETP-ALL) underwent allo-HSCT from his MRD (sister 42 years old) in CR1. He was conditioned with cyclophosphamide+13.2 Gy TBI, followed by PBSC graft and CsA/Mtx. On day + 28, he developed watery diarrhoea exceeding one litre in volume. Infective work-up (stool biofire, C. difficile, blood cultures, procalcitonin) was negative. He was started on IV methylprednisolone 2 mg/kg/day. By day-4 of steroids, there was an improvement in stool volume. However, by day-7 of steroids, there was again an increase in stool volume, worsening of consistency, and cholestasis. Hepatitis workup (Hepatitis-A, E, HBV-DNA, HCV-RNA) was negative. Colonoscopy revealed grade-3 GVHD. He was deemed to be steroid refractory, and ruxolitinib was initiated at a dose of 5 mg BD. He had a partial response by day + 28, and ruxolitinib was continued. He developed thrombocytopenia (platelet 10×10^9/L-20×10^9/L) and was initiated on weekly romiplostim. On day + 53 of ruxolitinib, he developed adenoviral reactivation with hepatitis. He was treated with four doses of cidofovir and he improved. After 3-months of ruxolitinib, he achieved a CR, and ruxolitinib was gradually tapered and stopped.

What's Known

In spite of its metabolic side-effects, corticosteroids are the first-line treatment of aGVHD. MMF, ATG, infliximab, daclizumab, sirolimus, and itacitinib have been added to corticosteroids as first-line treatment, albeit without benefit. The recommended steroid for aGVHD is IV methylprednisolone (1–2 mg/kg/day). Lower dose of 1 mg/kg methylprednisolone is used for skin or upper-gut GVHD. For patients with gut aGVHD, non-absorbable oral steroids like budesonide (9 mg/d) or beclomethasone (1.3–2.0 mg QID) are recommended. The conventional end-point for response in aGVHD studies has been day+28 ORR with CR rates. Other end-points include day+56 ORR, need of second-line therapy, NRM, and OS. Patients who have *progression in three days or absence of response in seven days* are termed sr-aGVHD [2]. Additionally, progression with a new organ involvement after prior treatment with therapeutic methylprednisolone or any recurrence that happens after/during the steroid taper is also called sr-aGVHD [31]. Sr-GVHD suffers from high NRM (upto 40% till 1-year) [32].

What's New

Do We Need Systemic Steroids for all Grades of GVHD?

An RCT of systemic steroids (methylprednisolone-1 mg/kg) versus no systemic treatment was conducted for patients with grade-1 GVHD. While steroids prevented progression to grade-2 GVHD, there was no difference in grade 3–4 GVHD or moderate-severe cGVHD in both arms. Importantly, infection rates were higher with systemic steroids. Hence, only topical steroids are recommended in patients with grade-1 GVHD. Systemic steroids are reserved for patients with ≥grade-2 GVHD [33].

Can We Tweak the Recommended Dose of Methylprednisolone for aGVHD?

Steroids are effective, but higher doses mean increased risk of infections. There is an unmet need for identifying the effective dose of steroids for the treatment of aGVHD at lower doses. An Italian RCT (1998) compared methylprednisolone 2 mg/kg/day versus 10 mg/kg/day, and did not find any difference in response rate, progression to higher-grade GVHD, or survival. Consequently, 2 mg/kg/day methylprednisolone became the approved dose [34]. In a landmark trial, physicians compared the utility of lower-dose steroids depending on the grade of aGVHD. Patients with grade-2a manifestations (upper-gut symptoms, diarrhoea <1.0 L/day, rash <50% BSA, no hepatic dysfunction; n = 102) were randomized to an initial prednisone dose at 1 mg/kg/day vs 0.5 mg/kg/day. On the other hand, those with grade-2b or higher manifestations (rash ≥50% BSA, diarrhoea ≥1.0 L/day or hepatic involvement; n = 62) were randomized to an initial prednisone dose of 2 mg/kg/day vs 1 mg/kg/day. Importantly, lower doses of steroids were effective for patients with grade-2a manifestations, but not for 2b manifestations. This implies that for patients with isolated upper-gut GVHD, grade-2 skin or gut-GVHD, an initial steroid dose of 0.5 mg/kg/day could be sufficient, especially if there is no hepatic involvement [35].

Combination Regimens for Newly Diagnosed aGVHD

The intent of combination regimens is to use either a lower dose of systemic steroids upfront, or plan a rapid steroid taper or devise steroid-free regimens, in order to escape its toxicities. Preliminary analysis of ruxolitinib + lower-dose methylprednisolone (1 mg/kg) showed encouraging day+28 CR rates of 82%. Absence of decline in REG3α levels at day 14 of treatment predicted refractoriness to this combination. Another RCT of extracorporeal photopheresis (ECP) + prednisone vs prednisone alone showed a marginally high benefit for day+56 outcomes in the ECP arm. ECP arm fared better for skin-only aGVHD, although the study was not powered for subgroup analysis. Importantly, the median steroid dose at day+28 and day+56 was similar in both arms. This meant that in spite of additive ECP, the steroid dose could not be tapered faster in the combination arm, thereby negating its marginal benefit [36].

40.5 Approved Therapies for srGVHD

Ruxolitinib

JAKs are a part of intracellular kinases which play an important role in the development of both innate and adaptive immunity. JAK family consists of four enzymes—JAK1, JAK2, JAK3, TYK2. Ruxolitinib is a selective JAK1/2 inhibitor that works in aGVHD by inhibiting cytokine-mediated tissue damage.

REACH1 was an open-label single-arm study of ruxolitinib for sr-aGVHD in patients ≥12 years of age, irrespective of HSCT type. More than half responded by day+28 (ORR 54.9%), and one-fourth (26.8%) achieved a CR. Importantly, ORR at any time was 73%, which meant that few patients responded after day +28. ORR/CR rates for grade-2, 3, 4 aGVHD were 82%/47%, 42%/20%, and 42%/7%, respectively. The likelihood of response also varied with organ involvement—skin (61%) > upper-gut/lower-gut (45%) > liver (26%), and the number of organs—2+ organs (47%) vs 1 organ (62%). Importantly, in spite of the acceptable response rates, the 12-month NRM rate was 52% [37].

Similarly, in a randomized multicentre study (REACH2) for sr-aGVHD, ruxolitinib was associated with a significantly better ORR (62% vs 39%) and CR rate (34% vs 19%) at day+28, and better durable ORR by day+56 (40% vs 22%). As expected, ORR was better for grade-2 (75%), than grade-3 (53%) and grade-4 (42%) GVHD. However, it should be noted that the 18-month incidence of NRM was 49%. This means that a proportion of patients lose their response to ruxolitinib. The finding of similar NRM in spite of better GVHD control reflects ruxolitinib's indirect effects (cytopenias, infections) on patient survival. Nonetheless, *ruxolitinib was the first FDA-approved drug for sr-aGVHD in patients ≥ 12 years of age in 2019* [38]. However, considering that 40% patients do not respond to ruxolitinib, and 10–20% patients lose their initial response, it is important to know the term "ruxolitinib-refractory". Refractoriness to ruxolitinib is defined as *progression after 5–10 days of ruxolitinib* or *lack of response after at least 2 weeks of ruxolitinib* or *any clinical worsening (increase in grade or new organ involvement) / increase in stage after initial improvement* [31].

Remestemcel

BM-derived mesenchymal stem cells (MSCs) have immunosuppressive properties. They have the ability to induce allogeneic tolerance and have been shown to decrease inflammatory biomarkers. A single-arm prospective study evaluated the role of remestemcel—allogeneic human BM-derived MSCs, which were expanded ex vivo, in paediatric patients below 12 years with sr-aGVHD. Importantly, MSCs express low-level MHC-class-1 molecules, and are negative for MHC-class-2 and costimulatory molecules. Hence, they can be administered without the need for HLA matching. They are expanded ex vivo in culture and cryopreserved in aliquots. Remestemcel was administered intravenously at a dose of $2x10^6$ MSCs/kg body weight, twice weekly, for 4 consecutive weeks (maximum 8 doses). Amongst 54 children, remestemcel resulted in a significant improvement by day 28, when compared with a pre-specified control (70% vs 45%). Importantly, unlike previous therapies, this 70% response was sustained through day+100, with an increase in CR rates from 29% to 44%. OS at day+180 was 68%, and remestemcel was well tolerated without any infusion reactions [39]. A recent update showed a 2-year OS benefit 51% vs 38%, remestemcel was approved by FDA in December 2024 for paediatric patients <12-years of age with sr-aGVHD [40]. Kebriaei et al. reported a randomized study of remestemcel in patients with sr-aGVHD between 6 months—70 years of age, but without any benefit. One limitation raised against this study is the primary end-point, which was "durability of CR of at-least 28 days". In the allo-HSCT field, achievement of CRs in sr-aGVHD is rare, and to keep "durable CRs" as the end-point was overzealous, which may have resulted in this study being a negative one. However, like the previous report, this study also highlighted the fact that paediatric patients, and those with liver involvement, had a better response [41].

Vedolizumab

Vedolizumab is a potential option for sr-aGVHD of the lower gut. Its day+28 ORR varies from 35–64%, with 6-month OS rates of 35–54%. Anecdotal reports describe its efficacy even in patients who are ruxolitinib refractory. However, prospective studies are lacking [36].

Faecal microbiota transplant (FMT)

Gut microbiota is linked to epithelial inflammation and immune response. In normal homeostasis, the GIT is colonized by *diverse* commensals like *Bacteroides*, *Lactobacillus*, *Bifidobacterium* etc. In allo-HSCT, multiple factors (chemotherapy, radiation, antibiotics, mucositis) lead to gut dysbiosis. Dysbiosis means a *less-diverse* microbial flora (overgrowth of pathogenic bacteria, and suppression of healthy commensals), which is causal in gut aGVHD. FMT means administering faecal suspension from a healthy donor, in order to restore the *diversity* of intestinal microflora, and thereby suppress the altered immune response in the GIT. FMT has been previously tried in conditions like refractory *C. difficile*, inflammatory bowel disease, and overgrowth of multi-drug-resistant bacteria [42].

The first report of FMT in sr-aGVHD was by the Japanese group. In four patients with sr-aGVHD, three patients had a CR. Notably, they also showed that these three responders had a partial change in their intestinal microbial flora to regular commensals, along with an increase in effector T-regulatory cells in peripheral blood. The latter finding laid an important hypothesis that FMT was capable of modulating a systemic anti-inflammatory response, which could thereby help even in non-gastrointestinal forms of aGVHD [43].

The first prospective study in this regard was published by the French team. Faecal material from 3–8 healthy donors was pooled and processed at a central facility, and cryopreserved at −80°celsius in 150 ml freeze-resistant bags, called as "MaaT013". MaaT013 was given via a rectal catheter, and a maximum of 3-weekly administrations were planned. Amongst 24 enrolled patients, day+28 ORR was 38%. Amongst 58 additional patients treated with compassionate use, day+28 ORR was 58%. 1-year OS was 25% and 38% in the trial and compassionate use patients, respectively [44]. Recently, a study from China reported FMT + ruxolitinib combination with encouraging day+28 ORR of 71%, and 6-month OS of 57% [45]. The benefits of FMT include its cheap cost, feasibility of administration, ready availability across HLA barriers, and minimal processing and administration cost. Hence, it has been recently tried in the field of GVHD prophylaxis, and its use is expanding [46].

The last two therapies are not FDA-approved for sr-aGVHD, but are promising.

40.6 Approach to a Case of Chronic GVHD

Case 40.4—How to diagnose and stage cGVHD

A 32-year-old gentleman underwent allo-HSCT for high-risk myelodysplastic syndrome with his MSD (sister, 29 years). He received Flu/Bu conditioning, PBSC-graft and CsA/Mtx. He had febrile neutropenia with grade-4 mucositis for which he received supportive care. He had oral lichen planus at 3 months post-transplant, which was managed with topical triamcinolone (steroids). Post 4-months, he presented with worsening exertional dyspnea along with sclerotic lesions over the upper limbs for 2 weeks. A skin biopsy suggested GVHD. CT-chest showed air trapping, and spirometry was suggestive of FEV1 45%. He was diagnosed with severe cGVHD lung with skin involvement. He was started on Inj Methylprednisolone 1 mg/kg BD along with topical betamethasone, Fluticasone/Azithromycin/Montelukast (FAM), and chest physiotherapy. By day + 8, there was improvement. Steroids were gradually tapered from week-2 onwards and over the next 4 weeks, and the patient was continued on FAM therapy and Cyclosporine. Patient continued to be in PR at 8-months on the last follow-up.

Risk factors for cGVHD in the above patient are PBSC graft, MAC, female donor for a male recipient [47].

Approach to a patient with suspected GVHD should include a careful clinical evaluation, including a close look at uninvolved organ systems for potential involvement. Infections should be ruled out as GVHD treated with systemic immunosuppression can worsen infections.

Symptoms of exertional dyspnea can be due to anemia, pleural/pericardial effusions, pneumonia, lung GVHD, etc. Hemogram, chest imaging, and 2D-ECHO can guide further evaluation.

Skin GVHD is a clinical diagnosis. Apart from GVHD, skin rash can be because of infections, drug reactions, nutritional deficiencies, etc. Biopsy supports the diagnosis. Based on the type of lesions, skin GVHD can be classified as acute, chronic, or overlap syndrome.

NIH Consensus Criteria provides a framework for the diagnosis and staging of cGVHD. Clinical features are classified as diagnostic or distinctive (Table 40.4). Diagnostic symptoms/signs refer to those manifestations that *establish the presence of cGVHD without the need for further testing or evidence of other organ involvement*. Distinctive signs and symptoms of cGVHD refer to those manifestations *that are not ordinarily found in aGVHD but are not considered sufficient in isolation to establish an unequivocal diagnosis of cGVHD*. Organs are scored (Table 40.5) and an overall severity (Table 40.6) is determined, which helps us understand the clinical relevance and morbidity of cGVHD across trials [48].

Table 40.4 Clinical features of chronic GVHD

Organ or site	Diagnostic (sufficient to establish the diagnosis of chronic GVHD)	Distinctive* (seen in chronic GVHD, but insufficient alone to establish a diagnosis)	Other features or unclassified entities	Common (seen with both acute and chronic GVHD)
Skin	Poikiloderma, Lichen planus-like features, Sclerotic features Morphea-like features, Lichen sclerosis-like features	Depigmentation, papulosquamous lesions	Sweat impairment, ichthyosis, keratosis pilaris, hypopigmentation, hyperpigmentation	Erythema, maculopapular rash, pruritus
Nails		Dystrophy, longitudinal ridging, splitting or brittle features, onycholysis, pterygium unguis, nail loss (usually symmetric, affects most nails)		
Scalp and body hair		New onset of scarring or nonscarring scalp alopecia (after recovery from chemoradiotherapy), loss of body hair, scaling	Thinning scalp hair, typically patchy, coarse, or dull (not explained by endocrine or other causes), premature gray hair	

(continued)

Table 40.4 (continued)

Organ or site	Diagnostic (sufficient to establish the diagnosis of chronic GVHD)	Distinctive* (seen in chronic GVHD, but insufficient alone to establish a diagnosis)	Other features or unclassified entities	Common (seen with both acute and chronic GVHD)
Mouth	Lichen planus-like changes	Xerostomia, mucoceles, mucosal atrophy, ulcers, pseudomembranes		Gingivitis, mucositis, erythema, pain
Eyes		New onset dry, gritty, or painful eyes, cicatricial conjunctivitis, Keratoconjunctivitis sicca, confluent areas of punctate keratopathy	Photophobia, periorbital hyperpigmentation, blepharitis (erythema of the eyelids with oedema)	
Genitalia	Lichen planus - like features, lichen sclerosus-like features	Erosions, fissures, ulcers		
Female	Vaginal scarring or clitoral/labial agglutination			
Males	Phimosis or urethral/ meatus scarring or stenosis			
GI tract	Esophageal web, strictures, or stenosis in the upper to mid third of the esophagus		Exocrine pancreatic insufficiency	Anorexia, nausea, vomiting, diarrhea, weight loss, failure to thrive (infants and children
Liver				Total bilirubin, alkaline phosphatase >2 upper limit of normal ALT >2 upper limit of normal

(continued)

Table 40.4 (continued)

Organ or site	Diagnostic (sufficient to establish the diagnosis of chronic GVHD)	Distinctive* (seen in chronic GVHD, but insufficient alone to establish a diagnosis)	Other features or unclassified entities	Common (seen with both acute and chronic GVHD)
Lung	Bronchiolitis obliterans diagnosed with lung biopsy (BOS)	Air trapping and bronchiectasis on chest CT	Cryptogenic organizing pneumonia restrictive lung disease	
Muscles, fascia, joints	Fasciitis joint stiffness or contractures secondary to fasciitis or sclerosis	Myositis or polymyositis	Oedema, muscle cramps arthralgia, or arthritis	
Hematopoietic and Immune			Thrombocytopenia, eosinophilia, lymphopenia, hypo- or hyper-gammaglobulinemia, autoantibodies (autoimmune hemolytic anemia, Immune thrombocytopenia)	
Others			Raynaud's phenomenon, pericardial or pleural effusions, ascites, peripheral neuropathy, nephrotic syndrome, myasthenia gravis, cardiac conduction abnormality or cardiomyopathy	

Abbreviations: *BOS* Bronchiolitis obliterans syndrome, *CT* Computerized tomogram

Table 40.5 Organ scoring of chronic GVHD

	Score 0	Score 1	Score 2	Score 3
Performance Score:	Asymptomatic and fully active (ECOG O; KPS or Lanksy PS 100%)	Symptomatic, fully ambulatory, restricted only in physically strenuous activity (ECOG 1; KPS or Lanksy PS 80–90%)	Symptomatic, ambulatory, capable of self-care >50% of waking hours out of bed (ECOG 2; KPS or Lansky PS 60–70%)	Symptomatic, limited self-care, >50% of waking hours in bed (ECOG 3–4; KPS or Lansky PS <60%)
			Of self-care, >50%	>50% of waking
SKIN SCORE % BSA *GVHD features to be scored by BSA:* Check all that apply: - Maculopapular rash/ erythema D Lichen planus-like features - Sclerotic features - Papulosquamous lesions or ichthyosis - Keratosis pilaris-like GVHD - SKIN features score	No BSA involved Sclerotic features	1–18% BSA	19–50% BSA Superficial sclerotic features "not hidebound" (able to pinch)	>50%BSA Deep sclerotic features "Hidebound" (unable to pinch) Impaired mobility Ulceration
Other skin GVHD features (NOT scored by BSA) Check all that apply: Hyperpigmentation Hypopigmentation Poikiloderma Severe or generalized pruritus Hair involvement Nail involvement Abnormality present but explained entirely by non-GVHD documented cause (specify): ____				
MOUTH				
Lichen planus like features present YES NO	No symptoms	Mild symptoms with disease signs not limiting oral intake significantly	Moderate symptoms with disease signs, partial limitation of oral intake	Severe symptoms with disease signs on examination with major limitation of oral intake
Abnormality present but explained entirely by non-GVHD documented cause specify):				

(continued)

Table 40.5 (continued)

	Score 0	Score 1	Score 2	Score 3
Eyes *Keratoconjunctivitis sicca (KCS) confirmed by ophthalmologist:* Yes No Not examined *Abnormality present but explained entirely by non-GVHD documented cause (specify):*	No symptoms	Mild dry eye symptoms not affecting ADL (requirement of lubricant eye drops 3 x per day)	Moderate dry eye symptoms partially affecting ADL (requiring lubricant eye drops >3 x per day or punctal plugs), **WITHOUT** new vision impairment due to KCS	Severe dry eye symptoms significantly affecting ADL (special eyewear to relieve pain) OR unable to work because of ocular symptoms OR loss of vision due to KCS
GI Tract				
Check all that apply: Oesophageal web/ proximal stricture or ring Dysphagia Anorexia Nausea Vomiting Diarrhea Weight loss>5% Failure to thrive	No symptoms	Symptoms without significant weight loss* (<5%)	Symptoms associated with mild to moderate weight loss* (5–15%) OR moderate diarrhea without significant interference with daily living	Symptoms associated with significant weight loss* >15%, requires nutritional supplements for most calorie needs OR esophageal dilatation OR Severe diarrhea with significant interference with daily living
*Abnormality present but explained entirely by non-GVHD documented cause (specify).:*________________.				
Liver	Normal total bilirubin and ALT or AP <3 x ULN	Normal total bilirubin and ALT ≥3 x ULN	Elevated total bilirubin but <3 mg/dl or ALT >5 times ULN	Elevated total bilirubin but <3 mg/dl
Lungs score %FEV1 Pulmonary function test Not performed	**%FEV1 ≥ 80%**	**%FEV1 60–79%**	**%FEV1 40–59%**	%FEV1 ≤ 39%
Abnormality present but explained entirely by non-GVHD documented cause (specify)				

(continued)

Table 40.5 (continued)

	Score 0	Score 1	Score 2	Score 3
Joints and facia P-ROM score Shoulder (1–7): _ Elbow (1–7): _ Wrist/finger (1–7): _ Ankle (1–4): _	No symptoms	Mild tightness of arms and legs, normal or mild decreased range of motion (ROM), and not affecting ADL	Tightness of arms or legs OR joint contractures, erythema, thought due to fasciitis, moderate decrease ROM AND mild to moderate limitation of ADL	Contractures WITH significant limitation of ADL (unable to tie shoes, button shirts, dress-self etc)
Genital tract (See Supplemental figure) Currently sexually active Yes No	*No signs*	*Mild signs and females with or without discomfort on exam*	*Moderate signs and may have symptoms with discomfort on exam*	**Severe signs with or without symptoms**
Abnormality present but explained entirely by non-GVHD documented cause (specify):				
Other indicators. Clinical features or complications related to chronic GVHD (check all that apply and assign a score to severity (0–3) based on functional impact where applicable none - 0, mild-1, moderate – 2, severe - 3)				
Ascites (serositis)		*Myasthenia gravis*		
Eosinophilia > 500 μL				
Pericardia! Effusion		*Peripheral neuropathy*		
Platelets < 100,000/μL				
Pleural effusion Polymyositis		*Others (specify)*		
Nephrotic syndrome		*Weight loss > 5% without GI symptoms*		
Overall GVHD Severity (Opinion of the evaluator)	No GVHD	Mild	Moderate	Severe

Abbreviations: *ADL* activities of daily living, *ALT* alanine transaminase, *AST* aspartate transaminase, *BSA* body surface area, *ECOG PS* Eastern co-operative oncology group performance status, *FEV1* forced expiratory volume in first second, *GI* gastrointestinal, *KCS* keratoconjunctivitis sicca, *KPS* Karnofsky performance status, *PROM* photographic range of motion, ULN—upper limit of normal

Table 40.6 NIH global severity of chronic GVHD

Mild chronic GVHD - 1 or 2 Organs involved with no more than score 1 *plus* - Lung score 0
Moderate chronic GVHD 3 or More organs involved with no more than score 1 OR At least 1 organ (not lung) with a score of 2 OR Lung score 1
Severe chronic GVHD At least 1 organ with a score of 3 OR Lung score of 2 or 3

Key points

In skin: higher of the 2 scores to be used for calculating global severity. In lung: FEV1 is used instead of clinical score for calculating global severity

If the entire abnormality in an organ is noted to be unequivocally explained by a non-GVHD documented cause, that organ is not included for calculation of the global severity

If the abnormality in an organ is attributed to multifactorial causes (GVHD plus other causes) the scored organ will be used for calculation of the global severity regardless of the contributing causes (no downgrading of organ severity score)

40.6.1 Management of Lung GVHD

Best management of lung GVHD lies in its early diagnosis (pre-emptive action) by doing spirometry post-allo-HSCT. Unfortunately, by the time patients develop dyspnoea, it has already progressed to BOS (Bronchiolitis obliterans syndrome). Management of Lung GVHD is best done in a clinical trial [49].

Treatment involves systemic immunosuppression with Methylprednisolone 1–2 mg/kg/day or Tab Prednisolone 0.5-1 mg/kg/day with CNI/MMF. Systemic steroids may be required for prolonged periods in lung GVHD. In case of steroid dependence, steroid-sparing agents like ruxolitinib, belumosidil may be considered. In addition, local BOS-directed therapy involves inhaled corticosteroids like the FAM protocol. Available data suggest early tapering of systemic immunosuppression in patients on FAM therapy [50]. Interestingly, there is data to suggest that prolonged azithromycin can lead to increased risk of relapse or secondary malignancy, however patients on azithromycin develop lesser infective exacerbations [51, 52].

Supportive treatment like chest physiotherapy, vaccination against influenza, COVID, pneumococcal, and Haemophilus influenzae-B (HiB) should be considered. Monitoring of IgG levels and IVIG prophylaxis can be considered if IgG levels are <400 mg/dL. Patients should be regularly monitored for the need for long-term oxygen therapy. As per ERS/EBMT guidelines, lung GVHD patients require regular follow-up with spirometry q3months or earlier as clinically indicated. As a last resort, lung transplantation may be considered [49].

40.7 Approach to Steroid-Refractory cGVHD (sr-cGVHD)

Case 40.5
A 52-year-old lady with B-acute lymphoblastic leukaemia underwent allo-HSCT from haploidentical donor (brother 45-years). She was conditioned using fludarabine + TBI 8Gy, PBSC graft and PTCy/Tac/MMF as GVHD prophylaxis. Post-transplant, she developed CMV reactivation at day + 27 which was treated with IV ganciclovir. She was gradually tapered off immunosuppression by 6 months. Post 8-months, she presented with tightness of joints and hyperpigmented skin lesions in bilateral upper and lower limbs, with dryness of eyes and yellowish discoloration of eyes and skin. Viral markers for hepatitis [Hepatitis A, E, HBV-DNA, HCV-RNA, Cytomegalovirus (CMV)] were negative. Liver biopsy was consistent with GVHD. She was diagnosed with moderate cGVHD involving the liver, skin, and eyes. She was initiated on systemic immunosuppression inj. Methylprednisolone 1 mg/kg BD along with systemic tacrolimus. Topical steroids, along with tacrolimus eye drops, were started. After 1-week of steroids, her liver parameters worsened marking steroid refractoriness. She was referred for further management. She was started on tab. Ruxolitinib 10 mg BD. Her liver parameters stabilized over the next 2 weeks. Her systemic steroids were tapered off, and she achieved PR after 2 months of therapy.

SR-aGVHD gets diagnosed by seeing the clinical dynamics of the patient in 1 week. In contrast, SR-cGVHD has been defined as *cGVHD progression while on prednisone at ≥1 mg/kg/day for 2 weeks, or stable cGVHD while on ≥0.5 mg/kg/day for 1–2 months*, and additional patients remain steroid-dependent with repeated symptom flares during taper of corticosteroids below 0.25 mg/kg/day [53]. Possible options for this patient outside of a clinical trial may be as follows.

Ruxolitinib
REACH3 was a phase 3, randomized, multi-centre trial (n = 329) for moderate-to-severe steroid-dependent or sr-cGVHD. Week-24 ORR: 50% (ruxolitinib) vs. 26% BAT ($p < 0.001$). The failure-free survival was better with ruxolitinib (not-reached vs. 5.7 months). There was a trend towards better OS, but not statistically significant at interim analysis. Common ≥grade-3 AEs were thrombocytopenia (15.2% vs 10.1%) and anaemia (12.7% vs 7.6%) in the ruxolitinib and control arms, respectively. The incidence of CMV reactivation was similar in the two groups [54].

Extra-Corporeal Photopheresis (ECP)
ECP involves leukapheresis, ex vivo treatment of harvested leukocytes (buffy-coat) with a photo-sensitizer (8-methoxy-psoralen) followed by ultraviolet-A (UVA) light administration, which primes the T-cells for apoptosis when reinfused back into the patient. These apoptotic lymphocytes are phagocytosed by macrophages, which consequently release anti-inflammatory mediators responsible for developing immune tolerance. Unlike others, ECP is "immune modulatory", and not immune-suppressive [55].

ECP has been assessed in both steroid-dependent and SR-cGVHD patients [56]. It has also shown significant response rates in patients with sclerodermatous and mucosal GVHD in previous studies, including a randomized phase-2 trial [56, 57]. ECP has the potential to increase T-regulatory cells, with favourable responses in difficult-to-treat sclerotic SR-cGVHD. ECP is associated with low rates of infectious complications and has a steroid-sparing effect [58]. It is usually administered twice weekly for the first month and then twice weekly every other week for 6–12 months. Once initiated, we also pursue steroid tapering as soon as possible, to reduce the impact on the treatment of fungal infection and to avoid new CMV reactivation episodes [59].

Ibrutinib

Ibrutinib inhibits BTK and IL-2-inducible T-cell kinase (ITK), reducing B-cell and T-cell activation, which are critical in cGVHD pathogenesis. This dual inhibition mitigates inflammatory and fibrotic processes, particularly in mucosal and cutaneous cGVHD [60]. It was tested in the iNTEGRATE study, which evaluated ibrutinib (420 mg daily) plus corticosteroids versus placebo plus corticosteroids in 193 patients with newly diagnosed moderate-to-severe cGVHD. Its primary end-point was 48-week ORR. ORR was 52% (ibrutinib) versus 39% (placebo) ($p = 0.04$), with higher CR rates in the ibrutinib group (15% vs 8%). It led to significant responses in skin (58%) and mouth (62%) in the ibrutinib arm, with modest effects in the liver and lung. Median PFS was not reached in the ibrutinib arm versus 15.9 months in the placebo arm (HR-0.65, $p = 0.02$). Lee-Symptom-Scale improvements were more frequent in the ibrutinib arm (41% vs 29% with ≥7-point reduction) [61].

Belumosudil

Belumosudil, a selective Rho-associated coiled-coil-kinase 2 (ROCK2) inhibitor, has emerged as a promising therapy for sr-cGVHD. Its pivotal ROCK-star study showed organ-specific response-rates - 37% (skin), 42% (eyes), 55% (mouth), 39% (liver), 26% (lungs), 71% (joints/fascia), 52% (upper-gut), 69% (lower-gut), and 45% (oesophagus). Median duration of response was 54 weeks; 62% of responders maintained their response at 12 months. Two-third (67%) of patients reduced corticosteroid doses, with 22% discontinuing steroids entirely. Lee-Symptom-Scale scores improved by ≥7 points in 38% of patients, indicating clinically meaningful symptom relief. Importantly, the low rates of grade ≥3 cytopenias and CMV infection rates are promising features of the safety profile of belumosudil [62].

Axatilimab

Axatilimab is an antibody against CSF1R that targets monocytes and macrophages. It was evaluated in a phase-2, multicentre RCT AGAVE-201 wherein 241 patients were analysed ($n = 80$ in the 0.3-mg dose group, $n = 81$ in the 1-mg dose group, and $n = 80$ in the 3-mg dose group). The primary end point was met in all the groups; ORR was 74% (0.3-mg dose), 67% (1-mg dose), and 50% (3-mg dose). More than 5-point reduction on the modified Lee-symptom-scale was reported in 60%, 69%, and 41% of the patients in the three dose groups, respectively. AEs leading to discontinuation occurred in 6% (0.3-mg), 22% (1-mg), and 18% (3-mg) [63].

Others

Baricitinib, a JAK-1/2 inhibitor FDA approved for rheumatoid arthritis has been tested both in sr-cGVHD and for GVHD prophylaxis [64]. ORR upto 90% has been observed in phase 1/2 studies. It has demonstrated response in ocular GVHD [65].

Of all the above drugs, ruxolitinib, ibrutinib, belumosudil, and axatilimab have been FDA approved for cGVHD, with ibrutinib being the first ever agent amongst these.

40.8 Long-Term Follow-Up of a cGVHD Patient

Case 40.6

A 45-year-old male with AML underwent allo-HSCT in CR1 with his fully-matched brother aged 54-years. He received Flu/Bu MAC, PBSC infusion and Tac/Mtx GVHD prophylaxis 18-months ago. Six months post-transplant, he developed moderate cGVHD involving skin (erythematous rash) and liver (elevated bilirubin and transaminases) managed with tacrolimus, low-dose prednisone and topical steroids. He reports complete resolution of GVHD symptoms. He was kept on a 3-monthly follow up for clinical evaluation. He was vaccinated as per the schedule (Table 40.7) after he was off immunosuppression.

1. Monitoring cGVHD

   A. Clinical and Laboratory Surveillance

      Multi-disciplinary evaluations: Conduct comprehensive assessments every 3–6 months, involving transplant haematology, dermatology, hepatology, and other subspecialties as indicated. Evaluate skin for rash/sclerosis/fasciitis (per NIH-2014 cGVHD criteria) and liver via serial bilirubin, alanine/aspartate aminotransferases (ALT/AST), and alkaline phosphatase levels.

      Tacrolimus Monitoring: Measure trough levels (target 5–10 ng/mL) biweekly initially, transitioning to monthly with stable dosing.

   B. Organ-Specific Testing

      Skin: Quantify BSA involvement and assess for sclerotic features using the modified Rodnan-score or Vienna-Skin-Score [66].

      Liver: Perform Doppler ultrasound or transient elastography (FibroScan) for persistent transaminitis elevation to exclude cirrhosis, especially those with chronic HBC/HCV. In patients with liver cirrhosis, monitor for hepatocellular carcinoma.

      Pulmonary: Annual spirometry to detect BOS. Monitoring can be more frequent once a patient develops GVHD [49].

      Ocular/Oral: Schirmer's test, slit-lamp exams every 6–12 months for ocular GVHD; dental evaluations for oral sicca or mucosal involvement [66].

Table 40.7 Vaccination schedule post HSCT

Vaccine	Timing post-transplant	Dosing schedule	Notes
Inactivated vaccines			
Influenza (Inactivated)	6 months	Annual dose (single dose)	Start as early as 4 months if community outbreak. Avoid live nasal vaccine
Pneumococcal conjugate vaccine (PCV13/PCV15/ PCV20)	6–12 months	PCV15 or PCV20: 3 doses (1 month apart) at 6–12 months; PCV20 may suffice as single dose later. If PCV13 is used, follow with PPSV23 at least 8 weeks later.	Adjust based on GVHD or immunosuppression. PCV20 preferred if available
Diphtheria, tetanus, pertussis (DTaP or Tdap)	6–12 months	3 doses (1–2 months apart); Tdap preferred for first dose, then DTaP or Td for others. Booster every 10 years.	Use acellular pertussis formulation
Haemophilus influenzae type b (Hib)	6–12 months	3 doses (1–2 months apart)	Essential for all patients, regardless of prior vaccination
Hepatitis B (HepB)	6–12 months	3 doses (0, 1, 6 months)	High-dose formulation (40 mcg) preferred. Check serology post-vaccination
Hepatitis A (HepA)	12 months	2 doses (6–12 months apart)	Recommended in high-risk areas or for travel
Inactivated polio (IPV)	6–12 months	3 doses (1–2 months apart)	Avoid oral polio vaccine (live)
Meningococcal (MenACWY)	12 months	2 doses (2 months apart); booster every 5 years	Consider Men-B in high-risk settings (2–3 doses based on brand)
Recombinant zoster (Shingrix)	12–24 months	2 doses (2–6 months apart)	For patients ≥18 years, off immunosuppression, and no active GVHD
COVID-19	3–6 months	Primary series (2–3 doses based on vaccine); boosters per local guidelines	Start as early as 3 months if high community prevalence
Live vaccines			
Measles, mumps, rubella (MMR)	24 months	2 doses (1–2 months apart)	Only if no active GVHD, off immunosuppression, and CD4 > 200/μL
Varicella (VAR)	24 months	2 doses (1–2 months apart)	Same criteria as MMR. Avoid in patients with ongoing immunosuppression

C. Diagnostic Confirmation

Biopsies: Reserve skin or liver biopsies for diagnostic uncertainty (e.g., drug-induced liver injury vs. GVHD) or progression despite therapy. Histopathology should assess for interface dermatitis (skin) or bile duct damage (liver).

Minimal Residual Disease: Monitor AML relapse risk with periodic BM aspirates or testing (e.g., flow cytometry, NGS) if clinical suspicion arises.

2. Quality of Life Assessment

Validated Instruments: Administer FACT-BMT (Functional Assessment of Cancer Therapy-Bone Marrow Transplant) scale, Lee cGVHD Symptom Scale, or SF-36 (Short-Form-Survey) every 6–12 months to quantify physical, functional, and emotional domains. Correlate scores with cGVHD severity to guide interventions [66–68].

Psychosocial Interventions: Refer to psycho-oncology for cognitive-behavioural therapy or mindfulness-based stress reduction to address post-transplant depression/anxiety (prevalence~20–40%) [66].

Vocational Rehabilitation: Assess return-to-work capacity via occupational therapy, addressing fatigue (common in 50% of survivors) or physical limitations [66].

3. Prevention and Management of Complications

Infectious Disease Prophylaxis

Antimicrobial Prophylaxis:

Pneumocystis jirovecii: Trimethoprim-sulfamethoxazole (800/160 mg thrice weekly) indefinitely while on immunosuppression.

Herpesviruses: Acyclovir/valacyclovir (400-800 mg BID) for CMV/VZV prophylaxis.

Fungal: Posaconazole or voriconazole for invasive fungal infection risk, particularly with augmented immunosuppression.

Vaccinations: Initiating inactivated vaccines (e.g., PCV13, influenza) at 6–12 months post-HSCT, avoiding live vaccines (e.g., MMR) until immunosuppression is discontinued as outlined in Table 40.7 [66].

Non-Infectious Complications

Secondary Malignancies: Annual dermatologic screening for squamous cell carcinoma (5–10% incidence post-HSCT) and adherence to age-appropriate screenings (e.g., colonoscopy at age 45). Second malignancies are rare events that need long-term follow-up. A study from India showed a 10-year C.I. of 5.6% [69].

Cardiovascular: Monitor lipids, blood pressure, and HbA1c every 6 months. Initiate statins or antihypertensives if clinically indicated.

Skeletal health: Perform DEXA scan at 1-year post-HSCT and every 1–2 years thereafter. Prescribe calcium (1000–1200 mg/day), vitamin D (800–2000 IU/day), and bisphosphonates for T-scores ≤ -2.5.

Endocrine dysfunction: Screen annually for hypothyroidism (TSH, free-T4), hypogonadism (testosterone, LH/FSH), and adrenal insufficiency (8 AM cortisol, ACTH-stimulation test).

Neurocognitive Effects: Assess for CNI-neurotoxicity (e.g., posterior reversible encephalopathy syndrome) with MRI if neurologic symptoms arise [66].

4. Patient-centred care and education

Survivorship-care plan: Develop an annually updated plan summarizing cGVHD status, complication screening, and QoL goals, shared with patient and local providers.

Education: Counsel on adherence to immunosuppression, sun protection (to reduce skin cancer risk), and symptom reporting. Provide written resources on cGVHD and post-HSCT care.

Lifestyle: Encourage Mediterranean diet, aerobic exercise (150 min/week as tolerated), and smoking cessation [66].

40.9 Conclusion

We have witnessed a paradigm shift in the field of HSCT in the last decade with respect to prevention of GVHD, early prognostication and risk stratification of acute GVHD, and newer therapeutic strategies for chronic GVHD. Management of steroid-refractory GVHD still remains a significant challenge; however, its outcomes have improved and are promising.

References

1. Jamy O, Zeiser R, Chen YB. Novel developments in the prophylaxis and treatment of acute GVHD. Blood. 2023;142(12):1037–46. https://doi.org/10.1182/blood.2023020073.
2. Malard F, Holler E, Sandmaier BM, et al. Acute graft-versus-host disease. Nat Rev Dis Primers. 2023;9(1):27. https://doi.org/10.1038/s41572-023-00438-1.
3. Holtan SG, DeFor TE, Lazaryan A, et al. Composite end point of graft-versus-host disease-free, relapse-free survival after allogeneic hematopoietic cell transplantation. Blood. 2015;125(8):1333–8. https://doi.org/10.1182/blood-2014-10-609032.
4. Kim HT, Logan B, Weisdorf DJ. Novel composite endpoints after allogeneic hematopoietic cell transplantation. Transplant Cell Ther. 2021;27(8):650–7. https://doi.org/10.1016/j.jtct.2021.05.005.
5. Gagelmann N, Ayuk F, Wolschke C, et al. Comparison of different rabbit anti-thymocyte globulin formulations in allogeneic stem cell transplantation: systematic literature review and network meta-analysis. Biol Blood Marrow Transplant. 2017;23(12):2184–91. https://doi.org/10.1016/j.bbmt.2017.08.027.
6. Notarantonio AB, Morisset S, Piucco R, et al. Differential clinical and immunological impacts of anti–T-lymphocyte globulin (ATLG) vs. anti-Thymocyte globulin (ATG) in preventing

graft-versus-host disease post-allogeneic hematopoietic stem cell transplantation: a comparative study. Am J Hematol. 2025;100:626–37. https://doi.org/10.1002/ajh.27619.
7. Luznik L, O'Donnell PV, Symons HJ, et al. HLA-haploidentical bone marrow transplantation for hematologic malignancies using nonmyeloablative conditioning and high-dose, posttransplantation cyclophosphamide. Biol Blood Marrow Transplant. 2008;14(6):641–50.
8. Bolaños-Meade J, Hamadani M, Wu J, et al. Post-transplantation cyclophosphamide-based graft-versus-host disease prophylaxis. N Engl J Med. 2023;388(25):2338–48. https://doi.org/10.1056/NEJMoa2215943.
9. Jurdi NE, Hoover A, O'Leary D, et al. Phase II study of myeloablative 7-8/8-matched allotransplantation with post-transplantation cyclophosphamide, tacrolimus, and mycophenolate mofetil. Transplant Cell Ther. 2023;29(9):576.e1–5. https://doi.org/10.1016/j.jtct.2023.06.008.
10. Takahashi T, Al-Kofahi M, Jaber M, et al. Higher abatacept exposure after transplant decreases acute GVHD risk without increasing adverse events. Blood. 2023;142(8):700–10. https://doi.org/10.1182/blood.2023020035.
11. Watkins B, Qayed M, McCracken C, et al. Phase II trial of costimulation blockade with abatacept for prevention of acute GVHD. J Clin Oncol. 2021;39(17):1865–77. https://doi.org/10.1200/JCO.20.01086.
12. Raghunandan S, Gorfinkel L, Graiser M, et al. Abatacept for the prevention of GVHD in patients receiving mismatched unrelated transplants: a real-world analysis. Blood Adv. 2023;7(16):4395–9. https://doi.org/10.1182/bloodadvances.2023010225.
13. Farag SS, Abu Zaid M, Schwartz JE, et al. Dipeptidyl peptidase 4 inhibition for prophylaxis of acute graft-versus-host disease. N Engl J Med. 2021;384(1):11–9. https://doi.org/10.1056/NEJMoa2027372.
14. Kandekar S, Punatar S, Khattry N, et al. Low levels of CD26 on certain cellular subtypes of donor harvest is associated with better clinical outcomes post allogeneic stem cell transplantation through regulation of NF-κB pathway and pro-inflammatory cytokines. Int Immunopharmacol. 2023;125(Pt A):111054. https://doi.org/10.1016/j.intimp.2023.111054.
15. Chen YB, Mohty M, Zeiser R, et al. Vedolizumab for the prevention of intestinal acute GVHD after allogeneic hematopoietic stem cell transplantation: a randomized phase 3 trial. Nat Med. 2024;30(8):2277–87. https://doi.org/10.1038/s41591-024-03016-4.
16. Luznik L, Pasquini MC, Logan B, et al. Randomized phase III BMT CTN trial of calcineurin inhibitor-free chronic graft-versus-host disease interventions in myeloablative hematopoietic cell transplantation for hematologic malignancies. J Clin Oncol. 2022;40(4):356–68. https://doi.org/10.1200/JCO.21.02293.
17. Al-Homsi AS, Cirrone F, Wo S, et al. PTCy, abatacept, and a short course of tacrolimus for GvHD prevention after haploidentical transplantation. Blood Adv. 2023;7(14):3604–11.
18. Al-Homsi AS, DeFor TE, Cole K, et al. CAST regimen for GvHD prophylaxis: a CIBMTR propensity score-matched analysis. Transplant Cell Ther. 2024;30(11):1092–8. https://doi.org/10.1016/j.jtct.2024.08.015.
19. Londono JAS, Cole K, Cirrone F, et al. LBA-3 - reducing Ptcy dose in patients receiving CAST for GvHD prevention results in accelerated engraftment at the cost of higher incidence of GvHD. Transplant Cell Therapy. 2024;30(2, Suppl):S488–9., ISSN 2666-6367. https://doi.org/10.1016/j.jtct.2024.02.010.
20. Abedin S, Furqan F, Runaas L, et al. Early safety and feasibility results from a phase II trial of De-escalated Ptcy and Ruxolitinib for Gvhd prophylaxis in older patients undergoing reduced intensity conditioning allogeneic HCT. Blood. 2024;144(Suppl 1):1039. https://doi.org/10.1182/blood-2024-200832.
21. Wu H, Shi J, Luo Y, et al. A multicenter randomized controlled trial of low-dose Ruxolitinib for Gvhd prophylaxis in Haploidentical hematopoietic stem cell transplantation. Blood. 2024;144(Suppl 1):1044. https://doi.org/10.1182/blood-2024-206823.
22. Meyer EH, Salhotra A, Gandhi AP, et al. Orca-T demonstrates improved survival free of chronic GvHD compared to conventional allogeneic hematopoietic stem cell transplant: a ran-

domized phase 3 trial in advanced hematologic malignancies. In: Presented at: 51st annual EBMT meeting. Florence, Italy; 2025. Abstract OS15-01.
23. Srour SA, Salhotra A, Lowsky R, et al. Safety and efficacy of orca-Q with Haploidentical donors for the treatment of advanced hematologic malignancies without the use of post-transplant cyclophosphamide. Blood. 2023;142(Suppl 1):773. https://doi.org/10.1182/blood-2023-189534.
24. Harris AC, Young R, Devine S, et al. International, multicenter standardization of acute graft-versus-host disease clinical data collection: a report from the Mount Sinai acute GVHD international consortium. Biol Blood Marrow Transplant. 2016;22(1):4–10. https://doi.org/10.1016/j.bbmt.2015.09.001.
25. Sharma N, Efebera Y. Acute graft-versus-host disease, prophylaxis and therapy. OBM Transplant. 2021;5(1) https://doi.org/10.21926/obm.transplant.2101139.
26. Major-Monfried H, Renteria AS, Pawarode A, et al. MAGIC biomarkers predict long-term outcomes for steroid-resistant acute GVHD. Blood. 2018;131(25):2846–55. https://doi.org/10.1182/blood-2018-01-822957.
27. MacMillan ML, Robin M, Harris AC, et al. A refined risk score for acute graft-versus-host disease that predicts response to initial therapy, survival, and transplant-related mortality. Biol Blood Marrow Transplant. 2015;21(4):761–7. https://doi.org/10.1016/j.bbmt.2015.01.001.
28. Ferrara JLM, Chaudhry MS. GVHD: biology matters. Blood Adv. 2018;2(22):3411–7. https://doi.org/10.1182/bloodadvances.2018020214.
29. Srinagesh HK, Ferrara JLM. MAGIC biomarkers of acute graft-versus-host disease: biology and clinical application. Best Pract Res Clin Haematol. 2019;32(4):101111. https://doi.org/10.1016/j.beha.2019.101111.
30. Etra A, El Jurdi N, Katsivelos N, et al. Amphiregulin, ST2, and REG3α biomarker risk algorithms as predictors of nonrelapse mortality in patients with acute GVHD. Blood Adv. 2024;8(12):3284–92. https://doi.org/10.1182/bloodadvances.2023011049.
31. Mohty M, Holler E, Jagasia M, et al. Refractory acute graft-versus-host disease: a new working definition beyond corticosteroid refractoriness. Blood. 2020;136(17):1903–6. https://doi.org/10.1182/blood.2020007336.
32. Martini DJ, Chen YB, DeFilipp Z. Recent FDA approvals in the treatment of graft-versus-host disease. Oncologist. 2022;27(8):685–93. https://doi.org/10.1093/oncolo/oyac076.
33. Bacigalupo A, Milone G, Cupri A, et al. Steroid treatment of acute graft-*versus*-host disease grade I: a randomized trial. Haematologica. 2017;102(12):2125–33. https://doi.org/10.3324/haematol.2017.171157.
34. Van Lint MT, Uderzo C, Locasciulli A, et al. Early treatment of acute graft-versus-host disease with high- or low-dose 6-methylprednisolone: a multicenter randomized trial from the Italian Group for Bone Marrow Transplantation. Blood. 1998;92(7):2288–93.
35. Mielcarek M, Furlong T, Storer BE, et al. Effectiveness and safety of lower dose prednisone for initial treatment of acute graft-versus-host disease: a randomized controlled trial. Haematologica. 2015;100(6):842–8. https://doi.org/10.3324/haematol.2014.118471.
36. Kujawska J, Zeiser R, Gil L. Recent advances in acute gastrointestinal graft versus host disease (aGvHD): aspects of steroid-resistant disease. Ann Hematol. 2025;104(2):855–65. https://doi.org/10.1007/s00277-024-05952-0.
37. Jagasia M, Perales MA, Schroeder MA, et al. Ruxolitinib for the treatment of steroid-refractory acute GVHD (REACH1): a multicenter, open-label phase 2 trial. Blood. 2020;135(20):1739–49. https://doi.org/10.1182/blood.2020004823.
38. Zeiser R, von Bubnoff N, Butler J, et al; REACH2 Trial Group. Ruxolitinib for glucocorticoid-refractory acute graft-versus-host disease. N Engl J Med. 2020;382(19):1800–1810. https://doi.org/10.1056/NEJMoa1917635.
39. Kurtzberg J, Abdel-Azim H, Carpenter P, et al; MSB-GVHD001/002 Study Group. A phase 3, single-arm, prospective study of Remestemcel-L, ex vivo culture-expanded adult human mesenchymal stromal cells for the treatment of pediatric patients who failed to respond to steroid treatment for acute graft-versus-host disease. Biol Blood Marrow Transplant. 2020;26(5):845–854. https://doi.org/10.1016/j.bbmt.2020.01.018.

40. FDA approves remestemcel-L-rknd for steroid-refractory acute graft versus host disease in pediatric patients. News release FDA; 2024. https://www.fda.gov/drugs/resources-information-approved-drugs/fda-approves-remestemcel-l-rknd-steroid-refractory-acute-graft-versus-host-disease-pediatric. Accessed December 18, 2024.
41. Kebriaei P, Hayes J, Daly A, et al. A phase 3 randomized study of Remestemcel-L versus placebo added to second-line therapy in patients with steroid-refractory acute graft-versus-host disease. Biol Blood Marrow Transplant. 2020;26(5):835–44. https://doi.org/10.1016/j.bbmt.2019.08.029.
42. Malard F, Gaugler B, Mohty M. Faecal microbiota transplantation in patients with haematological malignancies undergoing cellular therapies: from translational research to routine clinical practice. Lancet Haematol. 2022;9(10):e776–85. https://doi.org/10.1016/S2352-3026(22)00223-X.
43. Kakihana K, Fujioka Y, Suda W, et al. Fecal microbiota transplantation for patients with steroid-resistant acute graft-versus-host disease of the gut. Blood. 2016;128(16):2083–8.
44. Malard F, Loschi M, Huynh A, et al. Pooled allogeneic faecal microbiota MaaT013 for steroid-resistant gastrointestinal acute graft-versus-host disease: a single-arm, multicentre phase 2 trial. EClinicalMedicine. 2023;62:102111. https://doi.org/10.1016/j.eclinm.2023.102111.
45. Liu Y, Zhao Y, Qi J, et al. Fecal microbiota transplantation combined with ruxolitinib as a salvage treatment for intestinal steroid-refractory acute GVHD. Exp Hematol Oncol. 2022;11(1):96. https://doi.org/10.1186/s40164-022-00350-6.
46. Reddi S, Senyshyn L, Ebadi M, et al. Fecal microbiota transplantation to prevent acute graft-versus-host disease: pre-planned interim analysis of donor effect. Nat Commun. 2025;16:1034. https://doi.org/10.1038/s41467-025-56375-y.
47. Flowers MED, Inamoto Y, Carpenter PA, et al. Comparative analysis of risk factors for acute graft-versus-host disease and for chronic graft-versus-host disease according to National Institutes of Health consensus criteria. Blood. 2011;117(11):3214–9.
48. Lee SJ. Classification systems for chronic graft-versus-host disease. Blood. 2017;129(1):30–7. https://doi.org/10.1182/blood-2016-07-686642.
49. Bos S, Murray J, Marchetti M, et al. ERS/EBMT clinical practice guidelines on treatment of pulmonary chronic graft-versus-host disease in adults. Eur Respir J [Internet]. 2024 [cited 2025 May 1];63(3). Available from: https://publications.ersnet.org/content/erj/63/3/2301727
50. Williams KM, Cheng GS, Pusic I, et al. Fluticasone, azithromycin, and Montelukast treatment for new-onset bronchiolitis obliterans syndrome after hematopoietic cell transplantation. Biol Blood Marrow Transplant J Am Soc Blood Marrow Transplant. 2016;22(4):710–6.
51. Cheng GS, Bondeelle L, Gooley T, et al. Azithromycin use and increased cancer risk among patients with bronchiolitis obliterans after hematopoietic cell transplantation. Biol Blood Marrow Transplant J Am Soc Blood Marrow Transplant. 2020;26(2):392–400.
52. Vallet N, Le Grand S, Bondeelle L, et al. Azithromycin promotes relapse by disrupting immune and metabolic networks after allogeneic stem cell transplantation. Blood. 2022;140(23):2500–13.
53. Schoemans HM, Lee SJ, Ferrara JL, et al. EBMT-NIH-CIBMTR Task Force position statement on standardized terminology & guidance for graft-versus-host disease assessment. Bone Marrow Transplant. 2018;53(11):1401–15.
54. Zeiser R, Polverelli N, Ram R, et al. Ruxolitinib for glucocorticoid-refractory chronic graft-versus-host disease. N Engl J Med. 2021;385(3):228–38.
55. Cho A, Jantschitsch C, Knobler R. Extracorporeal photopheresis-An overview. Front Med. 2018;5:236.
56. Flowers MED, Apperley JF, van Besien K, et al. A multicenter prospective phase 2 randomized study of extracorporeal photopheresis for treatment of chronic graft-versus-host disease. Blood. 2008;112(7):2667–74.
57. Couriel DR, Hosing C, Saliba R, et al. Extracorporeal photochemotherapy for the treatment of steroid-resistant chronic GVHD. Blood. 2006;107(8):3074–80.
58. Lucid CE, Savani BN, Engelhardt BG, et al. Extracorporeal photopheresis in patients with refractory bronchiolitis obliterans developing after allo-SCT. Bone Marrow Transplant. 2011;46(3):426–9.

59. Wolff D, Fatobene G, Rocha V, et al. Steroid-refractory chronic graft-versus-host disease: treatment options and patient management. Bone Marrow Transplant. 2021;56(9):2079–87.
60. Miklos D, Cutler CS, Arora M, et al. Ibrutinib for chronic graft-versus-host disease after failure of prior therapy. Blood. 2017;130(21):2243–50.
61. Miklos DB, Abu Zaid M, Cooney JP, et al. Ibrutinib for first-line treatment of chronic graft-versus-host disease: results from the randomized phase III iNTEGRATE study. J Clin Oncol Off J Am Soc Clin Oncol. 2023;41(10):1876–87.
62. Cutler C, Lee SJ, Arai S, et al. Belumosudil for chronic graft-versus-host disease after 2 or more prior lines of therapy: the ROCKstar study. Blood. 2021;138(22):2278–89.
63. Wolff D, Cutler C, Lee SJ, et al. Axatilimab in recurrent or refractory chronic graft-versus-host disease. N Engl J Med. 2024;391(11):1002–14.
64. Holtzman NG, Im A, Ostojic A, et al. Efficacy and safety of Baricitinib in refractory chronic graft-versus-host disease (cGVHD): preliminary analysis results of a phase 1/2 study. Blood. 2020;136:1.
65. McManus T, Holtzman NG, Zhao A, et al. Systemic treatment with the Janus kinase inhibitor Baricitinib in ocular chronic graft-versus-host disease. Ophthalmol Sci. 2025;5(1):100627.
66. Rotz SJ, Bhatt NS, Hamilton BK, et al. International recommendations for screening and preventative practices for long-term survivors of transplantation and cellular therapy: a 2023 update. Transplant Cell Ther. 2024;30(4):349–85.
67. McQuellon RP, Russell GB, Cella DF, et al. Quality of life measurement in bone marrow transplantation: development of the functional assessment of cancer therapy-bone marrow transplant (FACT-BMT) scale. Bone Marrow Transplant. 1997;19(4):357–68.
68. Lee SJ, Cook EF, Soiffer R, et al. Development and validation of a scale to measure symptoms of chronic graft-versus-host disease. Biol Blood Marrow Transplant. 2002;8(8):444–52.
69. Mirgh S, Surendran A, Punatar S, et al. Second primary malignancies post autologous stem-cell transplant in multiple Myeloma from India—Knowing the Unknown. Indian J Hematol Blood Transfus. 2025; https://doi.org/10.1007/s12288-025-01984-2.

Chapter 41
The Role of Allogeneic Stem Cell Transplantation in Philadelphia Positive Acute Lymphoblastic Leukemia in the Era of Second- and Third-Generation TKI

Tommy Alfaro Moya and Rajat Kumar

Abstract Philadelphia-positive acute lymphoblastic leukemia (Ph + ALL) has historically been associated with a poor prognosis. The advent of tyrosine kinase inhibitors (TKIs) has significantly improved treatment outcomes, shifting the therapeutic landscape away from traditional chemotherapy-based approaches. Second-generation (dasatinib, nilotinib, bosutinib) and third-generation (ponatinib) TKIs have shown superior efficacy, deeper molecular responses, and improved survival rates. The role of allogeneic hematopoietic cell transplantation (allo-HCT) in the era of modern TKIs remains a subject of ongoing debate. Traditionally, allo-HCT was the only curative strategy; however, it was associated with transplant-related mortality (TRM) and graft-vs-host disease (GVHD), hence the survival benefit was controversial. Recent studies suggest that patients achieving deep molecular remission on TKI-based regimens may no longer require transplant. This chapter reviews the evolving role of allo-HCT in Ph + ALL, assessing its indications, timing, outcomes, and the integration of novel therapies such as monoclonal antibodies and chimeric antigen receptor T-cell (CAR-T) therapy. We discuss post-transplant TKI maintenance strategies, long-term complications, and emerging data on transplant-free approaches. A real-world clinical case is included to illustrate current decision-making in Ph + ALL.

Keywords Ph + ALL · Tyrosine kinase inhibitors · Allogeneic hematopoietic cell transplantation · Measurable residual disease

T. Alfaro Moya · R. Kumar (✉)
University of Toronto, Department of Medical Oncology and Hematology, Princess Margaret Cancer Centre, Toronto, ON, Canada
e-mail: tommy.alfaromoya@uhn.ca; rajat.kumar@uhn.ca

H. P. Pati et al. (eds.), *Clinical Hematology and Hemato-Oncology*,
https://doi.org/10.1007/978-981-92-1167-8_41

Learning Objectives

By the end of this chapter, readers will be able to

- Understand the role of second- and third-generation TKIs in Ph + ALL treatment.
- Discuss transplant-free approaches for select patients achieving deep molecular remission.
- Evaluate the necessity and optimal timing of allo-HCT in the TKI era.
- Recognize post-transplant challenges and the role of TKI maintenance therapy.
- Integrate novel immunotherapies into Ph + ALL management.

41.1 Introduction

Philadelphia-positive acute lymphoblastic leukemia (Ph + ALL) is a distinct subtype of ALL characterized by the t(9;22) translocation, it arises from a reciprocal translocation between the ABL1 oncogene located on the long arm of chromosome 9 and the breakpoint cluster region (BCR) on the long arm of chromosome 22, leading to the formation of the BCR-ABL fusion gene. This fusion gene encodes an oncogenic protein with constitutive tyrosine kinase activity, leading to uncontrolled cell proliferation, driving leukemogenesis, and is a key therapeutic target.

The Philadelphia chromosome (Ph) was the first cytogenetic abnormality identified in human cancer, specifically in chronic myeloid leukemia (CML) [1]. Ph + ALL is rare in children (<5% of cases), and it is significantly more prevalent in adults, with its incidence increasing with age [2]. The Philadelphia chromosome is the most common cytogenetic abnormality in adult ALL, occurring in 20–30% of cases. Its prevalence increases with age, affecting up to 50% of individuals over 50 [3–5]. Patients with Ph + ALL have a typical clinical presentation of bone marrow infiltration syndromes with pancytopenia; however, a higher incidence of central nervous system (CNS) disease and higher white blood cell count can be present at diagnosis [6]. Historically, Ph + ALL was associated with poor prognosis due to its aggressive nature and resistance to standard chemotherapy, making allogeneic hematopoietic cell transplantation (allo-HCT) the only curative treatment option for patients able to achieve a complete remission (CR). Despite the use of allo-HCT, the long-term outcomes of these patients were unfavorable due to high transplant-related mortality (TRM), graft-versus-host disease (GVHD), and relapse. Imatinib was the first TKI tested in Ph + ALL, improving prognosis by increasing the number of patients undergoing Allo-HCT in first complete remission (CR1) and reducing disease burden before transplant [7, 8]. The introduction of TKIs, initially developed for CML, has significantly improved outcomes for Ph + ALL patients by enabling deeper molecular responses and challenging the long-standing paradigm of routine allo-HCT for all eligible patients. More potent second- and third-generation TKIs, such as dasatinib, nilotinib, and ponatinib, have shown potential to improve outcomes even without allo-HCT, though no randomized trials comparing these TKIs in adults have been conducted [9–11]. Managing Ph + ALL involves careful decisions about TKI selection and timing, the use of chemotherapy, the need for allo-HCT, and monitoring measurable residual disease (MRD). This chapter covers key treatment principles, ongoing debates, challenges, and recent updates in adult Ph + ALL care.

41.2 Tyrosine Kinase Inhibitors in the Treatment of Ph + ALL

Ph + ALL is characterized by the BCR-ABL1 fusion protein, which drives leukemogenesis and makes the disease highly susceptible to TKIs. The introduction of TKIs has revolutionized Ph + ALL treatment, shifting the therapeutic approach from intensive chemotherapy-based regimens to TKI-based strategies that emphasize molecular response and targeted therapy [12]. The treatment of Ph + ALL involves a multi-phase strategy aiming for rapid remission, long-term disease control, and potential cure. Induction therapy is tailored to a patient's age, fitness level, and disease risk, balancing treatment intensity and toxicity. The primary goal is to achieve CR, minimizing disease burden, and inducing a deep molecular response.

41.3 The Role of TKIs in Frontline Therapy

Clinical trials have demonstrated that TKIs, either alone or combined with minimal chemotherapy, can induce remission in over 90% of patients with Ph + ALL [13]. TKIs are typically used alongside either low-intensity chemotherapy (e.g., steroids, vincristine) or intensive chemotherapy regimens such as hyperfractionated cyclophosphamide, vincristine, doxorubicin, dexamethasone (Hyper-CVAD) or Berlin-Frankfurt-Münster (BFM)-based protocols.

41.3.1 Imatinib: First-Generation TKI

Imatinib was the first TKI approved for Ph + ALL, significantly improving survival when combined with chemotherapy. The UKALLXII/ECOG2993 trial evaluated its role in treatment outcomes by comparing patients treated before and after its introduction [14]. The study included 266 patients in the pre-imatinib cohort and 175 in the imatinib cohort. CR rates improved from 82% to 92%, and four-year overall survival (OS) increased from 22% to 38%. Additionally, event-free survival (EFS) improved from 18% to 33%, and relapse-free survival (RFS) rose from 33% to 50%. The early introduction of imatinib led to better outcomes, increasing the rate of allo-HCT from 31% to 46%.

Despite its benefits, the study confirmed that allo-HCT remains essential for optimal long-term survival, as patients who underwent myeloablative allo-HCT had the highest survival rates. While imatinib improved early treatment response, its benefit beyond increasing transplant eligibility was modest. Imatinib remains approved by the US Food and Drug Administration (FDA) and the European Medicines Agency (EMA) for Ph + ALL but has largely been replaced by second- and third-generation TKIs.

41.3.2 Dasatinib: Second-Generation TKI

Dasatinib, a second-generation TKI, is frequently used in Ph + ALL due to its potency and ability to cross the blood-brain barrier, making it particularly useful for patients with CNS involvement.

A phase 2 study at MD Anderson Cancer Center investigated dasatinib combined with Hyper-CVAD as frontline therapy in 35 newly diagnosed patients (median age: 53) [15]. The CR rate was 94%, with a two-year OS of 64%. A long-term follow-up (expanded to 72 patients) confirmed the durability of response, with a CR rate of 96%, median disease-free survival (DFS) of 31 months, and OS of 47 months [16]. Major molecular response (MMR) was achieved by 93% of patients, with 94% achieving measurable residual disease (MRD) negativity within three weeks. Despite 39 deaths (19 due to relapse, seven post-allo-HCT), the study suggested that some patients might achieve long-term survival without transplantation, particularly with TKI maintenance.

The EWALL-PH-01 study evaluated dasatinib with low-intensity chemotherapy in elderly patients ($\geq$ 55 years). Among 71 enrolled patients, 96% achieved CR, and five-year OS was 36%, increasing to 45% when adjusting for non-disease-related deaths. Only seven patients underwent allo-HCT, indicating that dasatinib-based regimens may allow some older patients to avoid transplant [17]. However, 36 patients relapsed, and 75% of those tested post-relapse had the T315I mutation, which confers resistance to dasatinib.

41.3.3 Nilotinib: Alternative Second-Generation TKI

The Korean multicenter phase 2 trial assessed nilotinib with chemotherapy in 90 newly diagnosed patients with Ph + ALL (ages 17–71) [10]. The CR rate was 91%, and the cumulative complete molecular remission (CMR) rate reached 94%, with a two-year OS of 72%. Patients who failed to achieve early molecular remission had a significantly higher risk of relapse, emphasizing the importance of MRD monitoring.

The EWALL-PH02 trial, conducted by the European Working Group for Adult ALL, investigated nilotinib with low-intensity chemotherapy in elderly patients (≥55 years) [18]. Among 79 enrolled patients (72 evaluable), CR was achieved in 94.4%, with a four-year OS of 47%. Notably, patients who underwent allo-HCT (32% of the cohort) had a higher survival rate (61%) than those who did not (39%). These results highlight nilotinib-based regimens as an effective, less toxic alternative, although MRD monitoring remains critical for guiding transplant decisions.

41.3.4 Ponatinib: Third-Generation TKI

Ponatinib, a third-generation TKI, has demonstrated superior efficacy in achieving deep molecular responses, prolonging survival, and potentially reducing the need for allo-HCT, particularly in patients with the T315I mutation.

A meta-analysis by Jabbour et al. compared ponatinib-based therapy with first- and second-generation TKIs across 26 clinical trials [19]. Ponatinib achieved a complete molecular response (CMR) rate of 79%, significantly higher than earlier TKIs (34%). Two-year OS was also superior (83% vs. 58%), and three-year OS was 79% compared to 50% with earlier TKIs.

Jabbour et al. (2018) reported on a single-center phase 2 study with a median follow-up of 36 months [11]. Their findings demonstrated that all patients with active disease achieved complete remission, with 97% attaining major molecular response and 83% reaching complete molecular response. The estimated three-year event-free survival and overall survival rates were 70% and 76%, respectively. Notably, while 20% of patients underwent allo-HCT, the study found no significant survival advantage in those who received transplantation compared to those who did not. Cardiovascular toxicity, particularly arterial thrombotic events, emerged as a concern in patients receiving ponatinib at an initial dose of 45 mg daily. However, after protocol adjustments reducing the dose in a response-adapted manner, toxicity was mitigated without compromising efficacy.

Expanding on this research, Kantarjian et al. (2023) presented an updated long-term analysis with a median follow-up of 80 months, further substantiating the high efficacy of ponatinib in combination with hyper-CVAD [20]. Among 86 treated patients, all achieved complete remission, and 86% attained CMR. The estimated six-year EFS and OS rates were 65% and 75%, respectively. Importantly, only 23% of patients underwent allo-HCT, reinforcing prior findings that CMR achievement may negate the need for transplant in many cases. The study also confirmed that the implementation of a dose-modified ponatinib regimen (starting at 45 mg and reducing to 30 mg or 15 mg based on molecular response) effectively reduced the incidence of severe cardiovascular adverse events while maintaining the high remission rates. Compared to earlier generations of TKIs, ponatinib was shown to provide superior suppression of BCR-ABL1 T315I-mutated clones, which are associated with treatment resistance and disease relapse.

Both studies highlight the paradigm shift in the treatment of Ph + ALL, with ponatinib-based regimens offering an alternative to traditional TKI-chemotherapy approaches that required routine Allo-HCT. The high rates of durable molecular remission suggest that a significant proportion of patients can achieve long-term survival without transplantation. Moreover, optimized dosing strategies for ponatinib have mitigated cardiovascular risks, a critical consideration for long-term therapy.

41.3.5 Next-Generation TKIs

A phase 1 study conducted by Luskin et al. investigated the combination of asciminib, dasatinib, and prednisone for the treatment of newly diagnosed Ph + ALL and chronic myeloid leukemia in lymphoid blast crisis (CML-LBC) [21]. Given that resistance mutations frequently emerge in patients treated with dasatinib alone, the trial aimed to assess whether dual inhibition of BCR-ABL1 with asciminib, an allosteric inhibitor, could enhance responses and prevent the development of resistance. The study enrolled 24 patients, predominantly with de novo Ph + ALL, and determined that the recommended phase 2 dose of asciminib was 80 mg daily in combination with dasatinib 140 mg and prednisone. The regimen was well tolerated, with the primary dose-limiting toxicity being asymptomatic grade 3 pancreatic enzyme elevation. Hematologic and cytogenetic remission rates were high, with 100% of patients achieving complete hematologic remission at day 84, with 89% reaching MRD negativity by flow cytometry. Additionally, the study demonstrated that molecular responses deepened over time, with 74% of patients achieving a BCR-ABL1 transcript level of <0.1% by reverse transcription quantitative polymerase chain reaction (RT-qPCR).

The safety profile of this combination therapy was favorable, with no treatment-related mortality and minimal high-grade toxicities, aside from some cases of dasatinib-related pleural effusions. Importantly, the study found that dual BCR-ABL1 inhibition mitigated the development of resistance-associated mutations, a frequent challenge in Ph + ALL management. Although the study supported the effectiveness of this approach, several patients still required allo-HCT for long-term disease control.

Response to different TKIs, with or without transplant, is shown in Table 41.1.

Table 41.1 Response to TKIs with or without allo-HCT in Ph + ALL: key studies

Study	Number of patients and study type	Intervention	Main outcomes
Jabbour et al. (2018) [19]	Meta-analysis of 26 studies	Ponatinib + chemotherapy vs. earlier TKIs	Ponatinib + chemotherapy had higher CMR (79% vs. 34%) and 3-year OS (79% vs. 50%) compared to earlier TKIs
Foa et al. (2020) [27]	63 patients, phase 2 trial	Dasatinib + blinatumomab (chemo-free regimen)	Dasatinib + blinatumomab chemo-free regimen led to 60% molecular response and 3-year OS of 95%
Takiar et al. (2022) [35]	40 patients, retrospective cohort	TKI therapy pre- and post-allo-HCT	CMR before transplant improved EFS but not OS; high GVHD incidence (acute 62.5%, chronic 77.5%)
Kantarjian et al. (2023) [20]	86 patients, 80-month follow-up, prospective study	Ponatinib + hyper-CVAD	6-year OS/EFS: 75%/65%. No survival difference between allo-HCT and non-Allo-HCT groups
Chiaretti et al. (2023) [36]	74 patients, prospective study	Blinatumomab-based chemo-free regimen	High MRD-negative rates and long-term survival with minimal need for allo-HCT

ALL acute lymphoblastic leukemia; *Ph + ALL* Philadelphia positive acute lymphoblastic leukemia; *Allo-HCT* allogeneic hematopoietic cell transplantation; *CMR* complete molecular remission; *CR1* first complete remission; *EFS* event-free survival; *FTBI* fractionated total body irradiation; *GVHD* graft-versus-host disease; *MRD* measurable residual disease; *OS* overall survival; *RFS* relapse-free survival; *TKI* tyrosine kinase inhibitor; *Hyper-CVAD* hyperfractionated cyclophosphamide, vincristine, doxorubicin, and dexamethasone alternating with high dose methotrexate and cytarabine

41.4 The Evolving Role of Hematopoietic Stem Cell Transplantation in Ph + ALL

Allogeneic hematopoietic stem cell transplantation has long been considered the definitive curative approach for Ph + ALL, particularly for patients with MRD positivity following induction and consolidation therapy. The advent of TKIs has dramatically improved outcomes, reducing the historical dependence on transplantation [22]. However, allo-HCT remains an essential therapeutic strategy for many high-risk patients. The decision to proceed with transplant is primarily guided by MRD status, early treatment response, patient fitness, and donor availability.

Historically, allo-HCT was recommended for all patients achieving CR1 due to the high relapse rates associated with chemotherapy alone. With the introduction of more potent TKIs, many patients can now achieve deep molecular responses and long-term disease control without transplantation. As a result, transplant is increasingly reserved for high-risk patients, particularly those with persistent MRD after induction, poor early response, or additional cytogenetic abnormalities [23]. Allo-HCT is indicated in patients not achieving remission in a timely manner (indicating resistant disease) or in those relapsing after achieving remission, provided the transplant is safe and feasible.

Recent studies, including those by Ghobadi et al. and Nishiwaki et al., highlight the evolving role of MRD in transplant decision-making [22, 24]. Patients achieving deep MRD negativity (BCR-ABL1 transcript <0.01%) within three months of treatment may achieve long-term survival without allo-HCT, particularly when treated with ponatinib- or blinatumomab-based regimens [23]. In a study of 85 patients, those patients with CMR at 3 months had excellent long-term prognosis and likely did not require allo-HCT in first remission [25].

Conversely, persistent MRD positivity (>0.01%) at three months remains a high-risk feature associated with relapse and poor survival, reinforcing the need for allo-HCT [24].

The decision to transplant is based on a combination of factors. Beyond MRD status, age and comorbidities significantly influence transplant eligibility. Older patients (>60 years) often cannot tolerate myeloablative conditioning and may benefit from reduced-intensity conditioning or prolonged TKI therapy without transplant [23]. Frail patients may derive greater benefit from chemo-free regimens, such as blinatumomab-TKI combinations, which offer durable remissions without allo-HCT [26, 27].

41.5 Treatment-Free Remission in Non-transplanted Patients

In Ph + ALL, patients must continue TKIs lifelong. It is not known if some patients can stop TKIs and remain in remission. Treatment-free remission in chronic myeloid leukemia is a desired goal, but is it possible in Ph + ALL? In a study at MD Anderson Cancer Center, a retrospective analysis was performed on patients with Ph + ALL who achieved CR after chemotherapy along with TKIs, then achieved a complete molecular response and subsequently discontinued TKIs primarily due to side effects [28]. A total of 14 patients were identified. Their median duration of TKI treatment was 60 months, while the median duration of CMR before TKI discontinuation was 46.1 months. On follow-up of a median of 42.5 months, 11 patients (79%) remained in maintenance-free remission. Three patients relapsed, and two of these regained CMR on resuming TKI therapy. The study concluded that TKI discontinuation may be safe for highly selected patients in first CR who maintain CMR for at least 48 months [28].

41.6 Type of TKI Pre-allo-HCT

In the era of TKIs, most patients would have received a TKI during induction or consolidation, based on the standard of care, mutation status, and cost factors. The aim of these agents is to have the deepest molecular response pre-transplant, for the best outcomes. It is not clear if the type of TKI can influence the post-transplant outcomes. In a retrospective analysis of more than 600 patients who had

Table 41.2 Outcomes of allo-HCT in Ph + ALL in selected trials

Ref	Pre allo-HCT therapy	Patient numbers	Donor choice	Outcomes
Fielding et al. [14]	DNR/VCR/Pred/L-asp	75	MRD/MUD	5-yr OS MRD-44%; MUD 39%
Chiaretti et al. 2016 [40]	Imatinib +HAM	20	MRD/MUD/ Haplo	Benefit from Allo-HCT in OS and DFS
Ravandi et al. 2016 [9]	Dasatinib + HyperCVAD	41	MRD/MUD	12 m OS 87% 12 m RFS 83%
Ribera et al. 2024 [37]	Ponatinib + DNR/VCR/ Pred	26	MRD/MUD	3-yr OS 96% 3-yr EFS 70%
Ghobadi A et al. 2022 [22]	Imatinib/dasatinib/ ponatinib + HyperCVAD	98	MRD/MUD/ MMUD/cord blood	5-yr OS 58% 5-yr RFS 63%
Nishiwaki et al. 2024 [24]	Imatinib/dasatinib + chemotherapy	101	MRD/MUD/ MMUD/cord blood	5-yr OS 73% 5-yr RFS 70%

Adapted from Jamy O and Badar T [30] and Luskin MR 2024 [52]
allo-HCT allogeneic hematopoietic cell transplantation; *DNR* daunorubicin; *VCR* vincristine; *Pred* prednisolone; *L-asp* L-asparaginase; *HAM* cytarabine +mitoxantrone +G-CSF; *HyperCVAD* hyperfractionated cyclophosphamide, vincristine, doxorubicin, and dexamethasone alternating with high dose methotrexate and cytarabine; *MRD* matched related donor; *MUD* matched unrelated donor; *MMUD* mismatched unrelated donors; *OS* overall survival; *DFS* disease free survival; *RFS* relapse free survival; *EFS* event free survival.

undergone allo-HCT after receiving imatinib, dasatinib, or both, there was no advantage of one agent over the other in terms of survival. However, the use of dasatinib was associated with an increased risk of severe graft versus host disease [29].

Historically, allo-HCT was associated with high TRM, mainly in the form of GVHD and conditioning toxicity [30]. In the pre-TKI era, the main benefit of allo-HCT was a lower relapse, but a high TRM, hence there was no major benefit in overall survival. A summary of selected studies on allo-HCT is shown in Table 41.2. Over time, with better protocols for conditioning, GVHD prophylaxis, and control of disease with TKIs, the outcomes have improved [30].

41.7 Post-transplant TKIs

The risk of relapse after allo-HCT can be reduced or prevented using post-transplant TKIs. There is no consensus on the universal use of TKIs post-transplant, the agent of choice, or the duration of administration. TKIs can be used as prophylaxis when administration starts during complete molecular remission (CMR). Alternatively, these can be started on detection of MRD positivity. Prophylactic TKIs appear especially beneficial for patients not in CMR at the time of allo-HCT, while an

MRD-triggered TKI administration seems effective in low-risk patients [31]. Studies by Candoni et al. and Liu et al. demonstrate that ponatinib or dasatinib maintenance following transplant improves disease-free survival (DFS) by up to 50% [32, 33]. Patients with detectable MRD post allo-HCT should continue TKI therapy indefinitely to prevent relapse.

41.8 Future Directions

41.8.1 Optimizing Chemotherapy-Free Regimens for Ph + ALL

Chemotherapy-free regimens for Ph + ALL have advanced significantly over the past two decades. Early studies established the feasibility of TKIs as induction therapy, reducing reliance on cytotoxic agents. Vignetti et al. (2007) and Foà et al. (2011) demonstrated that imatinib or dasatinib plus steroids could achieve high remission rates without intensive chemotherapy, particularly in elderly patients [38, 39]. Subsequent studies refined TKI-based approaches, with Chiaretti et al. (2016) highlighting the role of MRD in treatment decisions, and Wieduwilt et al. (2021) supporting dasatinib plus dexamethasone induction, though allo-HCT remained a key strategy [49, 40]. More recent trials reinforced the shift toward targeted therapies. Sugiura et al. (2022) and Martinelli et al. (2022) showed that early molecular responders on dasatinib or ponatinib-based regimens might avoid allo-HCT [41, 42]. The landmark D-ALBA study (Foà et al., 2020) combined dasatinib with blinatumomab, achieving high molecular remission rates and reducing transplant need [27]. Jabbour et al. (2022) confirmed the effectiveness of dasatinib-blinatumomab and ponatinib-blinatumomab, reporting three-year OS of 80% and CMR rates of 86% [23].

Recent findings emphasize the durability and applicability of these regimens. Advani et al. (2023) validated dasatinib-blinatumomab as a viable option for elderly patients, with a three-year OS of 87% [43]. Foà et al. (2024) reaffirmed long-term response durability from the D-ALBA trial, reinforcing MRD's role in guiding therapy [44]. Meanwhile, Tang et al.(2024) introduced olverembatinib plus venetoclax, demonstrating promising molecular remission rates [45]. Chiaretti et al. (2023) compared dasatinib- and ponatinib-based chemo-free regimens, confirming both as highly effective with minimal toxicity [36].

41.8.2 Expanded Use of CAR-T Therapy

The integration of chimeric antigen receptor (CAR) T-cell therapy into the treatment paradigm for Ph + ALL represents a significant advancement in therapeutic strategies. The phase 2 study by Zhang et al. evaluated dasatinib in combination with CD19 and CD22 CAR-T cell therapy as a first-line treatment for newly diagnosed Ph + ALL [46]. This trial demonstrated high rates of CMR, with 72.2% of patients achieving CMR following CD19 CAR-T cell therapy, increasing to 76.9% after subsequent CD22 CAR-T cell therapy. Notably, no patients underwent allo-HCT, and the approach was associated with minimal toxicity, with no cases of severe cytokine release syndrome (CRS) or immune effector cell-associated neurotoxicity syndrome (ICANS). The findings suggest that dasatinib in combination with sequential CAR-T cell therapy offers a chemotherapy-free strategy capable of achieving deep and sustained remissions in Ph + ALL.

Similarly, a study by Yao et al. explored the role of CD19 CAR-T cell therapy in Ph + ALL patients who failed to achieve CMR at three months [47]. The study emphasized that persistent measurable residual disease is a predictor of poor long-term outcomes and that CAR-T cell therapy offers a potential salvage option. Among 13 patients treated with CD19 CAR-T cells, nine achieved CMR, and nine subsequently underwent allo-HCT, all achieving full donor chimerism. The study highlighted that early intervention with CAR-T therapy in patients with persistent MRD may improve long-term outcomes, although some patients still experienced antigen escapes or required further interventions. The findings underscore the need for continued refinement in CAR-T cell therapy strategies, particularly regarding optimizing timing and consolidation approaches.

Another study by Chen et al. investigated a novel consolidation strategy involving CD19 CAR-T cells, CD19+ feeding T cells (FTCs), and TKIs for Ph + ALL [48]. This phase 1 trial demonstrated that sequential administration of CD19 CAR-T cells with CD19+ FTCs resulted in durable responses, with 92% of patients achieving CMR and an OS rate of 83% at 27 months of follow-up. Importantly, the strategy avoided allo-HCT while maintaining strong efficacy. The study provided valuable insights into the durability of CAR-T cell responses and suggested that antigen stimulation via CD19+ FTCs could prolong CAR-T cell persistence, potentially reducing the risk of relapse. These findings contribute to an evolving shift in the management of Ph + ALL, where CAR-T therapy, particularly in combination with TKIs, may reduce dependence on allo-HCT.

41.9 A Clinical Case Example

A 35-year-old male was diagnosed with Philadelphia-positive B-ALL. He presented with fatigue and skin bruising. Clinical examination showed mild pallor, no lymphadenopathy, and spleen palpable 3 cm below the coastal margin. Blood counts revealed: Hb 100 g/l, WBC 2.8 × 10^9/L, platelets 20 × 10^9/L, neutrophils 0.5 × 10^9/L, lymphocytes 1.82 × 10^9/L and blasts present. A bone marrow aspirate showed a hypercellular marrow with 90% lymphoblasts. Cytogenetics: 46 XY, t(9;22) present. BCR-ABL1 positive; breakpoint p 190. CSF was clear. He was diagnosed with Ph + ALL. Treatment was commenced with the HyperCVAD protocol and Imatinib. He achieved complete remission (CR) in 6 weeks. BCR-ABL transcripts showed a 4.6 log reduction.

As there was a good molecular response, he was kept on the chemotherapy + imatinib 400 mg daily regimen. Due to hepatotoxicity, imatinib was changed to dasatinib 70 mg daily. BCR-ABL was undetectable in 3 months.

Three years later, he developed headaches. Investigations revealed a central nervous system (CNS) relapse. There was no hematologic relapse. BCR-ABL was detectable in blood and bone marrow. He was treated with Blinatumumab + Ponatinib 15 mg daily + CNS treatment (intrathecal triple therapy). CR was achieved and CNS was clear in 4 weeks.

He was referred for an allo-HCT. There was only a haplo-identical sibling donor available. He underwent a myeloablative conditioning (Etoposide + TBI 1200), with peripheral blood stem cells (PBSC) infused with an adequate $CD34^+$ cell dose of 7.4×10^6/Kg. Graft vs host disease prophylaxis consisted of post-transplant cyclophosphamide (PTCY) + anti-thymocyte globulin (ATG) + cyclosporine. He had neutrophil engraftment on day +18 and platelet engraftment on day +20.

Post transplant, he had multiple complications: acute GVHD grade III (gastrointestinal and skin) and chronic GVHD-extensive (skin, eyes, liver, and lungs). He required high doses of immune suppression, including intravenous methylprednisolone 2 mg/kg followed by tapering doses of steroids, cyclosporine, extracorporeal photophoresis (ECP), and ruxolitinib. He suffered from several infectious complications, the major ones being (a) EBV viremia and EBV colitis, requiring Rituximab, (b) Pseudomonas bacteremia, (c) BK virus hemorrhagic cystitis, (d) multiple episodes of bacteremia and pneumonia, (e) Covid −19 infection, and (f) RSV pneumonia. Due to the GVHD and organ dysfunction, he could not be started on TKI maintenance. Over the next three years, he gradually recovered. Immunosuppression was stopped.

At this point, he could have been started on prophylactic TKIs to reduce the risk of relapse. The risk was the potential side effects, especially due to the organ damage secondary to GVHD. It is also well known that chronic GVHD is associated with graft-versus-leukemia (GVL) effect, hence the risk of relapse would be presumed to be low.

Hence, it was debatable if the use of prophylactic TKI was required in his management. After discussion with the patient, assessing the risks and benefits, it was decided to monitor for MRD and initiate TKIs only if MRD was detectable. Patient remains in complete molecular remission. He is off all immunosuppression. He may be deemed as cured of his Ph + ALL but has sequelae of chronic GHVD.

41.10 Role of Allo-HCT

Despite these advances in precision medicine, allogeneic hematopoietic cell transplantation remains a powerful therapeutic option for patients with Ph + ALL. The decision to proceed to transplant versus continue with non-transplant therapy in first complete remission varies according to the policy of the concerned centre. The kinetics of response to primary treatment of Ph + ALL can provide guidance.

Monitoring the kinetics of MRD during therapy can predict the risk of relapse without transplant. Persistence of MRD, recurrence of MRD, additional genomic lesions (like IKZF1plus), ABL mutations, or frank relapse are clear indications of allo-HCT. The decision also depends on transplant-related factors: the patient's age, fitness, type of donor, caregiver support, and willingness to undergo allo-HCT with its risk of early TRM. These decisions are also influenced by the resources for MRD monitoring, availability of next-generation TKIs, immunotherapies like blinatumumab, and newer therapies like CAR-T cells. These novel therapies may be more challenging than an allo-HCT where there is a good donor, and the initial high cost of transplant may be less than prolonged monitoring and sequential TKIs and other innovative therapies. For any decision, the patient should be counselled on the different options, costs, risks, and benefits. A proposed algorithm is shown in Fig. 41.1. The decision to proceed to transplant should be a joint decision between the primary hematologist, transplant physician, and the patient.

In early allo-HCT trials, the donors were either limited to matched related or unrelated donors. With the advent of post-transplant cyclophosphamide (PTCY), it is now possible to utilise haploidentical donors for patients lacking a MRD or MUD donor [49]. There have been major advances in GVHD prophylaxis, especially with the use of PTCY [50]. Early trials used myeloablative conditioning, which was associated with high TRM. With the use of reduced intensity conditioning (RIC), older patients have less toxicity and TRM, resulting in better outcomes [51].

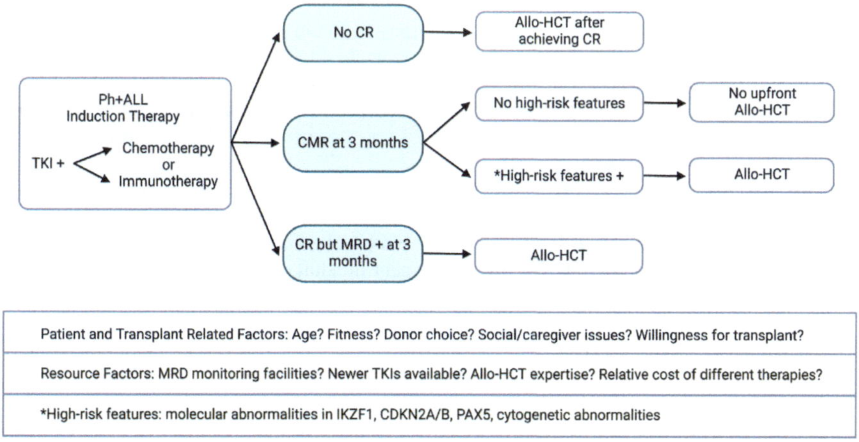

Fig. 41.1 Proposed algorithm for transplant in Ph + ALL

41.11 Conclusions

The management of Philadelphia chromosome-positive acute lymphoblastic leukemia has undergone a significant transformation with the advent of second- and third-generation tyrosine kinase inhibitors and the integration of immunotherapies. Historically, allo-HCT was considered the standard of care for long-term disease control. However, accumulating evidence from clinical trials suggests that patients achieving deep molecular remission with TKI-based regimens, particularly those incorporating ponatinib or blinatumomab, may not require allo-HCT.

Emerging chemo-free regimens, combining potent TKIs with immunotherapies such as blinatumomab, have reduced treatment-related toxicity, improved quality of life, and increased survival rates, further reshaping treatment paradigms. Additionally, CAR-T therapy and novel TKIs, such as asciminib, offer promising options for relapsed/refractory disease, reinforcing the trend toward precision medicine in Ph + ALL.

Moving forward, future research should focus on refining transplant-free strategies, optimizing MRD-based decision-making, and integrating novel immunotherapeutic agents to further improve outcomes while minimizing treatment-related morbidity. As clinical trials continue to define the optimal patient selection criteria for transplant omission, the management of Ph + ALL is shifting toward individualized, MRD-driven treatment approaches that balance efficacy and safety.

References

1. Nowell P, Hungerford D. A minute chromosome in human chronic granulocytic. Leuk Sci. 1960;132:1497.
2. Ribeiro R, Abromowitch M, Raimondi S, Murphy S, Behm F, Williams D. Clinical and biologic hallmarks of the Philadelphia chromosome in childhood acute lymphoblastic leukemia. Blood. 1987;70(4):948–53.
3. Burmeister T, Schwartz S, Bartram CR, Gökbuget N, Hoelzer D, Thiel E. Patients' age and BCR-ABL frequency in adult B-precursor ALL: a retrospective analysis from the GMALL study group. Blood. 2008;112(3):918–9.
4. Moorman AV, Chilton L, Wilkinson J, Ensor HM, Bown N, Proctor SJ. A population-based cytogenetic study of adults with acute lymphoblastic leukemia. Blood. 2010;115(2):206–14.
5. Appelbaum F. Impact of age on the biology of acute leukemia. In: 2005. p. 528–32.
6. Lazarus HM. Central nervous system involvement in adult acute lymphoblastic leukemia at diagnosis: results from the international ALL trial MRC UKALL XII/ECOG E2993. Blood. 2006;108(2):465–72.
7. Chalandon Y, Thomas X, Hayette S, Cayuela JM, Abbal C, Huguet F, et al. Randomized study of reduced-intensity chemotherapy combined with imatinib in adults with Ph-positive acute lymphoblastic leukemia. Blood. 2015;125(24):3711–9.
8. De Labarthe A, Rousselot P, Huguet-Rigal F, Delabesse E, Witz F, Maury S, et al. Imatinib combined with induction or consolidation chemotherapy in patients with de novo Philadelphia chromosome–positive acute lymphoblastic leukemia: results of the GRAAPH-2003 study. Blood. 2007;109(4):1408–13.

9. Ravandi F, Othus M, O'Brien SM, Forman SJ, Ha CS, Wong JYC, et al. US intergroup study of chemotherapy plus dasatinib and allogeneic stem cell transplant in Philadelphia chromosome positive ALL. Blood Adv 2016;1(3):250–9.
10. Kim DY, Joo YD, Lim SN, Kim SD, Lee JH, Lee JH, et al. Nilotinib combined with multiagent chemotherapy for newly diagnosed Philadelphia-positive acute lymphoblastic leukemia. Blood. 2015;126(6):746–56.
11. Jabbour E, Short NJ, Ravandi F, Huang X, Daver N, DiNardo CD, et al. Combination of hyper-CVAD with ponatinib as first-line therapy for patients with Philadelphia chromosome-positive acute lymphoblastic leukaemia: long-term follow-up of a single-centre, phase 2 study. Lancet Haematol. 2018;5(12):e618–27.
12. Liu-Dumlao T, Kantarjian H, Thomas DA, O'Brien S, Ravandi F. Philadelphia-positive acute lymphoblastic leukemia: current treatment options. Curr Oncol Rep. 2012;14(5):387–94.
13. Badar T, Alkhateeb H, Aljurf M, Kharfan-Dabaja MA. Management of Philadelphia chromosome positive acute lymphoblastic leukemia in the current era. Curr Res Transl Med. 2023;71(2):103392.
14. Fielding AK, Rowe JM, Buck G, Foroni L, Gerrard G, Litzow MR, et al. UKALLXII/ECOG2993: addition of imatinib to a standard treatment regimen enhances long-term outcomes in Philadelphia positive acute lymphoblastic leukemia. Blood. 2014;123(6):843–50.
15. Ravandi F, O'Brien S, Thomas D, Faderl S, Jones D, Garris R, et al. First report of phase 2 study of dasatinib with hyper-CVAD for the frontline treatment of patients with Philadelphia chromosome–positive (Ph+) acute lymphoblastic leukemia. Blood. 2010;116(12):2070–7.
16. Ravandi F, O'Brien SM, Cortes JE, Thomas DM, Garris R, Faderl S, et al. Long-term follow-up of a phase 2 study of chemotherapy plus dasatinib for the initial treatment of patients with P hiladelphia chromosome–positive acute lymphoblastic leukemia. Cancer. 2015;121(23):4158–64.
17. Rousselot P, Coude MM, Gokbuget N, Passerini CG, Hayette S, Cayuela JM, et al. Dasatinib and low-intensity chemotherapy in elderly patients with Philadelphia chromosome–positive ALL. 2016;128(6):10.
18. Ottmann OG, Pfeifer H, Cayuela JM, Spiekermann K, Jung W, Beck J, et al. Nilotinib (Tasigna®) and low intensity chemotherapy for first-line treatment of elderly patients with BCR-ABL1-positive acute lymphoblastic leukemia: final results of a prospective multicenter trial (EWALL-PH02). Blood. 2018;132(Supplement 1):31.
19. Jabbour E, DerSarkissian M, Duh MS, McCormick N, Cheng WY, McGarry LJ, et al. Efficacy of ponatinib versus earlier generation tyrosine kinase inhibitors for front-line treatment of newly diagnosed Philadelphia-positive acute lymphoblastic leukemia. Clin Lymphoma Myeloma Leuk. 2018;18(4):257–65.
20. Kantarjian H, Short NJ, Jain N, Sasaki K, Huang X, Haddad FG, et al. Frontline combination of ponatinib and HYPER-CVAD in Philadelphia chromosome-positive acute lymphoblastic leukemia: 80-months follow-up results. Am J Hematol. 2023;98(3):493–501.
21. Luskin MR, Murakami MA, Keating J, Flamand Y, Winer ES, Garcia JS, et al. Asciminib plus dasatinib and prednisone for Philadelphia chromosome–positive acute leukemia. Blood. 2025;145(6):577–89.
22. Ghobadi A, Slade M, Kantarjian H, Alvarenga J, Aldoss I, Mohammed KA, et al. The role of allogeneic transplant for adult Ph+ ALL in CR1 with complete molecular remission: a retrospective analysis. Blood. 2022;140(20):2101–12.
23. Jabbour E, Haddad FG, Short NJ, Kantarjian H. Treatment of adults with Philadelphia chromosome–positive acute lymphoblastic leukemia—from intensive chemotherapy combinations to chemotherapy-free regimens: a review. JAMA Oncol. 2022;8(9):1340.
24. Nishiwaki S, Sugiura I, Fujisawa S, Hatta Y, Atsuta Y, Doki N, et al. Utility of allogeneic stem cell transplantation for adult PH+ALL with complete molecular remission. Am J Hematol. 2024;99(5):806–15.
25. Short NJ, Jabbour E, Sasaki K, Patel K, O'Brien SM, Cortes JE, et al. Impact of complete molecular response on survival in patients with Philadelphia chromosome–positive acute lymphoblastic leukemia. Blood. 2016;128(4):504–7.

26. Chiaretti S, Foà R. How I treat adult Ph+ ALL. Blood. 2025;145(1):11–9.
27. Foà R, Bassan R, Vitale A, Elia L, Piciocchi A, Puzzolo MC, et al. Dasatinib–Blinatumomab for Ph-Positive Acute Lymphoblastic Leukemia in Adults. N Engl J Med. 2020;383(17):1613–23.
28. Kugler E, Kantarjian H, Jabbour E, Khaire N, Short NJ, Kadia TM, et al. Treatment-free remission in nontransplanted patients with Philadelphia chromosome-positive acute lymphoblastic leukemia. Cancer. 2025;131(5):e35773.
29. Giebel S, Labopin M, Peric Z, Passweg J, Blaise D, Salmenniemi U, et al. Impact of the Type of Tyrosine Kinase Inhibitor (imatinib or dasatinib) Used Before allo-HCT on Outcome of Patients with Philadelphia-Positive Acute Lymphoblastic Leukemia. A Study on Behalf of the Acute Leukemia Working Party of the EBMT. Transplant Cell Ther. 2025;31(1):14.e1–14.e10.
30. Jamy O, Badar T. Role of allogeneic hematopoietic stem cell transplantation for Philadelphia chromosome-positive B-cell acute lymphoblastic leukemia in the contemporary era. Cancer. 2024;17(1):104.
31. Nishiwaki S, Terakura S, Morishita T, Goto T, Inagaki Y, Miyao K, et al. Post-transplant TKIs for Ph+ ALL: practices to date and clinical significance. Int J Hematol. [Internet] 2025 [cited 2025 Mar 6]; Available from: https://link.springer.com/10.1007/s12185-025-03917-1
32. Candoni A, Chiusolo P, Lazzarotto D, Sartor C, Dargenio M, Chiaretti S, et al. Ponatinib as a prophylactic or pre-Emptive strategy to prevent cytological relapse after allogeneic stem cell transplantation in patients with Philadelphia chromosome-positive acute lymphoblastic leukemia transplanted in complete cytological remission. Cancer. 2024;16(11):2108.
33. Liu H, Xu H, Chi P, Feng Z, Xu X, Nie D, et al. A prophylactic tyrosine kinase inhibitor strategy based on measurable residual disease pre-transplantation for Ph^+ acute lymphoblastic leukemia undergoing allogeneic hematopoietic stem cell transplantation: a prospective multicenter cohort study. Am J Hematol. 2025;100(1):33–7.
34. Laport GG, Alvarnas JC, Palmer JM, Snyder DS, Slovak ML, Cherry AM, et al. Long-term remission of Philadelphia chromosome–positive acute lymphoblastic leukemia after allogeneic hematopoietic cell transplantation from matched sibling donors: a 20-year experience with the fractionated total body irradiation–etoposide regimen. Blood. 2008;112(3):903–9.
35. Takiar R, Foucar CE, Perissinotti AJ, Marini BL, Benitez-Colon L, Burke PW, et al. Real world outcomes in patients with Philadelphia chromosome positive acute lymphoblastic leukemia undergoing allogeneic stem cell transplantation–a single institution experience. Leuk Res Rep. 2022;18:100352.
36. Chiaretti S, Leoncin M, Elia L, Piciocchi A, Matarazzo M, Di Trani M, et al. Comparison between dasatinib-blinatumomab vs ponatinib-blinatumomab chemo-free strategy for newly diagnosed Ph+ acute lymphoblastic leukemia patients. Preliminary results of the Gimema ALLL2820 trial. Blood. 2023;142(Supplement 1):4249.
37. Ribera J, Morgades M, Ribera J, Montesinos P, Cano-Ferri I, Martínez P, et al. Ponalfil trial for adults with Philadelphia chromosome-positive acute lymphoblastic leukemia: long-term results. HemaSphere. 2024;8(4):e67.
38. Vignetti M, Fazi P, Cimino G, Martinelli G, Di Raimondo F, Ferrara F, et al. Imatinib plus steroids induces complete remissions and prolonged survival in elderly Philadelphia chromosome–positive patients with acute lymphoblastic leukemia without additional chemotherapy: results of the Gruppo Italiano Malattie Ematologiche dell'Adulto (GIMEMA) LAL0201-B protocol. Blood. 2007;109(9):3676–8.
39. Foà R, Vitale A, Vignetti M, Meloni G, Guarini A, De Propris MS, et al. Dasatinib as first-line treatment for adult patients with Philadelphia chromosome–positive acute lymphoblastic leukemia. Blood. 2011;118(25):6521–8.
40. Chiaretti S, Vitale A, Vignetti M, Piciocchi A, Fazi P, Elia L, et al. A sequential approach with imatinib, chemotherapy and transplant for adult Ph+ acute lymphoblastic leukemia: final results of the GIMEMA LAL 0904 study. Haematologica. 2016;101(12):1544–52.
41. Sugiura I, Doki N, Hata T, Cho R, Ito T, Suehiro Y, et al. Dasatinib-based 2-step induction for adults with Philadelphia chromosome–positive acute lymphoblastic leukemia. Blood Adv. 2022;6(2):624–36.

42. Martinelli G, Papayannidis C, Piciocchi A, Robustelli V, Soverini S, Terragna C, et al. INCB84344-201: Ponatinib and steroids in frontline therapy for unfit patients with Ph+ acute lymphoblastic leukemia. Blood Adv. 2022;6(6):1742–53.
43. Advani AS, Moseley A, O'Dwyer KM, Wood BL, Park J, Wieduwilt M, et al. Dasatinib/prednisone induction followed by blinatumomab/dasatinib in Ph+ acute lymphoblastic leukemia. Blood Adv. 2023;7(7):1279–85.
44. Foà R, Bassan R, Elia L, Piciocchi A, Soddu S, Messina M, et al. Long-term results of the Dasatinib-Blinatumomab protocol for adult Philadelphia-positive ALL. J Clin Oncol. 2024;42(8):881–5.
45. Tang H, Jia W, Jia S, Dong R, Gao S, Feng J, et al. A new chemotherapy-free regimen of olverembatinib in combination with venetoclax and dexamethasone for newly diagnosed Ph+ acute lymphoblastic leukemia: preliminary outcomes of a prospective study. Am J Hematol. 2024;99(6):1177–9.
46. Zhang M, Hu Y, Wei G, Fu S, Feng J, Hong R, et al. Dasatinib and CAR-T cell therapy for newly diagnosed Ph-positive acute lymphoblastic leukemia in adults. Blood. 2023;142(Supplement 1):891.
47. Yao Z, Gu B, Chen J, Xu Y, Chen F, Xue S, et al. CD19 chimeric antigen receptor T-cell therapy in adult patients with Philadelphia chromosome-positive acute lymphoblastic leukemia without complete molecular response at 3 months. Blood Cancer J. 2023;13(1):75.
48. Chen LY, Gong WJ, Li MH, Zhou HX, Xu MZ, Qian CS, et al. Anti-CD19 CAR T-cell consolidation therapy combined with CD19+ feeding T cells and TKI for Ph+ acute lymphoblastic leukemia. Blood Adv. 2023;7(17):4913–25.
49. Wieduwilt MJ, Yin J, Wetzler M, Uy GL, Powell BL, Kolitz JE, et al. Dasatinib and dexamethasone followed by hematopoietic cell transplantation for adults with Ph-positive ALL. Blood Adv. 2021;5(22):4691–700.
50. Bolaños-Meade J, Hamadani M, Wu J, Al Malki MM, Martens MJ, Runaas L, et al. Post-transplantation cyclophosphamide-based graft-versus-host disease prophylaxis. N Engl J Med. 2023;388(25):2338–48.
51. Tanaka J, Kanamori H, Nishiwaki S, Ohashi K, Taniguchi S, Eto T, et al. Reduced-intensity vs myeloablative conditioning allogeneic hematopoietic SCT for patients aged over 45 years with ALL in remission: a study from the Adult ALL Working Group of the Japan Society for Hematopoietic Cell Transplantation (JSHCT). Bone Marrow Transplant. 2013;48(11):1389–94.
52. Luskin MR. Ph+ ALL: new approaches for upfront therapy. Hematology. 2024;2024(1):78–85.

Chapter 42
Conditioning Regimen for Hematopoietic Stem Cell Transplant

Dharma Choudhary, Divya Doval, and Neelkumar Patel

Abstract HSCT remains a cornerstone in the management of a variety of hematological malignancies, bone marrow failure syndromes, benign and select inherited disorders. Conditioning serves a multifaceted role—eradicating residual malignant cells, immunosuppressing the host to prevent graft rejection, and creating space within the marrow microenvironment to facilitate engraftment of donor hematopoietic stem cells (Appelbaum, N Engl J Med 357(15):1472–1475, 2007).

Over the decades, conditioning regimens have evolved from high-intensity, MAC protocols to more nuanced approaches such as RIC and NMA, tailored to disease biology, patient age, comorbidities, and transplant platform. This evolution is driven by a growing recognition of the importance of balancing RRT with the need for effective disease control and long-term immune reconstitution (Copelan, N Engl J Med 354(17):1813–1826, 2006). MAC, typically involving high-dose alkylating agents such as busulfan or TBI, continues to be the standard for younger, fit patients with high-risk disease. However, these regimens are associated with substantial toxicity, including sinusoidal obstruction syndrome, interstitial pneumonitis, and long-term organ dysfunction, which limit their applicability in older or medically frail populations (Carreras and Diaz-Ricart, Bone Marrow Transplant. 46:1495–1502, 2011).

Conversely, RIC regimens, which emerged in the late 1990s, rely more on the GVT effect than on cytoreduction and thus aim to minimize regimen-related mortality while maintaining therapeutic efficacy. Agents such as fludarabine, melphalan, and low-dose TBI are frequently employed in these protocols, and they enable transplants in MAC-ineligible patients (Deeg and Sandmaier, Blood 116(23):4762–4770, 2010). Nonetheless, RIC may increase the risk of disease relapse, particularly in aggressive or chemo-resistant malignancies, necessitating careful patient and disease stratification.

Furthermore, the increasing application of novel transplant platforms—such as haploidentical transplantation with PTCy, and cord blood transplantation—has catalyzed further refinements in conditioning strategies. These newer modalities often

D. Choudhary (✉) · D. Doval · N. Patel
BLK-Max Super Speciality Hospital, New Delhi, India

H. P. Pati et al. (eds.), *Clinical Hematology and Hemato-Oncology*,
https://doi.org/10.1007/978-981-92-1167-8_42

require individualized conditioning approaches that integrate both immunologic considerations and the unique engraftment kinetics of the graft source (Luznik et al., Biol Blood Marrow Transplant J Am Soc Blood Marrow Transplant 14:641–650, 2008). In parallel, advances in pharmacokinetics-guided dosing, particularly with agents like busulfan, and the incorporation of targeted radiotherapeutics, such as radioimmunotherapy, have introduced a level of precision previously unattainable in conditioning regimen design.

Keywords Conditioning · MAC · RIC · NMA · PTCy

Abbreviations

ATG	Antithymocyte globulin
DFS	Disease-free survival
GVHD	Graft-versus-host disease
GVL	Graft-versus-leukemia
HSCT	Hematopoietic stem cell transplantation
MAC	Myeloablative conditioning
NMA	Non-myeloablative
NRM	Non-relapse mortality
OS	Overall survival
PTCy	Post-transplant cyclophosphamide
RIC	Reduced-intensity conditioning
RRT	Regimen-related toxicity
SOS	Sinusoidal obstruction syndrome
TLI	Total lymphoid irradiation
TMI	Total marrow irradiation
TRM	Transplant-related mortality

Learning Objectives

Clinical Decision-Making

- Factors influencing regimen selection
- Individualized approach to conditioning
- Socioeconomic and demographic considerations

Conditioning Regimen Intensity

- Myeloablative vs. reduced-intensity
- Toxicity versus relapse risk

Mechanisms of Action

- Myeloablation and lymphoablation roles
- Immunosuppressive effects of agents

Chemotherapeutic Agents
- Busulfan: properties and effects
- Cyclophosphamide: immunosuppressive role
- Fludarabine in conditioning regimens
- Treosulfan's low toxicity profile
- Thiotepa and CNS activity

Evolving Practices
- Emerging agents in SCT protocols

42.1 What Is a Conditioning Regimen and Its Role in Stem Cell Engraftment

A *conditioning regimen* is a preparatory therapeutic protocol administered prior to HSCT that serves to eliminate malignant cells, suppresses the host immune system, and creates hematopoietic space within the bone marrow niche to support successful donor stem cell engraftment. The regimen typically involves chemotherapy, radiotherapy, or a combination of both, with the choice tailored according to the underlying disease, transplant type (autologous vs. allogeneic), and patient-specific factors such as age and comorbidities [2].

The primary objectives of the conditioning regimen are threefold:

1. *Myeloablation*: Destruction of the recipient's existing hematopoietic system, especially in the setting of malignancy, to eradicate diseased or clonal hematopoietic cells
2. *Immunosuppression*: Suppression of the host immune system to prevent rejection of the incoming donor graft, particularly in allogeneic transplants
3. *Marrow Space Creation*: Elimination of host hematopoietic cells opens physical niches within the bone marrow, facilitating the homing, and engraftment of donor-derived HSCs

The effectiveness of stem cell engraftment is directly linked to the depth of immunoablation and niche availability. Without adequate suppression of host immunity, allogeneic grafts may be rejected through host-versus-graft immune responses. Conversely, insufficient marrow conditioning may result in graft failure due to limited niche availability or inadequate hematopoietic suppression [6].

Conditioning agents commonly used include TBI, cyclophosphamide, busulfan, fludarabine, and ATG, each with specific mechanisms of action. For example, busulfan induces DNA cross-linking, leading to marrow suppression, while fludarabine provides immunosuppression with lymphodepleting properties. By eliminating host hematopoietic elements and modulating immune tolerance, conditioning regimens remain a cornerstone of successful HSCT and long-term engraftment [4].

42.2 Hematopoietic Cell Transplantation-Specific Comorbidity Index (HCT-CI)

The HCT-CI is a validated prognostic tool developed to refine risk stratification for patients undergoing HSCT. It was introduced by Sorror et al. in 2005 to overcome the limitations of general indices such as the Charlson Comorbidity Index, which lacked specificity and prognostic relevance for transplant populations. It is designed to quantify the impact of pre-existing comorbidities on NRM and OS post-transplantation. By integrating comorbidity-related risks, the HCT-CI enables clinicians to make more informed decisions regarding patient eligibility, conditioning regimen intensity, and anticipated outcomes [7].

The index evaluates 17 comorbid conditions, each assigned a score based on its statistical association with increased transplant-related morbidity and mortality. The total score categorizes patients into low, intermediate, or high-risk groups (Table 42.1). These risk categories correlate with significantly different survival and NRM probabilities, thereby enhancing clinical decision-making.

Prospective Validation of the Predictive Power of the HCT-CI: A CIBMTR Study gave specific insights about the use of conditioning regimen and outcome [7].

- The HCT-CI is a validated tool predicting NRM and OS in both allo-HCT and ASCT (Tables 42.2, 42.3, and 42.4).
- Higher HCT-CI scores (≥3) consistently correlate with higher NRM and lower OS across transplant types.
- The age-adjusted HCT-CI (aaHCT-CI) further improves prognostication, especially when stratified by conditioning intensity.

Table 42.1 HCT-CI comorbidities and assigned scores [7]

Comorbidity	Score
Arrhythmia	1
Cardiovascular disease	1
Inflammatory bowel disease	1
Diabetes mellitus	1
Psychiatric disturbance	1
Mild hepatic dysfunction	1
Obesity (BMI >35)	1
Infection	1
Rheumatologic disease	2
Moderate/severe pulmonary	2
Renal dysfunction (Cr >2 mg/dL)	2
Peptic ulcer disease	2
Prior solid tumor	3
Moderate/severe hepatic	3
Heart valve disease	3

Table 42.2 Outcomes by HCT-CI score in Allo-HCT [7]

HCT-CI score	1-Year NRM	1-Year OS	3-Year NRM	3-Year OS
0	17%	69%	24%	54%
1–2	21%	62%	28%	47%
≥3	26%	56%	35%	38%

Table 42.3 Outcomes by HCT-CI score in ASCT [7]

HCT-CI score	1-Year NRM	1-Year OS	3-Year NRM	3-Year OS
0	3%	91%	5%	79%
1–2	3%	88%	6%	73%
≥3	5%	86%	9%	70%

Table 42.4 2-Year NRM and OS by age-adjusted HCT-CI and conditioning intensity (allo-HCT) [7]

aaHCT-CI score	Regimen	2-Year NRM	2-Year OS
0	NMA	5%	81%
	RIC	12%	87%
	MAC	10%	79%
1–2	NMA	9%	74%
	RIC	18%	70%
	MAC	20%	66%
3–4	NMA	17%	59%
	RIC	36%	50%
	MAC	37%	45%
≥5	NMA	35%	37%
	RIC	41%	35%
	MAC	49%	29%

42.2.1 Allogeneic HCT

- NRM increases and OS decreases progressively with rising HCT-CI scores.
- Even patients with moderate comorbidity burden (HCT-CI 1–2) show a significant decline in outcomes compared to score 0.
- Conditioning intensity modulates the impact: MAC has worse outcomes at higher scores compared to RIC/NMA.

42.2.2 Autologous SCT

- NRM remains low regardless of comorbidity score, but OS is negatively affected in patients with HCT-CI ≥3.
- Predictive power is stronger for mortality risk than toxicity, limiting its standalone use in ASCT planning.

42.2.3 Age and Regimen-Specific Findings

- Pediatric patients with HCT-CI ≥3 also show increased NRM and reduced OS, but not as drastically as in adults.
- NMA and RIC regimens show better tolerance and less comorbidity-driven outcome variability than MAC.

42.3 Classification of Conditioning Regimens

- *MAC*: High-dose regimens that cause irreversible bone marrow aplasia and require stem cell rescue. These are typically used in younger patients with aggressive diseases.
- *RIC*: Intermediate regimens that cause partial marrow ablation and rely more heavily on GVT effects for disease control.
- *NMA*: Minimal regimens that focus on immunosuppression, used primarily in older or comorbid patients where toxicity needs to be minimized.

42.3.1 Defining Conditioning Regimen Intensity

In an effort to bring clarity to the terminology surrounding preparative regimens, the CIBMTR convened a landmark workshop in 2006. This collaborative initiative brought together 56 transplant experts from 44 institutions across 9 countries, resulting in a consensus framework that refined the definitions of conditioning regimen intensity [8] (Fig. 42.1).

While traditional thinking emphasized the role of conditioning in simply creating physical space for donor stem cells, emerging insights underscore a more intricate reality. Engraftment is not merely a consequence of marrow depletion, but also involves the immune-mediated displacement of host lymphohematopoietic cells—a process shaped by complex immunological interactions that extend beyond cytotoxicity alone.

Traditionally, the regimen is called myeloablative when the agents are dosed as follows

- TBI at ≥5 Gy in a single fraction or ≥ 8 Gy when fractionated
- Busulfan >8 mg/kg orally or > 6.4 mg/kg intravenously
- Melphalan >150 mg/m^2
- Thiotepa >10 mg/kg
- Treosulfan >30 g/m^2

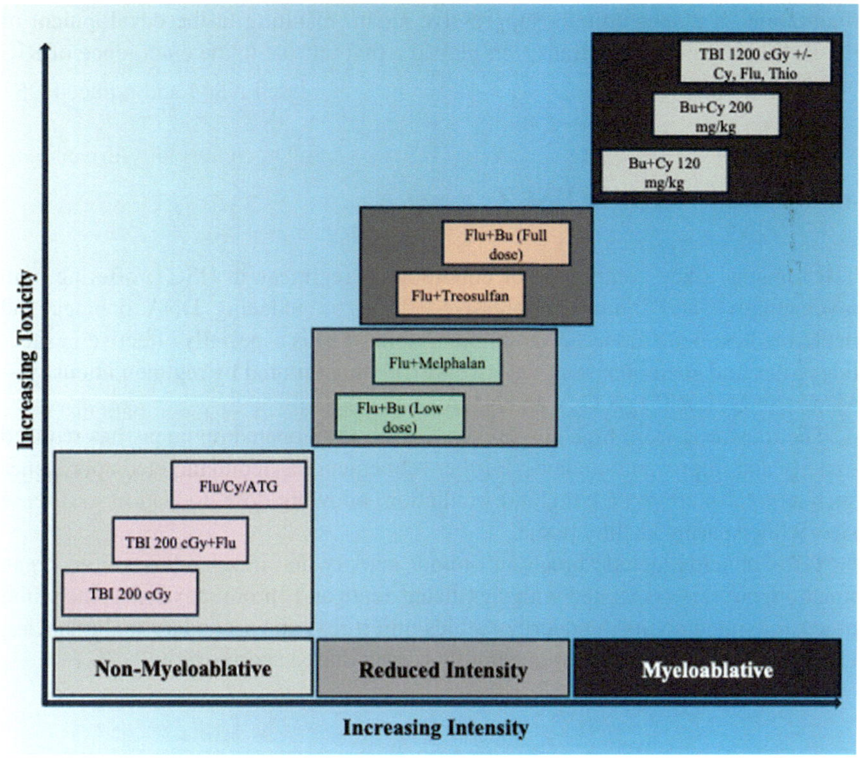

Fig. 42.1 Intensity of conditioning regimen

42.4 Evolution of Conditioning Regimens

Since the inception of HSCT, conditioning regimens have undergone continuous evolution, with the goal of minimizing non-hematopoietic toxicity while improving overall survival. Initially, myeloablation was achieved using TBI alone; however, its toxic effects prompted the combination of TBI with cyclophosphamide, establishing the first widely used myeloablative regimen (Cy/TBI) [9].

Challenges in delivering TBI across centers and the high TRM associated with early regimens led to the development of chemotherapy-based conditioning approaches. This shift introduced busulfan, an effective myeloablative alkylating agent, which was combined with (Bu/Cy) to enhance immunosuppression. However, the original Bu/Cy regimen was associated with significant toxicity, including hepatic SOS. Reductions in cyclophosphamide dosing helped mitigate toxicity, and the subsequent availability of intravenous busulfan improved pharmacokinetic consistency, reducing SOS risk.

Despite its myeloablative strength, busulfan has limited lymphoablative activity and thus requires combination with immunosuppressive agents. Ongoing efforts to reduce toxicity led to the replacement of cyclophosphamide with fludarabine, a potent immunosuppressive agent, resulting in the development of the Bu/Flu regimen. This transition played a pivotal role in the emergence of RIC and NMA strategies [10].

42.5 Role of TBI in HSCT

TBI remains a key component of conditioning regimens in HSCT, offering both myeloablative and immunosuppressive effects by inducing DNA damage and depleting host hematopoietic and immune cells. TBI is especially effective in sanctuary sites and chemoresistant disease, with dosing tailored by regimen intensity—MAC (≥8 Gy), RIC (≤8 Gy), and NMA (≤2 Gy) [11].

The transition from high single-dose TBI to fractionated regimens has reduced toxicity and improved outcomes. Further refinement has led to targeted approaches such as total marrow or lymphoid irradiation, allowing dose escalation to disease sites while sparing healthy tissue.

TBI's benefits include broad anti-tumor activity and independence from organ function, but it is associated with significant acute and chronic toxicities, including mucositis, pneumonitis, endocrinopathies, infertility, and secondary malignancies. Use in very young children is generally avoided due to neurotoxicity [12].

42.6 TBI-Based Myeloablative Regimens

TBI alone was first used for conditioning in patients with acute leukemia undergoing BMT in the 1950s. The addition of cyclophosphamide to TBI, introduced in the 1970s, improved outcomes. To mitigate extramedullary toxicity—particularly interstitial pneumonitis—Thomas and colleagues pioneered the use of fractionated TBI, demonstrating superior outcomes with 2 Gy/day over six days compared to a single 10 Gy dose. Fractionated or hyperfractionated TBI (multiple fractions per day) is now standard practice, offering reduced organ toxicity while maintaining antineoplastic efficacy [13].

Conditioning regimen intensity is a key determinant of disease control in MAC. Two prospective randomized trials comparing 12 Gy versus 15.75 Gy TBI showed a reduced risk of relapse at higher doses, but this was offset by significantly increased TRM, resulting in no survival benefit. Higher TBI doses were associated with increased incidence of SOS, pulmonary toxicity, renal failure, and grade ≥ 2 acute GVHD [14].

Various agents have been combined with high-dose TBI to enhance cytoreduction, including cytarabine, etoposide, melphalan, and busulfan. The EBMT acute leukemia working group compared outcomes in adults with ALL conditioned with etoposide–TBI versus cyclophosphamide–TBI. Etoposide–TBI was associated with superior 5-year leukemia-free survival (60% vs. 50%) and GVHD/relapse-free survival (43% vs. 33%), though there were no significant differences in NRM or incidence of acute or chronic GVHD. A CIBMTR study similarly reported a benefit with etoposide substitution or with escalating TBI dose >13 Gy in patients undergoing matched sibling allogeneic HCT for ALL in second complete remission. These data are limited by their retrospective nature, and no prospective randomized trials have addressed this question [15].

TBI delivery techniques include anteroposterior/posterior-anterior and parallel-opposed lateral fields. An EBMT survey of 57 centers highlighted substantial variation in TBI protocols. Most centers utilized linear accelerators (91%), in vivo dosimetry (93%), and lung shielding (84%). The total dose ranged from 8 to 14.4 Gy, administered in 1 to 8 fractions, with fraction sizes between 1.65 and 8 Gy.

TBI is associated with a spectrum of acute and chronic toxicities. Acute side effects include nausea (35–66%), vomiting, diarrhea, mucositis, parotitis, erythema, taste disturbances, anorexia, and fatigue. Late toxicities include pulmonary fibrosis, renal dysfunction, cataracts, infertility, osteoporosis, endocrine abnormalities, growth retardation in children, and secondary malignancies. Pulmonary toxicity—particularly interstitial pneumonitis—is the most common. Predictive factors include lung dose, total dose, fraction size, and concurrent use of cyclophosphamide or busulfan [16].

Endocrine and metabolic sequelae are particularly prevalent in survivors of childhood ALL treated with TBI-based conditioning. These include reduced β-cell reserve, insulin resistance, and increased risk of diabetes and metabolic syndrome. Cataracts affect up to 50% of patients at 10 years post-transplant, while thyroid dysfunction is observed in 20–57%. TBI-related bone loss, including osteopenia and osteoporosis, affects up to 31% of survivors [17].

Organ-sparing strategies, including dose reduction, fractionation, and shielding, are commonly employed to mitigate these toxicities. Lung blocks have proven effective in reducing radiation pneumonitis. Advances in radiation delivery—such as image-guided and intensity-modulated radiation therapy (IMRT)—enable homogenous dose distribution and minimize the risk of over- or underdosing. Improved patient selection, matched donor strategies, and supportive care have contributed to decreased TRM in recent years.

Emerging approaches such as TMI and TLI offer the promise of targeted, RIC. TMI focuses radiation on the skeletal system while sparing critical organs, facilitating dose escalation. In a phase I study, TMI at 15–18 Gy combined with fludarabine and cyclophosphamide yielded a 1-year OS of 42% and DFS of 22%, with acceptable toxicity. TLI, used in aplastic anemia for durable immunosuppression, is now being combined with TMI in total marrow and lymphoid irradiation (TMLI). A phase I study of TMLI dose escalation to 20 Gy with cyclophosphamide and etoposide for relapsed/refractory leukemia showed low non-relapse mortality at 100 days (3.9%) and 1 year (8.1%) [18].

42.7 Conditioning Regimens for Matched Donor HSCT

Allogeneic HSCT is a potentially curative therapy for various hematologic malignancies. In matched donor HSCT, traditionally, MAC has been employed; however, RIC approaches have gained popularity in patients with advanced age or comorbidities, with the goal of balancing disease control and treatment-related toxicity.

42.7.1 MAC Regimens

The most common MAC regimens in matched donor HSCT are cyclophosphamide with TBI(Cy/TBI) and busulfan with cyclophosphamide (Bu/Cy). TBI-based regimens provide superior CNS and sanctuary site penetration, making them a preferred option in ALL. Bu/Cy, conversely, avoids the long-term toxicities of radiation and is often used in AML [19].

Busulfan is typically administered as a pharmacokinetically adjusted intravenous infusion to reduce the risk of SOS, a serious complication of conditioning. Other agents, such as fludarabine, are increasingly incorporated to enhance immunosuppression while maintaining myeloablation, as seen in the Flu/Bu/Cy combination [20].

Outcomes with MAC are generally favorable in terms of relapse prevention, particularly in patients with high-risk disease. However, NRM remains a significant concern, especially in older patients and those with comorbidities.

42.7.2 RIC Regimens

RIC regimens induce less profound cytopenia and are designed for patients ineligible for MAC due to age or organ dysfunction. Common RIC regimens include Flu/Bu and Flu/Mel. These regimens rely more on GVL effects than direct cytotoxicity.

The Flu/Bu regimen uses a lower dose of Busulfan (6.4 mg/kg), which retains antileukemic activity while reducing toxicity. Flu/Mel is preferred in lymphoid malignancies and has demonstrated acceptable engraftment and GVHD rates [21].

Despite a higher risk of relapse, RIC regimens have shown comparable OS in select patient populations, primarily due to lower NRM [22].

42.7.3 Comparative Outcomes and Regimen Selection

Several studies have compared MAC and RIC in matched donor HSCT. A CIBMTR study involving patients with AML reported improved DFS with MAC in younger patients, but similar OS in older individuals due to higher NRM with MAC. Another large EBMT study found no OS difference between MAC and RIC in AML patients over 45 years.

Regimen choice is often based on disease risk, remission status, and patient-related factors. For example, patients with ALL in first complete remission (CR1) benefit most from TBI-based MAC regimens, whereas patients with MDS or AML with comorbidities may derive comparable benefit from RIC regimens.

42.7.4 Emerging Regimens and Novel Approaches

Treosulfan (Treo), a water-soluble busulfan analog, has gained attention for its reduced toxicity profile while maintaining myeloablative potential. A phase III trial comparing Flu/Treo to Flu/Bu in older patients with AML/MDS showed superior EFS and OS with Flu/Treo [23].

TMLI is also being investigated as a targeted radiation-based MAC platform, offering better tissue sparing and potential for RRT [18].

42.8 Conditioning Regimen for Haploidentical HSCT

Haplo-HSCT has emerged as a viable alternative to HLA-matched donor transplantation due to advances in GVHD prophylaxis, particularly PTCy. It has become increasingly utilized owing to nearly universal donor availability and the success of PTCy-based GVHD prophylaxis. The choice of conditioning regimen, ranging from NMA to MAC, significantly influences engraftment, relapse, and NRM outcomes [5].

Historically, haplo-HCT was associated with high rates of graft rejection due to HLA disparity between donor and recipient, particularly prior to the use of PTCY as GVHD prophylaxis. Early NMA regimens without cyclophosphamide resulted in frequent graft failure, prompting the inclusion of high-dose Cyclophosphamide in the conditioning phase. The Flu/Cy/TBI regimen was developed and widely adopted following improved engraftment outcomes reported by Johns Hopkins investigators [24].

Despite its efficacy, PTCy-based haplo-HSCT remains associated with concerns such as increased relapse risk due to potent GVHD suppression, hemorrhagic cystitis(HC), cardiotoxicity, and delayed immune reconstitution. HC may be mitigated by omitting busulfan from the conditioning regimen and recent studies suggest that reducing the PTCy dose (e.g., from 100 mg/kg to 80 or 70 mg/kg) may also decrease the incidence of HC and cardiac complications without compromising GVHD prophylaxis or OS [25]. Different studies are given in a comparative table (Table 42.5).

To improve engraftment and reduce rejection, especially in RIC settings, addition or escalation of TBI has been explored. Increasing TBI from 2 Gy to 4 Gy has led to improved donor chimerism and engraftment in patients with severe aplastic anemia and other hematologic malignancies.

42.8.1 MAC Regimens in PTCY-Based Haplo-HCT

Flu/TBI and Bu/Cy are the most commonly used MAC regimens in HLA-matched HSCT. In haploidentical HSCT with PTCY, multiple TBI- and Bu-based MAC regimens have been studied. Solomon et al. reported that Flu/Bu/Cy yielded 69% 1-year OS but had high rates of HC(75%) and mucositis, prompting dose reductions [20]. Flu/TBI(12 Gy) showed better tolerability, with 67% 4-year OS and only 2% grade $\geq$ 3 HC [10]. Chiusolo et al. found comparable OS between Flu/TBI and Flu/Bu/TBI in AML patients, with 4-year OS of 72% in CR and 26% in advanced disease. Sugita et al. reported 68% 2-year OS with Flu/TBI or Flu/Bu/TBI regimens. Symons et al. documented low GVHD rates and 54% 3-year OS with Cy/TBI or Bu/Cy [26].

Treosulfan-based MAC, with its reduced toxicity profile, has emerged as a viable alternative. Cieri et al. reported 56% 1-year OS and low GVHD rates with Treo/Flu/Mel. Saraceni et al., using EBMT data, found no significant differences between Treo and Flu/Bu/TBI-based MAC in AML patients in CR. Registry studies by Dholaria et al. showed TBI-based MAC had superior DFS and lower NRM in ALL, but not in AML. Swoboda et al. found no OS difference between Flu/TBI and Flu/Bu/TBI in ALL [27]. In an ATG-based haplo setting, Ling et al. found Flu/Bu had lower NRM and fewer grade $\geq$ 3 toxicities compared to Bu/Cy, with similar OS. Collectively, Flu/TBI and Flu/BU-based MAC regimens appear effective and safe for PTCY-based haplo-HCT, though the optimal regimen likely depends on disease and disease status.

42.8.2 RIC Regimens in PTCY-Based Haplo-HCT

Several RIC regimens have been evaluated in the context of PTCY-based haplo-HCT, aiming to balance reduced toxicity with adequate disease control. Flu/Bu and Flu/Mel are commonly used backbones, often combined with low-dose TBI [28]. The original Flu/Cy/TBI regimen has been compared with alternative RIC regimens in various studies. Devillier et al. found that Flu/Bu/TBI provided superior OS and DFS in AML patients aged <60 years, although associated with higher NRM in

Table 42.5 PTCy-based haploidentical HSCT with myeloablative conditioning (MAC): key studies

Author (Year)	N	Study type	Median age	Disease	MAC regimen	NRM	Relapse	Overall survival	Notes
Solomon et al., 2015	55	Single-center cohort	43	Advanced hematologic malignancies	Cy/TBI (12 Gy) + PTCy	7% (clin. sig. HC; grade ≥ 3 HC ~2%)*	NR	2y DFS superior to MUD in DRI low/ intermediate; OS NR	TBI-based MAC; favorable tolerability
Solomon et al., 2019	82	Single-center cohort	NR	Mixed malignancies	Flu/TBI (12 Gy) + PTCy	NRM 7% (1y); 13% (4y)	27% (4y)	67% (4y)	Low grade ≥ 3 HC (~2%) reported; good long-term tolerability
Symons et al., 2020	96	Prospective phase II	42	Mixed (adult+pediatric)	Busulfan-based or Flu/TBI MAC + PTCy	11% (1y)	43% (3y)	73% (1y); 54% (3y)	Low GVHD rates with marrow grafts
Chiusolo et al., 2018	150	Multicenter retrospective (AML)	51	AML	Modified PTCy MAC (various; Flu/TBI vs Flu/Bu/ TBI)	TRM 20% (4y)	24% (4y)	OS 72% (4y, CR) / 26% (4y, active)	Comparable survival across MAC subtypes in AML
Sugita et al., 2018/2019	50 (MAC arm)	Prospective multicenter	NR	Various	Flu/TBI or Flu/Bu/ TBI (MAC) + PTCy (PBSC)	10% (2y)	36% (2y)	68% (2y)	Good OS with PBSC; low NRM
Dholaria et al., 2021	427	EBMT/ ALWP registry (ALL)	32	ALL (adults)	Flu/TBI (MAC) vs TBF (MAC) + PTCy	21% vs 31% (2y)	34% vs 32% (2y)	51% vs 47% (2y)	TBI-based MAC favored for DFS/ NRM in ALL

(continued)

Table 42.5 (continued)

Author (Year)	N	Study type	Median age	Disease	MAC regimen	NRM	Relapse	Overall survival	Notes
Swoboda/ Labopin et al., 2022	236	EBMT ALWP (ALL)	NR	ALL (adults)	Flu/TBI (MAC) vs TBF (MAC) + PTCy	19.5% vs 31% (2y)	Trend ↓ with TBF (ns)	NR	No OS difference detected
Saraceni et al., 2023	284 (matched)	EBMT ALWP (AML CR)	NR	AML in CR	TBF (MAC) vs Treosulfan-based (MAC) + PTCy	Similar (matched)	Similar	Similar	No significant differences between Treo vs TBF in AML CR
Cieri et al., 2015	40	Single-center cohort	NR	High-risk malignancies	Treosulfan/ fludarabine/ melphalan (MAC) + PTCy/ Sir	17% (1y)	NR	56% (1y)	Low GVHD; Treo-based reduced toxicity
Duléry et al., 2019	51	Single-center cohort	NR	Myeloid/ lymphoid	TBF (MAC) + PTCy ± ATG	NR	NR	NR	Demonstrated safety of TBF + PTCy in haplo
Jaiswal et al., 2016	70	Prospective single-center (PBSC)	NR	Advanced leukemia	Flu/Bu/Mel (MAC) + PTCy (PBSC)	NR	26% (2y progression)	64% (2y)	Feasible with good engraftment; PBSC source

older patients. Sugita et al. demonstrated the feasibility of a Flu/Bu/TBI regimen, reporting 44% 2-year OS with manageable GVHD and low NRM in patients aged 50–60 years. Flu/Mel-based regimens have also shown encouraging results. Ciurea et al. observed 42% 2-year OS and low chronic GVHD with Flu/Mel combined with thiotepa or low-dose TBI, while Tanaka et al. reported 73% 2-year OS in adult T-ALL with Flu/Mel/TBI. Many studies are compared in Table 42.6.

Treosulfan, known for reduced extra-hematologic toxicity, has gained attention in reduced-toxicity conditioning regimens. A pivotal phase III trial by Beelen et al. in older or comorbid patients showed that Flu/Treo was superior to Flu/Bu in terms of EFS (59.5% vs. 49.7%) and OS (66.8% vs. 56.3%), with comparable relapse rates and lower NRM. These findings supported the regulatory approval of Flu/Treo and have led to its increasing use, including in PTCY-based haplo-HCT, where early data suggest comparable outcomes to conventional regimens [29].

Innovative approaches such as TMLI have also been explored. In a phase I study, Flu/Cy combined with TMLI yielded a 2-year OS of 83% in patients receiving 20 Gy, with acceptable toxicity and low NRM. Overall, Flu/Bu and Flu/Mel-based regimens, often combined with low-dose TBI, continue to be widely used. Emerging data suggest that Flu/Treo may offer a favorable toxicity profile and outcomes, particularly for patients ineligible for MAC [30].

42.8.3 MAC Versus RIC in PTCy-Based Haplo-HCT

To date, no randomized trials have directly compared MAC and RIC in the setting of PTCy-based haplo-HSCT. However, several retrospective studies have evaluated this question. Two single-center, propensity score–adjusted analyses yielded mixed results: Huselton et al. reported lower relapse incidence (RI) but higher NRM with MAC, resulting in similar OS, while Modi et al. found no significant differences in outcomes between MAC and RIC [31].

In a larger analysis using the CIBMTR database, Solomon et al. observed that among younger patients (18–54 years), MAC was associated with improved DFS and OS, albeit at the cost of higher NRM and lower RI; in older patients (55–70 years), there were no significant differences in RI, DFS, or OS, although RIC had a lower NRM. Similarly, an EBMT registry analysis by Santoro et al. in AML patients aged ≥45 years showed no significant differences in key outcomes between MAC and RIC, with most patients receiving PTCy [32].

Acuri et al. conducted a meta-analysis of 17 studies, including those with high PTCy usage, and found that MAC was associated with lower RI and higher NRM, without a significant OS advantage over RIC [33].

Currently, there is no clear consensus favoring MAC or RIC in PTCy-based haplo-HSCT. While MAC may reduce relapse risk, its potential benefits appear to be offset by increased toxicity. Prospective randomized trials are needed to better define the optimal conditioning intensity in this setting

Table 42.6 PTCy-based haploidentical HSCT with reduced intensity conditioning (RIC): key studies

Study	N	Study type	Median age (range), years	Disease	Conditioning regimen	NRM	Relapse	OS
Luznik et al.	68	Prospective	46 (1–71)	Various	Flu/Cy/TBI	15% (1 y)	51% (2 y)	36% (2 y)
Burroughs et al.	28	Retrospective	32 (14–62)	HL	Flu/Cy/TBI	9% (2 y)	40% (2 y)	58% (2 y)
Kasamon et al.	271	Retrospective	61 (50–75)	Various	Flu/Cy/TBI	12% (1 y)	46% (3 y)	46% (3 y)
Brammer et al.	22	Retrospective	46 (20–62)	Lymphoma	Flu/Mel + TT or TBI	19% (1 y)	27% (2 y)	54% (2 y)
Ciurea et al.	43	Retrospective	61 (55–69)	AML, MDS	Flu/Mel + TT or TBI	34% (2 y)	24% (2 y)	42% (2 y)
Sugita et al.	77	Prospective	58 (22–65)	Various	Flu/Bu/TBI	20% (2 y)	45% (2 y)	44% (2 y)
Castagna et al.	47	Prospective	43 (20–68)	Lymphoma	Flu/Cy/TT + TBI or TMLI	15% (4 y)	28% (4 y)	64% (4 y)
Tanaka et al.	18	Prospective	59 (27–64)	ATLL	Flu/Mel/TBI	11% (1 y)	28% (1 y)	73% (2 y)
Devillier et al. (<60 y)	97	Retrospective	52 (43–57)*	AML	Flu/Bu/TBI	18% (2 y)	43% (2 y)	51% (2 y)
Devillier et al. (>60 y)	117	Retrospective	68 (66–70)*	AML	Flu/Cy/TBI	23% (2 y)	28% (2 y)	55% (2 y)
Devillier et al. (TBF)	170	Retrospective	63 (61–68)*	AML	TBF (RIC)	30% (2 y)	22% (2 y)	54% (2 y)
Beelen et al. (Flu/Treo vs Flu/Bu)	570	Phase III randomized	62 (45–70)	AML, MDS	Flu/Treo vs Flu/Bu	Lower with Flu/Treo	Similar	66.8% vs 56.3% (2 y)
Al Malki et al.	31	Prospective	37 (21–58)	Various	Flu/Cy/TMLI	9% (1 y)	17% (1 y)	83% (1 y)
Kasamon et al. (update)	125	Prospective/Retrospective mix	NR	Various	Flu/Cy/TBI (modified)	NR	NR	NR
Ciurea et al. (multi-institution)	82	Prospective	NR	AML/MDS	Flu/Mel + low-dose TBI	NR	NR	NR

*Interquartile range

42.9 Conditioning Regimen in MUD Transplant

While MRD and MUD transplants often employ similar foundational conditioning regimens, key differences exist due to variations in immunologic risk, GVHD incidence, and engraftment kinetics.

Patients undergoing MUD transplantation are generally at higher risk for GVHD and graft rejection due to minor histocompatibility antigen disparities and greater HLA diversity compared to MRD recipients, even when a 10/10 HLA match is achieved. Consequently, conditioning regimens for MUD transplants often incorporate additional immunosuppressive agents such as ATG or alemtuzumab to mitigate these risks, which are less commonly required in MRD settings unless specific risk factors are present [34].

The intensity of the conditioning regimen may also differ. Both MRD and MUD transplants utilize MAC regimens such as Flu/Bu or Cy/TBI in younger, fit patients. However, for older patients or those with significant comorbidities, RIC is preferred. In MUD transplantation, RIC regimens are often supplemented with intensified immunosuppression to overcome the increased risk of graft failure and GVHD [35].

Furthermore, engraftment following MUD transplantation tends to be slower and less predictable, potentially necessitating adjustments in dosing or timing of conditioning agents. GVHD prophylaxis also tends to be more intensive in MUD settings, commonly incorporating calcineurin inhibitors with methotrexate, PTCy, or other agents depending on institutional protocols and graft source [24].

While the backbone of conditioning regimens remains largely similar across MRD and MUD allo-HSCT, the degree of immunosuppression and supportive care strategies are frequently escalated in the MUD setting to account for greater immunologic disparity. These modifications aim to balance the risks of graft rejection and GVHD while optimizing engraftment and OS.

42.10 Conditioning Regimen for Autologous Stem Cell Transplant

Conditioning regimens are an essential component of ASCT, serving multiple critical purposes that enhance the efficacy of the transplant. Primarily, high-dose chemotherapy, with or without TBI, is administered to achieve maximal cytoreduction of the underlying malignancy, thereby reducing tumor burden and the likelihood of relapse. Additionally, MAC creates marrow space to facilitate engraftment of the reinfused autologous HSC. Unlike in allo-HSCT, conditioning in ASCT does not aim to provide immunosuppression to prevent graft rejection or enable GVT effects; instead, its role is purely preparative and therapeutic. Tailoring the intensity and composition of the conditioning regimen based on disease type, patient fitness, and prior therapies is crucial to balancing efficacy with toxicity and optimizing transplant outcomes.

42.11 Conditioning Regimens for Multiple Myeloma

High-dose melphalan followed by ASCT remains a cornerstone of frontline therapy for eligible patients with newly diagnosed MM. This approach is typically reserved for patients aged ≤65–70 years with minimal comorbidities. The role of ASCT in the initial treatment of MM was established through randomized clinical trials conducted in the 1990s and early 2000s, which consistently demonstrated superior outcomes with ASCT compared to conventional chemotherapy regimens [36]. Most of these studies showed higher CR rates and improved PFS in patients receiving ASCT. However, only a few trials reported a significant OS benefit, likely due to the availability of effective salvage therapies at relapse [37].

Despite the advent of novel biologic agents and the implementation of consolidation and maintenance strategies, ASCT continues to be considered the standard of care in transplant-eligible patients. In a phase III trial conducted by the Italian GIMEMA group, patients were randomized to receive high-dose melphalan (200 mg/m^2) followed by ASCT or standard-dose melphalan with lenalidomide and prednisone. Following this, patients were re-randomized to receive either lenalidomide maintenance or a placebo [38]. The ASCT group demonstrated significantly prolonged PFS and OS, with the longest survival outcomes observed in patients who underwent ASCT followed by lenalidomide maintenance. Similarly, studies from the French Myeloma Group confirmed improved PFS in patients treated with ASCT following induction therapy incorporating proteasome inhibitors [39].

Several randomized studies have also investigated the optimal conditioning regimens for ASCT. Moreau et al. conducted a randomized trial comparing high-dose melphalan (200 mg/m^2) with a combination of melphalan (140 mg/m^2) and total body irradiation (TBI, 8 Gy) as conditioning regimens in newly diagnosed patients who had received VAD induction (vincristine, doxorubicin, dexamethasone). Patients in the melphalan-only arm experienced lower toxicity, shorter hospital stays, and faster hematologic recovery compared to those in the TBI-containing arm. Although no difference in EFS was noted, the 45-month OS was notably higher in the melphalan-only arm (66%) compared to the TBI arm (46%) [40].

The strategy of tandem transplantation has also been explored, most notably in the "Total Therapy" trials. In one such study, patients underwent VAD induction followed by stem cell mobilization with cyclophosphamide and a cycle of combination chemotherapy (EDAP: etoposide, dexamethasone, cytarabine, cisplatin). The first transplant used melphalan 200 mg/m^2 as conditioning, and patients achieving at least a partial response underwent a second transplant with the same regimen. Non-responders received a second transplant with melphalan 140 mg/m^2 and TBI. This was followed by interferon-based maintenance therapy. Approximately 70% of patients completed the second transplant, with CR rates improving from 5% post-induction to 41% after the second ASCT. Treatment-related mortality was 1% after the first and 4% after the second transplant, and the median 5-year actuarial survival was 58% [41].

The IFM conducted a pivotal trial assessing single versus double ASCT in patients younger than 60 years. Participants were randomized to receive either one ASCT with melphalan 200 mg/m^2 or two ASCTs—the second utilizing melphalan plus TBI within six months of the first. The double transplant strategy yielded superior outcomes, with 7-year OS (42% vs. 21%) and EFS (20% vs. 10%) favoring the tandem transplant arm. Benefits were most pronounced in patients who did not achieve a VGPR following the initial transplant. More recently, the EMN02/HO95 phase III trial demonstrated a benefit of tandem ASCT specifically in patients with high-risk disease [42].

Another approach under investigation is a sequential ASCT followed by an NMA allo-HSCT (auto-allo HCT). Meta-analysis of six randomized trials involving 1192 patients undergoing tandem ASCT and 630 patients receiving auto-allo HCT revealed higher CR rates and increased treatment-related mortality (TRM) in the auto-allo cohort, without a corresponding improvement in PFS or OS. However, a retrospective analysis from CIBMTR comparing post-relapse outcomes between 2000 and 2010 demonstrated superior 6-year OS in the auto-allo group (44% vs. 35%) [43]. Notably, the survival advantage became more evident beyond 12 months post-relapse, suggesting enhanced responses to salvage therapies within the donor-derived immune environment. Other factors associated with improved outcomes included trial participation, male sex, and the use of novel therapeutic agents.

42.12 Conditioning Regimen for Hodgkin Lymphoma

Approximately 10–20% of patients with cHL experience relapsed or refractory disease following first-line therapy. For transplant-eligible patients with chemosensitive disease, high-dose chemotherapy followed by autoHCT remains the standard of care, providing durable remission in approximately 50% of cases. Conditioning regimens used before autoHCT aim to eradicate residual tumor burden while allowing hematopoietic recovery through reinfusion of autologous stem cells.

42.12.1 Common Conditioning Regimens

BEAM, comprising carmustine, etoposide, cytarabine, and melphalan, is the most widely used conditioning regimen in autoHCT for cHL. Alternatives include CBV (cyclophosphamide, carmustine, etoposide), BuCy (busulfan, cyclophosphamide), and GemBuMel (gemcitabine, busulfan, melphalan). A CIBMTR analysis of 1012 patients with cHL undergoing autoHCT between 1995 and 2008 showed superior 3-year OS with BEAM (79%) compared to CBV (68–73%), BuCy (65%), and TBI-based regimens (47%) ($p < 0.001$). Multivariate analysis confirmed increased mortality risk with CBV (HR 1.53, $p = 0.003$), BuCy (HR 1.77, $p < 0.001$), and TBI (HR 3.38, $p < 0.001$), when compared to BEAM [44].

42.12.2 Alternative and Emerging Regimens

Due to pulmonary toxicity and availability concerns associated with carmustine, alternative regimens such as BeEAM (bendamustine replacing carmustine), TEAM (thiotepa, etoposide, cytarabine, melphalan), and TECAM (thiotepa, etoposide, cytarabine, cyclophosphamide, melphalan) have been explored. BeEAM demonstrated promising outcomes in a phase 1/2 study, including acceptable engraftment times and a median DFS of 19 months in patients with relapsed/refractory cHL. Retrospective and prospective studies of TEAM and TECAM have shown comparable PFS and OS to BEAM [45].

42.12.3 Toxicity Considerations

Carmustine and busulfan have been linked to pulmonary and renal toxicities, while melphalan commonly causes mucositis and gastrointestinal toxicity. Therefore, the choice of conditioning should be individualized based on comorbidities and prior treatments.

42.13 Conditioning Regimen for Non-Hodgkin Lymphoma

ASCT remains the standard of care in patients with relapsed or refractory lymphoma who respond to salvage chemotherapy. The foundation of this approach lies in the use of high-dose chemotherapy, which exhibits a steep dose-response curve and mediates a log-linear cell kill. This strategy was initially supported by the Skipper model, which demonstrated that the number of tumor cells killed is directly proportional to both the drug dose and the number of tumor cells present at the time of exposure.

42.13.1 Conditioning Regimens for DLBCL

DLBCL is the most common subtype of non-Hodgkin lymphoma. While frontline immunochemotherapy achieves long-term remission in a substantial proportion of patients, 30–40% experience relapse, and approximately 10% present with primary refractory disease.

ASCT is considered the standard of care for patients with relapsed or refractory DLBCL who demonstrate chemosensitive disease following salvage therapy. High-dose chemotherapy followed by ASCT offers the potential for long-term disease control and cure. Approximately 50% of patients undergoing ASCT for relapsed/

refractory DLBCL achieve durable remission, while the remaining 50% eventually relapse post-transplant [46].

The most commonly employed MAC for auto-SCT in DLBCL includes:

- *BEAM* (BCNU, etoposide, cytarabine, melphalan)
- *CBV* (cyclophosphamide, BCNU, etoposide)
- *Cy/TBI* (cyclophosphamide with total body irradiation)

Radiation-based regimens, while effective, are now less preferred due to the risk of secondary malignancies such as MDS and AML. As a result, BEAM and CBV remain the regimens of choice, with TBI used only for localized persistent disease. BEAM is the most widely adopted conditioning regimen owing to its efficacy and acceptable toxicity profile.

42.13.2 Conditioning Regimens in Follicular Lymphoma

Although both autologous and allogeneic HSCTs are effective in relapsed/refractory FL, they are underutilized. ASCT is recommended particularly in high-risk patients experiencing progression of disease within 24 months (POD24). In the GELA/GOELAMS study, patients with relapsed/refractory FL receiving high-dose therapy followed by ASCT had significantly better 3-year overall survival than those treated with conventional chemotherapy. ASCT is preferred in chemosensitive relapsed FL and should be considered as a standard option in early relapse. A conditioning regimen similar to that used in DLBCL has demonstrated durable responses in patients undergoing ASCT for follicular lymphoma.

42.13.3 Conditioning and Transplantation in Mantle Cell Lymphoma

Mantle cell lymphoma is a biologically aggressive B-cell lymphoma. Standard therapy includes cytarabine-containing induction followed by upfront auto-SCT consolidation in eligible patients. Historical regimens such as CHOP or R-CHOP had suboptimal outcomes, with remission rates below 35% and a short median PFS. Enhanced induction with R-hyperCVAD and the addition of bortezomib have improved response rates, with newer agents like ibrutinib and venetoclax showing activity in relapsed disease.

Current NCCN and ESMO guidelines recommend intensive induction therapy followed by upfront ASCT and maintenance rituximab in transplant-eligible patients. BEAM remains the most commonly used conditioning regimen in MCL. However, BeEAM has shown comparable efficacy with reduced pulmonary toxicity [47].

The optimal timing for ASCT in MCL is in the first complete or partial remission, as outcomes in second remission are inferior and relapse rates are higher. Even patients with low-risk disease are recommended to undergo upfront ASCT. Allo-SCT may be considered for patients relapsing after ASCT, with RIC preferred to minimize treatment-related mortality.

42.14 Primary Central Nervous System Lymphoma

ASCT is indicated in patients with newly diagnosed PCNSL who are fit and responsive to induction chemotherapy, typically based on high-dose methotrexate. Several studies, including randomized trials such as *IELSG32*, *PRECIS*, and *IELSG43*, have demonstrated the superiority of ASCT over WBRT or chemotherapy alone in this setting.

In the IELSG43 trial, ASCT as consolidation therapy resulted in a 3-year PFS of 79% compared to 53% with non-myeloablative chemotherapy. OS was also improved (86% vs. 71%). In the PRECIS study, the ASCT group demonstrated significantly better cognitive preservation and comparable survival outcomes to the WBRT arm.

ASCT is also considered in patients with relapsed or refractory PCNSL who are chemosensitive and otherwise eligible. However, this setting often involves older or more frail patients, limiting the feasibility and increasing the risk of toxicity.

An effective conditioning regimen for PCNSL must ensure high CNS penetration while minimizing systemic toxicity. The most widely accepted regimens include agents such as thiotepa, busulfan, and carmustine [48].

42.14.1 BCNU/Thiotepa

The combination of BCNU and thiotepa is the most commonly used regimen in PCNSL due to its excellent CNS bioavailability and tolerability. It has demonstrated favorable outcomes in multiple studies, with 5-year OS rates approaching 87%. This regimen typically includes BCNU 400 mg/m^2 and thiotepa 5 mg/kg on two consecutive days.

42.14.2 Thiotepa/Busulfan/Cyclophosphamide

The TBC regimen is associated with high response rates and long-term disease control but carries a significantly higher TRM, particularly in patients older than 60 years. TRM in some studies reached up to 19%.

42.14.3 Busulfan/Thiotepa

This alternative, which omits cyclophosphamide, offers moderate efficacy and lower toxicity, with a 2-year OS rate of 61%. It may be preferable in elderly or frail patients who cannot tolerate full-intensity regimens.

42.14.4 BEAM and LEED

BEAM (BCNU, etoposide, cytarabine, melphalan) and LEED (lomustine, etoposide, cytarabine, dexamethasone) are less favored due to their limited CNS penetration and suboptimal outcomes in PCNSL. Studies report 2-year OS rates around 60% with these regimens.

42.14.5 BuCyE (Busulfan, Cyclophosphamide, Etoposide)

Although this regimen is less toxic, it has been associated with high relapse rates (54%) and is not recommended as a standard conditioning protocol for PCNSL.

42.15 Conditioning Regimens in Autoimmune Diseases

ASCT in autoimmune diseases is primarily aimed at eradicating the self-reactive immune system. The primary objective to eliminate autoreactive lymphocytes and promote the regeneration of a self-tolerant immune system through immune reconstitution, rather than to ablate the entire hematopoietic system.

MAC regimens necessitate hematopoietic stem cell infusion to reestablish bone marrow function and prevent irreversible aplasia. In contrast, NMA regimens do not require stem cell support for hematopoietic recovery; however, stem cell infusion is routinely administered to expedite neutrophil recovery and reduce the duration of post-transplant neutropenia by approximately 4–5 days.

EBMT classifies conditioning regimens for autoimmune diseases into three categories based on intensity: low-, intermediate-, and high-intensity regimens [49].

(a) *Low-intensity regimens*

- High-dose cyclophosphamide (200 mg/kg) is the most commonly used low-intensity regimen for ASCT due to its potent immunosuppressive effects without significant myeloablation. Cyclophosphamide is often administered as 100 mg/kg for stem cell mobilization and repeated at 100 mg/kg for conditioning.

(b) *Intermediate-intensity regimens*

- *BEAM ± ATG*: The BEAM regimen with or without ATG, is classified as intermediate in intensity [50].
- *Cyclophosphamide and rabbit-ATG*: This combination is also considered intermediate intensity.

(c) *High-intensity regimens*

- *TBI-Cy-ATG*
- *BuCyATG*

Due to the increased risk of TRM, these high-intensity regimens are now rarely used and have largely been replaced by less intensive protocols.

Among intermediate regimens, BEAM in combination with ATG was previously the most widely accepted protocol. The addition of ATG aimed to achieve further depletion of residual T cells. However, current practice favors either high-dose cyclophosphamide alone or in combination with ATG as the conditioning regimen of choice. These approaches provide effective immunoablation with minimal myeloablative toxicity, making them both safe and efficacious for patients undergoing HSCT for autoimmune diseases.

42.16 Summary: Choosing Conditioning Regimen for SCT

- Multiple clinical and non-clinical factors influence regimen choice
- HCT-CI helps assess transplant-related risk
- Disease type and organ involvement must be evaluated
- Aim to minimize regimen-related toxicities and mortality
- Balance needed between relapse risk and toxicity (MAC vs. RIC)
- TBI provides myeloablation and immunosuppression, facilitating engraftment and disease eradication in HSCT
- Immunologic barriers and rejection risks must be addressed
- Genetic disorders (e.g., Fanconi anemia) require modified regimens
- MRD positivity favors myeloablative conditioning
- Anti-thymocyte globulin (ATG) reduces graft rejection and graft-versus-host disease by depleting recipient and donor T cells in HSCT
- GVHD risk should be balanced with potential GVL benefits
- Socioeconomic factors impact transplant access and outcomes

References

1. Appelbaum FR. Hematopoietic-cell transplantation at 50. N Engl J Med. 2007;357(15):1472–5.
2. Copelan EA. Hematopoietic stem-cell transplantation. N Engl J Med. 2006;354(17):1813–26.
3. Carreras E, Diaz-Ricart M. The role of the endothelium in the short-term complications of hematopoietic SCT. Bone Marrow Transplant. 2011;46(12):1495–502.

4. Deeg HJ, Sandmaier BM. Who is fit for allogeneic transplantation? Blood. 2010;116(23):4762–70.
5. Luznik L, O'Donnell PV, Symons HJ, Chen AR, Leffell MS, Zahurak M, et al. HLA-haploidentical bone marrow transplantation for hematologic malignancies using nonmyeloablative conditioning and high-dose, posttransplantation cyclophosphamide. Biol Blood Marrow Transplant. 2008;14(6):641–50.
6. Gyurkocza B, Sandmaier BM. Conditioning regimens for hematopoietic cell transplantation: one size does not fit all. Blood. 2014;124(3):344–53.
7. Sorror ML, Logan BR, Zhu X, Rizzo JD, Cooke KR, McCarthy PL, et al. Prospective validation of the predictive power of the hematopoietic cell transplantation comorbidity index: a Center for International Blood and Marrow Transplant Research Study. Biol Blood Marrow Transplant. 2015;21(8):1479–87.
8. Bacigalupo A, Ballen K, Rizzo D, Giralt S, Lazarus H, Ho V, et al. Defining the intensity of conditioning regimens: working definitions. Biol Blood Marrow Transplant. 2009 Dec;15(12):1628–33.
9. Thomas ED, Buckner CD, Banaji M, Clift RA, Fefer A, Flournoy N, et al. One hundred patients with acute leukemia treated by chemotherapy, total body irradiation, and allogeneic marrow transplantation. Blood. 1977;49(4):511–33.
10. Gooptu M, Kim HT, Ho VT, Alyea EP, Koreth J, Armand P, et al. A comparison of the myeloablative conditioning regimen fludarabine/busulfan with cyclophosphamide/total body irradiation, for allogeneic stem cell transplantation in the modern era: a cohort analysis. Biol Blood Marrow Transplant. 2018;24(8):1733–40.
11. Wong JYC, Filippi AR, Dabaja BS, Yahalom J, Specht L. Total body irradiation: guidelines from the international lymphoma radiation oncology group (ILROG). Int J Radiat Oncol Biol Phys. 2018;101(3):521–9.
12. Sabloff M, Tisseverasinghe S, Babadagli ME, Samant R. Total body irradiation for hematopoietic stem cell transplantation: what can we agree on? Curr Oncol Tor Ontol. 2021;28(1):903–17.
13. Thomas ED, Clift RA, Hersman J, Sanders JE, Stewart P, Buckner CD, et al. Marrow transplantation for acute nonlymphoblastic leukemic in first remission using fractionated or single-dose irradiation. Int J Radiat Oncol Biol Phys. 1982;8(5):817–21.
14. Clift RA, Buckner CD, Appelbaum FR, Bryant E, Bearman SI, Petersen FB, et al. Allogeneic marrow transplantation in patients with chronic myeloid leukemia in the chronic phase: a randomized trial of two irradiation regimens. Blood. 1991;77(8):1660–5.
15. Marks DI, Forman SJ, Blume KG, Pérez WS, Weisdorf DJ, Keating A, et al. A comparison of cyclophosphamide and total body irradiation with etoposide and total body irradiation as conditioning regimens for patients undergoing sibling allografting for acute lymphoblastic leukemia in first or second complete remission. Biol Blood Marrow Transplant. 2006;12(4):438–53.
16. Buchali A, Feyer P, Groll J, Massenkeil G, Arnold R, Budach V. Immediate toxicity during fractionated total body irradiation as conditioning for bone marrow transplantation. Radiother Oncol. 2000;54(2):157–62.
17. Leiper AD. Late effects of total body irradiation. Arch Dis Child. 1995;72(5):382–5.
18. Wong JYC, Filippi AR, Scorsetti M, Hui S, Muren LP, Mancosu P. Total marrow and total lymphoid irradiation in bone marrow transplantation for acute leukaemia. Lancet Oncol. 2020;21(10):e477–87.
19. Cornelissen JJ, Blaise D. Hematopoietic stem cell transplantation for patients with AML in first complete remission. Blood. 2016;127(1):62–70.
20. Solomon SR, Sizemore CA, Sanacore M, Zhang X, Brown S, Holland HK, et al. Haploidentical transplantation using T cell replete peripheral blood stem cells and myeloablative conditioning in patients with high-risk hematologic malignancies who lack conventional donors is well tolerated and produces excellent relapse-free survival: results of a prospective phase II trial. Biol Blood Marrow Transplant. 2012;18(12):1859–66.
21. Kekre N, Marquez-Malaver FJ, Cabrero M, Piñana J, Esquirol A, Soiffer RJ, et al. Fludarabine/busulfan versus fludarabine/melphalan conditioning in patients undergoing reduced-intensity conditioning hematopoietic stem cell transplantation for lymphoma. Biol Blood Marrow Transplant. 2016;22(10):1808–15.

22. Çiftçiler R, Göker H, Demiroğlu H, Aladağ E, Aksu S, Haznedaroğlu İC, et al. Comparison of myeloablative versus reduced-intensity conditioning regimens for allogeneic hematopoietic stem cell transplantation in acute myeloid leukemia: a cohort study. Turk J Hematol. 2019;36(2):88–96.
23. Beelen DW, Stelljes M, Reményi P, Wagner-Drouet EM, Dreger P, Bethge W, et al. Treosulfan compared with reduced-intensity busulfan improves allogeneic hematopoietic cell transplantation outcomes of older acute myeloid leukemia and myelodysplastic syndrome patients: final analysis of a prospective randomized trial. Am J Hematol. 2022;97(8):1023–34.
24. Luznik L, Bolaños-Meade J, Zahurak M, Chen AR, Smith BD, Brodsky R, et al. High-dose cyclophosphamide as single-agent, short-course prophylaxis of graft-versus-host disease. Blood. 2010;115(16):3224–30.
25. Sugita J, Yanada M. Current status of conditioning regimens in haploidentical hematopoietic cell transplantation. Hematology. 2024;29(1):2332866.
26. Symons HJ, Zahurak M, Cao Y, Chen A, Cooke K, Gamper C, et al. Myeloablative haploidentical BMT with posttransplant cyclophosphamide for hematologic malignancies in children and adults. Blood Adv. 2020;4(16):3913–25.
27. Swoboda R, Labopin M, Giebel S, Angelucci E, Arat M, Aljurf M, et al. Total body irradiation plus fludarabine versus thiotepa, busulfan plus fludarabine as a myeloablative conditioning for adults with acute lymphoblastic leukemia treated with haploidentical hematopoietic cell transplantation. A study by the Acute Leukemia Working Party of the EBMT. Bone Marrow Transplant. 2022;57(3):399–406.
28. Yanada M, Harada K, Shimomura Y, Arai Y, Konuma T. Conditioning regimens for allogeneic hematopoietic cell transplantation in acute myeloid leukemia: real-world data from the Japanese registry studies. Front Oncol. 2022;12:1050633.
29. Saraceni F, Labopin M, Raiola AM, Blaise D, Reményi P, Sorà F, et al. Thiotepa-busulfan-fludarabine compared to Treosulfan-based conditioning for haploidentical transplant with posttransplant cyclophosphamide in patients with acute myeloid leukemia in remission: a study from the acute leukemia working party of the EBMT. HemaSphere. 2023;7(10):e952.
30. Hui S, Brunstein C, Takahashi Y, DeFor T, Holtan SG, Bachanova V, et al. Dose escalation of total marrow irradiation in high-risk patients undergoing allogeneic hematopoietic stem cell transplantation. Biol Blood Marrow Transplant. 2017;23(7):1110–6.
31. Modi D, Kim S, Deol A, Ayash L, Ratanatharathorn V, Uberti JP. Comparison of myeloablative and reduced intensity conditioning regimens in haploidentical peripheral blood stem cell transplantation. Bone Marrow Transplant. 2021;56(3):741–4.
32. Solomon SR, St Martin A, Shah NN, Fatobene G, Al Malki MM, Ballen KK, et al. Myeloablative vs reduced intensity T-cell-replete haploidentical transplantation for hematologic malignancy. Blood Adv. 2019;3(19):2836–44.
33. Arcuri LJ, Hamerschlak N, Rocha V, Bonfim C, Kerbauy MN. Outcomes after haploidentical hematopoietic cell transplantation with post-transplantation cyclophosphamide: a systematic review and meta-analysis comparing myeloablative with reduced-intensity conditioning regimens and bone marrow with peripheral blood stem cell grafts. Transplant Cell Ther. 2021;27(9):782.e1–7.
34. Kröger N, Solano C, Wolschke C, Bandini G, Patriarca F, Pini M, et al. Antilymphocyte globulin for prevention of chronic graft-versus-host disease. N Engl J Med. 2016;374(1):43–53.
35. Ringdén O, Labopin M, Ehninger G, Niederwieser D, Olsson R, Basara N, et al. Reduced intensity conditioning compared with myeloablative conditioning using unrelated donor transplants in patients with acute myeloid leukemia. J Clin Oncol Off J Am Soc Clin Oncol. 2009;27(27):4570–7.
36. Fermand JP, Ravaud P, Chevret S, Divine M, Leblond V, Belanger C, et al. High-dose therapy and autologous peripheral blood stem cell transplantation in multiple myeloma: up-front or rescue treatment? Results of a multicenter sequential randomized clinical trial. Blood. 1998;92(9):3131–6.

37. Child JA, Morgan GJ, Davies FE, Owen RG, Bell SE, Hawkins K, et al. High-dose chemotherapy with hematopoietic stem-cell rescue for multiple myeloma. N Engl J Med. 2003;348(19):1875–83.
38. Palumbo A, Cavallo F, Gay F, Di Raimondo F, Ben Yehuda D, Petrucci MT, et al. Autologous transplantation and maintenance therapy in multiple myeloma. N Engl J Med. 2014;371(10):895–905.
39. Attal M, Lauwers-Cances V, Hulin C, Leleu X, Caillot D, Escoffre M, et al. Lenalidomide, bortezomib, and dexamethasone with transplantation for myeloma. N Engl J Med. 2017;376(14):1311–20.
40. Moreau P, Facon T, Attal M, Hulin C, Michallet M, Maloisel F, et al. Comparison of 200 mg/m(2) melphalan and 8 Gy total body irradiation plus 140 mg/m(2) melphalan as conditioning regimens for peripheral blood stem cell transplantation in patients with newly diagnosed multiple myeloma: final analysis of the Intergroupe Francophone du Myélome 9502 randomized trial. Blood. 2002;99(3):731–5.
41. Barlogie B, Jagannath S, Desikan KR, Mattox S, Vesole D, Siegel D, et al. Total therapy with tandem transplants for newly diagnosed multiple myeloma. Blood. 1999;93(1):55–65.
42. Attal M, Harousseau JL, Facon T, Guilhot F, Doyen C, Fuzibet JG, et al. Single versus double autologous stem-cell transplantation for multiple myeloma. N Engl J Med. 2003;349(26):2495–502.
43. Htut M, D'Souza A, Krishnan A, Bruno B, Zhang MJ, Fei M, et al. Autologous/allogeneic hematopoietic cell transplantation versus tandem autologous transplantation for multiple myeloma: comparison of long-term postrelapse survival. Biol Blood Marrow Transplant. 2018;24(3):478–85.
44. Maranzano M, Mead M. The role of transplantation in Hodgkin lymphoma. Front Oncol. 2022;12:1054314.
45. Sellner L, Boumendil A, Finel H, Choquet S, de Rosa G, Falzetti F, et al. Thiotepa-based high-dose therapy for autologous stem cell transplantation in lymphoma: a retrospective study from the EBMT. Bone Marrow Transplant. 2016;51(2):212–8.
46. Pettengell R, Radford JA, Morgenstern GR, Scarffe JH, Harris M, Woll PJ, et al. Survival benefit from high-dose therapy with autologous blood progenitor-cell transplantation in poor-prognosis non-Hodgkin's lymphoma. J Clin Oncol. 1996;14(2):586–92.
47. Dreyling M, Lenz G, Hoster E, Van Hoof A, Gisselbrecht C, Schmits R, et al. Early consolidation by myeloablative radiochemotherapy followed by autologous stem cell transplantation in first remission significantly prolongs progression-free survival in mantle-cell lymphoma: results of a prospective randomized trial of the European MCL Network. Blood. 2005;105(7):2677–84.
48. Steffanoni S, Calimeri T, Marktel S, Nitti R, Foppoli M, Ferreri AJM. Diagnosis and treatment using autologous stem-cell transplantation in primary central nervous system lymphoma: a systematic review. Cancer. 2023;15(2):526.
49. Sharrack B, Saccardi R, Alexander T, Badoglio M, Burman J, Farge D, et al. Autologous haematopoietic stem cell transplantation and other cellular therapy in multiple sclerosis and immune-mediated neurological diseases: updated guidelines and recommendations from the EBMT Autoimmune Diseases Working Party (ADWP) and the Joint Accreditation Committee of EBMT and ISCT (JACIE). Bone Marrow Transplant. 2020;55(2):283–306.
50. Gratwohl A, Passweg J, Bocelli-Tyndall C, Fassas A, van Laar JM, Farge D, et al. Autologous hematopoietic stem cell transplantation for autoimmune diseases. Bone Marrow Transplant. 2005;35(9):869–79.

Chapter 43
Haploidentical Hematopoietic Stem Cell Transplantation

M. Gopinathan and Rahul Naithani

Abstract Haploidentical hematopoietic stem cell transplantation (HSCT) is a curative option for various hematological conditions for patients who lack matched related donors. Haplo-HSCT is marked by key advancements in immunology, graft engineering, and post-transplant management, which have helped overcome the major challenges associated with human leukocyte (HLA) mismatches. In recent times, outcomes of haplo HSCT are similar to matched sibling donor transplants. There are several factors involved in appropriate donor selection. T-cell depletion has been a useful modality to reduce graft versus host disease (GVHD). Immune recovery is an important aspect of haplo HSCT and this is discussed. The recent Indian scenario is also presented.

Keywords Haploidentical · Transplant · India · T-cell depletion · Donor selection

Learning Objectives
Upon completion of this chapter, the reader will understand:

- HLA-haploidentical hematopoietic cell transplantation (HSCT) involves the transplantation of hematopoietic cells from a related donor who shares one HLA haplotype with the recipient while being mismatched for various HLA molecules on the haplotype that is not shared.
- There are various alternative sources for donors (such as haploidentical, mismatched unrelated donor, or umbilical cord blood) for patients who do not have a suitable HLA-matched sibling donor (MSD) or matched unrelated donor (MUD).

M. Gopinathan
Department of Hematology and Bone marrow Transplant, MGM Health Care & Cancer Institute, Chennai, India

R. Naithani (✉)
Department of Hematology and Bone Marrow Transplant, Artemis Hospital, Gurugram, India

H. P. Pati et al. (eds.), *Clinical Hematology and Hemato-Oncology*,
https://doi.org/10.1007/978-981-92-1167-8_43

- The primary benefits of haploidentical HSCT include the nearly universal availability of donors, the speed and reduced cost of the graft, a sufficient amount of hematopoietic stem cells for transplantation and immune reconstitution, as well as the ability to access the donor for additional donations or lymphocytes in the event of a relapse.
- The primary obstacles include host and donor T cells that react to HLA alloantigens, leading to significant bidirectional alloreactivity, as well as a high rate of fatal graft rejection or severe/fatal graft-versus-host disease (GVHD) unless appropriate preventive measures are taken.
- The selection process takes into account the donor's health, age, sex, relationship to the patient, HLA mismatch (in terms of both host-versus-graft and graft-versus-host), ABO blood group, cytomegalovirus (CMV) serostatus, and potentially matching for noninherited maternal antigens (NIMA) and natural killer cell alloreactivity.
- For patients with no other viable donors, desensitization procedures can be utilized to decrease the levels of circulating donor-specific HLA antibodies.
- There are various approaches for haploidentical hematopoietic stem cell transplantation (HSCT), both T-cell-depleted and T-cell-replete.
- *Immune reconstitution*–Kinetics of immune reconstitution are related to the transplantation platform.

43.1 Introduction

Bone marrow transplant (BMT) or hematopoietic stem cell transplantation (HSCT) is a curative option for various hematological conditions. Matched-related donors (MRD) are available for 25–30% of patients. For patients who do not have an HLA-matched sibling donor available, alternative graft sources include HLA-matched or partially mismatched unrelated adult donors, umbilical cord blood stem cells, and related donors who are partially HLA-mismatched (haploidentical donors) [1].

Sometimes clinicians are faced with a patient with severe aplastic anemia (SAA) or high-risk malignancies where an urgent transplant is required. In these situations, searching for a matched unrelated donor (MUD) and then confirmatory typing of the donor may not be feasible in a short period. Significant time delays can occur in the immediate availability of donors and the final delivery of hematopoietic stem cells (HSCs). A haploidentical (haplo) donor from a family is generally immediately available. This short time interval reduces the need for bridging therapies and reduces transfusion load and antimicrobial support. This is expected to improve transplant outcomes and reduce the financial burden for the family [2]. Haploidentical HSCT may also provide a stronger graft-versus-tumor (GVT) effect, a lower risk of graft-versus-host disease (GVHD), and the practical advantage of readily available donors for subsequent donor lymphocyte infusions or a second HSCT [3].

The history of haplo-HSCT is marked by key advancements in immunology, graft engineering, and post-transplant management, which have helped overcome the major challenges associated with HLA mismatches. The concept of haploidentical transplantation emerged in the 1970s as researchers sought alternatives for patients who did not have a matched sibling or unrelated donor. Early attempts at haplo-HSCT were largely unsuccessful due to high rates of graft rejection, severe graft-versus-host disease (GVHD), and transplant-related mortality (TRM). Initial haplo-HSCT attempts were based on the same protocols used for matched sibling donor (MSD) transplants, but these failed due to strong donor-recipient immune incompatibility. The lack of effective immunosuppression often resulted in graft rejection. In the 1980s and 1990s, T-cell depletion (TCD) emerged as a potential solution to prevent GVHD. Ex vivo depletion of T-cells from the graft significantly reduced GVHD but led to delayed immune reconstitution, increasing the risk of infections and relapse. Despite these early challenges, haplo-HSCT remained an area of interest, particularly for patients with urgent transplant needs. During the 1990s, advances in graft manipulation and immunosuppressive regimens improved haploidentical transplantation outcomes [4].

A breakthrough in haplo-HSCT occurred in the early 2000s with the development of post-transplant cyclophosphamide (PTCy) at Johns Hopkins University. This approach revolutionized haploidentical transplantation by selectively eliminating alloreactive T-cells while preserving regulatory T-cells, leading to lower GVHD rates without the need for extensive T-cell depletion, improved graft acceptance, and reduced risk of graft rejection with faster immune reconstitution, thereby reducing infection-related complications. In the last decade, haplo-HSCT has become an increasingly preferred option due to refined graft manipulation techniques like α/β T-cell depletion, NK-cell therapy, mesenchymal stem cell infusion, better conditioning regimens, and expanded use across diseases.

T-cell depletion has been a useful modality to reduce GVHD. Ex vivo T-cell–depletion strategies have progressively evolved, beginning with the selection of $CD34^+$ hematopoietic stem cell progenitors, followed by depletion of $CD3^+$ T cells, and more recently by selective removal of $\alpha\beta^+$ T cells with subsequent add-back of $CD45RO^+$ cells [5]. Ex vivo T-cell depletion strategies are technically demanding, costly, and consume a lot of time. A T-cell replete (TCR) haplo HSCT is superior to T-cell-depleted HSCT in adults with hematological malignancies in terms of overall survival (OS), non-relapse mortality (NRM), chronic GVHD (c GVHD), and immune reconstitution, which are important considerations in resource-constrained settings [6]. The use of post-transplant cyclophosphamide (PTCy) in T-cell–replete HSCT offers several inherent advantages, including procedural simplicity and ease of implementation, lower immediate costs related to donor processing and T-cell depletion, and the absence of complex logistics or specialized manufacturing facilities required for ex vivo T-cell depletion. Relapses and infections due to delayed immune reconstitution are common and are a major cause of death after haploidentical HSCT [7].

Advances in graft engineering and pharmacologic modulation of alloreactivity have led to reductions in GVHD and non-relapse mortality, while improving overall and progression-free survival, thereby establishing this graft source as a viable alternative for patients who lack an HLA-matched sibling or unrelated donor.

43.2 Advantages and Limitations of Haploidentical Donors

A key advantage of the HLA-haploidentical donor approach is the near-universal availability of closely related and highly motivated donors. These donors are usually immediately available. With peripheral blood stem cell apheresis increasing, adequate hematopoietic stem cells for transplantation and memory T cells for immune reconstitution are generally not an issue. There is a significant financial advantage to using a family donor as it saves the cost of procuring an unrelated donor or cord blood.

A haploidentical donor is readily available for post-transplant therapies like donor lymphocyte infusion (DLI) and, rarely, HLA-matched platelets. In patients with high-risk leukemia, a haploidentical HSCT may be associated with a stronger graft-versus-leukemia, leading to lower relapses and increased overall survival [8].

A major challenge in HLA-haploidentical HSCT is the high risk of graft rejection and GVHD resulting from bidirectional alloreactivity. Without effective prophylactic strategies, this can lead to a high incidence of fatal graft rejection or severe, potentially fatal GVHD [9].

43.3 Donor Selection for Haploidentical HSCT

Most centers have made molecular typing of the 10 HLA alleles—HLA-A, HLA-B, HLA-C, HLA-DRB1, and HLA-DQB1—the norm. At five years, the likelihood of OS may decrease by about 10% for every HLA mismatch [10]. Except for HLA-C antigen mismatches, which are often avoided since they seem to indicate a worse prognosis, the effects of HLA matching seem to be comparable for individuals undergoing unrelated peripheral blood hematopoietic cell (PBSC) transplants. Similar to bone marrow transplants, the outcome did not seem to be affected by HLA-DQB1 mismatch. The mismatched antigen's expression level may also affect the patient's outcome. For instance, elevated expression of the mismatched HLA-C was seen in a study of almost 2000 patients who received an unrelated donor graft with a single HLA-C mismatch where it was associated with increased risks of acute GVHD (a GVHD), non-relapse mortality, and overall mortality [11]. ABO-compatible donors, those with a cytomegalovirus (CMV) immunoglobulin G (IgG) serologic matching, younger adults over older adults, and male or nulliparous female donors over multiparous female donors for male recipients are given preference [12].

Donor-specific HLA antibodies Pregnancy, allogeneic transplantation, or previous blood transfusions can cause patients to develop sensitization to HLA alloantigens. Graft failure is more likely to occur when donor-specific HLA antibodies (DSA) are present [13]. It is recommended that the recipient be screened for donor-specific HLA antibodies. Desensitization to reduce DSA concentration and promote engraftment may be considered if no alternative graft source can be found [14]. Incorporating donor leukocyte irradiated buffy coat with a multimodality desensitization protocol demonstrated effectiveness in significantly reducing DSA levels before HSCT.

KIR gene haplotype The killer-cell immunoglobulin-like receptor (KIR) gene complex encodes up to 15 genes for natural killer (NK) cell immunoglobulin-like receptors that recognize epitopes on HLA-A, HLA-B, and HLA-C molecules, collectively referred to as KIR ligands.

KIR haplotypes can be activating or inhibitory. KIR haplotypes can be activated or inhibited. KIR-haplotype A mostly encodes inhibitory receptors with just one activating receptor, whereas KIR-haplotype B encodes multiple activating receptors. A study involving 1400 unrelated transplant donors providing grafts to patients with acute myeloid leukemia (AML) or acute lymphoblastic leukemia (ALL) demonstrated that KIR ligand status influenced outcomes in patients with AML but not in those with ALL [15].

Non-inherited maternal HLA antigens HLA-haploidentical siblings inherit either the paternal or the maternal HLA haplotype. Individuals who inherit the paternal HLA haplotype are mismatched for both the inherited and the non-inherited maternal HLA haplotypes. Exposure to maternal cells in utero may induce immunologic hyporesponsiveness to non-inherited maternal HLA antigens (NIMA), which can reduce alloreactivity against a NIMA-mismatched HLA-haploidentical sibling after hematopoietic cell transplantation (HCT). Mismatching with maternal antigens is more easily tolerated in haploidentical transplants than mismatching with paternal antigens [16].

Enhanced natural killer cell alloreactivity Natural killer (NK) cells might contribute to the prevention or treatment of relapse following HLA-haploidentical HSCT. The killer-cell immunoglobulin-like receptor (KIR) gene complex is responsible for encoding as many as 15 genes associated with NK cell immunoglobulin-like receptors that detect epitopes of HLA-A, HLA-B, and HLA-C, which are referred to as KIR ligands [17].

Following HLA-haploidentical hematopoietic cell transplantation (HCT), the presence of HLA mismatch between the donor and recipient results in a scenario where recipient leukemia cells do not express inhibitory "self" HLA ligands for KIRs on donor natural killer (NK) cells, which allows NK cells to exert a graft-versus-leukemia (GVL) response. The lack of HLA ligands on recipient cells for donor inhibitory KIRs (known as KIR ligand incompatibility) was found to predict NK cell alloreactivity in vitro and was linked to a strong anti-leukemia effect following T cell-depleted "megadose" HLA-haploidentical HSCT in cases of AML, but not in ALL. Conversely, the favorable impact of KIR ligand incompatibility was not observed following T cell-replete HLA-haploidentical HCT, likely because T cells that induce GVHD obscure the positive effects of NK cell alloreactivity [18].

43.4 Haploidentical Versus Other Donor Sources

MSD generally takes precedence over haplo donors due to long-term safety data, but certain scenarios that need reconsideration include:

1. Increasing donor age—comorbidities, concerns of mobilization, Clonal hematopoiesis of indeterminate potential (CHIP), etc.
2. MSD with carrier state in benign disorders like Primary immunodeficiency (PID), Inherited bone marrow failure syndrome, metabolic disorders, etc.
3. High-risk leukemias.

When transplanted for high-risk acute leukemias and lymphomas in partial remission, the graft versus leukemia effect is robust with haplo grafts, thus offering Leukemia relapse-free survival (LRFS) advantage with a balanced TRM. However, the risks should be weighed against the benefits, which is predicted in a precise manner with the use of the availability of KIR typing, selection based on NIMA mismatch, and use of online software for predicting vectors for graft versus host (GVH), host versus graft (HVG) direction.

Mehta et al. demonstrated comparable outcomes of haploidentical donors with MUD, MSD cohort of 661 patients [19]. Patients with haplo donors had better relapse-free survival (RFS) compared to MUD/MSD and GVHD-free, relapse-free survival (GRFS) compared to MUD donors, but a higher risk of viral reactivations and thereby NRM. On subset analysis, the NRM in the haplo cohort was mainly attributed to older recipients and donors. A Blood and Marrow Transplant Clinical Trials Network (BMT CTN) analysis revealed better transplant outcomes in AML between haplo TCR with PTCy versus MUD. The incidence of 3-month aGVHD (grade 2–4) rates was (16% vs 33%, $p < 0.0001$) in myeloablative conditioning (MAC) and (19% vs 28%, $p < 0.0001$) in reduced intensity conditioning (RIC), respectively, when compared with MUD [20]. Similarly, the 3-year incidence of cGVHD (30% vs 53%, $p < 0.0001$) was substantially lower with haplo than in the MUD cohort. Similarly, Xiao et al. demonstrated a pooled OS of 92.7% with thalassemia-free survival of 84.5% with both TCR/TCD approaches [21]. Since T-cell depletion always comes with a cost, even a TCR transplant with a PTCy backbone delivers an EFS of 68% and can be a game changer while dealing with PID [22].

43.5 Selection of Graft: Bone Marrow Versus Peripheral Blood Versus Umbilical Cord Blood

The major factors to be considered while selecting the source of graft include ease of collection, durability, and early engraftment while minimizing GVHD and a strong GVL with malignancies. While the peripheral blood (PB) source achieves early engraftment the cGVHD rates are slightly higher than the bone marrow (BM) source, though the NRM and OS were similar. Umbilical cord blood (UCB) has gone out of the landscape due to prolonged engraftment time, higher rejection, and delayed immune reconstitution thus defeating the purpose. The scientific basis for the above is a higher proportion of effector T cells (Teff) cells in the PB graft than regulatory T cells (Tregs) in the BM source, while the UCB source not only provides lesser nucleated cells, demanding higher processing with weight, but also lesser T cells and thereby permits more HLA mismatch. Table 43.1 summarizes the major features of the three stem cell sources.

In the setting of myeloid malignancies with MAC use, PB over BM achieves engraftment early, while the graft failure rates, NRM, and OS are similar between both groups [23]. A Center for International Blood and Marrow Transplant Research (CIBMTR) analysis using RIC for a variety of hematological malignancies reported higher acute and cGVHD, and lesser relapse with PB than BM though OS is the same [24]. The concluding note leans towards the use of PB for high-risk malignancies and MRD-positive disease, whereas the BM grafts can be restricted to experienced centers able to deliver higher nucleated cell dose and low-risk disease.

The limitations of using UCB in malignancies include a higher relapse risk compared to other sources due to lesser T cell dose and the preferred use of RIC to a larger extent [25]. Though HLA mismatch is permissible, the volumes required for adults are almost double that of children, placing them at a higher risk of GVHD [26]. UCB source remains a viable option in pediatric patients with metabolic/other benign disorders where a single unit suffices and when a suitable donor is not found [27].

Table 43.1 Sources of graft for haploidentical hematopoietic stem cell transplant

	Bone marrow	Peripheral blood	Cord blood
Composition	Tregs higher	Teff > Tregs	T naïve cells
Volume processed	10–20 ml/kg	150–400 ml	80–160 ml
CD34	3×10^6/kg	8×10^6/kg	0.2×10^6/kg
CD3	25×10^6/kg	250×10^6/kg	2.5×10^6/kg
Engraftment	Early than UCB, but slower than PB	Early and stable	Late
Graft failure	More than PB	Less	Highest
Acute GVHD	Lesser	Higher than BM	Least
Chronic GVHD	Lesser	Higher than BM	Least
Viral reactivations	Less than UCB	Less than UCB	Highest
Immune reconstitution	Early	Earliest than BM	Slowest
Preferred use	Benign>Malignancies	Malignancies	Benign>Malignancies

Tregs regulatory T cells; *Teff* effector T cells; *UCB* umbilical cord blood; *PB* peripheral blood; *BM* bone marrow; *GVHD* graft versus host disease

BM remains the preferred source in benign disorders like SAA, where GVHD is unacceptable, and GVL has no role. Though it is the preferred graft source in the United States, with improved immunosuppression, PB sources report similar GVHD rates on par with BM at an added advantage of earlier platelet engraftment with fewer graft failures [28]. Even in hemoglobinopathies with a good pretransplant immunosuppression and low-dose TBI as a part of conditioning, graft failure is reduced with PB than BM.

43.6 T-cell Reduction Strategies

The initial historical failures with haplografts helped us to decipher that successful engraftment needs bidirectional tolerance in overcoming the HLA barrier, which in turn is decided by the cell dose, composition, conditioning in the short term, and GVHD prophylaxis in the long term. Apart from absolute CD34, the role of donor T cells is well recognized in facilitating engraftment as well as triggering GVHD, with the resident host T cells mediating rejection. Thus, various T cell modulatory strategies have been devised and improvised over time [29]. Table 43.2 shows the comparison of T-cell-replete and T-cell-deplete platforms.

The initial TCD approaches using marrow grafts were conducted as early as 1980, with SCID transplants being successful with negligible GVHD rates, as there was a paucity of host T cells. This approach was marred with high rejection rates in malignancies due to the presence of resident T cells. Hence, a megadose CD34 strategy >10 × 10^6 cell/kg was introduced after a myeloablative total body irradiation (TBI) backbone, which resulted in engraftment close to 80% and 16% GVHD [30]. After several improvisations, α/β T-cell depletion is currently used with MAC, particularly in benign disorders, but of late, the RIC backbone is also developed. Since the neutrophil engraftment happens early compared to TCR transplant it can be adopted by elderly/frail individuals, patients with cardiac comorbidities to omit PTCy, and patients with infections. The challenges of graft failure, relapse, delayed immune reconstitution, and viral infections remain compared to TCR transplants, with added economic burden and availability of expertise.

The demonstration of PTCy in mice models by Luznik et al. opened the doorstep for a breakthrough in the haplotransplant space [31]. O Donnel et al. published the initial cohort of patients transplanted with BM using a RIC backbone of Fludarabine, TBI, which was later converted to MAC, facilitating higher engraftment [32]. The aGVHD rates were to the tune of 36%, with grade 3/4 in 6%, with safety analysis demonstrating lower cGVHD after two doses of cyclophosphamide. The 2-year EFS and OS were 36%, and 26% respectively, with this approach. Parallel BMT CTN 0603 and 0604 trials were comparing BM and UCB, with higher relapse rates in UCB, though EFS and OS were better in the BM source. To derive further efficacy, John Hopkins adapted the PTCy backbone with PB source and MAC conditioning with betterment in event-free survival (EFS), OS, GVHD rates, and reduction of relapse compared to the former approach [33].

Table 43.2 Comparison of T-cell replete and T-cell deplete platforms

	T-cell replete graft	T-cell deplete graft
Techniques	PTCy & GIAC strategy PTCy feasible	CD34 selection, CD3 depletion, TCR αβ depletion
Graft composition	CD34: 6–8 × 10^6 cells/kg CD3: 2–4 × 10^8 cells/kg	CD34: >10 × 10^6 cells/kg CD3 αβ: 0.04 × 10^6 cells/kg CD3 ϒδ: 7–55 × 10^6 cells/kg
Conditioning	MAC, RIC	MAC > RIC
GVHD prophylaxis	CNI + MMF	Nil or single agent CNI
aGVHD	Higher than TCD	Lesser than TCR
cGVHD	Comparable with PTCy	–
Graft failure	Less compared to TCD	Higher
Immune reconstitution	Fast Does not require addback	Slower Needs addback of memory cells
Usual causes of mortality	Disease relapse, toxicity, GVHD	Graft rejection, life threatening infections, relapse
Advantages	Low cost Faster immune reconstitution	Faster engraftment Avoid PTCy in elderly/ cardiac co-morbidities Feasible with active bacterial infections
Disadvantages	Longer duration of neutropenia, mucositis Delivering full dose in infants, elderly individuals, marrow failure syndromes, PIDs.	High cost Availability of expertise

PTCy post-transplant cyclophosphamide; *GIAC* granulocyte colony stimulating factor mobilization, intensive immunosuppression, antithymocyte globulin and combination of bone marrow and peripheral blood stem cell transplantation; *MAC* myeloablative conditioning; *RIC* reduced intensity conditioning; *TCR* T-cell replete; *TCD* T-cell deplete; *aGVHD* acute graft versus host disease; *cGVHD* chronic graft versus host disease *CNI* calcineurin inhibitor; *MMF* mycophenolate mofetil

Granulocyte colony stimulating factor mobilization, intensive immunosuppression, anti-thymocyte globulin, and a combination of BM and PB stem cell transplantation (GIAC) is an intense model of the TCR approach developed at Peking University with busulphan, cyclophosphamide, and semustine in conditioning. The initial studies with this strategy reported 100% engraftment and full chimerism and leukemia-free survival (LFS), aGVHD, and cGVHD rates similar to MUD. The median days of engraftment, NRM, and GVHD rates are better compared to PTCy, with survival benefit only in intermediate-risk disease [34]. However, with limitations in the accessibility of semustine and laborious post-transplant care due to intense immunosuppression, its use is restricted to a few centers.

Table 43.3 Time line of recovery [43]

Cell line	Time line
Monocytes	10–14 days
Neutrophils >0.5 × 10^9/L	~14 days for PBSC, ~21 days for BM, and ~ 30 days for CB
NK cells	30–100 days
T cells	100 days
CD19+ B cells	1–2 years

PBSC peripheral blood stem cell; *BM* bone marrow; *CB* cord blood

43.7 Immune Reconstitution in Haplo-Identical Transplant

The immune recovery follows a similar pattern of evolution, with innate immunity followed by adaptive immunity with adaptivity to a diverse antigenic repertoire. The timeline of immune recovery, as depicted in Table 43.3 remains crucial to derive the benefit of HSCT not only from primary hematopoietic recovery but also to extend graft versus leukemia effect and viral reactivations. The recovery of innate immunity is marked by an increase in monocytes with subsequent neutrophil engraftment and stabilization in the first month, followed by NK cell recovery in the first 100 days.

After a brief period of lymphopenia in the first month, the adaptive immunity recovers steadily over 2 years with complex interaction between T and B cell compartments, and is influenced by multiple factors, including

1. Donor and recipient age
2. MAC vs. RIC
3. Use of serotherapy
4. Source of graft
5. Graft composition—CD34/CD3
6. T cell depletion techniques
7. Type and duration of GVHD prophylaxis
8. Peripheral expansion of T cells after exposure to a variety of antigens
9. Thymic environment of the recipient
10. Concurrent use of myelosuppressive drugs
11. Active GVHD

The CD8 cytotoxic subset with a limited repertoire is followed by the memory T cell subset capable of wider recognition. The normal CD4/CD8 ratio is reversed until a year of transplant, and relative numbers are maintained by the cycling of mature lymphocytes [35]. The regulatory T cell subset helps to ameliorate inflammation through IL-10 and TGF-beta, preventing GVHD while preserving the GVL effect, which is thymus-dependent and is the last subset to expand. The B cell recovery happens a little later than T cells from 6 months and continues to stabilize till 2 years. It is imperative to remember that qualitative recovery follows quantitative recovery [36].

43.8 Methods of Assessment

The evaluation starts with a complete blood count, in particular, absolute lymphocyte count (ALC), and recovery of the same correlates with clearance of viral infections post-transplant. Immunoglobulin assay helps to determine the B cell functionality as well as aids the clinician in the replacement of intravenous immunoglobulin (IVIG), particularly in PID cohorts. Flow cytometric (FCM) enumeration of cell subset analysis demonstrates B, T, NK, myeloid as well as dendritic cell subsets.

43.9 Implications of Recovery

1. Mortality benefit with early immune reconstitution: Early immune recovery is associated with better infection-related mortality rates. ALC/CD3 at day 30, more than 300, 120 cells/microL, is associated with improved outcomes and stands as an independent predictor of PFS, and OS in transplant [37]. Treg improvement is seen better with post-transplant cyclophosphamide due to the expansion of myeloid-derived suppressor cells for abrogating GVHD while overcoming the HLA barrier.
2. Infections: The spectrum of infections follows the cell recovery with bacterial and fungal infections in the first 30 days, followed by viral infections. The diagnostic testing and duration of prophylaxis can be guided through analysis of immune recovery.
3. Timing of vaccination: With every vaccine given post-transplant, the host develops short and long-lived plasma cells for immediate and long-term response. Hence, the timing can be scheduled more logically, taking immune recovery into account.
4. Graft versus leukemia effect: The separation between GVHD and GVL is prominent over time; donor NK/T cells from the graft mainly contribute to disease control. In the absence of active GVHD, DLI can be timed preemptively to augment LFS in high-risk malignancies.

43.10 Indian Context

The number of haploidentical HSCTs increased to 683 (out of 1665 allogeneic HSCTs) in 2022. In that year, haploidentical transplants accounted for 26% of adult allogeneic HSCTs and 35% of pediatric allogeneic HSCTs. During the same period, the number of matched unrelated donor (MUD) transplants increased from 76 to 157. The expansion of transplant centers from 37 to 114 has significantly contributed to this growth [7].

Indian data on haploidentical HSCT is steadily expanding. With improvements in engraftment rates and reductions in the incidence of GVHD, haplo-HSCT has emerged as a viable and effective option for patients who otherwise have limited donor availability [38]. However, many of these studies are retrospective in nature, involve heterogeneous patient populations, and include both benign and malignant diseases. Consequently, they encompass a wide range of myeloablative and reduced-intensity conditioning regimens. While these achievements are noteworthy, further work remains to be done. Table 43.4 summarizes the Indian experience with haploidentical HSCT over the past five years [7].

Although the gap in the number of haploidentical transplants is gradually narrowing, another challenge remains. Internationally, outcomes following matched sibling donor (MSD), matched unrelated donor (MUD), and haploidentical HSCT are increasingly comparable [39, 40]. However, this parity has not yet been consistently observed in India. Some of the Indian studies summarized in Table 43.4 also have relatively shorter follow-up durations.

George et al. demonstrated a clear learning curve, with survival improving to 67% in more recent transplants compared with 25% during the 2010–2013 period [41]. While the single-center experiences reported in these studies are encouraging, continued research is necessary to optimize post-transplant cyclophosphamide (PTCy) administration and to identify patient-specific factors that may further improve treatment outcomes.

Table 43.4 Haplo-HSCT experience in India in the last five-years

Study (year)	Number	Median age (range)	Infections	Graft failure	Engrafted	GVHD	Cause of death	Survival
George et al. (2024)	Total: 127 Benign:61.5% AA: 46 PID: 21 Malignant: 38.5% AML: 15 ALL: 30	9.1 years (9 months-15 years)	92.7% Bact:31% Viral:76% Fungal:16%	Primary: 10.2%	113 (81.9%) Median: 16 days	Acute: 49.5% Chronic: 40.7%	Pre-engraftment: gram negative sepsis Day 100 NRM Malignant disease: 15.1% Benign disease: 31.7%	OS (2 years): 54.9%
Garg et al. (2024)	Total: 50 Benign: 12 (24%) AA: 6 Malignant: 38 (76%) AML: 16 ALL: 14	20 years (3–53 years)	GN-MDR: 19 (38%) Fungal: 2(4%) CMV reactivation: 33 (66%)	Primary: 3 (6%) Secondary: 5 (10%)	35 (70%) Neutrophil:16 days Platelet:18 days	Acute: 28% Chronic: 6%	Early TRM: 13 (26%) Late TRM: 7 (14%) Relapse related mortality @ day 100: 7 (14%)	OS (2 years): 43%
Arora et al. (2024)	Total: 51 Benign:25 Thalassemia-9 SCA 5 AA 6 FA 2 PID 3 Malignant: 26 ALL 15 AML 6	7.5 years (1–18 years)	–	15.6%	42 (82.3%)	Acute: 29% Chronic: 37%	Relapse: 8/15 Chronic GVHD:3/15 Others 4/15	OS (34.5 months): 70% RFS:55%

(continued)

Table 43.4 (continued)

Study (year)	Number	Median age (range)	Infections	Graft failure	Engrafted	GVHD	Cause of death	Survival
Jaiswal et al. (2024)	Total: 40 Benign: 40 AA: 24 PID: 2	10 years	CMV: 45%	5%	38 (95%)	Acute: 2.6% Chronic: 14.3%	NRM: 5%	OS: (4.6 years) 95%
Kharya et al. (2023)	Total: 79 AA: 79	10 years (1–4, 7–23)	Bacterial: 35(44.3%) Fungal: 5 (6.3%) Viral (non CMV): 12 (15.2%) CMV: 30 (37.9%)	Primary: 12 (16.43%) Secondary: 1 (1.63%)	Neutrophil:15 days Platelet: 18 days	Acute: 26.4% Chronic: 18.9%	TRM: 26 (33%) (all due to infectious complications)	OS (4 years): 61.6%
Lad et al. (2023)	Total: 33 AML/MDS: 15 (45%) ALL: 15 (45%)	28 years (15–35 years)	–	–	Neutrophil:14.5 day Platelet: 13 day	Acute: 27% Chronic: 71%	NRM 35%	OS (1.9 year): 52%
Mehta et al. (2023)	Total: 99 AML: 42 ALL: 28	31 years (9–62 years)	Culture positive: 42 (41.5%) CMV:65.3%	Primary: 9 (8.9%)	Neutrophil:15 day Platelet: 15.5 day	Acute: 33 (32.6%) Chronic: 71%	Sepsis: 27 (56.2%) Relapse: 10 (22.2%) GVHD: 4 (8.8%)	OS (1 year): 56.7%
Choudhary et al. (2021)	Total: 40 Thalassemia: 19 Sickle cell anemia: 21	7 years (1–29 years)	CMV: 42.5%	Primary: 4 (9%) Secondary: 6 (14%)	Neutrophil:14 day Platelet: 17 day	Acute: 22.5% Chronic: 20%	D + 100 TRM: 20% Sepsis: 6(15%) Acute GVHD: 2(5%)	OS (14.3 months): 80%

AA aplastic anemia; *ALL* acute lymphoblastic leukemia; *AML* acute myeloid leukemia; *CMV* cytomegalo virus; *FA* Fanconi anemia; *GVHD* graft versus host disease; *GN-MDR* Gram-negative multidrug resistant; *MDS* myelodysplastic syndrome; *NRM* non-relapse mortality, *OS* overall survival, *PID* primary immune deficiency; *RFS* relapse free survival; *SCA* sickle cell anemia; *TRM* transplant related mortality. Reproduced with permission from Springer Nature (License number 5980260459570)

43.11 Illustrative Cases

43.11.1 Case 1: Liver GVHD After Haploidentical HSCT for ETP ALL [41]

A 19-year-old male was diagnosed with early T-cell precursor acute lymphoblastic leukemia (ETP-ALL) and initiated on the BFM-95 regimen. His day-8 peripheral blood blast count was 12.1×10^9/L, and blasts persisted in the peripheral blood until day 22 of therapy. In view of the slow early response, oral venetoclax was added for 7 days (100 mg on day 1, 200 mg on day 2, 300 mg on day 3, and 100 mg from day 4 to day 7 in combination with oral posaconazole), while continuing the BFM regimen.

Post-induction bone marrow assessment on day 49 demonstrated morphologic remission but persistent measurable residual disease (MRD) of 0.99%. The patient subsequently received the HR1 phase of the BFM-95 protocol along with oral venetoclax (100 mg for 7 days with concomitant oral posaconazole). Bone marrow evaluation after HR1 showed <1% blasts with MRD negativity (<0.01%).

The patient did not have a matched sibling donor. A matched unrelated donor search identified six fully matched donors within India; however, none were willing to proceed with donation during the coronavirus pandemic.

The patient subsequently underwent a haploidentical allogeneic stem cell transplant with his father as the donor. The conditioning regimen consisted of fludarabine 30 mg/m^2 for three days (days −6, −5, and −4), followed by total body irradiation at 200 cGy twice daily for three days (days −3, −2, and −1). GVHD prophylaxis included tacrolimus, mycophenolate mofetil (MMF), and PTCy.

Neutrophil engraftment occurred on day +13 and platelet engraftment on day +10. The patient had persistently low tacrolimus trough levels and developed grade IV acute gastrointestinal GVHD on day +25 post-transplant, which responded to intravenous methylprednisolone. Chimerism analysis on day +30 demonstrated 99.14% donor chimerism. Bone marrow evaluation on day +60 showed morphologic remission with negative measurable residual disease (MRD <0.01%).

Later, the patient developed worsening liver function tests with hyperbilirubinemia. Hepatic GVHD was suspected, and steroid therapy was initiated; however, there was no clinical response. A liver biopsy subsequently revealed vanishing bile duct syndrome. Treatment with a combination of ruxolitinib, MMF, and steroids was initiated. At present, the patient has completed 5 years and 6 months of follow-up and remains in remission, doing well without any ongoing medications.

43.11.2 *Case 2: Refractory* **Clostridioides difficile** *Infection in a Child Post-haploidentical HSCT [42]*

A 2-year-old male with relapsed and refractory AML underwent haploidentical HSCT using his 5/10 HLA-matched sister as the donor. The conditioning regimen included cyclophosphamide, fludarabine, and melphalan. GVHD prophylaxis consisted of PTCy, MMF, and CSA.

On day +10 post-transplant, he developed grade IV acute GVHD involving the skin and gastrointestinal tract, presenting with rashes over the palms and trunk along with diarrhea. These symptoms responded to steroid therapy and resolved by day +15. The post-transplant course was further complicated by CMV reactivation on day +16, which was successfully treated with ganciclovir.

On day +19, the child developed severe diarrhea with 30–40 episodes of loose, watery stools per day. Stool testing by real-time polymerase chain reaction was positive for *Clostridioides difficile* infection (CDI), and treatment with metronidazole was initiated. At that time, the child was already receiving ciprofloxacin prophylaxis. Despite therapy, there was no improvement in stool frequency or consistency.

Oral vancomycin was added on day +25, and immunosuppression was reduced by discontinuing MMF and tapering the steroid dose, which was eventually stopped, while CSA was continued. The child subsequently developed per rectal bleeding lasting 2–3 days. A colonoscopy performed on day +29 revealed multiple colonic ulcers. Histopathological examination of the colonic biopsy showed mild architectural distortion with occasional crypt dropout. The crypts appeared dilated and atrophic and contained apoptotic debris, while the lamina propria did not show significant inflammatory infiltrate. No granulomas, parasites, viral inclusions, or eosinophils were identified. CMV testing became negative by day +32.

The child continued to experience persistent diarrhea and required parenteral nutrition for fluid and electrolyte support. Despite appropriate treatment with metronidazole for 6 days and oral vancomycin for 14 days, stool testing remained persistently positive for *C. difficile*.

On day +43, the child underwent fecal microbiota transplantation (FMT) using stool from his sister, who had also served as the hematopoietic stem cell donor. An upper gastrointestinal endoscopy was performed, and the fecal suspension was slowly instilled under direct visualization at the duodenojejunal junction. The patient was discharged 10 days after the FMT while receiving oral vancomycin and nasogastric feeding. Stool testing for *Clostridioides difficile* performed 16 days after FMT was negative, following which oral vancomycin was discontinued. At follow-up one year after HSCT and nine months after FMT, the child remained well with no recurrence of CDI, although he subsequently experienced a relapse of AML.

43.12 Future Directions

We now understand that younger donors may be associated with improved survival due to a lower incidence of GVHD and NRM. NK cell alloreactivity with a higher number of inhibitory KIRs with corresponding ligands in recipient cells may improve transplant outcomes. KIR gene typing for donor selection may be helpful in the future. Patients with high levels of DSA are at an advanced risk for engraftment failure and require desensitization. NK cells could augment the HSC graft of patients with myeloid malignancies, while CART cells could be administered during the early post HSCT period in patients with B-cell malignancies [43].

References

1. Batra A, Perumal Kalaiyarasi J, Kannan K, Mehra N, Ganesan P, Karunakaran P, Dhanushkodi M, Selvarajan G, Rajan AK, Kesana S, Ganesan T, Sagar TG, Radhakrishnan V. Haploidentical hematopoietic stem cell transplantation in leukemia's: experience from a cancer center in India. Indian J Hematol Blood Transfus. 2021;37(3):463–71.
2. Kleinschmidt K, Lv M, Yanir A, Palma J, Lang P, Eyrich M. T-cell-replete versus ex vivo T-cell-depleted haploidentical haematopoietic stem cell transplantation in children with acute lymphoblastic leukaemia and other haematological malignancies. Front Pediatr. 2021;24(9):794541.
3. Nagler A, Kanate AS, Labopin M, Ciceri F, Angelucci E, Koc Y, et al. Post-transplant cyclophosphamide versus anti-thymocyte globulin for graft-versus-host disease prevention in haploidentical transplantation for adult acute lymphoblastic leukemia. Haematologica. 2021;106:1591–8.
4. Meade MG, Bolaños-Meade J. The history of haploidentical stem cell transplantation: a trip from the bench to the bedside. Hematology. 2024;6(1):2346401. https://doi.org/10.1080/16078454.2024.2346401.
5. Bacigalupo A. T deplete or T replete: Which is better? https://library.ehaweb.org/eha/2015/20th/document?c_id=103621&type=article_review&media=6. Accessed 04 Feb 2025.
6. Ciurea SO, Mulanovich V, Saliba RM, Bayraktar UD, Jiang Y, Bassett R, Wang SA, Konopleva M, Fernandez-Vina M, Montes N, Bosque D, Chen J, Rondon G, Alatrash G, Alousi A, Bashir Q, Korbling M, Qazilbash M, Parmar S, Shpall E, Nieto Y, Hosing C, Kebriaei P, Khouri I, Popat U, de Lima M, Champlin RE. Improved early outcomes using a T cell replete graft compared with T cell depleted haploidentical hematopoietic stem cell transplantation. Biol Blood Marrow Transpl. 2012;18(12):1835–44.
7. Mishra K, Naithani R. Haploidentical hematopoietic stem cell transplantation in India-bridging the gap. Indian J Hematol Blood Transfus. 2024;40:371–4.
8. Nakamae H. Graft-versus-tumor effect of post-transplant cyclophosphamide-based allogeneic hematopoietic cell transplantation. Front Immunol. 2024;15:1403936. https://doi.org/10.3389/fimmu.2024.1403936.
9. Kongtim P, Vittayawacharin P, Zou J, Srour S, Shaffer B, Shapiro RM, Varma A, McGuirk J, Dholaria BR, McCurdy SR, DeZern AE, Bejanyan N, Bashey A, Furst S, Castagna L, Mariotti J, Ruggeri A, Bailen R, Teshima T, Xiao-Jun H, Bonfim C, Aung F, Cao K, Carpenter PA, Hamadani M, Askar M, Fernandez-Vina M, Girnita A, Ciurea SO. ASTCT consensus recommendations on testing and treatment of patients with donor-specific anti-HLA antibodies. Transplant Cell Ther. 2024;30(12):1139–54.

10. Fürst D, Müller C, Vucinic V, et al. High-resolution HLA matching in hematopoietic stem cell transplantation: a retrospective collaborative analysis. Blood. 2013;122:3220.
11. Petersdorf EW, Gooley TA, Malkki M, et al. HLA-C expression levels define permissible mismatches in hematopoietic cell transplantation. Blood. 2014;124:3996.
12. DeZern AE, Franklin C, Tsai HL, et al. Relationship of donor age and relationship to outcomes of haploidentical transplantation with posttransplant cyclophosphamide. Blood Adv. 2021;5:1360.
13. Gladstone DE, Zachary AA, Fuchs EJ, et al. Partially mismatched transplantation and human leukocyte antigen donor-specific antibodies. Biol Blood Marrow Transplant. 2013;19:647.
14. Zachary AA, Leffell MS. Desensitization for solid organ and hematopoietic stem cell transplantation. Immunol Rev. 2014;258:183.
15. Aversa F, Tabilio A, Velardi A, et al. Treatment of high-risk acute leukemia with T-cell-depleted stem cells from related donors with one fully mismatched HLA haplotype. N Engl J Med. 1998;339:1186.
16. van Rood JJ, Loberiza FR Jr, Zhang MJ, et al. Effect of tolerance to noninherited maternal antigens on the occurrence of graft-versus-host disease after bone marrow transplantation from a parent or an HLA-haploidentical sibling. Blood. 2002;99:1572.
17. Ruggeri L, Mancusi A, Capanni M, et al. Donor natural killer cell allorecognition of missing self in haploidentical hematopoietic transplantation for acute myeloid leukemia: challenging its predictive value. Blood. 2007;110:433.
18. Bishara A, De Santis D, Witt CC, et al. The beneficial role of inhibitory KIR genes of HLA class I NK epitopes in haploidentically mismatched stem cell allografts may be masked by residual donor-alloreactive T cells causing GVHD. Tissue Antigens. 2004;63:204.
19. Mehta RS, Saliba RM, Ghanem S, Alousi AM, Rondon G, Anderlini P, Al-Atrash G, Bashir Q, Hosing CM, Im JS, Kebriaei P, Khouri I, Marin D, Nieto Y, Olson A, Oran B, Popat UR, Qazilbash MH, Ramdial J, Saini N, Srour SA, Champlin RE, Rezvani K, Shpall EJ. Haploidentical versus matched unrelated versus matched sibling donor hematopoietic cell transplantation with post-transplantation cyclophosphamide. Transplant Cell Ther. 2022;28(7):395.e1–395.e11. https://doi.org/10.1016/j.jtct.2022.04.020.
20. Ciurea SO, Zhang M-J, Bacigalupo AA, Bashey A, Appelbaum FR, Aljitawi OS, Armand P, Antin JH, Chen J, Devine SM, Fowler DH, Luznik L, Nakamura R, O'Donnell PV, Perales M-A, Pingali SR, Porter DL, Riches MR, Ringdén OTH, Rocha V, Vij R, Weisdorf DJ, Champlin RE, Horowitz MM, Fuchs EJ, Eapen M. Haploidentical transplant with posttransplant cyclophosphamide vs matched unrelated donor transplant for acute myeloid leukemia. Blood. 2015;126(8):1033–40. https://doi.org/10.1182/blood-2015-04-639831.
21. Xiao H, Huang Q, Lai Y, Liu R. Haploidentical hematopoietic stem cell transplantation in pediatric transfusion-dependent thalassemia: a systematic review and meta-analysis. Transplant Cell Ther. 2025;31(2):101.e1–101.e12. https://doi.org/10.1016/j.jtct.2024.12.001.
22. Uppuluri R, Sivasankaran M, Patel S, Swaminathan VV, Ravichandran N, Ramanan KM, Vaidhyanathan L, Ramakrishnan B, Jayakumar I, Raj R. Haploidentical stem cell transplantation in children with benign disorders: improved survival and cost-effective care over 15 years from a single center in India. Indian J Hematol Blood Transfus. 2019;35(3):426–30. https://doi.org/10.1007/s12288-019-01087-9.
23. Shahzad M, Rehman G, Khan A, Amin MK, Ishaq MU, Akram U, Sadiq MH, Choudhary UIJI, Shamoon S, Khan BY, Chaudhary SG, Anwar I, Singh A, McGuirk JP, Mushtaq MU. Outcomes after bone marrow versus peripheral blood stem cells Haploidentical hematopoietic cell transplantation: a systematic review and meta-analysis. Blood. 2024;144(Supplement 1):7425.
24. Bashey A, Zhang MJ, McCurdy SR, St Martin A, Argall T, Anasetti C, Ciurea SO, Fasan O, Gaballa S, Hamadani M, Munshi P, Al Malki MM, Nakamura R, O'Donnell PV, Perales MA, Raj K, Romee R, Rowley S, Rocha V, Salit RB, Solh M, Soiffer RJ, Fuchs EJ, Eapen M. Mobilized peripheral blood stem cells versus unstimulated bone marrow as a graft source for T-cell-replete Haploidentical donor transplantation using post-transplant cyclophosphamide. J Clin Oncol. 2017;35(26):3002–9. https://doi.org/10.1200/JCO.2017.72.8428.

25. Cutler C, Ballen K. Reduced-intensity conditioning and umbilical cord blood transplantation in adults. Bone Marrow Transplant. 2009;44:667–71.
26. MacMillan ML, Weisdorf DJ, Brunstein CG, Cao Q, DeFor TE, Verneris MR, Blazar BR, Wagner JE. Acute graft-versus-host disease after unrelated donor umbilical cord blood transplantation: analysis of risk factors. Blood. 2009;113(11):2410–5.
27. Prasad VK, Mendizabal A, Parikh SH, Szabolcs P, Driscoll TA, Page K, et al. Unrelated donor umbilical cord blood transplantation for inherited metabolic disorders in 159 pediatric patients from a single center: influence of cellular composition of the graft on transplantation outcomes. Blood. 2008;112(7):2979–89.
28. Yang K, Gong S, Jiang T, Liang X, Hu J, Zhu P, Nie L, Xu Y, Fu B, Bone Marrow Failure Working Group of Hunan Province. Haploidentical peripheral stem cell transplantation for young patients with severe aplastic anemia using post-transplantation cyclophosphamide and methotrexate. Transplant Cell Ther. 2021;27:429.e1.
29. Hexner E. The role of T cells in hematopoietic stem cell engraftment. ScientificWorldJournal. 2006;6:246–53. https://doi.org/10.1100/tsw.2006.47. PMID: 16501826; PMCID: PMC5917223.
30. Aversa F, Tabilio A, Velardi A, Cunningham I, Terenzi A, Falzetti F, et al. Treatment of high-risk acute leukemia with T-cell-depleted stem cells from related donors with one fully mismatched HLA haplotype. N Engl J Med. 339:1186–93. https://doi.org/10.1056/NEJM199810223391702.
31. Luznik L, Engstrom LW, Iannone R, et al. Posttransplantation cyclophosphamide facilitates engraftment of major histocompatibility complex-identical allogeneic marrow in mice conditioned with lowdose total body irradiation. Biol Blood Marrow Transplant. 2002;8(3):131–8.
32. O'Donnell PV, Luznik L, Jones RJ, et al. Nonmyeloablative bone marrow transplantation from partially HLA-mismatched related donors using posttransplantation cyclophosphamide. Biol Blood Marrow Transplant. 2002;8(7):377–86.
33. DeZern AE, Zahurak M, Symons HJ, et al. Alternative donor BMT with posttransplant cyclophosphamide as initial therapy for acquired severe aplastic anemia. Blood. 2023;141(25):3031–8.
34. Tang F, Xu Y, Chen H, Xu L, Zhang X, Wang Y, Liu Q, Wu D, Huang X. Comparison of the clinical outcomes of hematologic malignancies after myeloablative haploidentical transplantation with G-CSF/ATG and posttransplant cyclophosphamide: results from the Chinese Bone Marrow Transplantation Registry Group (CBMTRG). Sci China Life Sci. 2020;63(4):571–81. https://doi.org/10.1007/s11427-019-9594-7.
35. Huttunen P, Taskinen M, Siitonen S, Saarinen-Pihkala UM. Impact of very early CD4+/CD8+ T cell counts on the occurrence of acute graft-versus-host disease and NK cell counts on outcome after pediatric allogeneic hematopoietic stem cell transplantation. Pediatr Blood Cancer. 2015;62(3):522–8. https://doi.org/10.1002/pbc.25347.
36. Small TN, Robinson WH, Miklos DB. B cells and transplantation: an educational resource. Biol Blood Marrow Transplant. 2009;15(1 Suppl):104–13. https://doi.org/10.1016/j.bbmt.2008.10.016.
37. Kim HT, Armand P, Frederick D, Andler E, Cutler C, Koreth J, Alyea EP 3rd, Antin JH, Soiffer RJ, Ritz J, Ho VT. Absolute lymphocyte count recovery after allogeneic hematopoietic stem cell transplantation predicts clinical outcome. Biol Blood Marrow Transplant. 2015;21(5):873–80. https://doi.org/10.1016/j.bbmt.2015.01.019.
38. Garg A, Trivedi M, Raj A, Shah K, Patel K, Vachhani A, Solanki H, Yadav R, Shah S. Haploidentical stem cell transplantation: half match but more hope!-single centre experience from Western India. Indian J Hematol Blood Transfus. 2024;40(3):385–91. https://doi.org/10.1007/s12288-023-01722-6.
39. Owattanapanich W, Leelakanok N, Sanpakit K, Buaboonnam J. A comparison of the clinical outcomes of haploidentical transplantation and other graft sources in acute lymphoblastic leukemia: a systematic review and meta-analysis. Clin Lymphoma Myeloma Leuk. 2022;22(3):174–91.

40. Srinivasan A, Raffa E, Wall DA, Schechter T, Ali M, Chopra Y, Kung R, Chiang KY, Krueger J. Outcome of haploidentical peripheral blood allografts using post-transplantation cyclophosphamide compared to matched sibling and unrelated donor bone marrow allografts in pediatric patients with hematologic malignancies: a single-center analysis. Transpl Cell Ther. 2022;28(3):158.e1–9.
41. Borah P, Dayal N, Pathak S, Naithani R. Short-course Venetoclax with standard chemotherapy is effective in early T-cell precursor acute lymphoblastic leukemia. J Pediatr Hematol Oncol. 2023;45(5):271–4. https://doi.org/10.1097/MPH.0000000000002672.
42. Borah P, Gautam V, Kumar V, Saikia B, Naithani R. Fecal microbiota transplantation for refractory *Clostridioides difficile* infection post Haploidentical transplant for pediatric acute myeloid leukemia. Blood Cell Ther. 2025;8(1):170–2. https://doi.org/10.31547/bct-2024-015.
43. Vittayawacharin P, Kongtim P, Ciurea SO. Future directions in haploidentical hematopoietic stem cell transplantation. Hematology. 2024;29(1):2366718. https://doi.org/10.1080/16078454.2024.2366718.

Part VII
CBC in Infection & Blood Component Therapy

Chapter 44
Automated Hemogram Analyzer Parameters in Diagnosis of Sepsis/Infections

Soundarya Ravi and Rakhee Kar

Abstract Application of robust diagnostic tools is pivotal for improving outcomes in sepsis management. High false-positive rates of sepsis screening tools remain a significant drawback. Microbiological culture, though considered the gold standard for diagnosing infections, typically takes 48–72 hours. Hence, recent research has focused on identifying reliable biomarkers, the most widely used being C-reactive protein, procalcitonin, and interleukin-6.

Complete blood count (CBC) sample processing using automated hematology analyzers (AHA) can provide numerous parameters useful in the diagnosis of sepsis and act as sepsis biomarkers. Inflammatory states in sepsis dysregulate iron metabolism and induce oxidative damage to RBCs, thereby leading to red cell distribution width (RDW) elevation, making it a valuable prognostic marker. Neutrophilic leukocytosis, monocytosis, and eosinopenia are reported in early sepsis, while severe sepsis or organ dysfunction may be indicated by leukopenia, lymphopenia, and monocytopenia. Among the various CBC-derived ratios, the neutrophil-to-lymphocyte ratio (NLR) is the most commonly studied in the context of sepsis. Less commonly studied ratios include the monocyte-to-lymphocyte ratio (MLR), platelet-to-lymphocyte ratio (PLR), and platelet count-to-mean platelet volume ratio (PC/MPV).

Cell population data (CPD) parameters in volume conductivity scatter (VCS) technology deranged in sepsis include increased mean neutrophil volume (MNV), mean monocyte volume (MMV), and volume distribution width (VDW), while mean neutrophil scatter (MNS) values are generally decreased. Monocyte distribution width (MDW), an emerging biomarker, reflects the heterogeneity in monocytes' size. Similarly, various leucocyte CPD generated by fluorescence flow cytometry also provide valuable information. The delta neutrophil index (DNI) reflects the immature granulocyte fraction in peripheral blood.

S. Ravi
Department of Hematology and Clinical Pathology, Manipal Hospitals, Bangalore, India

R. Kar (✉)
Department of Pathology, Jawaharlal Institute of Postgraduate Medical Education and Research, Puducherry, India

H. P. Pati et al. (eds.), *Clinical Hematology and Hemato-Oncology*,
https://doi.org/10.1007/978-981-92-1167-8_44

Thrombocytopenia is a common finding in sepsis. Elevated mean platelet volume (MPV), platelet distribution width (PDW), and immature platelet fraction (IPF), which reflect increased platelet turnover, serve as potential biomarkers for early sepsis detection and severity assessment.

Modern hematology analyzers generate novel research parameters to detect various infections. High fluorescence lymphocyte count (HFLC) is a valuable marker for distinguishing dengue from other febrile illnesses. In COVID-19, markers such as lymphopenia, neutrophilia, elevated NLR, eosinopenia, and CPD parameters like MDW and lymphocyte cell size and the width of dispersion (LY-WZ) provide insights into disease severity. Hemogram analyzers can detect malaria-infected RBCs directly using multi-angle polarized scatter separation (MAPSS) or fluorescence flow cytometry, or indirectly by identifying hallmark scattergram abnormalities.

Keywords Automated hematology analyzer · Biomarkers · Cell population data (CPD) · Immature granulocytes (IG) · Neutrophil-to-lymphocyte ratio (NLR) · Monocyte distribution width (MDW) · Multi-angle polarized scatter separation (MAPSS) · Platelet distribution width (PDW) · Red cell distribution width (RDW) · Total leukocyte count (TLC) · Sepsis · Volume conductivity scatter (VCS)

Learning Objectives

- Automated hematology analyzers (AHA) provide complete blood counts (CBC) and numerous other parameters useful for diagnosis and as biomarkers in sepsis.
- Red cell parameters like RDW, routine TLC, and DLC parameters, and various CBC-derived parameters like neutrophil-to-lymphocyte ratio (NLR), monocyte-to-lymphocyte ratio (MLR), platelet-to-lymphocyte ratio (PLR), and platelet count-to-mean platelet volume ratio (PC/MPV) have been used.
- Cell population data (CPD) in volume conductivity scatter (VCS) technology, such as mean neutrophil volume (MNV), mean monocyte volume (MMV), volume distribution width (VDW), and mean neutrophil scatter (MNS), along with monocyte distribution width (MDW), are emerging biomarkers.
- Similarly, numerous CPD parameters generated by fluorescence flow cytometry technology have also been used.
- Immature granulocyte (IG) fraction and delta neutrophil index (DNI) are also useful biomarkers.
- Thrombocytopenia, elevated platelet-derived indices such as mean platelet volume (MPV) and platelet distribution width (PDW), are often seen in sepsis. Immature platelet fraction (IPF) has emerged as a potential biomarker.
- Some parameters have been found useful in infections, such as high fluorescence lymphocyte count (HFLC) in differentiating dengue from other febrile illnesses; collective utility of parameters in COVID-19, and detection of malarial infection using multi-angle polarized scatter separation (MAPSS) and fluorescence flow cytometry, either by directly identifying infected red blood cells (i-RBCs) or indirectly by detecting hallmark scattergram abnormalities.

44.1 Introduction

44.1.1 Definition of Sepsis and Its Global Health Impact

Sepsis is a critical condition characterized by multi-organ dysfunction caused by an excessive and dysregulated inflammatory response to infection [1]. It continues to be a significant cause of morbidity and mortality in both adult and pediatric populations [2, 3]. Prompt detection of sepsis is essential for initiating early and appropriate treatment, thereby preventing irreversible organ damage and grave outcomes. Early recognition also minimizes the risk of long-term complications and reduces the chances of developing antibiotic resistance.

44.1.2 Screening Tools for Sepsis Diagnosis

Sepsis is diagnosed using a combination of clinical findings and laboratory investigations. Various screening tools, such as the systemic inflammatory response syndrome (SIRS) criteria, national early warning score (NEWS), quick sequential organ failure assessment (qSOFA), etc., are commonly used in clinical practice for preliminary diagnosis of sepsis and have evolved over time [1, 4, 5]. Recently, the 2021 Surviving Sepsis Guidelines introduced updated scoring systems, including the sequential organ failure assessment (SOFA) score and the quick SOFA (qSOFA) score, to facilitate rapid identification and prognostication [6]. However, these tools rely on clinical parameters that can be altered by non-infectious conditions, resulting in high false-positive rates and unnecessary interventions. Their lack of specificity and limited sensitivity in detecting early sepsis may also delay treatment [7].

44.1.3 Laboratory Diagnosis of Sepsis: Advancements and Limitations

Blood culture typically takes 48–72 hours. Treatment delays significantly increase the risk of morbidity and mortality, often necessitating the use of empirical antibiotic therapy, which can promote antibiotic resistance. Moreover, the accuracy of culture results depends on the quality and timing of sample collection, occasionally leading to diagnostic errors [8].

To overcome these limitations, recent research focuses on identifying reliable biomarkers for early sepsis detection, aiming to improve diagnostic accuracy and patient outcomes. Biomarkers are objectively measurable biological molecules or characteristics that reflect normal physiological processes, pathological changes, or responses to therapeutic interventions [9]. Commonly used sepsis biomarkers include C-reactive protein (CRP), procalcitonin (PCT), and interleukin-6 (IL-6) [10, 11]. Additional experimental biomarkers such as IL-8, IL-27, tumor necrosis factors (TNFs), immunoglobulins, presepsin, soluble urokinase plasminogen activator receptor (suPAR), etc., have also been evaluated for their diagnostic and prognostic utility [12, 13].

Sepsis biomarkers rise rapidly within a few hours and peak within 1–2 days [14]. These biomarkers also offer high negative predictive value, helping to rule out infection and reduce unnecessary antibiotic use. Additionally, they assist in stratifying patients by severity, guiding patient triage and treatment decisions. However, their diagnostic accuracy is limited by the risk of both false-positive and false-negative results. Apart from infections, some biomarker levels are elevated in non-infectious conditions such as inflammation, surgery, and trauma [15].

44.1.4 Role of Hematological Parameters in Infectious Diseases and Sepsis

Hematology plays an integral role in the diagnosis and management of sepsis and other infectious diseases. Critical changes in the body's immune response to infections are reflected as alterations in hematological parameters, which can be accurately analyzed using automated hematology analyzers (AHAs) [16]. They incorporate state-of-the-art technologies to assess both the morphological and functional characteristics of blood cells, generating detailed information, in the form of cell population data (CPD) [17]. CPD analysis enables the detection of subtle changes in blood cell characteristics, aiding in the diagnosis, monitoring of infections, and assessment of disease progression.

44.2 Overview of Automated Hematology Analyzers and Their Principles

Automated hematology analyzers (AHAs) are advanced, computerized devices designed to process blood samples efficiently, providing both numerical and graphical data for clinical analysis [18]. They operate using key principles like electrical impedance, optical light scattering, and fluorescence, for precise blood cell classification [19, 20]. Modern AHAs incorporate advanced technologies such as multi-angle polarized scatter separation (MAPSS™), volume conductivity scatter (VCS) technology, and fluorescence flow cytometry to generate detailed cell morphology data and specialized parameters like CPD [21, 22]. These systems can detect abnormalities, issue automated flags, and identify specialized cells, such as nucleated red blood cells (nRBCs) and immature white blood cells, without requiring additional samples.

44.3 Automated Hematology Analyzer Parameters in Sepsis

44.3.1 Red Blood Cell Parameters

Red blood cells (RBCs) play a critical role in transporting gases to and from tissues and maintaining the body's acid–base balance. Additionally, they exhibit antioxidant properties to protect tissues from damage, regulate vascular tone, and contribute to immune responses [23]. Systemic disorders like sepsis can alter RBC parameters through various mechanisms [24].

Red cell distribution width (RDW) is a key red cell parameter extensively studied in sepsis. RDW measures the variation in RBC volume, reflecting the degree of anisocytosis. It is calculated by hemogram analyzers as the ratio of the standard deviation (SD) of RBC volume to the mean corpuscular volume (MCV) and is expressed as a percentage. The normal RDW range is approximately 12% to 15%; but each laboratory has to establish its own reference range [25]. It also helps differentiate iron deficiency anemia, where RDW is elevated, from heterozygous beta thalassemia, where it remains normal [26].

Sepsis-induced inflammation dysregulates iron metabolism, impairing RBC production and maturation, while also causing oxidative damage to RBCs [27]. This leads to the premature release of immature RBCs, causing significant variations in cell size and elevated RDW levels. The extent of RDW elevation correlates with sepsis severity, making it a valuable and cost-effective prognostic marker, readily available in hemogram reports. Elevated RDW values, especially those above 15%, are associated with poor clinical outcomes and increased mortality in sepsis patients [28]. Furthermore, a rising RDW trend compared to baseline is recognized as a poor prognostic indicator. Tracking RDW levels during sepsis management can help monitor disease progression. In some studies, RDW has been incorporated into various scoring systems, alongside parameters such as the delta neutrophil index (DNI) and platelet count, to predict sepsis-related mortality [29].

Although RDW effectively highlights disease severity and predicts outcomes, its diagnostic accuracy for sepsis is limited due to its non-specificity [30]. Moreover, the lack of standardized RDW cut-off levels for sepsis further limits its diagnostic utility. Despite these limitations, combining RDW with other biomarkers like CRP or PCT can enhance its predictive utility [31].

44.3.2 White Blood Cell Parameters

During sepsis and infections, leukocytes are activated to perform phagocytosis or to mount immune responses against pathogens by producing cytokines and inflammatory mediators. This activation induces both qualitative and quantitative changes in the various leukocyte populations, which serve as effective sepsis indicators.

44.3.2.1 Total Leukocyte Count (TLC)

Leucocytosis (TLC levels >11 × 10^3/μL) is typically observed in sepsis, but also occurs in conditions like inflammation, stress, allergies, malignancies, or steroid use [32]. Normal TLC levels may be noted during early stages of sepsis, making it an unreliable marker in isolation [33]. In severe sepsis, TLC may drop below 4 × 10^3/μL (leukopenia), indicating a higher mortality risk [34].

44.3.2.2 Changes in the Differential Leukocyte Count (DLC)

Neutrophils, a cornerstone of innate immunity, combat pathogens through mechanisms such as phagocytosis, oxidative burst, and NET formation. The inflammatory response to sepsis triggers a significant increase in neutrophil count due to the premature release of neutrophils from the bone marrow into circulation. In addition, delayed neutrophil apoptosis during severe sepsis prolongs their survival [35]. However, severe sepsis can also cause myelosuppression and increased neutrophil consumption, leading to neutropenia [36].

Sepsis-induced immunosuppression causes lymphocyte apoptosis and depletion, resulting in lymphopenia, defined as an absolute lymphocyte count (ALC) below 1000 cells/μL [37]. This condition increases the risk of secondary infections and multi-organ dysfunction, making it a reliable prognostic indicator for mortality and adverse outcomes. Persistent lymphopenia (ALC ≤0.6 × 10^3/μL by day 4) is associated with a higher 28-day mortality in sepsis patients [38].

Monocytes play dual roles in innate and adaptive immunity during infections, acting as phagocytes and antigen-presenting cells (APCs). In sepsis, monocyte levels vary depending on disease stage and severity. Monocytosis occurs in the early stages as part of the immune response, while monocytopenia is associated with higher rates of bacteremia, disease severity, and organ dysfunction, indicating compromised defence mechanisms [39]. Although monocyte count has limited prognostic value, emerging markers like monocyte distribution width (MDW) show promise as sepsis biomarkers and will be discussed in subsequent sections [40].

A reduction in eosinophil count (eosinopenia) is commonly observed during acute infections, but its diagnostic accuracy remains inconsistent and is not superior to existing sepsis biomarkers [41]. Basophils, though being a part of the innate immune system, have a less-defined role in sepsis. One study found their absence in critically ill intensive care unit (ICU) patients to be an unfavorable prognostic indicator linked to higher mortality risk [42].

44.3.2.3 Immature Granulocytes (IG)

During sepsis, inflammatory mediators stimulate the bone marrow to produce and release immature myeloid precursors into circulation. As a result, peripheral blood may show the presence of promyelocytes, myelocytes, metamyelocytes, and band forms, collectively referred to as “left shift.” Modern AHAs such as the Sysmex (XE and XN series), Mindray etc. uses fluorescence flow cytometry to quantify these immature cells and generate a parameter known as the immature granulocytes (IGs) [43]. These analyzers employ a lysing agent, “Lysercell WDF,” to lyse the RBCs and stain the leukocytes with “Fluorocell WDF.” IGs are identified based on their granularity (SSC) and nucleic acid content (side fluorescence) in the white cell differential channel (WDF), forming a distinct cluster above neutrophils in the scattergram (Fig. 44.1). The IG fraction encompasses promyelocytes, myelocytes, and metamyelocytes, excluding band forms and myeloblasts [44]. Normally, IGs are absent or present under 1% in peripheral blood.

The IG parameter is increasingly used as an early sepsis marker, often detectable before CRP or PCT elevation [43]. An IG percentage above 3% is significant and correlated well with sepsis prediction, positive cultures, and higher mortality [45]. Conversely, low IG levels can aid in excluding sepsis [46]. In neonates, IG count combined with other parameters—such as the immature-to-total neutrophil (I/T) ratio, CRP, and blood culture—improves diagnostic accuracy for neonatal sepsis [47, 48].

Immature granulocytes (IG count and percentage) are economical and easily obtained via routine CBC and are a valuable parameter in ICU settings. However, elevated IG% is not specific to sepsis and occurs in conditions like inflammation, trauma, malignancies, steroid use, and myeloproliferative neoplasms (MPNs) [49]. Therefore, IG should be interpreted alongside clinical findings and other biomarkers for better accuracy.

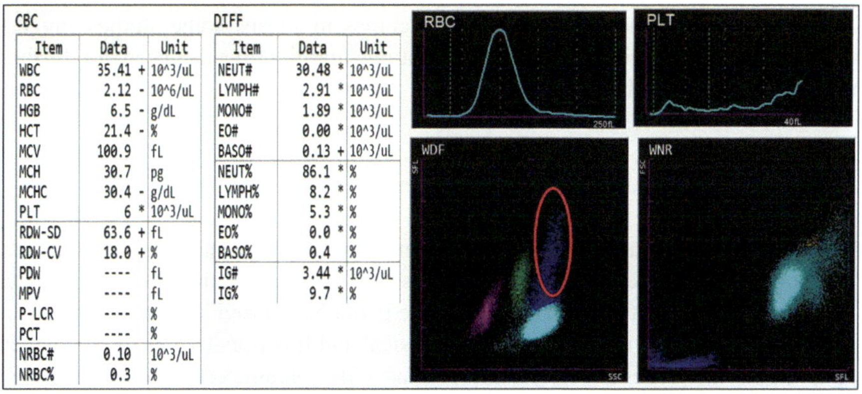
CBC

Item	Data		Unit
WBC	35.41	+	10^3/uL
RBC	2.12	-	10^6/uL
HGB	6.5	-	g/dL
HCT	21.4	-	%
MCV	100.9		fL
MCH	30.7		pg
MCHC	30.4	-	g/dL
PLT	6	*	10^3/uL
RDW-SD	63.6	+	fL
RDW-CV	18.0	+	%
PDW	----		fL
MPV	----		fL
P-LCR	----		%
PCT	----		%
NRBC#	0.10		10^3/uL
NRBC%	0.3		%

DIFF

Item	Data		Unit
NEUT#	30.48	*	10^3/uL
LYMPH#	2.91	*	10^3/uL
MONO#	1.89	*	10^3/uL
EO#	0.00	*	10^3/uL
BASO#	0.13	+	10^3/uL
NEUT%	86.1	*	%
LYMPH%	8.2	*	%
MONO%	5.3	*	%
EO%	0.0	*	%
BASO%	0.4		%
IG#	3.44	*	10^3/uL
IG%	9.7	*	%

Fig. 44.1 Hemogram report of a 39-year-old male with decompensated chronic liver disease (DCLD) and sepsis secondary to spontaneous bacterial peritonitis (SBP), analyzed on Sysmex XN-3000. The report reveals macrocytic anemia with elevated RDW, leukocytosis with neutrophilia, severe thrombocytopenia, and the presence of immature granulocytes (IGs), highlighted by a red circle in the WDF scatter plot

44.3.2.4 Ratio of the CBC Parameters

Among the various ratios derived from CBC parameters, the neutrophil-to-lymphocyte ratio (NLR) is widely studied in sepsis. NLR is calculated by dividing the absolute neutrophil count by the absolute lymphocyte count. As discussed earlier, during the acute phase of sepsis, neutrophil counts rise, and lymphocyte counts drop, leading to an elevated NLR. This elevation serves as a marker of acute inflammation in sepsis and infections, reflecting the dynamic interaction of the immune system. However, NLR values may fluctuate as sepsis progresses due to neutrophil migration to the infection site and lymphocyte depletion caused by immunosuppression, limiting its prognostic utility [50].

Elevated NLR is associated with poor outcomes and sepsis-related mortality [51]. Increasing NLR trends during serial monitoring can help assess sepsis severity and identify high-risk patients needing timely intervention [51]. Normal NLR values in the adult population range from 0.78 to 3.53 [52]. Cutoff values for predicting sepsis and mortality vary across studies, influenced by population, study objectives, analyzer type, and timing of measurement. A general cut-off is above 3.53, though some studies suggest thresholds above 5 or 10 [53]. Like other sepsis-related parameters, NLR lacks specificity and can be elevated in conditions like stress, coronary artery disease, malignancies, and during chemotherapy [54]. It should be interpreted cautiously alongside other biomarkers.

Other, less commonly studied CBC-derived ratios in sepsis include the monocyte-to-lymphocyte ratio (MLR), platelet-to-lymphocyte ratio (PLR), and platelet count-to-mean platelet volume ratio (PC/MPV) [55]. While increased MLR, PLR, and PC/MPV have been associated with poor outcomes in sepsis, some studies suggest these ratios are unreliable for prognostication, highlighting the need for further research to establish their clinical utility.

44.3.2.5 Leucocyte Cell Population Data

Modern hematology analyzers employ advanced technology and software to assess the morphological and functional properties of WBCs, generating quantitative data known as cell population data (CPD). These parameters provide precise, objective, and valuable insights into the real-time physical and functional states of leukocytes [17]. CPDs are generated alongside routine CBC parameters without requiring additional blood samples. Technologies such as VCS technology (Beckman Coulter Inc., USA) and fluorescence flow cytometry (Sysmex Corporation, Japan) commonly generate CPD, along with some other less commonly applied technologies. The different types of CPD and their utility in diagnosing and monitoring sepsis are outlined below:

Cell Population Data Generated by VCS Technology

Neutrophil and Monocyte Cell Population Data

VCS technology analyzes the physical properties of leukocytes, such as size, internal composition, and granularity, and expresses them quantitatively as CPD. The CPD parameters provided by the Beckman Coulter series of analyzers for neutrophils and monocytes include the following:

(i) Mean neutrophil volume (MNV)
(ii) Mean neutrophil conductivity (MNC)
(iii) Mean neutrophil scatter (MNS)
(iv) Mean monocyte volume (MMV)
(v) Mean monocyte conductivity (MMC)
(vi) Mean monocyte scatter (MMS)

Each parameter has its own standard deviation (e.g., MNV-SD) and derived indices, such as volume distribution width (VDW). Inflammatory states such as sepsis trigger immune activation, leading to measurable changes in neutrophil and monocyte properties, which are reflected in the corresponding CPD.

Increased MNV, MMV, and VDW are typically observed in sepsis, while MNS values decrease [56, 57]. For instance, an MNV >150 and MMV >170 helped to identify sepsis in adults with good diagnostic accuracy [57]. Similarly, Raimondi et al. [58] found MNV >148 predicted neonatal sepsis with high sensitivity (95%) and specificity (88%) [59]. One advantage of neutrophil CPD is that it can serve as an early sepsis indicator, even in the absence of leukocytosis or neutrophilia [56]. These parameters are now incorporated into clinical practice for differentiating sepsis from non-septic conditions, early sepsis detection, and treatment monitoring. Combining CPD with sepsis biomarkers like CRP improves diagnostic accuracy.

Monocyte Distribution Width (MDW)

Monocyte distribution width (MDW), an emerging sepsis biomarker, is a type of CPD that reflects monocyte size heterogeneity in peripheral blood. During bacteremia, pro-inflammatory signals such as pathogen-associated molecular patterns (PAMPs) activate monocytes, causing an increase in their size [59]. This infection-induced size variation, also known as early sepsis indicator (ESId), can be measured using VCS technology on Beckman Coulter analyzers (UniCel DxH800/900) [60]. MDW is derived from the standard deviation of monocyte cell volume values obtained during leukocyte differential counts [40]. Recent studies show that MDW is valuable for early sepsis prediction and identifying high-risk patients. With its high negative predictive value, MDW values below 20 effectively exclude sepsis, while values above 20, when combined with clinical and laboratory findings, indicate a high likelihood of sepsis [61]. However, MDW should not be used in isolation to diagnose or rule out sepsis.

In 2019, the FDA approved MDW for sepsis detection in adult emergency room (ER) patients [62]. Since then, its utility has been evaluated in settings like ICU and in infections such as COVID-19 [63]. Variations in MDW cutoff values (ranging from 20 to 27) have been attributed to differences in study designs, clinical settings (ER vs. ICU), calculation methods, or the type of anticoagulant used (K3-EDTA vs. K2-EDTA) [64, 65]. Notably, K2-EDTA anticoagulated samples tend to yield lower MDW levels than K3-EDTA samples.

Cell Population Data Generated by Fluorescence Flowcytometry

Analyzers utilizing fluorescence flow cytometry employ membrane surfactants and fluorescent dyes that bind to the cytoplasmic and nuclear components of leukocytes. Laser light interaction with these dyes enables the assessment of WBC morphological and functional properties [17]. Leukocyte CPD is generated based on the light scatter properties and emitted fluorescence.

Optical signals on the X-axis (side scatter or SSC) indicate a cell's internal complexity, such as granules and structures [66]. Fluorescence emitted along the Y-axis reflects a cell's nucleic acid content, while light scatter along the Z-axis (forward scatter or FSC) corresponds to cell size. For each leukocyte type, X, Y, and Z-axis parameters are recorded, along with the "width of dispersion" (WD), which describes the variability in signals, representing heterogeneity in cellular properties. Table 44.1 summarizes leukocyte CPD generated by fluorescence flow cytometry and their significance for each cell type.

In sepsis, increased neutrophil granularity (NE-X) and nucleic acid content (NE-Y) result from neutrophil activation and the premature release of immature myeloid cells into circulation. NE-Z serves as a combined marker of neutrophil activation, size, and nucleic acid content. Consequently, NE-X, NE-Y, and NE-Z values are significantly higher in sepsis patients than in healthy individuals [67]. Park et al. demonstrated that NE-SFL and NE-WY exhibit high diagnostic reliability for sepsis in adult patients (AUC: 0.909 and 0.905) [68]. Elevated NE-SFL, MO-WX, and MO-Y values were observed in pediatric sepsis patients upon PICU admission [69]. Moreover, NE-SFL and MO-X correlated strongly with disease severity and SOFA scores (AUC: 0.75 and 0.72) [70]. Urrechaga et al. developed a neutrophil and monocyte (NEMO) scoring system for sepsis prediction, incorporating NE-SFL, MO-X, and other CBC parameters [22].

Delta Neutrophil Index (DNI)

The delta neutrophil index (DNI), a reflection of the immature granulocyte fraction in peripheral blood, is generated by AHAs like the ADVIA 2120 (Siemens Healthcare Diagnostics). These analyzers employ a cytochemical myeloperoxidase (MPO) reaction combined with light beam reflection (to assess nuclear lobularity) to determine white blood cell differential counts [71]. DNI is calculated as the difference between

Table 44.1 The various leucocyte CPD and its significance pertaining to each cell type

S. No.	Parameter	Parameter description	Significance
Neutrophil parameters			
01	NE-SSC	Neutrophils complexity	Increases with more granules (e.g., toxic granules), vacuoles, or cytoplasmic inclusions; Decreases with lower cell complexity (e.g., hypogranular granulocytes)
02	NE-WX	Neutrophils complexity and its width of dispersion	Its increase reflects the degree of heterogeneity of neutrophils, compared to NE-SSC
03	NE-SFL	Neutrophils fluorescence intensity	Increases in proportion to the cellular DNA and RNA content, such as in immature granulocytes and band neutrophils
04	NE-WY	Neutrophils fluorescence intensity and its width of dispersion	Its increase reflects the degree of heterogeneity of neutrophils, compared to NE-SFL
05	NE-FSC	Neutrophils size	Changes in the presence of abnormally sized cells
06	NE-WZ	Neutrophils size and its width of dispersion	Its increase reflects the degree of heterogeneity of neutrophils, compared to NE-FSC
Lymphocyte parameters			
07	LY-X	Lymphocytes complexity	Its increase indicates abundant granules or vacuoles (e.g., large granular lymphocytes)
08	LY-WX	Lymphocytes complexity and its width of dispersion	Its increase reflects the degree of heterogeneity of lymphocytes, compared to LY-X
09	LY-Y	Lymphocytes fluorescence intensity	Increases in proportion to the cellular DNA and RNA content, such as in activated/abnormal lymphocytes and blasts
10	LY-WY	Lymphocytes fluorescence intensity and its width of dispersion	Its increase reflects the degree of heterogeneity of lymphocytes, compared to LY-Y
11	LY-Z	Lymphocytes size	Changes in the presence of abnormal-sized cells (e.g., increased in activated lymphocytes or a decrease in pyknotic lymphocytes)
12	LY-WZ	Lymphocytes size and its width of dispersion	Its increase reflects the degree of heterogeneity of lymphocytes, compared to LY-Z
Monocyte parameters			
13	MO-X	Monocytes complexity	Increases with more granules, vacuoles, and inclusions; Decreases with lower cell complexity
14	MO-WX	Monocytes complexity and its width of dispersion	Its increase reflects the degree of heterogeneity of monocytes, compared to MO-X
15	MO-Y	Monocytes fluorescence intensity	Increases in proportion to the cellular DNA and RNA content (e.g., activated monocytes, monoblasts)
16	MO-WY	Monocytes fluorescence intensity and its width of dispersion	Its increase reflects the degree of heterogeneity of monocytes, compared to MO-Y

(continued)

Table 44.1 (continued)

S. No.	Parameter	Parameter description	Significance
17	MO-Z	Monocytes size	Changes in the presence of abnormally sized cells
18	MO-WZ	Monocytes size and its width of dispersion	Its increase reflects the degree of heterogeneity of monocytes, compared to MO-Z

the total MPO-positive cells in peripheral blood and the mature polymorphonuclear cells. It is a proposed sepsis biomarker associated with increased complications and poor prognosis. It has also been combined with CBC parameters like RDW and platelet count in scoring systems for predicting sepsis-related mortality [29].

44.3.3 Platelet Parameters

Beyond their role in coagulation and hemostasis, platelets are pivotal in generating immune responses during inflammation. In sepsis, pathogens activate platelets via damage-associated molecular pattern (DAMP) receptors, triggering platelet aggregation to trap extracellular pathogens [72]. Severe sepsis causes endothelial dysfunction and tissue factor release, resulting in excessive platelet activation, consumption, and potentially disseminated intravascular coagulation (DIC). Thrombocytopenia is common in sepsis and is strongly associated with its severity and adverse outcomes. It can result from various mechanisms, including platelet consumption in DIC, decreased production, organ sequestration, immune-mediated destruction, and drug effects [73].

Platelet-derived indices, such as mean platelet volume (MPV) and platelet distribution width (PDW) are often elevated in sepsis due to increased platelet turnover [74]. Immature platelet fraction (IPF) is a potential biomarker for early sepsis detection and severity assessment [75]. Elevated IPF levels are associated with increased sepsis severity and mortality. Additionally, it may diagnose sepsis more quickly than conventional markers like CRP and lactate. However, evidence regarding its reliability remains mixed [55].

44.4 Automated Hematology Analyzer Parameters in Other Infections

44.4.1 Dengue Fever

Dengue fever, a viral hemorrhagic fever, causes notable hematological changes [76]. Leucopenia is the most frequent finding, resulting from transient myelosuppression due to virus-infected hematopoietic cells. However, early infection may show mild neutrophilic leukocytosis [77]. Dengue fever causes B-lymphocyte activation, leading to an increase in reactive/atypical lymphocytes in the peripheral blood, typically observed between days 5 and 9 of illness. Monocytosis is another frequent finding in these patients. Eosinophilia and occasional basophilia are observed during recovery. Older automated analyzers (e.g., Sysmex XE) can misclassify atypical lymphocytes as basophils, causing pseudobasophilia due to their increased resistance to lysis [78]. Thrombocytopenia is a hallmark of dengue, but elevated MPV and IPF during the acute phase indicate compensatory platelet production and predict recovery [79]. Plateletcrit is reduced during the thrombocytopenia phase of dengue. Increased hemoglobin and hematocrit levels in later stages reflect hemoconcentration, vascular permeability, and plasma leakage [76].

High fluorescence lymphocyte count (HFLC) and its percentage are research parameters that quantify activated lymphocytes using fluorescence flow cytometry (Sysmex Corporation, Japan; Mindray Bio-Medical Electronics, China) [80]. Activated B-lymphocytes exhibit high ribonucleic acid (RNA) content, resulting in high-intensity fluorescence signals when exposed to fluorescent dyes. These HFLC populations are detected in the WDF channel, located in the high-fluorescence region above the lymphocyte and monocyte areas (Fig. 44.2).

Elevated HFLC values are seen in viral infections, such as dengue and infectious mononucleosis, which are characterized by an increase in activated or atypical lymphocytes [81, 82]. Studies show HFLC is higher in dengue fever, especially in dengue hemorrhagic fever, compared to healthy individuals. Chhabra et al. reported that an HFLC cut-off of 1.75% can effectively distinguish dengue-positive from dengue-negative patients with 52% sensitivity and 90% specificity [83]. Thus, HFLC is useful for differentiating dengue from other acute febrile illnesses with thrombocytopenia [84]. It is inversely proportional to platelet count in dengue patients, with declining HFLC values potentially predicting platelet recovery and disease severity [81].

44.4.2 COVID-19 Infection

COVID-19 infection causes a spectrum of hematological changes, including altered blood counts and coagulation profiles [85]. Lymphopenia (lymphocyte count $\leq$1100/μL) is commonly observed, reflecting direct infection of lymphocytes by SARS-CoV-2. Lymphopenia serves as a biomarker for predicting disease severity and the need for ICU admission. Conversely, neutrophilia in severe COVID-19 infection leads to an elevated NLR, which acts as an inflammatory biomarker [85]. Eosinopenia ($<0.02 \times 10^9$ cells/L) occurs in nearly half of patients due to poor eosinophil mobilization from the marrow and interferon-induced apoptosis [86]. Other abnormalities include thrombocytopenia, anemia, and, occasionally thrombocytosis.

Similar to sepsis, elevated RDW, NLR, and PLR have been associated with a higher mortality risk and disease severity in COVID-19. Additionally, ratios such as

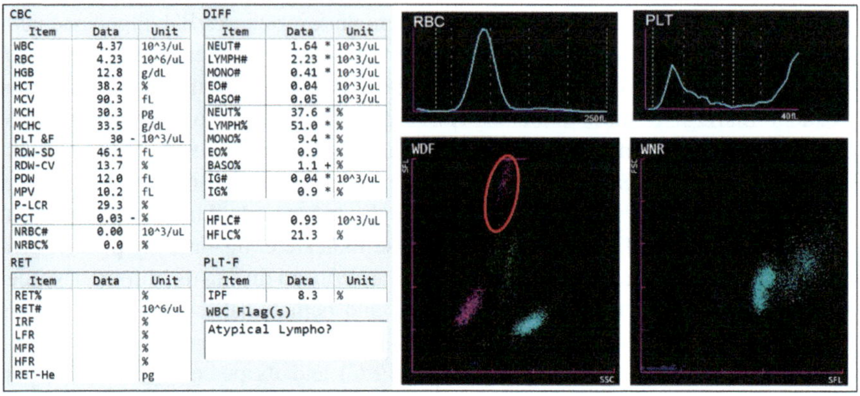

Fig. 44.2 Hemogram report of a 50-year-old female with acute febrile illness diagnosed as dengue infection (NS1 antigen positive), analyzed on Sysmex XN-3000. The report shows a normal total leukocyte count (TLC) with lymphocytic preponderance, thrombocytopenia, and an elevated high fluorescence lymphocyte count (HFLC%—21.3%), highlighted by a red circle in the WDF scatter plot, indicative of reactive lymphocytes

the neutrophil/CD4+ lymphocyte ratio (NCD4LR), neutrophil count to albumin ratio (NAR), lymphocyte/monocyte ratio (LMR), and neutrophil-to-platelet ratio (NPR), have been explored as potential biomarkers [85]. CPD variations have been studied in COVID-19, with MDW showing potential for predicting infection and correlating with severity [63]. Aberrant monocyte activation in COVID-19 causes heterogeneity in its morphology and function, leading to elevated MDW values. Lapic et al. demonstrated that most CPD parameters overlapped between COVID-19 and non-COVID-19 patients, except for LY-WZ, reflecting lymphocyte activation as part of the immune response to SARS-CoV-2 [87].

44.4.3 Malaria

Hematological abnormalities commonly reported in malaria include thrombocytopenia, anemia, and variations in leukocyte counts. Different hematology analyzers employ various technologies to detect malaria-related alterations in blood cells [88]. These changes can be identified through variations in scattergram patterns or leukocyte cell population data.

In Beckman Coulter hematology analyzers (DxH800 and LH750), significant differences were observed in the SD of lymphocyte and monocyte volumes between malaria-positive samples and healthy individuals. These parameters were used to derive a discriminant factor for malaria detection [49]. The Abbott Cell-Dyn series (CD4000) uses MAPPS technology to identify malarial infections in leukocytes by detecting hemozoin pigment in neutrophils and monocytes. This pigment depolarizes light, and the resulting light scattering pattern enables easy identification of parasitized WBCs. Other notable findings in malaria patients include pseudoreticulocytosis and spuriously elevated immature reticulocyte fraction (IRF) [89].

Sysmex analyzers (XE-2100) revealed various scattergram abnormalities in the WDF, WBC/BASO, and RET channels of malaria-positive cases [90]. The abnormalities detected in the WDF channel of malaria-positive cases are as follows: (1) Double neutrophil area/Split zone in the neutrophil region. (2) Merging of the neutrophil and eosinophil clusters. (3) Greying of the neutrophil-eosinophil region. (4) Pseudo-eosinophilia. The Sysmex XN-30 analyzers (Sysmex Corporation, Kobe, Japan) utilize fluorescence flow cytometry to detect malaria-infected red blood cells (i-RBCs) and white blood cells (i-WBCs) by staining malarial nucleic acid with Fluorocell M and lysing with Lysercell M [91]. When the stained cells are exposed to a 405 nm violet semiconductor laser, infected RBCs form a distinct cluster in the M scattergram (SFL-FSC axis), with parasitemia quantified as a percentage and absolute count. The analyzer can also detect gametocytic forms.

44.5 Conclusion

Global initiatives continue to focus on reducing the burden of sepsis by prioritizing early diagnosis and intervention to prevent the progression to multi-organ dysfunction and improve overall patient prognosis. Despite significant advancements, the ideal biomarker for sepsis remains elusive due to the complexity of the disease. Automated hematology analyzer parameters show great potential in aiding the early recognition, severity assessment, and monitoring of sepsis and other infections. While these parameters are readily available and cost-effective, they should always be interpreted alongside clinical findings and other laboratory results for accurate diagnosis and treatment. Future research should refine the role of CBC parameters, leveraging artificial intelligence (AI) and machine learning (ML) to identify novel patterns. Integrating CBC data with emerging biomarkers and clinical scoring systems could further enhance early detection and therapeutic monitoring, advancing sepsis management.

References

1. Singer M, Deutschman CS, Seymour CW, Shankar-Hari M, Annane D, Bauer M, et al. The third international consensus definitions for sepsis and septic shock (Sepsis-3). JAMA. 2016;315:801–10.
2. Reinhart K, Daniels R, Kissoon N, Machado FR, Schachter RD, Finfer S. Recognizing sepsis as a global health priority – a WHO resolution. N Engl J Med. 2017;377:414–7.
3. Fleischmann-Struzek C, Goldfarb DM, Schlattmann P, Schlapbach LJ, Reinhart K, Kissoon N. The global burden of paediatric and neonatal sepsis: a systematic review. Lancet Respir Med. 2018;6:223–30.

4. Smith GB, Redfern OC, Pimentel MA, Gerry S, Collins GS, Malycha J, et al. The National Early Warning Score 2 (NEWS2). Clin Med (Lond). 2019;19:260.
5. Seymour CW, Liu VX, Iwashyna TJ, Brunkhorst FM, Rea TD, Scherag A, et al. Assessment of clinical criteria for sepsis. JAMA. 2016;315:762–74.
6. Evans L, Rhodes A, Alhazzani W, Antonelli M, Coopersmith CM, French C, et al. Surviving sepsis campaign: international guidelines for management of sepsis and septic shock 2021. Intensive Care Med. 2021;47:1181–247.
7. Castello LM, Gavelli F. Sepsis scoring systems: mindful use in clinical practice. Eur J Intern Med. 2024;125:32–5.
8. Gupta S, Sakhuja A, Kumar G, McGrath E, Nanchal RS, Kashani KB. Culture-negative severe sepsis: nationwide trends and outcomes. Chest. 2016;150:1251–9.
9. Kataria Y, Remick D. Sepsis Biomarkers. Methods Mol Biol. 2021;2321:177–89.
10. Khassawneh M, Hayajneh WA, Kofahi H, Khader Y, Amarin Z, Daoud A. Diagnostic markers for neonatal sepsis: comparing C-reactive protein, interleukin-6 and immunoglobulin M. Scand J Immunol. 2007;65:171–5.
11. Sridharan P, Chamberlain RS. The efficacy of procalcitonin as a biomarker in the management of sepsis: slaying dragons or tilting at windmills? Surg Infect. 2013;14:489–511.
12. Kyriazopoulou E, Leventogiannis K, Tavoulareas G, Mainas E, Toutouzas K, Mathas C, et al. Presepsin as a diagnostic and prognostic biomarker of severe bacterial infections and COVID-19. Sci Rep. 2023;13:3814.
13. Kofoed K, Andersen O, Kronborg G, Tvede M, Petersen J, Eugen-Olsen J, et al. Use of plasma C-reactive protein, procalcitonin, neutrophils, macrophage migration inhibitory factor, soluble urokinase-type plasminogen activator receptor, and soluble triggering receptor expressed on myeloid cells-1 in combination to diagnose infections: a prospective study. Crit Care. 2007;11:R38.
14. Albrich WC, Harbarth S. Pros and cons of using biomarkers versus clinical decisions in start and stop decisions for antibiotics in the critical care setting. Intensive Care Med. 2015;41:1739–51.
15. Vincent JL, Teixeira L. Sepsis biomarkers. Value and limitations. Am J Respir Crit Care Med. 2014;190:1081–2.
16. McKenzie SB, Laudicina RJ. Hematologic changes associated with infection. Clin Lab Sci. 1998;11:239–51.
17. Urrechaga E. Reviewing the value of leukocytes cell population data (CPD) in the management of sepsis. Ann Transl Med. 2020;8:953.
18. Daves M, Roccaforte V, Lombardi F, Panella R, Pastori S, Spreafico M, et al. Modern hematology analyzers: beyond the simple blood cells count (with focus on the red blood cells). J Lab Precis Med [Internet]. 2024 [cited 2025 Feb 18];9. Available from: https://jlpm.amegroups.org/article/view/8320.
19. Coulter WH. Means for counting particles suspended in a fluid [Internet]. US2656508A, 1953 [cited 2025 Feb 19]. Available from: https://patents.google.com/patent/US2656508A/en
20. Groner W, George W. Method and apparatus for analysis of leukocytes using light scattered by each leukocyte at absorbing and non-absorbing wavelength [Internet]. US3781112A, 1973 [cited 2025 Feb 20]. Available from: https://patents.google.com/patent/US3781112A/en
21. Lehto T, Hedberg P. Performance evaluation of Abbott CELL-DYN Ruby for routine use. Int J Lab Hematol. 2008;30:400–7.
22. Urrechaga E, Bóveda O, Aguirre U. Role of leucocytes cell population data in the early detection of sepsis. J Clin Pathol. 2018;71:259–66.
23. Kuhn V, Diederich L, Keller TCS, Kramer CM, Lückstädt W, Panknin C, et al. Red blood cell function and dysfunction: redox regulation, nitric oxide metabolism, anemia. Antioxid Redox Signal. 2017;26:718–42.
24. Effenberger-Neidnicht K, Hartmann M. Mechanisms of hemolysis during sepsis. Inflammation. 2018;41:1569–81.
25. Lippi G, Pavesi F, Bardi M, Pipitone S. Lack of harmonization of red blood cell distribution width (RDW). Evaluation of four hematological analyzers. Clin Biochem. 2014;47:1100–3.

26. Piriyakhuntorn P, Tantiworawit A, Rattanathammethee T, Chai-Adisaksopha C, Rattarittamrong E, Norasetthada L. The role of red cell distribution width in the differential diagnosis of iron deficiency anemia and non-transfusiondependent thalassemia patients. Hematol Rep. 2018;10:7605.
27. Förhécz Z, Gombos T, Borgulya G, Pozsonyi Z, Prohászka Z, Jánoskuti L. Red cell distribution width in heart failure: prediction of clinical events and relationship with markers of ineffective erythropoiesis, inflammation, renal function, and nutritional state. Am Heart J. 2009;158:659–66.
28. Jandial A, Kumar S, Bhalla A, Sharma N, Varma N, Varma S. Elevated red cell distribution width as a prognostic marker in severe sepsis: a prospective observational study. Indian J Crit Care Med. 2017;21:552–62.
29. Kim YC, Song JE, Kim EJ, Choi H, Jeong WY, Jung IY, et al. A simple scoring system using the red blood cell distribution width, delta neutrophil index, and platelet count to predict mortality in patients with severe sepsis and septic shock. J Intensive Care Med. 2019;34:133–9.
30. Hu ZD, Lippi G, Montagnana M. Diagnostic and prognostic value of red blood cell distribution width in sepsis: a narrative review. Clin Biochem. 2020;77:1–6.
31. Wei X b, Liu Y h, He P c, Zhou Y l, Tan N, Chen J y, et al. Combined efficacy of C-reactive protein and red blood cell distribution width in prognosis of patients with culture-negative infective endocarditis. Oncotarget. 2017;8:71173–80.
32. Agnello L, Giglio RV, Bivona G, Scazzone C, Gambino CM, Iacona A, et al. The value of a complete blood count (CBC) for sepsis diagnosis and prognosis. Diagnostics (Basel). 2021;11:1881.
33. Seigel TA, Cocchi MN, Salciccioli J, Shapiro NI, Howell M, Tang A, et al. Inadequacy of temperature and white blood cell count in predicting bacteremia in patients with suspected infection. J Emerg Med. 2012;42:254–9.
34. Belok SH, Bosch NA, Klings ES, Walkey AJ. Evaluation of leukopenia during sepsis as a marker of sepsis-defining organ dysfunction. PLoS One. 2021;16:e0252206.
35. Shen X, Cao K, Jiang J, Guan W, Du J. Neutrophil dysregulation during sepsis: an overview and update. J Cell Mol Med. 2017;21:1687–97.
36. Farkas JD. The complete blood count to diagnose septic shock. J Thorac Dis. 2020;12:S16–21.
37. Wang Z, Zhang W, Chen L, Lu X, Tu Y. Lymphopenia in sepsis: a narrative review. Crit Care. 2024;28:315.
38. Drewry AM, Samra N, Skrupky LP, Fuller BM, Compton SM, Hotchkiss RS. Persistent lymphopenia after diagnosis of sepsis predicts mortality. Shock. 2014;42:383–91.
39. Chung H, Lee JH, Jo YH, Hwang JE, Kim J. Circulating monocyte counts and its impact on outcomes in patients with severe sepsis including septic shock. Shock. 2019;51:423.
40. Ciaccio AM, Agnello L, Sasso BL, Giglio RV, Iacona A, Gambino CM, et al. Monocyte distribution width (MDW) as a biomarker of sepsis: an evidenced-based laboratory medicine approach. Clin Chim Acta. 2023;540:117214.
41. Lavoignet CE, Le Borgne P, Chabrier S, Bidoire J, Slimani H, Chevrolet-Lavoignet J, et al. White blood cell count and eosinopenia as valuable tools for the diagnosis of bacterial infections in the ED. Eur J Clin Microbiol Infect Dis. 2019;38:1523–32.
42. Chen X, Zhu X, Zhuo H, Lin J, Lin X. Basophils absence predicts poor prognosis and indicates immunosuppression of patients in intensive care units. Sci Rep. 2023;13:18533.
43. Ayres LS, Sgnaolin V, Munhoz TP. Immature granulocytes index as early marker of sepsis. Int J Lab Hematol. 2019;41:392–6.
44. Bhansaly P, Mehta S, Sharma N, Gupta E, Mehta S, Gupta S. Evaluation of immature granulocyte count as the earliest biomarker for sepsis. Indian J Crit Care Med. 2022;26:216–23.
45. Jeon K, Lee N, Jeong S, Park MJ, Song W. Immature granulocyte percentage for prediction of sepsis in severe burn patients: a machine leaning-based approach. BMC Infect Dis. 2021;21:1258.

46. Nierhaus A, Klatte S, Linssen J, Eismann NM, Wichmann D, Hedke J, et al. Revisiting the white blood cell count: immature granulocytes count as a diagnostic marker to discriminate between SIRS and sepsis - a prospective, observational study. BMC Immunol. 2013;14:8.
47. Cimenti C, Erwa W, Herkner KR, Kasper DC, Müller W, Resch B. The predictive value of immature granulocyte count and immature myeloid information in the diagnosis of neonatal sepsis. Clin Chem Lab Med. 2012;50:1429–32.
48. Patel R, Banerji A, Patel D, Patel R. Study of immature granulocytes to total granulocytes ratio for detection of early onset neonatal sepsis. Int J Clin Diagn Pathol. 2024;7:87–90.
49. Briggs C, Kunka S, Fujimoto H, Hamaguchi Y, Davis BH, Machin SJ. Evaluation of immature granulocyte counts by the XE-IG master: upgraded software for the XE-2100 automated hematology analyzer. Lab Hematol. 2003;9:117–24.
50. Bhadade R, Naik I, Harde M, de Souza R. Neutrophil-to-lymphocyte ratio as a marker for diagnosis and prognostication of sepsis. J Assoc Physicians India. 2024;72:33–8.
51. Huang Z, Fu Z, Huang W, Huang K. Prognostic value of neutrophil-to-lymphocyte ratio in sepsis: a meta-analysis. Am J Emerg Med. 2020;38:641–7.
52. Forget P, Khalifa C, Defour JP, Latinne D, Van Pel MC, De Kock M. What is the normal value of the neutrophil-to-lymphocyte ratio? BMC Res Notes. 2017;10:12.
53. Wu H, Cao T, Ji T, Luo Y, Huang J, Ma K. Predictive value of the neutrophil-to-lymphocyte ratio in the prognosis and risk of death for adult sepsis patients: a meta-analysis. Front Immunol [Internet]. 2024 [cited 2025 Apr 9];15. Available from: https://www.frontiersin.org/journals/immunology/articles/10.3389/fimmu.2024.1336456/full.
54. Zahorec R. Neutrophil-to-lymphocyte ratio, past, present and future perspectives. Bratisl Lek Listy. 2021;122:474–88.
55. Liberski PS, Szewczyk M, Krzych ŁJ. Haemogram-derived indices for screening and prognostication in critically ill septic shock patients: a case-control study. Diagnostics (Basel). 2020;10:638.
56. Purohit AHL, Kumar P, Sharma S, Kapil A, Gupta A, Mukhopadhyay AK. Volume, conductivity, and scatter parameters as diagnostic aid to bacterial sepsis: a tertiary care experience. Indian J Pathol Microbiol. 2015;58:459–63.
57. Arora P, Gupta PK, Lingaiah R, Mukhopadhyay AK. Volume, conductivity, and scatter parameters of leukocytes as early markers of sepsis and treatment response. J Lab Physicians. 2019;11:29–33.
58. Raimondi F, Ferrara T, Capasso L, Sellitto M, Landolfo F, Romano A, et al. Automated determination of neutrophil volume as screening test for late-onset sepsis in very low birth infants. Pediatr Infect Dis J. 2010;29:288.
59. Wu J, Li L, Luo J. Diagnostic and prognostic value of monocyte distribution width in sepsis. J Inflamm Res. 2022;15:4107–17.
60. Beckman Coulter's Early Sepsis Indicator Receives 510(k) Clearance from the U.S. Food and Drug Administration [Internet]. [cited 2025 Apr 13]. Available from: httpss://www.beckmancoulter.com/about-beckman-coulter/newsroom/press-releases/2019/q2/2019-18-april-bec-esid-fda-clearance.
61. Polilli E, Frattari A, Esposito JE, Stanziale A, Giurdanella G, Di Iorio G, et al. Monocyte distribution width (MDW) as a new tool for the prediction of sepsis in critically ill patients: a preliminary investigation in an intensive care unit. BMC Emerg Med. 2021;21:147.
62. Sarani N, Dasgupta A, Enders M, Rowan L, Elsarraj H, Gralnek S, et al. Clinical utility of recently food and drug administration-approved intellisep test (sepsis biomarker) for early diagnosis of sepsis: comparison with other biomarkers. J Clin Med. 2024;13:4852.
63. Sharma P, Naseem S, Varma N, Khaire N, Jindal N, Sharma A, et al. Monocyte distribution width (MDW) in patients with COVID-19: an indicator of disease severity. Indian J Hematol Blood Transfus. 2023;40:1–5.
64. Agnello L, Lo Sasso B, Bivona G, Gambino CM, Giglio RV, Iacolino G, et al. Reference interval of monocyte distribution width (MDW) in healthy blood donors. Clin Chim Acta. 2020;510:272–7.

65. Malinovska A, Hernried B, Lin A, Badaki-Makun O, Fenstermacher K, Ervin AM, et al. Monocyte distribution width as a diagnostic marker for infection: a systematic review and meta-analysis. Chest. 2023;164:101–13.
66. Urrechaga E, Bóveda O, Aguirre U. Improvement in detecting sepsis using leukocyte cell population data (CPD). Clin Chem Lab Med. 2019;57:918–26.
67. Luo Y, Lin J, Chen H, Zhang J, Peng S, Kuang M. Utility of neut-X, neut-Y and neut-Z parameters for rapidly assessing sepsis in tumor patients. Clin Chim Acta. 2013;422:5–9.
68. Park SH, Park CJ, Lee BR, Nam KS, Kim MJ, Han MY, et al. Sepsis affects most routine and cell population data (CPD) obtained using the Sysmex XN-2000 blood cell analyzer: neutrophil-related CPD NE-SFL and NE-WY provide useful information for detecting sepsis. Int J Lab Hematol. 2015;37:190–8.
69. Biban P, Teggi M, Gaffuri M, Santuz P, Onorato D, Carpenè G, et al. Cell population data (CPD) for early recognition of sepsis and septic shock in children: a pilot study. Front Pediatr [Internet]. 2021 [cited 2025 Feb 16];9. Available from: https://www.frontiersin.org/journals/pediatrics/articles/10.3389/fped.2021.642377/full.
70. Buoro S, Seghezzi M, Vavassori M, Dominoni P, Apassiti Esposito S, Manenti B, et al. Clinical significance of cell population data (CPD) on Sysmex XN-9000 in septic patients with our without liver impairment. Ann Transl Med. 2016;4:418.
71. Ahn C, Kim W, Lim TH, Cho Y, Choi KS, Jang BH. The delta neutrophil index (DNI) as a prognostic marker for mortality in adults with sepsis: a systematic review and meta-analysis. Sci Rep. 2018;8:6621.
72. de Stoppelaar SF, van't Veer C, van der Poll T. The role of platelets in sepsis. Thromb Haemost. 2014;112:666–77.
73. Assinger A, Schrottmaier WC, Salzmann M, Rayes J. Platelets in sepsis: an update on experimental models and clinical data. Front Immunol [Internet]. 2019 [cited 2025 Apr 13];10. Available from: https://www.frontiersin.org, https://www.frontiersin.org/journals/immunology/articles/10.3389/fimmu.2019.01687/full.
74. Mangalesh S, Dudani S, Malik A. Platelet indices and their kinetics predict mortality in patients of sepsis. Indian J Hematol Blood Transfus. 2021;37:600–8.
75. Tauseef A, Zafar M, Arshad W, Thirumalareddy J, Sood A, Farooque U, et al. Role of immature platelet fraction (IPF) in sepsis patients: a systematic review. J Family Med Prim Care. 2021;10:2148–52.
76. Chaloemwong J, Tantiworawit A, Rattanathammethee T, Hantrakool S, Chai-Adisaksopha C, Rattarittamrong E, et al. Useful clinical features and hematological parameters for the diagnosis of dengue infection in patients with acute febrile illness: a retrospective study. BMC Hematol. 2018;18:20.
77. Azin FRFG, Gonçalves RP, Pitombeira MH d S, Lima DM, Branco IC. Dengue: profile of hematological and biochemical dynamics. Rev Bras Hematol Hemoter. 2012;34:36.
78. Manuel K, Ambroise MM, Ramdas A, Varghese RG. Pseudobasophilia as a screening tool in dengue: a single center study. J Lab Physicians. 2021;13:156–61.
79. Dadu T, Sehgal K, Joshi M, Khodaiji S. Evaluation of the immature platelet fraction as an indicator of platelet recovery in dengue patients. Int J Lab Hematol. 2014;36:499–504.
80. Tantanate C, Klinbua C. Performance evaluation of the automated nucleated red blood cell enumeration on Sysmex XN analyser. Int J Lab Hematol. 2015;37:341–5.
81. Ningombam A, Acharya S, Sarkar A, Kumar K, Brijwal M, Routray S, et al. Evaluation of sensitivity and specificity of high fluorescence lymphocyte count percentage of Sysmex XN analyzer in diagnosis of dengue. J Appl Hematol. 2022;13:132.
82. Huang T, Yang S, He Y, Li Q, Cui L. The clinical value of high fluorescent lymphocytes and smudge cells in the diagnosis of infectious mononucleosis. J Clin Lab Anal. 2021;35:e23965.
83. Chhabra G. Automated hematology analyzers: recent trends and applications. J Lab Physicians. 2018;10:15–6.

84. Oehadian A, Michels M, de Mast Q, Prihatni D, Puspita M, Hartantri Y, et al. New parameters available on Sysmex XE-5000 hematology analyzers contribute to differentiating dengue from leptospirosis and enteric fever. Int J Lab Hematol. 2015;37:861–8.
85. Gajendra S. Spectrum of hematological changes in COVID-19. Am J Blood Res. 2022;12:43–53.
86. Du Y, Tu L, Zhu P, Mu M, Wang R, Yang P, et al. Clinical features of 85 fatal cases of COVID-19 from Wuhan. A retrospective observational study. Am J Respir Crit Care Med. 2020;201:1372–9.
87. Lapić I, Brenčić T, Rogić D, Lukić M, Lukić I, Kovačić M, et al. Cell population data: could a routine hematology analyzer aid in the differential diagnosis of COVID-19? Int J Lab Hematol. 2021;43:e64–7.
88. Campuzano-Zuluaga G, Álvarez-Sánchez G, Escobar-Gallo GE, Valencia-Zuluaga LM, Ríos-Orrego AM, Pabón-Vidal A, et al. Design of malaria diagnostic criteria for the Sysmex XE-2100 hematology analyzer. Am J Trop Med Hyg. 2010;82:402–11.
89. Scott CS, Van Zyl D, Ho E, Ruivo L, Kunz D, Coetzer TL. Patterns of pseudo-reticulocytosis in malaria: fluorescent analysis with the Cell-Dyn CD4000. Clin Lab Haematol. 2002;24:15–20.
90. Juthani R, Gupta T, Basu D. Scatterplot variations seen in malaria using automated hematological analyzers: a series of ten cases. Int J Med Stud. 2021;9:21–4.
91. Pillay E, Khodaiji S, Bezuidenhout BC, Litshie M, Coetzer TL. Evaluation of automated malaria diagnosis using the Sysmex XN-30 analyser in a clinical setting. Malar J. 2019;18:15.

Chapter 45
Blood Component Therapy in Hematological Patients

Venkatesan Somasundaram and Akshaya Tomar

Abstract Blood component therapy is a cornerstone in managing hematological disorders, offering targeted transfusion strategies to optimize patient outcomes. This chapter explores the role of various blood components, including packed red blood cells (PRBCs), platelets, fresh frozen plasma (FFP), and cryoprecipitate, in treating anemia, thrombocytopenia, and coagulopathies. PRBC transfusions focus on restrictive strategies to balance oxygen delivery while minimizing risks such as iron overload and transfusion reactions. Platelet transfusions are essential in thrombocytopenia management, with strict guidelines to prevent transfusion refractoriness and alloimmunization. FFP plays a critical role in coagulation factor replacement, particularly in disseminated intravascular coagulation (DIC) and massive transfusion protocols. The chapter also highlights the complex transfusion needs of hematopoietic stem cell transplantation (HSCT) patients, emphasizing the importance of leukoreduction, irradiation, and ABO compatibility. Special considerations for autoimmune hemolytic anemia (AIHA) and fetal anemia due to Rh isoimmunization are discussed, underlining the challenges in immunohematology. Advances in blood component modifications, including leukoreduction, pathogen reduction, and extended antigen matching, continue to enhance transfusion safety and efficacy. The chapter stresses the importance of evidence-based transfusion thresholds, personalized treatment approaches, and emerging innovations to ensure optimal patient care.

Keywords Blood component therapy · Hematological disorders · Transfusion strategies · Platelet transfusion · Immunohematology · Coagulation management

---

V. Somasundaram (✉)
Department of Pathology, Armed Forces Medical College, Pune, India

A. Tomar
Department of Immunohematology and Blood Transfusion, Armed Forces Medical College, Pune, India

H. P. Pati et al. (eds.), *Clinical Hematology and Hemato-Oncology*,
https://doi.org/10.1007/978-981-92-1167-8_45

Learning Objectives
At end of reading this chapter, the reader should be able to understand and explain

- Basics of blood component therapy in managing hematological disorders
- Transfusion thresholds and best practices
- Transfusion administration protocols and guidelines
- Transfusion strategies under special circumstances
- Advances in blood component modifications

45.1 Introduction

Hematological disorders often lead to significant alterations in blood cell production, function, and survival. Blood component therapy is a cornerstone in the management of these disorders, aiming to correct deficiencies and mitigate complications arising from anemia, thrombocytopenia, and coagulation abnormalities. Unlike whole blood transfusion, component therapy allows targeted replacement of specific blood elements, thereby improving efficacy and reducing risks.

45.2 Packed Red Blood Cells (PRBCs)

45.2.1 Composition and Characteristics

Packed red blood cells (PRBCs) are prepared by removing most of the plasma from whole blood, resulting in a concentrated erythrocyte product. Each unit contains approximately 200–250 mL of red blood cells, a hematocrit of 55–65% (depends on the type of anticoagulant and preservative solution), and some residual leukocytes ($\sim 10^9$) and plasma.

45.2.2 Introduction to Anemia and Transfusion

Anemia is a common clinical condition requiring red blood cell (RBC) transfusion, particularly in surgical, critically ill, and hematology-oncology patients. Transfusion of packed red blood cells (PRBCs) is an essential therapeutic strategy aimed at restoring oxygen delivery to tissues, but the decision to transfuse should be based on clinical symptoms, hemoglobin levels, and patient comorbidities rather than arbitrary thresholds.

Historically, liberal transfusion strategies were used, but contemporary guidelines support a more restrictive approach to avoid unnecessary risks and complications [1].

45.2.2.1 Physiologic Adaptations in Anemia

The human body can compensate for moderate anemia through several adaptive mechanisms [2, 3]:

- Increased Cardiac Output: Cardiac output progressively increases as anemia worsens, primarily due to a rise in stroke volume. This adaptation helps maintain oxygen delivery despite reduced red blood cell levels. While heart rate can also contribute to the increase in cardiac output, its effect varies depending on individual physiological responses and the severity of anemia
- Increased 2,3-Diphosphoglycerate (2,3-DPG) Production: This enhances oxygen unloading at the tissue level.
- Redistribution of Blood Flow: Prioritizing oxygen delivery to vital organs such as the brain and heart.
- Enhanced Erythropoiesis: Stimulated by increased erythropoietin levels in chronic anemia.

These compensatory mechanisms allow for relatively low hemoglobin levels to be tolerated before symptoms manifest.

45.2.2.2 Effects and Risks of RBC Transfusion

Transfusion is beneficial for correcting anemia, but it also has associated risks:

- Infectious Risks: Despite modern screening, transfusion-transmitted infections, though rare, remain a concern.
- Immunologic Reactions: Allergic reactions, Hemolytic reactions, febrile non-hemolytic reactions, alloimmunization, TRALI (Transfusion-related Acute Lung Injury), and TRIM (Transfusion-related immunomodulation)
- Iron Overload: Chronic transfusions can lead to iron deposition in organs, necessitating iron chelation therapy.
- Volume Overload: Can contribute to transfusion-associated circulatory overload (TACO) in susceptible patients.

45.2.2.3 Current Transfusion Thresholds and Best Practices [4, 5]

- Hb <7 g/dL: Recommended threshold for transfusion in stable, hospitalized patients without significant cardiac disease.

- Hb <8 g/dL: Consider transfusion for post-operative patients and those with chronic cardiovascular conditions.
- Hb <9–10 g/dL: Appropriate for patients with acute coronary syndromes, stroke, or active bleeding with hemodynamic instability.
- Symptomatic Anemia: Transfusion is indicated regardless of Hb level in the presence of symptoms such as dyspnea, angina, tachycardia, or hypotension [29].

Decision-Making in Red Cell Transfusion (In Bleeding Patient)

<u>**Decision-Making in Red Cell Transfusion (In bleeding patient)**</u>

Assess the Degree of Blood Loss and Rate of Bleeding

- Conduct initial evaluation
- Address ABCs (airway, breathing, circulation)
- Identify severe hemorrhagic shock risks

↓

Perform Initial Examination and Rapid Assessment

- Check Heart Rate and Blood Pressure
- Examine for signs of massive bleeding (e.g., expanding abdomen, severe hematochezia)
- Consider comorbid conditions (e.g., cardiovascular disease)

↓

Obtain Emergency Laboratory Tests

- Complete Blood Count (CBC)
- Blood Type and Crossmatch
- Prothrombin Time (PT) and Partial Thromboplastin Time (PTT)

↓

Estimate Source and Rate of Bleeding

- Evaluate clinical findings and test results
- Decide on RBC transfusion rate and supportive measures

↓

Determine Need for Specialist Consultation

- ◇ Gastrointestinal bleeding → Gastroenterology and Surgery Consultation
- ◇ Postoperative bleeding → Consider angiography or exploratory surgery

↓

Assess Hemodynamic Status and Need for Emergency Intervention

- ◇ Administer crystalloids to maintain intravascular volume
- ◇ Provide red cell transfusions for oxygen-carrying capacity

↓

Monitor and Predict Further Blood Loss

- ◇ Estimate future bleeding and expected hemoglobin drop
- ◇ Perform expectant transfusion as needed

↓

Evaluate Clinical Symptoms and Vital Signs

- ◇ Monitor blood pressure and heart rate
- ◇ Assess anemia symptoms (e.g., cardiac ischemia, CHF symptoms, fatigue, dizziness)
- ◇ Measure hemoglobin at regular intervals

↓

Assess for Coronary Artery Disease (CAD) Risk

- ◇ Review the history of angina, MI, and CABG
- ◇ Examine ECG for ischemic changes
- ◇ Check chest X-ray for cardiomegaly, CHF signs

↓

Post-bleeding Management

- ◇ Conduct a thorough assessment of the bleeding source
- ◇ Stabilize and determine nadir hemoglobin level after equilibration

45.2.3 *Introduction to Hemoglobinopathies and their Management*

Hemoglobinopathies, such as sickle cell disease (SCD), thalassemia, and congenital hemolytic anemias, often require transfusions for both acute and chronic management. Transfusion therapy's goals in these conditions include preventing complications, reducing disease severity, and improving quality of life.

45.2.3.1 Transfusion Strategies in Hemoglobinopathies

1. *Sickle Cell Disease (SCD)* [6]

   - *Acute Indications*

     - Acute chest syndrome
     - Stroke or stroke prevention in children with high transcranial Doppler (TCD) velocities
     - Severe vaso-occlusive crises unresponsive to standard therapy

   - *Chronic Transfusion Therapy*

     - Used in patients with recurrent strokes or high-risk SCD complications.
     - Goal: Maintain HbS levels <30% to reduce complications.
     - Avoid over-transfusion (Hb >10 g/dL) to prevent hyperviscosity.

2. *Thalassemia*

   - *Transfusion-Dependent Thalassemia (TDT)* [7]

     - Regular transfusions maintain Hb ~9–10 g/dL to suppress ineffective erythropoiesis and prevent bone deformities.
     - Iron overload is a significant concern, requiring iron chelation therapy.

   - *Non-Transfusion-Dependent Thalassemia (NTDT)*

     - Occasional transfusions may be needed during periods of stress, infection, or pregnancy.

3. *Congenital Hemolytic Anemias (e.g., Hereditary Spherocytosis, G6PD Deficiency)* [8]

   - Transfusion is reserved for severe anemia or hemolytic crises.
   - Splenectomy may reduce transfusion dependence in hereditary spherocytosis.
   - In G6PD deficiency, oxidative stress should be avoided to prevent hemolysis.

45.2.3.2 Transfusion Administration Protocol

- *Dosing:* 1 unit PRBC increases Hb by ~1 g/dL.
- *Rate of Administration:*

  - 1–2 ml/min for initial 15 min, if no reactions are observed, can go up to 5 ml/min as tolerated by the patient (maximum time for transfusion is 4 h).
  - No need to warm the blood if the patient is not planned for massive transfusion (Transfusion of >20 units of PRBCs/blood components in 24 h)

- *Monitoring*
  - Pre- and post-transfusion hemoglobin levels.
  - Observe for transfusion reactions (fever, hypotension, hemolysis).
  - Iron status monitoring in chronically transfused patients.

45.2.4 Special Considerations

- *Leukodepleted RBCs* Leukocyte reduction enhances RBC storage by eliminating metabolically active white blood cells (WBCs), which would otherwise accelerate acidification of the storage bag. Additionally, WBCs release cytokines and, upon cold-induced lysis, secrete proteolytic, glycolytic, and lipolytic enzymes that compromise red cell integrity. However, the process is not without drawbacks—some red cells sustain damage, and a portion is lost during filtration, typically amounting to 15–35 mL, depending on filter size and whether whole blood or concentrated red cells are processed. Furthermore, RBCs from donors with sickle cell trait may obstruct the filters [9]. Despite these limitations, leukocyte reduction significantly enhances the 24-h in vivo recovery of transfused red cells by several percent, as indicated by the best available estimates.
- *Irradiated RBCs* prevent transfusion-associated graft-versus-host disease (TA-GVHD) in immunocompromised patients [10].
- *Washed RBCs:* Washing RBCs with saline to remove plasma results in minor red cell losses during bag transfers, along with the depletion of essential nutrients such as glucose, phosphate, and adenine. However, since washed RBCs are typically transfused within 6–24 h, the primary physiological concern is glucose loss. Although a small amount of glucose remains within the washed RBCs, it is rapidly metabolized, particularly if the cells are not promptly refrigerated. Without glucose, cellular metabolism ceases, making the red cells highly vulnerable to oxidative stress and erythro-apoptotic changes. There are no definite indications of Washed RBC use currently, except in IgA-deficient patients to prevent anaphylaxis [11].

45.3 Platelets

Composition and Types of Platelets

- Random Donor Platelets (RDP): Derived from multiple blood donors.
- Single Donor Platelets (SDP): Collected through an apheresis procedure.

Platelet transfusions play a crucial role in managing thrombocytopenia and controlling bleeding. The objective of these guidelines is to enhance the proper utilization of platelet transfusions, ensuring their use is appropriate while minimizing potential risks and reducing wastage. These recommendations are founded on an extensive review of existing literature and evidence-based best practices.

45.3.1 Classification of Platelet Transfusions

Platelet Transfusions are Categorized Into

1. Prophylactic Transfusions—Administered to patients with low platelet counts who are not actively bleeding (WHO bleeding score 0 or 1) to prevent potential hemorrhage.
2. Therapeutic Transfusions—Used to manage active bleeding in patients with a WHO bleeding score of 2 or higher.
3. Pre-Procedural Transfusions—Provided prior to surgical or invasive procedures to mitigate bleeding risks.

45.3.1.1 Indications for Platelet Transfusion [12–14]

1. *Prophylactic Platelet Transfusion*
   - Recommended for patients experiencing reversible bone marrow failure undergoing intensive therapy when platelet levels drop below 10×10^9/L.
   - Not typically required for individuals with chronic bone marrow failure unless persistent WHO grade ≥2 bleeding is observed.
   - Generally avoided in immune thrombocytopenia (ITP), thrombotic thrombocytopenic purpura (TTP), or heparin-induced thrombocytopenia (HIT) unless life-threatening bleeding occurs.
2. *Pre-Procedural Platelet Transfusion*
   - Lumbar puncture: Indicated if platelet count is below 40×10^9/L.
   - Percutaneous liver biopsy: Maintain platelet count above 50×10^9/L.
   - Major surgeries: Ensure platelet count exceeds 50×10^9/L.
   - Neurosurgical or posterior segment ophthalmic procedures: Maintain platelet count above 100×10^9/L.
3. *Therapeutic Platelet Transfusion*
   - Severe bleeding (WHO grade ≥3): Keep platelet count above 50×10^9/L.
   - Multiple trauma, brain injury, or intracerebral hemorrhage: Maintain platelet levels above 100×10^9/L.
   - Non-severe bleeding (WHO grade 2): Consider transfusion if platelet count is below 30×10^9/L.

45.3.1.2 Contraindications for Platelet Transfusion

- Thrombotic Thrombocytopenic Purpura (TTP): Not recommended unless life-threatening bleeding is present due to an increased risk of thrombosis.
- Immune Thrombocytopenia (ITP): Generally avoided unless critical bleeding or emergency surgery is required.
- Heparin-Induced Thrombocytopenia (HIT) and Post-Transfusion Purpura (PTP): Platelet transfusion is reserved for severe bleeding cases.

45.3.2 Platelet Transfusion in Special Cases

1. *Platelet Function Disorders (Congenital and Acquired)*
    - Glanzmann Thrombasthenia: Consider recombinant factor VIIa (rFVIIa) as the first-line treatment, especillay when there is platelet refractoriness/antibodies; platelet transfusion is used for severe bleeding.
    - Bernard-Soulier Syndrome and similar conditions: Prefer tranexamic acid (TXA) and desmopressin before opting for platelet transfusion.
    - Antiplatelet Therapy: Platelet transfusion should not be administered before procedures unless antiplatelet medications have been discontinued.
2. *Platelet Transfusion in Trauma and Surgery*
    - Early TXA administration is advisable for actively bleeding trauma patients, before opting for platelet transfusion.
    - In addition, Fibrinogen replacement (via cryoprecipitate or concentrate) is necessary in cases of severe trauma-related or perioperative bleeding when plasma fibrinogen levels drop below 1.5 g/L.

45.3.3 Risks and Adverse Reactions Associated with Platelet Transfusion

- Alloimmunization: May compromise future transfusion efficacy.
- Febrile Non-Hemolytic Transfusion Reactions (FNHTR): Occurs in approximately 1 in 6000 transfusions.
- Allergic Reactions: Estimated at a rate of 1 in 6000 transfusions.
- Bacterial Contamination and Sepsis: Rare due to stringent screening protocols but remains a risk.
- Hemolysis: Very uncommon (1 in 600,000 cases), but more frequent with ABO-incompatible transfusions.
- Transfusion-Related Acute Lung Injury (TRALI): A rare but severe complication.

45.3.4 Strategies to Mitigate Risks of Platelet Transfusion

- Prefer ABO-compatible platelets to enhance transfusion success.
- For RhD-negative females of childbearing age, RhD-negative platelets should be prioritized; if RhD-positive platelets are used, anti-D prophylaxis should be given.
- Platelet additive solutions (PAS) may help reduce allergic reactions.
- Hospitals should maintain standardized protocols for managing transfusion reactions, aligning with standard guidelines such as British Committee for Standards in Hematology (BCSH) guidelines.

45.3.5 Platelet Refractoriness and Alternative Treatments [15]

Platelet Refractoriness

- Patients with hypoproliferative thrombocytopenia who exhibit refractoriness to platelet transfusions should not receive HLA-matched platelets unless they have confirmed class I HLA antibodies.
- In cases unresponsive to HLA-selected platelets, human platelet antigen (HPA)-matched platelets may be considered.

Alternatives to Platelet Transfusion

- Tranexamic Acid (TXA): Recommended for patients with chronic bone marrow failure experiencing WHO grade ≥ 2 bleeding.
- Desmopressin (DDAVP): May be beneficial for patients with platelet function abnormalities.
- Thrombopoietin receptor agonists (e.g., Romiplostim, Eltrombopag) could be useful in select thrombocytopenia cases.

45.3.6 Platelet Transfusion During Shortages

Prioritization of platelet transfusion should be based on clinical urgency:

- Category 1: Emergency scenarios such as massive hemorrhage, critical care needs, or urgent surgical procedures.
- Category 2: Urgent cases requiring platelet support for planned surgeries.
- Category 3: Non-urgent situations, such as stable chronic bone marrow failure patients.

45.3.7 Conclusion

The guidelines emphasize the prudent administration of platelet transfusions, ensuring they are used only when medically necessary to minimize risks and preserve resources. Hospitals should implement strategies for ABO and RhD compatibility, manage transfusion-related reactions effectively, and utilize alternative therapies like TXA and desmopressin when applicable.

45.4 Fresh Frozen Plasma (FFP)

45.4.1 Composition and Characteristics

FFP contains clotting factors, fibrinogen, albumin, and immunoglobulins, making it crucial for coagulation support.

Difference between different types of plasma products [16–18]

	Fresh frozen plasma (from whole blood collection)	Fresh frozen plasma (from apheresis)	Cryoprecipitate plasma (cryo)	Cryosupernatant plasma (cryo-poor plasma)
Preparation	Whole blood undergoes high-speed centrifugation to facilitate the separation of its components, resulting in distinct layers: Plasma, red blood cells (RBCs), and the buffy coat, which contains platelets, white blood cells, residual RBCs, and some plasma. Plasma that is frozen within 8 h of collection is classified as fresh frozen plasma (FFP). If freezing occurs between 8 and 24 hours after collection, it is referred to as frozen plasma (FP)	Plasma is extracted from whole blood using a cell separator during apheresis. Typically, a single unit of fresh frozen plasma (FFP) collected through apheresis is roughly equivalent to two units of FFP obtained from whole blood donation. Both forms of FFP are considered interchangeable for clinical use	Plasma is frozen for 24 h and then thawed at a temperature of 1–6 °C, allowing insoluble proteins to precipitate. The mixture is then centrifuged to separate the cryoprecipitate, which is subsequently refrozen for storage	Plasma is frozen for 24 h and then thawed at a temperature of 1–6 °C, allowing insoluble proteins to precipitate. The mixture is then centrifuged to separate the supernatant, known as cryo-poor plasma, which is subsequently refrozen for storage

(continued)

	Fresh frozen plasma (from whole blood collection)	Fresh frozen plasma (from apheresis)	Cryoprecipitate plasma (cryo)	Cryosupernatant plasma (cryo-poor plasma)
Factors	Frozen plasma (FP) contains all coagulation factors, including labile factors such as Factor V (FV) and Factor VIII (FVIII:C). When prepared within 24 h of collection, FP has slightly lower FVIII:C levels compared to fresh frozen plasma (FFP) processed within 8 hours. However, the FVIII:C concentration remains at or above 0.50 IU/mL. FP is suitable for coagulation factor replacement, except in cases of isolated or severe FVIII deficiency	Includes all coagulation factors, including labile factors such as Factor V (FV) and Factor VIII:C (FVIII:C)	Cryoprecipitate is rich in factor VIII:C (FVIII:C), von Willebrand factor (vWF), fibrinogen, Factor XIII (FXIII), and fibronectin. Each unit of cryoprecipitate contains approximately *91 IU of FVIII:C, 113 IU of vWF, and 150 mg of fibrinogen* per bag	Lacks high molecular weight von Willebrand factor (vWF) multimers and has reduced levels of Factor VIII:C
Volume	Each bag = 1 unit (200—250 mL)	Each bag = 1 unit (400—600 mL)	Each bag = 1 unit (10–20 mL)	Each bag = 1 unit (>100 mL)
Dose	For adults, the standard plasma dosage is 10–15 mL per kilogram of body weight. The same dosage applies to pediatric patients. Plasma is typically infused over 2–3 h, or as clinically necessary. If there is no ongoing factor consumption or loss, this dosage can increase factor levels by approximately 25%	The recommended plasma dosage for both adults and pediatric patients is 10–15 mL per kilogram of body weight. It is typically administered over 2–3 h, or as needed based on clinical requirements. In the absence of ongoing factor consumption or loss, this dosage can increase coagulation factor levels by approximately 25%	For adults, the standard cryoprecipitate dosage is 1 unit per 5 kg of body weight, with a maximum total dose of 10 units (bags). In pediatric patients, the recommended dose is 1 unit per 5–10 kg of body weight or 5–10 mL/kg. If there is no ongoing fibrinogen consumption or loss, this dosage can increase fibrinogen levels by approximately 0.5 g/L	Plasma exchange (PLEX) generally involves replacing 1.0–1.5 times the patient's plasma volume per session. It is specifically used as a replacement fluid in PLEX for the management of thrombotic thrombocytopenic purpura (TTP)

45.4.2 Indications for FFP Transfusion (Based on BCSH Guidelines)

1. Single-Factor Deficiencies
   FFP is indicated when no factor-specific concentrate is available, particularly for Factor V deficiency.
2. Multiple-Factor Deficiencies and Disseminated Intravascular Coagulation (DIC)
   - Used in patients with severe bleeding and multiple-factor deficiencies.
   - Should be combined with treatment for the underlying cause.
   - Grade C recommendation (Level IV evidence).
3. Thrombotic Thrombocytopenic Purpura (TTP)
   - Cryosupernatant plasma or FFP may be used in plasma exchange.
   - Treatment should be guided by a hematology consultant.
   - Grade B recommendation (Level Ib evidence).
4. Urgent Reversal of Warfarin Effect
   - FFP is used in emergencies such as life-threatening bleeding.
   - Should be combined with intravenous vitamin K.
   - Grade B recommendation (Level III evidence).
5. Liver Disease and Coagulopathy
   - FFP is indicated for coagulopathy with severe bleeding or prior to invasive procedures.
   - Routine prophylactic transfusion is not recommended.
   - Grade B recommendation (Level IIa evidence).
6. Massive Transfusion Protocols
   - FFP may be used to maintain INR and PTT values at less than 1.5 times the reference range.
   - Clinical judgment and coagulation tests should guide transfusion.
   - Grade B recommendation (Level IIb evidence).
7. Neonatal Considerations
   - Used in hemorrhagic disease of the newborn or severe coagulopathy.
   - Recommended dose: 10–15 mL/kg body weight.
   - Grade C recommendation (Level IV evidence).

45.4.3 Inappropriate Uses of FFP [19]

FFP should not be used for:

1. Hypovolemia—Crystalloids or volume expanders are preferred.
2. Reversal of Prolonged INR Without Bleeding—Vitamin K administration is sufficient.
3. Prevention of Intraventricular Hemorrhage in Preterm Infants—No proven benefit.
4. Treatment of Immunodeficiency—Intravenous immunoglobulin (IVIG) should be used instead.
5. Wound Healing, Nutritional Support, or Protein-Losing Conditions—Not indicated.

45.4.4 General Considerations for FFP Transfusion

- Informed consent is required before transfusion.
- ABO compatibility should be ensured, but Rh compatibility is not necessary.
- Plasma should be transfused immediately after thawing.
- Close monitoring of coagulation tests (INR, PTT, fibrinogen) is essential.

45.4.5 Conclusion

The existing guidelines on FFP emphasize a rational approach to the use of FFP based on clinical evidence. Adherence to these recommendations will optimize patient safety, reduce unnecessary transfusions, and conserve blood product resources. Clinicians should ensure proper assessment before prescribing FFP to avoid inappropriate use.

45.5 Cryoprecipitate Transfusion Guidelines [20]

45.5.1 Introduction

- Cryoprecipitate is a plasma-derived product obtained by thawing fresh frozen plasma (FFP) at 4 °C.
- It is rich in Factor VIII, von Willebrand Factor (vWF), and fibrinogen, making it crucial for managing coagulopathies.
- Limited indications exist for its use, primarily for restoring fibrinogen levels in bleeding patients.

45.5.2 Indications for Cryoprecipitate Transfusion [21]

- Disseminated Intravascular Coagulation (DIC): When fibrinogen is <1 g/L with active bleeding.
- Liver Disease with Bleeding: Preoperative or active bleeding with fibrinogen <1 g/L.
- Hypofibrinogenemia due to Thrombolytic Therapy: To restore clotting potential.
- Massive Transfusion Protocols: To maintain fibrinogen >1.5 g/L.
- Renal or Liver Failure with Abnormal Bleeding: When DDAVP is not appropriate.
- Congenital Hypofibrinogenemia: When specific fibrinogen concentrates are unavailable.
- Prophylactic Use: Considered when fibrinogen is <1.0 g/L in patients undergoing invasive procedures.
- Not Recommended: In patients without active bleeding or surgical risk.

45.5.3 Dosage and Administration

Dosage Guidelines
- Adults: 2 pooled units (each containing 5 donor units), providing 3–3.5 g of fibrinogen, increasing plasma fibrinogen by ~1 g/L.
- Pediatrics: 5–10 mL/kg, up to a maximum of 2 pooled units.

Administration
- Must be thawed at 30–37 °C for 20–30 min before use.
- Infused using a 170-200 μm filter to remove clots.
- Must be administered immediately after thawing and within 4 h.
- Infusion rates:
  - Adults: Over 20–30 minutes, or rapidly in emergencies.
  - Pediatrics: 10–20 mL/kg/hr.

Compatibility and Safety Considerations
- ABO group matching is preferred, but non-group-matched cryoprecipitate can be used if no high-titer anti-A or anti-B is present.
- RhD positive cryoprecipitate may be given to RhD-negative females of childbearing potential, and anti-D prophylaxis is not required.
- All patients must wear an ID band for correct identification before transfusion.

Risks and Adverse Reactions
- Common Reactions:
  - Febrile (fever-related) reactions.
  - Urticaria (hives).
  - Anaphylaxis.

  - Bacterial contamination risks.
  - Transfusion-Related Acute Lung Injury (TRALI).
- Monitoring Protocol:
  - Baseline vitals.
  - 15-min check after infusion starts.
  - Post-transfusion assessment for any adverse reactions.

45.5.4 Conclusion

Cryoprecipitate is a specialized blood component mainly used to restore fibrinogen in bleeding or surgical patients. Proper dose calculation, ABO compatibility, and adherence to safety guidelines are essential to prevent complications

45.6 Transfusion Support for Hematopoietic Stem Cell Transplant (HSCT) Patients

45.6.1 Introduction

Hematopoietic stem cell transplantation (HSCT) is an increasingly utilized treatment for a range of conditions, including:

- Hematological malignancies (e.g., leukemia, lymphoma).
- Bone marrow failure syndromes (e.g., aplastic anemia).
- Solid tumors requiring high-dose chemotherapy.
- Metabolic and autoimmune disorders.

Transfusion support plays a critical role in pre-, peri-, and post-transplant care, addressing challenges like cytopenias, alloimmunization, ABO incompatibility, and transfusion-related infections [22].

45.6.2 Types of HSCT and Their Impact on Transfusion Needs

By Donor Type

- Autologous HSCT (patient's own stem cells).
- Allogeneic HSCT (stem cells from a matched or mismatched donor, related or unrelated).

By Stem Cell Source:

- Bone marrow-derived stem cells—high red blood cell (RBC) and plasma content.

- Peripheral blood stem cells (PBSCs)—lower RBC content, reducing risk of hemolysis.
- Cord blood—small volume, usually ABO-compatible.

Each type influences transfusion requirements and risks, especially regarding ABO mismatches and graft rejection.

45.6.3 Key Transfusion Considerations for HSCT

1. Pre-transplant Blood Product Selection
   HSCT patients require special blood product modifications to minimize transfusion-related complications:

   - Leukoreduction (LR)—Removes white blood cells (WBCs), reducing alloimmunization, and non-hemolytic febrile reactions.
   - Irradiation—Prevents transfusion-associated graft-versus-host disease (TA-GVHD).
   - Cytomegalovirus (CMV) seronegative blood—Reduces CMV transmission in immunosuppressed patients.

   CMV Risk and Blood Products

   - CMV resides in WBCs, making leukoreduction a CMV-safe alternative.
   - AABB guidelines consider LR equivalent to CMV-negative products, but some centers use both LR and CMV-negative blood for high-risk patients.

2. ABO Incompatibility in HSCT
   Major ABO Incompatibility
   Occurs when the recipient has preformed antibodies against donor RBCs (e.g., an O recipient receiving an A or B graft).

   - Risk: Acute hemolysis from recipient's anti-A/B antibodies attacking donor RBCs.
   - Prevention: RBC depletion of the graft via apheresis or plasma exchange.

   Minor ABO Incompatibility
   Occurs when the donor has preformed antibodies against recipient RBCs (e.g., an O donor for an A or B recipient).

   - Risk: Delayed hemolysis due to donor lymphocytes producing anti-A/B antibodies post-engraftment.
   - Management: Plasma depletion of the graft and close post-transplant monitoring.

   Bidirectional ABO Incompatibility
   Occurs when both donor and recipient have incompatible ABO antigens.

   - Prevention: Both RBC and plasma depletion of the graft.
   - Monitoring: Watch for both acute and delayed hemolysis.

Post-transplant Blood Type Considerations

- Recipient's original RBCs and antibodies may persist for months post-transplant.
- Transfused RBCs must be compatible with both donor and recipient plasma.
- Platelet transfusions must avoid ABO incompatibility to prevent hemolysis.

3. Preventing Alloimmunization and TA-GVHD
   Alloimmunization and Platelet Refractoriness

   - 10–15% of HSCT patients develop alloantibodies against HLA antigens.
   - Leukoreduction reduces but does not eliminate the risk.
   - HLA-matched platelets are required if patients become refractory.

   TA-GVHD Prevention via Irradiation

   - TA-GVHD occurs when transfused donor lymphocytes attack the recipient's tissues.
   - Mortality is >90%.
   - Prevention: Irradiated blood products for all HSCT patients.
   - Irradiation is required throughout the pre-, peri-, and post-transplant periods, potentially lifelong.

45.6.4 Transfusion Management at Different HSCT Stages

Pre-transplant Phase

- Optimize hemoglobin and platelet levels before transplant.
- Avoid excessive transfusions to minimize alloimmunization risk.
- Select ABO-compatible or modified blood products.
- Consider erythropoiesis-stimulating agents (ESAs) to reduce transfusion dependence.

Peri-transplant Phase

- Monitor for bleeding due to thrombocytopenia.
- Use antifibrinolytics (e.g., aminocaproic acid) in high-risk cases.
- Transfuse based on clinical need, not just hemoglobin levels.

Post-transplant Phase

- Monitor for delayed engraftment, hemolysis, and immune complications.
- Adjust transfusion protocols based on evolving donor cell engraftment.
- Continue irradiated and CMV-safe blood products until immune reconstitution is confirmed.

45.6.5 Post-transplant Complications and Management

1. Delayed Engraftment and Cytopenias
    - Prolonged pancytopenia increases transfusion dependence.
    - Graft failure requires continued RBC and platelet support.
2. Immune Hemolysis
   Occurs due to ABO incompatibility or immune dysregulation post-HSCT.
    - Acute hemolysis: Immediate RBC destruction from residual recipient antibodies.
    - Delayed hemolysis: Occurs as donor lymphocytes begin producing antibodies against recipient RBCs.
    - Management: Close monitoring, transfusing type O RBCs, and possibly RBC exchange transfusion.
3. Passenger Lymphocyte Syndrome (PLS)
    - Occurs when donor lymphocytes produce antibodies against host RBCs.
    - Onset: 1–2 weeks post-transplant.
    - Management: Transfusion of antigen-negative RBCs, immunosuppressive therapy.
4. Pure Red Cell Aplasia (PRCA)
    - Major ABO mismatch leads to persistent suppression of RBC production.
    - May require RBC transfusions for over a year.
    - Management: Reducing immunosuppression, plasma exchange, or donor lymphocyte infusions.
5. Platelet Refractoriness
    - Failure to achieve expected platelet count increments after transfusion.
    - Causes: Alloimmunization (immune) vs. sepsis, splenomegaly (non-immune).
    - Management: HLA-matched platelets, crossmatched platelets, alternative agents like recombinant Factor VIIa.

Key Take Home Points
HSCT patients require specialized transfusion protocols to mitigate risks associated with ABO incompatibility, TA-GVHD, alloimmunization, and delayed engraftment.

- Leukoreduction, irradiation, and CMV-negative products are essential.
- Pre- and post-transplant monitoring for hemolysis, immune complications, and cytopenias is critical.
- Future research will refine transfusion thresholds and improve transplant outcomes.

45.7 Autoimmune Hemolytic Anemia (AIHA)

45.7.1 Introduction

Autoimmune hemolytic anemia (AIHA) is a rare disorder characterized by the production of autoantibodies that target and destroy red blood cells, leading to hemolysis. The incidence of AIHA has been reported to range from 1 in 80,000 to 1 in 25,000 annually, with variability attributed to differing diagnostic criteria. AIHA affects individuals across all age groups but is more prevalent in adults, particularly those over 40 years, with peak incidence observed after 70 years. This distribution is closely linked to the increased risk of lymphoproliferative malignancies and secondary AIHA in older individuals.

AIHA is classified based on the nature of autoantibodies and underlying etiology. Primary (idiopathic) AIHA occurs in isolation without an identifiable cause, whereas secondary AIHA arises due to immune dysregulation associated with conditions such as autoimmune diseases, malignancies, and infections. The prevalence of AIHA subtypes varies based on patient demographics and comorbid conditions. Warm-reactive autoantibodies are responsible for approximately 70% of AIHA cases, followed by cold agglutinins (15%) and drug-induced antibodies (12%). Secondary AIHA is defined by a higher incidence of hemolysis in patients with associated disorders, resolution of anemia upon successful treatment of the primary disease, and an underlying immunologically mediated pathophysiology [23, 24].

This case highlights the complexities of AIHA, emphasizing the importance of early diagnosis, immunohematological workup, and a multidisciplinary approach for optimal management. Understanding the classification and underlying mechanisms of AIHA is crucial for tailoring treatment strategies and improving patient outcomes.

45.7.2 Real Case History and Presentation

Initial Symptoms and Clinical History

A 47-year-old male with no known comorbidities presented with complaints of a non-productive cough for 3 months associated with low-grade fever with chills, malaise, and significant unintentional weight loss. He also complained of reduced appetite for 2 months

Diagnostic Workup (Only Significant Findings)

Investigation	Findings
Chest X-ray (PA view)	Large lobulated mass in the right hilum, likely due to lymphadenitis
MSCT thorax	6.4 × 6.1 × 8.8 cm mildly heterogeneously enhancing lesion in the anterior mediastinum
CT-guided biopsy	Diagnosis: Thymoma type AB

- *Admission Laboratory Reports:*
  - *Hemoglobin*: 13.2 g/dL
  - *TLC*: 9100/cumm (DLC—50/36/7/7)
  - *Platelets*: 2.73 lakhs/cumm
  - *All other investigations*: Within normal limits
  - *Plan*: Excision via median sternotomy (since it is a major surgery with risk of bleeding, prophylactic demand for PRBC was made)

Blood Transfusion Challenges

- *Blood requirement:* Six units of Packed Red Blood Cells (PRBC)
- *Blood group:* B Rh D positive
- *Issue encountered:* Initial cross-matching incompatibility

Immunohematological Workup

Investigation	Room temperature	4 °C	37 °C	Remarks
ICT	2+	1+	4+	
DCT	3+			
Autocontrol	2+	1+	3+	
Monospecific DCT	IgG predominant shows 3+ reaction			
3 cell panel	Pan agglutination			
11 cell panel	Pan agglutination			

45.7.3 *Further Laboratory Workup*

Antibody Identification—Elution Technique

Methodology

1. Red cells (DCT positive) were washed with saline and DiaCidel wash solution.
2. The supernatant eluate was tested for antibody identification.

Results of Elution and Indirect Coombs Test

- The eluate and ICT confirmed the presence of warm autoantibodies, consistent with AIHA.

Autoantibody Adsorption Studies

Auto-adsorption Technique

1. Red cells were washed three times with saline and supernatant removed.
2. Patient serum was incubated with autologous RBCs at 37 °C for 45–60 min.
3. Centrifugation and testing for ICT and antibody specificity.

Findings
- Multiple cycles of adsorption were required.
- If agglutination persisted, further adsorption was necessary.
- Three to six aliquots of RBCs were used to remove autoantibodies.

Management and Transfusion Strategy

Preoperative Management
- *Elective surgery deferred* due to high antibody levels.
- *First-line therapy:* Corticosteroids to reduce antibody production.

Blood Transfusion Approach

1. *Phenotype-matched units* (Rh and Kell matched).
2. *Rh D-negative or best-matched units* used.

Key Considerations
- *Allogeneic vs. Autologous Transfusion:* Survival of allogeneic RBCs in AIHA is similar to autologous RBCs.
- *Alloantibody exclusion required* before finalizing transfusion strategy.

45.7.4 Conclusion

This case highlights the complex transfusion challenges associated with AIHA, secondary to thymoma. A multidisciplinary approach involving hematology, immunohematology, and transfusion medicine is essential to ensure safe and effective management.

Key Takeaways
- AIHA should be suspected in cross-match incompatibility cases.
- Advanced immunohematology techniques (elution, adsorption) are critical for antibody identification.
- Corticosteroids serve as the first-line management approach.
- Phenotypically matched RBCs and autologous donation are key strategies for transfusion.

45.8 Pediatric Transfusion Guidelines with Dosage Recommendations [25]

45.8.1 Introduction

The pediatric transfusion guidelines outline best practices for administering blood components to infants and children. Given the variability in clinical conditions, transfusions should be individualized rather than based solely on laboratory thresholds. The document provides dosage recommendations for different blood components based on age, weight, and clinical status.

45.8.2 Pretransfusion Testing and Compatibility

Infants (<4 Months)
- ABO and Rh typing required.
- Antibody screening using maternal or infant serum.
- Compatibility testing not required unless:
  - Direct antiglobulin test (DAT) is positive.
  - Unexpected antibodies are detected.

Older Children (≥ 4 Months)
- ABO/Rh typing and antibody screening are mandatory.
- Compatibility testing required if alloantibodies are present.

Red Blood Cell (RBC) Transfusion

Indications
- Hb <7 g/dL with anemia symptoms.
- Hb <8 g/dL pre-surgery, with bone marrow failure or symptomatic anemia.
- Hb <13 g/dL for patients with severe cardiopulmonary disease or on ECMO.
- Acute blood loss ≥15–20% of blood volume.

Dosage
- 10–15 mL/kg per transfusion, infused over 2–4 h.
- Expected Hb Increase:
  - 3 g/dL for CPD/CPDA-1 RBCs (Hct ~80%).
  - 2 g/dL for additive solution RBCs (Hct ~60%).

Volume Calculation Formula

$$\text{Volume required} = \frac{\text{Total Blood Volume}(\text{TBV}) \times (\text{Desired Hct increase})}{\text{Hct of RBC Unit}}$$

- *TBV:* 85–100 mL/Kg for newborns, 75 mL/Kg for older children

Sickle Cell Disease (SCD) and Hemoglobinopathies

Goals of Transfusion

- Improve oxygen delivery.
- Reduce circulating sickle cells.
- Prevent stroke and other complications.

Methods of Transfusion

1. Simple Transfusion: 10–15 mL/kg RBCs, avoiding Hb >10 g/dL.
2. Chronic Transfusion: Maintain HbS <30% for stroke prevention.
3. Exchange Transfusion: Rapidly reduces HbS to <30%, preventing viscosity-related complications.

Complications in SCD Transfusion

- Alloimmunization: Requires antigen-matched RBCs.
- Hyperhemolytic Syndrome: Managed with IVIG and steroids.

45.8.3 Platelet Transfusion

Indications

Patient condition	Transfusion Threshold
Stable, non-bleeding	<10,000/μL
Bleeding or invasive procedure	<50,000/μL
Major surgery, neurosurgery, ECMO	<80,000-100,000/μL

Dosage

- 5–10 mL/kg per transfusion (pooled or apheresis platelets).
- Expected platelet increase: 50,000-100,000/μL per dose.

Corrected Count Increment (CCI) Formula

$$\mathrm{CCI} = \frac{\left(\text{Post transfusion Platelet count} - \text{Pre transfusion Platelet count}\right) \times \text{BSA}\left(\text{m}^2\right)}{\text{Number of Platelets Transfused}}$$

** Poor response (<7.5 × 10^9/L) indicates Platelet refractoriness, requiring HLA-matched platelets*

45.8.4 Plasma Transfusion

Indications

- Bleeding or surgery with coagulation factor deficiency.
- Disseminated intravascular coagulation (DIC).
- Liver disease with coagulopathy.
- Thrombotic thrombocytopenic purpura (TTP) while awaiting plasma exchange.

Dosage

- 10–15 mL/kg per transfusion.
- Expected clotting factor increase: ~15–20%.

45.8.5 Cryoprecipitate Transfusion

Indications

- Hypofibrinogenemia (<100 mg/dL) with bleeding.
- Von Willebrand disease (if factor concentrate is unavailable).

Dosage

- 1–2 units per 10 kg body weight.
- Expected fibrinogen increase: 60–100 mg/dL.

45.8.6 Granulocyte Transfusion

Indications

- Severe neutropenia (< 500/μL) with infections unresponsive to antibiotics.
- Inherited neutrophil dysfunction syndromes.

Dosage

- 1×10^{10} cells daily for 5 days.

Special Considerations in Pediatric Transfusion

RBC Storage and Preservatives

- Fresh RBCs (<7 days) preferred for neonates to reduce potassium risk.
- Washed RBCs may be needed for hyperkalemia risk.

CMV Risk Reduction

- Leukoreduced or CMV-negative blood for:
  - Neonates <1200 g birth weight.
  - Immunocompromised children.
  - Transplant recipients.

Irradiated Blood Requirements

- Required for:
  - Premature infants <1200 g birth weight.
  - Patients with congenital immunodeficiencies.
  - Intrauterine transfusions.
  - Hematopoietic stem cell transplantation (HSCT) recipients.

Minimizing Donor Exposures

- Single-donor or sterile aliquot blood units reduce exposure in neonates.

Blood Relatives as Donors

- Not recommended due to the risk of transfusion-associated graft-versus-host disease (TA-GVHD).

45.9 Fetal Anemia in Rh Isoimmunized Pregnancy

45.9.1 Introduction

- Rh isoimmunization occurs when an Rh-negative mother develops antibodies against fetal Rh-positive blood, leading to hemolytic disease of the fetus and newborn (HDFN) [26].
- This can result in neonatal jaundice, kernicterus, cerebral palsy, hydrops fetalis, intrauterine death, or the need for exchange transfusions.
- Anti-D immunoglobulin has significantly reduced the incidence, but in India, many women do not receive prophylaxis due to home deliveries, high costs, or negligence.
- Intrauterine transfusion (IUT) is the primary treatment for severe fetal anemia caused by Rh isoimmunization.

45.9.2 Prerequisites for planning IUT

- Indirect Coombs Test (ICT) >1:16 was considered a critical threshold for fetal anemia risk.
- Fetal monitoring included:
  - Ultrasound (USG) for hepatomegaly, placentomegaly, cardiomegaly, hydrops, and ascites.
  - Middle cerebral artery peak systolic velocity (MCA-PSV) via Doppler for anemia detection.
- IUT was performed if Hb <10 g/dL or hematocrit <30%, starting from 16 weeks (intraperitoneal) and 21 weeks (intravascular) gestation.

45.9.3 Indications for Intrauterine Transfusion (IUT) [27]

- Severe fetal anemia (Hb <10 g/dL, Hct <30%).
- Fetal hydrops on ultrasound (ascites, pleural effusion, skin edema).
- MCA-PSV >1.5 MoM indicating fetal anemia.
- Fetuses under 32–34 weeks that cannot be safely delivered.

45.9.4 Techniques of IUT [28]

Intravascular Transfusion (IVT)
- Preferred method, especially for hydropic fetuses.
- Blood is directly transfused into the umbilical vein at the cord insertion site.
- Post-transfusion hematocrit checked immediately.

Volume Calculation Formula

$$\text{Donor Hct} - \text{Desired Hct} \times \text{Feto} - \text{placental blood volume} \div \left(\text{Desired Hct} - \text{Fetal Hct}\right)$$

Intraperitoneal Transfusion (IPT)
- Used when IVT is difficult (e.g., posterior placenta, maternal obesity, early gestation).
- Blood is injected into the fetal peritoneal cavity, from where it is absorbed. Volume transfused: (gestational age in weeks—20) × 10 mL.

45.9.5 Procedure of IUT

- Fetus is paralyzed using vecuronium (0.3 mg/kg fetal weight) to prevent excessive movement.
- A 20G needle is inserted under ultrasound guidance into the umbilical vein (IVT) or peritoneal cavity (IPT).
- Packed O-negative RBCs (Hct 75–80%) are transfused at 10 mL/min using a 10–20 mL syringe.
- Continuous monitoring of fetal heart rate for tachycardia or bradycardia.
- Repeat transfusions are scheduled based on an expected post-transfusion hematocrit fall of 1% per day.

45.10 Discussion

- Ultrasound-guided IUT is a life-saving technique in severe fetal anemia.
- Success rates have improved due to advances in Doppler ultrasound and fetal monitoring.
- Comparison with global data:
  - Survival rate in AIIMS study: 85.6% (IUT cases).
  - Comparable to international centers where survival ranges from 75% to 88%.
- More experienced centers have higher success rates due to operator expertise.
- Early referrals to specialized centers are crucial for optimal outcomes.

45.10.1 Conclusion

- IUT is the only effective treatment for severe fetal anemia in Rh-isoimmunized pregnancies.
- High survival rates (85.6%) prove its effectiveness.
- Early diagnosis, Doppler ultrasound monitoring, and specialized fetal medicine units are critical for optimal outcomes.
- More training and availability of IUT services in India are needed to improve perinatal survival.

45.11 Summary

Blood component therapy remains a cornerstone in the management of hematological disorders, providing precise and individualized transfusion support for patients with anemia, thrombocytopenia, coagulopathies, and immune-mediated conditions. Restrictive transfusion strategies have gained prominence, particularly in PRBC transfusions, to optimize oxygen delivery while preventing iron overload, alloimmunization, and transfusion-related complications. Similarly, platelet transfusions are reserved for critical cases, ensuring minimal exposure to donor antigens and reducing the risk of refractoriness.

Coagulation disorders, whether acquired or congenital, require carefully calibrated transfusions of fresh frozen plasma (FFP) and cryoprecipitate. These components play a vital role in massive transfusion protocols, disseminated intravascular coagulation (DIC), and liver failure-associated coagulopathies. The balance between coagulation support and avoidance of volume overload remains crucial in transfusion decisions.

The challenges of transfusion in high-risk patient groups such as hematopoietic stem cell transplantation (HSCT) recipients and individuals with autoimmune hemolytic anemia (AIHA) underscore the need for advanced immunohematological techniques. The use of leukoreduced, irradiated, and HLA-matched blood components has significantly improved outcomes in HSCT patients, reducing complications such as transfusion-associated graft-versus-host disease (TA-GVHD) and alloimmunization. Meanwhile, AIHA requires meticulous antibody identification and phenotype-matched transfusions to mitigate hemolysis risks.

For fetal anemia due to Rh isoimmunization, ultrasound-guided intrauterine transfusion (IUT) remains the only life-saving intervention. Early detection through Doppler ultrasound and fetal monitoring has greatly enhanced survival rates, allowing pregnancies to be carried to safer gestational ages.

With continuous advancements in transfusion medicine, such as extended antigen matching, pathogen reduction, and artificial blood substitutes, blood component therapy is evolving toward more precise, patient-specific approaches. The ongoing refinement of transfusion guidelines will ensure better safety, efficacy, and long-term outcomes for patients requiring blood support.

References

1. World Health organiation Information sheet for clinicians. The appropriate clinical use of blood and blood products.
2. Tuman KJ. Tissue oxygen delivery: the physiology of anemia. Anesthesiol Clin North Am. 1990;8(3):451–69.
3. Brecher ME, Zylstra-Halling VW, Pineda AA. Rejuvenation of erythrocytes preserved with AS-1 and AS-3. Am J Clin Pathol. 1991;96(6):767–9. Available from: https://pubmed.ncbi.nlm.nih.gov/1746494/.
4. Klein HG, Spahn DR, Carson JL. Red blood cell transfusion in clinical practice. Lancet. 2007 Aug 4;370(9585):415–26. Available from: https://pubmed.ncbi.nlm.nih.gov/17679019/.
5. Hébert PC, Wells G, Blajchman MA, Marshall J, Martin C, Pagliarello G, et al. A multicenter, randomized, controlled clinical trial of transfusion requirements in critical care. Transfusion Requirements in Critical Care Investigators, Canadian Critical Care Trials Group. N Engl J Med. 1999;340(6):409–17. Available from: https://pubmed.ncbi.nlm.nih.gov/9971864/.
6. Chou ST, Alsawas M, Fasano RM, Field JJ, Hendrickson JE, Howard J, et al. American Society of Hematology 2020 guidelines for sickle cell disease: transfusion support. Blood Adv. 2020;4(2):327–55. Available from: https://doi.org/10.1182/bloodadvances.2019001143.
7. Bain A. Management of transfusion dependent thalassaemia (TDT) a short guide.
8. Sharon BI. Transfusion therapy in congenital hemolytic anemias. Hematol Oncol Clin North Am. 1994;8(6):1053–86.
9. Kumar H, Gupta P, Mishra D, Sarkar R, Jaiprakash M. Leucodepletion and Blood Products. Med J Armed Forces India. 2011;62(2):174. Available from: https://pmc.ncbi.nlm.nih.gov/articles/PMC4921955/.
10. Moroff G, Luban NLC. The irradiation of blood and blood components to prevent graft-versus-host disease: technical issues and guidelines. Transfus Med Rev. 1997;11(1):15–26.
11. Cardigan R, New HV, Tinegate H, Thomas S. Washed red cells: theory and practice. Vox Sanguinis. 2020;115:606–16.
12. Capraru A, Jalowiec KA, Medri C, Daskalakis M, Zeerleder SS, Taleghani BM. Platelet transfusion—insights from current practice to future development. J Clin Med. 2021;10

13. Meledeo MA, Thomas KA, Bynum JA, Reddoch-Cardenas KM, Getz TM, Pidcoke HF, et al. Platelet Transfusion. Trauma Induced Coagulopathy. 2024;391–428. Available from: https://www.ncbi.nlm.nih.gov/books/NBK560632/.
14. Estcourt LJ, Birchall J, Allard S, Bassey SJ, Hersey P, Kerr JP, et al. Guidelines for the use of platelet transfusions. Br J Haematol. 2017;176(3):365–94.
15. Cohn CS. Platelet transfusion refractoriness: how do I diagnose and manage? Hematology. 2020(1):527. Available from: https://pmc.ncbi.nlm.nih.gov/articles/PMC7727584/.
16. Green L, Bolton-Maggs P, Beattie C, Cardigan R, Kallis Y, Stanworth SJ, et al. British Society of Haematology Guidelines on the spectrum of fresh frozen plasma and cryoprecipitate products: their handling and use in various patient groups in the absence of major bleeding. Br J Haematol. 2018;181(1):54–67.
17. Wong MP, Droubatchevskaia N, Chipperfield KM, Wadsworth LD, Ferguson DJ. Guidelines for frozen plasma transfusion a new document from the transfusion medicine advisory group of BC describes appropriate use of frozen plasma, fresh-frozen plasma, and cryosupernatant. BC Med J. 49. Available from: www.bloodlink.bc.ca.
18. Duguid J, O'Shaughnessy DF, Atterbury C, Maggs PB, Murphy M, Thomas D, et al. Guidelines for the use of fresh-frozen plasma, cryoprecipitate and cryosupernatant. Br J Haematol. 2004;126:11–28.
19. Health International F. Appropriate Use of Blood and Blood Products.
20. (UK) NCGC. Cryoprecipitate: thresholds and targets. 2015; Available from: https://www.ncbi.nlm.nih.gov/books/NBK338779/.
21. York N. New York State Council on Human Blood and Transfusion Services Guidelines for the administration of cryoprecipitate Fourth Edition 2012 New York State Council on Human Blood and Transfusion Services. Available from: www.wadsworth.org/labcert/blood_tissue.
22. Jekarl DW, Kim JK, Han JH, Lee H, Yoo J, Lim J, et al. Transfusion support in hematopoietic stem cell transplantation. Blood Res. 2023;58(Suppl 1):S1. Available from: https://pmc.ncbi.nlm.nih.gov/articles/PMC10133853/.
23. Binsfeld M, Devey A, Gothot A. Transfusion support and pre-transfusion testing in autoimmune haemolytic anaemia. Vox Sang. 2024;119(10). Available from: https://pubmed.ncbi.nlm.nih.gov/38922929/.
24. Versino F, Revelli N, Villa S, Pettine L, Zaninoni A, Prati D, et al. Transfusions in autoimmune hemolytic anemias: Frequency and clinical significance of alloimmunization. J Intern Med. 2024 ;295(3):369–74. Available from: https://onlinelibrary.wiley.com/doi/full/10.1111/joim.13753.
25. York N. New York State Council on Human Blood and Transfusion Services Guidelines for transfusion of pediatric patients 2016 New York State Council on Human Blood and Transfusion Services. Available from: www.wadsworth.org/labcert/blood_tissue.
26. Hall V, Vadakekut ES, Avulakunta ID. Hemolytic Disease of the Fetus and Newborn. Handbook of Pediatric Transfusion Medicine. 2025;191–208. Available from: https://www.ncbi.nlm.nih.gov/books/NBK557423/.
27. Delaney M, Matthews DC. Hemolytic disease of the fetus and newborn: managing the mother, fetus, and newborn. Hematology.2015(1):146–51.
28. New H V, Berryman J, Bolton-Maggs PHB, Cantwell C, Chalmers EA, Davies T, et al. Guidelines on transfusion for fetuses, neonates and older children. [cited 2025 Mar 23]; Available from: http://www.bcshguidelines.com/BCSH_PROCESS/EVIDENCE_LEVELS_AND_GRADES_.
29. Jeffry L. Carlson & Paul Hebert. 2016. Anemia and blood transfusion, Rossi's principles of transfusion medicine, Pg 110–125, Wiley Blackwell

GPSR Compliance

The European Union's (EU) General Product Safety Regulation (GPSR) is a set of rules that requires consumer products to be safe and our obligations to ensure this.

If you have any concerns about our products, you can contact us on ProductSafety@springernature.com

In case Publisher is established outside the EU, the EU authorized representative is:

Springer Nature Customer Service Center GmbH
Europaplatz 3
69115 Heidelberg, Germany

Batch number: 10889553

Printed by Printforce, the Netherlands